PEDIATRIC SECRETS

PEDIATRIC SECRETS

Third Edition

RICHARD A. POLIN, MD
Professor of Pediatrics
College of Physicians and Surgeons
Columbia University
New York, New York

Director, Division of Neonatology
Children's Hospital of New York
New York, New York

MARK F. DITMAR, MD
Assistant Chief, Department of Pediatrics
Southern Ocean County Hospital
Manahawkin, New Jersey

Assistant Clinical Professor of Pediatrics
Yale University School of Medicine
New Haven, Connecticut

HANLEY & BELFUS, INC./Philadelphia

Publisher: HANLEY & BELFUS, INC.
Medical Publishers
210 South 13th Street
Philadelphia, PA 19107
(215) 546-7293; 800-962-1892
FAX (215) 790-9330
Web site: http://www.hanleyandbelfus.com

***Note to the reader*:** Although the information in this book has been carefully reviewed for correctness of dosage and indications, neither the authors nor the editor nor the publisher can accept any legal responsibility for any errors or omissions that may be made. Neither the publisher nor the editor makes any warranty, expressed or implied, with respect to the material contained herein. Before prescribing any drug, the reader must review the manufacturer's current product information (package inserts) for accepted indications, absolute dosage recommendations, and other information pertinent to the safe and effective use of the product described.

Library of Congress Cataloging-in-Publication Data

Pediatric secrets / edied by Richard A. Polin, Mark F. Ditmar.—3rd ed.
p. ; cm—(The Secrets Series®)
Rev. ed. of: Pediatric secrets / Richard A. Polin, Mark F. Ditmar. 2nd. c1997.
Includes bibliographical references and index.
ISBN 1-56053-456-7 (alk. paper)
1. Pediatrics—Examinations, questions, etc. I. Polin, Richard A. (Richard Alan), 1945- II. Ditmar, Mark F. III. Series.
[DNLM: 1. Pediatrics—Examination Questions. WS 18.2 P3702 2001]
RJ48.2 .P65 2001
618.92'0076—dc21

2001024151

PEDIATRIC SECRETS, 3rd edition ISBN 1-56053-456-7

Last digit is the print number: 9 8 7 6 5 4 3 2 1

CONTENTS

CONTRIBUTORS

Peter C. Adamson, M.D.
Associate Professor, Pediatrics, Department of Oncology, Children's Hospital of Philadelphia and University of Pennsylvania, Philadelphia, Pennsylvania

Kwame Anyane-Yeboa, M.D.
Associate Professor of Clinical Pediatrics, Division of Genetics, Department of Pediatrics, Columbia University; Associate Attending Pediatrician, The New York Presbyterian Hospital, New York, New York

Richard Aplenc, M.D.
Instructor, Pediatrics, University of Pennsylvania, Children's Hospital of Philadelphia, Philadelphia, Pennsylvania

Balu H. Athreya, M.D.
Professor of Pediatrics, Thomas Jefferson University, Philadelphia, Pennsylvania; Pediatric Rheumatologist, DuPont Hospital for Children, Wilmington, Delaware

JoAnn Bergoffen, M.D.
Chief, Department of Genetics, Kaiser Permanente Northern California Region, Santa Teresa Medical Center, San Jose, California

Gerard T. Berry, M.D.
Professor, Pediatrics, University of Pennsylvania School of Medicine; The Children's Hospital of Philadelphia, Philadelphia, Pennsylvania

Peter M. Bingham, M.D.
Assistant Professor of Pediatrics, University of Pennsylvania School of Medicine; Attending Physician, Division of Neurology, Children's Hospital of Philadelphia, Philadelphia, Pennsylvania

Nathan J. Blum, M.D.
Assistant Professor of Pediatrics, Division of Child Development and Rehabilitation, University of Pennsylvania School of Medicine; Children's Hospital of Philadelphia, Philadelphia, Pennsylvania

Elizabeth Chalom, M.D.
Chief, Pediatric Rheumatology, Saint Barnabas Medical Center, Assistant Director of Medical Education for St. George's, Saint Barnabas Medical Center, Livingston, New Jersey; Director, Pediatric Rheumatology, Children's Hospital of New Jersey, Newark Beth Israel Medical Center, Newark, New Jersey

Barbara A. Chini, M.D.
Assistant Professor, Pulmonary Medicine, Allergy, and Clinical Immunology, University of Cincinnati College of Medicine; Children's Hospital Medical Center, Cincinnati, Ohio

Robert R. Clancy, M.D.
Professor of Neurology and Pediatrics, Division of Neurology, University of Pennsylvania School of Medicine; Children's Hospital of Philadelphia, Philadelphia, Pennsylvania

Bernard J. Clark III, M.D.
Associate Professor of Pediatrics, University of Pennsylvania School of Medicine; Medical Director, Heart Transplantation Program, Children's Hospital of Philadelphia, Philadelphia, Pennsylvania

Mark C. Clayton, M.D.
Developmental Pediatrics, Children's Hospital, Greenville Hospital System, Greenville, South Carolina

James Coplan, M.D.
Clinical Associate Professor of Pediatrics, Division of Child Development and Rehabilitation, University of Pennsylvania School of Medicine, Children's Hospital of Philadelphia, Philadelphia, Pennsylvania

Cori L. Daines, M.D.
Assistant Professor, Pulmonary Medicine, Allergy, and Clinical Immunology, University of Cincinnati College of Medicine; Children's Hospital Medical Center, Cincinnati, Ohio

Richard S. Davidson, M.D.
Associate Professor of Orthopaedic Surgery, University of Pennsylvania School of Medicine; Attending Surgeon, Division of Orthopaedic Surgery, Children's Hospital of Philadelphia, Philadelphia, Pennsylvania

Mark F. Ditmar, M.D.
Assistant Chief, Department of Pediatrics, Southern Ocean County Hospital, Manahawkin, New Jersey; Assistant Clinical Professor of Pediatrics, Yale University School of Medicine, New Haven, Connecticut

Alan E. Donnenfeld, M.D.
Clinical Associate Professor of Obstetrics and Gynecology, University of Pennsylvania School of Medicine; Acting Chief, Section of Maternal Fetal Medicine and Genetics, Pennsylvania Hospital, Philadelphia, Pennsylvania

John P. Dormans, M.D.
Associate Professor of Orthopaedic Surgery, University of Pennsylvania School of Medicine; Chief, Division of Orthopaedic Surgery, Children's Hospital of Philadelphia, Philadelphia, Pennsylvania

Andrew H. Eichenfield, M.D.
Clinical Associate Professor of Pediatrics, Mount Sinai School of Medicine; Chief, Division of Pediatric Rheumatology, The Mount Sinai Hospital, New York, New York

Alexis M. Elward, M.D.
Instructor in Pediatrics, Pediatrics/Infectious Diseases, Washington University, St. Louis Children's Hospital, St. Louis, Missouri

Anders Fasth, M.D., Ph.D.
Professor in Pediatric Immunology, Department of Pediatrics, Göteborg University; The Queen Silvia Children's Hospital; Göteborg, Sweden

Maria C. Garzon, M.D.
Assistant Professor, Dermatology and Pediatrics, Columbia University; Director of Pediatric Dermatology, Children's Hospital of New York, New York, New York

Daniel E. Hale, M.D.
Associate Professor of Pediatrics, University of Texas Health Science Center at San Antonio; Senior Physician, Pediatric Endocrinology, Santa Rosa Children's Hospital, San Antonio, Texas

William D. Hardie, M.D.
Assistant Professor, Pulmonary Medicine, Allergy, and Clinical Immunology, University of Cincinnati College of Medicine; Children's Hospital Medical Center, Cincinnati, Ohio

Mary Catherine Harris, M.D.
Associate Professor, Department of Pediatrics, University of Pennsylvania School of Medicine; Attending, Children's Hospital of Philadelphia, Philadelphia, Pennsylvania

Constance J. Hayes, M.D.
Professor of Clinical Pediatrics, Division of Pediatric Cardiology, Columbia University; Children's Hospital of New York, New York Presbyterian Hospital, New York, New York

Robert Hayman, M.D.
Attending, Department of Pediatrics, Schneider Children's Hospital, North Shore–LIJ Health System, New Hyde Park, New York

Fred M. Henretig, M.D.
Professor of Pediatrics and Emergency Medicine, University of Pennsylvania School of Medicine; Director, Section of Clinical Toxicology, Children's Hospital of Philadelphia; Medical Director, The Poison Control Center, Philadelphia, Pennsylvania

Georg A. Holländer, M.D.
Professor in Pediatrics, Department of Research, University of Basel; The University Children's Hospital, Basel, Switzerland

Allan J. Hordof, M.D.
Professor of Clinical Pediatrics, Division of Pediatric Cardiology, Department of Pediatrics, Columbia University; Children's Hospital of New York, New York Presbyterian Hospital, New York, New York

David A. Hunstad, M.D.
Fellow in Pediatric Infectious Diseases and Molecular Microbiology, Pediatrics/Infectious Diseases and Molecular Microbiology, Washington University; St. Louis Children's Hospital, St. Louis, Missouri

Joshua E. Hyman, M.D.
Assistant Professor of Orthopaedic Surgery, Columbia University College of Physician and Surgeons; Children's Hospital of New York, New York Presbyterian Hospital, New York, New York

Ellen B. Kaplan, M.D.
Chief, Pediatric Pulmonology Section, Hackensack University Medical Center, Hackensack, New Jersey; Assistant Professor of Pediatrics, University of Medicine and Dentistry of New Jersey–New Jersey Medical School, Newark, New Jersey

Kent R. Kelley, M.D.
Assistant Professor of Clinical Neurology and Clinical Pediatrics, Epilepsy Center/Neurology Department, Northwestern University; Children's Memorial Hospital, Chicago, Illinois

Thomas L. Kennedy, M.D.
Professor of Clinical Pediatrics, Yale University School of Medicine, Section of Pediatric Naphrology, Yale University and University of Connecticut, New Haven, Connecticut; Chairman, Department of Pediatrics, Bridgeport Hospital, Bridgeport, Connecticut

Leonard Kristal, M.D.
Clinical Assistant Professor of Dermatology and Pediatrics, State University of New York at Stony Brook, Stony Brook, New York

Peter B. Langmuir, M.D.
Instructor, Division of Oncology, The Children's Hospital of Philadelphia and University of Pennsylvania School of Medicine; Attending Physician, Children's Hospital of Philadelphia, Philadelphia, Pennsylvania

Jane M. Lavelle, M.D.
Associate Professor of Pediatrics, University of Pennsylvania School of Medicine; Associate Director, Emergency Medical Services, Children's Hospital of Philadelphia, Philadelphia, Pennsylvania

Francis Y. Lee, M.D.
Assistant Professor, Orthopaedic Surgery, Columbia University College of Physicians and Surgeons; Children's Hospital of New York, New York Presbyterian Hospital, New York, New York

Chris A. Liacouras, M.D.
Associate Professor of Pediatrics, Director of Pediatric Endoscopy, Division of Gastroenterology and Nutrition, University of Pennsylvania School of Medicine; Children's Hospital of Philadelphia, Philadelphia, Pennsylvania

Mark R. Magnusson, M.D., Ph.D.
Assistant Professor of Pediatrics, University of Pennsylvania School of Medicine; Medical Director, Children's Hospital Home Care and Case Management; Co-Director, Diagnostic Center, Children's Hospital of Philadelphia, Philadelphia, Pennsylvania

Peter Mamula, M.D.
Assistant Professor, Department of Pediatrics, Division of Gastroenterology and Nutrition, University of Pennsylvania, Children's Hospital of Philadelphia, Philadelphia, Pennsylvania

Jonathan E. Markowitz, M.D.
Attending Physician, Assistant Professor, Department of Pediatrics, Division of Gastroenterology and Nutrition, University of Pennsylvania, Children's Hospital of Philadelphia, Philadelphia, Pennsylvania

Peter J. Marro, M.D.
Assistant Professor of Pediatrics, Division of Neonatology, University of Vermont College of Medicine; Barbara Bush Children's Hospital, Portland, Maine

Steven E. McKenzie, M.D., Ph.D.
Professor of Medicine and Pediatrics, Director, Cardeza Foundation for Hematologic Research and Division of Hematology, Thomas Jefferson University, Philadelphia, Pennsylvania

Steve Miller, M.D.
AP Gold, Associate Professor of Clinical Pediatrics, Director, Pediatric Emergency Medicine, Children's Hospital of New York, Columbia University, College of Physicians and Surgeons; Director, Pediatric Emergency Medicine, Children's Hospital of New York, New York, New York

Jeffrey E. Ming, M.D., Ph.D.
Assistant Professor of Pediatrics, University of Pennsylvania School of Medicine; Attending Physician, Division of Human Genetics and Molecular Biology, Children's Hospital of Philadelphia, Philadelphia, Pennsylvania

Douglas R. Nordli, Jr., M.D.
Associate Professor of Clinical Neurology and Clinical Pediatrics, Epilepsy Center/Neurology Department, Northwestern University; Children's Memorial Hospital, Chicago, Illinois

Michael E. Norman, M.D.
Clinical Professor, Pediatrics, University of North Carolina School of Medicine, Chapel Hill, North Carolina; Immediate Past Chairman and Consultant, Department of Pediatrics, Carolinas Medical Center, Charlotte, North Carolina

Sharon E. Oberfield, M.D.
Professor of Pediatrics, Professor and deputy Director, Pediatric Endocrinology, Columbia University College of Physicians and Surgeons, New York, New York

Carlos Ramon Perez, M.D.
Associate in Pediatrics, Pediatric Pulmonology, Geisinger Medical Center, Danville, Pennsylvania

David A. Piccoli, M.D.
Professor, Department of Pediatrics, University of Pennsylvania School of Medicine, Gastroenterology and Nutrition, University of Pennsylvania School of Medicine and The Children's Hospital of Philadelphia, Philadelphia, Pennsylvania

Richard A. Polin, M.D.
College of Physicians and Surgeons, Columbia University; Director, Division of Neonatology, Children's Hospital of New York, New York, New York

James William Prebis, M.D.
Assistant Professor of Clinical Pediatrics, Division of Pediatric Nephrology, Northeastern Ohio Universities College of Medicine; Children's Hospital Medical Center of Akron, Akron, Ohio

Anne F. Reilly, M.D.
Assistant Professor of Pediatrics, Division of Oncology, University of Pennsylvania School of Medicine; Children's Hospital of Philadelphia, Philadelphia, Pennsylvania

Carlos D. Rose, M.D.
Associate Professor of Pediatrics, Thomas Jefferson University School of Medicine; Attending Physician, Division of Rheumatology, Alfred I duPont Hospital for Children, Wilmington, Delaware

Philip Roth, M.D., Ph.D.
Associate Professor of Pediatrics, Neonatology, State University of New York–Downstate Medical School, Brooklyn, New York; Director of Neonatology, Staten Island University Hospital, Staten Island, New York

David P. Roye, Jr., M.D.
Livingston Professor, Orthopaedic Surgery, Columbia University; Children's Hospital of New York, New York Presbyterian Hospital, New York, New York

Joseph W. St. Geme, III, M.D.
Associate Professor of Pediatrics and Molecular Microbiology, Pediatrics/Infectious Diseases, Washington University/St. Louis Children's Hospital, St. Louis, Missouri

F. Meredith Sonnett, M.D.
Assistant Professor of Clinical Pediatrics, Associate Director, Pediatric Emergency Medicine, Columbia College of Physicians and Surgeons, Children's Hospital of New York, New York, New York

Thomas J. Starc, M.D., M.P.H.
Professor of Clinical Pediatrics, Division of Pediatric Cardiology, Department of Pediatrics, Columbia University; Children's Hospital of New York, New York Presbyterian Hospital, New York, New York

Carlos R. Vega-Rich, M.D.
Associate Professor of Clinical Pediatrics, Division of Neonatology, Department of Pediatrics, Albert Einstein College of Medicine; J.D. Weiler Hospital of the Albert Einstein College of Medicine, Children's Hospital at Montefiore Medical Center, Bronx, New York

Steven J. Wassner, M.D.
Professor and Vice-Chair for Education, Pediatrics, Pennsylvania State College of Medicine; Chief, Division of Pediatric Nephrology, M.S. Hershey medical Center, Hershey, Pennsylvania

Robert W. Wilmott, M.D.
Professor, Pulmonary Medicine, Allergy, and Clinical Immunology, University of Cincinnati College of Medicine, Children's Hospital Medical Center, Cincinnati, Ohio

Mark Yudkoff, M.D.
Professor, Pediatrics–Child Development, University of Pennsylvania School of Medicine; Children's Hospital of Philadelphia, Philadelphia, Pennsylvania

Elaine H. Zackai, M.D.
Professor of Pediatrics and Genetics, University of Pennsylvania School of Medicine; Director, Clinical Genetics Center, Children's Hospital of Philadelphia, Philadelphia, Pennsylvania

PREFACE TO THE THIRD EDITION

The third edition of *Pediatric Secrets* attempts to continue the premise of the previous editions by providing updated discussions of varied topics in both primary and specialized pediatric care that occur in the context of inpatient and outpatient practice. We have tried to be both current and concise, to distinguish science from style in areas of clinical contention and to allow for more expanded explanations when appropriate. In this edition, we have also tried to incorporate aspects of alternative and complementary medicine, which are growing areas of interest both to pediatric researchers and to parents.

We are indebted to the chapter authors, particularly for their efforts in tackling a wider array of controversial topics; to Linda Belfus and Tom Stringer for their editorial diligence and malleable deadlines; and, very specially, to Helene, Allison, Mitchell, Jessica and Greg and to Nina, Erin and Cara for always leaving the light on.

Richard A. Polin, M.D.
Mark F. Ditmar, M.D.

In Memoriam
This book is dedicated to the memory of
Drs. David Cornfeld and Edward Charney

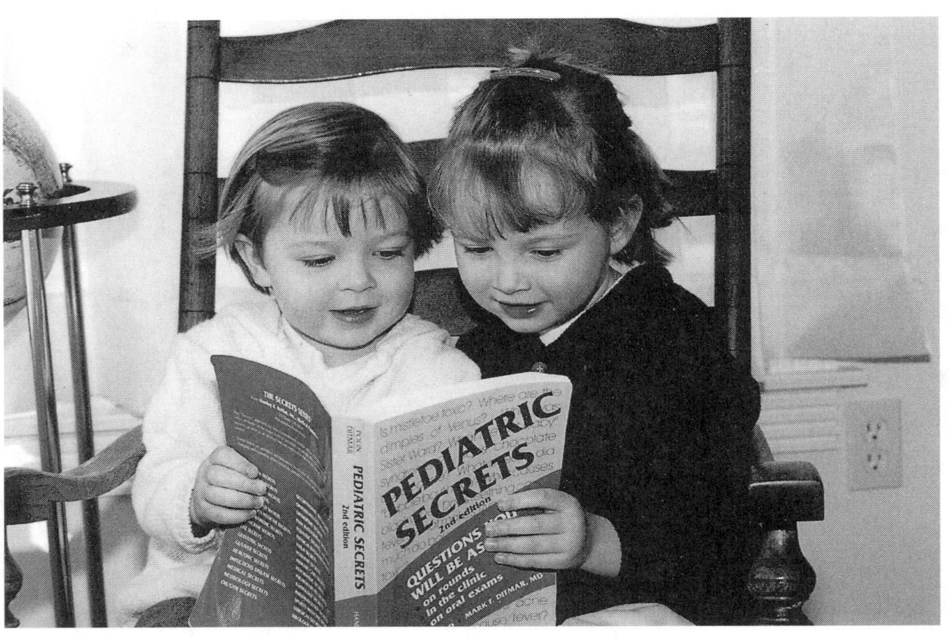
THE SECRETS SERIES
POLIN
DITMAR
PEDIATRIC SECRETS
2nd edition
PEDIATRIC
SECRETS
2nd edition
on rounds
in the clinic
on oral exams
MARK F. DITMAR, MD

1. ADOLESCENT MEDICINE

Mark F. Ditmar, M.D.

CLINICAL ISSUES

1. What are the major health risks for adolescents?

Behavioral and social rather than biomedical. ***Unintentional injury*** (particularly alcohol-related automobile accidents) and ***violence*** (i.e., suicide, homicide) account for about 80%-85% of deaths in 15-19-year olds and 60%-70% of deaths in 10-14-year olds in the U.S. Substance abuse has risen steadily in the 1990s after over a decade of steady decline. More than two-thirds of high school seniors have had sexual intercourse. One quarter of the approximate 11-13 million cases of sexually-transmitted disease reported annually to the CDC involve adolescents. Of the one million adolescent pregnancies annually, 85%-90% are unintended.

2. Name the four major risk factors associated with injuries to adolescents.

1. Use of ***alcohol*** while engaged in activities (e.g., driving, swimming, boating)—20% of all adolescent deaths are alcohol-related car crashes.
2. Failure to use ***safety devices*** (e.g., seat belts, motorcycle or bicycle helmets)—Seat belt use among adolescents is the lowest of any age group (30-50%) and fewer than ten pecent use bicycle helmets.
3. Access to ***firearms***—50% of deaths of black male teenagers and 20% of deaths of white male teenagers are due to firearms, primarily handguns.
4. ***Athletic*** participation—Most injuries are reinjuries, highlighting the importance of proper rehabilitation.

Elster AB, Kuznets NJ (eds): AMA Guidelines for Adolescent Preventive Services (GAPS). Baltimore, Williams & Wilkins, 1994, pp. 29-40.

3. How sleepy are adolescents?

Chronic sleep deprivation appears to be a widespread problem. In a survey of 3120 high school students in Rhode Island, only 15% slept more than 8.5 hours on a school night. Those with significant sleep deprivation (defined as less than 6¾ hours on school nights) had increased daytime sleepiness, depressive mood and sleep/wake behavior problems.

Wolfson AR, Carskadon MA: Sleep schedules and daytime functioning in adolescents. Child Dev 69:875-887, 1998.

4. Which adolescents are at increased risk for anemia?

Approximately 10% of U.S. teenagers (and up to 40-50% of black, urban female teenagers) are anemic (defined as a hemoglobin less than 12.0 g/dL for girls, less than 12.5 g/dL for boys ages 12-14 and less than 13.0 for boys ages 15-17). The major cause is iron deficiency because of increased requirements during pubertal growth spurts, increased losses in menstruation and poor dietary habits. Greater-than-average risk factors include:

- Low socioeconomic background
- Menorrhagia
- Pregnancy
- Malabsorption
- Vegetarian or "fad" diets
- Intense lengthy physical training
- Chronic disease
- Family history of anemia or bleeding disorder

Hord JD: Anemia and coagulation disorders in adolescents. Adolescent Medicine: State of the Art Reviews 10(3): 359-367, 1999.

5. How do you evaluate a breast lump noted by a teenage girl on self-examination?

Although the incidence of cancerous lesions is extremely low in adolescents, it is not zero, and breast lumps do require careful follow-up. *Fibrocystic changes* (i.e., proliferation of stromal and epithelial elements, ductal dilatation, cyst formation) are common in later adolescence and are characterized by variations in size and tenderness with menstrual periods. The most common tumor (up to 95%) is a *fibroadenoma*, which is a firm, discrete, rubbery, smooth mass usually found laterally. Other causes of masses include lipomas, hematomas, abscesses, and, rarely, adenocarcinoma (especially if a bloody nipple discharge is present).

The size, location and other characteristics of a mass should be documented and reevaluated over the next one to three menstrual periods. A persistent or slowly growing mass should be evaluated with ***fine-needle aspiration***. ***Ultrasound*** can be helpful in distinguishing cystic from solid masses. ***Mammography*** is a very poor tool for identifying distinct pathologic lesions in teenagers because the breast density of adolescents makes interpretation difficult.

Neinstein LS: Breast disease in adolescents and young women. Pediatr Clinic North Am 46(3): 607-629, 1999.

6. Should teenage girls be instructed on breast self-examination (BSE) as part of a routine health maintenance exam?

This remains controversial. Data on the effectiveness of BSE in younger women are very limited, especially given the lower incidence of cancer in this group. While learning the techniques may increase body awareness and lower apprehension during future clinical exams, concern exists about false positive BSEs with increased patient anxiety and reduction in time available during an office encounter for other health promotion efforts with proven effectiveness.

U.S. Preventive Services Task Force: Screening for breast cancer. In Guide to Clinical Preventive Services, 2nd ed. Baltimore: Williams & Wilkins, 1996, pp. 73-87.

7. What causes should be considered in a teenage girl with galactorrhea?

- *Drug-induced*—including oral contraceptives, amphetamines, cocaine, marijuana, opiates, phenothiazines, reserpine, methyldopa
- *Pregnancy-associated*—postabortion or postmiscarriage (may persist up to 3 months), postpartum (if term delivery, may persist up to 1 year)
- *Malignancy*—including pituitary adenoma (more likely if serum prolactin is very elevated), hypothalamic craniopharyngioma, hypothalamic infiltrative disease (e.g., histiocytosis, sarcoidosis)
- *Hypothyroidism*
- *Chronic renal disease* (in part due to delayed clearance of prolactin)
- *Chest wall factors*—nipple manipulation, surgery, herpes zoster

8. What is the most common cause of chronic pelvic pain in adolescents without a history of pelvic inflammatory disease?

Endometriosis. This condition results from implantation of endometrial tissue at ectopic locations within the peritoneal cavity. The pain is both noncyclic (may occur with intercourse or defecation) and cyclic (often most severe just before menses) and poorly controlled by non-steroidal anti-inflammatory medications or oral contraceptives. Intermenstrual bleeding is common. Although adult women classically have tender nodules noted in the posterior vaginal fornix and along the uterosacral ligaments, nodularity is rare in adolescents, which often masks clinical diagnosis. Definitive diagnosis is by laparoscopy and biopsy. Therapy can be medical (e.g., danazol) and/or surgical (e.g., excision, coagulation, laser vaporization).

Laufer M, Propst A: Diagnosing and treating adolescent endometriosis. Contemp Pediatr 9: 71, 2000.

9. Why should you ask teenage girls about their cola consumption?

High consumption of carbonated cola beverages (and low milk intake) appears to be associated with increased likelihood of fractures in teenage girls. In addition, significant data are emerging that a predisposition to osteoporosis in later life may be strongly influenced by bone changes in childhood and adolescence. Thus, simple nutritional changes, such as decreasing carbonated cola intake, may be valuable.

Wyshak G: Teenaged girls, carbonated beverage consumption, and bone fractures. Arch Pediatr Adolesc Med 154:610-613, 2000.

Fassler A-L, Bonjour J-P: Osteoporosis as a pediatric problem. Pediatr Clin North Am 42(4):811-824, 1995.

10. What should be suspected in teenagers with chronic somatic complaints?

Children and adolescents with chronic stomach aches, musculoskeletal pain and headaches are common in pediatric practice. These symptoms may be manifestations of more serious psychiatric problems. In a four-year study of 4500 patients, certain clinical presentations had a higher incidence of underlying psychopathology. Girls with frequent musculoskeletal pains (≥3 times weekly) *or* headaches (at least on a weekly basis lasting a minimum of one hour) or both headaches *and* stomach aches had higher likelihoods of depression and anxiety disorder. Boys with complaints of chronic headaches *and* stomach aches had higher likelihoods of disruptive behavior disorders (i.e., conduct disorder, oppositional defiant disorder or attention-deficit/hyperactivity disorder).

In an earlier study of teenagers with psychosomatic musculoskeletal pain, 75% were female, the median age was 13 years, and the median duration of symptoms was 1 year. Multiple sites of pain were common, and hyperesthesia occurred in 45%. Nearly all maintained a cheerful affect when complaining of severe pain. Two types of families were seen. One was cohesive, stable and organized but intolerant of separation and autonomy. The other was chaotic and emotionally unsupportive with high levels of conflict. Nearly all responded favorably to intensive physical and occupational therapy along with individual or family psychotherapy.

Egger HL, et al: Somatic complaints and psychopathology in children and adolescents: Stomach aches, musculoskeletal pains, and headaches. J Am Acad Child Adolesc Psychiatry 38:852-860, 1999.

Sherry DD, et al: Psychosomatic musculoskeletal pain in children: Clinical and psychological analyses of 100 children. Pediatrics 88:1093-1099, 1991.

11. Should an athlete be allowed back into a game following a concussion?

A concussion is defined by the Center for Disease Control and Prevention as an alteration in mental status caused by head trauma. Loss of conciousness may or may not be involved. Concern exists that if an athlete is allowed to return prematurely to competition, then minor head trauma may elicit a "second impact syndrome" with significant neurologic deterioration. Recommendations of the American Academy of Neurology regarding the return to sports activity after a concussion are as follows:

Grade 1 Concussion

Definition: transient confusion, no loss of consciousness, mental status abnormalities for ≤ 15 minutes.

Management: return to sports activities same day only if all symptoms resolve within 15 minutes; if a second grade 1 concussion occurs, no sports activity until asymptomatic for 1 week.

Grade 2 Concussion

Definition: transient confusion, no loss of consciousness, mental status abnormalities for > 15 minutes.

Management: no sports activity until asymptomatic for 1 full week; if a grade 2 concussion occurs on the same day as a previous grade 1 concussion, no sports activity for 2 weeks.

Grade 3 Concussion

Definition: concussion involving loss of consciousness

Management: no sports activity until asymptomatic for 1 week if loss of consciousness was brief (seconds), or for 2 weeks if loss of consciousness was prolonged (minutes or longer)
Second grade 3 concussion, no sports activity until asymptomatic for 1 month
Any abnormality on computed tomography or magnetic resonance imaging, no sports activity for remainder of season; patient should be discouraged from any future return to contact sports

Centers for Disease Control and Prevention: Sports-related recurrent brain injuries—United States. MMWR 1997;46:224-227.

12. Which teenagers get "stingers"?

Most commonly, ***football players***. Stingers, also called burners, are traumatic injuries to the brachial plexus (brachial plexus neuropraxia). They usually result from a head-on collision, as in tackling, which stretches or compresses the brachial plexus with resultant are pain (such as stinging or burning), paresthesia, or weakness. Although typically transient, recurrent stingers suggest cervical spine pathology.

13. What diagnoses require mandatory disclosure regardless of confidentiality?

In most states:

- Notification to child welfare authorities under state ***child-abuse*** (physical and sexual) reporting laws
- Notification to law enforcement officials of ***gunshot*** and ***stab wounds***
- Warning from a psychotherapist to a reasonably identifiable victim of a patient's ***threat of violence***
- Notification to parents or other authorities if a patient represents a reasonable threat to himself or herself (i.e., ***suicidal ideation***)

14. What techniques can increase compliance in the adolescent?

- Simplify the regimen
- Make the patient responsible
- Discuss potential side effects
- Use praise liberally
- Educate the patient
- Enlist cooperation
- Work together with parents without giving them complete control

15. When can teenagers give their own consent for medical care or procedures?

Teenagers who are married, parents themselves, members of the armed forces, living apart from their parents or high school graduates may fit the definition of an emancipated or "mature minor." However, that definition varies from state to state. For certain services, many states waive the legal requirement of emancipation, and any individual under age 18 may obtain services without parental permission. These include care for sexually transmitted diseases, contraception services, pregnancy-related care, substance abuses treatment, mental health services, and treatment for rape or sexual assault.

16. How does the "HEADSS" system assist in adolescent interviewing?

This mnemonic, devised at the Children's Hospital of Los Angeles, allows a systematic approach to multiple health issues and risk factors affecting teenagers.

***H*—Home** (living arrangements, family relationships)
***E*—Education** (school issues, employment)
***A*—Activities** (friends, exercise, television time)
***D*—Drugs** (personal use, peer use)
***S*—Sex** (orientation, contraception, abuse)
***S*—Suicide** (ideation, attempts)

EATING DISORDERS

17. What types of dieting raise concern for the development of an eating disorder?

Dieting that is associated with:

- Decreasing weight goals
- Increasing criticism of body image
- Increasing social isolation
- Amenorrhea or oligomenorrhea

Woodside DB: A review of anorexia nervosa and bulimia nervosa. Curr Prob Pediatr 25:69, 1995.

18. How is the diagnosis of anorexia made?

Anorexia nervosa constitutes a spectrum of psychological, behavioral, and medical abnormalities. The 1996 Diagnostic and Statistical Manual for Primary Care (DSM-PC): Child and Adolescent Version criteria list five components:

1. Refusal to maintain body weight or body mass index (BMI) at or above minimal norms for age and height (less than 85% of expected weight for height or a BMI of less than 18).
2. Intense fear of gaining weight or becoming fat
3. Disturbances of perception of body shape and size
4. Denial of seriousness of weight loss or low body weight
5. In postmenarchal girls, amenorrhea (i.e., the absence of at least three consecutive menstrual cycles)

19. What are good and bad prognostic indicators for recovery from anorexia?

Good: Early age at onset, high educational achievement, improvement in body image after weight gain, emotionally well-adjusted, supportive family

Poor: Late age at onset, continued overestimation of body size, self-induced vomiting or bulimia, laxative abuse, family dysfunction, male

20. What hormonal abnormalities may be seen in anorexia nervosa?

Amenorrhea is seen in most cases due to hypothalamic/pituitary dysfunction with very low levels of LH and FSH. Twenty-five percent of affected girls experience amenorrhea before significant weight loss occurs, suggesting the psychological effect on physiology. Symptoms suggestive of ***hypothyroidism***, such as constipation, cold intolerance, dry skin, bradycardia, and hair or nail changes, are common. Thyroid studies, however, have relatively normal results, except for a low triiodothyronine (T_3) and increased reverse T_3 (rT_3), a less active isomer.

The T_3/rT_3 reversal is also seen in conditions associated with weight loss, possibly indicating it is a physiologic means of adapting to a lower energy state. Other abnormalities include a loss of diurnal variation in ***cortisol***, diminished plasma ***catecholamine*** levels, normal or increased ***growth hormone*** levels, and flattened glucose tolerance curve.

21. How common is laxative abuse in anorexia nervosa?

Self-reported use is approximately 10%, but when urine screening is done, it has been found to be 20-30%. Biochemical urine screening can be done using high-performance thin-layer chromatography, especially if laxatives have been ingested within 36 hours. Direct toxicity of laxatives can lead to steatorrhea and occasionally to fat-soluble vitamin malabsorption. Fat globules in stool suggest laxative abuse.

Turner J, et al: Detection and importance of laxative use in adolescents with anorexia nervosa. J Am Acad Child Adolesc Psychiatry 39:378-385, 2000.

22. Describe the psychologic profile of a typical patient with anorexia nervosa.

- Moody and irritable
- Driven to excel in sports
- Perfectionistic
- Introverted, emotionally inhibited
- Obsessive-compulsive
- Poor self-esteem
- Preoccupied with thoughts of food
- Chronic sleep disturbances
- Depressed

23. What causes sudden death in anorectics?

Chronic emaciation affects the myocardium. Anorectics develop depressed cardiovascular function and an altered conduction system. ECG changes are common. Patients with anorexia have significantly lower heart rates (averaging 20 beats/min less than peers), lower R values in V6, and longer QRS intervals. These ECG changes often occur without underlying electrolyte abnormalities. The arrhythmogenic potential is heightened if electrolytes (specifically potassium) are distorted by excessive vomiting or laxative abuse. Sudden death is likely due to the culmination of chronic myocardial injury in emaciated patients (> 35-40% below ideal weight) with resultant heart failure and dysrhythmia.

Panagiotopoulos C, et al: Electrocardiographic findings in adolescents with eating disorders. Pediatrics 105:1100-1105, 2000.

24. Do males with anorexia nervosa have a similar clinical profile compared with females?

It is estimated that less than 5% of anorexia nervosa involves boys. Males are more likely to:

- Have been obese before the onset of symptoms
- To be ambivalent regarding the desire to gain or lose weight
- Have more issues regarding gender and sexual identity
- Involve dieting with sports participation
- Engage in "defensive dieting" (avoiding weight gain after a athletic injury)

Farrow JA: The adolescent male with an eating disorder. Pediatr Ann 21: 769-774, 1992.

25. How is the diagnosis of bulimia nervosa made?

Bulimia nervosa is a syndrome of voracious, high-caloric overeating and subsequent forced vomiting (by gagging or ipecac) and/or other purging methods (e.g., laxatives, diuretics), often done during periods of frustration or psychological stress. Its incidence is felt to be higher than that of anorexia nervosa, and males are rarely involved. The diagnosis is made by ***history***.

26. List the medical complications of bulimia nervosa.

***Electrolyte abnormalities*:** hypokalemia, hypochloremia, and metabolic alkalosis. The hypokalemia can cause a prolonged QT interval and T-wave abnormalities.

***Esophageal*:** acid reflux with esophagitis and (rarely) Mallory-Weiss tear

***Cardiac*:** use of ipecac can result in cardiomyopathy (due to a toxic effect of one its principal components, the alkaloid emetine).

***CNS*:** neurotransmitters can be affected, causing changes in perceptions of satiety

***Miscellaneous*:** enamel erosion, salivary gland enlargement, cheilosis, and knuckle calluses (signs of recurrent vomiting)

27. How do anorexia nervosa and bulimia nervosa differ?

ANOREXIA NERVOSA	BULIMIA NERVOSA
Vomiting or diuretic/laxative abuse uncommon	Vomiting or diuretic/laxative abuse
Severe weight loss	Less weight loss; avoidance of obesity
Slightly younger	Slightly older
More introverted	More extroverted
Hunger denied	Hunger pronounced
Eating behavior may be considered normal and a source of self-esteem	Eating behavior is egodystonic
Sexually inactive	Sexually active
Obsessional fears with paranoid features	Histrionic features
Amenorrhea	Menses irregular or absent
Death from starvation/suicide	Death from hypokalemia/suicide

From Shenker IR, Bunnell DW: Bulimia nervosa. In McAnarmey ER, et al (eds): Textbook of Adolescent Medicine. Philadelphia, W.B. Saunders, 1993, p. 545; with permission.

28. What modalities are used to treat eating disorders?

- ***Nutritional rehabilitation***—very large caloric intakes (e.g., 3000-4000 kcal/day) may be needed to achieve adequate gain. Controversy exists regarding strict versus lenient inpatient protocols. Routine use of appetite stimulants, nasogastric feedings, or hyperalimentation is not recommended.
- ***Medication***—prokinetic agents (e.g., domperidone) are used to minimize postprandial bloating. Antidepressants, including serotonin-specific reuptake inhibitors, are more commonly used in bulimia nervosa.
- ***Psychotherapy***, including family therapy

Woodside DB: A review of anorexia nervosa and bulimia nervosa. Curr Probl Pediatr 25:67-89, 1995.

29. Name the three features that constitute the "female athletic triad."

Disordered eating, amenorrhea, and ***osteoporosis***. These three distinct yet interrelated disorders are often seen in active girls and young women. All female athletes are at risk for developing this triad, with 15—60% of female athletes demonstrating abnormal weight-control behaviors. Diagnosis is based on history, physical examination, and laboratory evaluation. The basic lab workup should include urine hCG, TSH, prolactin, FSH, LH, testosterone, DHEA-S and progesterone challenge test. Ongoing counseling is often indicated, as well as nutritional and hormonal intervention. Treatment commonly includes calcium supplements and oral contraceptives.

American Academy of Pediatrics, Committee on Sports Medicine and Fitness: Medical concerns in the female athlete. Pediatrics 106:610-613, 2000.

30. What are the risk factors for obesity in teenagers?

- ***Positive family history***: With one obese parent, probability of obesity is 40%; with two obese parents, this increases to 70-80%
- ***Degree of obesity as a child:*** More severe obesity is likely to persist
- ***Socioeconomic status:*** Generally, higher socioeconomic status confers a higher likelihood of obesity. This trend is maintained in adulthood for boys, but reverses in late adolescence for girls.
- ***Television viewing:*** Increased TV viewing appears to correlate with higher likelihood of obesity.
- ***Race:*** More common among whites than blacks.
- ***Family size:*** Obesity decreases as family size increases and has the greatest prevalence among single children.

Robinson TN: Reducing children's television viewing to prevent obesity. JAMA 282:1561-1567, 1999.

31. Which is a better tool to estimate body fat in an adolescent—body mass index (BMI) or triceps skinfold?

BMI *(weight in kg/height in m^2)* above the 85th percentile has been used to define obesity. However, it can be evelated in individuals with large frames ("big-boned") who are overweight but not overfat.

Triceps skinfold (TSF) correlates better with percent body fat and total body fat in adolescents. A TSF > 85% for age, sex, and race is the most widely accepted criterion for obesity. Of note, a problem with the TSF is the variability of technique, which limits the reproducibility of results.

32. Do obese children and adolescents become obese adults?

Only 25-50% in most tracking studies have become obese adults, but in some studies it has ranged as high as 75%. The most important risk factors for persistence of obesity are later age of onset and increased severity of obesity at any age. The problem is very significant and worsening. Multiple studies indicate about 15-30% of U.S. children are overweight.

Gauthier BM, et al: High prevalence of overweight children and adolescents in the Practice Partner Research Network. Arch Pediatr Adolesc Med 154:625-628, 2000.

Mokdad AH et al: The spread of the obesity epidemic in the United States, 1991-1998. JAMA 282:1519-1522, 1999.

33. What cardiac risk factors are present in obese adolescents?

Elevated triglycerides, elevated total cholesterol, decreased HDL cholesterol, hypertension, diminished maximum work capacity, and strong family history of coronary artery disease. The incidence of these associations is not small. Large percentages of obese adolescents may have at least three risk factors present.

34. What is the long-term outlook for the obese teenager?

Obesity in adolescence is associated with medical, economic, and social consequences. Obese teenagers, especially females, have lower rates of school completion, lower rates of marriage, lower household incomes, and higher rates of poverty. Even if weight corrections occur later, the early obesity is associated with increased atherosclerotic heart disease in men and women, with colorectal cancer and gout in men, and with arthritis in women.

Gortmake SL, et al: Social and economic consequences of overweight in adolescence and young adulthood. N Engl J Med 327:1008-1012, 1992.

Must A, et al: Long-term morbidity and mortality of overweight adolescents: A follow-up of the Harvard Growth Study of 1922-1935. N Engl J Med 327:1350-1355, 1992.

35. Are fat distribution measurements of any prognostic value in adolescents?

In adults, the distribution of body fat rather than percent excess of body fat seems to be a better indicator of potential morbidity. For example, when the waist-hip circumference ratio is measured, an adult with a higher ratio (increased abdominal fat or "android" habitus) has a higher frequency of hypertension, diabetes, and hyperlipidemia compared with an equally obese individual with a lower ratio (increased pelvic fat or "gynecoid" habitus). However, prospective long-term data are not available to indicate whether fat distribution measurements have any prognostic significance in adolescents.

36. How effective are intervention and treatment for obesity in adolescents?

Weight reduction regimens, involving behavior modification and dietary therapy, are modestly effective in short-term results, but notoriously ineffective in achieving long-term weight loss.

Spieth LE, et al: A low-glycemic index diet in the treatment of pediatric obesity. Arch Pediatr Adolesc Med 154: 947-951, 2000.

Gortmaker SL, et al: Reducing obesity via a school-based interdisciplinary intervention among youth. Arch Pediatr Adolesc Med 153:409-418, 1999.

Haddock DK, et al: Treatments for childhood and adolescent obesity. Ann Behav Med 16:235-244, 1994.

MENSTRUAL DISORDERS

37. What is the difference between primary and secondary amenorrhea?

Primary amenorrhea: no onset of menses by age 16, or within 3 years of onset of secondary sex characteristics, or within 1 year of Tanner V breast/pubic hair development

Secondary amenorrhea: no menses for 3 months after previous establishment of regular menstrual periods

38. What causes primary amenorrhea?

The key feature in the differential diagnosis is whether the amenorrhea is associated with the development of secondary sex characteristics.

Amenorrhea without secondary sex characteristics
- Chromosomal or enzymatic defects (e.g., Turner syndrome, chromosomal mosaics, 17α-hydroxylase deficiency)
- Congenital absence of uterus
- Gonadal dysgenesis (with elevated gonadotropins)
- Hypothalamic-pituitary abnormalities (with diminished gonadotropins)

Amenorrhea with secondary sex characteristics
- Dysfunction of hypothalamic release of GnRH (e.g., stress, excessive exercise, weight loss, chronic illness, polycystic ovary disease, medications, hypothyroidism)
- Abnormalities of pituitary gland (e.g., tumor, empty sella syndrome)
- Ovarian dysfunction (e.g., irradiation, chemotherapy, trauma, viral infection, autoimmune inflammation)
- Abnormalities of genital tract (e.g., cervical agenesis, imperforate hymen, testicular feminization with absent uterus)
- Pregnancy

39. How can estrogen influence be evaluated on vaginal or cervical smears?

Vaginal smear: In patients with normal estrogen, 15–30% of cells are superficial (small pyknotic nuclei with large cytoplasm), and the remainder are intermediate (larger nuclei with visible nucleolus, but still with cytoplasm predominant). If parabasal cells are noted (nuclear:cytoplasmic ratio of ≥ 50:50), relative estrogen deficiency should be suspected.

Cervical smear: Cervical mucus is smeared onto a glass slide and allowed to dry. If a fern pattern appears, estrogen is normal (since salts crystallize only if estrogen is unopposed by progesterone). No fern pattern occurs in the second half of menses after ovulation due to the presence of progesterone. Absence of ferning in pregnancy is also due to higher progesterone levels.

40. What is the value of a progesterone challenge test in a patient with amenorrhea?

If bleeding ensues within 2 weeks after administration of oral medroxyprogesterone (10 mg daily for 5 days) or intramuscular progesterone in oil (50-100 mg), the test is postitive. This indicates that the endometrium has been primed by estrogen and that the pituitary-hypothalamic-ovarian axis and outflow tract are functioning.

41. A 14-year-old girl has Tanner III features and monthly abdominal pain but no onset of menstrual flow. What is the likely diagnosis?

An ***anatomic abnormality of the vagina*** (e.g., imperforate hymen or transverse vaginal septum) or cervix (e.g., agenesis).

42. An obese 16-year-old has oligomenorrhea, hirsutism, acne and an elevated LH/FSH ratio. What condition is likely?

Polycystic ovary syndrome. This disorder is characterized by the triad of *menstrual irregularities* (amenorrhea/oligomenorrhea), *hirsutism,* and *acne* which begins during puberty. Obesity is common. In these individuals, there is an apparent gonadotropin-dependent, functional ovarian hyperadrogenism with elevated LH (or LH:FSH ratio >3:1) and insulin resistance. A dysregulation of ovarian synthesis of androgens and estrogen is likely. Studies of mainly white, European females have found that 60% of teens with oligomenorrhea have endocrine signs compatible with polycystic ovary syndrome. Endocrine evaluation should strongly be considered in oligomenorrheic adolescents before reassurance is given or before prescriptions are written for oral contraceptives.

Stashwick CA: Amenorrhea and acne in the adolescent girl: Is it polycystic ovary syndrome? Contemp Pediatr 17: 38, 2000.

van Hooff MHA et al: Endocrine features of polycystic ovary syndrome in a random population sample of 14-16 year-old adolescents. Hum Reprod 14:2223-2229, 1999.

43. What are the range of complications of polycystic ovary sydrome?

- Infertility
- Type 2 diabetes
- Cardiovascular disease
- Abnormal lipid metabolism
- Endometrial cancer

Solomon CG: The epidemiology of polycystic ovary syndrome: Prevalence and associated disease risks. Endocrinol Metab Clin North Am 84;1897:1999.

44. What constitutes excessive menstrual bleeding in an adolescent?

As a rule, most menstrual periods do not last >8 days, do not occur more frequently than every 21-40 days, and are not associated with >80 ml of blood loss. The quantitation can be difficult, as pad or tampon numbers correlate poorly with total blood loss. Blood clots or a change in pad numbers appears to have more reliability. Suspicion of excessive loss should prompt an evaluation of hematocrit and/or reticulocyte count.

45. How common are anovulatory menstrual periods in adolescents?

Anovulatory cycles (and with them, an increased likelihood of irregular periods) occur in 50% of adolescents for up to 2 years after menarche and in up to 20% after 5 years (the rate in adults). Anovulatory cycles result in unopposed estradiol production which can cause (1) breakthrough bleeding at varying intervals due to insufficient hormone to support a thickened endothelium, and (2) heavy and prolonged menstrual flow due to lack of progesterone. However, most anovulatory menstrual cycles are normal because the intact negative feedback loop (rising estradiol lowers FH and LSH which, in turn, lower estradiol) does not allow prolonged elevated estrogren with endometrial proliferation.

46. Describe the evaluation for a patient with dysfunctional uterine bleeding.

Dysfunctional uterine bleeding is abnormal bleeding in the absence of structural pelvic pathology. It remains a diagnosis of exclusion. Depending on the age of the patient and history of sexual activity, the following studies should be considered:

- Speculum exam for evidence of trauma, vaginal foreign body, DES-induced adenosis
- Bimanual exam for ovarian mass, uterine fibroid, signs of pregnancy or pelvic inflammatory disease
- Pap smear for cervical dysplasia
- Pregnancy test
- Serum prolactin
- Thyroid function tests
- Coagulation studies (especially for von Willebrand disease)

47. How can the *timing* of abnormal uterine bleeding help identify the most likely cause?

Abnormal bleeding at the normal time of cyclic shedding
Blood dyscrasia (especially von Willebrand disease)
Endometrial pathology (e.g., submucous myoma, intrauterine device)
Abnormal bleeding at any time in the cycle, but normal cycles
Vaginal foreign body
Trauma
Endometriosis
Infection
Uterine polyps
Cervical abnormality (e.g., hemangioma)
Noncyclic bleeding or abnormal cyclic bleeding (<21 days or >45 days, usually associated with anovulatory cycles)
Physiologic (especially in early adolescence)
Polycystic ovary disease
Psychosocial pathology
Excessive exercise
Endocrine disorders
Adrenal/ovarian tumors
Ovarian failure

Adapted from Kozlowski K, et al: Adolescent gynecologic conditions presenting in emergency settings. Adolesc Med State Art Rev 5:65, 1993; with permission.

48. How should dysfunctional uterine bleeding be managed?

Management depends on the estimated blood loss as determined by hemoglobin (Hb) concentration and signs of ortthrostatic hypotension:

- ***No acute hemorrhage, no anemia***
  Expectant management, consider oral contraceptive
  Use of menstrual calendar
  Begin iron supplementation
- **No acute hemorrhage, mild anemia** (Hb 10–12 gm/dl)
  Oral contraceptive: potent progestin (e.g., norgestrel/ethinyl estradiol) or cyclic medroxyprogesterone (e.g., 10 mg for 5?7 days every 35–40 days) with change to a less potent progestin when flow is lighter
  Begin iron supplementation
- **No acute hemorrhage, moderate anemia** (Hb < 10 gm/dl)
  Oral contraceptive: high-dose estrogen (50 μg)–potent progestin combination, since severe bleeding may have left little endometrium on which the progestin can act
  Begin iron supplementation
- **Acute hemorrhage, significant anemia** (Hb 7–9 gm/dl), no orthostatic changes
  Oral contraceptive: high-dose estrogen (50 μg)–potent progestin combination every 6 hrs for 2 days tapered over 1 wk, with longer-term use likely (after estrogen tapered)
  Consider hospitalization if bleeding is severe
  Clotting studies due to higher likelihood or underlying coagulopathy
- ***Acute hemorrhage, severe anemia*** (<7 gm/dl), orthostatic changes
  Hospitalize for high-dose estrogen intravenously (e.g., 25 mg every 4 hrs for 24 hrs) with concurrent oral high-dose progestin
  Consider transfusion
  Unresponsive bleeding may require dilation and curettage
  Clotting studies

49. Why is dysmenorrhea more common in *late* rather than *early* adolescence?

Dysmennorhea occurs almost entirely with ovulatory cycles. Menses shortly after the onset of menarche is usually anovulatory. With the establishment of more regular ovulatory cycles after 2-4 years, primary dysmenorrhea becomes more likely.

50. In a teenager with dysmenorrhea, what factors suggest an underlying identifiable pathologic problem rather than primary dysmenorrhea?

Primary dysmenorrhea is painful menses without identifiable pelvic pathology and accounts for the vast majority of cases in teenagers. However, underlying pathology is more likely if any of the following conditions is present: ***menorrhagia*** (excessive volume or duration of menses); ***intermenstrual bleeding***; ***pain*** at times ***other than menses*** (suggesting outflow obstruction); or ***abnormal uterine shape*** on exam (suggesting uterine malformation).

51. What classes of medications are used for dysmenorrhea?

***Prostglandin inhibitors*:** evidence strongly suggests a key role for prostaglandins in pain production (especially $PGF_{2\alpha}$ and $PGE_{2\alpha}$). Non-steroidal anti-inflammatory agents can limit local production. Naproxen, ibuprofen and mefanamic acid are all effective. Side effects of indomethacin and phenylbutazone limit their use. Aspirin is no more effective than placebo.

***Oral contraceptives*:** OCPs act by reducing endometrial growth, which limits total production of endometrial prostaglandin. Ovulation is suppressed which also minimizes pain. A 30-35 μg combined estrogen-progestin pill is preferred. After 4-6 months, OCPs may be stopped and symptoms reassessed if the need for contraception is not an issue.

Central-acting analgesic: Tramadol acts by binding to m-opioid receptors and inhibiting reuptake of norepinephrine and serotonin. It is neither an NSAID or a narcotic and appears to be non-addictive.

Alternative medicines: Herbal teas, fruits and vegetables may be beneficial.

Laufer MR, Goldstein DP: Dysmenorrhea, pelvic pain and the premenstrual syndrome. In Emans SJ, et al (eds): Pediatric and Adolescent Gynecology, 4th ed. Lippincott-Raven, Phildadelphia, 1998, pp. 363-410.

SEXUAL DEVELOPMENT

52. What are the ranges of normal in the stages of pubertal development in boys?

Dr. James Tanner in 1969-70 categorized the progression of stages of puberty, dividing pubertal development in boys into pubic and genital development. Nearly all boys begin puberty with testicular enlargement, followed in about 6 months by pubic hair and then about 6-12 months later by phallic enlargement. For boys, puberty lasts on average 3.5 years.

Tanner Stages of Sexual Maturation in Boys

STAGE	DESCRIPTION	MEAN AGE	AGE RANGE 5–95%
	Pubic Hair		
I	None	—	—
II	Countable; straight; increased pigmentation and length; primarily at base of penis	12	10–14
III	Darker; begins to curl; increased quantity	13	11.25–15
IV	Increased quantity; coarser texture; covers most of pubic area	13.75	12–15.75
V	Adult distribution; spread to medial thighs and lower abdomen	14.5	13–17.5
	Genital Development		
I	Prepubertal	—	—
II	Testicular enlargement (>4 ml volume); slight rugation of scrotum	11.5	9.5–13.75
III	Further testicular enlargement; penile lengthening begins	12.5	10.25–14.5
IV	Testicular enlargement continues; increased rugation of scrotum; increased penile breadth	13.25	11.25–15.5
V	Adult	14.25	12.5–17

53. What are the ranges of normal in the stages of pubertal development in girls?

Tanner divided pubertal development in girls according to pubic hair and breast development. About 85% of girls begin puberty with initiation of breast enlargement, while 15% have axillary hair as the first sign. Menarche usually occurs about 18-24 months after the onset of breast development. For girls, the duration of puberty is longer than boys and averages 4.5 years. There is evidence accumulating that the onset of puberty is occurring earlier in girls and that these standards may need to be revised (see Endocrinology, question 87).

Tanner Stages of Sexual Maturation in Girls

STAGE	DESCRIPTION	MEAN AGE	AGE RANGE 5–95%
	Pubic Hair		
I	None	—	—
II	Countable; straight; increased pigmentation and length; primarily on medial border of labia	11.25	9–13.5
III	Darker; begins to curl; increased quantity on mons pubis	12	9.5–14.25
IV	Increased quantity; coarser texture; labia and mons well covered	12.5	10.5–15
V	Adult distribution with feminine triangle and spread to medial thighs	14	12–16.5
	Breast Development		
I	Prepubertal	—	—
II	Breast bud present; increased areolar size	11	9–13
III	Further enlargementof breast; no secondary contour	12	10–14
IV	Areolar area forms secondary mound on breast contour	13	10.5–15.5
V	Mature; areolar area is part of breast contour; nipple projects	15	13–18
Menarche		12.8	11–14.5

54. When do boys develop the ability to reproduce?

The average age of spermarche (as demonstrated by the presence of spermatozoa in first morning urine) is 13.3 years. Unlike in girls in whom menarche follows the peak height velocity, in boys spermarche occurs before the growth spurt.

55. When is delayed sexual development a concern?

The first easily recognizable sign of puberty in most females is a breast bud, which occurs at a mean age of 11 years. In boys, it is testicular enlargement, which on average begins at 11.5 years. Evaluation should be considered in girls with no breast development by 13 years or no menarche by 15 years and in boys with no testicular enlargement by age 14. By statistical definition, this is 3% of teenagers. If the norms for the onset of puberty are adjusted, the timing of concerns for delayed development may also change.

56. Why should the sense of smell be tested in a teenager with delayed puberty?

Kallman syndrome is characterized by a defect in GnRH with resultant gonadotropin deficiency and hypogonadism. Maldevelopment of the olfactory lobes occurs, with resultant anosmia or hyposmia. Less commonly, cleft palate, congenital deafness, and color blindness can occur. These patients require hormonal therapy to achieve puberty and fertility.

57. Which tests should you consider in a boy or girl with delayed puberty?

If history or physical examination do not suggest an underlying cause (e.g., anorexia nervosa), tests should include LH, FSH, testosterone (male), and bone age. These tests will help categorize the condition as hypergonadotropic (implying possible gonadal defects, androgen insensitivity, or enzyme defects) or hypogonadotropic (implying constitutional delay or primary hypothalamic-pituitary problems).

Further testing is predicated on the results of these intitial tests. For example, a 14½-year-old male with a bone age of 11.5 years and a total testosterone of 23 ng/dl (normal prepubertal level is <10) will probably begin to show outward evidence of puberty within the next few months. Therefore, no further studies are warranted. On the other hand, if this boy has a bone age of 12.5 years, testosterone <10 ng/dl, and no elevation of FH and LSH, specific testing of the hypothalamic-pituitary axis is indicated.

58. Can puberty be safely accelerated?

In some teenagers, more commonly boys, the constitutional delay in puberty has significant psychological effects. Studies have shown that in **boys**, puberty can be accelerated without any compromise in expected adult height. In boys aged >14 years with plasma testosterone levels of <10 ng/dl, testosterone enanthate, 50-100 mg IM, can be given monthly for 4-6 months. Treatment for **girls** who are constitutionally-delayed is less well studied. Conjugated estrogen, 0.3 mg (e.g., Premarin), or ethinyl estradiol (5-10 ug) daily for 2-3 months has been used in girls >13 years without breast buds.

59. When do lesbians and gay males begin to personalize homosexuality?

During ***adolescence***. For this reason, health providers need to be sensitive not to assume sexual identities during their interactions with teenagers.

Friedman RC, Downey JI: Homosexuality. N Engl J Med 331:923-930, 1994.

SEXUALLY TRANSMITTED DISEASES

60. How does the prevalence of sexually transmitted diseases (STDs) in adolescents compare with that in adults?

Among sexually active individuals, adolescents have a ***higher likelihood*** than adults of being infected with an STD. About 25% of adolescents will contract at least one STD by the time of high school graduation. Reasons for the increased susceptibility include:

- Cervical ectropion: *Neisseria gonorrhoeae* and *Chlamydia trachomatis* more readily infect columnar epithelium, and the adolescent ectocervix has more of this type of epithelium than does that of an adult.
- Cervical metaplasia in the transformation zone (for columnar to squamous epithelium) is more susceptible to human papillomavirus infection.
- Less frequent use of barrier methods of contraception

61. What is considered the most common STD in teenagers in the U.S.?

Human papillomavirus (HPV) affects 20-40% of sexually active adolescent females. More than 80 HPV types have been identified, with variable presentations including anogenital condyloma acuminatum and cervical infection which may lead to cervical dysplasia. In the latter infection, the association of HPV with the potential for cervical carcinoma increases the urgency of screening for HPV in sexually active teenagers. Visualization of anogenital warts can be enhanced by wetting the area with 3-5% acetic acid (vinegar), which whitens the lesions. HPV is also a cause of non-sexually transmitted disease, including deep plantar warts, palmar warts, and common warts.

62. What is the effect of douching of the incidence rate of STDs?

Douching is practiced by about 15% of teenage girls and up to 37% of black teenage girls. It associated with pathogenic changes in the vaginal flora and an increased risk of PID and ectopic pregnancy. The practice favors the development of bacterial vaginosis and should be discouraged. Of note, microflora levels return to normal within 72 hours unless bactericidal douching agents are used.

Merchant JS et al: Douching: A problem for adolescent girls and young women. Arch Pediatr Adolesc Med 153:834-837, 1999.

63. Is the presence of an ectropion noted on pelvic exam a concern?

An *ectropion* is the outward rolling of a margin. A cervical ectropion is the extension of the erythematous columnar epithelium from the os onto the duller, pink cervix. It is a relatively common finding in adolescents. However, large ectropions extending to the vaginal wall or abnormal cervical shape can be associated with diethylstilbestrol (DES) exposure *in utero* or chronic cervicitis.

64. Which teenage girls should have Pap smears done?

Although carcinoma is rare in teenagers, cervical dysplasia is not. This is due in large part to the widespread acquisition of HPV, of which a number of subtypes are oncogenic. Most national organizations recommend that females who are sexually active and/or ≥ 18 years of age should have at least an annual Pap test. Because the false-negative rate of the test can be up to 30%, those teenagers at particularly high risk (e.g., multiple sexual partners, recurrent STDs) should be considered for more frequent testing. There is controversy in this area, however. Since the incidence of *in situ* carcinoma is very low in teenagers, debate centers around whether the specter of a pelvic exam may be a deterrent to teenagers initially seeking reproductive health care.

Perlman SE, et al: Should pelvic examinations and Papanicolaou cervical screening be part of preventive health care for sexually active adolescent girls? J Adolesc Health 23:62-67, 1998.

Shafer MB: Annual pelvic examination in the sexually active adolescent female: What are we doing and why are we doing it? J Adolesc Health 23:68-73, 1998.

65. How can you minimize the chance of a false-negative Pap smear?

- Lubricate the speculum with warm water only (avoid lubricating gels)
- Obtain endocervical specimen with cytobrush rather than cotton-tipped swab for greater collection of cells
- Fix slides immediately to avoid drying artifacts
- Paired cervical smears increase the yield (but also the cost)

66. What is the best way to screen for STDs?

The gold standard for STDs, particularly in any cases of possible sexual abuse, remains *culture*. However, nonculture techniques involving amplification of nucleic acid (e.g., polymerase chain reaction, ligase chain reaction and transcription-mediated amplification), are widely used and widely studied. The CDC (and the courts) view the nonculture techniques as having a greater potential for false positivity and the result of a single nonculture test is presumptive.

67. Are pelvic exams with specula always required to obtain specimens in teenagers?

A number of studies have been done demonstrating that:

- *Urine testing* for chlamydia and gonorrhea using nucleic acid amplification techniques approaches the sensitivity and specificity of specimens obtained using a speculum
- Vaginal specimens obtained without use of a specula have a high screening validity for trichomonas, bacterial vaginosis and yeast infections
- *Self-collection* by teenagers of vaginal specimens yielded comparable PCR results to physician-obtained cervical and vaginal specimens.

Future trends in screening for STDs in teenage girls may shift from endocervical sampling to urine-based and vaginal self-collection.

Shafer MB: Is the routine pelvic examination needed with the advent of urine-based screening for sexually transmitted diseases? Arch Pediatr Adolesc Med 153:119-25, 1999.

Polaneczy M, et al: Use of self-collected vaginal specimens for detection of Chlamydia trachomatis infections. Obstet Gynecol 91:375-378, 1998.

Blake DR, et al: Evaluation of vaginal infectious in adolescent women: Can it be done without a speculum? Pediatrics 102: 939-944, 1998.

68. Describe the appearance of condylomata acuminata.

Condyloma acuminata (anogenital warts) are soft, fleshy, wet, polypoid or pedunculated papules that appear in the genital and perianal area. They may coalesce and take on a cauliflower appearance.

69. How do you treat condylomata and human papillomavirus (HPV) infection?

A common approach for mucosal involvement is 25% podophyllin resin in benzoin applied carefully to the lesion and a 2-3 mm margin of surrounding skin and washed off completely in 3–6 hours. Reapplications can be done, but failure rates can be >50%. Other approaches, particularly on nonmucosal surfaces, include liquid nitrogen, 85% trichloroacetic acid, topical 5-fluorouracil, alpha-interferon, imiquimod cream 5% and ablative therapy (e.g., laser, surgical excision).

70. A sexually active 17-year-old woman with adnexal and right-upper-quadrant (RUQ) tenderness likely has what condition?

Fitz-Hugh—Curtis syndrome. This is a perihepatitis caused by gonococci or, less commonly, chlamydiae. It should be suspected in any patient with pelvic inflammatory disease (PID) who has RUQ tenderness. It may be mistaken for acute hepatitis or cholecystitis. The pathophysiology is felt to be the direct spread from a pelvic infection along the paracolic gutters to the liver, where inflammation develops and capsular adhesions form (the so-called violin string adhesions seen on surgical exploration). If RUQ pain persists despite treatment for PID, ultrasonography should be done to rule out a perihepatic abscess.

71. A teenage girl develops migratory polyarthritis, fever, and scattered petechial lesions several days prior to menses. What condition should be suspected?

Gonococcal-arthritis-dermatitis syndrome (GADS). After a migratory polyarthritis or polyarthralgia, the arthritis settles in one or two large joints. The patient then develops painful tenosynovitis over the tendon sheaths, in addition to a characteristic crop of embolic skin lesions over the trunk and extremities. Diagnosis is confirmed by culturing gonococci from blood, synovial fluid, and/or rectal or genitourinary sites.

72. What are the clinical criteria for pelvic inflammatory disease?

All three of the following must be present:

1. Lower abdominal tenderness
2. Cervical motion tenderness
3. Adnexal tenderness

Plus one or more of the following:

- Oral temperature >38.3° C (101° F)
- Abnormal cervical or vaginal discharge (particularly with leukocytes)
- Elevated erythrocyte sedimentation rate (usually >15 mm/hr)
- Elevated C-reactive protein
- Cervical infection with *Neisseria gonorrhoeae* or *Chlamydia trachomatis* (the former by culture, the latter by nonculture tests, such as nucleic acid amplification)

As no single clinical aspect or laboratory test is definitive for PID, a constellation of findings is used to support the diagnosis.

American Academy of Pediatrics: Pelvic inflammatory disease. In Pickering LK (ed): 2000 Red Book, 25th ed. Elk Grove Village, IL, American Academy of Pediatrics, 2000, p. 432.

73. How is the diagnosis of PID *definitively* made?

- *Endometrial biopsy* with histopathologic evidence of endometritis
- *Transvaginal or abdominal ultrasonography* revealing tubo-ovarian abscess or consistent fallopian tube abnormalities (e.g., thickened, fluid-filled fallopian tubes with or without free pelvic fluid)
- *Laparoscopy* revealing abnormalities consistent with PID

American Academy of Pediatrics: Pelvic inflammatory disease. In Pickering LK (ed): 2000 Red Book, 25th ed. Elk Grove Village, IL, American Academy of Pediatrics, 2000, p. 432.

74. What are the sequelae of pelvic inflammatory disease (PID)?

Twenty-five percent of patients with a history of PID will have one or more major sequelae of the disease, including:

- *Tubo-ovarian abscess*—approximately 15-20% of all adolescents with PID
- *Recurrent infection*
- *Chronic abdominal pain*—may include exacerbated dysmenorrhea and dyspareunia related to pelvic adhesions, which occur in approximately 20% of patients with PID
- *Ectopic pregnancy*—risk is increased 3-7-fold
- *Infertility*—up to 11% after 1 episode of PID, 30% after 2 episodes, and 55% after ≥3 episodes

Lawson MA, Blythe MJ: Pelvic inflammatory disease in adolescents. Pediatr Clin North Am 46(4): 767-781, 1999.

75. Which adolescents with PID should be hospitalized for intravenous antibiotics?

- *Surgical emergency*, such as appendicitis or ectopic pregnancy (or if such a diagnosis cannot be excluded)
- *Severe illness:* pelvic or tubo-ovarian abscess, overt peritonitis
- *Immunodeficiency:* (HIV infection with low CD4 lymphocyte count, immunosuppressive therapy)
- *Pregnancy*
- *Expected unreliable compliance or follow-up or inability to tolerate outpatient regimen*
- *Failure of outpatient therapy*

American Academy of Pediatrics: Pelvic inflammatory disease. In Pickering LK (ed): 2000 Red Book, 25th ed., Elk Grove Village, IL, American Academy of Pediatrics, 2000, p. 433.

76. When do the symptoms of endocervicitis occur in relation to menses?

Gonorrhea is much more likely to present during menstruation. Of patients with gonorrhea, 85% develop symptoms during the first 7 days of menses compared with only 33% with chlamydial infections.

77. How are the genital ulcer syndromes differentiated?

Genital ulcers may be seen in herpes simplex, syphilis, chancroid, lymphogranuloma venereum, and granuloma inguinale (donovanosis). Herpes and syphilis are the most common, and granuloma inguinale is very rare. Although there is overlap, clinical distinction is as follows:

Differentiation of Genital Ulcer Syndromes

	HERPES SIMPLEX	SYPHILIS (PRIMARY, SECONDARY)	CHANCROID	LYMPHOGRANULUM VENEREUM (LGV)
Agent	Herpes simplex virus	*Treponema pallidum*	*Haemophilus ducreyi*	*Chlamydia trachomatis*
Primary lesions	Vesicle	Papule	Papule-pustule	Papule-vesicle
Size (mm)	1–2	5–15	2–20	2–10
Number	Multiple, clusters (coalesce ±)	Single	Multiple (coalesce ±)	Single

Depth	Sperficial	Superficial or deep	Deep	Superficial or deep
Base	Erythematous, nonpurulent	Sharp, indurated, nonpurulent	Ragged border, purulent, friable	Varies
Pain	Yes	No	Yes	No
Lymphade-	Tender, bilateral	Nontender, bilateral	Tender, unilateral, may suppurate, unilocular fluctuance	Tender, unilateral, may suppurate, multilocular fluctuance

From Shafer MA: Sexually transmitted disease syndromes. In McAnarmey ER, et al (eds): Textbook of Adolescent Medicine. Philadelphia, W.B. Saunders, 1992, p. 708, with permission.

78. What is the value of oral acyclovir, famciclovir and valacyclovir in the treatment of genital herpes infections in immunocompetent hosts?

- Useful mainly in primary episode of disease
- Lessens duration of pain and itching (especially with initiation of therapy within 6 days of onset of disease)
- May lessen systemic symptoms of headache, fever, myalgia and malaise
- Shortens viral shedding (and thus may shorten period of contagion)
- If history of ≥6 episodes/year, delays and reduces frequency of recurrences while on therapy

Acyclovir appears to be safe when used in adults for up to 10 years, but longer-term studies of its toxicity remain to be done. Thus, chronic administration should not be used for prophylaxis in individuals who have mild disease. Discontinuation of prophylactic medication is recommended at 1 year to reassess need.

79. How are the three most common causes of postpubertal vaginitis clinically distinguished?

Candidal vaginitis: vulvar itching and erythema, vaginal discharge (thick, white curdlike)

Trichomonas vaginitis: vulvar itching and erythema, vaginal discharge (gray, yellow-green, frothy; rarely malodorous)

Bacterial vaginosis: minimal erythema, vaginal discharge (malodorous; thin white discharge clings to vaginal walls)

80. How does the vaginal pH help indicate the cause of a vaginal discharge?

Ordinarily, the vaginal pH of a pubertal girl is <4.5 (compared with 7.0 in prepubertal girls). If the pH is >4.5, infection with *Trichomonas* or bacterial vaginosis should be suspected.

81. How does evaluation of the vaginal discharge help to identify the etiology?

	CANDIDAL VAGINITIS	TRICHOMONAS VAGINITIS	BACTERIAL VAGINOSIS
pH	≤ 4.5	≥ 5.0	≥ 5.0
KOH prep	Mycelia pseudohyphae	Normal	Fishy odor (Pos. "whiff" test)
NaCl prep	Few WBCs	Many WBCs Motile trichomonads	Few WBCs

82. What are "clue cells"?

Clue cells are vaginal epithelial cells to which are attached many bacteria. This gives the cell a stippled appearance when viewed in a normal saline preparation. Clue cells are characteristic, but not diagnostic, of bacterial vaginosis.

83. What is the etiology of bacterial vaginosis?

Formerly called nonspecific, *Gardnerella*, or *Haemophilus* vaginitis, bacterial vaginosis is the replacement of normal vaginal lactobacilli with a variety of bacteria, including *Gardnerella vaginalis*, genital mycoplasmas, and an overgrowth of anaerobic species. *G. vaginalis* can be found in small numbers in up to 30% of nonsexually active adolescents, so vaginal cultures are of limited value.

84. Is there an effective treatment for bacterial vaginosis?

Optimal management remains unclear. Acceptable treatment options include oral metronidazole (Flagyl), 0.075% metronizadole gel or 2% clindamycin cream. Treatment failure is about 15%. Relapse rates as high as 30% may occur within 3 months.

Nyirjesy P: Vaginitis in the adolescent patient. Pediatr Clin North Am 46:733-745, 1999.

85. What is the most common STD in sexually active teenage males?

Urethritis, both gonococcal and nongonococcal. Nongonococcal urethritis, particularly that due to *Chlamydia trachomatis*, is more common and is often asymptomatic. Other less common causes of nongonococcal urethritis include *Ureaplasma urealyticum, Trichomonas vaginalis*, herpes simplex, human papillomavirus, and yeast

86. How should asymptomatic, sexually active teenage males be screened for urethritis?

Chlamydia trachomatis is the most common cause of *asymptomatic* urethritis. The most definitive screening method is to obtain urethral swabs for culture, although this method is invasive and not cost-effective. Non-culture methods (e.g., enzyme immunoassay, direct fluorescent antibody, PCR, LCR) can also be done on the swabbed specimen. A less invasive strategy is to test centrifuged, first-void urine for infection by culture or non-culture methods. A third strategy is to obtain 15 ml of unspun first-void urine and test it for leukocyte esterase (a dipstick test for the presence of WBCs). If positive, more specific studies can be done for *C. trachomatis* on spun urine or a urethral swab. This approach is about 70% sensitive. Precise guidelines on screening remain controversial. Generally, unless a precise STD exposure is known, studies for gonorrhea are not done because this organism is more commonly associated with symptoms (dysuria or penile discharge).

Report of U.S. Preventive Services Task Force. Chlamydial Screening. Guide to Clinical Preventive Services, 2nd ed. Baltimore, Williams & Wilkins, 1996, pp. 325-334.

SUBSTANCE ABUSE

87. What are the four types of alcohol and drug abuse by teenagers?

1. ***Experimental***—weekend beer or marijuana use at parties; a curiosity factor
2. ***Recreational***—weekday use and progression to harder drugs, liquor; driven by peer acceptance and pressure
3. ***Problematic***—daily use; personality changes noted; difficulties at school and with family; constant need to experience pleasure
4. ***Compulsive***—most of the time under the influence of drugs or alcohol; frequent legal problems; a true addiction with need to avoid abstinence effects

Comerci GD, Schwebel R: Substance abuse: An Overview. Adol Med: State of Art Rev 11:87, 2000.

88. What is the CRAFFT screen?

A 9-item screening test for adolescent substance abuse. Two or more "yes" answers indicate a greater than 90% sensitivity and greater than 80% specificity for significant substance abuse. A number of screening instruments are available for interviewing adolescents, and the search for alcohol or drug use should be part of routine medical care.

Knight JR et al: Reliabilities of short substance abuse screening tests among adolescent medical patients. Pediatrics 105: 948S-953S, 2000.

Knight JR et al: A new brief screen for adolescent substance abuse. Arch Pediatr Adolesc Med 153:591-196, 1999.

89. When should drug users be referred for professional evaluation and counseling?

Referral or more extensive evaluation depends on the age and development of the adolescent. At any age, the recreational, problematic, or compulsive user warrants professional intervention. The younger adolescent may also benefit from evaluation at the experimental stage, if only in an effort to postpone such behavior.

90. Are teens who drink excessively likely to become adults who drink excessively?

In a study of 940 adolescents evaluated at ages 14-18 and at age 24, a majority of those with problematic use of alcohol as a teenager had the problem persisting into early adulthood.

Rohde P et al: Natural course of alcohol use disorders from adolescence to young adulthood. J Am Acad Adolesc Psychiatr 40:83-90, 2001.

91. Should an adolescent be screened for drug abuse without his or her consent?

This is an area of contention. The official position of the American Academy of Pediatrics is that testing not be done without consent in a competent older adolescent, even if a parent wishes otherwise. Others have argued that a teenager's right to privacy and confidentiality does not supersede potential risks of serious damage from drug abuse, particularly if there is strong clinical suspicion or parental concerns. The legal ramifications are evolving and vary from state to stage. In 1995, the U.S. Supreme Court ruled that random drug testing of high school athletes was legal.

92. A teenager who is being screened for drug abuse submits a suspicious urine specimen for testing. How can you tell if it is urine?

- pH should be 4.6–8.0.
- Temperature should range between 90.5 and 98.6°F (32.5–37°C).
- Urine submitted at body temperature will exceed 90.5°F (32.5°C) for 15–20 minutes. If the temperature is below this level in first 4 minutes, the specimen should be considered suspect.
- Urine creatinine concentration should exceed 0.2 mg/ml.
- Urine specific gravity should be not < 1.003.

93. How long do illicit drugs remain detectable in urine specimens?

There is variability depending on a patient's hydration status and method of intake, but as a rule, metabolites can be detected after ingestion as follows:

Amphetamines:	48 hrs	*Marijuana*:	3 days for light smoker 21–27 days for heavy smoker
Barbiturates (short acting):	24 hrs		
Benzodiazepines:	3 days	*Morphine*:	48 hours
Cocaine:	2–3 days	*Phencyclidine*:	3 days for casual use 8 days for heavy use

Of note, most urine screens are very sensitive and may detect drugs up to 99% of the time in concentrations established as analytic cutoff points. However, the screens can be much less specific, sometimes with false-positive rates up to 35%. Therefore, second tests utilizing the analytic methodology most specific for the suspected drug should be used.

AAP Task Force on Substance Abuse: Substance Abuse: A Guide for Health Professionals. Elk Grove Village, IL: American Academy of Pediatrics, 1988, p 55.

94. What factors increase the likelihood of teenage alcohol and/or drug abuse?

- ***Peer use***
- ***School problems*** (school failure, poor school achievement)
- ***Psychologic problems*** (rebelliousness, early antisocial behavior)
- ***Age at first experimentation*** (particularly age < 15 yrs associated with later drug use)

95. What types of drinking behavior are concerning for the development of alcoholism in teenagers?

Patterns of drinking: drinking before going to a party, morning drinking to overcome a hangover, frequent loss of control with drinking, drinking at school, drinking more than peers, mixing of drugs with alcohol to achieve a stronger high

Drinking-related behaviors: marked personality changes while drinking, development of blackouts or temporary amnesia, drinking-related arrests, drinking-related fights, guilt about drinking

Werner MJ, Adger HA: Early identification, screening and brief intervention for adolescent alcohol use. Arch Pediatr Adolesc Med 149:1241–1248, 1995.

96. What is the genetic predisposition of alcoholism?

A male child of an alcoholic father is four times more likely to become an alcoholic. If a *monozygotic twin* is an alcoholic, the likelihood of the other twin becoming an alcoholic is ***55%;*** for *dizygotic twins*, it is ***25%.***

97. Which type of substance abuse is more common in younger adolescents than older adolescents?

Inhalants. Up to 20% of 8th graders in some surveys report recent use of inhalants (or "huffing"), compared with about 15% of 12th graders. Household products are typically abused, including aliphatic hydrocarbons (e.g., gasoline, butane in cigarette lighters), aromatic hydrocarbons (e.g., benzene and toluene in glues and acrylic paints), alkyl halides (e.g., methylene chloride and trichloroethylene in paint thinners and spot removers) and ketones (e.g., acetone in nail polish remover). Inhalant abusers appear to have a greater risk of long-term substance abuse compared with other psychoactive drugs. Of note, inhalants have short durations of action and usually cannot be detected by toxic screen. They can cause cerebral atrophy and death (by asphyxiation or cardiac arrhythmia).

Neumark YD, et al: The epidemiology of adolescent inhalant drug involvement. Arch Pediatr Adolesc Med 152:781-786, 1998.

98. What are the toxicities of chronic marijuana use?

***Pulmonary*:** Decreased pulmonary function. Compared to cigarette smoke, marijuana smoke contains more carcinogens and respiratory irritants and produces higher carboxyhemoglobin levels and greater tar deposition. Long-term studies will determine if there is a link between chronic marijuana smoke exposure and lung cancer.

***Endocrine*:** Associated with decreased sperm count and motility. May interfere with hypothalamic/pituitary function and increase likelihood of anovulation. Antagonizes insulin, which may affect diabetic management.

***Behavioral*:** Short-term memory impairment, interference with learning, possible "amotivational syndrome."

99. Teenagers who report the use of "peace pills," "angel dust," or "gorilla biscuits" are likely referring to what illicit drug?

Phencyclidine (PCP). Related to the anesthetic drug ketamine, PCP is categorized as an hallucinogen. It should be considered as a possible cause if a teenager presents with a distorted thought process and signs of nystagmus, hypertension, ataxia, and miotic pupils.

100. What is ecstasy?

Ecstasy or "X" is methylenedioxymethamphetamine (MDMA), an analogue of amphetamine. It has become increasing popular among adolescents and college students due to its ease of availability and reputation as an aphrodisiac.

101. List the potential side effects of anabolic steroids.

Endocrine:	In males—testicular atrophy, oligospermia, gynecomastia; In females—hirsutism, masculinization
Musculoskeletal:	Premature epiphyseal closure
Dermatologic:	Acne, alopecia, temporal hair recession
Hepatic:	Impaired excretory function with cholestatic jaundice, elevated LFTs, peliosis hepatitis (a form of hepatitis in which hepatic lobules have microscopic pools of blood), benign and malignant tumors
Cardiovascular:	Hypertension, decreased HDL cholesterol, increased LDL cholesterol
Psychologic:	Aggressive behavior, mood swings, increased libido

Bagatell CJ, Bremner WJ: Androgens in men: Uses and abuses. N Engl J Med 334:707–714, 1996.

102. Is androstenedione a safe, natural way for teenagers to increase muscle mass?

No. "Andro," a precursor to testosterone, is normally produced in the adrenal glands and testes and converted in the peripheral tissues by 17-beta-hydroxysteroid dehydrogenase. It is a compound also found in plants and in highly-publicized homerun hitters. However, studies show that it is more likely to result in increases in serum estradiol than testosterone or muscle mass. If teenage males know that breasts, rather than biceps, are more likely to emerge, they will likely steer clear of androstenedione.

Leder BZ, et al: Oral androstenedione administration and serum testosterone concentrations in young men. JAMA 283:778-782, 2000.

King DS, et al: Effect of oral androstenedione on serum testosterone and adaptations to resistance training in young men: a randomized controlled trial. JAMA 281:2020-2028, 1999.

103. What are the risks of smokeless tobacco?

Due to the decreased gingival blood flow caused by nicotine, chronic ischemia and necrosis can occur. Chronic use results in ***gingival recession*** and ***inflammation***, ***periodontal disease***, and ***oral leukoplakia*** (a premalignant change). The risk of oral and pharyngeal cancer is increased. Although more commonly used by males, smokeless tobacco used by pregnant females may be associated with low-birthweight infants and premature birth. Smokeless tobacco, as with cigarettes, is also addictive.

104. When does cigarette smoking begin?

In the U.S., about three-quarters of daily adult smokers began between the ages of 13 and 17. Worldwide, the average age is lower. Cigarette smoking remains the major preventable cause of premature death in the world. Clearly, the development of effective early intervention programs for adolescents is vital.

105. Are adolescents in the U.S. smoking less?

On the contrary, data from the CDC indicate that percentage of younger people smoking cigarettes increased dramatically in the 1990s. From 1991 to 1997, 9th graders increased from 23% to 33%, 10th graders from 25% to 35%, 11th graders from 32% to 37% and high school seniors from 30% to 39%. Efforts to reverse this trend have included broad-based public education, increased prices on tobacco products, tighter restrictions on tobacco marketing and promotion, limitations on adolescents' access to tobacco products and increasing funding for tobacco cessation programs.

Committee on Substance Abuse, American Academy of Pediatrics: Tobacco's toll: Implications for the pediatrician. Pediatrics 107:794-798, 2001.

U.S. Department of Health and Human Services: Youth Risk Behavior Surveillance System. Atlanta, GA, Centers for Disease Control and Prevention, National Center for Chronic Disease Prevention and Health Promotion, Office on Smoking and Health, 1999.

106. How does nicotine withdrawal present in teenagers?

Nicotine withdrawal can occur abruptly, within 2 hours of last use, peaking at 24 hours and persisting for weeks. Symptoms include a strong desire for nicotine, irritability, frustration, anger, anxiety, depression, difficulty in concentrating, restlessness, increased appetite, headache, and GI disturbances. Signs include decreased heart rate, weight gain, slow waves on electroencephalogram, decreased catecholamine levels, decreased metabolic rates, and alteration of REM sleep patterns. Nicotine is a reinforcing and addicting drug, and in teenagers (as in adults), attempts at discontinuing cigarettes have multiple physiologic consequences. Therefore, in addition to behavior-modifying techniques, pharmacologic treatments (e.g., nicotine replacement patches) should be considered.

Miller NS, Cocores JA: Nicotine dependence: Diagnosis, chemistry, and pharmacologic treatments. Pediatr Rev 14:275–279, 1993.

107. How effective are school-based youth smoking cessation programs?

In general, success rates are low (5-17%) when looking at cessation at 6-7 months post-intervention with a variety of programs: structured educational courses, nicotine replacment therapy and computer-based education. Clearly, this is an area where new approaches and strategies are needed.

Lovato C, Shoveller J: Youth smoking cessation: school-based approaches. In Moyer VA, et al (eds): Evidence Based Pediatric and Child Health. London, BMJ Books, 2000, pp. 154-160.

Jorenby DE: New developments in smoking cessation. Curr Opin Pulm Med 4:103-106, 1998.

TEENAGE MALE DISORDERS

108. How common is gynecomastia in teenage boys?

As many as 75% of boys aged 12–14.5 years have some breast development. In about 25%, it lasts for > 1 year, and in 7%, for > 2 years. It occurs most commonly during Tanner genital stage II–III and usually consists of subareolar enlargement (breast bud). It may be unilateral or bilateral. The breast bud may be tender, indicating recent rapid growth of tissue. Obese boys often have breast enlargement due to the deposition of adipose tissue, and differentiation from gynecomastia (true breast budding) is sometimes difficult.

109. Why does gynecomastia occur so commonly?

Early in puberty, production of estrogen (a stimulator of ductal proliferation) increases relatively faster than that of testosterone (an inhibitor of breast development). This slight imbalance causes the breast enlargement. In obese teenagers, the enzyme aromatase, found in higher concentrations in adipose tissue, converts testosterone to estrogen.

110. What drugs are associated with gynecomastia?

***C*:** **C**alcium-channel blockers: verapamil, nifedipine
***H*:** **H**ormonal medications: anabolic steroids, oral contraceptives
***E*:** **E**xperimental/illicit drugs: marijuana, heroin, amphetamines, methadone
***S*:** p**S**ychoactive drugs: phenothiazines, tricyclic antidepressants, diazepam
***T*:** **T**estosterone antagonists: spironolactone, ranitidine, cimetidine, ketoconazole

111. What other entities besides drugs are associated with gynecomastia?

The overwhelming majority of cases of gynecomastia in adolescent males occur as part of normal pubertal development. In addition to drugs, other causes include:

- Recovery from chronic disease
- Inadequate androgen production—Klinefelter syndrome, testicular failure, isolated LH deficiency (fertile eunuch)
- Excess estrogen production—feminizing tumors (usually adrenal)
- Pseudo-gynecomastia—carcinoma of the breast, neurofibromatosis, hemangiomas, lipomas, abscess, bruise
- Other—pituitary tumor, testicular tumor, hypo- or hyperthyroidism, liver disease

Braunstein GD: Gynecomastia. N Engl J Med 492:490–495, 1993.

112. Which boys with gynecomastia warrant further evaluation?

- Prepubertal boys
- Pubertal-age boys with little or no virilization and small testes
- Hepatomegaly or abdominal mass palpated
- Child with CNS complaints

Evaluations may include testing for hypothalamic or pituitary disease, feminizing tumors of the adrenal or testes, and genetic abnormalities (e.g., Klinefelter syndrome). Of note, although breast cancer is nearly reportable if it occurs in boys and is extremely rare in men (0.2%), in patients with Klinefelter syndrome, the rate increases to 3–6%.

113. What treatment options are available for developmental gynecomastia?

Treatment usually depends on the amount of breast tissue present and the degree of psychological problems that this causes. There are three primary options:

- ***Reassurance.*** Explanation of the process and expected resolution usually suffices for most adolescents. They should be told that resolution can take up to 24 months.
- ***Medications.*** These may include antiestrogens (clomiphene citrate, tamoxifen), aromatase inhibitors (testolactone), non-aromatizable androgens (dihydrotestosterone), and weak androgens (danazol).
- ***Surgery.*** This should be done by a plastic surgeon who has experience in breast reduction.

114. What are the clinical manifestations of testicular torsion?

Testicular torsion in adolescents usually presents with acute-onset hemiscrotal pain that radiates to the groin and lower abdomen. Nausea and vomiting are common, but fever is rare. The testis is acutely tender and swollen and may be high-riding. The cremasteric reflex is absent. Many patients report previous episodes of severe acute scrotal pain. Radionuclide imaging of the scrotum with Tc-99m pertechnetate and/or color Doppler ultrasound demonstrates low or absent blood flow and can be helpful in equivocal cases. However, testis salvage depends on timely restoration of blood flow, and obtaining such studies should not delay a highly suspect case from surgical exploration. The spermatic cord sometimes can be untwisted manually, giving temporary relief, but surgical exploration is still required for fixation to prevent recurrence. Both testes may be secured since the underlying suspension defect is often bilateral.

115. How is testicular torsion clinically differentiated from other causes of the acute painful scrotum?

Epididymitis: Usually slower in onset; pain initially localized to epididymis, but as inflammation spreads, whole testis may become painful; not usually associated with vomiting; pain does not usually radiate to the groin; usually associated with dysuria, pyuria, and discharge; often caused by *Neisseria gonorrhoeae* and *Chlamydia trachomatis;* history of STDs is suggestive; unusual in prepubertal boys and in nonsexually active teenagers

Orchitis: Usually slower in onset; often systemic symptoms (nausea, vomiting, fever, chills) secondary to diffuse viral infection; in mumps, occurs about 4–6 days after parotitis; bilateral involvement more common

Torsion of appendix testis: Sudden onset of pain; localized tender nodule at upper pole (often with bluish discoloration); nausea and vomiting uncommon

Incarcerated hernia: Acute onset; pain not localized to hemiscrotum; usually palpable inguinal mass; testes not painful; symptoms and signs of bowel obstruction (vomiting, abdominal distension, guarding, rebound tenderness)

Kadish HA, et al: A retrospective review of pediatric patients with epididymitis, testicular torsion, and torsion of testicular appendages. Pediatrics 102:73-76, 1998.

116. How does the Prehn sign help distinguish between epididymitis and testicular torsion?

Classically, relief of pain with elevation of the testis (*negative Prehn sign*) is associated with epididymitis, while persistent pain (*positive Prehn sign*) is more indicative of testicular torsion. However, there is considerable overlap, and this relatively nonspecific sign should be interpreted in the context of other signs and symptoms.

117. If complete testicular torsion has occurred, how long before irreversible changes develop?

Irreversible changes develop in ***4–6 hours***. However, it is clinically impossible to distinguish partial from complete torsion, and thus duration of symptoms should not be used as a gauge for determining viability. Duration of symptoms does correlate with abnormal testicles on follow-up examination, underscoring the need for prompt diagnosis. Two-thirds of patients with testicles salvaged between 12 and 24 hours after the onset of symptoms have palpable evidence of testicular atrophy on follow-up, compared with only 10% when the diagnosis is made in <6 hours.

118. What is the most frequent solid cancer in older adolescent males?

Testicular cancer. The most common type is a seminoma, which, if detected when confined to the testicle (stage I), has a cure rate of up to 97% with orchiectomy and radiation. Although its overall effectiveness is debated, most authorities recommend that all adolescent males be taught testicular self-examination so that irregularities or changes in size can be noted early.

119. What is the significance of a varicocele in a teenager?

A *varicocele* is an enlargement of either the pampiniform or cremasteric veinous plexus of the spermatic cord which results in a boggy enlargement ("bag of worms") of the upper scrotum. About 15% of boys aged 10–15 years have a varicocele, and in 2%, the varicoceles are very large. Most are asymptomatic. Longitudinal studies of adolescents show that large varicoceles may interfere with normal testicular growth and result in decreased spermatogenesis. Surgical correction can prevent the progressive damage. If a varicocele is very large, causing pain, or associated with asymmetric testicular volume, surgical referral is advisable.

Kass EJ, Reitelman C: Adolescent varicocele. Urol Clin North Am 22:151–159, 1995.

120. On which side do varicoceles more commonly occur?

The ***left*** side. The left spermatic vein drains into the left renal vein, and the right spermatic vein drains into the inferior vena cava. These hemodynamics favor higher left-sided pressures, which predispose to left-sided varicoceles. Unilateral left-sided varicoceles are the most common types, occurring in 90% of patients, with the remainder bilateral. A unilateral right-sided lesion is rare. Many experts consider its finding a reason to search for other causes of venous obstruction, such as a renal or retroperitoneal tumor, with ultrasound, CT or MRI.

121. An adolescent who boasts of his overpowering "hircismus" is likely in need of what corrective action?

Both a dictionary and a shower. Hircismus is offensive axillary odor.

TEENAGE PREGNANCY

122. How common is teenage pregnancy in the United States?

About 1 in 10 girls and young women under age 20 years become pregnant each year (about 1 million pregnancies). The likelihood that an adolescent will become pregnant before age 20 is about 1 in 4. Up to 90% are unplanned. About 50% of pregnancies progress to delivery, 35% are terminated by abortion, and 15% end by miscarriage.

123. What factors make it more likely that a teenager will become pregnant?

- ***Early initiation of sexual intercourse***: Risk factors for early initiation include low socioeconomic status, low future-achievement orientation, and academic difficulties
- ***Influence from peers and sisters*:** If surrounded by sexually active friends and siblings, teenager is more likely to be permissive with regard to sexual behavior and pregnancy itself. Many teens do not view pregnancy as a negative experience.
- ***Family history of early parenting***
- ***Lack of family support and structure***
- ***Improper use or nonuse of contraceptives***
- ***History of repeated negative pregnancy tests***
- ***Race:*** Blacks and Hispanics have higher rates than whites, although rates significantly vary by race according to socioeconomic status

Emans SJ, et al: Teenage pregnancy. In Emans SJ, et al (eds.): Pediatric and Adolescent Gynecology, 4th ed. Philadelphia, Lippencott-Raven, 1998, pp. 675-713.

124. What factors are associated with a later initiation of sexual intercourse in adolescents?

- Emphasis on abstinence
- Parental consistency and firmness in discipline
- Goal orientation
- High academic achievement
- Regular attendance at a place of worship

American Academy of Pediatrics, Committee on Adolescence: Contraception and adolescents. Pediatrics 104:1161-1166, 1999.

125. If a teenager has been pregnant once, how likely is she to become pregnant again during her teenage years?

Repeat adolescent pregnancy is common. Up to 30% become pregnant again within 1 year, and 25–50% during the second year. Factors associated with a likely second teen pregnancy include age < 16 years at first conception, boyfriend > 20 years, school dropout, below expected grade level at the time of first pregnancy, welfare dependency after the first pregnancy, complications during the first pregnancy, and departure from the hospital without birth control.

126. What are the risks for infants of teenage mothers?

Teenage mothers have a disproportionately increased risk of having babies who are ***low-birth-weight***, ***premature***, or ***small-for-gestational age***. In addition, infant mortality is two to three times greater for infants of teenage mothers. Studies conflict as to whether these risks are due to inherent biologic difficulties with pregnancy at a young age or due to sociodemographic factors associated with teenage pregnancy (e.g., poverty, inadequate prenatal care).

Fraser AM, et al: Association of young maternal age with adverse reproductive outcomes. N Engl J Med 332:1113–1117, 1995.

127. How soon after conception will a urine pregnancy test be positive?

Human chorionic gonadotropin (hCG) is a glycoprotein (with α and β subunits) produced by trophoblastic tissue. Urine levels of 25 mIU/ml are detectable by the most sensitive methods (i.e., radioimmunoassay or enzyme immunoassay to the β subunit) by about 7 days after fertilization. Although many home pregnancy tests can detect these low levels, some are less sensitive and detect levels of hCG of around 1500 mIU/ml. This occurs on average about 3 weeks after fertilization (or 1 week after the missed menstrual period).

128. In what setting should ectopic pregnancy be suspected?

Amenorrhea with unilateral abdominal or pelvic ***pain*** and irregular ***vaginal bleeding*** is ectopic pregnancy until proven otherwise. Sequential hCG levels can help in determining an ectopic from an intrauterine pregnancy. Ordinarily, the doubling time of hCG levels is about 48 hours. In ectopic pregnancy, there is usually a significant lag. Other causes of lag include missed abortion and spontaneous abortion. Abdominal or transvaginal ultrasound is also useful in diagnosis. Laparoscopy may be necessary if the diagnosis remains unclear.

129. What is the mechanism of action of oral contraceptive pills (OCPs)?

- ***Interference with hypothalamic GnRH***, with suppression of pituitary FSH and LH and subsequent lack of ovulation
- ***Changes in cervical mucus***, with less volume, but thicker and more tenacious, acting as a barrier to sperm
- ***Histologic changes in endometrium***, with atrophy and decreased glycogen content, affecting implantation

130. List the absolute contraindications to OCP use.

- History of thromboembolic disease (e.g., thrombophlebitis, stroke)
- Abnormal liver function
- Estrogen-dependent neoplasia
- Breast cancer
- Undiagnosed vaginal or uterine bleeding
- Pregnancy

131. After OCPs are discontinued, how long is amenorrhea likely to persist?

OCPs suppress the hypothalamic-pituitary axis, and this suppression can continue for a few months following discontinuation. If amenorrhea continues for > 6 months, secondary causes of amenorrhea should be sought.

132. What is the risk to the fetus if a teenager is pregnant and is begun inadvertently on OCPs?

The most common risk is masculinization of female infants, which occurs rarely (< 1%) but especially with the use of OCPs with higher concentrations of progestational agents. The development of pseudohermaphroditism is not a problem. Maternal use of the OCPs is associated with higher bilirubin levels in the newborn. Suspected (but unproven) associations have included congenital heart disease (e.g., transposition of the great arteries, ventricular septal defects, tetralogy of Fallot), CNS malformations, and limb reduction anomalies.

133. Is there an association between urinary tract infections and certain contraceptives?

Use of the diaphragm and spermicide with nonoxynol-9 appear to be significant risk factors.

134. What oral treatment is effective for emergency postcoital contraception (e.g., rape)?

The most commonly used "morning-after" pill is Ovral (50 μg ethinyl estradiol, 0.5 mg norgestrel) which is given as two tablets at the time of evaluation and two tablets 12 hours later. It is most effective when given within 72 hours of intercourse. A pregnancy test should be done before administration of the pills and 3 weeks after treatment to assess for failure. Nausea is the most common side effect.

135. Describe the implantable (Norplant) and injectable (Depo-Provera) methods of contraception.

Both are progestin-only contraceptive methods with extended duration, which minimizes problems with compliance. **Norplant** (levonorgestrel), following surgical implantation, provides contraception for 5 years. Side effects include menstrual irregularities (prolonged bleeding, irregular bleeding, intermenstrual spotting) and weight gain (usually secondary to increased appetite). Amenorrhea is common in the first year but diminishes with time. The devices may be visible under the skin, and surgical removal can be difficult and associated with scarring. Its effect is reversible immediately upon surgical removal, with relatively rapid return of fertility.

Depo-Provera (depot medroxyprogesterone acetate), following intramuscular injection, provides contraception for 3 months. Menstrual irregularities and weight gain are common, with amenorrhea being very common. Following discontinuation, there may be a prolonged period of infertility (up to 24 months).

136. In evaluating a teenager, what is the progression of cervicouterine changes that suggest pregnancy?

4–6 wks: Softening of the lower uterine segment (*Hegar sign*) and softening of the cervix (Goodell's sign)

6 wks: Vagina and cervix assume a bluish hue (*Chadwick sign*)

Uterine size changes

Nongravid	Lemon
8 wks	Tennis ball or orange
10 wks	Baseball
12 wks	Softball or grapefruit (unless uterus retroflexed)
>12 wks	Palpable above the symphysis
16 wks	Palpable between the symphysis and umbilicus
20 wks	Level of the umbilicus

TEENAGE SUICIDE

137. How commonly do adolescents attempt suicide in the U.S.?

About 2000 teenagers die from suicide each year, but data on the frequency of attempts are hampered by underreporting. For each death by suicide, there are an estimated 50–200 attempts that fail, placing the number of attempts between 250,000–1,000,000 in the United States. From 1950 to 1990, the suicide rate for adolescents in the 15- to 19-year old group increased by 300% compared with a 17% increase for the general population.

138. Who are more likely to attempt suicide, males or females?

Up to nine times as many females as males attempt suicide. However, males (particularly white males) are much more likely to succeed, due in large part to the choice of more lethal methods (especially firearms). Females more commonly try ingestions or wrist slashing.

139. What are the most common major stressors of teenagers?

- Failing grades in school
- Increasing arguments between parents
- Serious family illness or death
- Failing relationship with boyfriend or girlfriend
- Problem with sibling(s)

Green JW, et al: Stressful life events and somatic complaints in adolescents. Pediatrics 75:19–22, 1985.

140. Which adolescents are at increased risk for suicide?

- ***History of previous attempts***, especially those involving very lethal methods and those within the past 2 years (1–10% of failed suicides will be successful in future attempts)
- ***Signs of major depression*** (fatigue, sadness, loss of appetite, sleep irregularities)
- ***Substance abuse*** (up to 50% of victims aged 18–24 years have blood alcohol levels ≥ 0.10%)
- ***Family history of psychiatric problems***, including suicide and depression
- ***Personal history of "acting out" behavior*** (delinquency, truancy, sexual promiscuity)
- ***Living out of the home*** (in a correctional facility or group home)
- ***History of physical or sexual abuse***

American Academy of Pediatrics, Committee on Adolescence: Suicide and suicide attempts in adolescents. Pediatrics 105:871-874, 2000.

141. Which adolescents who have attempted suicide should be hospitalized?

Although many programs admit all patients, even if medically stable, those adolescents with failed attempts who strongly should be considered for inpatient evaluation include:

- All with recurrent attempts
- Evidence of psychosis or persisting pervasive wish to die
- Method other than ingestion (e.g., jumping, use of firearm, attempted asphyxiation by hanging or carbon monoxide inhalation)
- Attempt at remote location (with less likelihood of discovery)
- Inadequate home, social, and supervisory situation

2. BEHAVIOR AND DEVELOPMENT

Nathan J. Blum, M.D., Mark Clayton, M.D., and James Coplan, M.D.

ATTENTION DEFICIT HYPERACTIVITY DISORDER

1. What is the most commonly diagnosed behavior disorder in children in the U.S.?

Attention deficit hyperactivity disorder (ADHD) is a chronic neurodevelopmental/behavioral disorder that is diagnosed based on the number, severity, and duration of three clusters of behavioral problems: *inattention*, *hyperactivity*, and *impulsivity*. It is the most commonly diagnosed behavior disorder in children, affecting 4-12% of school-aged children. According to the latest Diagnostic and Statistical Manual of Mental Disorders (DSM-IV), written in 1994, symptoms of inattention, hyperactivity, and impulsivity must have lasted for > 6 months and be inconsistent with developmental level. These symptoms have to involve more than one setting and result in significant impairment at home, school, or in social settings. Some symptoms must have begun before age 7.

2. How is ADHD classified in DSM-IV?

ADHD is currently considered to be a single disorder with three subtypes: ***Predominantly Inattentive Type, Predominantly Hyperactive-Impulsive Type,*** *and* ***Combined Type***. There is a separate category, ADHD Not Otherwise Specified, which can be used in cases where the symptoms are prominent but do not meet the exact criteria for one of the ADHD subtypes.

3. Is there a system for classifying children with hyperactivity or inattention whose symptoms are not severe enough to meet criteria for ADHD?

Yes. In 1996, the American Academy of Pediatrics (AAP) published the Diagnostic and Statistical Manual for Primary Care (DSM-PC)—Child and Adolescent Version, which allows for developmental and behavioral concerns to be classified as normal "Variations" or "Problems" that do not meet criteria for a specific psychiatric disorder. Therefore, a child may be considered to have a Hyperactive/Impulsive Variation or Problem as well as an Inattention Variation or Problem.

4. Does ADHD exist in girls?

Yes, although boys are diagnosed with ADHD 3-4 times more frequently than girls. Some of this difference may be related to the fact that boys with ADHD are more likely to exhibit disruptive behaviors and thus be referred for diagnostic evaluation. Compared with female controls, girls with ADHD are more likely to have conduct, mood and anxiety disorders and more impairment on measures of social, school and family functioning. Because of this increased comorbidity with mood and anxiety disorders, they are less likely to demonstrate a therapeutic response to stimulant medications.

Biederman J et al: Clinical correlates of attention deficit hyperactivity disorder in females: Findings from a large group of pediatrically and psychiatrically referred girls. J Am Acad Child Adolesc Psychiatry 38:966-978, 1999.

5. Is there a genetic predisposition to ADHD?

Family, twin, and adoption studies have all shown a ***high rate of heritability*** for ADHD, with both autosomal dominant transmission (without full penetrance) and X-linked recessive transmission proposed. Studies of family-based associations have found differences in susceptibility based on both the dopamine transporter locus (DAT) and dopamine D4 receptor locus (DRD4). ADHD has also been found in specific genetic disorders, such as fragile X syndrome, William syndrome (chromosome 7) or the 22q11 deletion syndromes (e.g., velocardiofacial syndrome, DiGeorge syndrome).

6. What is the neuroanatomic or neurochemical basis for ADHD?

Abnormalities involving the neurotransmitters *dopamine* and *norepinephrine* have been linked to ADHD. Evidence for the importance of these neurotransmitters comes from both the production of ADHD-like behavior in animals when such systems are altered as well as the findings that the medications used primarily in treating ADHD have their effects on these neurotransmitters.

Anatomic evidence has come from neuroradiographic imaging and nuclear scanning techniques and has suggested differences in cortical, subcortical, and cerebellar areas between both children and adults with ADHD and control groups. Perhaps because of the heterogeneity of the disorder, anatomic differences that are consistently present and specific for ADHD have not been identified.

7. What conditions can mimic ADHD?

Medical: lead toxicity, iron deficiency, thyroid dysfunction, visual/hearing impairment, sleep disorders, mass lesions (e.g., hydrocephalus), seizures, complex migraines, neurofibromatosis, tuberous sclerosis, and various medications (cold preparations, steroids, recreational drugs)

Developmental or learning disorders: mental retardation, autistic spectrum disorders (e.g., PDD, Asperger syndrome), and specific learning disabilities. Central auditory processing difficulties have also been investigated, though it is still unclear as to whether such difficulties are a different disorder or represent the cognitive deficits seen in ADHD.

Behavioral or emotional disorders: affective disorders (dysthymia, bipolar disorder), anxiety disorders, stress reactions (e.g., post-traumatic stress disorder, adjustment disorder), other disruptive behavior disorders (e.g., oppositional defiant disorder), and personality disorders.

8. What are the comorbid disorders commonly seen with ADHD?

Children with ADHD often have additional problems as outlined in the table below. These problems often interfere with the child's ability to function in home, school, or social situations and the treatment plan must address these issues as well as the ADHD symptoms.

COMORBID DISORDER	RATE	COMMENTS
Oppositional defiant disorder	Up to 70% in boys; 40% in girls	
Conduct disorder	20% (boys) & 10% (girls)	
Depression	20%	
Bipolar disorder	10–15%	
Anxiety	30% (boys) & 40% (girls)	
Tic disorders	10–20%	50–70% of children with chronic tic disorders will have ADHD
Mental retardation	3–10%	
Academic problems	~20% with learning disability (LD)	Even if no LD, over 50% require tutoring, 30% repeat a grade, and 30–40% will receive special education. 10–35% will drop out before graduating
Sleep problems	50–60% (without meds)	Controls have rates up to 35%.
Language problems	50% R/E; 60% pragmatics	R/E = receptive/expressive

9. Is there a definitive diagnostic test for ADHD?

No, there is not a biological test that is sensitive or specific enough to diagnose ADHD. Systematic observation of the child at home or school is very helpful, but often not available. Office observations and office-based tests of attention are not reliable as many children with ADHD will be able to control their symptoms during a brief office visit. Standardized rating scales completed by parents and teachers allow clinicians to compare a teacher's or parent's rating of a child's attention or activity level to that of other children. However, rating scales can be subject to biases of the rater and do not assess duration of symptoms or degree of impairment and thus should not be considered diagnostic instruments in themselves.

Mercugliano M., Power TJ, & Blum NJ: The Clinician's Practical Guide to Attention-Deficit/Hyperactivity Disorder. Baltimore, Paul H. Brookes, 1999.

10. How should ADHD be treated?

A multimodal approach is recommended, which may include psychotropic medication, behavioral therapies, family education and counseling, and educational interventions.

American Academy of Pediatrics. Clinical practice guideline: diagnosis and management of the child with attention-deficit/hyperactivity disorder. Pediatrics 105:1158-1170, 2000.

National Institutes of Health Concensus Development Conference Statement: Diagnosis and treatment of attention deficit hyperactivity disorder (ADHD). J Am Acad Child Adolesc Psychiat 39:182-193, 2000.

11. Are psychostimulants the best medications for treating ADHD?

The stimulant medications are the first choice in treating ADHD. They are the medications that are most effective in improving attention span and decreasing distractability. They tend to have fewer side effects than alternative medications, although pemoline is infrequently used because it has been associated with hepatic failure. Stimulants (e.g., methylphenidate [e.g., Ritalin]) have been used since the late 1930s for behavioral problems. They will provide a significant response to the core ADHD symptoms in roughly 70 to 80 percent of affected children. There may also be a positive response in the child's social interactions, self-esteem, aggression, memory, and academic performance. Some experts have recommended a double-blind placebo trial with Ritalin to more objectively verify the beneficial response. There is controversy about the possible overuse of stimulants in children of all ages.

Accardo P, Blondis TA: What's all the fuss about Ritalin? J Pediatr 138:6-8, 2001.

Kent MA et al: Double-blind methylphenidate trials. Arch Pediatr Adolesc Med 153:1292-1296, 1999.

12. What are the side effects of the stimulants?

Common complaints with stimulant usage include ***appetite suppression, sleep disturbance, headaches,*** and ***abdominal pain***. Rarer problems include nervous habits or OCD features, hallucinations, dysphoria, and drowsiness. Liver failure has been reported with pemoline. Slight increases in heart rate and blood pressure occur, but usually are not clinically significant. Stimulants do not require any specific cardiovascular monitoring. New onset of tics may occur with stimulant use, but compared with placebo, stimulants do not always make tics worse. Dysphoria and "rebound hyperactivity" are occasionally noted by parents at the conclusion of a dosing interval when the stimulant is losing its behavioral effects. Longer-acting, time-release stimulants (e.g., Concerta) may have less rebound effects.

Law SF, Schachar RJ: Do typical doses of methylphenidate cause tics in children treated for attention-deficit hyperactivity disorder. J Am Acad Child Adolesc Psychiatry 38:944-951, 1999.

13. What medications other than stimulants can be used to treat ADHD?

Tricyclic antidepressants (TCAs) have been used in the treatment of ADHD, with significant therapeutic responses seen in about 60% of affected children. Newer antidepressants such as ***bupropion*** and ***venlafaxine*** have been reported to have some benefit for ADHD symptoms. The ***alpha-2 adrenergic agonists*** clonidine and guanfacine may help decrease hyperactivity and impulsivity in some children.

14. What do the pharmacologic treatments of cigarette smoking and ADHD have in common?

Bupropion has been demonstrated to be effective for ADHD symptoms. It is also marketed under the name Zyban for the treatment of cigarette smoking.

15. Is a positive response to stimulant medication diagnostic of ADHD?

A positive response is ***not*** diagnostic because (a) children without symptoms of ADHD given stimulants demonstrate positive responses in sustained and focused attention, and (b) observer bias (i.e., parent or teacher) can be considerable. Thus, many experts recommend a placebo-controlled trial when stimulant medication is used.

Zametkin AJ, Ernst M: Problems in the management of attention deficit-hyperactivity disorder. N Engl J Med 340:40-46, 1999.

16. How young is "too young" to diagnose ADHD and prescribe stimulant medications?

The diagnosis is considered difficult to make in children less than ages 4-6 because the validity and reliability of the diagnosis of ADHD in these age groups have not been demonstrated. Methylphenidate carries a warning against its use in children less than 6 years of age. Concerns exist regarding the unproven treatment of children as such a young age and the potential deleterious effect of psychotropic drugs on brain development. However, there has been a dramatic increase in the "off-label" use of stimulant medication in the 1990s for children ages 2–4. The evaluation and most ideal treatment of these younger children remains a challenge.

Zito JM et al: Trends in the prescribing of psychotropic medications to preschoolers. JAMA 283:1025-1030, 2000.

Coyle JT: Psychotropic drug use in the very young child. JAMA 283:1080:2000.

Rappley MD et al: Diagnosis of attention-deficit/hyperactivity disorder and the use of psychotropic medication in very young children. Arch Pediatr Adolesc Med 153:1039-1045, 1999.

17. Is chronic use of stimulants by patients with ADHD associated with increased rates of substance abuse as adolescents?

On the contrary, untreated ADHD has been found to be a significant risk factor for future substance abuse. Pharmacotherapy has been associated with an 85% reduction in risk in adolescents with ADHD.

Biederman J et al: Pharmacotherapy of attention-deficit/hyperactivity disorder reduces risk for substance use disorder. Pediatrics 104:e20, 1999.

18. Is the Feingold diet of any value in the treatment of ADHD?

Dr. Benjamin Feingold hypothesized in the early 1970s that hyperactivity in children was due to the ingestion of low-molecular weight chemicals, such as salicylates and artificial additives for color and flavor. He recommended a diet devoid of these substances and claimed up to a 50% improvement in children on such a diet. Few controlled studies, however, have been able to demonstrate such an effect.

19. Does sugar make children hyperactive?

Although it would be gratifying if complex behavioral problems could be attributable solely or in large measure to dietary causes, this has not been shown to be the case. In a double-blind controlled trial involving excessive dietary intakes of sucrose or aspartame (Nutrasweet), no adverse behavioral or cognitive changes were noted.

Wolraich ML, et al: Effect of sugar on behavior or cognition in children. JAMA 274:1617–1621, 1995.

20. Do children with ADHD become adults with ADHD?

Ongoing observations of children initially diagnosed with ADHD note that ***70-80%*** will continue to have symptoms present during adolescence and up to ***60%*** will show symptoms as adults. These adolescents and adults also have continued problems with anxiety and depression as well as with tobacco and substance use. Motor vehicle infractions, employment difficulties, and intimate relationships have also been described as problematic for adults. Children and adolescents with symptoms of conduct disorder as well as ADHD are at the highest risk for severe problems as adults.

Accardo PJ et al (eds): Attention Deficits and Hyperactivity in Children and Adults: Diagnosis, Treatment, and Management, 2nd ed. New York, Marcel Dekker, 2000.

BEHAVIOR PROBLEMS

21. How much do babies normally cry each day?

In Brazelton's oft-quoted 1962 study of 80 infants, it was found that at 2 weeks of age, the average crying time was nearly 2 hours per day, increasing to nearly 3 hours at 6 weeks and then declining to about 1 hour at 12 weeks.

Brazelton TB: Crying in infancy. Pediatrics 29:579-586, 1962.

22. What characterizes infantile colic?

Colic is excessive crying or fussiness, which occurs in 10–20% of infants, and is one of the most frequent problems encountered in early pediatric office visits. For study purposes, it is defined as paroxysms of crying in an otherwise healthy infant for > 3 hours/day on > 3 days/week. The typical picture is a baby (usually ages 2 wks to 3 mos) who cries intensely for several hours at a time usually in the late afternoon or evening. Often the infant appears in pain and has a slightly distended abdomen with legs drawn up.
Occasional temporary relief occurs if gas is passed.

The symptoms nearly always resolve by 3 to 4 months of age, but the problem can have repercussions, including early discontinuation of breastfeeding, multiple formula changes, heightened maternal anxiety and distress, diminished maternal-infant interaction, and increased risks for child abuse.

23. Does the cry of colic have distinct acoustic characteristics?

At four in the morning, parents would swear so, but actual acoustic analyses of the cries infants with clinically-defined colic did not differ from the cries of "non-colicky" infants with pre-feeding hunger.

St. James-Roberts I: What is distinct about infants' "colic" cries? Arch Dis Childhood 80:56-62, 1999.

24. Explain the origins of colic.

Studies have not revealed a unifying explanation for colic. In many cases its origin seems to lie in the interaction of infant characteristics and parental handling. The infants may have a predisposition towards being more irritable, more sensitive, and more intense (temperament characteristics) in combination with ineffective parental responses to the crying (increased stimulation when the baby is tired). Inexperience or anxiety may exacerbate these problems. Other theories that may explain some cases of colic include:

Gastrointestinal: cow milk protein intolerance, lactose intolerance, immature GI system with hyperperistalsis and excessive gas, faulty feeding techniques (especially overfeeding)

Hormonal (causing enterospasm): increased motilin levels, increased circulating serotonin, progesterone deficiency

25. Are any treatments useful for colic?

The most effective treatment for colic is ***counseling***. The counseling usually emphasizes that crying is a way for infants to communicate their needs. The types of needs that a healthy infant may have are reviewed: to eat, to have a diaper changed, to be held, to suck, to play, or to sleep. Encouraging parents to try each of these for a few minutes when the infant is crying will usually decrease the duration of crying. ***Other interventions*** that have been tried, but tend *not* to be very effective for most infants, include treatment for possible GI causes such as dietary changes to eliminate cow milk in the infant's or nursing mother's diet, formula changes to soy or protein hydrolysates or the use of simethicone to decrease intestinal gas. Other medications, such as phenobarbital and diphenhydramine, are used empirically in clinical practice for severe cases of crying. They may be helpful due to their sedating qualities, but large double-blind studies have not been done and long-term use is not encouraged. Dicyclomine HCl had been used for colic in earlier decades, but was associated with apnea and is now contraindicated for infants. Interventions which increase vestibular stimulation (e.g., increased carrying, real or simulated automobile rides) have not been shown to be consistently beneficial.

Lucassen PL et al: Effectiveness of treatments for infantile colic: systematic review. BMJ 316:1563-1569, 1998.

26. What are the most common types of behavioral problems in children?

- ***Problems of daily routine*** (e.g., food refusal, sleep abnormalities, toilet difficulties)
- ***Aggressive-resistant behavior*** (e.g., temper tantrums, aggressiveness with peers)
- ***Overdependent-withdrawing behavior*** (e.g., separation upset, fears, shyness)
- ***Hyperactivity***
- ***Undesirable habits*** (e.g., thumb-sucking, head banging, nail biting, playing with genitals)
- ***School problems***

Chamberlin RW: Prevention of behavioral problems in young children. Pediatr Clin North Am 31:332, 1984.

27. What percentage of 2-3 year old children will have temper tantrums more than once a day?

In research studies, severe tantrums are usually defined as 3 or more tantrums per day or one tantrum per day lasting at least 15 minutes. Approximately ***5%*** of 2-3 year old children have severe temper tantrums.

28. How should children be punished?

There is no one right way to punish a child, but there are wrong ways. The goal of punishment should be to teach children that a specific behavior was wrong and to discourage the behavior in the future. To meet this goal, punishment should be consistent and relatively brief. It should be carried out in a calm manner as soon as possible after the infraction. Time-out from ongoing activity and removal of privileges are two punishment techniques that can be used. Corporal punishment is not recommended as it is too often used by parents when the parent is angry and teaches that hitting is an appropriate response when one is angry at another person.

29. How valid is the proverb "spare the rod and spoil the child" as a defense for corporal punishment?

The actual biblical proverb (Proverbs 13:24) reads, "He who spares the rod hates his son, but he who loves him is careful to discipline him." While the proverb has often been used as a justification for spanking, in actuality it does not refer to specific discipline strategies but rather the need for love and discipline. In addition, the rod may refer to the shepherd's staff, which was used to guide, rather than hit, sheep. Most developmental authorities advise against corporal punishment as a means of discipline.

Recent studies have suggested that slapping and spanking during childhood correlates linearly with lifetime prevalence of anxiety disorder, alcohol abuse or dependence and externalizing problems.

MacMillan HL et al: Slapping and spanking in childhood and its association with lifetime prevalence of psychiatric disorders in a general population sample. Can Med Assoc J 161:805-809, 1999.

Carey TA: Spare the rod and spoil the child: Is this a sensible justification for the use of punishment in child rearing? Child Abuse Negl 18:1005–1010, 1994.

30. True or False: "Time out" is an effective punishment because it allows the child to think about what he or she did wrong.

False. The full name of "time out" is *time out from positive reinforcement.* When a child is placed in "time out," he or she is briefly removed from the opportunity to participate in fun activities. It is the loss of this opportunity that makes time out an effective punishment. In situations where the children are asked to do something they do not want to do, time out may not be very effective because it allows children to avoid the activity in which they do not want to participate. Time out may provide the opportunity for the child to think about what he or she did wrong, but it is not what makes time out an effective punishment.

31. What is negative reinforcement?

Negative reinforcement refers to a situation in which a behavior occurs more frequently because it results in avoiding at unpleasant activity. For example, if a child tantrums when asked to clean the room, and the parents stops asking the child to clean the room then the tantrum is being negatively reinforced. The tantrum is likely to occur again when the child is asked to clean the room. A teacher who gives children no homework on Friday night if they have completed all the homework on Monday to Thursday is using negative reinforcement to increase homework completion during the week. Negative reinforcement is often confused with punishment, but they are very different. Punishment decreases the frequency of a behavior, but negative reinforcement increases the frequency of the behavior.

32. How often are toddlers in child care bitten?

Very frequently. ***Fifty percent*** of toddlers in child-care will be bitten at least 3 times per year.

33. Is physical injury a concern in children with head banging?

Although a common problem occurring in 5–15% of normal children, head banging rarely results in physical injury, and then usually in children with autism or other developmental disabilities. Normal children often show signs of bliss as they bang away. The activity usually resolves by 4 years of age. It may resume spontaneously during national board exams.

34. At what age does continued use of transitional objects or security blankets become abnormal?

Use of transitional objects varies with age and between cultures. Their use is common in toddlers and decreases during the preschool years. While most school-aged children do not use transitional objects during the day, a study of over 900 seven-year-olds in New Zealand found the 13% still had strong attachments to a transitional object at bedtime.

35. What is the difference between a "blue" breathholding spell and a "white" breathholding spell?

Actually, there are far more similarities than differences. Both are syncopal attacks occurring commonly in children age 6 month to 4 years, peaking between ages 1½ and 3. The *blue* or *cyanotic spell* is more common. Vigorous crying provoked by physical or emotional upset leads to apnea at end expiration. This is followed by cyanosis, opisthotonus, rigidity, and loss of tone. Brief convulsive jerking may occur. The episode lasts from 10–60 seconds. A short period of sleepiness may ensue. The *white* or *pallid spell* is similar except that they are more commonly precipitated by an unexpected event that frightens the child. These children on testing demonstrate increased responsiveness to vagal maneuvers. This parasympathetic hypersensitivity may cause cardiac slowing, diminished cardiac output, and diminished arterial pressure, resulting in a pale appearance.

Blum NJ: Repetitive behavior. In Levine MD, Carey WB, Crocker AC (eds): Developmental-Behavioral Pediatrics, 3rd ed. Philadelphia, WB Saunders, 1999, p 430-442.

36. When should a diagnosis of seizure disorder be considered rather than a breath-holding spell?

- Precipitating event is minor or nonexistent.
- History of no or minimal crying or breathholding.
- Episode lasts > 1 minute.
- Period of post-episode sleepiness lasts > 10 minutes.
- Convulsive component of episode is prominent and occurs before cyanosis.
- Occurs in child < 6 months or > 4 years old.

37. Does treatment with iron decrease the frequency of breath-holding spells?

The relationship between anemia, iron deficiency, and breath-holding spells is unclear. In the 1960s it was observed that children with breath-holding spells had lower hemoglobin levels than controls. Treatment with iron has decreased the frequency of breath-holding spells in some children. Interestingly, some of the children whose breath-holding spells respond to iron are not anemic and the mechanism by which iron decreases breath-holding spells is not known.

Mocan H et al: Breath-holding spells in 91 children and response to treatment with iron. Arch Dis Child 81:261-262, 1999.

38. Does thumb-sucking vary with race and culture?

Yes. Various studies found that 45% of American children < 4 years of age suck their thumbs (boys and girls equally) compared with 30% of Swedish children, 17% of Indian children, and 1% of Eskimo children. Eskimo children probably don't need to suck their thumbs because they are usually carried in their mothers' backpacks with a bottle close at hand. Most thumb-sucking stops spontaneously by age 4.

39. When does prolonged thumb-sucking warrant intervention?

If frequent thumb-sucking persists ***beyond 4–5 years*** or ***when permanent teeth begin to erupt***, treatment is usually indicated. Treatment commonly has two components: application of a substance with an unpleasant taste at frequent intervals (such products are commercially available), or modification with positive reinforcement (small rewards) given when a child is observed not sucking his or her thumb. Occlusive dental appliances are generally not needed. Persistent thumb-sucking after eruption of permanent teeth can lead to malocclusion.

40. When should "toilet training" be started?

When the child is physically and emotionally ready. The physical prerequisite of neurologic maturation of bladder and bowel control usually occurs between 18 and 30 months of age. The child's emotional readiness is often influenced by his or her temperament, parental attitudes, and parent-child interactions. The "potty chair" should be introduced sometime between 2 and 3 years of age. Most children will achieve daytime bladder and bowel control by 3½ years.

41. Are girls or boys toilet-trained earlier?

On average, ***girls*** are toilet-trained earlier than boys. With regard to most other developmental milestones in the first years of life, however, there do not seem to be significant sex differences (e.g., in walking or running, sleep patterns, or verbal ability). Girls do show more rapid bone development.

42. A 10-month-old infant who is demonstrating frequent self-gagging behavior has what likely diagnosis?

Rumination syndrome is a rare disorder characterized by the regurgitation and reswallowing of food. It typically occurs in infants between 2 and 12 months of age after a period of normal feeding. The infant may be noted to be gagging himself or herself with the tongue or hand while alone. A chaotic family situation often exists. If gastrointestinal pathology has been eliminated as a cause of the problem, treatment consists of improving family interaction and instituting antireflux measures (e.g., thickened feedings).

43. When is masturbation in a child considered pathologic?

Masturbation, or the rhythmic self-manipulation of the genital area, is considered a normal part of sexual development. However if masturbation occurs to the exclusion of other activities, if it occurs in public places beyond 6 years of age, or if the child engages in activities that mimic adult sexual behavior, evaluation for sexual abuse, CNS abnormalities, or psychological pathology would be appropriate.

44. When is a child's laughter nothing to sneer at?

Pathologic laughter is that which occurs without a stimulus, is not in response to the environmental surroundings, and has no associated emotional feelings. Causes can include Angelman syndrome, gelastic epilepsy, multiple sclerosis, Wilson disease and mood-altering drugs (e.g., hallucinogens, alcohol, benzodiazepines, nitrous oxide).

Nirenberg SA: Normal and pathologic laughter in children. Clin Peditar 30:630-632, 1991.

CRANIAL DISORDERS

45. How many fontanels are present at birth?

Although there are ***6*** fontanels present at birth (2 anterior lateral, 2 posterior lateral, 1 anterior, and 1 posterior), only 2 (the anterior and posterior fontanels) are usually palpable on physical examination.

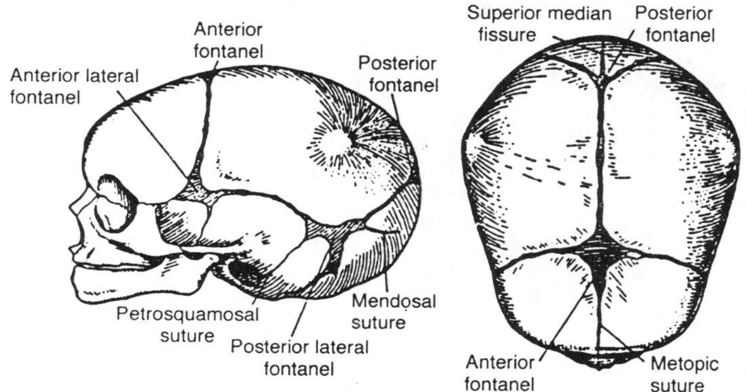

The cranium at birth, showing major sutures and fontanels. No attempt is made to show molding or overlapping of bones, which sometimes occurs at birth. (From Silverman FN, Kuhn JP (eds): Caffey's Pediatric X-ray Diagnosis, 9th ed. St. Louis, Mosby, 1993, p 5; with permission.)

46. When does the anterior fontanel close?

Usually ***between 10 and 14 months*** of age. However, it may not be palpable as early as 3 months, or it may remain open until 18 months of age.

47. Which conditions are associated with premature or delayed closure of the fontanel?

Premature closure: Microcephaly, high calcium/vitamin D ratio in pregnancy, craniosynostosis, hyperthyroidism, or it may be a normal variant.

Delayed closure:

Skeletal disorders	**Chromosomal abnormalities**	**Other conditions**
Acondroplasia	Down syndrome	Athyrotic hypothyroidism
Aminopterin-induced syndrome	Trisomy 13 syndrome	Hallermann-Streiff syndrome
Alpert syndrome	Trisomy 18 syndrome	
Cleidocranial dysostosis	Malnutrition	
Hypophosphatasia	Progeria	
Kenny syndrome	Rubella syndrome	
Osteogenesis imperfecta	Russell-Silver syndrome	
Pyknodysostosis		
Vitamin D deficiency rickets		

48. When is an anterior fontanel too big?

The size of the fontanel can be calculated using the formula: (length + width)/2, where length = anterior-posterior dimension and width = transverse dimension. Although there is wide variability in the normal size range of the anterior fontanel, designation of normal upper limits is helpful in identifying disorders in which a large fontanel may be a feature (e.g., hypothyroidism, hypophosphatasia, skeletal dysplasias, increased intracranial pressure). Of note, the *posterior fontanel* normally is fingertip size or smaller in 97% of full-term newborns.

49. What are the types of primary craniosynostosis?

Craniosynostosis is the premature fusion of various cranial suture lines, resulting in ridging of the sutures, asymmetric growth, and deformity of the skull. Suture lines (with resultant disorders listed in parentheses) include sagittal (scaphocephaly or dolichocephaly), coronal (brachycephaly), unilateral coronal or lambdoidal (plagiocephaly), and metopic (trigonocephaly). Multiple fused sutures can result in a high and pointed skull (oxycephaly or acrocephaly).

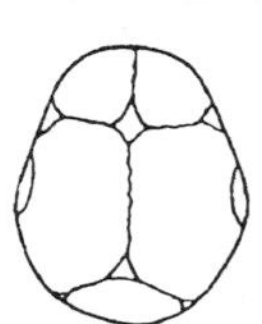

Normocephaly

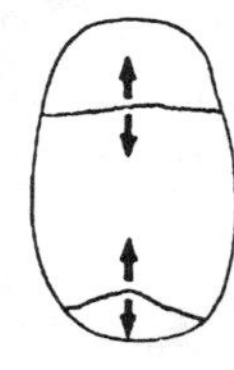

Dolichocephaly

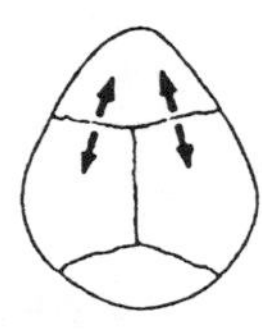

Trigonocephaly

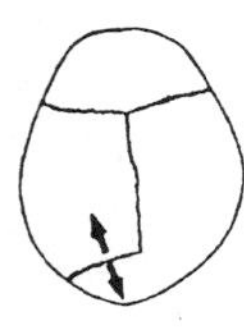

Plagiocephaly

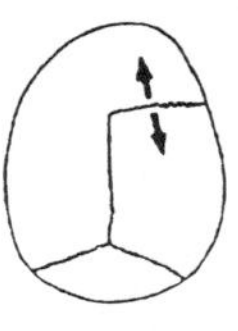

Plagiocephaly

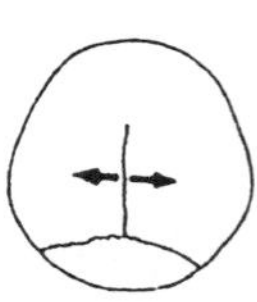

Brachycephaly

From Gorlin RJ: Craniofacial defects. In Oski FA, et al (eds): Principles and Practice of Pediatrics, 2nd ed. Philadelphia, J.B. Lippincott, 1994, p 508; with permission.

50. What is the most common type of primary craniosynostosis?

Sagittal (60%). Coronal synostosis accounts for 20% of cases.

51. What causes craniosynostosis?

Most cases of isolated craniosynostosis have no known etiology. *Primary* craniosynostosis may be observed as part of craniofacial syndromes, including Apert, Crouzon, and Carpenter syndromes. *Secondary* causes can include abnormalities of calcium and phosphorus metabolism (e.g., hypophosphatasia, rickets), hematologic disorders (e.g., thalassemia), mucopolysaccharidoses, and hyperthyroidism. Inadequate brain growth, as in microcephaly, can lead to craniosynostosis.

52. Who develops positional plagiocephaly?

Since the implementation of the "back-to-sleep" program by the AAP in 1992 to reduce the risk for SIDS, a larger percentage of infants have developed occipital flattening (posterior plagiocephaly) due to transient calvarial deformation from prolonged supine sleeping positions. Positional plagiocephaly rarely has ridging of the suture lines. Simple positional modifications usually suffice for correction.

53. What features suggest significant pathologic plagiocephaly rather than simple positional plagiocephaly?

- Patients presenting before the age of 3 months
- Significant compensatory frontal changes (i.e., ipsilateral frontal prominence or bossing with anterior or inferior displacement of tragus)
- Significant facial asymmetry and/or mandibular malalignment
- Progession despite conservative treatment regimens (e.g., positional modifications)
- Evidence of possible intracranial effects or increased pressure (e.g., papilledema, falling head circumference percentiles, delay in milestones)

Keating RF: Craniosynostosis: diagnosis and management in the new millennium. Pediar Ann 26:600-612, 1997.

54. Which syndrome of craniosynostosis most commonly has exophthalmos as a constant finding?

Crouzon syndrome. In this syndrome, the craniosynostosis is associated with midface hypoplasia and shallow orbits. This leads to prominent ocular proptosis and associated hypertelorism, strabismus, and exposure conjunctivitis.

55. What conditions are associated with skull softening?

- Cleidocranial dysostosis
- Craniotabes
- Lacunar skull (associated with spina bifida, major CNS anomalies)
- Osteogenesis imperfecta
- Multiple wormian bones (associated with hypothyroidism, hypophosphatasia, chronic hydrocephalus)
- Rickets

56. What is the significance of craniotabes?

In this condition, abnormally soft, thin skull bones buckle under pressure and recoil like a ping-pong ball. It is best elicited on the parietal or frontal bones and is often associated with rickets in infancy. It may also be seen in hypervitaminosis A, syphilis, and hydrocephalus. Craniotabes may be a normal finding during the first 3 months of life.

57. Which imaging study is preferable in the evaluation of microcephaly, CT or MRI?

MRI has superior ability to:

- Differentiate gray and white matter
- Identify abnormalities of neuronal migration, sulcation, and gyration
- Identify patterns of myelin deposition or demyelination
- Provide greater details of the basal ganglia, brainstem, and cerebellum

DeMyer W: Microcephaly, micrencephaly, megalocephaly, and megalencephaly. In Swaiman K (ed): Pediatric Neurology, 2nd ed. St. Louis, Mosby-Year Book, 1999, p 303.

58. In addition to careful sequential charting of head circumference, what other features on history or examination should raise suspicion for the later development of microcephaly?

- Infants up to age 6 months whose chest circumference exceeds head circumference (unless infant is very obese)
- Delayed developmental milestones
- Neurologic abnormalities (e.g., seizures, spasticity)
- Marked backward slope of forehead (seen in familial microcephaly)
- Occipital flattening not related to positioning
- Early closure of anterior fontanel
- Significantly prominent suture lines

Moe PG, Seay AR: Neurologic and muscular disorders. In Hay WW, et al (eds): Current Pediatric Diagnosis and Treatment, 14th ed. Norwalk, Appleton & Lange, 1999, pp 662-663.

59. What are the three main general causes of macrocephaly?

1. ***Increased intracranial pressure*:** from dilated ventricles (e.g., progressive hydrocephalus of various causes), subdural fluid collections, intracranial tumors, benign increased intracranial pressure (i.e., pseudotumor cerebri) from various causes
2. ***Thickened skull*:** cranioskeletal dysplasias (e.g., osteopetrosis), various anemias
3. ***Megalencephaly*** (enlarged brain): familial, syndromic (e.g., Sotos syndrome), storage diseases, leukodystrophies, neurocutaneous disorders (e.g., neurofibromatosis)

DENTAL DEVELOPMENT AND DISORDERS

60. When do primary and secondary teeth erupt?

Mandibular teeth usually erupt first. The central incisors appear by 5–7 months, with approximately 1 new tooth per month thereafter until 23–30 months, at which time the second molars (and thus all 20 primary or deciduous teeth) are in place. Of the 32 secondary teeth, the central incisors erupt first between 5 and 7 years, and the third molars are in place by 17–22 years.

61. What is the significance of natal teeth?

Although the first primary tooth usually erupts by 6–12 months of age, occasionally teeth are present at birth (natal teeth) or erupt within 30 days after birth (neonatal teeth). When x-rays are taken, 95% of natal teeth are primary incisors and 5% are supernumerary teeth or extra teeth. Very sharp teeth which can cause tongue lacerations and very loose teeth which can be aspirated should be removed. Females are affected more commonly than males, and the prevalence is 1:2000–3500. Most cases are familial and without consequence, but natal teeth can be associated with genetic syndromes, including the Ellis–van Creveld and Hallermann-Streiff syndromes.

62. How common is congenital absence of teeth?

Congenital absence of primary teeth is very rare, but up to 25% of individuals may have absence of one or more third molars, and up to 5% may have absence of another secondary or permanent tooth (most commonly the maxillary lateral incisors and mandibular second premolar).

63. What are mesiodentes?

These are ***peg-shaped supernumerary teeth***, occurring in up to 5% of individuals, which most commonly are situated in the maxillary midline. They should be considered for removal because they interfere with the eruption of permanent incisors.

64. What constitutes the 32 permanent teeth?

Upper and lower central incisors, lateral incisors, cuspids, first bicuspids, second bicuspids, first molars, second molars, third molars.

65. What is a ranula?

A large ***mucocele***, usually bluish, painless, soft, and unilateral, that occurs under the tongue. Most self-resolve. If large, surgical marsupialization can be done. If recurrent, excision may be needed.

66. What causes tooth discoloration?

COLOR	CAUSE	COLOR	CAUSE
Generalized		*Localized*	
Bluish-brown	Dentinogenesis iperfecta	Yellow	Trauma
Yellow	Amelogenesis imperfecta		Chromogenic bacteria
	Tetracycline ingestion	Gray	Trauma
Reddish-brown	Porphyria	Black/blackish-brown	Trauma
	Fluorosis		Liquid iron supplements
			Tobacco
Blue/bluish-green	Rh incompatibility		Tea or other foods
Brown	Tetracycline ingestion		Chromogenic bacteria
Gray	Tetracycline ingestion	Pink	Internal resorption

From Kula K: Dental problems. In Oski FA, et al (eds): Principles and Practice of Pediatrics, 2nd ed. Philadelphia, J.B. Lippincott, 1994, p 864; with permission.

67. Where are Epstein pearls located?

These white, superficial, mobile nodules, usually midline and often paired, are present on the ***hard palate*** in many newborns. They are keratin-containing cysts that are asymptomatic, do not increase in size, and usually exfoliate spontaneously within a few weeks.

68. How common is dental caries in children?

Very common. By 17 years of age only 15-20% of individuals are free from dental caries and the average child has 8 decayed, missing, or filled tooth surfaces. Prevention of dental caries involves decreasing the frequency of tooth exposure to carbohydrates (frequency is more important than total amount), use of fluoride, toothbrushing, and the use of sealants.

69. How does fluoride minimize the development of dental caries?

- Topical fluoride from toothbrushing is thought to increase remineralization of enamel.
- Bacterial fermentation of sugar into acid plays a major role in the development of caries, and fluoride inhibits this process.
- As teeth are developing, fluoride incorporates into the hydroxyapatite crystal of enamel, making it less soluble and less susceptible to erosion.

70. Should fluoride supplements be given with or without food?

Fluoride absorption is reduced by 30–40% in infants when it is given with formula or food. Thus, the recommendation is to give fluoride on an empty stomach.

71. How long should fluoride supplementation be continued?

Fluoride supplementation should continue until 14–16 years of age, when the third molar crowns are completely calcified.

72. How effective are dental sealants in preventing cavities?

Dental sealants may reduce the development of caries by up to 80% when compared to rates in untreated teeth. Although fluoride acts primarily by protecting smooth surfaces, dental sealants (commonly bisphenol A and glycidyl methacrylate) act by protecting the pits and fissures of the surface, especially in posterior teeth. Reapplication may be needed every 2 years. As a preventive dental procedure, it is relatively underutilized.

73. Which children are susceptible to periodontitis?

The periodontium consists of the gingiva, alveolar bone, and periodontal ligament that connects the two. Periodontitis is the triad of hypertrophied gingiva, loose teeth (due to loss of alveolar bone), and purulent exudate. It is rare in children but may be seen in adolescents with chronically poor periodontal hygiene. Juvenile periodontitis is a disease of rapid alveolar bone loss due to colonization by bacteria pathogenic to the periodontium. It is mainly seen in children with disorders of neutrophil function (e.g., Chediak-Higashi syndrome, cyclic neutropenia).

74. How common is gingivitis in children?

Gingivitis is extremely common, affecting nearly 50% of children. The disorder is usually painless and is manifested by bluish-red discoloration of gums, which are swollen and bleed easily. The cause: bacteria in plaque deposits between teeth. The cure: improved dental hygiene and daily flossing.

75. What is the largest health related expense before adulthood for normally developing children?

Dental braces. Over 50% of children have dental malocclusions that could be improved with treatment, but only 10-20% have severe malocclusions that require treatment. For others the cost and benefits of braces need to be weighed individually. Besides the financial expense, the costs of braces include physical discomfort and some increases in the risk for tooth decay and periodontal disease.

76. What causes halitosis is children?

Halitosis, or bad breath, is usually due to oral factors, including microbial activity on the dorsal tongue and between the teeth. Conditions associated with postnasal drip including chronic sinusitis, upper and lower respiratory tract infections and various systemic diseases are also causes.

Amir E, et al: Halitosis in children. J Pediatr 134:338-343, 1999

DEVELOPMENTAL ASSESSMENT

77. Why do infants have primitive reflexes, and when should they disappear?

Primitive reflexes are *automatisms*, usually triggered by an external stimulus: such as rooting, triggered by touching the corner of the mouth and the asymmetric tonic neck (ATNR), triggered by rotating the head. Some, such as the rooting, sucking or grasp reflexes, have obvious survival value, enabling an otherwise helpless newborn to suckle (or, in the case of our primate relatives, to cling to the mother). Others, such as the ATNR or tonic labyrinthine (TL) reflex, have no obvious purpose. Most primitive reflexes disappear in a cephalocaudad (head to tail) direction. For example, the palmar grasp reflex disappears by three to six months, while the plantar grasp reflex may not disappear until nine to 12 months. The ATNR and TL never disappear, although they are effectively suppressed except when the adult applies great amounts of body tone (for example, most people yawn using an ATNR or TL).

78. What three primitive reflexes, if persistent beyond 4–6 months, can interfere with the development of the ability to roll, sit, and use both hands together?

Moro reflex: Sudden neck extension results in extension, abduction, and then adduction of upper extremities with flexion of fingers, wrists, and elbows.

Asymmetric tonic neck reflex: In a calm supine infant, turning of the head laterally results in relative extension of the arm and leg on the side to the turn and flexion of both on the side away from the turn (the "fencer" position).

Tonic labyrinthine reflex: In an infant being held suspended in the prone position, flexion of the neck results in shoulder protraction and hip flexion, while neck extension causes shoulder retraction and hip extension.

79. What do babies and baby oaks have in common?

Both have a trunk, limbs and want to be vertical, relative to gravity. In infants, this quest for verticality is demonstrated by the emergence of *righting reactions* and *protective extension*. Head righting emerges in the first 4 months of life (in the anterior-posterior plane at 2-3 mo, and in the lateral plane at 3-4 mo), followed by trunk righting in sitting (4-5 months). Protective extension (PE) with the upper extremities from the sitting position follows a progression: anterior PE 5 months, lateral PE 6-7 months, downward PE ("parachute," when held under the axillae and by the examiner and thrust toward the floor) at 9 months, and posteriorly in sitting to form a "tripod" at 12 months.

80. At what age do children develop handedness?

Usually by ***18–24 months***. Hand preference is usually fixed after 5 years of age. Handedness before 1 year of age may be indicative of a problem with the non-preferred side (e.g., hemiparesis, brachial plexus injury).

81. What are the major developmental landmarks for motor skills during the first 2 years of life?

DEVELOPMENTAL LANDMARK	MONTHS
Major gross motor	
Steadiness of head when placed in supported position	1–4
Transfers objects from hand to hand	5–7
Sits without support for > 30 sec	5–8
Cruises or walks holding on	7–13
Stands alone	9–16
Walks alone	9–17
Walks up stairs with help	12–23
Major fine motor	
Grasp	2–4
Reach	3–5
Transfers objects from hand to hand	5–7
Fine pincer grasp with index finger and thumb apposition	9–14
Spontaneous scribbling	12–24

82. What are the most common causes of gross motor delay?

Normal variation is the most common, followed by ***mental retardation***. ***Cerebral palsy*** is a distant third, and all other conditions combined (spinal muscular atrophy, myopathies, etc) run a distant fourth. The most common pathological cause of gross motor delay is mental retardation, even though most children with MR have normal gross motor milestones.

83. Do infant walkers promote physical strength or development of the lower extremities?

No. On the contrary, published data confirm that infants in walkers actually manifest mild but statistically significant gross motor *delays*. Infants with walkers were found to sit, crawl and walk later than those without walkers. Safety hazards can include head trauma, fractures, burns, finger entrapments and dental injuries. Most of the serious injuries involve falls down stairs. The American Academy of Pediatrics has recommended a ban on the manufacture and sale of mobile infant walkers.

Siegel AC, et al: Effects of baby walkers on motor and mental development in human infants. Development 20:355-361, 1999.

84. What is the "developmental quotient (DQ)"?

(***Developmental age/chronologic age***) × 100.

85. How predictive is infant developmental testing?

For infants with DQ's in the *normal* range (above 70), infant testing has *minimal* predictive value (other than to suggest that repeat testing later in childhood will also yield results >70): testing in normal infants cannot predict who will be a slow, average, or bright student. For infants with *abnormal* DQ's of 50 or less, however, the predictive validity is *high*, indicating a significant risk of developmental disability in childhood.

86. Do premature infants develop at the same rate as term infants?

For the most part, premature infants do develop at the same rate as term infants. In ongoing developmental assessments, they eventually "catch up" to their chronologic peers not by accelerated development, but through the arithmetic of time. As they age, their degree of prematurity (in months) becomes less a percentage of their chronologic age. Early in life, the extent of prematurity is key and must be taken into account during assessments. Such "correction factors" are generally unnecessary after age two-three years, depending on the degree of prematurity.

87. When can an infant smell?

The sense of smell is present ***at birth***. Newborn infants show preferential head turning toward gauze pads soaked with their mother's milk, as opposed to the milk of another woman.

88. What are the best measures of cognitive development?

Ideally, cognitive development should be assessed in a fashion that is free of motor requirements. ***Receptive language*** is the best measure of cognitive function. Even an eye blink, or voluntary eye gaze, can be used to assess cognition independently of motor disability. Adaptive skills such as tool use (spoon, crayon) are also useful, although they may be delayed because of purely motoric reasons. Gross motor milestones, such as walking, raise concerns about MR if delayed, but normal gross motor milestones cannot be used to infer normal cognitive development.

89. What do the stages of play tell us about a child's development?

A well-taken history of a child's play is a valuable adjunct to more traditional milestones such as language and adaptive skills:

AGE RANGE	PLAY ACTIVITY	UNDERLYING SKILLS
3 mo	Midline hand play	Sensorimotor; self-discovery
4-5 mo	Bats at objects	Ability to effect environment
6-7 mo	Directed reaching; transfers	
7-9 mo	Banging and mouthing objects	

12 mo	Casting ("I throw it down, and you pick it up for me"); explores objects by visual inspection and handling, rather than orally	Object permanence; social reciprocity; use of pointing, joint attention (eye gaze), and simple language to effect response in caregiver
16–18 mo +	Stacking and dumping; exploring; lids; light switches; simple mechanical toys (jack-in-the-box; shape ball)	Means-ends behavior: experimenting with causality
24 mo	Imitative play ("helping" with the dishes; doll play with a physical doll)	Language and socialization; development of "inner language"
36 mo	Make-believe play (doll play with a pillow to represent the doll, for example)	Distinguish between "real" and "not real"
48 mo	Simple board games, rule-based play ground games such as "Tag"	Concrete operations (Piaget)

90. What can one learn about a child's developmental level with a crayon?

A lot. Below 9 months, the infant will use it as a teething object. Between 10 and 14 months, the infant will make marks on a piece of paper, almost as a byproduct of holding the crayon and "banging" it against the paper. By 14 to 16 months, the infant will make marks spontaneously, and by 18 to 20 months, vigorous scribbling. By 20 to 22 months, an infant will begin copying specific geometric patterns as presented by the examiner:

Age	***Task***
20-22 mo	Alternates from scribble to stroke on imitation of examiner
27-30 mo	Alternates from horizontal to vertical on imitation of examiner
36 mo	Copies circle from illustration
3½ yr	Copies cross
4 yr	Copies square
5 yr	Copies triangle
6 yr	Copies "Union Jack"

The ability to execute these figures requires visual-perceptual, fine motor, and cognitive ability. Delay in the ability to complete these tasks suggests difficulty with one or more of these underlying streams of development.

91. When does a child learn to unbutton and button-up clothing?

By ***3 years*** of age, approximately ***50%*** of children can button. About ***90%*** can do so by ***4 years***. Unbuttoning precedes buttoning up by 3 to 6 months. In these days of Velcro, it is important to ascertain that the child has had adequate opportunities to practice the technique. Unbuttoning and buttoning up are driven by a combination of fine motor and cognitive ability.

92. What is the value of the Goodenough-Harris drawing test?

This "draw-a-person" test is a screening tool used to evaluate a child's cognition and intellect, visual perception, and visual-motor integration. The child is asked to draw a person, and a point is given for each body part drawn with pairs (such as legs) considered 1 part. An average child aged 4 yr, 9 mo will draw a person with 3 parts, and most children by 5 yr, 3 mo will draw a person with 6 parts.

93. Do twins develop at a rate comparable to infants of single birth?

Twins exhibit ***significant verbal and motor delay*** in the first year of life. The difficulty lies not in the lack of potential but in the relative lack of individual stimulation. In general, children who are more closely spaced in a family have slower acquisition of verbal skills. Twins with significant language delay or with excessive use of "twin language" (language understood only by the twins themselves) may be candidates for interventional therapy.

Groothius JR: Twins and twin families. Clin Perinatol 12:467–468, 1985.

94. What percentage of children are left-handed?

Various studies put the prevalence at between ***7 and 10%.*** However, in former premature infants without cerebral palsy, the rate increases to 20–25%. While antecedent brain injury has been hypothesized to account for this increase in prevalence of left-handedness, studies of unilateral intraventricular hemorrhage and handedness have not demonstrated a relationship. Of note, animals such as mice, dogs, and cats show paw preferences, but in these groups, 50% prefer the left paw and 50% the right paw.

Marlow N, et al: Laterality and prematurity. Arch Dis Child 64:1713–1716, 1989.

MENTAL RETARDATION

95. How is mental retardation defined?

Mental retardation is defined as *significantly subaverage intellectual functioning* (minus 2 SD on a standardized measure) **plus** deficits in *two or more* of the following areas: communication, self-care, home living, social skills, community use, self-direction, health, or safety. The American Association on Mental Retardation stipulates that this definition "refers to … limitations in *present functioning*" (emphasis added), thereby stripping the definition of MR of prognostic value. In fact, however, IQ and adaptive scores show sufficient stability over time (especially among individuals functioning in the mentally retarded range), that the diagnosis of MR does, in fact, carry prognostic value as well (see comments on infant developmental testing, above).

Gillberg C: Practitioner review: physical investigations in mental retardation. J Child Psych Psychiatr 38: 889-897, 1997.

Batshaw ML: Mental retardation. Pediatr Clin North Am 40:507-522, 1993.

96. How is intelligence classified with IQ scores?

Most IQ tests are constructed to yield a mean IQ of 100, and a standard deviation of 15 points:

IQ	STANDARD DEVIATION	CATEGORY
> 130	> +2 SD	Very superior
116–130	+1 to +2	High average to superior
115–85	Mean +/– 1 SD	Average
84–70	–1 to –2 SD	Low average to borderline
69–55	–2 to –3	Mild MR
54–40	–3 to –4	Moderate MR
39–25	–4 to –5	Severe MR
< 25	< –5 SD	Profound MR

97. Worldwide, what is the most common preventable cause of mental retardation?

Iodine deficiency leads to maternal and fetal hypothyroxinemia during gestation, which causes brain developmental injury. Severe endemic iodine deficiency can cause cretinism (characterized by deaf-mutism, severe intellectual deficiency, and often hypothyroidism) and may occur in 2–10% of isolated world communities. Moderate iodine deficiency, even more common, leads to milder degrees of cognitive impairment.

Xue-Yi C, et al: Timing of vulnerability of the brain to iodine deficiency in endemic cretinism. N Engl J Med 331:1739–1744, 1994.

98. What features can indicate cognitive problems in infants and young children?

In younger infants and toddlers, fine motor and especially language development are the usual best correlates of cognitive achievement. As the child ages, the various milestones can be evaluated. Significant sequential delay should warrant referral for formal developmental testing to evaluate the possibility of mental retardation.

2–3 mos	Not alerting to mother with special interest
6–7 mos	Not searching for dropped object
8–9 mos	No interest in peek-a-boo
12 mos	Does not search for hidden object
15–18 mos	No interest in cause-and-effect games
2 yrs	Does not categorize similarities (e.g., animals vs vehicles)
3 yrs	Does not know own full name
4 yrs	Cannot pick shorter or longer of two lines
4½ yrs	Cannot count sequentially
5 yrs	Does not know colors or any letters
5½ yrs	Does not know own birthday or address

First LR, Palfrey JS: The infant or young child with developmental delay. N Engl J Med 330: 478–483, 1994.

99. What findings in a child with mental retardation should prompt a cranial MRI?

- Cerebral palsy or motor asymmetry
- Abnormal head size or shape
- Craniofacial malformation
- Loss or plateau of developmental skills
- Multiple somatic anomalies
- Neurocutaneous findings
- Seizures
- IQ < 50

Palmer FB, Capute AJ: Mental retardation. Pediatr Rev 15:473–479, 1994.

LANGUAGE DEVELOPMENT AND DISORDERS

100. What is the difference between speech and language?

Language includes any symbol system for the storage or exchange of information. *Speech* is one subset of language. When parents bring a child for evaluation of "delayed speech," the examiner must determine whether the child has isolated speech delay, expressive plus receptive delay, or across the board language delay (expressive, receptive, and visual). Different disabilities give rise to different patterns of delay.

Wang PP, Baron MA: Language: A Code for Communicating. In Batshaw ML: Children with Disabilities. Baltimore, Brookes Publishing, 1997.

101. What are average times for development of expressive, receptive and visual language milestones?

AGE	EXPRESSIVE	RECEPTIVE	VISUAL
0-3 mo	Coo	Alerts to voice	Recognizes parents; visual tracking
4-6 mo	Monosyllabic babbling, laugh, "raspberry"	Turns to voice and sounds	Responds to facial expressions
7-9 mo	Polysyllabic babbling; Mama/dada, nonspecific	Recognizes own name; inhibits to command "No"	Imitates games (patty cake; peek-a-boo)
10 mo	Mama/dada specific	Follows at least one 1-step command without a gestural cue ("Come here"; "Give me," etc.)	Points to desired objects
12 mo	First word other than mama/dada or names of other family members or pets		
16–18 mo	Uses words to indicate wants	Follows many 1-step commands; points to body parts on command	
22–24 mo	Two-word phrases	Follows 2-step commands	
30 mo	Telegraphic speech	Follows prepositional commands	
36 mo	Simple sentences		

102. What are the warning signs of delayed language development?

Signs of Language Problems Needing Further Evaluation

0– 6 mos	Child does not respond to sounds or turn toward the speaker who is out of sight.
	Child makes only crying sounds (no cooing or comfort sounds).
1 yr	Child shows only inconsistent responses to sound.
	Child has stopped babbling or does not babble yet.
2 yrs	Child does not understand or attend when spoken to.
	Child does not use any words.
	Vocabulary is minimal (less than eight to 10 words) and is not growing.
	Speech primarily echoes what others say.
$2\frac{1}{2}$ yrs	Child is not combining words.
	Child has difficulty following commands or answering simple questions.
3 yrs	Child still echoes
	Sentences are not used.
	Vocabulary is less than 100 words.
4 yrs	Child has difficulty formulating statements and questions.
	Child has deficient conversational skills and has difficulty learning concepts and/or sequences, such as numbers and the aphabet.
	Language usage is deviant and not used appropriately for social interaction.
5 yrs	Child cannot retain and follow verbal directions.
	Child has difficulty learning sound-symbol relationships.
	Sentence structure is noticeably faulty, and word order in sentences is poor.
	Child cannot describe an event or outing.

Blum NJ, Baron M: Speech and language disorders. In: Schwartz MW, Curry TA, Sargent J, et al (eds): Pediatric Primary Care: A Problem Oriented Approach. Philadelphia, Mosby, 1997: 845-849.

103. Should all newborns be screened for hearing impairment?

In 1993, The National Institutes of Health (NIH) recommended that all newborns be screened by a device that measures otoacoustic emissions (OAEs). OAEs are acoustic echoes from the cochlea when a sound is introduced into the external auditory canal. Abnormal results warrant testing using the more specific auditory brainstem response, which uses scalp electrodes to determine responses to broad-band auditory stimuli. The NIH recommendation was made to identify hearing disability as early as possible. Average age at detection for these infants is usually delayed until 14 months. Such disability occurs in 1-3/1,000 children, but testing only those children with high-risk criteria identifies only 50% of infants with hearing impairment. The recommendation for universal screening has been criticized because of the poor specificity and poor positive-predictive value of abnormal test results in the newborn period as well as unclear cost-benefit analyses.

In 1999, the AAP endorsed the implementation of universal newborn hearing screening and many states in the U.S. are mandating this approach.

American Academy of Pediatrics, Task Force on Newborn Hearing and Screening: Newborn and infant hearing loss: Detection and intervention. Pediatrics 103:527-530, 1999.

104. Do deaf infants babble?

Yes. Babbling begins at about the same time in deaf and hearing infants, but deaf infants stop babbling without the normal progression to meaningful communicative speech.

105. At what age does a child's speech become intelligible?

Intelligibility increases by about 25% per year. A 1-year-old has about 25% intelligibility, a 2-year-old 50%, a 3-year-old 75%, and a 4-year-old 100%. Significantly delayed intelligibility should prompt a hearing and language evaluation.

106. What are the most common causes of so-called "delayed speech"?

The most common causes of speech or langauge delay include: developmental language disorders (normal cognition, impaired intelligibility, delayed emergence of phrases, sentences, and grammatical markers); mental retardation, hearing loss, and autistic spectrum disorder.

107. Which of the following can cause speech or language delay: birth order, bilingual upbringing, tongue-tie or laziness?

None of the above should be considered a primary cause of language difficulty in a toddler or child with significant delay.

108. What do ELM Scale, CLAMS, REEL, and PPVT have in common?

All are ***screening tests*** that can be used for in-office screening when language delay is suspected: Early Language Milestone Scale (ELMS), Clinical Linguistic and Auditory Milestone Scale (CLAMS), Bzoch-League Receptive Emergent Language (REEL) Scale, and the Peabody Picture Vocabulary Test (PPVT). Failure on one of these tests should prompt referral for an audiologic and cognitive assessment.

109. What causes flat tympanograms?

Tympanometry is an objective measurement of the compliance of the tympanic membrane and the middle ear compartment that involves varying the air pressure in the external ear canal from approximately –200 to +400 mm H_2O while measuring the reflected energy of a simultaneous acoustic tone. A normal tracing looks like an inverted V with the peak occurring at an air pressure of 0 mm H_2O, indicating a functionally normal external canal, an intact tympanic membrane, and a lack of excess of middle ear fluid. Flat tympanograms occur with ***perforation of the tympanic membrane***, ***occlusion of the tympanometry probe*** against the wall of the canal, ***obstruction of the canal*** by a foreign body or impaction by cerumen, or ***large middle ear effusion***. Flat tympanograms due to middle ear effusion are usually associated with a 20 to 30 decibel conductive hearing loss, although in occasional instances the loss may be as great as 50 dB.

110. Does otitis media with effusion (OME) cause speech delay?

Probably. But data establishing delay with how many days with OME, and at what ages, remain elusive.

111. Which children should be considered for a formal hearing test?

Parental concern that the child does not hear normally. (This is listed first because although it is often the earliest sign of hearing problems, it unfortunately is often overlooked by the pediatrician.)

Medical

- Birth weight < 1500 gm
- Hyperbilirubinemia at level exceeding indications for exchange transfusion
- Neonatal ICU care (regardless of indication)
- Congenital infection (e.g., cytomegalovirus, rubella, herpes, toxoplasmosis, syphilis)
- Bacterial meningitis

Genetic

- Malformations of the first or second branchial arch (microtia or dysplastic ears; mandibular hypoplasia, etc)
- Neonatal abnormalities of the neural crest (widely spaced eyes; iris heterochromia, white forelock)
- Family history of childhood-onset hearing loss

Developmental

- Delay in acquisition of language and/or speech
- Any other developmental disability (MR, CP, autism)

112. What methods are used to test hearing at different ages?

The gold standard remains pure tone testing under headphones (usually not achievable until about 30 months of age), but there are clinically valid methods that can be used at any age. Hearing testing should never be put off "until the child is older" if an indication for audiologic evaluation exists.

AGE	METHOD	COMMENT
Any	Otoacoustic emissions	Useful for newborn screening; occasional false positives
Any	Brainstem auditory evoked response	Sensitive, specific. Often requires sedation in younger children
0–6 months	Alerting to sound	Sound-field; assesses hearing in the better of the two ears, if an asymmetry exists
6–18 months	Conditioned orienting	Sound-field; assesses hearing in the better of the two ears, if an asymmetry exists
24 +	Play audiometry	Picture pointing, etc. Tests speech reception threshold.
30 +	Pure tones under headphones	Tests each ear separately

113. A toddler with a bifid uvula and hypernasal speech most likely has what condition?

Velopharyngeal insufficiency with a possible submucosal cleft palate. The velum, or soft palate, moves posteriorly during swallowing and speech, separating the oropharynx from the nasopharynx. Velopharyngeal insufficiency exists when this separation is incomplete, as may occur after cleft palate repair or following adenoidectomy (usually transient). In severe cases, nasopharyngeal regurgitation of food may occur. In milder cases, the only manifestation may be hypernasal speech due to nasal emission of air during phonation. If a bifid uvula is present, one should palpate the palate carefully for the presence of a submucous cleft.

114. What advice should be given to parents whose child stutters?

Stuttering is a common characteristic of the speech of preschool children. However, the vast majority of children do not persist with stuttering beyond 5 or 6 years of age. Preschoolers at increased risk for persistence of stuttering include those with a positive family history of stuttering and those with anxiety-provoking stress related to talking. A child older than 5 or 6 years who stutters should be referred to a speech-language pathologist for assessment and treatment. The pediatrician can help guide parents of children < 5 years of age with stuttering by making the following suggestions:

- Do not give the child directives about how to deal with his or her speech (e.g., "slow down" or "take a breath").
- Provide a relaxed, easy speech model in your own manner of speaking to the child.
- Reduce the need/expectations for the child to speak to strangers, adults, or authority figures or to compete with others (such as siblings) to be heard.
- Listen attentively to the child with patience and without showing concern.
- Seek professional guidance if speech is not noticeably more fluent in 2–3 months.

115. How do cluttering and palilalia differ from stuttering?

Cluttering is speech so rapid that it is often intelligible. There is repetition and omission of sounds, syllables, and whole words. Unlike stuttering, cluttering may benefit from advising a child to consciously slow his or her speech. *Palilalia* is intelligible speech in which whole words or phrases are repeated rapidly. This can be associated with neurologic diseases such as pseudobulbar palsy or Tourette syndrome.

116. Which infants with "tongue-tie" should have surgical correction?

"Tongue-tie," or *partial ankyloglossia*, is the restriction of mobility of the tongue due to a short or thickened lingual frenulum. In theory, partial ankyloglossia can interfere with breastfeeding and speech. The vast majority of infants, particularly those who can extend the tip of the tongue past the lips, accommodate and eventually develop normal lingual mobility. Indications for surgical correction are imprecise, but children with persistent speech problems after 2–4 years should be considered.

117. List the three essential features of autism.
Autism is a behaviorally defined developmental disorder. Children diagnosed with this disorder must have significant problems in three areas:

1. ***Impaired social interactions***, such as failure to make eye contact or show interest in interacting with others
2. ***Absent*** or ***abnormal speech*** and language development
3. ***Narrow range of interest*** and ***stereotyped or repetitive response*** to objects

Although most children with autism also have mental retardation, about 25% have an IQ > 70.

118. Which behaviors of children should arouse suspicion of possible autism?

- Avoidance of eye contact during infancy
- Relating to only part of a person's body (i.e., lap) rather than to whole person
- Failure to acquire speech or speech acquisition in an unusual manner, such as echolalia (repeating another person's speech)
- Repetition of TV commercials and singing out of context and without communicative purpose
- Spending long periods of time in repetitive activities and fascination with movement (i.e., spinning records, dripping water)
- Interest in small visual details or patterns
- Unusual abilities, such as early letter and number recognition
- Early reading with minimal comprehension

Coplan J: Counseling parents regarding prognosis in autistic spectrum disorder. Pediatrics 105:e65, 2000.

119. Is there a biochemical or neurologic basis for autistic behavior?

The early hypothesis that autism resulted from parental coldness, rejection, or mishandling is incorrect. The current belief is that autistic behavior arises from neurodevelopmental dysfunction of the CNS. Unfortunately, neither the biochemical basis nor the anatomic abnormality for autism is known.

120. Parents complain that their daughter has poor communication skills, decreased social interaction, marked periodic breathing, and loss of purposeful hand movements. What diagnosis should be suspected?

Rett syndrome. This X-linked neurodegenerative disorder affects girls exclusively. After a normal birth and early infancy, developmental arrest begins around 7–18 months of age, followed by severe decline of cognitive skills and loss of purposeful hand movements. Profound dementia, microcephaly, ataxia, spastic paraparesis, seizures, and characteristic hand-wringing and respiratory stereotypies develop progressively. Genetic testing for Rett syndrome is now available in some laboratories.

SCHOOL PROBLEMS

121. How is learning disability defined?

The term "learning disability" dates back to 1963 when Dr. Samuel Kirk used it to refer to children with normal intelligence who had difficulties with learning academic skills. Various definitions have since been proposed; a currently accepted one was proposed by the National Joint Committee on Learning Disabilities in 1990. According to the NJCLD, the term learning disability "... refers to a heterogenous group of disorders manifest by significant difficulties in the acquisition and the use of listening, speaking, reading, writing, reasoning, or mathematics abilities." The NJCLD notes that these disorders are lifelong and "intrinsic to the individual." Such difficulties are not due to visual, hearing, or motor handicaps, emotional problems, mental retardation, or environmental or socioculturoeconomic issues.

122. How are the learning disabilities (LD) classified?

Various classification systems have been proposed. DSM-IV lists 4 types of LD: ***reading***, ***mathematics***, ***writing***, and ***"not otherwise specified."*** Often a distinction is made between verbal (language) and nonverbal (performance) abilities, though there can be considerable overlap in a child. Social-emotional disabilities are often considered part of the nonverbal grouping. Neuropsychologists investigate the role of specific brain processes such as memory, attention, phonemic awareness and others in creating difficulties with learning disabilities.

Capin DM: Developmental learning disorders: Clues to their diagnosis and management. Pediatr Rev 17:284-290, 1996.

123. What distinguishes dyslexia, dyscalculia and dysgraphia?

Dyslexia is a reading learning disability. It is the most common learning disability effecting 2–10% of school-aged children. Characterized by problems decoding single words, it is usually be due to deficits in phonological processing. Reading disabilities are heritable in many cases, though the mode of transmission appears variable; linkage studies have found loci on chromosomes 1 and 6.

Dyscalculia, or specific mathematics disability, affects 1-6% of children. Mathematics disabilities involve difficulties in computation, math concepts, and/or application of those concepts to everyday situations.

Dysgraphia, or disorder of written expression, affects 2-8% of children. Difficulties with writing have several possible etiologies, including problems with: fine motor control, linguistic abilities, visual-spatial skills, attention, memory, and sequencing.

Beitchman JH, Young AR: Learning disorders with a special emphasis on reading disorders: A review of the past 10 years. J Amer Acad Child Adol Psych 36: 1020-1032, 1997.

124. What are executive functions?

Executive functions are cognitive abilities involved in the regulation of behavior. They include goal-directed processes such as planning, organization of information, memory, and inhibition of emotions or impulsive responses. Problems with executive function have been implicated in both LD and ADHD.

125. In addition to learning disabilities, what factors may contribute to academic underachievement?

- Hearing or visual problems
- Mental retardation
- Developmental language disorders
- ADHD
- Emotional/psychiatric disorders
- Disorganized home environment
- Lack of social support
- Sleep problems
- Chronic medical conditions
- Medications (e.g., anticonvulsants, antihistamines)

126. Is waiting until a child is older to start school a problem?

Although parents and schools often want to delay the start of school for children who have difficulty learning academic skills or who have problems with behavioral regulation, studies suggest that this is not usually an effective intervention. In contrast, if delayed school entry results in the child being older than most classmates, this has been associated with later behavioral and school problems.

127. Is the term school phobia outdated?

Yes. There are multiple reasons why children refuse to go to school, and most of them are not related to phobias. Both separation anxiety disorder and generalized anxiety disorder are associated with school avoidance in children and should be considered. Depression, learning problems, and family stressors may also contribute to refusal to go to school. Understanding these underlying factors is important in developing an intervention that is likely to be successful.

128. How much of a problem are the bullies?

Bullying is defined as "unintentional, unprovoked abuse of power by one or more children to inflict pain or cause distress to another child on repeated occasions." It is a universal problem in schools worldwide. The victims frequently experience a range of psychological, psychosomatic and behavioral problems that include anxiety, insecurity, low self-esteem, sleeping difficulties, bedwetting, sadness, frequent bouts of headache and abdominal pain.

Nansel TR, et al: Bullying behaviors among US youth: prevalence and association with psychosocial adjustment. JAMA 285:2094-2100, 2001.

Pearce JH, Thompson AE: Practical approaches to reduce the impact of bullying. Arch Dis Child 79:528-531, 1998.

129. What is IDEA?

Not just a good idea, it is the law. The ***Individuals with Disabilities Education Act*** (IDEA) of 1990 (PL 101-476) entitled all children with disabilities to a free an appropriate educational experience. IDEA mandates that a child is entitled to receive an individual diagnostic evaluation to establish academic, behavioral, and social-emotional strengths and weaknesses. An Individualized Education Plan (IEP) can then be formed as a contract between the school system and the child/family to define the services that will be provided and how the child's progress will be monitored. Families are entitled to due process procedures if they and the school cannot agree on a plan or the plan is not implemented.

Craig SE: Special education services for children with disabilities. In Levine MD, Carey WF, Crocker AC (eds): Developmental-Behavioral Pediatrics, 3rd ed. Philadelphia: WB Saunders, pp. 781-792.

130. What is Section 504?

Section 504 of the Rehabilitation Act of 1973 is a civil rights law that stipulates that individuals with disabilities must be provided access to any services that receive government funding. Since public schools receive government funding this law mandates that school must make accommodations to provided for the needs of children with disabilities. It may offer an option for a child not considered eligible under the provisions of IDEA.

PSYCHIATRIC DISORDERS

131. What is the prevalence of childhood psychiatric disorders?

Overall, ***17–22%*** of children aged 4–20 in community samples are diagnosed with a specific psychiatric disorder. The most common disorders are:

Attention deficit hyperactivity disorder (4–10%)
Oppositional disorder (5–10%)
Conduct disorder (1–5%)
Separation anxiety (3–5%)
Overanxious disorder (2–5%)
Depression (2–6%)

132. If a parent has an affective disorder, what is the likelihood that an offspring will have similar problems?

20-25% of these children will develop a major affective disorder, and as many as ***40–45%*** will have a psychiatric problem.

133. How does mania differ in children and adolescents?

Mania occurs in approximately 0.5 to 1% of adolescents and occurs less frequently in prepubertal children. *Younger children* may present with extreme irritability, emotional lability, and aggression. Dysphoria, hypomania and agitation may be intermixed. Hyperactivity, distractibility, and pressured speech often occur in all age groups. Symptoms in *adolescents* more closely resemble those in adults. They include: elated mood, flight of ideas, sleeplessness, bizarre behavior, delusions of grandeur, paranoia, or euphoria.

134. What are the essential features of a conversion reaction in children?

A *conversion reaction* is the presence of symptoms (suggestive of a physical disorder) that cannot be explained by a known physical disorder and instead are thought to be an expression of psychological conflict or need, particularly in settings of anxiety or depression. However, these distinctions are often not so clear. In many cases the symptoms develop in conjunction with a medical illness or injury that may explain at least some of the symptoms. In addition, adults and children diagnosed with conversion disorders are, not uncommonly, later found to a medical condition that may explain some of the symptoms. Thus, when a conversion disorder is suspected medical and psychological evaluation and treatment should occur concurrently. Conversion disorder should be distinguished from malingering in which the individual is intentionally producing the symptoms.

135. What ritualistic behaviors are common in children with obsessive-compulsive disorder (OCD)?

The most common rituals involve ***excessive cleaning***, repeating ***gross motor rituals*** (e.g., going up and down stairs), and repetitive ***checking behaviors*** (e.g., checking that doors are locked or that homework is correct). Obsessions most commonly deal with fear of contamination. Symptoms tend to wax and wane in severity, and the specific obsessions or compulsions change over time. Most children attempt to disguise their rituals. Anxiety and distress that interfere with school or family life can occur when children fail in efforts to resist the thoughts or activities. Counseling and serotonin-reuptake-inhibiting medications (e.g., clomipramine, fluoxetine, sertraline, paroxetine, fluvoxamine, citalopram) can be beneficial.

136. What distinguishes a conduct disorder from an oppositional defiant disorder?

Both are disruptive behavior disorders of childhood and early adolescence. *Conduct disorder* is the more serious disorder in that it is diagnosed when the child's behaviors violate the rights of others (e.g., assault) or major societal norms (e.g., stealing, truancy, fire setting). Children with conduct disorder are at risk for developing the antisocial personality disorder of adults. *Oppositional defiant disorder* is characterized by recurrent negativistic, defiant behaviors toward authority figures.

137. What are common symptoms of depression in a child?

Young children with depression tend to look sad and be tearful. They may have somatic symptoms and they tend to describe themselves negatively such as "I am stupid," and "nobody loves me." Lack of concentration, deteriorating school performance, loss of interest in activities, and suicidal ideation occur in children and adolescents. Psychomotor retardation, change in appetite, hopelessness, sleep problems or hypersomnia, delusions, and drug use are more common in adolescents.

138. How are organic and psychiatrically-based psychoses differentiated?

Psychosis is the manifestation of marked abnormalities in mental functions with diminished grasping of reality and can present in a variety of ways, including disoriented thought, rapidly fluctuating moods, or violent behavior. *Organic psychosis* refers to abnormal behavior and mentation that has a known underlying cause (e.g., illicit drugs). *Psychiatrically based psychosis* does not have an identifiable cause and includes diagnoses such as childhood and adolescent schizophrenia, and severe manic-depressive illness.

	ORGANIC PSYCHOSIS	PSYCHIATRICALLY BASED PSYCHOSIS
Onset	Acute	Insidious, previous episodes
Premorbid state	Normal (history of substance abuse)	Poor social, sexual development
Mental status	Depressed sensorium	Normal sensorium
Orientation	Disoriented	Usually normal
Memory	Recent memory loss	Usually normal
Vital signs	Abnormal (tachycardia, fever)	Usually normal
Hallucinations	Visual, tactile, olfactory	Auditory
Response to therapy	Dramatic	Less dramatic

139. What are the most common side effects of selective serotonin reuptake inhibitors (SSRIs) in children?

- ***Gastrointestinal***: Nausea and anorexia are usually transient and can be minimized by taking the medication with food.
- ***Sleep***: Daytime sedation, insomnia, vivid and frightening dreams. SSRIs decrease total sleep time and the duration of rapid-eye-movement sleep.
- ***Sexual***: Delayed orgasm, anorgasmia, and decreased libido. Boys may develop gynecomastia, and girls may develop mammoplasia.
- ***Behavioral***: Restlessness, hyperactivity, social disinhibition. Reduction in dose usually decreases these symptoms. Abrupt discontinuation can cause similar symptoms, so assess compliance.

Walsh KH, McDougle CJ: When SSRIs make sense. Contemp Pediatr 12:83-105, 2000.

140. What is the serotonin syndrome?

Serotonin syndrome is a rare but serious side effect of SSRIs. It is characterized by fever, muscular rigidity, hyper-reflexia, and mental status changes. Rhabdomyolysis, seizures, and disseminated intravascular coagulation may occur. This side effect is life-threatening and requires abrupt discontinuation of the medication and emergent treatment in an intensive care setting.

141. What cardiac parameters need to monitored in children on tricyclic antidepressants?

Tricyclic antidepressants affect cardiac conduction and thus the ECG should be monitored for children on antidepressants. Tricyclic antidepressants should be stopped if any of the following parameters are exceeded:

PR interval:	More than 210 milliseconds
QRS interval:	Widening by more than 30% over baseline
QTc interval:	More than 450 milliseconds
Heart rate:	More than 130 beats per minute
Systolic BP:	More than 130 mm Hg
Diastolic BP:	More than 85 mm Hg

Viesselman JO: Antidepressant and antimanic drugs. In Werry JS, Aman MG (eds): Practitioner's Guide to Psychoactive Drugs for Children and Adolescents, 2nd ed. New York, Plenum Medical Book, 1999, pp. 249-296.

PSYCHOSOCIAL FAMILY ISSUES

142. How likely is it that children in the U.S. will experience the separation or divorce of their parents?

More than 50% of first marriages end in divorce. It is estimated that nearly 75% of black children and 40% of white children born to married parents will experience their parents' divorce before they reach 18 years of age. And the flip side of this stressor is that 50% of individuals who divorce will remarry within five years, creating another major family transition for a child.

Emery RE, Coiro MJ: Divorce: consequences for children. Pediatr Rev 16:306-310, 1995.

143. How do children of different ages vary in their response to parental divorce?

Preschool (ages 2 1/2–5): Most likely to show regression in developmental milestones (e.g., toilet training); irritability; sleep disturbances; preoccupation with fear of abandonment; demanding with remaining parent.

Early school-age (6–8): Most likely to demonstrate open grieving; preoccupied with fear of rejection and of being replaced; half may have a decrease in school performance.

Later school-age (ages 9–12): More likely to demonstrate profound anger at one or both parents; more likely to distinguish one parent as the culprit causing the divorce; deterioration in school performance and peer relationships; sense of loneliness and powerlessness.

Adolescents: Significant potential for acute depression and even suicidal ideation; acting-out behavior (substance abuse, truancy, sexual activity); self-doubts about own potential for marital success.

Kelly JB: Children's adjustment in conflicted marriage and divorce: A decade review of research. J Am Acad Child Adolesc Psychiatry 39:963-973, 2000.

144. What factors are central to a good outcome following a divorce?

- Ability of parents to set aside or resolve conflicts without involving children
- Emotional and physical availability of custodial parent to the child
- Parenting skills of custodial parent
- Extent to which child does not feel reject by noncustodial parent
- Child's temperament
- Presence of supportive family network
- Absence of continuing anger or depression in the child

Wallerstein JS: Separation, divorce, and remarriage. In Levine MD, et al (eds): Developmental-Behavioral Pediatrics, 3rd ed. Philadelphia, W.B. Saunders, 1999, pp 149–161.

145. Is it preferable for children of divorced parents to live with their mother or father?

Early research suggested that boys had a more difficult time adjusting to divorce than girls, but in most cases the children were living with their mothers. Some current research suggests that children may initially do better when living with the same sex parent, but that children living with the same sex parent may be more likely to have difficulties when they are trying to establish relationships with members of the opposite sex.

146. How much does chronic illness increase the risk of emotional and behavioral problems?

Children with a variety of chronic illnesses have been shown to have an approximately 2-fold increased risk of behavioral or emotional disorders. The increased risk is even greater if the chronic illness involves the central nervous system.

147. What is the "vulnerable child syndrome"?

The *vulnerable child syndrome* is characterized by excessive parental concern about the health and development of their child. It usually occurs after a medical illness in which the parents are understandably upset or worried about the health of their child (e.g., prematurity, congenital heart disease). However, this concern persists despite the child's recovery. Problems of the syndrome can include pathologic separation difficulties for parent and child, sleep problems, overprotectiveness, and overindulgence. Children are at risk for behavior, school, and peer relationship problems.

148. Is a child aware of his or her own fatal illness?

Many studies have demonstrated that even young children are cognizant that a medical condition is life-threatening and experience increased levels of anxiety and isolation compared to children with nonfatal illnesses.

149. How does the cognitive understanding of death evolve?

Toddler (< 3 yrs):	Death as separation, abandonment, or change
Preschool (3–6 yrs):	Prelogical thought with magical and egocentric beliefs that child may be responsible for death; death as temporary and reversible
School-age (6–11 yrs):	Concrete logical thinking; death as permanent and universal but due to a specific illness or injury rather than as a biologic process; death something that occurs to others
Adolescence (12+ yrs):	Abstract logical thinking; more complete comprehension of death; death as a possibility for self

American Academy of Pediatrics, Committee on Psychosocial Aspects of Child and Family Health: The pediatrician and childhood bereavement. Pediatrics 105:445-447, 2000.

150. When do symptoms of grief peak for children who have experienced the death of a parent?

Approximately half of children will have peak symptoms in the month after the death of the parent. One third will not have peak symptoms until 6 months after the death and 15-20% will not have peak symptoms until 12 months after the death.

151. Are thoughts of wanting to die abnormal in children who have experienced the death of a parent?

No. Children who have experienced the death of a parent often feel that they would be better off dead or that they should have died with the deceased person. In addition, they may express the hope of dying to visit the deceased parent. The risk of attempting suicide is much lower in this group than in depressed children with suicidal ideation.

Siegel BS: Bereavement and loss. In: Parker S, Zuckerman B (eds): Behavioral and Developmental Pediatrics. Boston, Little, Brown, & Co., 1995, pp 343–347.

152. Should adopted children be informed of their adoption?

Yes. It should not occur as a one-time event, but increasing amounts of information can be given over time. Most preschool children will not understand the process or meaning of adoption, and for them disclosure should be guided by what the child wants to know. School-age children should be aware of their adoption and feel comfortable discussing it with their parents.

153. Do adopted children have more emotional and behavioral problems than other children?

Probably, but it may not be due to the adoption process. Studies suggest that adopted children are referred for psychiatric intervention about twice as frequently as would be expected. However, multiple factors contribute to this including: biological or social influences prior to adoption, differences in parental or referrer tendency to refer adopted children, frequency of evaluation prior to adoption and other experiences. Thus it is very difficult to determine whether the adoption process itself contributes to increased behavioral or emotional problems.

154. How common is domestic violence?

Statistics indicate that 10-40% of families are afflicted by domestic violence. The potential impact on children in these families is enormous, including behavioral problems, developmental delay and abuse. The AAP has recommended that all pediatricians incorporate screening for domestic violence as part of anticipatory guidance.

Siegel RM, et al: Screening for domestic violence in the community pediatric setting. Pediatrics 104:874-877, 1999.

155. Does having gay or lesbian parents affect a child's gender identity or sexual orientation?

Children with gay or lesbian parents do not seem to differ from children with heterosexual parents in their gender identity or sex role behaviors. There is not an increased incidence of homosexuality in these children.

156. Does participation in day care during the infancy and toddler years have negative effects on cognitive development?

This question has been examined in a large multi-site study funded by the National Institute of Child Health and Human Development. At 24 and 36 months there has been no relationship between the number of hours in care and any of the measures of cognitive or language development. However, child care of higher quality was consistently associated with better language and cognitive outcomes. The frequency of language stimulation in the child care setting seemed to be the most important variable.

157. What are the consequences of being a "latchkey" child?

The term refers to the millions of children < age 18 who are in unsupervised care after school due to families where one or two parents work. Because of the enormous variability of circumstance, the consequences may be positive (e.g., increased maturity, self-reliance) or negative (e.g., isolation, feelings of neglect). Increased after-school programs may minimize negative consequences.

158. Does adult television programming depict more acts of violence than children's programming?

No. Adult programming depicts about five violent acts per hour, but children's Saturday morning programming depicts 20-25 acts of violence per hour. By age 18, a typical child will have witnessed over 200,000 acts of violence on television and over 18,000 murders.

Shapiro HL: Electronic media. In Levine MD, et al (eds): Developmental-Behavioral Pediatrics, 3rd ed. Philadelphia, W.B. Saunders, 1999, pp 188-191.

159. What are the effects of heavy television watching in children?

At one point or another, TV viewing has been blamed for many of the problems facing children today. Studies have documented effects of heavy television viewing in the following areas: increased aggressive behavior, increase in general level of arousal, desensitization to violence, increased obesity, and decreased school performance. There does not seem to be a large effect of television viewing on cognition or attention.

SLEEP PROBLEMS

160. What is the average daily sleep requirement by age?

Birth—16 hrs	*4 yrs*—11.5 hrs
6 mos—14.5 hrs	*6 yrs*— 9.5 hrs
12 mos—13.5 hrs	*12 yrs*—8.5 hrs
2 yrs—13 hrs	*18 yrs*—8 hrs

161. What is the typical pattern of napping?

Naps decline from 2 per day at age 1 year to 1 per day at 2 years and then to .5 at age 5 years. A two-year-old typically naps for 2.3 hours and five-year-old for 1.7 hours. Most children no longer take naps beginning between ages 4 and 5, although there is wide variance.

162. What are the effects of sleep deprivation on humans?

Residency and newborns are particularly well designed to educate one about these effects, which include: decreased attention, decreased motivation, increased problems with emotional self-regulation, and problems with short-term memory and memory consolidation. In preschoolers, the amount of night and 24-hour sleep is clearly related to daytime behavior problems. Sleeping less at night is correlated with DSM-III-R diagnostic problems, including "acting out" behaviors—hyperactivity, oppositional or noncompliant behavior and aggression ("externalizing behavior problems"). No relationship has been noted between sleep and internalizing behavior problems (e.g., anxiety) in younger children.

Lavigne JV et al: Sleep and behavior problems among preschoolers. J Dev Behav Pediatr 20:164-169, 1999.

163. How do the sleep-wake patterns of breastfed infants compare with non-breastfed infants?

Breastfed infants tend to sleep for shorter times and wake more frequently during the night. This may be related to the fact that gastric emptying is more rapid with breast milk than with formula.

164. Why is the supine sleeping position recommended for infants?

In countries that have advocated the supine sleeping position as a preventive measure for sudden infant death syndrome (SIDS), there have been dramatic decreases in the incidence of SIDS. Hypotheses on why the prone position is more dangerous for infants have included the potential for airway obstruction and the possibility of rebreathing carbon dioxide, particularly when soft bedding is used.

Willinger M: Sleep position and sudden infant death syndrome. JAMA 273:818–819, 1995.

165. Do infants sleep better prone or supine?

Although the supine position is recommended to minimize the chance of SIDS, infants sleep longer (by 16%), have fewer and shorter arousals (by 40%), and spend greater time in non-REM sleep (by 25%) in the ***prone*** position.

Kahn A, et al: Prone or supine body position and sleep characteristics in infants. Pediatrics 91:1112, 1993.

166. When do infants begin to sleep through the night?

By ***about 3 months*** of age, about ***70%*** of infants (slightly more for bottlefed and slightly less for breastfed babies) will not cry or awaken their parents between midnight and 6 am. By ***6 months***, ***90%*** of infants fit this category, but between 6 and 9 months the percent of infants with night awakenings increases.

167. Does feeding infants cereal before bedtime promote their sleeping through the night?

It is important to have current references on hand when debating a knowledgeable grandmother because most will insist it is so. Although there is some conflicting data, recent studies suggest that early introduction of cereal does not promote sleeping through the night.

Macknin ML, et al: Infant sleep and bedtime cereal. Am J Dis Child 143:1066–1068, 1989.

168. What advice to parents may minimize the problem of night waking?

- After a parental-child bedtime routine, place the infant in the sleep setting while awake (e.g., do not rock an infant to sleep).
- Parent should not be present as the child falls asleep.
- Gradually eliminate night feedings (infants by 6 months receive sufficient daytime nutrition to allow this).
- Transitional objects (e.g., blanket, teddy bear, etc.) may minimize separation issues.

Blum NJ, Carey WB: Sleep problems among infants and young children. Pediatr Rev 17:87–93, 1996.

169. Are problems associated with parents and infants sleeping in the same bed together?

Parents and children sleeping together has been a common practice throughout human history and is still the norm in many cultures today. Concern about cosleeping has focused on two areas. First children under 1 year of age or severely disabled children sleeping in adult beds are at risk for suffocation due to entrapment in the bed structure or overlying by the adult. Second, some studies have found that cosleeping is associated with behavior problems. When co-sleeping is the cultural norm it does not appear to be associated with an increase in behavior or sleep problems. However, if cosleeping is a response to a child's sleep problems it may serve to maintain the sleep problems and in some cases (if the parents don't want the child in their bed) it may be indication that the child's parents are having difficulty setting limits for the child. In these situations co-sleeping is likely to be associated with other behavior problems.

Latz S, Wolf AW, Lozoff B: Cosleeping in context: Sleep practices and problems in young children in Japan and the United States. Arch Pediatr Adoles Med 153:339-346, 1999.

170. How common are sleep problems in elementary school-aged children?

40% of children ages 7-12 experience sleep-onset delay, 10% night awakening and 10% have significant daytime sleepiness. Of note, some studies have shown that the extent of sleep is also inversely related to teacher-reported psychiatric symptoms.

Owens JA: Sleep habits and sleep disturbances in elementary school-aged children. J Dev Behav Pediatr 21:27-36, 2000.

Aronen ET et al: Sleep and psychiatric symptoms in school-aged children. J Am Acad Child Adolesc Psychiatr 39:502-508, 2000.

171. What is the role of melatonin in the treatment of sleep problems of children?

The most common sleep-wake cycle disorder in children appears to be sleep fragmentation with difficulties in both sleep induction and maintenance. Melantonin, in both fast-release and slow-release forms, appears to be a safe medication in preliminary studies in children. As it cannot be patented, there are potential problems of the quality of the product as purchased in health food stores.

Jan JE et al: Melatonin treatment of sleep-wake cycle disorders in children and adolescents. Develop Med Child Neurol 41:491-500, 1999.

172. What are parasomnias?

Parasomnias are ***undesirable physical phenomena*** that occur during sleep. Examples include: night terrors, nightmares, sleepwalking, sleeptalking, nocturnal enuresis, sleep bruxism, somniloquy and body rocking. Between the ages of 3-13 years, nearly 80% of all children will have had at least one parasomnia.

Laberge L et al: Development of parasomnias from childhood to early adolescence. Pediatrics 106:67-74, 2000.

173. At what age do sleepwalking and sleeptalking occur?

Sleepwalking occurs most commonly between ages 5 and 10. As many as 15% of children aged 5–12 may have somnambulated once, and as many as 10% of 3-10-year-old children may sleeptalk regularly. The sleepwalking child is clumsy, restless, and nonpurposeful. The episode is not remembered. Injury is common during this outing.

Sleeptalking is monosyllabic and often incomprehensible. Both conditions usually end before age 15. Severe cases may benefit from diazepam or imipramine therapy.

174. What is the difference between night terrors and nightmares?

Nightmares are frightening dreams that occur during REM sleep, usually in the last half of the night, and may be readily recalled on awakening. The child is aroused without difficulty and is usually easily consolable, but returning to sleep after a nightmare may be problematic. *Pavor nocturnus* (Latin for fear of the night) is more commonly known as ***night terrors.*** These are brief episodes which occur in non-REM stage IV sleep. They usually last 30 seconds to 5 minutes during which a child sits up, screams, and appears aroused, often staring and sweating profusely. The child cannot be consoled, rapidly goes back to sleep, and does not recall the episode in the morning. Onset of night terrors in an older child or persistent multiple attacks may indicate more serious psychopathology.

175. What recommendation should be given to a parent whose child is having night terrors?

Often, an explanation of the phenomenon to the parent, with emphasis on the fact that the child is still asleep during the episode and should not be awakened is all that is needed. If stress or sleep deprivation coincide with the night terrors, these factors should be addressed. If this is not successful, other approaches may be considered.

- When night terrors occur at the same time each night, the parent may awaken the child 15 minutes before the anticipated event over a 7-day period and keep him or her awake for at least 5 minutes. This often disrupts the sleep cycle and results in resolution of the problem.
- Rarely, for severe night terrors, a short course of diazepam will suppress REM sleep, reset the sleep cycles, and result in cessation of the problem.

176. What percent of children snore?

5-10 % of preadolescent children are reported by their parents to snore at night.

177. What is the restless legs syndrome?

The *restless legs syndrome* involves myoclonus that occurs during rest and light sleep. The leg movements may disrupt sleep. Dysesthesias may be present when the child is awake. The disorder is inherited as an autosomal trait.

178. What is the classic tetrad of symptoms seen in narcolepsy?

1. ***Excessive daytime sleepiness***: episodes of sleep may occur without warning, usually during sedentary or monotonous activities.
2. ***Cataplexy***: sudden, reversible decrease in muscle tone that is usually precipitated by emotions such as anger, laughter, or fear.
3. ***Sleep paralysis***: an inability to move, talk, or open ones eyes that occurs near the onset of sleep or as one is waking from sleep.

4. ***Hypnagogic hallucinations***: auditory of visual hallucinations that occur near the onset of sleep or as one is waking from sleep.

Children with narcolepsy may not manifest all 4 of these features. Excessive daytime sleepiness often occurs a few years before cataplexy is seen. Sleep paralysis and hynagogic hallucinations may be seen in children who do not have narcolepsy.

VISUAL DEVELOPMENT/DISORDERS

179. When does the eye develop, and what happens if that development is arrested?

The eye, which is derived from both ectoderm and mesoderm, begins to develop at about the 22nd day of gestation and will be completed over the next 6-8 weeks. Anomalies due to arrested ocular development will therefore depend on the timing of the interference. Failure of the optic vesicle to form, seen prior to day 22, may lead to *anophthalmia* or *cyclopia*. This has been reported in such syndromes as trisomy 13 and Klinefelter syndrome. Interference during the third week, such as failure of invagination, may lead to a *congenital cystic eye* or nonattachment of the retina. Failure of closure, around the sixth week, may produce colobomas of the lens, iris, or chorioretinal area.The eyelids are fused until roughly 25–27 weeks, though may remain closed up to 32 weeks gestation. Failure of the eyelids to separate is known as *cryptophthalmos*.

180. How well does a newborn see?

The visual perception system functions in a fairly complex manner at the time of birth, and as early as 36 hours after birth many infants can both discriminate a number of facial expressions and imitate them. Due to the short diameter of the eye as well as retinal immaturity, a newborn's visual acuity is roughly ***20/200 to 20/400***. The human face is the most preferred object of fixation in early infancy. The light sense is one of the most primitive of all visual functions and is present by the 7th fetal month. Studies have shown however that while the majority of newborns are hyperopic, roughly 25% are myopic at birth. The finding of myopia increases in premature infants, especially those with retinopathy of prematurity.

181. Do babies make tears?

Alacrima, or the absence of tear secretion, is not uncommon in the newborn period, although some infants may produce reflexive tearing at birth. In most others, tearing is delayed and typically not seen until the infant is ***2-4 months old***. Persistent lack of tearing is seen in Riley-Day syndrome, or familial dysautonomia. This is a rare genetic syndrome seen in the Ashkenazi Jewish population, affecting 1 in 10,000 newborns. Other symptoms include diaphoresis, skin blotching or marbling, hyporeflexia, and indifference to pain.

182. At what age does an infant's eye color assume its permanent color?

A neonate's eyes will never be lighter than they are at birth. The pigmentation of the iris in all races increases over the first 6-12 months. The eye color is usually defined by sixth months and always by one year.

183. A two-week-old infant with intermittent eye discharge and clear conjunctiva has what likely diagnosis?

Nasolacrimal duct obstruction, seen in roughly 5% of newborns, is typically due to an intermittent blockage at the lower end of the duct. Massaging the area and watchful waiting are generally all that is needed. Almost all (95%) resolve by 6 months and a few thereafter. Ophthalmologic referral in the first 6 months is usually unnecessary, unless there are multiple episodes of acute dacrocystitis or a large congenital mucocele. Most ophthalmologists advise referral between 6 and 13 months, because during this period simple probing of the duct is curative in 95% of patients. After 13 months, the cure rate by probing alone falls to 75%, and silicone intubation of the duct is often necessary.

Chiesi C, et al: Congenital nasolacrimal duct obstruction: Therapeutic management J Pediatr Ophthalmol Strabismus 36:326-330, 1999.

Katowitz JA, Welsh M: Timing of initial probing and irrigation in congenital nasolacrimal duct obstruction. Ophthalmology 94:698-705, 1987.

184. What is the most common congenital oculomotor anomaly?

Duane syndrome (or Duane retraction syndrome). This involves a limitation in abduction and /or adduction, with retraction of the globe and narrowing of the palpebral fissure seen on attempted adduction. Up or down eye movements may also be seen on attempted adduction, including the cornea "disappearing." It is usually unilateral, with the left eye more likely to be affected. Its etiology typically is due to variations in innervation of the affected eye's lateral rectus muscle. Most cases are sporadic, though a familial pattern can exist; Duane syndrome may also be associated with other syndromes, such as Goldenhar or Klippel-Feil. As the patient typically develops a head turn to compensate, management depends on the severity of the head turn as well as the other findings (e.g., orbital retraction, up or down eye movements).

185. What is normal visual acuity for children?

Birth–6 mos:	Improves from 20/400 to 20/80 gradually
6 mos–3 yrs:	Improves from 20/80 to 20/50
2–5 yrs:	Improves to 20/40 or better and a < 2-line difference between left and right eyes on visual charts
> 5 yrs:	20/30 or better and < 2-line difference between eyes on visual charts

It should be noted that almost 20% of the pediatric population require eyeglasses for correction of refractive errors prior to adulthood.

186. When do binocular fixation and depth perception develop in children?

Binocularity of vision depends primarily on adequate coordination of the extraocular muscles and is normally established by 3–6 months of age. At about 6–8 months, early evidence of depth perception is seen, but it is still poorly developed. Depth perception becomes very accurate at 6 or 7 years and continues to improve through the early teens.

Hartmann EE et al: Preschool vision screening: Summary of a task force report. Pediatrics 106:1105-1112, 2000.

Committee on Practice and Ambulatory Medicine, Section on Ophthalmology, American Academy of Pediatrics: Eye examination and vision screening in infants, children, and young adults. Pediatrics 98: 153-157, 1996.

187. How does refractive capacity vary with age?

The newborn infant is typically slightly hyperoptic (far-sighted). The mild hyperopia actually increases slowly for about the first 8 years. Hyperopia then decreases gradually until adolescence, when vision is emmetropic (no refractive error). After 20 years, there is a tendency for myopia (near-sightedness).

188. How are the degrees of blindness classified?

The World Health Organization defines blindness as:

- *Visual impairment*: Snellen visual acuity ≤ 20/60 (best eye corrected)
- *Social blindness*: Snellen visual acuity ≤ 20/200 or a visual field ≤ 20°
- *Virtual blindness*: Snellen visual acuity < 20/1200 or visual field ≤ 10°
- *Total blindness*: No light perception

189. Can cortically blind infants see?

Yes. *Cortical blindness*, now often referred to as *cortical visual impairment* (*CVI*), involves a disruption of vision due to injuries or delayed development in the geniculostriate pathways. Infants with CVI will typically have a normal ocular examination, including an intact pupillary light reflex, but will have variable visual function, including loss of peripheral field vision. CVI has many etiologies, including hypoxic-ischemic encephalopathy, head trauma, hydrocephalus, CNS infections, and metabolic diseases. In some cases, vision recovery may be rapid, though for many the course is protracted and only partial recovery occurs.

190. A two-month old baby is noted to have eyes that appear to turn outward rather than looking forward. Is this strabismus?

Yes, but intervention is not needed unless the symptom persists beyond 3-4 months of age. Strabismus is defined as any deviation from perfect ocular alignment. However, the majority of infants will be found to have an *exodeviated* alignment, i.e., looking somewhat out, rather than an *orthotropic*, or straight, alignment. The majority of infants will become orthotropic by 4 months of age.

191. Name the four most common types of childhood strabismus.

Strabismus is the misalignment of the eyes with either an in-turning (esotropia), out-turning (exotropia), or up-turning (hypertropia) of one eye. Four types most commonly occur:

1. ***Strabismus of visual deprivation***: occurs when normal vision in one or both eyes is disrupted by any cause. The most serious varieties occur with tumors (e.g., retinoblastoma). In children with ocular tumors, strabismus may be the presenting sign.

2. ***Infantile** or **congenital esotropia***: occurs within the first few months of life, usually as an isolated conditions. Corrective surgery is usually required.

3. ***Accommodative esotropia***: commonly occurs between ages 2 and 4 in very far-sighted (hyperopic) children. These children use extra lens accommodation because of their visual problems, leading to persistent convergence. Eyeglasses to correct the hyperopia usually correct the esotropia.

4. ***Childhood exotropia***: appears between ages 2 and 5 as intermittent misalignment, often brought on by fatigue, visual inattention, or bright sunlight. There is a strong hereditary component. Surgery is often necessary after correction of refractive errors and elimination of any pathology that might have caused visual deprivation.

Trobe J: Physician's Guide to Eye Care, 2nd ed. San Francisco, Foundation of the American Academy of Ophthalmology, 2nd ed, 2001, p 182.

192. What separates pseudostrabismus from true strabismus?

Often a cause of unnecessary ophthalmologic referrals, *pseudostrabismus* is the appearance of ocular misalignment (usually esotropia) that occurs in children with a broad and flat nasal bridge and prominent epicanthal folds. The iris appears shifted to the midline with differing amounts of white sclera on each side. This is a common condition that may occur in up to 30% of newborns. No treatment is required. It may be distinguished from true esotropia, or *strabismus*, by observation of full extraocular movements, by symmetric reflections of a flashlight on the cornea from a distance of about 12 in (although this test as a measure of strabismus is more accurate in infants ≥ 6 months), and by normal visualization of red reflexes by direct ophthalmoscopy.

Infants do not focus well because the macula and fovea are poorly developed at birth. Therefore, it is not uncommon for infants occasionally to have an inward crossing of the eyes or for their eyes to be turned slightly outward to 10° or 15°. Persistent in-turning of the eyes for more than a few seconds or outward deviation > 10–15° requires ophthalmologic referral.

Romano PE: Vision/eye screening: Test twice and refer once. Pediatr Ann 19:359–367, 1990.

193. How is amblyopia different from strabismus?

Amblyopia refers to decreased visual acuity in one eye due to decreased visual stimulation of that eye. The visual cortex adheres to the concept of: "if you don't use it, you lose it." Amblyopia is the most common cause of vision loss in children less than 6 years old, and occurs in 1–2% of this age group. *Strabismus* is one cause of amblyopia, as the child will use the "straight" eye to fixate and will ignore the visual input from the other eye. Another type is *anisometropic amblyopia*, which is due to a significant difference in refraction between the two eyes. Amblyopia can also be due to *deprivation*, such as from congenital cataracts or ptosis. *Occlusion amblyopia* is typically iatrogenic in etiology, with prolonged covering of the preferred eye to treat amblyopia in the other eye causing changes in visual acuity in the preferred eye. The treatment of amblyopia involves getting the child to use the weaker eye. This commonly is done by covering the strong eye, such as with a patch. Patching has been described since the 18th century as a treatment for amblyopia.

194. How common are cataracts in children?

A *cataract* is an opacification of the lens and can occur in one or both eyes. In general, cataracts affect approximately 1 in 1000 children. They are, however, one of the leading causes of blindness in children, and up to 20% of children enrolled in schools for the blind have had cataracts. Cataracts can occur sporadically. This is seen in one-third of the cases. Other causes include heredity, genetic syndromes, infectious exposures *in utero*, intrauterine hypoxia, trauma, retinoblastoma, congenital glaucoma, uveitis, exposure to ionizing radiation and prolonged use of corticosteroids.

195. What is ectopia lentis?

Ectopia lentis refers to the displacement or dislocation of the lens. It may be due to trauma, but has also been associated with systemic diseases such as Marfan syndrome, homocystinuria, and congenital syphilis.

196. What diseases may present with a white pupil?

Leukocoria, or white pupil, may due to any mass behind the pupillary space. This includes cataracts, retinoblastoma, and infants with retinopathy of prematurity that develop retinal detachment. It should be noted that, in retinoblastoma, the incidence of leukocoria is 60-70% rather than 100%.

197. What produces the cherry red spot?

The *cherry red spot* often seen in various lipid storage disorders (e.g., Tay-Sachs, Niemann-Pick, Farber) is actually the normal red macular area surrounded by abnormal retinal changes, typically involving loss of choroidal detail and color (i.e., gray).

198. Do crocodile tears really exist?

Not for crocodiles; they do not have tear glands. In Shakespeare, the term is an indicator of false or hypocritical sorrow, but in the world of ophthalmology, crocodile tears refers to *paradoxic lacrimation*, such as tearing while eating. It may be congenital or acquired, most commonly seen in aberrant regeneration of the facial nerve after a Bell palsy.

199. How common is physiologic anisocoria?

Anisocoria refers to unequalness in pupillary size, which is a relatively common condition. ***Up to 20%*** of individuals without any illness will have a difference > 0.4 mm in the size of their pupils.

200. Is heterochromia normal?

It can be. *Heterochromia* (different colored irises) can be familial, usually transmitted as an autosomal dominant trait. It is also seen in the Waardenburg syndrome (white forelock, congenital deafness, and partial albinism). However, changes in color can occur from trauma, hemorrhage, inflammation (uveitis, iridocyclitis), malignancy (retinoblastoma, neuroblastoma), or glaucoma.

201. Which children are at high risk for visual abnormalities?

- Prematurity (birth weight < 1250 gm)
- Family history of congenital ocular abnormality (e.g., cataract, retinoblastoma), strabismus, or amblyopia
- Maternal intrauterine or cervicovaginal infection or substance abuse
- Systemic condition with vision-threatening ocular manifestations

Trobe J: Physician's Guide to Eye Care, 2nd ed. San Francisco, Foundation of the American Academy of Ophthalmology, 2001, p 19.

202. How is color blindness inherited?

Color blindness typically involves variable loss of the ability to distinguish colors, especially red, green, and blue. The defects can be partial (anomaly) or complete (anopia). Defects in appreciating red or green color are transmitted in an X-linked recessive manner and affect up to 1% and 6%, respectively, of the male population. Blue color blindness is an autosomal dominant phenomenon and occurs in 0.1% of the population.

203. What visionary in pediatric medicine was also an Olympic gold medalist?

Dr. Benjamin Spock. At the Paris Olympics in 1924, he was a member of the Yale University rowing team that won the gold medal in the eight-oared shell with coxswain. His book, *The Common Sense Book of Baby and Child Care*, has helped many parents stay afloat and has sold over 25 million copies since its original publication in 1945.

3. CARDIOLOGY

Thomas J. Starc, M.D., M.P.H., Allan J. Hordof, M.D., Constance J. Hayes, M.D., and Bernard J. Clark, III, M.D.

CLINICAL ISSUES

1. Is mitral valve prolapse (MVP) always pathologic?

It is debated, but in all likelihood the answer is no. Some studies show that up to 13% of normal children have some degree of posterior leaflet prolapse on echocardiography. Probably, there is a spectrum of anatomic abnormalities, the most minor of which are a variation of normal. Those children with clinical features of mitral valve insufficiency constitute the pathologic category. Whenever auscultation reveals the classic findings of MVP, referral to a pediatric cardiologist is recommended. This allows evaluation of the child for possible accompanying cardiac abnormalities (e.g., mitral insufficiency, secundum atrial septal defects) and confirmation of the diagnosis.

2. What connective tissue diseases may be associated with MVP?

Marfan syndrome, Ehlers-Danlos syndrome, pseudoxanthoma elasticum, osteogenesis imperfecta, Hurler syndrome.

3. Do patients with MVP require prophylaxis against subacute bacterial endocarditis (SBE)?

This is controversial. The incidence of endocarditis in patients with MVP *and* systolic murmur is 1/2000 per annum. Three factors—***male gender*, *advanced age*,** and the presence of *systolic murmur*—seem to be associated with an increased risk of endocarditis in patients with MVP. Some experts argue that all should receive treatment and others recommend selectively treating only patients with MVP *and* systolic murmur (mitral regurgitation) or thickened leaflets.

4. Which cardiac conditions lead to Eisenmenger syndrome?

Eisenmenger syndrome refers to cardiac right-to-left or bi-directional shunting that results from the development of high pulmonary resistance due to obstructive pulmonary vascular disease. The resultant right-to-left shunting can cause chronic hypoxia with cyanosis, polycythemia, right ventricular hypertrophy, and right ventricular failure, depending on the size of the shunt. Congenital heart lesions with elevated pulmonary blood flow and elevated pulmonary artery pressure (e.g., large VSD, A-V canal defect, large PDA) may lead to pathologic changes in pulmonary arterioles and arteries with medial and intimal thickening. These changes eventually become irreversible, and the cardiac shunt direction changes from the initial left-to-right to right-to-left with accompanying cyanosis.

5. Can a patient with heart disease simultaneously be polycythemic and iron deficient?

Yes, patients with *cyanotic* heart disease may develop both clinical entities. Initially, as a response to cyanosis, the hematocrit rises and will remain elevated and the mean corpuscular volume (MCV) will be lower than normal. Detailed studies of iron stores often reveal a concurrent deficiency. Those children with a history of poor nutrition and blood loss (e.g., previous surgery) are especially at-risk for developing iron deficiency.

6. What are the most common vascular rings and slings?

Vascular rings occur when the trachea and/or esophagus are encircled by aberrant vascular structures. *Vascular slings* are compressions, typically anterior, caused by nonencircling aberrant vessels.

	FREQUENCY	SYMPTOMS	TREATMENT
"Complete" rings			
Double aortic arch	50%	Respiratory difficulty, worse by feeding or exertion (onset < 3 mos)	Surgical division of a smaller arch (usually the left)
Right aortic arch with left ligamentum arteriosum	45%	Mild respiratory difficulty (onset later in infancy) Swallowing dysfunction	Surgical division of ligamentum arteriosum
"Incomplete" rings (slings)			
Anomalous innominate artery	< 5%	Stridor and/or cough in infancy	Conservative management or surgical suturing of artery to the sternum
Aberrant right subclavian artery	< 5%	Occasional swallowing dysfunction	Usually no treatment necessary
Vascular sling or anomalous left pulmonary artery (LPA)	Rare	Wheezing and cyanotic episodes in first weeks of life	Surgical division of anomalous LPA (from RPA) and anastomosis to the MPA

Adapted from Park MK: Cardiology for Practitioners, 3rd ed. St. Louis, Mosby-Year Book, 1995.

7. What evaluations may be done if a vascular ring is suspected?

- *Chest x-ray*: for detection of possible right-sided aortic arch
- *Barium esophagram*: considered the gold standard for diagnosis at present; confirms external indentation of esophagus in up to 95% of cases
- *MRI*: non-invasive and used in some centers initially (rather than esophagram) as primary diagnostic modality
- *Rigid bronchoscopy*: may confirm diagnosis by detecting pulsatile indentation of trachea
- *Arteriogram*: precise delineation of vascular anatomy, especially prior to surgery
- *Echocardiogram*: not helpful in identifying the ring itself, but important in evaluating for possible congenital heart disease, which occurs in up to 25% of patients with vascular rings

8. Describe four categories of cardiomyopathy in children.

1. ***Dilated cardiomyopathy*** is the most common type of cardiomyopathy, and the etiology is usually unknown. Anatomically, the heart is normal, but both ventricles are dilated. Older children present with symptoms of congestive heart failure, including malaise, edema, weight gain, and respiratory distress. Infants present with poor weight gain, feeding difficulty, and respiratory distress. In all pediatric age groups, a more acute presentation with shock can occur. Treatment includes inotropic support, diuretics, and afterload-reducing agents. In progressive forms, cardiac transplant is the only definitive treatment.
2. ***Hypertrophic cardiomyopathy with LV outflow obstruction*** is also known by terms such as idiopathic hypertrophic subaortic stenosis (IHSS) or asymmetric septal hypertrophy. Of these patients, the majority have some degree of LV outflow tract obstruction secondary to abnormal hypertrophy of the subaortic region of the intraventricular septum. Most are inherited in an autosomal dominant fashion. This cardiomyopathy is associated with ventricular dysrhythmias and sudden death. Treatment usually includes beta-blockers (e.g., propranolol) or calcium channel blockers (e.g., vera-

pamil). Occasionally, the surgical myomectomy of the obstructing portion of the septum is needed. Recent advances in the treatment of this disease also include placement of an implantable defibrillator to prevent sudden death due to arrhythmias.

3. ***Hypertrophic cardiomyopathy without LV outflow obstruction*** is also usually of unknown etiology. However, it may be associated with systemic metabolic disease, particularly storage disease. Pompe disease (glycogen storage disease type II) and mitrochondrial enzyme deficiency diseases are typical. Patients may present with failure to thrive or acutely in shock. Cardiomegaly is a constant feature. Pompe disease may have associated hypoglycemia. Treatment generally includes inotropic support, diuretics, and dietary manipulation to treat the underlying metabolic problems.
4. ***Restrictive cardiomyopathy***. The major hemodynamic problem is abnormal diastolic function of the ventricles. The ventricles may be of normal size, or hypertrophied, with normal systolic function. The atria are typically enlarged. The etiology is usually unknown, but may be due to storage disease.

Towbin JA: Pediatric myocardial disease. Pediatr Clin North Am 46:289-311, 1999.

9. What deficiency causes Keshan disease?

Selenium. Keshan disease is a reversible cause of dilated cardiomyopathy due to selenium deficiency. The condition is associated with left ventricular dilatation and decreased function and may present as cardiogenic shock or chronic congestive heart failure. In the U.S., the disease has been described in patients on unusual selenium-restricted diets and in malnourished patients with increased gastrointestinal losses (e.g., HIV infections). The condition derives its name from the Keshan Province in mainland China, where the disease is endemic because of decreased selenium content in the soil.

10. What are the cardiac causes of sudden cardiac death in young athletes?

Sudden death occurs because of ventricular fibrillation in the setting of myocardial or coronary abnormalities or primary rhythm disorders. The main structural causes are hypertrophic cardiomyopathy (particularly with extreme LVH), anomalies of the coronary artery, Marfan syndrome, and arrhythmogenic RV dysplasia. Abnormal coronary arteries as a sequelae of Kawasaki syndrome may be a consideration. Prolonged QT syndrome and Wolff-Parkinson-White syndrome have also been implicated. Children with repaired congenital heart disease (especially aortic stenosis, tetralogy of Fallot, transposition of the great vessels, and Ebstein anomaly) are at higher risk for sudden death.

Despite the notoriety of sudden death (especially in professional or college athletes), it should be noted that this is relatively rare in younger athletes. Of the approximately 5 million high schoolers who participate in athletics each year, only 25 (or 1/200,000) die of atraumatic causes during sports.

Wren C, et al: Sudden death in children and adolescents. Heart 83:410-413, 2000.

Spirito P, et al: Magnitude of left ventricular hypertrophy and risk of sudden death in hypertrophic cardiomyopathy. N Engl J Med 342:1778-1785, 2000.

Liberthson RR: Current concepts: Sudden death from cardiac causes in children and young adults. N Engl J Med 334:1039–1044, 1996.

11. How can the preparticipation sports physical identify patients at risk for sudden death?

History

- Some common causes of sudden death may be associated with *previous symptoms* of exertional chest discomfort, dizziness or prolonged dyspnea with exercise, syncope, or palpitations.
- *Family history of cardiovascular disease* at an early age or sudden death. For example, although 40%of cases of hypertrophic cardiomyopathy are sporadic, 60% are inherited in an autosomal dominant fashion.

- *History of seizures* may be associated with prolonged QT syndrome.

Physical exam

- *Marfanoid features*: tall and thin habitus, hyperextensible joints, pectus excavatum, click and murmur suggestive of MVP.
- *Pathologic murmurs*, particularly a systolic murmur that increases with expiration and standing or decreases with squatting and is associated with an increased LV impulse (e.g., hypertrophic cardiomyopathy) or one associated with a suprasternal thrill (e.g., valvular aortic stenosis).
- *Dysrhythmia* present.

Berger S, et al: Sudden cardiac death in infants, children and adolescents. Pediatr Clin North Am 46:221-234, 1999.

McCaffrey FM, et al: Sudden cardiac death in young athletes. Am J Dis Child 145:177–183, 1991.

12. In which patients is syncope more likely to be of a cardiac nature?

Syncope is suspicious for a cardiac cause if it includes:

- Sudden onset without any prodromal period of dizziness or imminent awareness
- Syncope during exercise
- Complete loss of awareness and muscle tone so that fall results in injury, usually head trauma
- History of palpitations or abnormal heartbeat prior to event
- Very fast or very slow heart rate after event
- Family history of sudden death

Dysrhythmias are the most common cause of cardiac syncope, particularly supraventricular tachycardia, ventricular tachycardia and heart block. The causes can be primary (e.g., Wolff-Parkinson-White, prolonged QT syndrome, heart block) or secondary (e.g., prescription medications, illicit drugs, postsurgical, Lyme disease). Other causes include hypertrophic cardiomyopathy, congenital heart disease (although syncope is very rare as an initial presentation), and rarely tumors (particularly if syncope occurs while recumbent).

Lewis DA, Dhala A: Syncope in the pediatric patient: the cardiologist's perspective. Pediatr Clin North Am 46:205-219, 1999.

Gersony WM: The older child and adolescent with chest pain, mitral valve prolapse, syncope. In Gessner IH, Victoria BE (eds): Pediatric Cardiology: A Problem-Oriented Approach. Philadelphia, W.B. Saunders, 1993, pp 147–154.

13. What is the most common cause of syncope in children?

In otherwise healthy children, ***vasodepressor syncope***. This entity goes by a number of terms including *vasovagal syncope* and *neurocardiogenic syncope*. Individuals who experience an orthostatic challenge may paradoxically respond with a decreased heart rate and increased peripheral vasodilation, which results in hypotensive syncope, often recurrent. Treatment for recurrent episodes may involve mineralocorticoids, salt and extra fluids, beta-blockers and disopyramide. In one study, patients who drank 64 ounces of noncaffeinated fluid per day (in an effort to expand plasma volume) had a syncopal reduction rate of 90%.

Younoszai AK, et al: Oral fluid therapy: A promising treatment for vasodepressor syncope. Arch Pediatr Adolesc Med 152:165-168, 1998.

14. Can tilt-table testing help in evaluating children with unexplained syncope?

Tilt-table testing is used to evaluate possible vasodepressor syncope and involves monitoring of cardiovascular responses and symptoms when an individual is transitioned from supine to head-up positioning. Different centers use different protocols regarding provocative stimuli, duration and extent of tilting and types of medications studied if testing is abnormal. Since orthostatic stress can precipitate pre-syncopal or syncopal episodes, tilt-table testing in theory is designed to identify those individuals with an abnormal physiologic response. Although its use in children and teenagers has increased significantly in the past decade, it still remains unclear if it is primarily a research or clinical tool.

Salim MA, et al: Syncope recurrence in children: Relation to tilt-test results. Pediatrics 102:924-926, 1998.

15. Which clinical and laboratory findings are suggestive of transient myocardial ischemia in a neonate?

Transient myocardial ischemia is usually encountered in a term infant with a history of hypoxic stress. Respiratory difficulty and signs of congestive heart failure (e.g., tachycardia, cardiomegaly, and a gallop rhythm) are frequently present. A systolic murmur due to tricuspid or mitral regurgitation is also a common finding. The severity of the clinical picture may vary from mild to circulatory shock. The ECG frequently demonstrates features of subendocardial ischemia with generalized flattening of T waves and ST-segment depression. During recovery, abnormal Q waves may also be observed. On echocardiography, decreased ventricular shortening and Doppler findings of mitral and/or tricuspid regurgitation occur. Serum levels of creatinine kinase (MB fraction) are characteristically elevated, particularly in the presence of tricuspid regurgitation.

16. What are the most common clinical signs of coarctation of the aorta in older children?

- Differential blood pressure—arms > legs: *virtually universal*
- Systolic murmur or bruit in the back: *almost always*
- Systolic hypertension in the upper extremities: *almost always*
- Diminished femoral or lower extremity pulses: *usual*
- Absent femoral or lower extremity pulses: *uncommon*

Ing FF, et al: Early diagnosis of coarctation of the aorta in children: A continuing dilemma. Pediatrics 98: 378-382, 1996.

17. How valuable is the pediatric autopsy?

As diagnostic technology has developed, the percentage of autopsies performed has declined in both adult and pediatric medicine. However, in one review of autopsies of 193 children, 10% of cases revealed an unexpected finding that, had it been known, might have changed management with possibilities of cure or significantly prolonged survival. Another 18% had unexpected major findings that would not have changed management.

Stambouly JJ, et al: Correlation between clinical diagnoses and autopsy findings in critically ill children. Pediatrics 92:248–251, 1993.

CONGENITAL HEART DISEASE

18. What are the proven etiologies for congenital heart disease (CHD)?

Only a small percentage of cases have identifiable causes:

- *Primary genetic factors* (e.g., chromosomal abnormalities or single gene abnormalities) 10%
- *Environmental factors* (e.g., chemicals, drugs such as isotretinoin, viruses such as rubella, and maternal disease) 3–5%
- *Genetic-environmental interactions* (i.e., multifactorial) 85%

19. What prenatal maternal factors may be associated with cardiac disease in the neonate?

PRENATAL HISTORICAL FACTOR	ASSOCIATED CARDIAC DEFECT
Diabetes mellitus	LV outflow obstruction (asymmetric septal hypertrophy, aortic stenosis), D-transposition of great arteries, ventricular septal defect
Lupus erythematosus	Heart block, pericarditis, endomyocardial fibrosis

Rubella	Patent ductus arteriosus, pulmonic stenosis (peripheral)
Alcohol abuse	Pulmonic stenosis, ventricular septal defect
Trimethadione usage	Ventricular septal defect, tetralogy of Fallot
Lithium usage	Ebstein anomaly
Aspirin abuse	Persistent pulmonary hypertension syndrome
Coxsackie B infection	Myocarditis

From Gewitz MH: Cardiac disease in the newborn infant. In Polin RA, Yoder MC, Burg FD (eds): Workbook in Practical Neonatology, 3rd ed. Philadelphia, W.B. Saunders, 2001, p. 269; with permission.

20. In a cyanotic newborn, how can you distinguish pulmonary disease from cyanotic congenital heart disease?

The ***hyperoxia test***. The infant is placed in 100% oxygen, and an arterial blood gas is obtained. A PaO_2 > 100 mmHg is usually achieved in infants with primary lung disease, whereas a PaO_2 < 100 mmHg is characteristic of heart disease. Typically, children with cyanotic heart disease also have low or normal pCO_2 whereas children with lung disease have elevated pCO_2. Unfortunately, the hyperoxia test does not usually distinguish children with cyanotic heart disease from those with persistent pulmonary hypertension of the newborn.

21. During the first day of life, which congenital heart lesions commonly present with cyanosis?

Independent pulmonary and systemic circulations (severe cyanosis)
  Transposition of great arteries with an intact ventricular septum
Inadequate pulmonary blood flow (severe cyanosis)
  Tricuspid valve atresia
  Pulmonary valve atresia with intact ventricular septum
  Tetralogy of Fallot
  Ebstein anomaly of the tricuspid valve
Admixture lesions (moderate cyanosis)
  Total anomalous pulmonary venous return
  Hypoplastic left heart syndrome
  Truncus arteriosus

Victoria BE: Cyanotic newborns. In Gessner IH, Victoria BE (eds): Pediatric Cardiology: A Problem Oriented Approach. Philadelphia, W.B. Saunders, 1993, p 101.

22. In the patient with suspected heart disease, what bony abnormalities seen on a chest x-ray increase the likelihood of CHD?

- *Hemivertebrae, rib anomalies*: associated with tetralogy of Fallot, truncus arteriosus, VACTERL syndrome
- *11 ribs*: seen in Down syndrome
- *Skeletal chest deformities* (scoliosis, pectus excavatum, narrow AP diameter): associated with Marfan syndrome, mitral valve prolapse
- *Bilateral rib notching*:coarctation of the aorta (usually older children)

23. How do pulmonary vascular markings on a chest x-ray help in the differential diagnosis of a cyanotic newborn with suspected cardiac disease?

In a moderately or severely cyanotic newborn with suspected anatomic heart disease, the chest x-ray may help to differentiate the types of congenital heart defects. The increase or decrease in pulmonary vascular markings is indicative of pulmonary blood flow:

Decreased pulmonary markings *(inadequate pulmonary blood flow)*
  Ebstein anomaly
  Pulmonary atresia or severe stenosis
  Tetralogy of Fallot

Tricuspid atresia, severe stenosis or insufficiency

Increased pulmonary markings *(increased pulmonary blood flow)*

Transposition of great arteries

Total anomalous pulmonary venous return

Truncus arteriosus

24. What ECG findings are considered characteristic for various congenital heart malformations?

Left axis deviation: atrial septal defect (primum), endocardial cushion defect, tricuspid atresia

Wolff-Parkinson-White: Ebstein anomaly, L-transposition of great arteries

Complete heart block: L-transposition of great arteries, polysplenia syndrome

25. What chest x-ray findings are considered characteristic for various congenital heart diseases?

Boot-shaped heart: Tetralogy of Fallot, tricuspid atresia

Egg-shaped heart: Transposition of great arteries

Snowman silhouette: Total anomalous pulmonary venous return

Rib notching: Coarctation of the aorta (older children)

26. Which are the ductal-dependent cardiac lesions?

Ductal-dependent pulmonary blood flow

- Critical pulmonic stenosis
- Pulmonary atresia
- Tricuspid atresia with pulmonary stenosis or pulmonary atresia

Ductal-dependent systemic blood flow

- Coarctation of the aorta
- Hypoplastic left heart syndrome
- Interrupted aortic arch

27. Which types of CHD are associated with right aortic arch?

Tetralogy of Fallot with pulmonary atresia	50%
Truncus arteriosus	35%
Classic tetralogy of Fallot	25%
Double outlet right ventricle	25%
Single ventricle	12.5%

Crowley JJ, et al: Telltale small signs of congenital heart disease. Radiol Clin North Am 31:573–582, 1993.

28. Which genetic syndromes are most commonly associated with CHD?

SYNDROME	PATIENTS WITH CHD	PREDOMINANT HEART DEFECT(S)
Down	50%	ECD, VSD, TOF
Turner	20	CoA
Noonan	65	PS, ASD, ASH
Marfan	60	MVP, AoAn, AR
Trisomy 18	90	VSD, PDA
Trisomy 13	80	VSD, PDA
DiGeorge	80	IAA-B, TA
Williams	75	SVAS, peripheral PS

AoAn = aortic aneurysm; AR = aortic regurgitation; ASD = atrial sepal defect; ASH = asymmetric septal hypertrophy; CoA = coarctation of the aorta; ECD = endocardial cushion defect; IAA-B = interrupted aortic arch, type B; MVP = mitral valve prolapse; PDA = patent ductus arteriosus; PS = pulmonic stenosis; SVAS = supravalvular aortic stenosis; TA = truncus arteriosus; TOF = tetralogy of Fallot; VSD = ventricular septal defect.

From Frias JL: Genetic issues of congenital heart defects. In Gessner IH, Victoria BE: Pediatric Cardiology: A Problem Oriented Approach. Philadelphia, W.B. Saunders, 1993, p 238; with permission.

29. Which infants with CHD should be evaluated for other anomalies?

In the evaluation of the newborn with heart disease, several known associations between CHD and other anomalies should be considered, especially for the patient with more complex disease. Syndromes such as CHARGE or VACTERL may first be detected by the presence of heart disease and one other anomaly. The association between conotruncal defects (tetralogy of Fallot, truncus arteriosus, and interrupted aortic arch) and deletion in chromosome 22 is often subtle. Some of these patients may have DiGeorge syndrome or velo-cardio-facial syndrome, but others may have only minimal palatal dysfunction. For this reason, patients with conotruncal cardiac defects should undergo screening for deletions in chromosome 22, and if found, these patients should be referred to a geneticist for special testing and evaluation.

30. Why does the ductus arteriosus close after birth?

Patency of the ductus arteriosus in the neonate is regulated by the opposing actions of oxygen (constrictor) and prostaglandin E_2 (dilator). In addition, several mediators (bradykinin, acetylcholine, histamine, and 5-hydroxytryptamine) have been demonstrated to constrict the ductus *in vitro*. Most of these substances, however, are not active *in vivo*. Permanent closure is brought about by destruction of the endothelium and proliferation of the subintimal layers. Ultimately, connective tissue is formed which seals the lumen.

31. Describe the clinical manifestations of a large patent ductus arteriosus (PDA).

- Tachypnea and tachycardia
- Bounding pulses
- Hyperdynamic precordium
- Systolic murmur or systolic and diastolic murmur
- Wide pulse pressures
- Labile oxygenation (premature infant)
- Apnea (premature infant)

32. How commonly do PDAs occur in premature infants?

30% in infants weighing 501 to 1500 grams.

33. When should indomethacin be administered to newborns with a PDA?

Indomethacin is effective in closing a PDA within the first 10 days of life and may be most effective during the first 24–48 hours of life. Indomethacin is indicated in preterm infants with a hemodynamically significant PDA, defined as one in which there is deteriorating respiratory status (e.g., tachypnea, apnea, CO_2 retention, increased ventilatory support, failure to wean ventilatory support) or evidence of congestive heart failure. For infants < 1000 gm, indomethacin treatment should be initiated at the first sign of a clinical PDA. An asymptomatic murmur will develop into a large hemodynamically significant shunt in 80% of these babies. Infants > 1000 gm have a higher rate of spontaneous closure, and only 30% will develop a hemodynamically significant shunt. For these infants, a PDA murmur may be followed, without treatment, but therapy should be initiated as soon as symptoms of a significant shunt occur.

Clyman RI: Recommendations for the postnatal use of indomethacin: An analysis of four separate treatment strategies. J Pediatr 128:601–607, 1996.

34. How often does a PDA reopen after indomethacin therapy?

Reopening following successful closure with indomethacin occurs in approximately 25% of infants (33% of infants < 1000 gm). The ductus is more likely to reopen when indomethacin therapy is initiated beyond the first week of life. In most cases, permanent constriction does not occur after a single dose; second and third doses are recommended 12 and 36 hours following the initial one. Of note, the response to indomethacin does not, in general, depend on the peak concentration or duration of therapy. Recurrence is also independent of the initial concentrations or duration of administration. The rate of reopening is the same whether the drug is given continuously for 36 hours or over 5–7 days.

35. What is the role of ibuprofen in the treatment of PDA?

Because of the possible side effects of indomethacin, ibuprofen is under study as an alternative pharmacologic treatment. Recent studies indicate that when administered on the third day to premature infants with RDS, it is as effective as indomethacin and is significantly less likely to induce oliguria.

Van Overmeire B, et al: A comparison of ibuprofen and indomethacin for closure of patent ductus arteriosus. N Engl J Med 343:674-681, 2000.

36. When should the ductus arteriosus be surgically ligated?

Surgical ligation is generally indicated in infants who have failed two courses of medical management, including indomethacin. In infants in whom indomethacin is contraindicated (e.g., BUN > 30 mg/dl, creatinine > 1.8 mg/dl, platelet count < 60,000/mm^3, evidence of bleeding diathesis) and decompensation has occurred secondary to the PDA, surgical ligation should be performed.

37. Does phototherapy increase the incidence of PDA in premature infants?

In vitro studies have demonstrated that exposure of isolated ductal rings to light resulted in photorelaxation and prevention of constriction despite stimulation with oxygen. While a significant reduction in the incidence of PDA with shielding of the chest wall from phototherapy has been reported in premature infants, the use of shielding remains very controversial and should not be done routinely.

38. How do an ostium primum and an ostium secundum defect differ?

A variety of atrial septal defects exist, categorized in large part by their location. Defects may be isolated to the atrial septum itself or may extend into the ventricles (e.g., endocardial cushion defects). An *ostium secundum* is an isolated defect that involves a persistently enlarged opening at the fossa ovalis, which is approximately in the center of the septum. An *ostium primum* defect is located more inferiorly and is part of an atrioventricular canal defect, often in association with a regurgitant mitral valve.

39. How do the presentations of VSD and ASD differ?

Ventricular septal defect: In an infant with a *large* VSD, signs indicative of congestive heart failure generally appear at 4–8 weeks of age, as the pulmonary vascular resistance drops and pulmonary blood flow increases. Congestive heart failure can occasionally be seen at 1–2 weeks of age in infants with large shunts in whom vascular resistance falls more quickly. The child with a *small* VSD may present with a systolic murmur in the first few days of life. These infants do not develop congestive heart failure and spontaneous closure occurs in most.

Atrial septal defect: Most children with an isolated ASD are not diagnosed until they are 3-5 years of age. The majority are asymptomatic at the time of diagnosis. Rarely, infants with an ASD demonstrate signs of congestive heart failure during the first year of life. The congestive heart failure is due to a large left-to-right shunt and increased pulmonary blood flow and may be associated with failure to thrive or recurrent lower respiratory infections.

40. What occurs during a "Tet spell"?

Tet spells are cyanotic and hypoxic episodes that occur in patients with classic tetralogy of Fallot (TOF) anatomy (i.e., VSD, pulmonic stenosis, aorta overriding the ventricular septum and right ventricular hypertrophy). They may also occur in children with TOF with pulmonary atresia, and in those with complex anatomy and TOF "physiology" (such as double-outlet right ventricle with pulmonary stenosis). The exact pathophysiology is a subject of much discussion, but felt to be related to a change in the balance of systemic to pulmonary vascular resistance. Spells may be initiated by events which cause a *decrease in systemic vascular resistance* such as fever, crying, and hypotension, or events which cause an *increase in pulmonary outflow tract obstruction*. Both types of events will cause more *right-to-left shunting* and *increased cyanosis*. Hypoxia and cyanosis lead to metabolic acidosis and systemic vasodilatation, which cause a further increase in cyanosis. Anemia may be a predisposing factor. While most episodes are self-limited and last < 30 minutes, a prolonged Tet spell can lead to stroke or death. Therefore, a Tet spell is an indication for surgery.

41. How do you treat a Tet spell?

- Try to calm and to soothe the patient.
- Patient should assume a squatting or knee-chest position to increase systemic vascular resistance, often best achieved by being held by a parent.
- Supplemental oxygen should be given.
- Morphine, 0.1 mg/kg IM or IV
- If prolonged, NaHCO3, 1.0 mEq/kg IV
- If prolonged, volume expansion
- If prolonged, phenylephrine, 50-100 µg/kg IV bolus, followed by continuous infusion.
- If prolonged, propranolol 0.1 mg/kg IV.

42. After what age does a presumed peripheral pulmonic branch stenosis murmur deserve more detailed study?

The murmur of peripheral pulmonic branch stenosis, a low-intensity systolic ejection murmur heard frequently in newborns, is due to the relative hypoplasia of the pulmonary arteries as well as the acute angle of the branching of pulmonary arteries in the early newborn period. This murmur usually persists until ***3–6 months of age***.

43. What should parents be told about the risk of recurrence for common heart defects?

Recurrence risks for cardiovascular anomalies vary from 1–4% and are usually higher with the more common lesions (e.g., the recurrence risk for VSD is 3%, and the recurrence risk for Ebstein anomaly is 1%). The risk of CHD in pregnancies after the birth of one affected child is about 1–4%. With 2 affected first-degree relatives, the risk is tripled. With 3 affected children, the family may be considered at even higher risk.

CONGESTIVE HEART FAILURE

44. Identify the clinical signs and symptoms associated with congestive heart failure (CHF) in children.

They may be grouped into three categories:

- Signs/symptoms of ***impaired myocardial performance***: cardiomegaly,* tachycardia,* gallop rhythm,* cold extremities or mottling,* pulsus alternans, growth failure,* sweating with feeding*
- Signs/symptoms of ***pulmonary congestion:*** tachypnea,* wheezing,* rales, cyanosis, dyspnea, cough
- Signs/symptoms of ***systemic venous congestion***: hepatomegaly,* neck vein distention, peripheral edema

(* = often seen in infants)

45. What acid-base changes are associated with CHF?

Mild CHF: *respiratory alkalosis*, as a result of tachypnea (stimulation of J receptors 2° to increasing pulmonary edema)

Moderate or severe CHF: *respiratory acidosis*, as a consequence of pulmonary edema and reduced compliance, and *metabolic acidosis*, as a result of decreased tissue perfusion

46. In infancy, how does the likely cause of CHF vary by age?

At birth	• Hypoplastic left heart syndrome • Severe birth asphyxia (hypoxia + acidosis) • Volume overload lesions Severe tricuspid or pulmonary insufficiency Large systemic AV fistula
First week	• PDA in small premature infants • Transposition of great arteries • Hypoplastic left heart syndrome • Total anomalous pulmonary venous return, particularly with pulmonary venous obstruction • Others: Systemic AV fistula Critical aortic or pulmonic stenosis
1–2 wk	• Coarctation of the aorta (preductal, with associated anomalies) • Critical aortic stenosis • Large left-to-right shunt lesions (VSD, PDA) in premature infants • All other lesions listed above
4–6 wk	• Some left-to-right shunt lesions such as complete AV canal defect
6 wk–4 mo	• Large VSD • Large ASD • Others (e.g., anomalous left coronary artery from the pulmonary artery)

From Park MK:Pediatric Cardiology for Practitioners, 3rd ed. St. Louis, Mosby, 1995; with permission.

47. If a patient develops CHF and cardiomegaly but no murmur is heard, what is the differential diagnosis?

Newborns

- *Myocarditis*
- *Cardiomyopathy* secondary to asphyxia, hypoglycemia, or hypocalcemia
- *Glycogen storage disease* (Pompe disease)
- *Cardiac dysrhythmia*
  Paroxysmal supraventricular tachycardia
  Congenital heart block
- *Atrial flutter and/or fibrillation*
- *Arteriovenous malformations*, e.g., CNS (vein of Galen)
- *Sepsis*

Outside newborn period

- *Myocardial diseases*
  Endocardial fibroelastosis
  Myocarditis (viral or idiopathic)
  Glycogen storage disease (Pompe disease)
- *Coronary artery diseases* resulting in myocardial insufficiency
  Anomalous origin of LCA from pulmonary artery
  Collagen disease (periarteritis nodosa)
  Kawasaki syndrome (mucocutaneous lymph node syndrome)

Calcification of the coronary arteries
Medial necrosis of coronary arteries

- *CHD with severe heart failure*
  Coarctation of the aorta in infants
  Ebstein anomaly

48. When should afterload reduction be used in children?

In settings of low cardiac output (CO) due to myocardial dysfunction with increased peripheral vascular resistance (cool extremities and poor capillary refill) and pulmonary congestion, afterload reduction can decrease overall cardiac work and myocardial O_2 consumption while increasing CO and oxygen delivery. It is often used to aid a failing heart in the immediate postoperative period and also may be of value in children with chronic ventricular dysfunction and those with mitral and/or aortic regurgitation or systemic-to-pulmonic shunts. Agents can be used that preferentially dilate arterioles (e.g., hydralazine), veins (e.g., nitrates), or both (e.g., sodium nitroprusside, captopril and other ACE inhibitors). As a rule, arteriolar vasodilators tend to increase CO, and venous dilators tend to lessen pulmonary congestion. Afterload reduction may be of little use in shock states due to causes other than myocardial failure. If the blood pressure remains unacceptably low (i.e., unstable shock), there is no role for afterload reduction. Volume replacement and inotropic support should first be used. Afterload reduction may also be of little benefit in the "warm phase" of septic shock when CO is actually increased and there is peripheral vasodilation.

DIAGNOSTIC STUDIES AND PROCEDURES

49. What are normal pressures and saturations as measured in cardiac catheterizations?

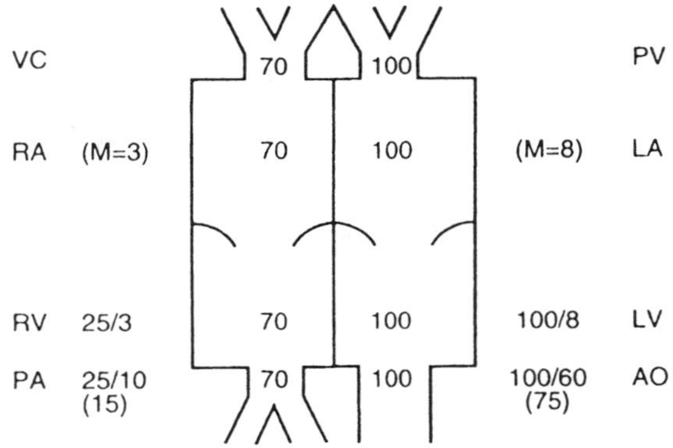

Normal pressure and oxygen saturation values in children. AO, aorta; LA, left atrium; LV, left ventricle; PA, pulmonary artery, PV, pulmonary veins; RA, right atrium; RV, right ventricle; VC, vena cava. (From Stromberg D: Cardiac catheterization. In Taeusch HW, et al (eds): Pediatric and Neonatal Tests and Procedures. Philadelphia, W.B. Saunders, 1966, p 242, with permission.)

50. What is the significance of the Qp/Qs ratio?

Qp/Qs is the ratio of pulmonary blood flow (Qp) to systemic blood flow (Qs), thus *quantifying the amount of intracardiac shunt.* A quick way of estimating Qp/Qs is to take the difference of O_2 saturations in the pulmonary vein and artery (assuming the pulmonary vein to be fully saturated) and divide this by the difference of the aortic and mixed venous saturations.

$$Qp/Qs = (PV\ sat - PA\ sat)/(Ao\ sat - Mixed\ Venous\ sat)$$
$$Qp/Qs = (100\text{-}70)/(100\text{-}70) = 30/30 = 1/1 \text{ (in a normal patient)}$$

44. How is shortening fraction calculated by echocardiography?

$$[(LVED - LVES)/LVED] \times 100$$

where LVED= left ventricular end-diastolic dimension, and LVES= left ventricular end-systolic dimension. The normal range is *28–38%.*

52. Is echocardiography helpful in diagnosing a patent ductus arteriosus?

With the use of high-resolution, two-dimensional echocardiography, PDA is detectable in the vast majority of preterm infants. This sensitivity increases to virtually all patients with the addition of color Doppler and pulsed Doppler to detect reversal of blood flow in the descending aorta during diastole. When the diagnosis of PDA is in doubt, the echocardiogram can help to confirm the diagnosis. The mere presence of a PDA is insufficient to determine the appropriate therapy for an infant with a PDA, and *clinical* assessment is needed to guide therapeutic decisions.

53. What are the indications for endomyocardial biopsy (EMB)?

- *Cardiac transplant rejection*: EMB is still the most reliable technique for diagnosing rejection, even though cyclosporine has altered biopsy findings.
- *Doxorubicin cardiotoxicity*: EMB is the most sensitive method for determining the extent of myocardial injury.
- *Other* potential uses for EMB: myocarditis, glycogen storage disease, cardiac tumors, and rheumatic carditis.

54. When is exercise testing indicated in a child?

Exercise testing is generally performed on children >7 years of age, since coordination and cooperation are needed for the treadmill or bicycle ergometer.

Potentially Useful Indications

- Diagnosis of exercise-induced symptoms, such as syncope, chest pain, or palpitations
- Evaluation of patients with known or suspected dysrhythmias; usually tachydysrhythmias or ectopy
- Evaluation of exercise tolerance, especially postoperatively
- Assessment of potential myocardial ischemia, as in LV outflow tract obstruction, cardiomyopathies, or coronary artery diseases
- Assessment of blood pressure responses, especially in coarctation of the aorta

Relative Contraindications

- Active inflammatory cardiac disease
- Acute heart failure
- Critical cardiac outflow obstruction
- Known ischemic disease with angina
- Severe pulmonary vascular disease
- Severe hypertension
- Serious rhythm disturbance

Graham TP, et al:Recommendations for use of laboratory studies for pediatric patients with suspected or proven heart disease. Circulation 72:207, 443A–450A, 1987.

55. What is the most common indication in children for a pacemaker?

Symptomatic bradycardia. Bradycardia may be due to a variety of reasons, including complete heart block, sick sinus syndrome, or the use of cardiac medications that cause bradycardia (e.g., propranolol). Other indications include the use of pacemakers to better control certain types of ventricular dysrhythmias, such as those due to prolonged QT syndrome.

56. Explain the code system used to describe pacemakers.

The most commonly used code for pacemakers remains the 3-letter code. The first letter refers to the chamber being *paced* (***V***entricle, ***A***trium, ***D***ual), the second to the chamber being *sensed* (***V***entricle, ***A***trium, ***D***ual), and the third to the *mode of action* (***I***nhibit, ***T***rigger, ***D***ual). Thus, a VVI unit indicates a paced ventricle and sensing of spontaneous ventricular activity that can inhibit the pacer.

ECG AND DYSRHYTHMIAS

57. What are the characteristic features of the ECG of a premature infant?

In the premature infant, there is less RV dominance, since the RV growth occurs during the third trimester (which has not been completed). The R wave may be small in the right precordial leads, and there may be no significant S wave over the left precordium. The electrical axis is often in the normal quadrant (0 to 90 degrees).

58. What are the most helpful clues for diagnosing right ventricular hypertrophy by ECG in a newborn?

- Pure R wave (with no S wave) in V_1 > 10 mm
- R in V_1 > 25 mm or R in aVR > 8 mm
- A qR pattern in V_1 (also present in 10% of normal newborns)
- Upright T in V_1 after 7 days of age
- RAD > +180°

59. How does the ECG in an infant differ from that in the older child?

- The ECG at birth reflects RV dominance. The QRS complex consists of a tall R wave in the right precordial leads (V_1-V_2), and an S wave in the left precordial leads (V_5-V_6). The axis is also rightward (120 to 150 degrees).
- In the toddler age group (2 to 4 years), there is an axis shift from the right to the normal quadrant, and the R wave diminishes over the right precordial leads. The S wave disappears from the left precordium.
- The school age child has a nearly adult tracing, with a small R and a dominant S in the right precordial leads, and an axis in the normal quadrant.

60. Describe the ECG abnormalities associated with potassium and calcium imbalances.

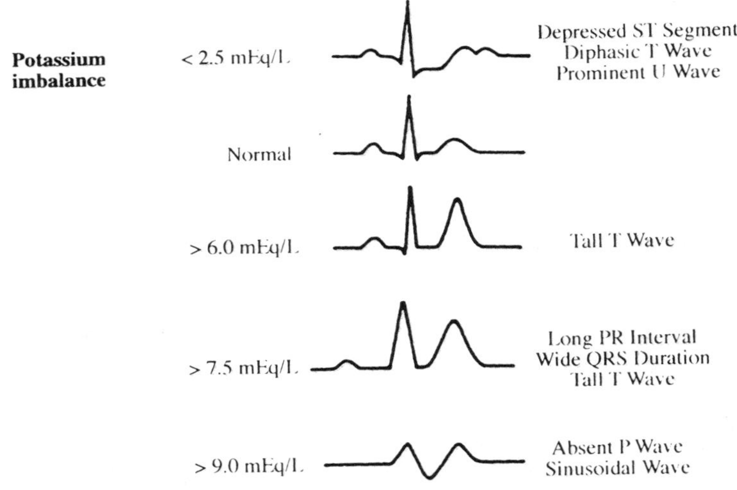

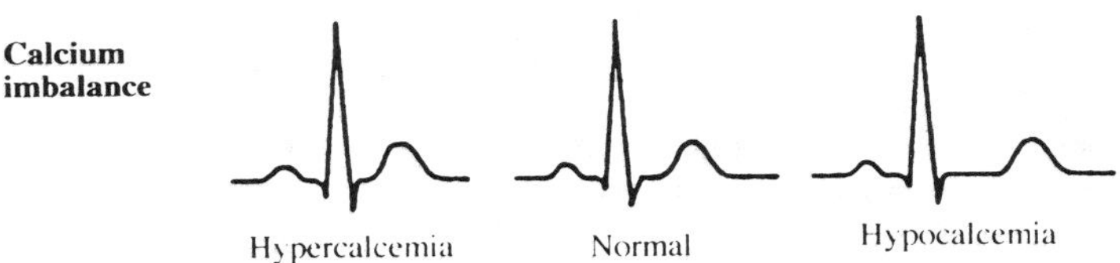

From Park MK, Guntheroth WG: How to Read Pediatric ECGs, 3rd ed. St. Louis, Mosby, 1992, pp 106–107; with permission.

61. What is the corrected QT interval (QT_C)?

The QT interval represents the time required for ventricular depolarization and repolarization. It spans the onset of the QRS complex to the end of the T wave. This interval varies with the heart rate. The QT_C adjusts for heart rate differences. As a rule, a prolonged QT_C interval is diagnosed when the QT_C exceeds 0.44 sec.

$$QT_C = QT\ (in\ sec) / \sqrt{RR\ (in\ sec)}$$

62. What causes a prolonged QT interval?

Congenital long QT syndrome

- *Hereditary form*
  - Jervell-Lange-Nielsen syndrome (associated with deafness)
  - Romano-Ward syndrome
- *Sporadic type*

Acquired long QT syndrome

- *Drug-induced*
  - Antidysrhythmic agents (esp. quinidine, procainamide, amiodarone, sotolol)
  - Phenothiazines
  - Tricyclic antidepressants
  - Lithium
  - Cisapride
- *Metabolic/electrolyte abnormalities*
  - Hypocalcemia
  - Very-low-energy diets
- *CNS and autonomic nervous system disorders* (esp. after head trauma or stroke)
- *Cardiac disease*
  - Myocarditis
  - Coronary artery disease
- *Short QT interval*
  - Hypercalcemia
  - Digitalis effect

63. How abnormal are premature atrial contractions (PACs)?

Premature atrial beats are usually benign, with two exceptions:

1. Children have a small risk of developing supraventricular tachycardia or atrial flutter if PACs occur frequently.
2. In children on digoxin, PACs rarely may be an early sign of digoxin toxicity.

64. How does supraventricular tachycardia in children differ from physiologic sinus tachycardia?

SVT typically has:

- Persistent ventricular rate of > 180 bpm
- Fixed or almost fixed RR interval on ECG

- Abnormal P-wave shape or axis, or absent P waves
- Little change in heart rate with activity, crying, or breathholding

65. What are common causes of atrial flutter and fibrillation in childhood?

- Intra-atrial surgery (Mustard, Fontan, ASD repair)
- Congenital heart disease (Ebstein anomaly)
- Heart disease with dilated atria (AV valve regurgitation)
- Idiopathic with an otherwise normal heart
- Cardiomyopathy
- Myocarditis

66. When are isolated premature ventricular contractions (PVCs) usually benign in the otherwise healthy school-aged child?

- Structurally normal heart
- ECG intervals, especially QT_C, are normal.
- No paired or multiform PVCs or "R-on-T" phenomena
- No evidence of myocarditis, cardiomegaly, or ventricular tumor
- No history of drug use
- Electrolytes and glucose are normal.
- PVCs decrease with exercise

67. Name the two most common mechanisms of supraventricular tachycardia (SVT).

1. Wolff-Parkinson-White syndrome (due to an accessory bypass tract)
2. AV nodal re-entry

68. What are the settings in which atrial arrhythmia (and SVT) may occur?

- *Structurally normal heart*: accessory bypass tract or AV nodal re-entry
- *Congenital heart disease* (pre- or post-operatively): Ebstein anomaly, L-TGA with VSD and PS; following Mustard, Senning, Fontan procedures
- *Hypertrophic cardiomyopathy*
- *Dilated cardiomyopathy*
- *Drug-induced*: sympathomimetics (e.g., cold medications, theophylline, beta-agonists)
- *Infections*: myocarditis or fever
- *Hyperthyroidism*

69. What are some of the causes of a wide QRS?

- Premature ventricular contraction or ventricular tachycardia.
- Premature atrial contraction with aberrancy or supraventricular tachycardia with aberrancy
- Bundle branch blocks.
- Pre-excitation syndromes (Wolff-Parkinson-White).
- Electronic ventricular pacemaker.

70. What vagal maneuvers are used to treat paroxysmal supraventricular tachycardia (PSVT) in children?

Infants

- Placement of an ice-soaked wet washcloth or rubber cloth filled with crushed ice over forehead and nose
- Insertion of rectal thermometer
- Gagging with tongue blade

Older children, adolescents

- Above methods
- Unilateral carotid massage

- Valsalva maneuver (abdominal straining while holding breath)
- Doing a headstand

In general, Valsalva maneuver and carotid massage are not effective for children under age 4. Ocular pressure is not recommended because it has been associated with retinal injury. Vagal stimulation slows conduction in the AV node and prolongs refractoriness of the AV node, interrupting the re-entrant circuit.

Kaminer SJ, Strong WB: Cardiac arrhythmias. Pediatr Rev 15:437–439, 1994.

71. Other than vagal maneuvers, what treatments are used acutely in managing SVT?

If a patient's clinical condition has deteriorated rapidly, synchronized direct-current (DC) ***cardioversion*** is indicated. In patients who are stable and have failed vagal maneuvers, ***adenosine*** has replaced digoxin and verapamil as the first drug of choice. An initial bolus of 50–100 microgm/kg will exert an effect in 10–20 sec by blocking conduction through the AV node. If ineffective, the dose can be increased in increments of 50–100 microgm/kg every 1–2 min, up to 300 μg/kg. The usual adult dose of adenosine is 6 and then 12 mg IV push. Adenosine has a very short half-life (< 10 sec), and minimal side effects (e.g., minor flushing, headache, dyspnea). Because it may provoke or exacerbate bronchospasm, it is relatively contraindicated in asthmatics. It should be used with caution in patients following cardiac transplantation. Patients who have had a Fontan procedure tend to need the higher dose for a therapeutic effect. Digoxin is ordinarily *not* used in acute situations because of its delayed onset of action. Intravenous verapamil is felt to be contraindicated in infants < 6-12 months of age.

Etheridge SP, Judd VE: Supraventricular tachycardia in infancy: Evaluation, management and follow-up. Arch Pediatr Adolesc Med 153:267-271, 1999.

72. Which children are candidates for transcatheter ablation techniques for supraventricular tachycardia (SVT)?

In transcatheter ablation, a high-frequency alternating electrical current is applied to endocardial tissue. This results in a destructive thermal lesion directly at the focus of abnormal electrical activity or accessory pathway. Ablation therapy is used most commonly in children with dysrhythmias refractory to medical management and in those with life-threatening symptoms or possible lifelong medication requirements. Ablation is now commonly performed in children who are symptomatic from WPW or AV node re-entrant tachycardia. Recommendations for transcatheter ablation are changing as increased experience with the safety and efficacy of the procedure are gathered. Recommendations vary with the age of the patient, severity of the arrhythmia, type of lesion, difficulty with medical control of the arrhythmia, and skill of the operator.

Villain E: Drugs and ablation in the treatment of supraventricular tachyarrhythmias in children. Curr Opin Pediatr 5:606–610, 1993.

73. How is Wolff-Parkinson-White (WPW) syndrome diagnosed on ECG?

An accessory pathway bypasses the AV node, resulting in early ventricular depolarization (pre-excitation). It is the most common cause of SVT in children. In infants and younger children with rapid heart rates, the delta wave may not be evident. Additional clues which may be suggestive of WPW include:

- PR interval < 100 msec
- QRS duration of > 80 msec
- No Q wave in left chest leads
- Left axis deviation

Perry JC, et al: Clues to the electrocardiographic diagnosis of subtle Wolff-Parkinson-White syndrome in children. J Pediatr 117:871-875, 1990.

INFECTIOUS AND INFLAMMATORY DISORDERS

74. How many blood cultures should be obtained to rule out subacute bacterial endocarditis?

At least three separate blood cultures should be obtained. In 10–30% of children, the first two cultures may be negative. In addition, the use of multiple sites may decrease the likelihood of mistaking a contaminant for the true etiologic agent. In low-level bacteremia, additional specimen volume (at least 3 ml) may increase the likelihood of positivity.

75. Why might properly collected blood cultures be negative in the setting of clinically suspected bacterial endocarditis?

- *Prior antibiotic use*
- The bacterial endocarditis may be *right-sided.*
- *Nonbacterial* infection: fungal (e.g., aspergillus, candida) or unusual organisms (e.g., rickettsia, chlamydia)
- *Unusual bacterial* infection: slow-growing organisms or anaerobes
- Lesions may be *mural, nonvalvular* (less likely to be hematogenously seeded)
- *Nonbacterial thrombotic* endocarditis (sterile platelet–fibrin thrombus formations following endocardial injury)
- *Incorrect diagnosis*

Starke JR: Infectious endocarditis. In Feigin RD, Cherry JD (eds): Textbook of Pediatric Infectious Diseases, 4th ed. Philadelphia, W.B. Saunders, 1998, p 321.

76. Which cardiac lesions are at increased risk for bacterial endocarditis?

- Cyanotic heart disease with a surgical shunt (e.g., Tetralogy of Fallot with a Blalock-Taussig shunt)
- AV valve insufficiency (e.g., mitral insufficiency)
- Semilunar valve disease (e.g., aortic stenosis)
- Intracardiac shunts (e.g., ventricular septal defect, patent ductus arteriosus)
- Coarctation of the aorta
- Artificial valves

77. How reliable is the echocardiogram for diagnosing bacterial endocarditis (BE)?

Echocardiography can sometimes identify an intracardiac mass attached either to the wall of the myocardium or to part of the valve itself. Although the yield of echocardiography for diagnosing BE is low, the likelihood of a positive finding is increased under certain conditions: *indwelling catheters*, *prematurity*, *immunosuppressed patients*, and evidence of *peripheral embolization*. BE is still a clinical and laboratory diagnosis (physical examination and blood cultures, respectively) and *not* an "echocardiographic" diagnosis. A negative study does not rule out BE.

78. How do Osler nodes and Janeway lesions differ?

Both types of lesions are noted in individuals with bacterial endocarditis. Pain is a key discriminator. *Osler nodes* are painful, tender nodules found primarily on the pads of the fingers and toes. *Janeway lesions* are painless, nontender, hemorrhagic nodular lesions seen on the palms and soles, especially on thenar and hypothenar eminences. Both lesions are rare in children with endocarditis.

Farrior JB, Silverman ME: A consideration of the differences between a Janeway's lesion and an Osler's node in infectious endocarditis. Chest 20:239–243, 1976.

79. When should myocarditis be suspected?

The presentation of myocarditis can be variable, ranging from subclinical to rapidly progressive CHF. It should be considered in any patient who presents with unexplained heart failure. Clinical signs include tachycardia out of proportion to fever, grunting respirations with relatively clear lungs to auscultation, a quiet precordium, and hepatomegaly.

80. What conditions are associated with the development of myocarditis?

Infections

Bacterial: diphtheria
Viral: coxsackie B (most common), coxsackie A, HIV, echoviruses, rubella
Mycoplasmal
Rickettsial: typhus
Fungal: actinomycosis, coccidioidomycosis, histoplasmosis
Protozoal: trypanosomiasis (Chagas disease), toxoplasmosis

Inflammatory

Kawasaki disease, systemic lupus erythematosus, rheumatoid arthritis

Chemical/physical agents

Radiation injury
Drugs: doxorubicin
Toxins: lead
Animal bites: scorpion, snakes

81. When should steroids be given to a child with myocarditis?

The use of steroids in myocarditis depends on the underlying etiology and may be controversial. Some authorities feel that the use of steroids may inhibit interferon synthesis and increase viral replication. If the inflammatory process is secondary to rheumatic disease, however, steroids may be indicated.

82. A child visiting from Mexico presents with unilateral eye swelling and new-onset acute CHF. What is a likely diagnosis?

Acute myocarditis due to ***Chagas disease*** (American trypanosomiasis). Seen in 25–50% of patients in endemic areas with early Chagas disease, Romaña sign is unilateral, painless, violaceous, palpebral edema often accompanied by conjunctivitis. The swelling occurs near the bite site of the parasitic vector, the reduviid or *Triatomine* bug. Chagas disease, a protozoan infection, is the most common cause of acute and chronic myocarditis in Mexico, Central and South America.

83. What are the common clinical symptoms and signs of pericarditis?

***Symptoms*:** chest pain, fever, cough, palpitations, irritability, abdominal pain

***Signs*:** friction rub, pallor, pulsus paradoxus, muffled heart sounds, neck vein distention, hepatomegaly

84. What are the possible infectious causes of pericarditis in a child?

Purulent

Bacterial: *Staphylococcus aureus, Haemophilus influenzae,* streptococci, *Neisseria meningitidis, Streptococcus pneumoniae,* anaerobes, *Francisella tularensis, Salmonella,* enteric bacilli, *Pseudomonas, Listeria, Neisseria gonorrhoeae, Actinomyces, Nocardia*
Tuberculosis
Fungal: histoplasmosis, coccidioidomycosis, aspergillosis, candidiasis, blastomycosis, cryptococcosis

Viral

Coxsackie virus B
Other: influenza A and B, mumps, echoviruses, adenoviruses, Epstein-Barr virus, hepatitis viruses, measles, cytomegalovirus

Other

Rickettsial: typhus, Q fever
Mycoplasmal: *Mycoplasma pneumoniae*
Parasitic: *Entamoeba histolytica,* echinococcus
Spirochetal: syphilis, leptospirosis
Chlamydial: psitticosis
Protozoal: toxoplasmosis

From Pinsky WW, et al: Infectious endocarditis. In Feigin RD, Cherry JD (eds): Textbook of Pediatric Infectious Diseases, 4th ed. Philadelphia, W.B. Saunders, 1998, p 339; with permission.

85. What are noninfectious causes of pericarditis?

- *Postpericardiotomy syndrome*
- *Rheumatic fever*
- *Connective tissue disorders*: juvenile rheumatoid arthritis, systemic lupus erythematosus, dermatomyositis, periarteritis nodosa
- *Trauma*: blunt or penetrating
- *Metabolic*: uremia, myxedema
- *Hypersensitivity*: serum sickness, pulmonary infiltrates with eosinophilia, Stevens-Johnson syndrome, drugs (hydralazine, procainamide, chemotherapy)
- *Neoplasm*: leukemia, metastatic disease
- *Postirradiation*

From Pinsky WW, et al: Infectious endocarditis. In Feigin RD, Cherry JD (eds): Textbook of Pediatric Infectious Diseases, 4th ed. Philadelphia, W.B. Saunders, 1998, p 339; with permission.

86. What are the principal diagnostic criteria for Kawasaki disease?

The mnemonic ***My HEART*** may be helpful:

M **M**ucosal changes, especially oral and upper respiratory; dry and chapped lips; "strawberry tongue"
H **H**and and extremity changes, including reddened palms/soles, edema, desquamation from fingertips and toes (late findings)
E **E**ye changes, primarily a bilateral conjunctival injection without discharge
A **A**denopathy, usually cervical, often unilateral, of at least 1.5 cm in diameter
R **R**ash, usually a truncal exanthem without vesicles or crusts
T **T**emperature elevation, often to 104°F or above, lasting for > 5 days

The presence of fever and at least 4 of the other 5 features are needed for the classic diagnosis. However, a significant number of cases of atypical Kawasaki disease (20-60% of total) have been reported which feature <5 of the criteria, accompanied by the typical coronary artery changes. A high index of suspicion is important, as Kawasaki disease has replaced acute rheumatic fever as the leading cause of identifiable acquired heart disease in children in the United States.

87. If untreated, what percentage of children with Kawasaki disease will develop coronary artery ectasia or aneurysms?

15%-25%.

88. What is the typical ages of children with Kawasaki disease?

The majority of patients are ***between 1 and 8 years***. However, cases can occur in infants and teenagers. Both of these groups appear to be at increased risk of developing coronary artery sequelae. The diagnosis is often delayed particularly in infants because signs and symptoms of the illness may be atypical, subtle or absent.

89. Why should all children with Kawasaki disease receive gammaglobulin therapy?

IV gammaglobulin has been demonstrated to decrease the incidence of coronary artery abnormalities in children with Kawasaki disease. Additionally, fever and laboratory indices of inflammation resolve more quickly after treatment. Early trials used a dose of 400 mg/kg/day for 4 consecutive days. More recent studies demonstrate that a single infusion over 12 hours of 2 g/kg is at least as effective as the 4-day regimen in preventing aneurysms and is better at hastening defervescence.

IVIG improves outcome with coronary artery dilation developing in <5% and giant coronary aneurysms <1% of patients. At present, there is no reliable means of predicting which children with Kawasaki disease will develop coronary artery abnormalities. Therefore, all children with Kawasaki disease should receive parenteral gammaglobulin. The efficacy of this therapy has not been evaluated in children who have been ill for > 10 days. However, treatment in this situation is reasonable if the child remains symptomatic. Some recent studies suggest that patients with increased levels of C-reactive protein, LDH or gamma-GTP before therapy or elevation of wbc counts and C-reactive protein following therapy are at increased risk for sequelae and might benefit from more aggressive therapy.

Mori M, et al: Predictors of coronary artery lesions after intravenous gammaglobulin treatment in Kawasaki disease. J Pediatr 137:177-180, 2000.

Fukunishi, M et al: Predictors of non-responsiveness to high-dose gammaglobulin therapy in patients with Kawasaki disease at onset. J Pediatr 137:172-176, 2000.

90. Is aspirin therapy of benefit in children with Kawasaki disease?

By itself, high-dose aspirin (80 – 100 mg/kg/day divided every 6 hours) is effective in decreasing the degree of fever and discomfort in patients during the acute stages of illness up to about 14 days. It is unclear if high-dose aspirin has an additive effect in decreasing the incidence of coronary artery abnormalities when used in conjunction with gammaglobulin. Aspirin may be beneficial when administered in low dose after resolution of fever, due to its effects on platelet aggregation and prevention of the thrombotic complications seen in children with Kawasaki disease. Therefore, aspirin in low dose (3–5 mg/kg/day) is advised for about 6–8 weeks. If a follow-up echocardiogram at that time reveals no coronary abnormalities, therapy is usually discontinued. If abnormalities are present, therapy is continued indefinitely.

91. When are corticosteroids indicated in the treatment of Kawasaki disease?

This is an area of marked controversy. Early reports suggested that methylprednisolone decreased the incidence of cardiac abnormalities in children with Kawasaki disease. Some subsequent evaluations failed to confirm this finding and, in fact, in some studies the incidence of coronary artery abnormalities actually increased in children who received prednisone versus placebo. As a result, steroids were contraindicated in the treatment of this disease. Recently, there has been a resurgence of interest in the use of steroids in the treatment of Kawasaki disease, especially in the more difficult cases. Therefore, the final resolution of this question is unclear.

92. What causes Kawasaki disease?

Despite considerable progress in understanding the pathogenesis of this syndrome, the inciting agent remains undiscovered. Toxic agents, such as mercury and lead, and allergic and immunologic causes have been studied as potential causative factors. Numerous case reports and clinical series report infectious agents associated with Kawasaki disease, including rickettsiae, *Klebsiella pneumoniae, Escherichia* sp., parainfluenza virus, Epstein-Barr virus, retrovirus, *Propionibacterium acnes*, retroviruses, and toxic shock syndrome toxin 1 (TSST-1) staphylococci. The association between Kawasaki disease and shampooing or spot-cleaning rugs or carpets has been studied, as well as the importance of mites.

Mason WH, Takahashi M: Kawasaki syndrome. Clin Infect Dis 28:169-185, 1999.

93. How do the clinical stages of Kawasaki disease correlate with the arterial pathologic changes?

Kawasaki Syndrome: Disease Phases, Complications, and Degree of Arteritis

	ACUTE (1–11 DAYS)	SUBACUTE (11–21 DAYS)	CONVALESCENT (21–60 DAYS)	CHRONIC (? YEARS)
Clinical findings	Fever, conjunctivitis, oral changes, extremity changes, irritability	irritability persists; prolongation of fever may occur; normalization of most clinical findings; palpable aneurysms may develop	Most clinical findings resolve; aneurysmal dilation of peripheral vessels may persist; conjunctivitis may persist	—
Arterial correlates	Perivasculitis, vasculitis of capillaries, arterioles, and venules; inflammation of intima of medium and larger arteries	Aneurysms, thrombi, stenosis of medium-sized arteries, panvasculitis, and edema of vessel wall; myocarditis less prominent	Vascular inflammation decreases	Scar formation; intimal thickening

From Hicks RV, Melish ME: Kawasaki syndrome. Pediatr Clin North Am 33:1115–1175, 1986; with permission.

94. How is Kawasaki disease distinguished from measles?

These two entities can have a large degree of clinical overlap, and in countries where measles is more prominent, the need for clinical distinction is not rare. As a rule, the conjunctivitis of Kawasaki disease is nonexudative; in measles, it is exudative. Koplik spots seen in measles are discrete oral lesions, whereas in Kawasaki disease the mucosal erythema is more diffuse. The rash of measles usually begins on the face and hairline; in Kawasaki disease on the trunk and extremities. In measles, a low total WBC count and ESR are the norm, whereas both are usually elevated in Kawasaki disease.

95. What factors are most strongly associated with the development of coronary artery disease in patients with Kawasaki disease?

- Duration of fever > 16 days
- Recurrence of fever after an afebrile period of ≥ 48 hours
- Dysrhythmias (other than first-degree heart block)
- Cardiomegaly
- Male gender
- Age < 1 year

PHARMACOLOGY

96. How valuable are digoxin levels?

Digoxin levels may not be helpful in children because of the presence of endogenous digoxin-like immunoreactive substances, which cross-react with immunoassay antibodies to digoxin. Also, in children, the concentration of digoxin is much higher in the myocardium than in the plasma. Digoxin levels may be helpful, however, in older children (especially in presence of dysrhythmias).

97. How long before oral digoxin begins to work?

Oral digoxin reaches peak plasma levels 1–2 hours after administration, but a peak hemodynamic effect is not evident until 6 hours after administration (vs. 2–3 hours for IVdigoxin).

98. An infant with Wolff-Parkinson-White (WPW) syndrome and supraventricular tachycardia (SVT) is given digoxin, and the attending cardiologist is dismayed. Why?

Digoxin can enhance conduction through a bypass tract while slowing conduction through the AV node. *Ventricular fibrillation* has been reported in patients with WPW treated with digoxin. This effect is believed to be due to enhanced conduction down the bypass tract. For this reason, propranolol has replaced digoxin as the drug of choice in the treatment of children with SVT and WPW.

99. What are the indications for prostaglandin E_1 (PGE_1) in the neonate?

PGE_1 is indicated in cardiac lesions with *ductal dependent blood flow* to either the pulmonary circulation (e.g., pulmonary atresia with intact ventricular septum, tricuspid atresia with intact ventricular septum, critical pulmonary stenosis) or systemic circulation (e.g., critical coarctation of the aorta, interrupted aortic arch, hypoplastic left heart syndrome). In infants with *suspected CHD* in whom a specific diagnosis is not known (e.g., prior to transport to a tertiary care center), PGE_1 is clinically indicated in cases of profound cyanosis, poor perfusion, and/or metabolic acidosis.

100. What are the major side effects of PGE_1?

Apnea, fever, cutaneous flushing, seizures, hypotension, bradycardia/tachycardia.

101. Are there any conditions during the newborn period in which PGE_1 use is contraindicated?

PGE_1 maintains the patency of the ductus arteriosus and is usually most effective in infants <96 hours of age. The use of PGE_1 may have *adverse* physiologic effects under certain situations:

- Transposition of the great arteries with a restrictive atrial septal defect
- Tetralogy of Fallot without a patent ductus arteriosus
- Total anomalous pulmonary venous return
- Persistent pulmonary hypertension of the newborn

102. What are the side effects of indomethacin in the neonate?

- Mild but usually transient renal dysfunction
- Hyponatremia
- Hypoglycemia
- Platelet dysfunction, producing a prolonged bleeding time
- Occult blood loss from gastrointestinal tract
- Spontaneous perforation of the intestine

103. How do alpha, beta, and dopaminergic receptors differ?

Alpha: in vascular smooth muscle, cause vasoconstriction

Beta$_1$: in myocardial smooth muscle, increase inotropic (contractile force) and chronotropic (cardiac rate) effect

Beta$_2$: in vascular smooth muscle, cause vasodilation

Dopaminergic: in renal and mesenteric vascular smooth muscle, cause vasodilation

104. How do relative receptor effects differ by drug type?

DRUG	ALPHA	BETA$_1$	BETA$_2$	DOPAMINERGIC
Epinephrine	+++	+++	+++	0
Norepinephrine	+++	+++	+	0
Isoproterenol	0	+++	+++	0
Dopamine	0 to +++ (dose-related)	++ to +++ (dose-related)	++	+++
Dobutamine	0 to +	+++	+	0

Effect of medication: 0 = none, + = small, ++ = moderate, +++ = large.

For dopamine, at low doses (2–5 μg/kg/min), dopaminergic effects predominate. At high doses (5–20 μg/kg/min), increased alpha and beta effects are seen. At very high doses (> 20 μg/kg/min), a markedly increased alpha effect with decreased renal and mesenteric blood flow occurs. For dobutamine, $beta_1$ inotropic effects are more pronounced than chronotropic effects.

105. How are emergency infusions for cardiovascular support prepared?

CATECHOLAMINE	MIXTURE	DOSE
Isoproterenol Epinephrine Norepinephrine	0.6 mg × body wt (in kg), added to diluent to make 100 ml	1 ml/hr delivers 0.1 μg/kg/min
Dopamine Dobutamine	6 mg × body wt (in kg), added to diluent to make 100 ml	1 ml/hr delivers 1 μg/kg/min

PHYSICAL EXAMINATION

106. Which cardiac conditions accentuate or diminish the intensity of the first heart sound?

The intensity of the S_1 depends mainly on the position of the mitral leaflets at the time when the left ventricle begins to contract. The loudness is greatest in situations that cause wide separation of the leaflets at the beginning of systole: short PR interval, left-to-right shunts, tachycardia, short cycle lengths in atrial fibrillation, mitral stenosis with mobile cusps, high-output states, and mobile left atrial myxoma. Fibrosis or calcification of the mitral valve cusps cause a faint S_1, as does bradycardia and first-degree AV block.

107. In what settings can an abnormal second heart sound be auscultated?

Widely split S_2

- Prolonged right ventricular (RV) ejection time:
  RV volume overload—atrial septal defect, partial anomalous pulmonary venous return
  RV pressure overload—mild pulmonary stenosis
  RV conduction delay—right bundle branch block
- Shortened left ventricular (LV) ejection time
  Early aortic closure—mitral regurgitation

Single S_2

- Presence of only one semilunar valve—aortic or pulmonary atresia, truncus arteriosus
- P2 not audible—tetralogy of Fallot, transposition of great arteries, pulmonary stenosis, pulmonary hypertension
- A2 delayed—severe aortic stenosis
- May be normal in a newborn

Paradoxically split S_2 (A2 follows P2): present in severe aortic stenosis, left bundle branch block, pulmonary hypertension

Loud P2

- Pulmonary hypertension
- Dilation of nonhypertensive pulmonary artery, as in atrial septal defect

108. When can S_3 and S_4 be considered a normal finding during a pediatric cardiac examination?

An S_3 occurs early in diastole. It may be benign but can be abnormal in children with dilated ventricles and decreased compliance (as in CHF). An S_4 occurs late in diastole. It is usually abnormal in children.

109. What are the possible etiologies of an ejection click?

An ejection click occurs at the onset of ventricular ejection, follows S_1, and is best heard at the base of the heart. Possible etiologies include:

- *Stenosis of semilunar valves*: aortic stenosis or pulmonary stenosis
- *Dilation of great arteries*: tetralogy of Fallot (dilated aorta), truncus arteriosus, hypertension, or coarctation of the aorta
- *Mitral valve prolapse* (produces midsystolic click)
- *Other* (rare): cardiac tumors, atrial septal aneurysms, and dissecting aortic aneurysms

110. How can the likelihood of finding mitral valve prolapse (MVP) on auscultation be increased?

In MVP, the leaflets of the mitral valve apparatus billow into the left atrium. The characteristic midsystolic click of MVP may represent the snapping of the chordae tendineae or redundant portions of the cusps themselves. The crescendo, late systolic murmur represents mitral insufficiency. Maneuvers that *decrease LV size and volume* (and thus increase the relative size of the leaflets) increase the likelihood of hearing the click or murmur. These include the straining phase of a Valsalva maneuver, inspiration, and change from a supine to sitting position or from a squatting to standing position. The left lateral decubitus position may also be facilitative.

111. What is the difference between pulsus alternans and pulsus paradoxus?

Pulsus alternans is a pulse pattern in which there is alternating (beat-to-beat) variability of pulse strength due to decreased ventricular performance (sometimes seen in CHF).

Pulsus paradoxus indicates an exaggeration of normal reduction of systolic blood pressure during inspiration. Associated conditions include cardiac tamponade (effusion or constrictive pericarditis), respiratory illness (asthma or pneumonia), and myocardial disease affecting wall compliance (endocardial fibroelastosis or amyloidosis).

112. How is pulsus paradoxus measured?

To measure a pulsus paradoxus, determine the systolic pressure by noting the first audible Korotkoff sound. Then, retake the blood pressure by raising the manometer pressure to at least 25 mmHg higher than the systolic pressure, and allow it to fall very slowly. Stop as soon as the first sound is heard. Note that the sound disappears during inspiration. Lower the pressure slowly and note when all pulsed beats are heard. The difference between these two pressures is the pulsus paradoxus. Normally, in children, there is an 8–10 mmHg fluctuation in systolic pressure with different phases of respiration.

113. As a screening tool for coarctation of the aorta (COA) in infants and older children, how reliable is palpation for absent femoral pulses?

The detection of decreased lower extremity pulses seen in coarctation can be subtle, variable and ultimately unreliable. In some *infants*, a patent ductus arteriosus may provide blood flow to the lower extremities, bypassing a severe coarctation. Upper and lower pulses may be equal as long as the ductus remains open. As the ductus closes, signs of coarctation of the aorta may appear with respiratory distress and cardiac failure. Decreased or absent pulses may then be noted. In *older children*, simultaneous palpation of upper and lower extremity pulses is important. If collaterals have developed, a delay in pulse rather than diminished volume may be noted. In a study of older patients (>1 year) with documented coarctation, only 20% had absent pulses and distinguishing differences between UE and LE blood pressures by palpation alone was unreliable. Thus, it is recommended that screening for COA be done by measuring both upper extremity and one lower extremity blood pressure in infancy.

Ing FF, et al: Early diagnosis of coarctation of the aorta in children: A continuing dilemma. Pediatrics 98: 378-382, 1996.

114. What is the differential diagnosis for a systolic murmur in each auscultatory area?

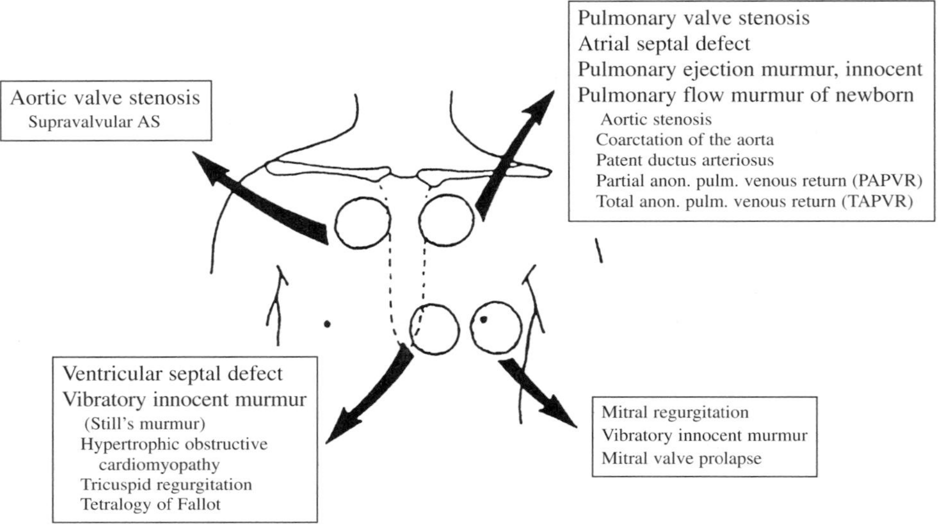

Systolic murmurs audible at various locations. Many may radiate to other areas. Less common conditions are shown in smaller type. Adapted from Park MK: Pediatric Cardiology for Practitioners, 3rd ed. St. Louis, Mosby-Year Book, 1995, with permission.

115. What are the most common innocent murmurs?

TYPE (TIMING)	DESCRIPTION OF MURMUR	COMMON AGE GROUP
Classic vibratory murmur (Still murmur) (systolic)	Maximal at MLSB or between LLSB and apex Grade 2–3/6 Low-frequency vibratory, "twanging string," or musical	3–6 yr Occasionally in infancy
Pulmonary ejection murmur (systolic)	Maximal at ULSB Early to midsystolic Grade 1–2/6 in intensity	8–14 yr
Pulmonary flow murmur of newborn (systolic)	Maximal at ULSB Transmit well to left and right chest, axillae, and back Grade 1–2/6 intensity	Premature and full-term newborns Usually disappears by 3–6 mos of age
Venous hum (continuous)	Maximal at right (or left) supra- and infraclavicular areas Grade 1–2/6 intensity Inaudible in supine position Intensity changes with rotation of head and compression of jugular vein	3–6 yr
Carotid bruit (systolic)	Right supraclavicular area and over carotids Grade 2–3/6 intensity Occasional thrill over a carotid artery	Any age

MLSB, mid-left sternal border; LLSB, lower-left sternal border; ULSB, upper-left sternal border.

116. What features are suggestive of a pathologic murmur?

- Diastolic murmurs
- Pansystolic murmurs
- Murmurs associated with a thrill
- Late systolic murmurs
- Continuous murmurs
- Associated cardiac abnormalities (e.g., asymmetric pulses, click, abnormal splitting)

McCrindle BW, et al: Cardinal clinical signs in the differentiation of heart murmurs in children. Arch Pediatr Adolesc Med 150:169–174, 1996.

Rosenthal A: How to distinguish between innocent and pathologic murmurs in childhood. Pediatr Clin North Am 31:1229–1240, 1984.

117. If a murmur is detected, what noncardiac factors suggest that the murmur is pathologic?

- Evidence of growth retardation (most commonly seen in murmurs with large left-to-right shunts)
- Associated dysmorphic features (e.g., valvular disease in Hurler syndrome, Noonan syndrome)
- Exertional cyanosis, pallor, or dyspnea, especially if associated with minor exertion such as climbing a few stairs (may be sign of early CHF)
- Short feeding times and volumes in infants (may be sign of early CHF)
- Syncopal or presyncopal episodes (may be seen in hypertrophic cardiomyopathy)
- History of IVdrug abuse (risk factor for endocarditis)
- Maternal history of diabetes mellitus (associated with asymmetric septal hypertrophy, VSD, d-transposition), alcohol use (associated with pulmonic stenosis and VSD), other medications
- Family history of congenital heart disease

118. How skillful are pediatric residents at distinguishing innocent from pathologic murmurs?

The batting average is about one-third. Utilizing a computerized simulator, the diagnostic accuracy of residents at Duke University in distinguishing valvular PS, VSD, ASD, AS and innocent murmurs was 33%. Practice (and training) does make perfect (or near perfect). Pediatric cardiologists correctly identified 84%.

Gaskin PRA, et al: Clinical auscultation skills in pediatric residents. Pediatrics 105:1184-1187, 2000.

SURGERY

119. Name the major shunt operations for congenital heart disease (CHD).

Shunts between a systemic artery and pulmonary artery are used to improve oxygen saturation in patients with cyanotic CHD and diminished pulmonary blood flow. Veno-arterial shunts which connect a systemic vein and the pulmonary artery are also used for similar purposes.

- The ***Blalock-Taussig*** shunt consists of an anastomosis between a subclavian artery and the ipsilateral pulmonary artery. The subclavian artery can be divided, and the distal end anastomosed to the pulmonary artery (*classic BT shunt*), or a prosthetic graft can be interposed between the two arteries (*modified BT shunt*).
- The ***Waterston*** shunt is an anastomosis between the ascending aorta and right pulmonary artery.
- The ***Potts*** shunt is an anastomosis between the descending aorta and left pulmonary artery.
- The *classic* **Glenn** anastomosis is a connection between the distal right pulmonary artery and the superior vena cava, which is ligated below the site of the anastomosis.
- In the *bi-directional* **Glenn** operation, the SVC is anastomosed to the right pulmonary artery. However, the right pulmonary artery is left in continuity with the left pulmonary artery. SVC blood flow can go either to the left or right pulmonary artery.

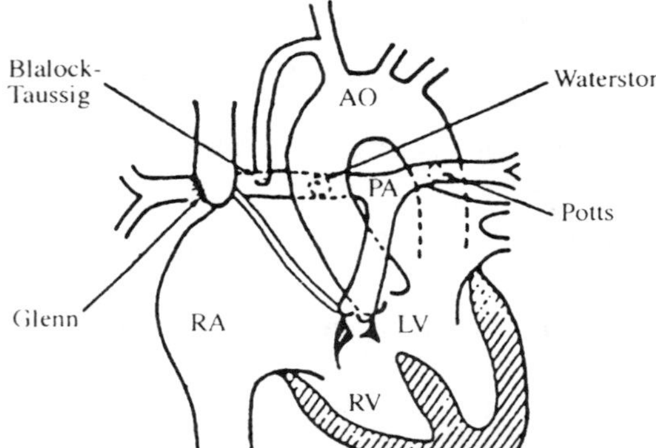

From Park MK: Pediatric Cardiology for Practitioners, 3rd ed. S. Louis, Mosby-Year Book, 1995; with permission.

120. Which factors are associated with more favorable outcomes with the Fontan procedure?

The *Fontan procedure*, initially done in 1971 for tricuspid atresia, establishes a direct continuity between the systemic venous channels (right atrium/superior vena cava/inferior vena cava) and pulmonary arteries. It thus bypasses the need for a functioning ventricle to pump blood to the lungs and also minimizes the need for conduits and valves. Favorable outcomes are more likely if:

- Pulmonary artery pressure is normal
- Pulmonary vascular resistance is normal
- Pulmonary arteries are of adequate size
- End-diastolic pressure is low

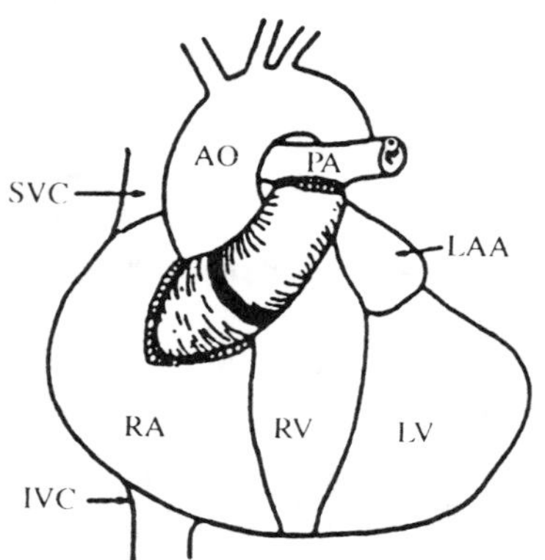

Adapted from Park MK: Pediatric Cardiology for Practitioners, 3rd ed. St. Louis, Mosby-Year Book, 1995; with permission.

121. For which congenital heart disorder is the "switch operation" done?

Transposition of the great arteries (TGA). This procedure restores the aorta and the pulmonary artery to their correct anatomic positions It involves reimplantation of the coronary arteries. The first successful operation of this type was reported by Jatene in 1976.

122. What are the indications for surgical repair of ASD and VSD?

***Ventricular septal defect*:** Infants with a large VSD refractory to medical therapy, causing failure to thrive and/or repeated lower respiratory tract infections, should be referred for surgery. Pulmonary hypertension is another indication for surgery. In older children with normal pulmonary artery pressure, but with significantly increased pulmonary blood flow or left ventricular dilatation, surgical closure is sometimes advised.

***Atrial septal defect*:** Asymptomatic children should be scheduled for repair during the first 5 years of life. The rare infant with a symptomatic ASD should undergo surgery at the time of diagnosis.

123. Is there any surgical therapy for hypoplastic left heart syndrome (HLHS)?

Two surgical options are available: ***heart transplantation*** and the ***Norwood procedure***. In HLHS, severe underdevelopment of the left ventricle, mitral valve, aortic valve, and ascending aortic arch occurs. Newborns usually develop signs of severe CHF. The *Norwood procedure* was reported initially in 1983. Long-term survival is significantly better with heart transplantation, but donor shortages are major problems and 20–30% of infants die awaiting transplant.

124. What are the three stages of the Norwood procedure?

Stage I: The proximal main pulmonary artery is transected, and with additional homograft material, it is used to help rebuild the aorta. This creates a univentricular systemic pumping chamber and changes the physiology from aortic atresia to pulmonic atresia. The distal main pulmonary artery is oversewn, and a systemic-to-pulmonary shunt placed between the innominate artery and right pulmonary artery to correct pulmonary flow.

Stage II: (performed at about age 6 months) seeks to regulate pulmonary blood flow by changing to a bidirectional Glenn anastomosis (superior vena cava to distal right pulmonary artery).

Stage III: One to 2 years later, a Fontan procedure is performed (right atrium to pulmonary artery) which ultimately separates the venous and arterial sides.

125. What is the long-term prognosis for heart transplantation in infancy and childhood?

Survival statistics have improved dramatically over the last 10 years with the use of newer and safer immunosuppressive agents such as cyclosporine and FK506. However, children who receive transplanted hearts are at increased risk for cardiac rejection, infection, accelerated coronary artery disease, and lymphoproliferative syndromes. Recent estimated 5-year survival rates vary between 65-70%.

126. What are the most common cardiothoracic postoperative syndromes?

- ***Postcoarctectomy syndrome***: arteritis in the mesenteric circulation causing abdominal pain (2–8 days after surgery)
- ***Postpericardiotomy syndrome***: immunologic phenomenon leading to pericardial effusion, chest pain, fever, irritability, and elevated ESR (1–3 weeks following surgery).

4. DERMATOLOGY

Maria C. Garzon, M.D., Robert Hayman, M.D., and Leonard Kristal, M.D.

ACNE

1. What is the most common skin disorder of adolescence?

Acne. Some would say it is the most common medical disorder of adolescents. Up to 85% of teenagers will develop at least a few lesions of acne. Despite the condition's widespread prevalence, it is important not to underestimate the psychologic (as well as at times dermatologic) significance of the condition. Problems of embarrassment, social inhibition, and depression are highly associated with acne. In addition, treatment of noninflammatory acne before the development of inflammation and possible scarring is vital.

2. When is acne most likely to develop?

The development of microcomedones is typically the earliest sign of acne. Studies have shown that comedones occur in three-fourths of premenarchal girls at an average age of 10 years and about half of 10-11 year-old boys. They may herald (or predate) the onset of puberty.

3. What factors are involved in the pathogenesis of acne vulgaris?

Acne is a *multifactoral disorder* that arises within the sebaceous follicles of the skin. Factors include: (a) *altered keratinization* in the follicle with the development of a denser keratin plug; (b) *increased sebum production* modulated by androgens; (c) *bacterial proliferation* (*Propionibacterium acnes*) within the plugged, lipid-rich follicle; and (d) *increased inflammation* provoked by bacterial lipases and chemotactic factors.

4. How do a "blackhead" and a "whitehead" differ histopathologically?

Both lesions are produced by obstruction and distention of the sebaceous follicle with sebum and cellular debris. When the follicular contents tent the overlying skin but are not exposed to the atmosphere, a **whitehead** occurs. If the contents project out of the follicular opening, oxidation of the exposed mass of debris produces a color change and a **blackhead**.

5. What is the difference between neonatal acne and infantile acne?

Occurring in up to 20% of newborns, *neonatal acne* is a variant of acne vulgaris that presents at birth or in the first few weeks. It is attributed to the transient elevation of androgenic hormones, both maternally derived and endogenous, that are present in a newborn infant. The lesions typically resolve within 1–3 months as androgen levels fall.

A smaller number of infants develop acne on a delayed basis (3–6 months) characterized by greater degrees of inflammatory papules and pustules. This *infantile* acne may persist for years. The cause is unknown. Most have no evidence of precocious puberty or increased hormonal levels, although severe acne in this age group warrants evaluation for hyperandrogenism. Systemic therapy is sometimes required.

Mengesha YM, Hansen RC: Toddler-age nodulocystic acne. J Pediatr 134:644-648, 1999.

6. Is a newborn with acne more likely to be a teenager with acne?

The presence or severity of acne in an infant less than three months is not felt to correlate with an increased likelihood of adolescent acne. However, delayed acne between 3 and 6 months of age (especially if persistent and severe) does have a higher correlation with the likelihood of more severe adolescent acne. Family history of severe acne also increases the likelihood of future problems.

7. What are the severest forms of acne?

Acne fulminans is a rare but severe disorder that has also been called acute febrile ulcerative acne. It occurs in teenage boys as extensive inflammatory, ulcerating lesions on the trunk and chest usually associated with fever, malaise, arthralgia and leukocytosis. The etiology remains unclear, but immune complexes are thought to be involved. Treatment is systemic: antibiotics, glucocorticoids, and retinoids.

Acne conglobata is a severe form of acne that presents with comedones, papules, pustules, nodules and abscesses. It is associated with significant scarring. It often arises in early adulthood, more typically in females. Systemic retinoid therapy is the treatment of choice.

8. What is the therapeutic approach to acne?

Acne therapies, including *comedolytics, antibacterial agents, and hormonal modulators,* target various factors involved in the pathogenesis of acne. Topical agents including erythromycin, clindamycin, erythromycin–benzoyl peroxide, benzoyl peroxide and azaleic acid reduce the population of *P. acnes*. Systemic antibiotics (e.g., tetracycline and its derivatives) most frequently are used for moderate-to-severe papulopustular acne. The topical retinoid tretinoin (Retin-A, Avita) is comedolytic and prevents the formation of new keratin plugs. The systemic retinoid isotretinoin (Accutane) is used in cases of severe acne vulgaris. The exact mechanism of action of isoretinoin is not known but appears to be related to inhibition of sebaceous gland activity. Other agents used in severe acne include intralesional glucocorticoids and systemic glucocorticoids. Hormonal modulation is most commonly accomplished with oral contraceptive pills, although antiandrogenic agents (e.g., spironolactone) are used in teenage females with premenstrual flares, hirsutism and male-pattern alopecia.

Mancini AJ: Acne vulgaris: A treatment update. Contemp Pediatr 17:122-133, 2000.

9. What side effects are associated with topical retinoids?

Agents that bind to the retinoid receptor (e.g., Retin-A, Avita, Differin) are effective agents for acne. The most common side effects are *irritation* (erythema, burning) and *excessive dying* of the skin. An *increased susceptibility to sunburn* is also reported, and non-comedogenic sunscreens are recommended if exposure to ultraviolet light is unavoidable. Treatment is usually begun with a low strength. Liquid and gel forms tend to be more drying than creams. Patients should be instructed to apply only a pea-sized amount every other night prior to bedtime about ½ hour after washing; the dose may be increased to nightly application if they are not becoming irritated.

10. When is the use of oral isotretinoin indicated in teenagers with acne?

Isotretinoin, which is 13-*cis*-retinoic acid (Accutane), is most appropriately used for nodulocystic acne, acne conglobata, or severe scarring acne that has been unresponsive to standard modes of treatment (including oral/topical antibiotics and topical retinoins). Its most dangerous side effect is teratogenicity, and rigorous monitoring and definitive contraceptive counseling are mandatory.

11. In what situations should the use of azelaic acid be considered?

Approved by the FDA in 1996, azelaic acid (Azelex) is a naturally occurring dicarboxylic acid derived from the fungus *Pityrosporum ovale*. It is comedolytic and may be helpful in decreasing hyperpigmentation (particularly vilaceous hues of healing) in individuals predisposed to such changes. It can be effective as a monotherapy in mild disease or in combination therapy with systemic antibiotics in moderate-to-severe disease.

12. What serious side effects may be associated with systemic minocycline therapy for acne?

Tetracyclines, including the derivative minocycline, are the most widely prescribed oral antibiotics for acne and have been used safely over long periods of time. They are contraindicated for patients less than the age of 8 years due to the potential for permanent dental staining. Rare reactions particularly to minocycline have included pneumonitis, autoimmune hepatitis, drug-induced lupus, serum-sickness like reactions and severe hypersensitivity reactions.

Sturkenboom MCJM, et al: Minocycline and lupuslike syndrome in acne patients. Arch Intern Med 159:493-497, 1999.

Eichenfield AH: Minocycline and autoimmunity. Curr Opin Pediatr 11:447, 1999.

13. What guidelines can help to maximize the compliance of teenagers with therapy for acne?

- Reassure the teenager that acne is both common and treatable.
- Explain that acne cannot be scrubbed away.
- Do not overload teens with data. A few "take-home" messages are optimal.
- Allow teenagers to ask questions.
- Remember to treat the teenager's back and chest if they are involved, not just the face.
- Give the teenager choices whenever possible (e.g., Retin-A versus benzoyl peroxide).
- Be aware of the cost of medications.
- Do not take noncompliance personally.

Strasburger VC: Acne: What every pediatrician should know about treatment. Pediatr Clin North Am 44: 1519-20, 1997.

CLINICAL ISSUES

14. What skin findings are suggestive of occult spinal dysraphism (OSD)?

Intraspinal anomalies without a detectable back mass may present with skin findings. Midline dermatologic findings in the lumbosacral area concerning for OSD include:

- Lipoma
- Hypertrichosis
- Pits: dermal dimples or sinuses about the intergluteal cleft (particularly with lateral deviation of the cleft)
- Vascular lesions (hemangioma, port wine stain, telangiectases)
- Pigmentation variants (hyper-, including lentigo and melanocytic nevus, and hypo-)
- Aplasia cutis congenita
- Appendages (skin tags, tail)

Howard R: Congenital midline lesions: Pits and protuberances. Pediatr Ann 27:150-160, 1998.

15. What is the characteristic rash of hepatitis B virus infection?

Circulating immune complexes contribute to the pathogenesis of cutaneous manifestations of hepatitis B. The most common cutaneous associations are ***urticaria*** and ***Gianotti-Crosti syndrome*** (papular acrodermatitis of childhood).

Urticaria, or "hives," may be the major feature of the prodrome of hepatitis B. The rash may precede the arthralgias and icterus and may last several days; it may also be maculopapular or petechial.

Gianotti-Crosti syndrome consists of nonpruritic, erythematous, 1–5-mm papules arranged symmetrically on the face, buttocks, and extremities. The lesions erupt over a few days and do not become confluent (remember, the trunk is spared!). They may last for 3 weeks; lymphadenopathy may persists for months. This rash is classically associated with anicteric hepatitis, which develops at the same time as the rash or weeks later. The association is more common in Europe, where hepatitis B Adw serotype is more common than in the U.S., where the Ayw serotype predominates. Other viruses, such as Epstein-Barr virus, may also be associated with these cutaneous findings.

16. What is the natural history of molluscum contagiosum?

Molluscum contagiosum is a common skin infection caused by a poxvirus. Lesions are small pink- tan dome-shaped papules often with a dimpled (or umbilicated) center. They are usually asymptomatic but may associated with an eczematous dermatitis and itch.. Suprainfection may complicate the course, require antibiotic therapy and increase the likelihood of scarring after resolution. In healthy children, the course is self-limited but may last for up to 2-4 years. Persistent and widespread molluscum may require screening for congenital or acquired immunodeficiences.

17. What is the best way to eradicate molluscum contagiosum?

If watchful waiting is not desired, therapeutic options rely primarily on destructive methods. Curettage (with core removal), cryotherapy, and peeling agents (salicyclic and lactic acid preparations) can be utilized. An increasingly popular method is the use of cantharidin, a blistering agent, applied to individual lesions.

Silverberg, NB et al: Childhood molluscum contagiosum: Experience with cantharidin in 300 patients. J Am Acad Dermatol 43:503-507, 2000.

18. Describe the characteristic clinical picture of erythema nodosum.

A prodrome of fever, chills, malaise, and arthralgia may precede the typical skin findings. Crops of red to blue tender nodules appear over the anterior shins. Lesions may be seen on the knees, ankles, thighs, and, occasionally, lower extensor forearms and face. They may evolve through a spectrum of colors that resemble a bruise. Often, the changes are misdiagnosed as cellulitis or secondary to a traumatic event.

19. What infectious and noninfectious conditions are associated with erythema nodosum?

Infectious	**Noninfectious**
Group A β-hemolytic streptococci	Sarcoidosis
Tuberculosis	Ulcerative colitis
Yersinia	Regional ileitis
Coccidioidomycosis	Hodgkin disease
Histoplasmosis	Lymphosarcoma
North American blastomycosis	Leukemia
Psittacosis	Behçet syndrome
Lymphogranuloma venereum	Sulfonamides
Ornithosis	Halogens
Cat-scratch fever	Contraceptives
Measles	

20. What is the most effective way to treat warts?

The mode of therapy depends on the type and number of warts, location on the body, and age of the patient. No matter what treatment is used, warts can always recur; there are no absolute cures. The major goal is to remove warts without residual scarring. Of course, a major option is no treatment at all because most warts self-resolve in 1–2 years.

Flat warts	Liquid nitrogen (lightly)
	Topical tretinoin cream
	Cantharidin, if not facial
Filiform warts	Liquid nitrogen
	Curettage and electrodesiccation

Common warts	Liquid nitrogen Cantharidin Salicylic acid preparations Curettage and electrodesiccation, if solitary
Plantar warts	Salicylic acid preparations, including 40% plaster Liquid nitrogen (gently) Cantharidin Curettage and electrodesiccation (may scar) Podophyllin (concentration and contact time can be varied)

Some dermatologists also use intralesional bleomycin for recalcitrant warts, carbon-dioxide and pulsed-dye lasers, topical formaldehyde or glutaraldehyde, and other chemical mixtures. In some case reports, oral cimetidine has been effective, perhaps due to its immunomodulatory activity.

Siegfried EC: Warts on children: An approach to therapy. Pediatr Ann 25:79–90, 1996.

21. What are the most common causes of lumps and bumps in the skin of children?

While most parents fear malignancy, nodules or tumors in the skin are very rarely malignant. A study of 775 excised and histologically-diagnosed superficial lumps in children revealed the following :

- *Epidermal inclusion cysts*—59%
- *Congenital malformations* (pilomatrixoma, lymphangioma, hemangioendothelioma, brachial cleft cyst)—17%
- *Benign neoplasms* (neural tumors, lipoma, adnexal tumors)—7%
- *Benign lesions of undetermined etiology* (xanthomas, xanthogranulomas, fibromatosis, fibroma)—6%
- *Self-limited processes* (granuloma annulare, urticaria pigmentosa, persistent insect bite reaction)—6%
- *Malignant tumors*—1.4%
- *Miscellaneous*—4%

Wyatt AJ, Hansen RC: Pediatric skin tumors. Pediatr Clin North Am 47:937-963, 2000.

Knight PJ, Reiner CB: Superficial lumps in children: What, when and why? Pediatrics 72:147,1983.

22. An eight-year-old who presents with a hard, nontender, freely mobile nodule of the neck with a slightly bluish hue of the skin about it has what likely diagnosis?

Pilomatrixoma. Also called the benign calcifying epithelioma of Malherbe, this is a benign tumor of children and adolescents of typically the face and the neck. It is usually not confused with a malignant condition and treatment is excisional for cosmetic reasons. located on the head and neck. The overlying skin frequently shows a bluish discoloration.

23. What condition classically is diagnosed by the Darier sign?

Mastocytoma. This is a benign lesion composed of mast cells that arises at birth or in early infancy. It appears as a pink/tan plaque or nodule, often with a peau d'orange surface. *Darier sign* refers to the eliciting of erythema and an urticarial wheal by stroking/rubbing the lesion. The skin changes are caused by the release of histamine from the mechanically traumatized mast cells.

24. What disorder can present as "freckles" associated with hives?

Urticaria pigmentosa (mastocytosis). Presenting at birth or early infancy, multiple mastocytomas appear as brown macules, papules or plaques (vesicle formation can also occur) and are often mistaken for freckles or melanocytic nevi. Lesions may be only cutaneous or can affect other organ systems (e.g., lungs, kidney, GI tract, central nervous system). The Darier sign is a key feature of diagnosis.

25. Is topical or systemic therapy better for impetigo?

Impetigo is a superficial skin infection caused by staphylococcus aureus or group A streptococcus. Historically, streptococcus was the most prevalent agent. However, over the last few decades, *S. aureus* appears to be the predominant organism, although mixed infections may also occur. Bullous impetigo is usually caused by *S. aureus.*

Consequently, treatment usually requires an antibiotic that is active against both streptococci and staphylococci. Topical antibiotics (mupirocin) can be used in localized disease. Systemic antibiotics are usually indicated for extensive involvement, outbreaks among household contacts, schools or athletic teams or if topical therapy has failed. Cephalosporins (e.g., cephalexin, cefadroxil), amoxicillin-clavulanate and dicloxicillin are most effective. Erythromycin may effective in some cases, but increasing numbers of staphylococci are resistant and local resistance patterns should determine its usage.

26. Should the honey-colored crusts of impetigo be soaked and removed to facilitate healing?

While local custom may say otherwise, vigorous scrubbing does not seem to help.

27. Does treatment of streptococcal skin infections prevent post-streptococcal glomerulonephritis?

No study has ever demonstrated that treatment of impetigo or pyoderma prevents renal complications in the index case. Clearly, acute rheumatic fever does not occur following the skin infections, and glomerulonephritis is limited to a few serotypes, especially 49, 55, 57, and 60, which appear to be less prevalent in recent years. However, treatment lessens the likelihood of contagious spread to other hosts who may be susceptible to renal complications.

Of note, glomerulonephritis occurs about 7–21 days after the onset of the skin infection. Serum antistreptolysin (ASO) titers, which are elevated after streptococcal pharyngeal infections, are usually not elevated following skin infections. Therefore, to confirm the diagnosis of an antecedent skin infection, antihyaluronidase (AHT) and anti-DNase B are more appropriate titers to obtain.

28. A perianal rash in a child with a sore throat is suggestive of what condition?

***Perianal streptococcal (GABHS) dermatitis*.** This should be considered in any younger infant, toddler or child who presents with rectal pain, itching or blood-streaked stools. Most do not have symptomatic pharyngitis. Physical exam may reveal tender perianal erythema, sometimes with a red, psoriasiform rash. A rectal swab for rapid antigenic detection and/or culture reveals GABHS. Throat swabs are concurrently positive in two-thirds. Treatment is similar to that for GABHS pharyngitis. Differential diagnosis includes psoriasis, seborrheic dermatitis, pinworms, candidiasis, sexual abuse and inflammatory bowel disease.

Krol AL: Perianal streptococcal dermatitis. Pediatr Dermatol 7:97-100, 1990.

29. What dermatologic sign starts from scratch?

Dermographism occurs when the skin is stroked firmly with a pointed object. The result is a *red line*, followed by an *erythematous flare*, which is eventually followed by a *wheal*. This "triple response of Lewis" usually occurs within 1–3 minutes. Dermographism (or skin writing) is an exaggerated triple response of Lewis and is seen in patients with urticaria. The tendency to be dermographic can appear at any age and may last for months to years. The cause is often unknown. White dermographism is seen in patients with an atopic diathesis, in whom the red line is replaced by a white line without a subsequent flare and wheal.

30. Do geographic tongues vary in the northern and southern hemispheres?

Despite the Hubble telescope, more research awaits. *Geographic tongue* refers to the benign condition in which denudations of the filiform papillae on the lingual surface occur, giving the tongue the appearance of a relief map. The patterns change over hours and days, and the histopathology resembles that of psoriasis. The patient is usually asymptomatic. No treatment is effective or necessary since self-resolution is the rule. Etiology in any hemisphere is unknown.

ECZEMATOUS DISORDERS

31. In the land of medicolinguistics, what is the difference between eczema and atopic dermatitis?

The term *eczema* derives from the Greek word *exzein*, to erupt—*ex* (out) plus *zein* (to boil). To most physicians, eczema is synonymous with atopic dermatitis, a chronic skin disease manifested by intermittent skin eruption. **Eczema** is primarily a morphologic term used to describe an erythematous, scaling, inflammatory eruption with itching, edema, papules, vesicles, and crusts. There are other "eczematous eruptions" (nummular eczema, allergic contact dermatitis), but "garden variety" eczema is certainly the most common.

Atopic dermatitis is a broader allergic tendency with multiple dermal manifestations mostly secondary to pruritus. Jacquet stated that atopic dermatitis is an "itch that rashes, not a rash that itches." Its manifestations are dry skin, chronic and recurrent dermatitis, low threshold to pruritus, hyperlinear palms, eyelid pleats (Dennie lines), pityriasis alba, and keratosis pilaris, among others.

32. What is the usual distribution of rash in eczema?

Infant:	Cheeks, trunk and extensor surfaces of extremities, knees and elbows
Child:	Neck, feet, and antecubital and popliteal fossae
Older child:	Neck, hands and feet, antecubital and popliteal fossae

33. Describe the five key battle plans to treat atopic dermatitis.

Atopic dermatitis is a chronic disorder for which there is no cure. (This must be explained to parents, who often expect that once their child is clear, he or she will remain clear.) Key features of therapy include:

1. ***Reduce pruritus***. It is important to break the itch-scratch cycle and to prevent new lesions from forming. Topical corticosteroids, oral antihistamines and bland emollients help reduce pruritus. Some children may need higher than the recommended doses of Atarax and Benadryl.

2. ***Hydrate the skin***. Emollients (petrolatum and unfragranced lotions and creams) prevent evaporation of moisture via occlusion and are best applied right after bathing, when the skin is maximally hydrated, to "lock-in"moisture. There us no general consensus about the appropriate frequency of bathing for children with atopic dermatitis. Some patients benefit for using humidifiers, particularly in cold climates during the winter months. If a humidifier is used, ongoing cleaning is necessary to minimize the growth of molds and other allergens that may exacerbate other allergic conditions that often coexist with atoptic dermatitis.

3. ***Reduce inflammation***. Topical steroids are invaluable as anti-inflammatory agents and can hasten clearing of eruptions that are erythematous (inflamed). Medium-strength corticosteroids can be used on areas other than the face and occluded regions (diaper area); low-strength steroids (such as 1% hydrocortisone) may be used in these thin-skinned areas. Newer immunomodulators are currently under investigation.

4. ***Control infection***. Superinfection with *Staphylococcus aureus* is extremely common. Skin can be cultured and sensitivities obtained. Erythromycin and cephalosporins are the usual antibiotics of choice for infected atopic dermatitis. Resistance to erythromycin occurs frequently.

5. ***Avoid irritants***. Gentle fragrance-free soaps and shampoos should be used; wool and tight synthetic garments should be avoided; tight non-synthetic garments may help minimize the "itchy" feeling; consider furniture, carpeting, pets, and dust mites as possible irritants and/or trigger factors.

Kristal L, Klein PA: Atopic dermatitis in infants and children: an update. Ped Clin North Am 47:877-896, 2000.

34. What role might tacrolimus play in the treatment of atopic dermatitis?

Tacrolimus (or FK506) is an immunosuppressive agent with a spectrum of activity similar to cyclosporine. In topical ointment form, it is minimally absorbed with no detectable blood levels. It has been effective in limited clinical trials.

Goguniewicz M et al: A randomized, vehicle-controlled trial of tacrolimus ointment for treatment of atopic dermatitis in children. J Allergy Clin Immunol 102:637-644, 1998.

35. Does massage therapy help children with atopic dermatitis?

It appears so. Stress and anxiety have been associated with increasing severity of dermatitis in children, possibly by alterations of the immune system. Massage may serve to lessen stress levels, increase peripheral blood supply and increase vagal activity.

Schachner L et al: Atopic dermatitis symptoms decreased in children following massage therapy. Pediatr Dermatol 15:390-395, 1998.

36. Do soaps or clothes make any difference in atopic dermatitis?

Soaps: Less drying, nondetergent soaps, such as Dove, Tone, and Caress, are better than more drying soaps such as Ivory. Other mild soaps include Cetaphil, Purpose, Aveeno, and Basis; the latter is a superfatted soap.

Clothing: Avoid woolen clothes—the fibers can irritate the skin and trigger the itch-scratch cycle. If woolens must be used, they should be lined. Soft fibers are the least irritating and itchy (cotton jerseys).

Knoell KA, Greer KE: Atopic dermatitis. Pediatr Rev 20:46-52, 1999.

37. Is there a genetic basis for atopic dermatitis?

It is likely that both genetic and environmental factors play a role. Although specific genetic information is lacking, it has been strongly suggested that an individual's genotype determines whether he or she will develop atopic dermatitis. Many children with atopic dermatitis have a family history of atopy. If one parent has an atopic diathesis, 60% of offspring will be atopic; if two parents do, 80% of children are affected. Monozygotic twins are often concordant for atopic disease.

38. Are there consistent immunologic alterations in children with atopic dermatitis?

Humoral changes include elevated IgE levels and a higher-than-normal number of positive skin tests (type I cutaneous reactions) to common environmental allergens. Cell-mediated abnormalities have been found only during acute flares of the dermatitis. These include mild to moderate depression of cell-mediated immunity, a 30–50% decrease in lymphocyte-forming E-rosettes, decreased phagocytosis of yeast cells by neutrophils, and chemotactic defects of polymorphonuclear and mononuclear cells.

39. What other skin conditions mimic atopic dermatitis?

- Seborrheic dermatitis
- Scabies
- Contact dermatitis
- Langerhans cell histiocytosis
- Xerotic eczema (dry skin)

- Immunodeficiency disorders (e.g., Wiskott-Aldrich syndrome, Hyper IgE syndrome, severe combined immunodeficiency)
- Nummular eczema
- Metabolic disorders (e.g., phenylketonuria, essential fatty acid deficiency, biotinidase deficiency)

40. In patients with atopic dermatitis, what condition causes the bumps on the cheeks, upper arms and thighs?

Keratosis pilaris. Associated both with atopic dermatitis and ichthyosis vulgaris, this condition runs in families and is asymptomatic. It is characterized by spiny follicular papules, giving involved areas a "chicken skin" or "gooseflesh" feel. Usual treatment is with bland emollients or emollients containing a mild peeling agent such as alpha hydroxy acid.

41. What features help to differentiate seborrheic from atopic dermatitis in infancy?

	SEBORRHEIC DERMATITIS	ATOPIC DERMATITIS
Color	Salmon	Pink, red (if inflamed)
Scale	Yellowish, greasy	Whiter, nongreasy
Age	Infants < 6 mos or adolescents	May begin at 2–12 mos and continue through childhood
Itching	Not present	May be severe
Distribution	Face, postauricular scalp, axillae and groin	Cheeks, trunk, and extensors of extremities
Associated features	None	Dennie pleats, allergic shiners, palmar creases
Lichenification (thickening of skin with exaggerated skin markings)	None	May be prominent
Response to topical steroids	Rapid	Slower

42. How should parents cope with cradle cap?

Seborrheic dermatitis of the scalp (or "cradle cap") in infancy presents as a yellow greasing scaling adherent rash on the scalp which may extend to the forehead, eyes, ears, eyebrows, nose, and back of head. It appears in the first few months of life and generally resolves in several weeks to a few months. Treatment includes application of mineral oil follwed by shampooing with a mild anti-dandruff shampoo containing selenium (e.g., Selsun Blue, Sebulex). A mild potency topical steroid such as hydrocortisone (1%-2.5%) may be needed for inflamed lesions. Families should be advised not to scrub or pick off the scale, as the underlying skin is often tender and inflamed.

43. What are the causes of irritant contact diaper rash?

A variety of local factors are involved. Diapers contribute to the chafing of the skin and the prevention of moisture evaporation increasing epidermal hydration and permeability to irritants. Proteolytic enzymes in urine and stool and ammonia in urine irritate chafed skin. Of note, ammonia (and urine itself) will not negatively affect intact skin. Seasoned pediatricians will advise that alcohol-based diaper wipes also feed the flames of diaper rash.

44. What features of diaper rashes suggest more sinister diseases?

- Marked tenderness, rapid onset (staphylococcal scaled skin syndrome)
- Deep ulcerations, vesicles (herpes simplex)
- Beefy red, erosive, extensive (particularly intertriginous), poorly responsive to topi-

cal steroids and antifungals (Langerhans cell histiocytosis, acrodermatitis enteropathica, immunodeficiency states)

- Extensive, severe with pungent odor (abuse or neglect with infrequent changing)

Boiko S: Making rash decisions in the diaper area. Pediatr Ann 29:50-56, 2000.

45. Are cloth diapers "better" than disposables?

There is no clear answer here, though there are parties who would swear by one or the other. Studies, however, have shown (1) a decreased incidence of diaper rash with disposable diapers, and (2) a documented decrease in skin moisture and incidence of rash with superabsorbent diapers due to decreased leakage and less alkaline pH. The adjective "better" implies a value judgment, and other factors such as cost, environmental impact, and convenience must be considered. More than 97% of the diapers used in the U.S. are of the disposable variety.

46. Are topical steroid/antifungal preparations useful for treating children with diaper dermatitis?

Most diaper dermatitis is usually diagnosed as either irritant contact dermatitis or candidal dermatitis. Irritant diaper dermatitis responds well to mild topical corticosteroids (due to their anti-inflammatory properties) and a topical barrier such as zinc oxide ointment. Candidiasis of the diaper area responds well to topical antifungal preparations; sometimes, an oral anticandidal medication is also necessary. In both types of diaper dermatitis, frequent diaper changes, exposure to air, and avoidance of excessive moisture are helpful. Combination preparations containing both antifungal and corticosteroid medications are not recommended to treat diaper dermatitis, as the strength of the steroid molecule in these products is usually too high for use in the diaper area.

Kazaks EL, Lane AT: Diaper dermatitis. Pediatr Clin North Am 47:909-920, 2000.

47. What is the differential diagnosis of dermatoses of the feet in children?

The seven wonders of the foot: (1) juvenile plantar dermatosis, (2) allergic contact dermatitis, (3) tinea pedis, (4) scabies, (5) psoriasis, (6) granuloma annulare, and (7) plantar warts.

48. Which dietary deficiencies may be associated with an eczematous dermatitis?

Zinc, biotin, essential fatty acids, histidine, and protein (kwashiorkor).

49. How does the vehicle used in a dermatologic preparation affect therapy?

In general, *acute lesions* (moist, oozing) are best treated with aqueous, drying preparations. *Chronic, dry lesions* fare better when a lubricating, moisturizing vehicle is used. As a rule, any vehicle that enhances hydration of the skin enhances percutaneous absorption of topical medications (most of which are water-soluble). Thus, in preparations of equal concentration, the potency relationship is ointment > cream > gel > lotion.

Drying vehicles

Lotion: A suspension of powder in water. Therapeutic powder remains after aqueous phase evaporates. Useful in hairy areas, particularly the scalp.

Gel: Transparent emulsion that liquifies when applied to skin. Most useful in acne preparations and tar preparations for psoriasis.

Pastes: Combination of powder (usually cornstarch) and ointment which is stiffer than ointment.

Moisturizing vehicles

Creams: Mixture of oil in a water emulsion. More useful than ointments when environmental humidity is high and in naturally occluded areas. Less greasy than ointment.

Ointments: Mixture of water in an oil emulsion. Also has an inert petroleum base. Longer lubricating effect than cream.

50. What other skin findings are associated with atopic dermatitis?

Hyperlinear palms, pityriasis alba, keratosis pilaris, ichthyosis vulgaris, lichen spinulosis, eyelid pleats (Dennie-Morgan folds).

51. What are the two main types of contact dermatitis?

Irritant and allergic. *Irritant contact dermatitis* arises when agents, such as harsh soaps, bleaches, or acids, have direct toxic effects upon contact with the skin. *Allergic contact dermatitis* is a T-cell mediated inflammatory immune reaction requiring sensitization to a specific antigen.

52. What type of agents can cause allergic contact dermatitis in children?

Allergic contact dermatitis can occur in all age groups but is often under recognized in pediatric patients. Sensitizers include plant resins (poison ivy, sumac or oak), nickel in jewelry, metal snaps and belts, topical neomycin ointment, preservatives (formaldehyde releasers) and materials used in shoes including adhesives, rubber accelerators and leather tanning agents.

53. When does the rash in poison ivy appear relative to exposure?

Poison ivy, or rhus dermatitis, is a typical delayed hypersensitivity reaction. The time between exposure and cutaneous lesions is usually ***2–4 days***. However, the eruption may appear as late as a week or more after contact (this explains why lesions continue to erupt after the initial "outbreak" of rash)

.

54. Are the vesicles in poison ivy contagious?

No. The contents of blisters do not contain the allergen. Washing the skin removes all surface oleoresin and prevents further contamination.

55. What is the "id" reaction?

Your superego will be stroked if you identify the "id" reaction in a confusing dermatologic case. This reaction is the generalization of a local inflammatory dermatitis (e.g., contact dermatitis, tinea capitis following treatment) to sites that have not been directly involved with the offending agent. The exact mechanism remains unclear, but may be immune complex–mediated.

FUNGAL INFECTIONS

56. If Serpico has serpigo, what is his disease?

In medieval times, *tinea* or a cutaneous fungal infection, particularly involving skin, hair and nails, was known as serpigo. The term is no longer used. *Tinea* is a general term used to describe a dermatophytic infection, with specific terminology based usually on location.

57. What are ways to diagnose tinea infections?

While microscopic examination of KOH preparations is employed in search of hyphae, the use of *dermatophyte test medium* is reliable, simple, inexpensive and more definitive. Samples from hair, skin or nails are obtained by scraping with a scalpel, cotton-tip applicator or toothbrush (the latter especially for tinea capitis) and inoculated directly onto the test medium. After approximately 1-2 weeks, a color change from yellow to red in the agar surrounding the dermatophyte colony indicates positivity. If the most definitive diagnosis is needed, culture on Sabouraud medium is the test of choice.

Friedlander SF et al: Use of the cotton swab method in diagnosing tinea capitis. Pediatrics 104:276-279, 1999.

58. What are the clinical presentations of tinea capitis?

Endemic in the black community in the U.S., tinea can present with *scalp scaling, "black dot" tinea, inflammation* or a *kerion*. Scalp scaling can occur without hair loss and should not be attributed to seborrheic dermatitis after infancy and before puberty. The "black dot" presentation occurs when the infected hair shaft breaks at the surface of the scalp leaving a bald patch with black dots (or lighter dots depending on hair color). Some patients will present with inflammatory papules, pustules, erythema and scaling or as a kerion (a boggy, tender mass). Regional adenopathy is very common with inflammatory tinea.

Hubbard TW: Predictive value of symptoms in diagnosing childhood tinea capitis. Arch Pediatr Adolesc Med 153:1150-1153, 1999.

59. How do the features of tinea capitis vary by cause?

Organisms Responsible for Tinea Capitis

FEATURE	*M. CANIS*	*T. TONSURANS*
Source	Cats and dogs	Other children
Fluorescence	Yellow-green	None
Contagious	Not very	Yes, very
Hair loss	Yes	Yes
Kerion	Yes	Yes
Children infected	Rural and suburban	Urban
Cinical patterns	Thickened hairs	Black-dot, dandruff-like, or multiple areas of alopecia

Adapted from Weston WL, Lane AT: Color Textbook of Pediatric Dermatology. St. Louis, Mosby, 1991, p 57; with permission.

60. Is a Wood lamp helpful in screening for tinea capitis?

In 1930, yes. In the new millennium, no. The reason is the changing epidemiology of tinea. Previously, more cases were caused by *Microsporum canis*, which is an exothrix fungus (stays on the outside of the hair shaft) and fluoresces yellow-green with Wood light. Now, more cases are caused by *Trichophyton tonsurans*, which is an endothrix fungus (invades the inner part of the hair shaft) and does not fluoresce. In certain scenarios, a Wood lamp can be helpful, but as a screening tool, it is not.

61. Why is topical therapy alone insufficient for tinea capitis?

The dermatophytes (i.e., fungi) that cause tinea can thrive deep in the hair shaft beyond the reach of topical therapy alone. Recommended therapy is a combination of oral griseofulvin (microsize or ultramicrosize preparation), which is given after milk, ice cream or a fatty meal to facilitate absorption, and biweekly shampooing with 1% or 2.5% selenium sulfide or ketoconazole shampoo to decrease the spread of spores. Of note, relative resistance by tinea to griseofulvin is being increasingly observed and higher, longer dosing may be needed to achieve clinical cure. Although newer systemic antifungals are available and have been used in selective cases, they are currently not approved for the treatment of tinea capitis in children.

Elewski BE: Tinea capitis: A current perspective. J Am Acad Dermatol 42:1-20, 2000.

62. How should children receiving griseofulvin for tinea capitis be monitored?

The incidence of hepatitis or bone marrow suppression from griseofulvin in children is rare. Children who are undergoing an acute course of treatment (6–8 weeks) do not need obligatory blood counts or LFTs. However, a history of hepatitis or its risk factors would warrant a pretreatment evaluation of liver function and intermittent monitoring. For those rare cases in which griseofulvin is going to be used for > 2 months, one should consider obtaining complete blood counts and LFTs on an every-other-month basis.

63. Is a kerion a bacterial or fungal entity?

A *kerion* is a fluctulant and tender mass that occurs in some cases of tinea capitis. Occipital or posterior cervical lymph nodes are often enlarged. A kerion is felt to be primarily an excessive inflammatory response to tinea, and thus initial treatment consists of antifungal agents, principally griseofulvin and selenium sulfide shampoo. However, bacterial cultures of kerions will demonstrate *Staphylococcus aureus* or a mixture of gram-negative bacteria in two-thirds of cases. Since most kerions resolve without antibiotics, the role of these bacteria in the pathogenesis is unclear. Short courses of oral steroids are indicated in those lesions that are exquisitely painful.

Honig PJ, Caputo GL, et al: Microbiology of kerions. J Pediatr 123:422–424, 1993.

64. What puts the "versicolor" in tinea versicolor?

A very common superficial disorder of the skin, tinea versicolor is caused by the fungus *Pityrosporum orbiculare* (formerly known as *Malassezia furfur*). It presents as multiple macules and patches, with fine scales, over the upper trunk, arms, and occasionally the face and other areas. Lesions are "versatile" in color (light tan, reddish or white) and "versatile" by season (lighter in summer and darker in winter compared with surrounding skin). The fungus interferes with melanin production, possibly by disruption of tyrosinase activity, at the involved sites. Diagnosis can be confirmed by KOH preparation of a scraping from involved skin, which has characteristic fungal hyphae and a grape-like spore pattern referred to as "spaghetti and meatball" appearance. Wood's light will also display fluorescence (yellow-brown).

65. What is the treatment for tinea versicolor?

- Selenium sulfide 2.5% lotion or 1% shampoo is the primary treatment of choice and is applied over the affected area overnight multiple times during the first week, with decreasing frequency over the ensuing weeks.
- Other topicals: 25% sodium thiosulfate (Tinver lotion), various antifungal topicals (often quite expensive)
- Oral ketoconazole and fluconazole in a single one-time dose and oral itraconazole once daily for five days are effective in adults and may be considered for use in older adolescents, although side effects may occur.

There are reports that this fungus causes central-line sepsis in neonates on hyperalimentation. So interest in this fungus isn't only skin deep.

66. After the sneaker is removed, how do you distinguish between "shoe dermatitis" and "athlete's foot"?

Allergic contact dermatitis (shoe dermatitis) involves the dorsa of the toes and distal third of the foot. The rash is red, scaly, and vesicular. KOH preparations of scrapings are negative. In ***tinea pedis*** (athlete's foot), presentations can include redness and scaling primarily on the instep or entire weight-bearing surface or ertythema and maceration between the toes, especially the third and fourth web spaces. A less common presentation is one in which vesicular lesions develop. The nails may be yellowed and thickened. The KOH preparation is positive for hyphae. Tinea pedis is very uncommon in prepubertal children.

HAIR AND NAIL ABNORMALITIES

67. How fast does hair grow?

About a centimeter per month.

68. What causes alopecia in children?

Some hair loss is due to disorders of the hair itself—follicles, sebaceous glands, growing phase, etc. Others are secondary to diseases of the scalp. A useful approach is to classify loss by pattern (diffuse vs localized) and time of presentation (congenital vs acquired):

Congenital localized
Sebaceous epidermal nevi
Melanocytic nevi
Hemangiomas
Lymphangiomas
Aplasia cutis
Incontinentia pigmenti
Focal dermal hypoplasia
Chondrodysplasia punctata
Intrauterine trauma (e.g., scalp electrodes)
Infection (e.g., herpes, gonococcal)

Congenital diffuse
Hair shaft abnormalities
Trichorrhexis nodosa
Pili torti
Trichorrhexis invaginata
(Netherton syndrome)
Menkes' syndrome
Trichoschisis
Loose anagen syndrome
Genetic syndromes
(e.g., ectodermal dysplasia)

Acquired localized
Tinea capitis
Alopecia areata
Traumatic scarring (e.g., trichotillomania)
Seborrheic dermatitis
Androgenic alopecia
Langerhans cell histiocytosis
Neonatal lupus
Acne keloidalis
Linear scleroderma

Acquired diffuse
Telogen effluvium
Anagen effluvium
Proximal trichorrhexis nodosa
Lamellar ichthyosis
Acrodermatitis enteropathica
Endocrinopathies
(e.g., hypothyroidism)

Adapted from Datloff J, Esterly NB: A system for sorting out pediatric alopecia. Contemp Pediatr 3:53–56, 1986; with permission.

69. How can alopecia areata be differentiated from tinea capitis?

In *tinea capitis* the fungal organism invades the hair shaft but is also present in the epidermis, the top layer of the skin. There are usually changes of scaling and inflammatory lesions, intermingled with black dots representing broken hairs. In *alopecia areata*, the scalp is smooth although there may be a pink discoloration. Some hairs within the patch may have a tapered appearance with the wider end distally and a thinner end at the base of the scalp (the "exclamation point hair"). There is no lymphadenopathy in alopecia areata, but this is not uncommon in tinea capitis.

70. What are poor prognostic indicators for recovery of hair in alopecia areata?

Atopy, presence of other immune disease, family history of alopecia areata, young age at onset, nail dystrophy and extensive hair loss

Madani S, Shapiro J: Alopecia areata update. J Am Acad Dermatol 42:549-566, 2000.

71. Are most hairs growing or resting?

Most infants and children have about 90% of scalp hair in the growing (anagen) and about 10% in the resting (telogen) state. On average, a single scalp hair will grow for about 3 years, rest for 3 months, and then, upon falling out, is replaced by a new growing hair.

72. What is the likely diagnosis in a child who develops diffuse hair loss 3 months after major surgery?

Telogen effluvium. This is the most common cause of diffuse acquired hair loss in children. In a healthy individual, most hairs are present in a growing (anagen) phase. After a physical or emotional stress such as a significant fever, illness, pregnancy, birth, surgery or large weight loss, a large number of scalp hairs can convert to the resting (telogen) phase.

Two to five months after the stressful event, the hair begins to shed, at times coming out in large clumps. The condition is temporary and usually does not produce more than 50% of hair loss. When the hair roots are examined there is a characteristic lighter colored root bulb characterizing a telogen hair. The hair loss can continue for 6 to 8 weeks, at which time new, short regrowing hairs should be visible.

Anagen effluvium, the loss of growing hairs, is most commonly seen during radiation and chemotherapy treatments for cancer.

73. What puzzling cause of asymmetric hair loss in a child will sometimes cause an intern to pull his or her hair out?

Trichotillomania is hair loss due to self-manipulation, such as rubbing, twirling, or pulling. Hair loss is asymmetric. The most common physical finding is *unequal hair lengths* in the same region *without evidence of epidermal changes* of the scalp. Parents often do not observe the causative behavior, and convincing them of the likely diagnosis may take some effort. Behavior modification, along with application of petroleum or oil to the hair to make pulling more difficult, is the treatment of choice. Rarely, a child will swallow the hair and develop vomiting because of the formation of a gastric trichobezoar (hairball).

74. Which dermatologic diseases are commonly associated with nail abnormalities?

Psoriasis:	Nail pitting, longitudinal ridging, onycholysis (separation of nail plate from nailbed at distal margin), thickening of the nailplate, oil spots (yellowish-red discolorations of the nailbed), yellowish-white subungual hyperkeratosis
Lichen planus:	Longitudinal grooves, rough surface, thinning of nailplate, pterygium formation, scarring and loss of nailplate
Alopecia areata:	Nail pitting, often in a grid-like pattern
Darier disease:	Red and white longitudinal streaks, breaks at distal edges resulting in V-shaped notches, wedge-shaped subungual hyperkeratosis
Atopic dermatitis:	Nail ridging (if chronic periungual inflammation)

75. How should ingrown toenails be managed?

Soaks, open-toed sandals, properly fitting shoes, topical or systemic antibiotics, incision and drainage, or surgical removal of the lateral portion of the nail may all be utilized. Control is obtained best by letting the nail grow beyond the free end of the toe. Dental floss wedged between the nail and the lateral nailfold may help to prevent the nailplate from cutting into the skin and setting up a foreign body reaction. Proper instruction on nail care, including straight rather than arc trimming, is mandatory.

76. Which pathogens are responsible for paronychia?

Acute paronychia (inflammation of the nailfold usually with abscess formation) is most commonly caused by *Staphylococcus aureus*. The proximal or lateral nailfolds become intensely erythematous and tender. If a collection of pus develops at this site, it should be incised and drained. The treatment of acute paronychia includes oral administration of antistaphylococcal antibiotics.

Chronic paronychia is caused most often by *Candida albicans* and often involves a history of chronic water exposure (e.g., dishwashing, thumbsucking). Although rarely inflamed, there is edema of the nailfolds and separation of the folds from the nailplate. The nails may become ridged and develop a yellow-green discoloration. A bacterial culture may reveal a variety of gram-positive and gram-negative organisms. Therapy includes topical antifungal agents and avoidance of water. There is no place for griseofulvin in the treatment of chronic paronychia.

77. A healthy second grader who develops progessive yellowing and increasing friability of all nails over a period of twelve months likely has what condition?

Twenty nail dystrophy (trachonychia). The progressive development of rough nails with longitudinal grooves, pitting, chipping, ridges and discoloration, occurring in isolation in school age children, has been given this name, although not all nails need be involved. The etiology remains unclear, and a majority of cases resolve spontaneously without scarring. The nail changes, however, may herald other conditions such as alopecia areata, lichen planus and psoriasis. A twenty-one gun salute will be given to the identifier of the cause of the idiopathic variety.

78. Is griseofulvin effective for treating fungal nail infections?

Griseofulvin is used less frequently for treating fungal nail infections because cure rates are very low and requires very long periods of treatment. Griseofulvin is also ineffective for treating yeasts that also cause some nail infections. When a child presents with a nail abnormality, it is important to consider dermatophytosis as well as candidal nail infections and dermatoses that present with nail findings. Newer agents including terbinifine and itraconazole are currently being evaluated for treatment of children with nail infections but are not yet approved for this indication.

INFESTATIONS

79. How do lice differ?

There are three main types of lice that infest humans, feeding primarily on human blood and causing pruritus and excoriations.

1. **Pediculosis capitis** (head lice). *Pediculus capitis*, the smallest and most common of the three human lice, is an obligate human parasite. Spread occurs directly by contact with an infected individual or indirectly through use of shared combs, brushes, or hats. For unknown reasons, infestation is nearly 35 times more likely in whites than blacks.

2. **Pediculosis corporis** (body lice). *Pediculus humanus*, the largest (2–4 mm) of the three types, is usually associated with poor hygiene. It does not live on the body but instead in the seams of clothing. It can be a vector for other diseases, such as epidemic typhus, trench fever, and relapsing fever.

3. **Pediculosis pubis** (pubic lice). *Phthirus pubis* is also known as the crab louse because it is a broad insect with legs that look like claws. It is sometimes mistaken for a brown freckle. Acquisition is primarily through sexual contact.

80. Can prepubertal children acquire pubic lice?

Though a relatively common infestation in adolescents and adults, in whom it is acquired through sexual contact, pediculosis pubis can occur in prepubertal children. Because of its predilection for hairy, nonscalp regions, the eyelashes are the most common location. The pubic louse can be transmitted via contaminated items such as towels, but its discovery on a child should raise the suspicion of sexual abuse.

81. What are the clinical findings of head lice infestation?

Scalp pruritus is most common, but many children are ***asymptomatic***. A search for lice should be made in any school-age child presenting with scalp itching. On physical examination, an actual louse (wingless, grayish insects about 3-4 mm) may be difficult to find, although one should easily be able to find nits (eggs). The nits are attached to the hair close to the surface of the scalp and are oval and flesh-colored. Those that have not hatched are not easily removed from the hair shaft (as compared with hair casts, dander and external debris). Overdiagnosis is common. Microscopic evaluation of a few hairs can confirm the diagnosis. When the louse emerges, the empty egg case, or nit, appears white in color. Nits are found in greatest density on the parietal and occipital areas. There may also be a rash present at the nape of the neck. Excoriations from scratching and secondary bacterial infections with adenopathy can occur.

One other nit note is that the female louse usually attaches the nits to the hair about 3-4 mm from the scalp. Measuring the distance of the nits from the scalp allows the approximate dating of the initiation of the infestation (with hair growth at 1 cm/month).

Pollack RJ et al: Overdiagnosis of head lice infestations in North America. Pediatr Infect Dis J 19:689-693, 2000.

82. What types of treatment are available for head lice?

- ***Permethrin***, 1% (e.g., Nix): A synthetic pyrethroid applied as a 10-minute creme rinse. It has higher residual and ovicidal activity than lindane and no risk for neurotoxicity. It is the drug of choice, although there increasing resistance to this medication has been reported in numerous countries. Repeat application in 7–10 days is strongly advised. Longer duration of application (up to a few hours) can also be considered. A 5% permethrin preparation (e.g., Elimite) may be used in patients not responding to the 1% preparation.
- ***Pyrethrins*** (e.g., RID, A-200, R&C): Natural plant extracts mixed with piperonyl butoxide. These are applied as 10-minute shampoos and have lower ovicidal activity than Nix and no residual activity. Repeat application in 7–10 days is required to kill newly hatched lice. Treatment failures are common.
- ***Malathion***, 0.5% (e.g., Ovide): Applied as an 8–12-hour lotion, it has better ovicidal activity and less toxicity than lindane. Malathion has an alcohol vehicle and a risk of flammability. If ingested, it may cause severe respiratory distress.
- ***Lindane***, 1% (e.g., Kwell): applied as a 10-minute shampoo. Ovicidal activity is low and repeat application is necessary. Resistance has been reported. If improperly used (e.g., ingestion or prolonged use), neurotoxicity is possible, especially in infants.
- ***Asphyxiants***: *petroleum jelly (Vaseline), mayonnaise, olive oil.* Left on the scalp overnight, these popular treatments attempt to suffocate the lice.
- ***Hair Clear 1,2,3:*** A combination product of Ylang Ylang, anise, coconut oil, isopropyl alcohol, rubbing alcohol.
- ***Trimethoprim-sulfamethoxazole:*** After taken orally by the patient, the antibiotic is ingested by the lice during a blood feeding and may kill symbiotic bacteria required for nutrition and reproduction.

Meinking TL, et al: Comparative efficacy of treatments for pediculosis capitis infections: update 2000. Arch Dermatol 137:287-292, 2001.

83. Should parents nit pick?

Once an infestation of lice has been properly treated, the nits are not viable or contagious. Despite this, many schools will not allow children with nits to attend, although this nit-free policy has not been shown to be of benefit in controlling outbreaks. Increasing resistance to therapy may make removal more important to avoid diagnostic confusion. Manual removal (nit picking) is the most effective method, although it is time consuming and tedious. Fine-toothed combs, especially the LiceMeister comb available through the National Pediculosis Association (www.headlice.org), aid in the removal. Commercial nit-removal solutions or soaking the hair with 3–5% acetic acid (white vinegar) and applying a towel dampened with the same solution for 30–60 minutes may loosen the attachments of nits to the hair allowing for easier removal.

84. How is a skin scraping for scabies done?

Since the highest percentage of mites are usually concentrated on the hands and feet, the web spaces between digits are the best places to look for the characteristic linear burrows. Moisten the skin with alcohol or mineral oil, scrape across the area of the burrow with a small rounded (e.g., #15) scalpel blade, and place the scrapings on a glass slide with a drop of KOH (or additional mineral oil if used) and a cover slip. Burrows, if unseen, can be more precisely localized by rubbing a washable felt-tip marker across the webspace and removing the ink with alcohol. If burrows are present, ink will penetrate through the stratum corneum and outline the site. Under the microscope, mites, eggs, and/or scybala (mite feces), may be seen.

85. What treatment eliminates the scabies' babies?

The treatment of choice for treating scabies is permethrin 5% cream (Elimite, Acticin). It may be used in children as young as two months. It is more effective than Lindane, the previously accepted treatment for scabies, and has a much lower risk of neurotoxicity . Crotamiton and sulfur are also less effective treatments. It must be stressed that all family members and close contacts should be treated simultaneously.

The cream is applied from the neck to the toes at night with removal after 8-14 hours by bathing or showering. Retreatment in 1 week may be considered. Thick crusting in debilitated and immunosuppressed individuals may protect the mites and prevent adequate therapy, so removal of these crusts is essential. Physicians must make patients aware of the fact that lesions and pruritus may linger for 1–2 weeks after effective therapy. One must be supportive during this time to prevent unnecessary retreatment by parents. Antihistamines and low potency topical steroids may help control symptoms.

86. What was the first human disease whose cause had a precise identification?

Scabies. The etiologic agent, *Sarcoptes scabiei*, was first identified in 1687. The itch for knowledge, it seems, initially was stronger than the thirst for knowledge.

NEONATAL CONDITIONS

87. What are the most common dermatologic findings in the newborn?

Sebaceous hyperplasia: multiple pinpoint yellowish papules seen in areas that have numerous sebaceous glands such as the nose, cheeks, upper lip, and forehead. These lesions resolve spontaneously.

Milia: epidermal inclusion cysts presenting as 1-2 mm white papules commonly seen on the nose, cheeks and forehead. They usually resolve within the first month.

Skin peeling: commonly seen on the ankles, feet, and hands in normal newborns. Postmature infants (>42 weeks gestation) have a more widespread peeling usually on the hands, feet, and lower trunk.

88. What is the most common birthmark?

Two varieties of birthmarks compete for this title, depending on the race of the infant.

Salmon patches (vascular stains or nevi): faint pink red, macular, patches, composed of distended dermal capillaries, found on the glabella, eyelids, and the nape of the neck. Seen in 70% of white infants and 60% of black infants. Uusually fade, but may persist indefinitely, becoming more prominent during crying.

Mongolian spots (dermal melanosis): blue-black macules found on the lumbosacral area and occasionally on shoulders and backs. Seen in 80–90% of oriental, black, and Native American babies but ≤ 10% of white infants. Most Mongolian spots fade by age 2 and disappear by age 10.

89. How concerning are pustular lesions in the newborn period?

When presented with pustules in the newborn, it is very important to rule out infectious etiologies as some may be life-threatening. The purulent material should be evaluated with a Gram stain, KOH, Tzanck preparation, and bacterial and viral cultures. A Wright stain will reveal the presence of neutrophils or eosinophils.

90. What is the differential diagnosis of vesicles or pustules in the newborn?

Noninfectious	***Infectious***
Miliaria	Candidiasis
Erythema toxicum	Staphylococcal folliculitis
Transient neonatal pustular melanosis	Herpes simplex
Infantile acropustulosis	Congenital syphilis
Incontinentia pigmenti	Varicella
Langerhans cell histiocytosis	Bacterial sepsis

From Roberts LJ: Dermatologic diseases. In McMillan JA, et al (eds): Oski's Pediatrics, Principles and Practice, 3rd ed. Philadelphia, Lippincott Williams & Wilkins, 1999, p. 376; with permission.

91. What is the significance of midline dermatologic lesions in the newborn period?

When lesions (vascular, sinusoid, nodular) are present in the midline of the scalp, face or back, there is the possibility underlying central nervous system malformations. Before any midline lesion is considered for surgical removal, appropriate imaging studies should be considered to document the true extent of the lesion.

92. Should a newborn with a sharp red line down the center of the body prompt a call to the NICU?

Not unless the caller wants to be red-faced. This is likely the ***"harlequin color"*** change, a relatively common entity seen in up to 10% of newborns, particularly premature infants. It consists of reddening of one side of the body with a sharp line of demarcation along the midline. The change occurs only when the child is lying on one side. The superior half is light, whereas the dependent half is dark and subfused. The cause is thought to be an imbalance in autonomic regulation of peripheral blood vessels. If the infant is flipped, the color pattern reverses. If the infant is placed prone or supine, the color change disappears.

93. What is the medical significance of cutis marmorata?

Cutis marmorata is the bluish mottling of the skin often seen in infants and young children exposed to low temperatures or chilling. The reticulated marbling effect is due to dilated capillaries and venules causing darkened areas on the skin. This disappears with warming. Cutis marmorata is of no medical significance and no treatment is indicated. However, persistent cutis marmorata is associated with trisomy 21, trisomy 18, and Cornelia de Lange syndromes. There is also a congenital vascular anomaly, termed cutis marmorata telangiectatic congenita, that has persistent blue reticulate mottling of the skin.

94. A healthy infant with multiple reddish nodules most likely has what entity?

Subcutaneous fat necrosis consists of sharply circumscribed, indurated nodular lesions usually seen in healthy term newborns and infants in the first few days to weeks of life. The stony hard areas of panniculitis are generally movable and slightly elevated, and the overlying skin is a reddish, violaceous color. While the cause is unknown, it is thought that obstetric trauma and pressure on bony prominences may contribute to the problem. The usual sites (cheeks, back, buttocks, arms, and thighs) are consistent with this. Histologically, the lesions display extensive inflammation in the subcutaneous tissue with large fat lobules. Most lesions are self-limiting and require no therapy. However, occasionally they may extensively calcify and spontaneously drain with subsequent scarring. Remember that significant hypercalcemia may be present in a small number of patients. Therefore, a serum calcium should be ordered whenever the disorder is suspected and rechecked periodically until the condition resolves.

95. What should the family of a newborn with a yellow, cobblestoned, hairless patch be advised to do?

The lesion is likely a ***nevus sebaceous***. This hamartomatous neoplasm presents usually as a yellow- pink hairless plaque on the scalp (or face) at the time of birth and is composed primarily of malformed sebaceous glands. Under the influence of androgens at puberty, the glands may hypertrophy and lead to the development of other neoplasms (e.g., basal cell carcinoma). The risk of neoplastic (usually benign) development is 10-15%. Some experts advise excision in the pre-teen, prepubertal years. Careful monitoring of the lesion (for new growths or nonhealing ulcerations) at all ages is advised, especially in adolescence.

96. What is the long-term outcome for the collodion baby?

A *collodion baby* is the term used to describe babies born encased in a translucent membrane (like saran-wrap). Generally, this membrane heralds ichthyosis. Two-thirds of affected infants develop lamellar ichthyosis or, less frequently, X-linked ichthyosis, epidermolytic hyperkeratosis, Netherton syndrome, or Conradi syndrome. However, many infants with collodion membranes also end up with normal skin.

97. Cutis aplasia of the scalp is commonly associated with which chromosomal abnormality?

Aplasia cutis congenita (congenital absence of the skin) presents on the scalp as solitary or multiple well-demarcated ulcerations or atrophic scars. Of variable depth, the lesions may be limited to epidermis and upper dermis or occasionally extend to the skull and dura. While most children with this lesion are normal without multiple anomalies, other associations include epidermolysis bullosa, placental infarcts, teratogens, sebaceous nevi and limb anomalies. Scalp cutis aplasia has been classically associated with ***trisomy 13 syndrome.***

98. What is the "hair collar" sign?

This is a scalp finding in some infants with aplasia cutis congenita consisting of a thin, translucent glistening membrane with a ring of hypertrichosis, usually midline. When it is associated with an exophytic nodule, it is suggestive of cranial dystraphism.

99. What is the appearance and distribution of transient neonatal pustular melanosis?

Consisting of small vesicopustular lesions, 3–4 mm in size, *transient pustular melanosis* occurs in almost 5% of black and < 1% of white newborns. It may be present at birth or appear shortly after birth. The lesions most often cluster on the neck, chin, palms, and soles, although they may occur on the face and trunk. The pustules rupture easily and re progress to brown pigmented macules with a fine collarette of scale. Microscopic examination of the contents of the pustules reveals neutrophils with no organisms. There are no associated systemic manifestations and the eruption is self-limited, although the hyperpigmentation may last for months.

100. Is erythema toxicum neonatorum really toxic?

Not in the least. *Erythema toxicum* is a common eruption composed of erythematous macules, papules, and pustules occurring in newborns usually in the first few days of life. The lesions may start as irregular, blotchy, red macules, varying in size from millimeters to several centimeters. They often develop into 1–3-mm, yellow-white papules and pustules on an erythematous base, giving a "flea-bitten" appearance. They occur all over the body except on the palms and soles, which are spared because the lesions occur in pilosebaceous follicles, which are absent on the palmar and plantar surfaces. The rash is less common in premature infants, with incidence proportional to gestational age and peaking at 41–42 weeks. While it may be seen at birth, it is most common in the first 3–4 days of life and is occasionally noted as late as 10 days of life. Erythema toxicum usually lasts 5–7 days and heals without pigmentation. Other than the rash, the newborn appears healthy.

101. How is the diagnosis of erythema toxicum confirmed?

Erythema toxicum is often confused with a variety of other skin disorders, including impetigo neonatorum, herpes simplex, transient neonatal pustular melanosis, milia, and miliaria. The diagnosis can be confirmed by staining the contents of a pustule with Wright or Giemsa stain. Clusters of eosinophils confirm the presence of erythema toxicum.

102. How are the most common neonatal papular lesions distinguished?

	NEONATAL ACNE	MILIA	ERYTHEMA TOXICUM
Distribution	Face	Face +	Face +
Appearance	Papule or pustule	Yellow or white papule	Yellow or white papule
Erythematous	+	–	+
Contents on smear	PMNs	Keratin + sebaceous material	Eosinophils
Incidence	Occasional	40–50% of term infant	30–50% of term infants
Course	Last several months	Disappear in 3–4 wks	Disappear in 2 wks

PMN, polymorphonuclear cells.

103. For academic purposes (and ICD-9-CM coding), is it possible to be more scientific about the diagnosis of "prickly heat"?

The scientific name for this condition is *miliaria rubra*. It is due to sweat retention, and its clinical morphology is determined by the level at which sweat is trapped. Sweat trapped at a superficial level produces clear vesicles without surrounding erythema (*sudamina or crystallina*); miliaria rubra (prickly heat, erythematous papules, vesicles, papulovesicles) is produced by sweat trapped at a deeper level; pustular lesions (*miliaria pustulosa*) and even abscesses (*miliaria profunda*) are produced with sweat retention at the deepest of levels (infants rarely develop these types). With the advent of air conditioning, miliaria rarely occurs in newborn nurseries.

PAPULOSQUAMOUS DISORDERS

104. What diseases are associated with the Koebner reaction?

Koebnerization is a response to local injury whereby skin lesions are found at the sites of trauma (e.g.. linear lesions at the sites of scratching). This is seen in *psoriasis* as well as in other conditions such as *lichen planus* and *flat warts*.

105. A skin scale that easily bleeds on removal is characteristic of what condition?

The appearance of punctate bleeding points after removal of a scale is the *Auspitz sign*. It is seen primarily in ***psoriasis*** and is related to the rupture of capillaries high in the papillary dermis near the skin surface.

106. What is the typical pattern of lesions in childhood psoriasis?

Psoriasis presents as well-circumscribed, erythematous plaques with overlying white scale in children and adults. These occur on the *scalp*, *elbows*, *knees*, *sacrum* and *genitalia*. Psoriasis may also present with guttate (drop-like) lesions over the trunk and extremities.

These children may have group A beta hemolytic streptococcus infection as an underlying precipitating factor.

107. What percentage of children with psoriasis have nail involvement?

Nail changes, most commonly with pitting, may be the only manifestation of psoriasis. Approximately ***80%*** of children with psoriasis demonstrate pitting of the nails. Other nail changes include onycholysis (separation of the nailplate from nailbed at distal margin) and thickening of the nailplate, often with white-yellow discoloration. Subungual debris may occur.

108. Which joints are classically involved in psoriatic arthritis?

The ***distal interphalangeal joints*** of the hands and feet. Juvenile psoriatic arthritis (in patients < 16 years old) often presents as an acute monoarthritis. Joint changes often precede the skin changes. Psoriatic arthritis is more common in patients who have severe psoriasis. Flares are unrelated to the skin condition. Uveitis may also complicate the disease.

109. What are treatment modalities for psoriasis?

Various therapies have been used to treat psoriasis. The choice of treatment will depend upon the extent of involvement, previous treatments and the age of the patient. Topical treatments include topical corticosteroids, calcipotriene (a vitamin D analog), retinoids and tar. Other treatment modalities include UVA/UVB phototherapy and, rarely, systemic retinoids and methotrexate.

110. Why are systemic corticosteroids contraindicated in childhood psoriasis?

Following the discontinuation of the steroids, erythroderma or pustular psoriasis may result. Fever and hypoalbuminemia can also occur.

111. What are the 8 Ps of lichen planus?

Papules—usually 2–6 mm in diameter, which often are seen linearly due to the Koebner reaction

Plaques—commonly generated from a confluence of papules with exaggerated surface markings of the overlying skin (Wickham striae)

Planar—individual lesions, usually flat-topped

Purple—distinctly violaceous

Pruritus—often intensely itchy

Polygonal—borders of papules are often angulated

Penis—common site of involvement in children

Persistent—chronic with remissions and exacerbations up to 18 months

112. How is pityriasis rosea distinguished from secondary syphilis?

Often with difficulty. Both are primarily papulosquamous rashes. *Pityriasis rosea* classically consists of oval lesions which organize in parallel fashion on the trunk (the "Christmas tree" distribution) and are preceded in 40–80% of cases by a large annular erythematous lesion (herald patch). *Secondary syphilis* lesions occur 3–6 weeks after the chancre, and in comparison to pityriasis rosea, they have more involvement of the palms, soles, and mucous membranes and have accompanying lymphadenopathy. However, because atypical presentations are common, testing for syphilis should be considered in any sexually active individual who is diagnosed with pityriasis rosea.

113. What is the treatment for pityriasis rosea?

A wide range of treatments are used: dapsone, ketotifen, sunlight/UV light. In a recent clinical study, erythromycin has been shown to be beneficial.

Sharma PK et al: Erythromycin in pityriasis rosea: A double-blind, placebo-controlled clinical trial. J Am Acad Dermatol 42:241-244, 2000.

PHOTODERMATOLOGY

114. Why is limiting excessive sun exposure in children important?

Most people receive 80% of their lifetime sun exposure before age of 18. Years of unprotected sun exposure will lead to freckling, wrinkling and skin cancer formation, including melanoma. In an era of rising rates of melanoma (lifetime risk of 1:75), squamous and basal cell carcinomas, use of sun protection strategies (e.g., sunscreens) during the pediatric years could lower the risk to an individual by 80%. Broad-spectrum sunscreens may attenuate the number of nevi in white children, especially if they have freckles.

Gallagher RP et al: Broad-spectrum sunscreen use and the development of new nevi in white children: A randomized clinical trial. JAMA 283:2955-2960, 2000.

115. What are good strategies for protection against sun exposure?

- Avoid sun if possible during peak hours (10 AM-3 PM) or seek shade
- Apply sunscreen at least 30 minutes before sun exposure
- Use a broad spectrum sunscreen of at least SPF 30
- Apply liberal amounts of sunscreen (2 mg/body cm or about 30 ml for an adult, 15 ml for a 7-year-old)
- Wear protective clothing, hats and sunglasses

116. What types of sunscreens are available?

Physical sunscreens are composed of zinc oxide or titanium dioxide and function by scattering ultraviolet light. Although they are opaque, newer micronized preparations are easier to apply and more acceptable to patients. *Chemical sunscreens* absorb either ultraviolet A (UVA) or ultraviolet B (UVB) light. Most commercially available sunscreens are combinations of various agents. In order for sunscreens to function well they must be applied on all exposed surfaces in adequate quantities and reapplied throughout the day.

117. How is the SPF of a sunscreen determined?

SPF is the *"sun protection factor."* It measures the effectiveness of a sunscreen to protect against ultraviolet B light. It is not a measurement of ultraviolet A protection. It is a ratio of the dose of ultraviolet light needed to produce minimal redness on sun protected skin to the dose of ultraviolet light need to produce minimal redness on unprotected skin. Ergo, an SPF of 15 means a person can spend 15 times longer in the sun without burning.

118. Should sunscreens be avoided in infants?

This is controversial. There are concerns that the skin of infants less than six months has different absorptive characteristics and that biologic systems that metabolize and excrete drugs may not be fully developed. However, there is no evidence that the limited use of sunscreen in infants is problematic. Physical protection (e.g., clothing, hats, shade and *sunglasses*) is most ideal, but if an infant's skin is not adequately protected, it may be reasonable to apply sunscreen to small areas, such as the face and the back of the hands.

Committee on Environmental Health: Ultraviolet light: A hazard to children. Pediatrics 104:328-333, 1999.

119. Which "lime" disease is not transmitted by ticks?

Limes contain psoralens that react with ultraviolet light and can produce erythema, vesicles and/or hyperpigmentation on areas of the skin that have come in contact with lime juice. This is known as *phytophotodermatitis* and is seen with other psoralen-containing plants, such as celery and figs. Additionally, berloque dermatitis (*berloque* is French for pendant, which some lesions can resemble) is an irregularly patterned hyperpigmentation of the neck due to photosensitization by furocoumarins (i.e., psoralens) in perfumes. It is caused by fragrances that contain oil of bergamot, an extract from the peel of an orange grown in southern France and Italy. Oil of bergamot contains 5-methoxypsoralen, which enhances the erythematous and pigmentary response of UVA light.

120. Which conditions are associated with marked sun sensitivity?

Inherited disorders: porphyrias, xeroderma pigmentosum, Bloom syndrome, Rothmund-Thomson syndrome, Hartnup disorder

Exogenous agents: drug-induced (e.g.tetracyclines, thiazides), photoallergic contact dermatitis (associated with PABA esters, perfumes)

Systemic disease: lupus erythematosus, dermatomyositis

Idiopathic disorders: polymorphous light eruption, solar urticaria, actinic prurigo, hydroa vacciniforme

Garzon MC, DeLeo VA: Photosensitivity in the pediatric patient. Curr Opin Pediatr 9:377-387,1997.

121. What is the appearance of polymorphous light eruption (PMLE)?

The most common pediatric photodermatosis, PMLE is characterized by itchy red papules, plaques or papulovesicles that appear several hours to days after UV light exposure. It can be diagnosed by phototesting (induction of lesions by intentional UV light exposure) and by skin biopsy. It is usually suggested by the classic history and exclusion of other photosensitivity disease.

122. Are steroids effective in the treatment of severe sunburn?

Steroids may be useful in treating severe sunburn. A short course of prednisone (1–2 mg/kg/day) with tapering after 4–8 days may abort severe sunburn reactions and provide relief.

123. Is a child with sun sensitivity protected by sitting behind a window?

Yes and no, depending on the reason for the sensitivity. UV light is divided into 3 wavelength groups: UVC (200–290 nm), UVB (290–320 nm), and UVA (320–400 nm). UVC light is cytotoxic and can cause retinal injury, but fortunately it is almost completely absorbed by the ozone layer. UVB light causes sunburn, dermatologic flares (e.g., in patients with lupus erythematosus), and with chronic exposure, skin cancer. UVA light (which is also emitted from the fluorescent lamps used in most schools) is responsible for psoralen and drug phototoxicity and porphyria flares. Windows block UVB light, but not UVA. Thus, children with the latter kinds of disorders would not be protected.

PIGMENTATION DISORDERS

124. What disorders of childhood are associated with areas of hypopigmentation?

Hypopigmentation is caused by a decrease, not total absence, of pigmentation or melanin Conditions that feature hypopigmented lesions include tuberous sclerosis, tinea versicolor, pityriasis alba, hypomelanosis of Ito, leprosy, and postinflammatory hypopigmentation.

125. Is treatment helpful in children with postinflammatory hypopigmentation?

In children with pityriasis alba (postinflammatory hypopigmentation associated with atopic dermatitis), low potency topical steroids and careful sun exposure (controversial) can make skin color more uniform. Treatment does not seem to help in other cases of postinflammatory hypopigmentation, such as following infection, abrasions or burns.

126. What treatments are available for vitiligo?

Vitiligo is a disorder of depigmentation (total absence of pigmentation). The etiology is unknown but may be autoimmune in nature. There are rare associations with other autoimmune conditions including thyroiditis and juvenile onset diabetes. Treatment is often unsatisfactory. Potent topical steroids have been used for localized areas. Ultraviolet light therapy has been employed for some children with severe extensive disease. Dyes (including self-tanning agents) and coverage cosmetics are often helpful to camouflage skin lesions.

127. What conditions are associated with albinism?

Albinism constitutes a number of clinical syndromes characterized by disorders of melanin synthesis that may affect the skin, hair and eyes. *Localized (partial) albinism* or piebaldism is congenital depigmentation of the skin often with a white forelock of hair, caused by a genetic mutation that differs from generalized albinism. Localized congenital depigmentation associated with congenital deafness characterizes Waardenburg syndrome. *Generalized (oculocutaneous) albinism* is often complicated by ocular abnormalities including visual impairment, photophobia and nystagmus.

128. What are the metabolic causes of hyperpigmentation?

- Hepatobiliary disorders
- Hemochromatosis
- Addison disease
- Hyperthyroidism
- Hypothyroidism
- Acromegaly
- Cushing syndrome
- Heavy metals (silver, gold, mercury)
- Drugs (thorazine, antimalarials)
- Fixed drug eruptions (phenolphthalein, barbitu rates, busulfan, cyclophosphamide, aspirin, phenacetin, phenytoin, gold, arsenic, trimeto-prim-sulfamethoxazole, tetracycline)
- Porphyria cutanea tarda, variegate porphyria
- Gaucher disease
- Niemann-Pick disease
- B_{12} deficiency
- Wilson disease
- Hyperparathyroidism

129. What is the likely diagnosis if a patient taking trimethoprim-sulfamethoxasole develops an erythematous, sharply marginated, round lesion which leaves an area of hyperpigmentation upon resolution?

Fixed drug eruption. These 2-10 cm plaques, soliatary or multiple, are red to violaceous inflammatory reactions that occur following medication ingestion, commonly antibiotics, especially trimethoprim-sulfamethoxazole and tetracycline. The are commonly mistaken for urticaria or erythema multiforme. The resultant hyperpigmentation helps to make the distinction.

Morelli JG et al: Fixed drug eruptions in children. J Pediatr 134:365-367, 1999.

130. Why are Spitz nevi and malignant melanoma often confused?

The *Spitz nevus* can appear suddenly and grow rapidly. Histologically, it has many pleomorphic cells and mitotic figures which can be mistaken for malignancy. It actually was previously referred to as benign juvenile melanoma. Benign is the key word for this red to brown, dome-shaped papule, which usually appears on the face or extremity. Because malignant melanoma is rare in children, beware of the misdiagnosed Spitz nevus.

131. What are the clinical features of familial dysplastic nevus syndrome?

The syndrome, also known as the familial atypical mole syndrome (FAMS), is the term used for families who have acquired nevi that develop into melanoma. These nevi are 5–15 mm in diameter and are round to oval in shape. Furthermore, they have irregular and indistinct margins, exhibit variation in color within the same lesion, and have both macular and elevated components. They tend to occur in sun-protected areas.

132. In children with pigmented nevi, what factors increase the risk of melanoma?

Melanoma is rare during childhood. If there is a family history of melanoma or atypical moles, history of severe sunburns before age 18 or the child has a giant congenital nevus, the risk is greater. Estimated risks vary for different sized congenital nevi. The projected lifetime risk for a melanoma developing in a small congenital nevus is 0.02%; for a giant nevus, 2–3%. Acquired nevi very rarely develop melanomas.

Ceballos PI, et al: Melanoma in children. N Engl J Med 332:656–662, 1995.

133. What is the differential diagnosis of yellow-brown or orange nodules in children?

- Nevus sebaceous
- Juvenile xanthogranuloma (JXG)
- Solitary mastocytoma
- Urticartia pigmentosa
- Benign cephalic histiocytosis
- Langerhans cell histiocytosis
- Spitz nevus
- Connective tissue nevus

134. What are the characteristic findings of urticaria pigmentosa?

The characteristic lesions are red-brown, brown, yellow-brown, or yellow macules, papules, plaques, or nodules that have rippled surface (peau d'orange). The lesions are oval or round and frequently are mistaken for pigmented nevi or xanthoma. They vary in size from several millimeters to many centimeters. They occur on any portion of the skin surface but tend to concentrate on the trunk. The diagnosis is clinched by stroking the lesion, a maneuver which causes degranulation of the collection of mast cells, release of histamine, and urtication (Darier sign).

VASCULAR DYSPLASIAS

135. Describe the life history of hemangiomas.

Hemangiomas are common benign vascular tumors. They are rarely fully developed at birth, but precursor lesions (an area of pallor, telangiectasia, or "bruise") may be detected on close inspection within the first few days of life. They may have superficial (capillary) and/or deep (cavernous) components. Hemangiomas undergo a growth phase until age 6-12 months, at which time they start to involute. This process of involution occurs over several years at a rate of approximately 10% resolution each year. There still may be residual skin changes (e.g. skin redundancy, pallor, atrophy, telangiectasia) after the hemangioma has resolved. As 90-95% resolve spontaneously, it is important to avoid the temptation of plastic surgery, cryotherapy, radiation therapy, or sclerosing agents, which can hasten resolution but lead to a higher likelihood of scarring.

Drolet BA, Esterly Frieden IJ: Hemangiomas in children. N Engl J Med 341:173-181, 1999.

136. What are the major goals in the management of hemangiomas?

The decision regarding which hemangiomas require treatment and the best therapeutic modality may not always be an easy one. The major goals of management are:

- Prevent or reverse life-threatening or function-threatening complications
- Treatment of ulcerated hemangiomas
- Prevent permanent disfigurement caused by a rapidly enlarging lesion
- Minimize psychosocial stress for the family and patient
- Avoid overly aggressive procedures that may result in scarring in lesions that have a good likelihood of involuting without significant residual lesions

137. Which hemangiomas are especially worrisome?

- *Multiple cutaneous hemangiomas*—may be associated with visceral hemangiomas (e.g., liver)
- *Large hemangiomas*—may cause significant disfigurement of underlying structures and may be associated with congestive heart failure

- *"Beard" hemangiomas*—may be a marker for underlying laryngeal or subglottic hemangioma that may impair respiratory function
- *Midline spinal hemangiomas*—may be a marker underlying spinal cord abnormality
- *Head/neck hemangiomas*- usually larger lesions, may be associated with other congenital anomalies including CNS, cardiac, and ocular defects (e.g., PHACE syndrome).
- *Vulnerable anatomic locations*—impair vital functions, cause disfigurement, (e.g. periocular, neck, lip, nasal tip)
- *Ulcerated hemangiomas*—increased risk of suprainfection, cause pain and lead to scarring.

Metry DW, Hebert AA: Benign cutaneous vascular tumors of infancy: When to worry, what to do. Arch Dermatol 136:905-914, 2000.

138. When are systemic corticosteroids indicated in the treatment of cavernous or capillary hemangiomas?

While the approach to palpable hemangiomas generally involves observation over time, indications for systemic corticosteroids (prednisone, 2–4 mg/kg/day, tapered over 2–4 months) include:

- Kasabach-Merritt syndrome with severe persistent thrombocytopenia (e.g., 40,000 platelet/mm^3)
- Lesions that interfere with normal physiologic functioning (breathing, hearing, eating, vision), especially periocular hemangiomas (to prevent ambylopia)
- Recurrent bleeding, ulceration, or infection
- A rapidly growing lesion that distorts facial features
- High-output congestive heart failure

Wahrman JE, Honig PJ: Hemangiomas. Pediatr Rev 15:266–271, 1994.

139. If intralesional or systemic steroids have failed as options for hemangiomas requiring treatment, what else may be of benefit?

- ***Pulsed dye laser:*** May be used with other modalities; minimal scarring, but limited penetration (2 mm) restricts use to superficial lesions.
- ***Interferon (alpha):*** Used subcutaneously, it may act by blocking endothelial cell motility and inhibit angiogenesis.
- ***Chemotherapeutic agents (cyclophosphamide, vincristine):*** Usually used for life-threatening hemangiomas with failure of other modalities.
- ***Embolization***
- ***Surgery***

140. Why is an infant with a hemangioma and new-onset thrombocytopenia so worrisome?

This can indicate the development of the ***Kasabach-Merritt syndrome*** *(or phenomenon),* a life-threatening condition of rapidly enlarging vascular tumors and progressive coagulopathy. Platelets are sequestered within the lesion(s), forming thrombi and consuming coagulation factors. Ecchymoses may develop initially around the hemangioma, but a disseminated coagulopathy with microangiopathic hemolytic anemia can result. Aggressive therapy (systemic steroids, alpha-interferon, and surgery) is frequently needed.

Recent evidence suggests that the features seen in this syndrome are not usually seen with the common hemangiomas of infancy, but rather with rare vascular tumors (Kaposiform hemangioendothelioma and tufted angioma).

141. How do strawberry hemangiomas differ from port-wine stains?

Strawberry hemangiomas are superficial, palpable, vascular nevi that usually involute with time. *Port-wine stains,* sometimes called nevus flammeus or salmon patches, are flat vascular malformations that do not involute.

Strawberry hemangiomas	***Port-wine stains***
Palpable	Flat, macular
Common (up to 10% in children age < 1)	Less common (0.1–0.3%)
Often inapparent at birth (more visible at 2–52 wks)	Present at birth
Bright red	Pale pink to blue-red (darkens with age)
Well-defined borders	Borders variable
Predilection for head and neck (40–60%)	May be anywhere but increased percentage on head and face
Pathology: proliferating angioblastic endothelial cells with variable blood-filled capillaries	Pathology: dermal capillary dilation
90–95% involute spontaneously by age 9	No involution: may worsen with darkening and hypertrophy
Rapid growth phase	Proportionate growth (as child grows)
Suggested therapy: watchful waiting active treatment for some lesions	Suggested therapy: flash lamp pulsed-dye laser in children

VESICOBULLOUS DISORDERS

142. What is the Nikolsky sign?

This sign demonstrates "epidermal fragility."

When pressure is applied to
a blister, it enlarges laterally.
This is seen in epidermal
blistering diseases such as
pemphigus vulgaris and
scalded skin syndrome.

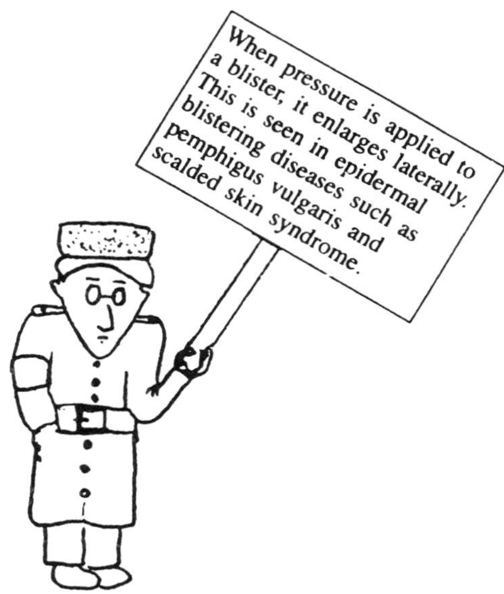

143. What are causes of skin blistering in childhood?

Infectious:	Bacterial-bullous impetigo, staphylococcal scalded skin syndrome Viral-HSV, varicella
Contact dermatitis:	Poison ivy, phytophotodermatitis

Inherited disorders:	Epidermolysis bullosa, bullous congenital ichthyosiform erythroderma
Autoimmune disorders:	Linear IgA disease, bullous pemphigoid, pemphigus vulgaris
Other:	Erythema multiforme, toxic epidermal necrolysis, thermal injury (burns)

144. How is staphylococcal scalded skin syndrome (SSSS) differentiated from toxic epidermal necrolysis (TEN)?

Both are diffuse bullous diseases. *SSSS* commonly arises in young children less than five years of age and develops after a localized staphylococcal infection with diffuse cutaneous disease caused by an exfoliative toxin. *TEN* is felt to be a hypersensitivity reaction (often to a drug), perhaps representing the most severe end of the spectrum of erythema multiforme, and occurs in all age groups.

Differentiation between SSSS and TEN

	SSSS	TEN
Etiology	Infectious; group II staphylococci	Immunologic; usually drug related
Morbidity/mortality	Low	High
Mucous membrane involvement	Rare	Frequent
Nikolsky sign	Present	Absent
Target Lesions	Absent	Often present
Level of blister	Upper epidermis (below stratum corneum)	Subepidermal
Histopathology	No epidermal necrosis or dermal Inflammation	Full thickness epidermal necrosis; prominent perivascular dermal inflammation

Adapted from Roberts LJ: Dermatologic diseases. In McMillan JA, et al (eds): Oski's Pediatrics, Principles and Practice, 3rd ed. Philadelphia, Lippincott Williams & Wilkins, 1999, p. 379; with permission.

145. What is epidermolysis bullosa (EB)?

Epidermolysis bullosa is a heterogeneous group of inherited disorders characterized by blister formation, either spontaneously or at sites of trauma. There are three general categories of EB: simplex, junctional and dystrophic. The extent of blistering and degree of scarring roughly correlates to the level of blister formation in the epidermis or dermis.

146. What should be considered in an individual who develops EB later in life?

This disorder is very similar to the inherited form of EB. It is seen first during adolescence or adulthood. Immunoelectron microscopy localizes the immune deposits below the basement membrane. Therefore the split is in a location similar to the dominantly inherited *dystrophic* form of EB. These patients blister following trauma. Scarring, milia formation, and nail dystrophy occur. Other diseases associated with acquired EB and thought to be possible precipitants include: amyloidosis, dermatitis herpetiformis, Ehlers-Danlos syndrome, impetigo, ingestions (arsenic, penicillamine, sulfonamides), inflammatory bowel disease, poison oak, porphyria, scarlet fever, and tuberculosis.

147. How might neonatal foreskin be involved in a potential major advance in the treatment of epidermolysis bullosa?

Apligraf is a tissue-engineered bilayered human skin equivalent which has been developed from keratinocytes of neonatal foreskin. These cells are allowed to differentiate *in* vitro and simulate a normal epidermis. They are supported by an underlying artificial dermis of bovine collagen impregnated with human fibroblasts. Apligraf is believed to be immunologically inert because it does not contain Langerhans cells, endothelial cells and certain cell surface cell surface markers. It has been approved for venous ulcers and acute wounds and has shown promise as an epidermal replacement therapy in EB. A true cure will require gene therapy.

Falabella AF et al: Tissue-engineered skin (Apligraf) in the healing of patients with epidermolysis bullosa wounds. Arch Dermatol 136:1225-1230, 2000.

148. What distinguishes erythema multiforme major versus minor?

Erythema multiforme (EM) is a hypersensitivity reaction that develops most commonly as a response to infection or drugs. It is characterized by target lesions, which are round lesions with dusky centers as a result of epidermal necrosis. These lesions typically last longer than one week. This helps distinguish them from urticaria, where individual lesions resolve within 24 hours of onset. EM is divided into minor and major variants, depending on the extent of skin and mucosal involvement. If the condition has minimal mucosal or cutaneous denudation, it is *minor*. Widespread mucosal involvement, including ocular surfaces, and large surface desquamation connote *major*. Cutaneous erythema multiforme lesions and involvement of two or more mucosal surfaces may be termed Stevens-Johnson syndrome.

149. Is steroid therapy beneficial in the treatment of Stevens-Johnson syndrome or toxic epidermal necrolysis?

A continuing area of controversy. Studies are inconclusive. Treatment may be considered early in the course of illness in a toxic patient if multiple mucosal surfaces are involved, but skin denudation is limited. The potential for steroids to increase medical complications (e.g., hemorrhage, infection) must be taken into account. If initiated, clinical response (or lack thereof) should be carefully followed and steroids discontinued if no benefits are accruing. Since the majority of cases will spontaneously resolve, other therapies are vital: skin care, nutritional support, ophthalmologic care and treatment of secondary bacterial infections.

Leaute-Labreze C, et al: Diagnosis, classification and management of erythema multiforme and Steven-Johnson syndrome. Arch Dis Child 83:347-352, 2000.

150. What infectious agent is most commonly associated with recurrent EM minor?

Herpes simplex virus infection.

151. What disease should be considered if a child has chickenpox that is not resolving?

Pityriasis lichenoides. This describes a spectrum of disease comprised of both acute and chronic forms. Erythematous papules and vesicles often with necrotic centers characterize *pityriasis lichenoides et varioliformis acuta* (PLEVA) or Mucha-Habermann disease. (Generally speaking, the longer the name assigned to a particular dermatologic entity, the less likely a clear etiology has been established.) This is the form that is most commonly misdiagnosed as chickenpox (or impetigo, vasculitis, or scabies). Diagnosis is by biopsy. The chronic form, *pityriasis lichenoides chronica* (PLC), may be preceded by the acute form or characterized by red/brown scaly papules without the necrotic lesions seen in PLEVA. Both forms may respond to treatment with oral erythromycin or ultraviolet light.

5. EMERGENCY MEDICINE

Steve Miller, M.D., *Meri Sonnett,* M.D., *Fred Henretig,* M.D.,
Jane M. *Lavelle,* M.D., *and Mark* F. *Ditmar,* M.D.

CHILD ABUSE AND SEXUAL ABUSE

1. What is the most common cause of severe closed head trauma in infants < 1 year of age?

Shaken impact or shaken baby syndrome. Remember, this injury is more likely to occur from severe shaking and impact, hence the dual terminology. Violent shaking of an infant with sudden impact can result in subdural hematomas, subarachnoid hemorrhages, and cerebral infarcts. The diagnosis is suggested by the lack of a corroborating mechanism of injury in the face of a symptomatic child, or rarely, a confession by the perpetrator. Physical exam reveals retinal hemorrhages in many cases. Other signs of trauma are usually lacking. Diagnosis is confirmed by CT or MRI scanning. If a lumbar puncture is performed, the fluid may be bloody or xanthochromic. The prognosis is grim for an infant presenting in coma from this abuse: 50% die and nearly half of the survivors have significant neurologic sequelae.

2. What important historical and physical findings are indicators of child abuse?

Historical

- Multiple previous hospital visits for injuries
- History of untreated injuries
- Cause of trauma not known or inappropriate for age or activity
- Delay in seeking medical attention
- History incompatible with injury findings
- Parents unconcerned about injury or more concerned about unrelated minor problem (e.g., cold, headache)
- History of abused siblings
- Lack of detail regarding events preceding injury
- Premature or problem child
- Changing or inconsistent stories to explain injury
- No consistent primary care giver

Physical examination

- Signs of general neglect, poor hygiene, or failure to thrive
- Withdrawn or explosive personality
- Burns, especially cigarette, or immersion burns on buttocks or perineum
- Genital trauma or sexually transmitted infection
- Signs of excessive corporal punishment (welts, belt or cord marks, bites)
- Frenulum lacerations in young infants (associated with forced feeding)
- Multiple lesions in various stages of resolution
- Neurologic injury associated with retinal or scleral hemorrhages
- Fractures suggestive of abuse
- Old injuries, fractures, burns or bruises

Kottmeier P:The battered child. Pediatr Ann 16:343–351, 1987.
Fontana V: The maltreatment syndrome of children. Pediatr Ann 13:740, 1984.

3. A 2-month-old brought in full cardiac arrest following a seizure is later found to have retinal hemorrhages. What is the likelihood the hemorrhages are secondary to seizures or chest compressions from resuscitative efforts?

Unlikely, although this remains controversial. In a prospective study of inpatient hospital pediatric arrests, only one of 43 patients was found to have acute retinal hemorrhages. These were multiple punctate hemorrhages, which differ from the larger hemorrhages seen in patients with shaken impact syndrome. In addition, this patient was thrombocytopenic and had undergone prolonged cardiac chest massage. Other studies involving seizures have found no associated retinal findings. Therefore, the finding of retinal hemorrhages should make one highly suspicious of non- accidental trauma.

Odom A et al: Prevalence of retinal hemorrhages in pediatric patients after in-hospital cardiopulmonary resuscitation: a prospective study. Pediatrics 99:e3, 1997.

Tyagi AK et al: Can convulsions alone cause retinal haemorrhages in infants? Br J Ophthalmol 62:659-660, 1998.

4. When should child abuse be considered in the event of an unexplained death of a child?

Always. Sudden infant death syndrome (SIDS) should be a diagnosis of exclusion in any unexplained death. Deaths due to SIDS usually occur in the first year of life, most commonly (90%) in children less than 7 months of age. All children who die suddenly of unclear causes should have a complete physical exam looking for signs of external trauma such as bruises, injury to the genitalia, as well as an ophthalmologic exam looking for retinal hemorrhages.

5. What are the causes of sudden and unexpected deaths (SUDS) in infancy?

Sudden infant death syndrome (SIDS) accounts for about 85%-90% of cases. As the incidence of SIDS has been falling since more infants began sleeping in the supine position, the percentage of non-SIDS deaths has increased. In a 10-year study of 669 infants in Quebec, other causes included: infection (7%), cardiovascular disease (2.7%), child abuse or neglect (2.6%) and metabolic diseases or genetic disorders (2.1%). The percentage of non-SIDS cases was significantly higher in ages atypical for SIDS: <1 month and > 6 months of age.

Cote A et al: Sudden unexpected death in infants: What are the causes? J Pediatr 135:437-443, 1999.

American Academy of Pediatrics, Committee on Child Abuse and Neglect: Distinguishing sudden infant death syndrome from child abuse fatalities. Pediatrics 94:124-126, 1994.

6. Which conditions with ecchymoses can be mistaken for child abuse?

Mongolian spot (dermal melanosis): Commonly mistaken for bruises, especially when they occur elsewhere than the classic lumbosacral area; unlike bruises they do not fade with time.

Coagulation disorders: In 20% of cases of hemophilia, there is no family history of disease; bruising may be noted on unusual places in response to minor trauma.

Folk medicine: Southeast Asian practices of spoon rubbing (*quat sha*) or coin rubbing (*cao gio*) can produce ecchymoses; practice of cupping (inversion of heated cup on back) produces circular ecchymoses.

Moxibustion: Southeast Asian practice of burning an herbal substance on the child's abdomen to cure disease.

Neuroblastoma: May present with unilateral or bilateral periorbital ecchymoses.

Ehlers-Danlos: Marked blood vessel fragility with easy bruising; suspect diagnosis if skin is very hyperextensible and joints are hypermobile.

Infectious/Inflammatory: Multiple entities (such as erythema multiforme, Henoch-Schönlein purpura, meningococcemia) usually have other clinical features.

Dyes: Clothing dyes, especially from jeans, sometimes mimic bruising; are easily removed by topical alcohol.

7. How do the color changes in an ecchymosis progress?

Visual aging of bruises is an inexact science with significant variability. Bruises on the face or genitalia heal more quickly than bruises on other parts of the body as there is increased blood supply to these regions. In general, the better the blood supply and the more superficial the wound, the faster it will heal. It takes roughly 5-7 days for a bruise to become greenish yellow. The following table should only be used as a guideline.

0–1 day	Red/blue	*8–10 days*	Yellow/brown
1–5 days	Blue/purple	*1.5–4 weeks*	Resolution
5–7 days	Green/yellow		

Schwartz AJ, Ricci LR: How accurately can bruises be aged in abused children? Literature review and synthesis. Pediatrics 97:254–257, 1996.

8. How are fractures dated radiographically in children?

Following a fracture:

1–7 days	Soft-tissue swelling; fat and fascial planes blurred; sharp fracture line
7–14 days	Periosteal new bone formation as soft callus forms; blurring of fracture line; occurs earlier for infants, later for older children
14–21 days	More clearly defined (i.e., hard) callus forming as periosteal bone converts to lamellar bone
21–42 days	Peak of hard callus formation
≥ 60 days	Remodeling of bone begins with reshaping of deformity (up to 1–2 years)

If the timing of an injury does not correlate with the dating of a fracture, or if fractures at multiple stages of healing are present, child abuse should be suspected.

9. What fractures are suggestive of child abuse?

Spinal fractures, posterior and anterior rib fractures, skull fractures, metaphyseal chip fractures, and vertebral, femoral, pelvic, or scapular fractures. These are fractures that commonly result from twisting (spiral fractures), throwing, and beating. Metaphyseal chip fractures are the result of the forceful jerking of an extremity. Anterior and posterior rib fractures occur with severe side-to-side compression of the thorax. They are almost never caused by CPR! The description and forcefulness of injury should be consistent with the fracture. One should be especially suspicious if such fractures occur in a child not yet walking.

Wissow LS: Child abuse and neglect. N Engl J Med 332:1425–1431, 1995.

10. What constitutes the "skeletal survey"?

Skeletal injuries, particularly multiple healed lesions, are strong indicators of a pattern of abuse, particularly in the absence of sufficient clinical evidence to justify such a diagnosis. The skeletal survey is a multiple-imaging series that includes anteroposterior (AP), posteroanterior (PA) and other views of:

1. *Appendicular skeleton:* humeri (AP views), forearms (AP), hands (oblique PA views), femurs (AP), lower legs (AP), feet (AP)
2. *Axial skeleton:* thorax (AP and lateral), pelvis (AP, including mid and lower lumbar spine), lumbar spine (lateral), cervical spine (lateral), skull (frontal and lateral)

"Body grams" (studies that encompass the entire child in 1 or 2 exposures) are not felt to be of sufficient sensivity to be useful. Of note, if abuse is highly suspected and the initial study is normal, a follow-up series in two weeks will increase the diagnostic yield.

Section on Radiology. American Academy of Pediatrics: Diagnostic imaging of child abuse. Pediatrics 105:1345-48, 2000.

11. When are burn injuries suspicious for child abuse?

Burn injuries account for about 5% of cases of physical abuse. As with other injuries, the description of the incident causing the burn should be consistent with the child's development and the extent and degree of the burn observed. The following types are suspicious for abuse:

Immersion burns: Sharply demarcated lines on the hands and feet ("stocking glove" distribution), buttocks, and perineum with a uniform depth of burn; the immersion of a child in a hot bath is a classic example.

Geographic burns: Burns usually of second or third degree in a distinct pattern, such as circular cigarette burns or steam iron burns.

Splash burns: Pattern with droplet marks projecting away from the most involved area. Splash marks on the backside of the body usually require another person and may or may not be accidental.

12. How do you recognize Munchausen syndrome by proxy?

In this form of child abuse, adults inflict illness on a child or falsify symptoms in order to obtain medical care for a child. Features include:

- Recurrent episodes of a confusing medical picture
- Multiple diagnostic evaluations at medical centers ("doctor shopping")
- Unsupportive marital relationship, often with maternal isolation
- Compliant, cooperative, overinvolved mother
- Higher level of parental medical knowledge
- Parental history of extensive medical treatment or illness
- Conditions resolve with surveillance of child in hospital
- Findings correlate to presence of the parent

Ludwig S: Child abuse. In Fleisher GR, Ludwig S (eds): Textbook of Pediatric Emergency Medicine, 4th ed. Baltimore, Lippincott Williams & Wilkins, 2000, p 1679.

13. How often is sexual abuse committed by an individual known previously by the child or adolescent?

75–80%. Relatives are the perpetrators in 50% of cases.

14. Following documentation of history and a careful physical exam, what evidence should be collected in suspected sexual abuse or assault of a postpubertal female?

If suspected history of sexual contact, loss of consciousness, or poor history:

1. ***Evidence of sexually transmitted disease*** (STD)
   - Gonococcal cultures of pharynx, vagina or cervix, and rectum
   - Chlamydial cultures of pharynx, vagina or urethra, and rectum
   - RPR or VDRL test for syphilis; if positive, confirm with specific antibody testing
   - Other studies for STDs if clinically suspected
2. ***Pregnancy testing*** if postmenarchal
3. ***Evidence of sexual contact***, including 2–3 swabbed specimens from each area of assault for:
   - Sperm (motile/nonmotile)
   - Acid phosphatase (secreted by prostate and a component of seminal plasma)
   - P_{30} (prostate glycoprotein present in seminal fluid)
   - Blood group antigens
4. ***Evidence to document perpetrator***
   - Foreign material on clothing
   - Suspected nonpatient hairs
   - DNA testing (controversial)

15. What options should be offered to a postpubertal female following a sexual assault involving vaginal penetration?

After a negative pregnancy test, the following issues should be discussed:

1. *Gonococcal prophylaxis*: Especially if abuse occurring less than 48 hours prior to evaluation (due to organism incubating and potential for false negative cultures).
2. *HIV testing/prophylaxis*: Consensus guidelines do not exist regarding HIV testing and post-exposure prophylaxis and must be individualized depending on a variety of factors (e.g., extent of sexual contact, status of perpetrator, parental wishes). Prophylaxis is not indicated if >72 hours has passed since the known exposure.
3. *Pregnancy prophylaxis*: Oral contraceptives (e.g, Ovral, 2 tablets x 2 given 12 hours apart) within 72 hours of the sexual contact.

16. How long does forensic evidence of sexual abuse persist after contact?

	Type of Evidence			
SITE	MOTILE SPERM	NONMOTILE SPERM	ACID PHOSPHATASE	P 30
Pharynx	0.5–6 hrs	6 hrs (?)	6 hrs (?)	Unknown
Rectum	0.5–8 hrs	24 hrs	24 hrs (?)	Unknown
Vagina	0.5–8 hrs	7–48 hrs	12–48 hrs	12–48 hrs
Clothing	< 0.5 hr	Up to 12 mos	Up to 3 yrs	Up to 12 yrs

Of note, lack of cervical mucus in prepubertal girls decreases survival of motile sperm and the utility of body swabbing in prepubertal girls is very low after 24 hours. Data are very limited on pharyngeal persistence of nonmotile sperm and pharyngeal and rectal persistence of acid phosphatase. Both acid phosphatase and P_{30} can persist indefinitely on clothing if it is kept dry and not washed.

From Reece RM: Child Abuse: Medical Diagnosis and Management. Philadelphia, Lea & Febiger, 1994, p 234; with permission.

Christian CW et al: Forensic evidence findings in prepubertal victims of sexual assault. Pediatrics 106:100-104, 2000.

17. What is the best predictor of *Neisseria gonorrhoeae* infection in children aged < 12 years examined for sexual abuse?

Vaginal or ***urethral discharge***. Without evidence of discharge, the likelihood of a culture result being positive is near zero.

Sicoli RA, et al: Indications for Neisseria gonorrhoeae cultures in children with suspected sexual abuse. Arch Pediatr Adolesc Med 149:86–89, 1995.

18. If a patient is diagnosed with an infection caused by an STD-associated organism, how likely is sexual abuse the reason for acquisition?

ORGANISM	INCUBATION	SEXUAL ABUSE
Neisseria gonorrhoeae	2–7 days	Certain
Treponema pallidum (syphilis)	10–90 days (avg 3 wks)	Certain
Chlamydia trachomatis	Variable (min 1 wk)	Probable
Trichomonas vaginalis	4–20 days (avg 1 wk)	Probable
Herpes simplex virus, type II	2–14 days	Probable
Human papillomavirus (condylomata accuminatum)	Unknown; may range from 3 mos to several years	Possible
Hepatitis B	45–160 days (avg 120 days)	Possible
Herpes simplex virus, type I (genital location)	2–12 days	Possible
HIV	Variable (months to years)	Possible
Bacterial vaginosis (nonspecific vaginosis or *Gardnerella*-associated vaginosis)	Unknown	Uncertain
Ureaplasma urealyticum	10–20 days	Uncertain
Candida albican	Unknown	Unlikely

All of these organisms can be acquired perinatally, complicating the diagnosis of sexual abuse in infants. As infants grow to prepubertal children, newly diagnosed acquisition of these organisms makes sexual abuse more likely.

American Academy of Pediatrics: Sexually transmitted diseases. In Pickering LK (ed): 2000 Red Book, 25th ed. Elk Grove Village, IL, American Academy of Pediatrics, 2000, p143.

Committee on Child Abuse and Neglect: Guidelines for the evaluation of sexual abuse in children. Pediatrics 87:254–260, 1991.

19. Is the size of the hymenal opening an important finding in the diagnosis of sexual abuse?

The hymenal opening is measured with a child in the supine, frog-leg position, and various studies have attempted to determine a size which most likely correlates with sexual abuse. The ranges have been from 4–10 mm, but variations in technique, positioning, and relative relaxation of the patient have limited the value of absolute numbers. In addition, there is considerable overlap in diameter between sexually abused and nonabused girls. Thus, the size of the hymenal opening has been deemphasized as a diagnostic or confirmatory test, particularly as an isolated finding. More important in the exam is inspection for scarring and tears of the hymen and surrounding tissues. Recent studies have reexamined the concept of hymenal size as a screening tool for abuse.

Pugno PA: Genital findings in prepubertal girls evaluated for sexual abuse: A different perspective on hymenal measurements. Arch Fam Med 8:403-406, 1999

Heger A, Emans SJ: Introital diameter as the criteria for sexual abuse. Pediatrics 85:222–223, 1990.

20. What is the most common finding on physical exam of a child who has been sexually abused?

A ***normal physical exam*** is the most common physical finding. It is crucial to know that a normal physical exam does not rule out sexual abuse.

ENVIRONMENTAL EMERGENCIES

21. How do fresh and salt water drownings differ?

Fresh water injures the lung primarily by disrupting surfactant, leading to alveolar collapse. Damage to the alveolar membranes leads to transudation of fluid into the air spaces and pulmonary edema. *Salt water* pulls fluid into the air spaces directly by creating a strong osmotic gradient, and the accumulated water washes away surfactant leading to alveolar collapse. By either mechanism, patients develop ventilation-perfusion mismatch and hypoxemia which may require agressive mechanical support. Severe pulmonary involvement may be evident during initial resuscitation. Other children may initially have normal lung exams, chest x-rays and blood gases, but develop pulmonary edema and progressive respiratory failure over the ensuing 12 to 24 hours.

22. What is the effect of water temperature on drowning victims?

Hypothermia is common in submersion victims, because water conducts heat away from the body 32 times more effectively than air. At normal temperature, anoxia causes irreversible damage to the brain after approximately 5 minutes. Hypothermia can protect the brain against the effects of prolonged hypoxia. In one study, children in full cardiopulmonary arrest after drowning had a uniformly dismal neurological outcome (death or persistent vegetative state) if their temperature was greater than 33ºC, while four of fourteen children in full arrest whose temperature was less than 33ºC survived neurologically intact. Hypothermia will develop more rapidly and thus protect more effectively in smaller children with proportionally larger surface areas, in colder water submersions and when the child struggles vigorously or swallows large amounts of water.

Biggart M, Bohn D: Effect of hypothermia and cardiac arrest on outcome of near-drowning accidents in children. J Pediatr 117:179-183, 1990.

23. What cardiovascular changes occur as body temperature falls?

31–32° C: Elevated HR, cardiac output, and blood pressure; peripheral vasoconstriction and increased central vascular volume; normal ECG

31–28° C: Diminished HR, cardiac output, and blood pressure; ECG irregularities include PVCs, supraventricular dysrhythmias, atrial fibrillation, and T-wave inversion

< 28° C: Severe myocardial irritability; ventricular fibrillation, usually refractory to electrical defibrillation; often absent pulse or blood pressure; J waves on ECG

24. How should CPR be modified in the hypothermic patient?

The myocardium becomes very irritable below 30° C, and even mild stimulation can provoke ventricular fibrillation. On the other hand, due to drastically slowed metabolic rates, very slow but perfusing rhythms are better-tolerated in hypothermic patients. Therefore it is advised that chest compressions be performed only for truly pulselsess patients. If ventricular fibrillation does occur, it will often be unresponsive to usual defibrillation until the core temperature rises above 30° C. Medications generally used in cardiopulmonary resuscitation, such as atropine and lidocaine, will often be ineffective as long as the patient remains profoundly hypothermic. Due to decreased metabolism, they may accumulate to toxic levels if given in multiple doses to a hypothermic patient. Patients with profound hypothermia may appear clinically dead with absent pulse and respirations and unreactive pupils and yet may still be successfully resuscitated with little or no lasting neurological impairment. Resuscitative efforts should usually continue until the temperature has risen to 36° C ("no one is dead until warm and dead").

25. What are the hazards of externally rewarming a hypothermic patient too rapidly?

- ***Core temperature "afterdrop"***—External rewarming causes peripheral vasodilation and return of cold venous blood to the core.
- ***Hypotension***—Peripheral vasodilation increases total vascular space. Furthermore, hypothermia is often a hypovolemic state because of cold-induced diuresis and cold-induced renal tubular and concentrating dysfunction in the setting of depressed myocardial function.
- ***Acidosis***—Lactic acid returns from the periphery, resulting in rewarming acidosis.
- ***Dysrhythmias***—Rewarming alters acid-base and electrolyte status in the setting of an irritable myocardium.

26. What are acceptable rewarming methods for the hypothermic child?

For mild hypothermia (32-35° C) passive rewarming by removing cold clothing and placing the patient in a warm, dry environment with blankets is generally sufficient. Active external rewarming involves the use of heating blankets, hot water bottles, overhead warmers, etc. Patients should be given warmed, humidified oxygen by facemask or endotracheal tube. More aggressive core rewarming techniques include gastric or colonic irrigation with warm fluids, peritoneal dialysis, pleural lavage, and extracorporeal blood rewarming with partial bypass. Intravenous and other fluids should be heated to 43(C.

27. Should the Heimlich maneuver be done as the first step in near-drowning resuscitation?

No. The Heimlich maneuver has no demonstrable effect in removing water from the lung or improving oxygenation. Because of laryngospasm, relatively small amounts of water are aspirated into the victim's lungs during drowning. Asphyxia results from cessation of respiration and obliteration of surfactant activity. The Heimlich maneuver may even be counterproductive. During the panic stage of drowning, the victim typically swallows a significant amount of water. Abdominal thrusts may cause regurgitation and complicate airway management.

28. What systems malfunction in heatstroke?

Heatstroke is a medical emergency of multisystem dysfunction caused by very high fever (usually > 41.5° C). Profound *CNS* disturbance—confusion, seizures, loss of consciousness—is the hallmark of the condition. Other problems include (1) *hypotension* due to volume depletion, peripheral vasodilation, and myocardial dysfunction; (2) *acute tubular necrosis* and *renal failure* with marked electrolyte abnormalities; (3) *hepatocellular injury* and dysfunction; (4) *abnormal hemostasis*, often with signs of disseminated intravascular coagulation; and (5) *rhabdomyolysis*.

29. What is the "critical thermal maximum"?

42° C. This is the body temperature at which cell death begins as physiologic processes unravel. Enzymes denature, lipid membranes liquefy, mitochondria misfire, and protein production fails.

30. Discuss the important considerations in the pulmonary and airway management of children with suspected smoke inhalation.

1. *How extensive are the signs of smoke inhalation?* Physical exam may reveal carbonaceous sputum, singed nasal hairs, facial burns, or pulmonary abnormalities. These make development of pneumonia more likely.

2. *Are there symptoms/ signs of impending airway obstruction due to mucosal injury and edema?* These include hoarseness, stridor, increasing respiratory distress and difficulty handling secretions. If present (along with PE signs as noted above), the airway should be directly visualized by bronchoscopy or laryngoscopy. If significant swelling, erythema or blistering is seen, intubation should be performed electively to protect the airway from progressive obstruction.

3. *Are there signs of carbon monoxide poisoning and tissue hypoxia?* Possibilities include headache, confusion, irritability, visual changes, and other CNS abnormality. Their presence warrants aggressive oxygen therapy, including consideration of hyperbaric oxygen if available.

31. Which laboratory studies are needed in suspected carbon monoxide poisoning?

- ***Blood carboxyhemoglobin*** (HbCO) level

0–1%	Normal (smokers may have up to 5–10%)
10–30%	Headache, exercise-induced dyspnea, confusion
30–50%	Severe headache, nausea, vomiting, increased HR and respirations, visual disturbances, memory loss, ataxia
50–70%	Convulsions, coma, severe cardiorespiratory compromise
> 70%	Usually fatal

- ***Hemoglobin level***—to evaluate correctable anemia
- ***Arterial pH***—to elevate acidosis
- ***Urinalysis*** for myoglobin—Patients with CO poisoning are susceptible to tissue and muscle breakdown with possible acute renal failure resulting from renal deposition of myoglobin.

32. What are the key aspects in treatment of CO poisoning in children?

- ***Very close monitoring***
- ***100% oxygen*** until HbCO falls to 5%. The half-life of HbCO is 4 hours if the patient is breathing room (at sea level), 1 hour in 100% oxygen (at sea level), and < 1 hour in a hyperbaric oxygen chamber with 100% oxygen.
- ***Correct metabolic acidosis***, especially when pH< 7.2. Although correcting the acidosis shifts the oxyhemoglobin dissociation curve to the left (theoretically decreasing oxygen delivery to the tissues), a blood pH < 7.2 can compromise cardiac performance.

- Refer for use of ***hyperbaric oxygen*** if: (a) history of coma, seizure, or abnormal mental status at the scene or in the emergency department; (b) persistent metabolic acidosis; (c) neonate; (d) pregnant woman; or (e) HbCO level > 25%, even if the patient is neurologically intact.

33. Why is carbon monoxide such a deadly toxin?

- It is odorless and invisible and can overwhelm a patient without warning.
- It is a product of partial combustion of nearly all fossil fuels, so it is ubiquitous in daily living, ranging from running cars to heating homes to barbecuing with charcoal.
- Often misdiagnosed as flu-type illness because of subacute presentation of headache, dizziness, and malaise.
- Nearly irreversible binding to hemoglobin (with affinity 200–300 times that of oxygen) which shifts the oxyhemoglobin dissociation curve to the left and changes its shape from sigmoidal to hyperbolic (with greatly diminished O_2 tissue release).
- Strong binding to other heme-containing proteins, particularly in the mitochondria, leading to metabolic acidosis and cellular dysfunction (especially cardiac and CNS tissues).

34. If a victim of smoke inhalation has a severe and persistent metabolic acidosis despite therapy, what diagnosis should be suspected?

Cyanide poisoning. Hydrogen cyanide (HCN) gas results from the thermal decomposition of nitrogen-containing materials (e.g., polyurethane, silk, plastics). The short half-life of HCN (approximately 1 hour) can make the diagnosis difficult. In one study, elevated blood lactate levels = 10 mmol/L correlated with toxic levels of blood cyanide when no other causes of acidosis existed. Many authorities recommend routine treatment for possible cyanide toxicity with sodium thiosulfate during the initial resuscitation of a fire victim. If the patient remains critically ill with coma, seizure, acidemia, and elevated lactate levels, treatment with sodium nitrate should be considered. Although this treatment detoxifies cyanide, it does result in the formation of methemoglobin, which decreases the O_2-carrying capacity of hemoglobin.

Baud FJ, et al: Elevated blood cyanide concentrations in victims of smoke inhalation. N Engl J Med 325:1761–1766, 1991.

35. What are the different degrees of burn injuries?

Classification of Burn Wounds

DEGREE	DEPTH	INCHES	CLINICAL APPEARANCE	CAUSE
1°	Epidermis	0.002	Dry, erythematous	Sunburn, scald
2°	Superficial dermis	0.02	Blisters, moist, erythematous	Scald, immersion, contact
	Deep dermis	0.035	White eschar	Grease, flash fire
3°	Subcutaneous	0.040	Avascular—white or dark, dry, waxy (yellow)	Prolonged immersion, flame, contact, grease, oil
4°	Muscle		Charred, skin surface cracked	Flame

From Coren CV: Burn injuries in children. Pediatr Ann 16:328-339, 1987.

Alternatively, burns can be described as either superficial (first degree), partial (second degree) or full thickness (third and fourth degree).

36. How does the "rule of nines" apply in children?

The "rule of nines" is a device to estimate the extent of burns. For example, in adults, the entire arm is 9% of total body surface area (TBSA), the front of the leg is another 9%, etc. The resulting estimate of the extent of burns is particularly helpful in calculating fluid requirements. Correction for age is necessary with this formula because of differing body proportions. Of note, the surface of a patient's palm represents about 1% of TBSA.

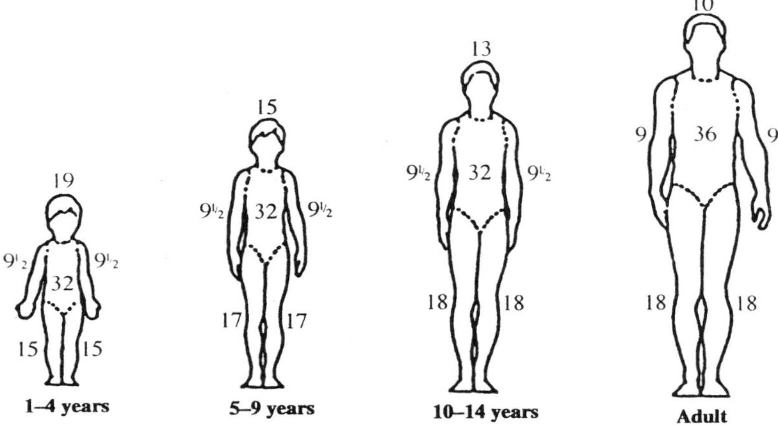

From Carajal HF: Burn injuries. In Behrman RE, et al (eds): Nelson Textbook of Pediatrics, 14th ed. Philadelphia, W.B. Saunders, 1992, p 235; with permission.

37. Which burn injuries are indications for hospitalization?

- Second-degree burns covering > 10% of BSA
- Third-degree burns covering > 2% of BSA
- Significant burns involving hands, feet, face, joints or perineum
- Self-inflicted burns
- Burns resulting from suspected child abuse
- Electrical burns
- Circumferential burns (which may predispose to vascular compromise)
- Explosion, inhalation, or chemical burns (where other organ trauma may be involved)
- Significant burns in children with chronic metabolic or connective tissue diseases (in whom healing may be compromised with the increased risk of secondary infection)
- Significant burns in children younger than age 2 years

Rodgers GL: Reducing the toll of childhood burns. Contemp Pediatr 17:152-173, 2000.

38. How is the Parkland formula utilized in the fluid management of children with burns?

Burns jeopardize the intravascular volume status of children in several ways: (a) direct surface loss from burned area, (b) edema froom increased capillary permeability and leakage of oncotically-active proteins, and (c) release of mediators which can cause third-spacing. Some of these mediators may also depress cardiac function and hamper the body's ability to compensate for a decreased intravascular volume. For all these reasons, burn victims require aggressive fluid resuscitation.

The Parkland formula is a commonly used method for estimating the fluid requirements of burn victims. It recommends giving 4 mL/kg of crystalloid per % body surface area affected over the first 24 hours, in addition to usual maintenance requirements. The first half of the additional fluid is provided over the first 8 hours and the remainder over the next 16. This and other similar formulas are only initial fluid estimates. It is essential to monitor urine output and other signs of intravascular volume, sometimes including invasive intravascular monitoring.

39. Why are alkali burns worse than acid burns of the eye?

Alkali burns are caused by lye, such as in Drano or Liquid Plumber, or by lime, or ammonia among others. They are characterized by *liquefaction necrosis*. They are worse than acid burns because the damage is ongoing. When spilled in the eye, *acid* is quickly buffered by tissue and limited in penetration by precipitated proteins; *coagulation necrosis* results, which is usually limited to the area of contact. Alkali, however, has a more rapid and deeper advancement, causing progressive damage at the cellular level by combining with membrane lipids. This underscores the importance of extended irrigation of the eyes, particularly in alkali burns.

40. How do the injuries produced by lightning and high-voltage wires differ?

Lightning consists of direct current (DC) of extremely high voltage (200,000 to 2 billion volts) delivered over milliseconds. In contrast, high-voltage wires deliver alternating current (AC) of lower voltage (rarely exceeding 70,000 V) over a longer period of time. *Lightning* exposure causes massive electrical countershock with asystole, respiratory arrest, and minimal tissue damage. *High-voltage* exposure causes ventricular fibrillation and deep tissue injury. Resultant muscle necrosis can lead to substantial myoglobin release and renal failure.

41. In electrical injury, is AC or DC more hazardous?

At low voltages, such as those found in household electrical devices, alternating current is more dangerous than direct. Exposure to *AC* can provoke tetanic muscle contractions, so that the victim who has grasped an electrical source is unable to let go, prolonging the exposure and producing greater tissue injury. Direct current or high-voltage *AC* typically cause, a single forceful muscular contraction that will push or throw the victim away from the source.

42. If a toddler suffers a full-thickness burn to the corner of the mouth after biting on an electrical cord, what complications are possible?

Severe burns of the oral commissure can become markedly edematous within the first several hours. An eschar develops at the site, which can detach with significant bleeding from the labial artery 1 to 3 weeks later. Scarring can be extensive, and plastic surgeons should be consulted early in the management of this kind of injury.

43. What agents are the most common causes of anaphylaxis seen in U.S. emergency rooms?

Food. *Peanuts, tree nuts* (e.g., almonds, hazelnuts) and *seafood* head the list and are twice as common as bee stings as a trigger. Severe reactions occur 1-2 hours after exposure. Anaphylaxis may occur without a skin reaction, so a high index of suspicion is needed in a child with unexplained, sudden bronchospasm, laryngospasm, severe GI symptoms or poor responsiveness. In some adolescents, certain foods (e.g., wheat, celery, shellfish), if ingested within 4 hours of exercise, can lead to food-dependent, exercise-induced anaphylaxis. Risk factors for fatal anaphylactic reactions: *history of asthma, delayed diagnosis, delayed administration of epinephrine.*

Sampson HA: Fatal food-induced anaphylaxis. Allergy 53S:125, 1998.

44. How does one distinguish between poisonous and nonpoisonous snakes?

Preferably by turning the pages of *National Geographic*. North America has 41 groups of snakes, but nearly all of poisonous bites are caused by four groups: rattlesnakes, moccasins, copperheads, and coral snakes. Distinguishing features include:

- Elliptical and vertically oriented pupils (in moccasins and copperheads) compared with round pupils (in nonpoisonous snakes)
- Curved fangs that can fold against the palate

- Triangular head contrasted with more oval-shaped head of harmless snakes
- Bodies are more stout and sausage-like compared with slender bodies of harmless snakes
- Distal tail scales arranged in a single row compared to the double-row scales of non-venomous snakes
- Coral snakes with rings of yellow, red, and black with the red always touching the yellow but never the black. As the herpetologists sing: "Red touch yellow—kill a fellow/ Red touch black, a poison lack."

Roever JM: Snake Secrets. New York, Walker & Company, 1979, pp 39–43.

LACERATIONS

45. What telephone advise should be given regarding transport of an avulsed digit?

Wrap the severed piece in a dry gauze (sterile if possible). Place the wrapped piece in a small, sealed plastic bag to minimize contact with water. Place this bag in a container filled with ice. It is incorrect to place the avulsed piece in any liquid, as this causes tissue swelling. Direct contact with ice is to be avoided to prevent tissue necrosis.

46. Which eyelid lacerations warrant ophthalmologic evaluation?

- Full-thickness lacerations
- Lacerations involving the lid margin
- Deep lower-lid lacerations that may involve damage to the tear-drainage system
- Ptosis of the involved lid
- Significant tissue avulsion
- Associated eyeball injury

Levin AV: Eye trauma. In Fleisher GR, Ludwig S (eds): Textbook of Pediatric Emergency Medicine, 4th ed. Baltimore, Lippincott Williams &Wilkins, 2000, p 1403.

47. Which lacerations should be repaired by a surgeon?

- Large complex lacerations
- Stellate or flap lacerations
- Lacerations with questions of tissue viability
- Lacerations involving lip margins (vermilion border)
- Deep lacerations with nerve or tendon damage
- Lacerations that evoke intention tremors in the medical house officer

48. How many days should sutures remain in place?

Blood supply dictates healing, the more the better. In general, as the site of laceration proceeds, from head to toe, the length of time of suture placement increases: *eyelids*—3 days; *face*—5 days; *trunk and upper extremities*—7 days; and *lower extremities*—10 days.

49. When should a nerve injury be suspected in a finger laceration?

- ***Abnormal testing of sensation*** (diminished pain or two-point discrimination)
- ***Abnormal autonomic function*** (absence of sweat or lack of skin wrinkling after soaking in water)
- ***Diminished range of motion of finger*** (may also indicate joint, bone, or tendon disruption)
- ***Pulsating blood emerging from wound*** (on flexor aspect, nerve is superficial to digital artery and arterial flow implies nerve damage)

50. What should be done if nerve damage is suspected?

For injuries to major nerves, such as the brachial plexus, immediate consultation is necessary. If the digital nerve is injured, immediate repair is not essential, and this is not a true emergency. Delayed nerve repair is very satisfactory, particularly in younger children. If an operating suite and personnel are not poised to proceed, skin closure can be done and the operation deferred (after surgical consultation). Care must be taken not to stop the arterial bleeding with a hemostat or other clamp, as this may further damage the nerve. Simple pressure, often for extended periods, generally suffices.

51. Which lacerations should not be sutured?

Lacerations at high risk for infection should be considered for healing by secondary intention or delayed primary closure. As a general rule, these include *cosmetically unimportant puncture* wounds, *puncture wounds*, *human bites,* lacerations involving *mucosal surfaces* (e.g., mouth, vagina), and wounds with a *high probability of contamination* (e.g., acquired in a garbage bin). Many authorities in the past recommended that wounds untreated for more than 6-12 hours on the arms and legs and 12-24 hours to the face not be sutured. However, the type of wound and risk for infection are more important than any absolute time criterion. For example, a non-contaminated laceration to the face should be considered for suturing even 24 hours after the injury.

52. Dog bites or cat bites: which are at greater risk for infection?

Generally, infection rates are ***higher in cat bites*** because of the greater likelihood of a puncture wound rather than a laceration injury. Additionally, *Pasteurella multocida*, the most common pathogen responsible for infection, is present in higher concentrations in cat bites. Wounds caused by cat and dog bites usually contain multiple other organisms, including *Staphylococcus aureus, Moraxella, Streptococcus, Neisseria* species. and anaerobes.

Talon DA, et al: Bacteriologic analysis of infected dog and cat bites. N Engl J Med 340:85-92 1999.

53. Should antibiotic prophylaxis be given for dog, cat, and human bites?

This is a controversial topic. Studies indictate that antibiotic prophylaxis is not indicated for "low-risk" dog bites, but should be considered for "high-risk" injuries such as cat and human bites, hand and foot wounds, puncture wounds and wounds treated initially after 12 hours. Equally or more important is that all such wounds should first be irrigated under pressure, cleaned, and debrided as necessary.

Fleisher GR: The management of bite wounds. N Engl J Med 340: 138-140, 1999.

Cummings P: Antibiotics to prevent infection in patients with dog bite wounds: A meta-analysis of randomized trials. Ann Emerg Med 23: 535-540, 1994.

54. Following a laceration or penetrating injury, how long before a tetanus infection usually develops?

Rarely, tetanus has been reported within a day of injury or > 60 days after injury. However, > 80% of tetanus cases occur from 3–14 days after the acute injury, and > 90% occur within 2–21 days. The average onset of symptoms is day 7. Following repeat immunization, protective concentrations of antibody appear in the vast majority of patients within 4–7 days after vaccination.

Wassilak SG:Timing of tetanus immunoprophylaxis in wound management. Pediatr Infect Dis J 9:67–68, 1990.

55. What are recommendations for tetanus prophylaxis in a child with a lacertion?

NO. OF PREVIOUS VACCINATIONS	MOST RECENT BOOSTER	TYPE OF WOUND	RECOMMENDATION FOR CHILDREN ≥ 7 YEARS OF AGE
Unclear or < 3	—	Clean minor	Adult –type tetanus vaccine
		Tetanus-prone	Adult-type tetanus vaccine plus tetanus immunoglobulin

≥ 3	> 10 years	Clean, minor	Adult –type tetanus vaccine
		Tetanus-prone	Adult –type tetanus vaccine
≥ 3	5-10 years	Clean, minor	None
		Tetanus-prone	Adult-type tetanus vaccine
≥ 3	< 5 years	Clean, minor	None
		Tetanus-prone	None

In children < 7 years of age, other tetanus-containing vaccines (DtaP, DT) should be given rather than the adult-type tetanus vaccine (td), depending on the immunization status and previous reactions. *Clean, minor wounds gene*rally are defined as wounds that are <6 hours old; not infected or contaminated with feces, soil or saliva; superficial enough to permit irrigation and debridement; and surrounded by viable tissues. Most are linear. *Tetanus-prone wounds* include all other wounds but especially those caused by puncture, crush injury, burns, or frostbite.

56. Since 1980, what two animals have caused the most cases of rabies in the United States?

From 1980 to 1996, 32 cases of human rabies were reported to the Centers for Disease Control and Prevention. Twenty of these cases were believed to be the result of ***bat*** exposure while the other twelve cases were variants of rabies likely due to exposure to ***dogs*** contacted outside the United States (i.e. exotic dogs). There were no reported cases due to dog exposures clearly occurring within United States. None of the 32 patients received a complete rabies prophylaxis series.

Noah DL, Drenzek CL, Smith JS, et al: Epidemiology of human rabies in the United States, 1980 to 1996. Ann Int Med 128:922-930, 1998.

57. If at a local petting zoo, a playful 20-month-old is bitten by a duck, scratched by a rabbit (breaking skin), spit on by a camel, and licked on the face by a horse, should rabies prophylaxis be given?

In general, no prophylaxis is needed for any of these animal wounds unless the animal is actively rabid. The local health department should be contacted if there is any question. Immediate rabies vaccination and rabies immune globulin is recommended for bites or scratches (which break the skin) from bats, skunks, raccoons, foxes and most other carnivores. Bites from dogs and cats generally do not necessitate prophylaxis if the animal is healthy and can be observed closely for a 10 day period. No case in the U. S. has been attributed to a dog or cat that has remained healthy for the confinement of 10 days.

American Academy of Pediatics: Rabies. In Pickering LK (ed): 2000 Red Book, 25th ed. Elk Grove Village, IL, 2000, p 475-482.

58. If irrigation under pressure with normal saline is the method of choice to clean a laceration, how much pressure should be used?

Copious irrigation of a wound at high pressure markedly lowers bacterial counts in the wound. It is not clear what the most optimal degree of pressure should be, but the recommended standard is between 5-8 lbs/sq inch. This amount of pressure is expected to wash out debris without damaging tissue. The method often used of punching a hole in the top of a plastic normal saline bottle does not provide enough pressure while a 19-gauge needle attached to a 20 ml syringe may produce too much pressure. A 16-gauge needle/catheter attached to a 60 ml syringe may be a good choice, especially for wounds which have a low likelihood of contamination.

Singer AJ, et al. Pressure dynamics of various irrigation techniques commonly used in the emergency department. Ann Emerg Med 24:36-40, 1994.

59. What are some of the ingredients in the alphabet soup of topical anesthetics?

LET (**l**idocaine, **e**pinephrine, **t**etracaine), ***TAC*** (**t**etracaine, **a**drenaline, **c**ocaine), ½ ***TAC*** (with a lower percentage of cocaine), ***V-TAC*** (**v**iscous TAC), ***PLP*** (**p**rilocaine, **l**idocaine, **p**henylephrine), ***EMLA*** (**e**utectic **m**ixture of **l**ocal **a**nesthetics) and other combinations. TAC was among the first developed, but its higher costs and safety concerns (due to the cocaine component) have resulted in others, primarily LET, replacing it as first-line therapy.

Stewart GM et al: Use of topical lidocaine in pediatric laceration repair: A review of topical anesthetics. Ped Emerg Care 14:419-423, 1998.

60. In what situations is EMLA cream useful?

EMLA stands for **E**utectic **M**ixture of **L**ocal **A**nesthetics, which are lidocaine and prilocaine. EMLA is very useful in anesthetizing the skin prior to venipuncture, IVplacement, injection, lumbar puncture, or circumcision. The cream is placed on the site and covered with an occlusive dressing for 1–2 hours. Obviously, its most practical use is for anticipated procedures.

61. What are methods for decreasing the pain of local lidocaine infiltration?

- Infiltration into the subcutaneous layer
- Infiltration at a slow rate
- Buffering the anesthetic (e.g., with bicarbonate)
- Warming the anesthetic to body temperature
- Using a small gauge needle (e.g. 30-gauge)
- Distracting the patient / hypnosis / biofeedback

Noeller T, Cydulka RK: Laceration repair techniques. Emerg Med Reports 17:207-217, 1996.

62. When is the use of lidocaine with epinephrine contraindicated as an anesthetic?

When there is question of tissue viability and in any instance in which vasoconstriction might produce ischemic injury to an "end organ" without an alternative blood supply (e.g., tip of nose, margin of ear, tip of finger or toe).

63. Is the "DPT lytic cocktail" a thing of the past?

With the development of newer anesthetic and analgesic agents, it should be. **DPT** stands for **D**emerol (meperidine), **P**henergan (promethazine), and **T**horazine (chlorpromazine), and for many years, it has been a mainstay of pediatric sedation and analgesia. The combination of two phenothiazines and a long-acting narcotic runs counter to the ideal of rapid onset of action with reversibility that should characterize these types of medications. Problems with the DPT cocktail include its administration (IM), delayed onset of action, prolonged (up to 6 hours) sedation, hypotension, and respiratory depression.

Committee on Drugs: Reappraisal of lytic cocktail Demerol, Phenergan, and Thorazine (DPT) for the sedation of children. Pediatrics 95:598–602, 1995.

64. How is conscious sedation best managed in children?

There is no single best method for conscious sedation of pediatric patients for diagnostic, radiologic, or minor surgical procedures. Surveys indicate a wide variety of approaches are used in emergency rooms and radiology suites, including chloral hydrate, opioids (morphine, meperidine, fentanyl, butorphanol), benzodiazepines (diazepam, midazolam), barbiturates (pentobarbital, thiopental), and the DPT lytic cocktail.

Although conscious sedation by definition is a state of medically controlled depressed consciousness with a patent airway, maintained protective reflexes, and appropriate responses to stimulation on verbal command, the potential for rapidly developing problems should be anticipated. These can include hypoventilation, apnea, airway obstruction, or cardiorespiratory collapse. Consequently, keys to any pharmacologic method of conscious sedation are administration under supervised conditions (eliminating home treatment prior to office or hospital arrival), competent personnel capable of resuscitation, ongoing monitoring (especially the use of pulse oximetry), and sufficient equipment for resuscitation (e.g, positive pressure oxygen delivery system, suction apparatus).

Linzer JF: Conscious sedation: What you should know before and after. Clin Pediatr Emerg Med 1:306-310, 2000.

RESUSCITATION

65. How does the CPR technique differ between an infant and a child?

The general resuscitation principles of **ABC** (airway-breathing-circulation) remain the same. However, the following modifications and caveats regarding pediatric CPR should be noted:

• After determining unresponsiveness in the pediatric patient, CPR should first proceed for one minute (20 breaths, or 20 cycles, if both ventilations and compressions are needed) before activating EMS.

• Avoid inadvertently obstructing the pediatric airway by compressing the more pliable soft tissues of the neck when performing the head tilt-chin lift maneuver to open the airway.

• In an infant, the heart is lower in relation to the external chest than in a child. Thus the proper position for chest compression is 1 finger-breadth below the intersection of the intermammary line. The rescuer should use 2 or 3 fingers to compress the sternum to a depth of 0.5–1.0 inches at a rate of at least 100 times/minute. The infant should be ventilated at a rate of 20 breaths/minute.

For older children (> 1 year old), the rescuer places the heel of the hand 2 finger-breadths above the sternal notch. Depth of compression is optimally 1.0–1.5 inches with a recommended rate of 80 times/minute. The older child should be ventilated at a rate of 16 breaths/minute.

66. What is the Thaler technique for infant CPR?

This is the technique of encirclement. The rescuer clasps the fingers together beneath the thoracic spine, encircles the chest with the hands and compresses with the thumbs. Care should be taken to minimize the limitation of chest movement during ventilation.

67. Can CPR cause rib fractures in infants?

Very unlikely. In one study of 91 infants who underwent autopsy and postmortem x-rays following CPR, none had rib fractures. Child abuse must always remain at the top of a list when rib fractures are identified.

Spevak MR, et al: Cardiopulmonary resuscitation and rib fractures in infants: A postmortem radiologic-pathologic study. JAMA 272:617–618, 1994.

68. Is there any use for the "precordial thump" in pediatric CPR?

Even in witnessed and documented ventricular fibrillation, the thump is felt *not* to be more effective than routine external compression in terms of converting the abnormal rhythm, and there is increased risk of internal organ damage.

69. Are fixed and dilated pupils a contraindication to resuscitation in a patient in cardiac arrest?

No. Pupillary dilatation begins 15 seconds after cardiac arrest and is complete at approximately 1 minute 45 seconds. It may only be a sign of transient hypoxia. The only absolute contraindications to resuscitation are rigor mortis, corneal clouding, dependent lividity, and decapitation.

70. Why is the airway of an infant or child more prone to obstruction than that of an adult?

- An infant has less margin of safety because of the smaller airway diameter. Because airflow is inversely proportional to the airway radius raised to the fourth power (the oft-cited Poiseuille law), small changes in the diameter of the trachea can result in very large drops in airflow.
- The tracheal cartilage of an infant is softer and can result in collapse upon hyperextension. This is particularly important if CPR is performed with vigorous extension of the neck. Air exchange may then be obstructed.
- In an infant, the lumen of the oropharynx is relatively smaller due to the larger size of the tongue and smaller size of the mandible.
- Lower airways are smaller and less developed in children. The typical peanut and an infant's mainstem bronchus always seem to fit hand-in-glove.

71. How can size and depth of endotracheal tubes (ETT) be estimated?

1. For choosing a tube size, a good rule of thumb is:

$$\text{ID (mm)} = \frac{16 + \text{age (yrs)}}{4}$$

For example, a 2-year-old would warrant a 4.5-mm tube by this formula. Since this is an approximation, the next smaller or larger size tubes should be available. To convert internal diameter (ID) size to French catheter size, multiply by 4 (e.g., a 5.0 tube is 20 French).

2. Another good guide is the rule of "pinky," the infant or child's pinky approximates the internal diameter of the correct sized tube.
3. Following insertion of the ETT, appropriate depth (measured by markings at the gum line) can be approximated by the following formula for children > 1 year:

$$\frac{\text{Age in years}}{2} + 12 \text{ cm}$$

72. At what ages should cuffed vs. uncuffed ETTs be used?

In adolescents and adults, cuffed ETTs are used and inflated just enough to obliterate any audible air leak. However, *in children less than 8 years*, an uncuffed ETT is advised, as the cricoid cartilage is the narrowest part of the airway and serves as a functional cuff. Therefore, an uncuffed ETT should allow minimal air leak at the cricoid ring. Absence of an air leak indicates there may be excessive pressure at the cricoid cartilage.

73. What emergency drugs can be given via an endotracheal tube?

E-LAINE (***E***ndotracheally—***L***idocaine, ***A***tropine, ***I***soproterenol, ***N***aloxone, and ***E***pinephrine).

74. Is there ever an indication for intracardiac epinephrine?

Outside of televised dramas, epinephrine is very rarely administered via the intracardiac route. Other methods of administration (peripheral or central IV, intraosseous or endotracheal tube) should be readily available. The use of intracardiac epinephrine interrupts CPR and can cause tamponade, coronary artery laceration, or pneumothorax. If epinephrine is accidentally given into the cardiac muscle rather than the ventricular chamber, intractable ventricular fibrillation or cardiac standstill may result.

75. What is the role of high-dose epinephrine in pediatric resuscitations?

Animal studies, anecdotal reports, and a small clinical trial in children showed that the use of epinephrine in higher doses (100–200 times normal) facilitated the return of spontaneous circulation better than the standard lower dose. Larger prospective studies in adults did not show an advantage. One retrospective study of pediatric out-of-hospital cardiopulmonary arrests also did not document any benefits. While the evidence accumulates, the American Heart Association recommends that after the first standard dose of IVor intraosseous epinephrine (0.01 mg/kg of a 1:10,000 solution), subsequent higher doses (0.1–0.2 mg/kg of a 1:1000 solution) might be effective. In the scenario of a witnessed cardiac arrest, the use of high-dose epinephrine should strongly be considered.

Gueuginaud PY, et al: A comparison of repeated high doses versus repeated standard doses of epinephrine for cardiac arrest out of the hospital. New Engl J Med 339:1595-1601.1999.

Patterson M, et al: High dose epinephrine in pediatric cardiopulmonary arrest [abstract]. Pediatr Res 43:69, 1998.

Dieckmann RA, Vardis R: High-dose epinephrine in pediatric out-of-hospital cardiopulmonary arrest. Pediatrics 95:901–913, 1995.

76. How effective is intratracheal epinephrine?

Epinephrine is poorly absorbed from the lung, and if available, intraosseous or IVadministration is preferable. If epinephrine is to be given via an endotracheal tube in an acute setting, it should be mixed with 1–3 ml of normal saline and instilled with a catheter or feeding tube beyond the end of the endotracheal tube to facilitate dispersal. The ideal endotracheal dose in unclear, but because of the poor absorption, initial higher doses (0.1–0.2 mg/kg of a 1:1000 solution) should be used.

77. When is atropine indicated during a resuscitation?

Atropine may be administered to the child with symptomatic bradycardia after other resuscitative measures (i.e., oxygenation and ventilation) have been initiated. It is useful in breaking the vagally mediated bradycardia associated with laryngoscopy and may have some benefit during the initial treatment of atrioventricular block. The deleterious effects of a slow heart rate are more likely to occur in a younger child, whose cardiac output is more dependent on rate changes than volume or contractility changes. Atropine is no longer routinely recommended in the treatment of asystole.

78. What risks are associated with administering an inappropriately low dose of atropine?

If the dose of atropine is too small, paradoxically worsening bradycardia may result. This is due to atropine's central stimulating effect on the medullary vagal nerve at lower doses, which slows atrioventricular conduction and heart rate. Standard dosing of atropine in a setting of bradycardia is 0.02 mg/kg IV. However, at least 0.1 mg should be used even in the youngest patient.

79. When is the use of calcium indicated during a resuscitation?

Routine use of calcium is no longer recommended during a resuscitation. There is evidence that calcium may increase postischemic injury in the intracranial reperfusion phase following resuscitation. Calcium use may be justified in three settings of resuscitation: (1) an overdose of a calcium channel blocker, (2) hyperkalemia resulting in cardiac dysrhythmia, and (3) infants and children with low serum calcium.

80. If pulseless electrical activity (PEA) is suspected, what should be done ASAP?

PEA exists when there is organized electrical activity on ECG without evidence of effective myocardial contraction (i.e., absent blood pressure or nonpalpable pulse). The electrical rate can be fast or slow, and the complexes narrow or wide. PEA is caused either by myocardial disease (hypoxic/ischemic myocardium due to respiratory arrest is most common in children) or by causes extrinsic to the heart. If prolonged myocardial ischemia is the cause of PEA, the prognosis is poor.

However, rapid diagnosis of an extracardiac cause and its treatment may be life-saving. The extracardiac causes of PEA include hypovolemia, tension pneumothorax, cardiac tamponade, hypoxemia, acidosis, and pulmonary embolus. The treatment of PEA begins with the initiation of chest compressions and ventilation with 100% oxygen, followed by the administration of epinephrine and sodium bicarbonate if the patient is acidotic. Extracardiac causes are treated with fluid administration, pericardiocentesis, or thoracentesis as indicated. Empiric administration of calcium is no longer felt to be of value.

81. Why should one bone up on the technique of intraosseous infusions?

Because of the difficulty and delays in establishing IV access in pediatric resuscitations, intraosseous infusions have become the very early second-line of therapy in emergency settings. Failure to achieve intravenous access in three attempts or 90 seconds (whichever is shorter) is an indication for intraosseous access. An intraosseous line is a rapid means of vascular access and utilizes the marrow cavity of bone, which drains into the central venous system. All medications and fluids that can be given intravenously can be given by the intraosseus route, at the same rate and dosages, with comparable distribution. The technique is straightforward and involves placing a styleted needle, bone marrow needle, or intraosseous needle into the proximal tibia approximately 1–3 cm below and medial to the tibial tuberosity. Distal tibial and proximal femoral sites are less commonly used.

82. What features indicate that an intraosseous needle has been correctly placed?

- A soft pop should be felt as you break through the cortex.
- The needle should be very stable.
- There should be free flow of intravenous fluids without infiltration of the subcutaneous tissues.
- Bone marrow aspiration, while confirming placement, may not always be possible even when needle placement is correct. Therefore, if one cannot aspirate marrow you should rely on signs #1-3 for determination of placement.

83. Is capillary refill still a useful clinical sign?

Capillary refill is the return to normal color of the pulp of the finger or fingernail after it has been compressed. In healthy children, a normal value is approximately 2 seconds. In theory, a normal refill time is a measure of adequate peripheral perfusion and thus normal cardiac output and peripheral vascular resistance. It has been used as a measure of perfusion in the settings of trauma and possible dehydration. However, it must be utilized in conjunction with other clinical features, because studies of its usefulness as a sole indicator of dehydration have shown it to have a low sensitivity and specificity. In one study of children with 5–10% dehydration, only 50% had prolonged capillary refill. In addition, lower ambient temperature has a significant effect on delaying capillary refill. Capillary refill should be measured in the upper extremity.

Baraff LJ: Capillary refill: Is it a useful clinical sign? Pediatrics 92:723–724, 1993.

84. When are MAST trousers of potential value in pediatric resuscitation?

Pneumatic anti-shock garments (PASGs), or the *MAST (Military Anti-Shock Trousers) suit*, is a pneumatic device that inflates around the lower extremities, pelvis, and abdomen. The MAST became standard prehospital therapy in the late 1970s for patients in hypovolemic shock based on anecdotal reports of efficacy. While there is no doubt that application of MAST often raises blood pressure, most likely through a rise in systemic vascular resistance, there is no evidence that MAST improves outcome. In the presence of shock associated with chest trauma, MAST use may increase hemorrhage severity and mortality. It is absolutely contraindicated in pulmonary edema. Thus, enthusiasm for MAST has begun to wane except for patients with unstable pelvic fractures, for whom it may stabilize the fractures and tamponade retroperitoneal bleeding.

85. Are steroids indicated in the treatment of shock in children?

No. The controversy has related primarily to the role of steroids in treating septic shock. There are data in animals that steroids given prior to, or concomitantly with, endotoxin can improve survival. However, in multiple clinical trials in adults, early steroids have not been shown to decrease long-term mortality and actually may have contributed to increased mortality because of higher secondary infection rates in steroid-treated patients compared with controls. Data in children are lacking. However, by extrapolation, steroids at present are not indicated.

86. Following a motor vehicle accident, an 8-year-old presents with right-sided pain, a heart rate of 150, a blood pressure of 110/80 and capillary refill time of 3.5 seconds. How should his initial fluid therapy be managed?

It is important to recognize that this child is in shock, despite a normal blood pressure for age. For children in shock, changes in blood pressure are often late and precipitous. Findings of tachycardia, prolonged capillary refill, and diminished pulses are indicative of hypovolemia in this patient, requiring aggressive fluid resuscitation. Isotonic crystalloid (saline or lactated Ringer's solution) should be given in boluses of 20 ml/kg as quickly as possible. There is controversy about giving colloid solutions (such as albumin, hydroxyethyl starch, dextran) in fluid resuscitation, although there does not seem to be any clear benefit and there is little information on their use in children. If, after 40 ml/kg of crystalloid, hemodynamic measures have not improved or have worsened, blood products should be given in 10 ml/kg boluses. Typed and cross-matched blood would be the ideal choice, but it is usually not ready in time to be used. Type-specific packed red blood cells should be available within 15 minutes and are the next option. O-negative packed red blood cells should be reserved for those in profound shock or with exsanguinating hemorrhage.

87. What initial ventilator settings would be recommended for a 16-year-old, 50 kilogram patient who has just been intubated and placed on a mechanical ventilator?

The normal tidal volume (TV) of a child is *7 ml/kg*. When mechanically ventilated, an increased TV of *10ml/kg* is used in order to compensate for the increased dead space in the ventilator circuit. The initial inspired oxygen concentration (FIO_2) of an intubated patient should always be 100% until ABG results are obtained. The respiratory rate should approximate the normal respiratory rate of the patient for his or her age. Thus, in our example, the following initial ventilator settings would be appropriate: TV = 500ml, FIO_2 = 100%, and RR = 15/minute. Ventilator settings should then be appropriately readjusted according to ABG results.

A notable exception to this rule occurs in the intubated asthmatic. These patients suffer from airtrapping and require increased exhalation time. They are initially ventilated at higher flow rates, increased inspiratory:expiratory breath ratios (at least 1:3) and reduced ventilation rates of 6-10 breaths/minute. This is called controlled mechanical hypoventilation or permissive hypercapnia.

88. What is the proper treatment if a large bolus of air is accidentally injected into a 6-year-old child?

The main problem is that the air can block the right ventricular outflow tract or main pulmonary artery. This is similar to "vapor lock" in automobiles, in which air in the carburetor prevents fuel from flowing and a stall results. The patient should be placed in a steep head-down position with the right side up to trap air in the upper right ventricular chamber and prevent passage to the outflow tract. Therapeutic options include:

- 100% oxygen
- Careful monitoring, including ECG
- Observation for symptoms or signs of dysrhythmia, hypotension, or cardiac arrest
- If air is auscultated in the heart, a right ventricular tap should be considered.
- If arrest occurs, standard CPR should be initiated, as manual compression may help to dislodge air emboli.

89. What is the effect of body temperature on arterial blood gases (ABGs)?

CO_2 and O_2 are more soluble and exert less partial pressure at lower temperatures. Therefore, blood sampled from a hypothermic patient and warmed to the standard 37° in the blood gas analyzer will have a higher partial pressure than exists in the patient. Similarly, blood sampled from the hyperthermic patient and cooled to 37° will have a lower partial pressure than exists in the patient. For each 1° C difference from 37°, the PaO_2 changes by about 7% and the $PaCO_2$ by about 4.5%. Although much debate exists whether to use the "corrected" (patient body temperature) or "uncorrected" (37° C of blood gas analyzer) value, the difference in most clinical scenarios is not significant. In cases of extreme temperature differences (e.g., hypothermia in cold-water near-drowning), the difference may be considerable.

90. How do pediatric and adult defibrillation differ?

- ***Smaller dosing***: 2 W-sec/kg and then doubled as needed
- ***Smaller paddles***: Standard pediatric paddles are 4.5 cm in diameter compared with 8.0 cm in adults
- ***Rarer use***: Ventricular fibrillation is uncommon in children

91. What is the difference between livor mortis and rigor mortis?

Livor mortis or dependent lividity is the gravitational pooling of blood that results in a line of mauve staining in the dependent half of a recently deceased body. It usually is noticeable 30 minutes after death and is very marked at 6 hours. *Rigor mortis* is the muscular stiffening and shortening that result from ongoing cellular activity and depletion of ATP after death, with increasing lactate and phosphate and salt precipitation. Neck and facial changes begin at 6 hours, shoulder and upper extremities at 9 hours, and trunk and lower extremities at 12 hours. Livor mortis and rigor mortis are absolute indications not to initiate a resuscitation. They should be looked for during the initial rapid assessment. In the confusion of the moment, they may be easily overlooked.

92. When should a failing resuscitation be stopped?

Studies have suggested that when *more than two rounds of medication* (i.e., epinephrine and bicarbonate) have been given and/or > *20 minutes* have elapsed since the initiation of resuscitation without clinical cardiovascular or neurologic improvement, the likelihood of death or survival with neurologic devastation greatly increases. Unwitnessed out-of-hospital arrests are nearly always associated with a poor outcome. In settings of hypothermia, asystolic patients should be rewarmed to 36° before resuscitation is discontinued.

Schindler M, et al: Outcome of out-of-hospital cardiac or respiratory arrest in children. N Engl J Med 335:1473-1479, 1996.

93. What factors are predictive of good or bad outcomes for pediatric ED resuscitation?

PREDICTORS OF GOOD OUTCOME AFTER PEDIATRIC CARDIAC ARREST	PREDICTORS OF BAD OUTCOME AFTER PEDIATRIC CARDIAC ARREST
Witnessed arrest	Unwitnessed arrest
Bystander CPR	No bystander CPR

EMS arrival time <10 minutes	Resuscitation efforts >30 minutes before ROSC*
Resuscitation effort <20 minutes	≤ 2 doses epinephrine before ROSC*
Rhythm of VF* or VT*	>2 doses of epinephrine before ROSC*
Prehospital ROSC*	Rhythm of PEA or asystole
Cause of arrest submersion	Cause of arrest sepsis, trauma, or SIDS

*ROSC=Return of spontaneous circulation; *VF=Ventricular fibrillation; *VT=Ventricular tachycardia.

94. Why is resuscitation less successful in children than in adults?

Adults more commonly experience collapse and arrest from primary cardiac disease and associated dysrhythmias—ventricular tachycardia and fibrillation. These are more readily reversible and carry a better prognosis. Children, however, have cardiac arrest as a secondary phenomenon from other processes, such as respiratory obstruction or apnea, often associated with infection, hypoxia, acidosis, or hypovolemia. Primary cardiac arrest is rare. The most common dysrhythmia associated with pediatric cardiac arrest is asystole. It is less frequently reversible, and by the time a child has cardiac arrest, severe neurologic damage is almost always present.

95. Endotracheal intubation in a 1-year-old: straight or curved blade?

Children under 3 years of age tend to have an "anterior" larynx with a small oropharynx relative to a large tongue. The epiglottis is also relatively long and narrow compared to that of an older child or adult and it is angled to obscure the vocal cords. A straight blade (e.g., Miller or Wis-Hipple) with an anteriorly directed tip is designed to pick up the epiglottis directly, which is more useful for visualizing the vocal cords of the young child. It is harder to pull the long and narrow epiglottis out of the way with the curved blade (e.g., Macintosh), as it does not directly lift the entire epiglottis out of the way. As with most procedures, practice makes perfect.

96. What are the top ten errors in running a resuscitation?

One subjective list is as follows:

1. Leader of code not clearly designated
2. Failure to place nasogastric tube
3. Failure to give proper medications in response to situation
4. Failure to periodically assess breath sounds, pupils, pulses
5. Delay in access before attempting intraosseous line or other
6. Leader of code too involved with individual procedure
7. Failure to assign roles
8. Failure to assess patient initially
9. Failure to observe adequate cardiac compressions
10. Failure to respect mechanical errors when patient crashes.

TOXICOLOGY

97. What are the most common poisonings in children under 6 years of age?

The most common ingestion, though non-toxic, in younger children is the silica gel that is often used for packaging. The most common toxic ingestions in this population are dishwasher detergents. About 4 million people in the US are poisoned every year. Children under age 6 years account for about 60% of all poisonings. More children less than age 4 years die of accidental poisonings at home than are accidently killed with guns in the home. Approximately 60% of reported poisonings are nonpharmaceuticals and 40% are pharmaceuticals. In descending order of frequency, the most common are:

Nonpharmaceuticals	*Pharmaceuticals*
Cosmetics and personal care products	Analgesics
Cleaning substances	Cough and cold preparations
Plants, including mushrooms and tobacco	Topical agents
Battery, toy and other foreign bodies	Vitamins
Insecticides, pesticides and rodenticides	Antimicrobials

Litovitz TL, et al: 1999 Annual Report of the American Association of Poison Control Centers Toxic Exposure Surveillance System. Am J Emerg Med 18 (5): 517-574, 2000.

98. What is the role of ipecac in the treatment of acute poisonings and overdoses?

Syrup of ipecac is becoming obsolete. Previously a favored means of gastric emptying, the efficacy of ipecac-induced emesis has been questioned. In 1997, the American Academy of Clinical Toxicology stated (a) that ipecac should not be administered routinely in the management of poisoned patients; (b) there is no evidence from clinical studies that it improves the outcome of poisoned patients; and (c) its routine administration in the ED should be abandoned. Ipecac may delay the administration or reduce the effectiveness of activated charcoal, oral antidotes, and whole bowel irrigation. In addition, ipecac can be sedating itself and can confuse the exam of a patient who has ingested a sedative hypnotic agent. Some experts argue it may be useful in young children who have small particle ingestions (e.g., plant parts, seeds, mushrooms) in whom gastric lavage may be less successful. However, ipecac is no longer routinely recommended for home use.

Quang LS, Woolf AD: Past, present and future role of ipecac syrup. Curr Opin Pediatr 12(2):153-162, 2000.

American Academy of Clinical Toxicology, European Association of Poisons Centres and Clinical Toxicologists: Position statement: Ipecac syrup. J Toxicol Clin Toxicol 35:699-709, 1997.

99. When is ipecac-induced vomiting contraindicated?

Coma, ***C***onvulsions, ***C***austics, and household hydro***C***arbons.

100. When is gastric lavage indicated?

Gastric lavage involves the passage of a large orogastric tube (e.g., 24-Fr orogastric for a toddler, 36-Fr orogastric for a teenager) with sequential administration and aspiration of small volumes of normal saline (50-100 ml in smaller children, 150-200 ml in teenagers) with the intent of removing toxic substances present in the stomach. Efficacy remains unproven, and complications are possible (e.g., laryngospasm, esophageal injury, aspiration pneumonia). Its use is reserved for patients with a potentially life-threatening quantity of poisonous ingestion occurring within 60 minutes of evaluation.

American Academy of Clinical Toxicology, European Association of Poisons Centres and Clinical Toxicologists: Position statement: Gastric lavage. J Toxicol Clin Toxicol 35:711-719, 1997.

101. What are the indications for whole bowel irrigation (WBI) in acute ingestions?

This is a method of GI decontamination using a large volume of polyethylene glycol–balanced electrolyte solution such as Colyte or GoLYTELY. These solutions are not known to cause electrolyte imbalance because neither are they significantly absorbed nor do they exert osmotic effect. WBI is indicated for *iron overdose*, *sustained-release medications* and *ingestion of crack vials or cocaine packets.* The usual recommended dosing is 500 ml/hour in toddlers and 2 L/hour in adolescents and adults (by mouth in cooperative patients or by nasogastric tube in uncooperative patients).

102. Should activated charcoal be given to a sleepy 2-year-old who consumed half a bottle of a liquid antihistamine 2 hours prior to evaluation?

This would not be a good idea because of a potentially compromised airway (sleepy child) and the delay in administration. The effectiveness of activated charcoal decreases with time. In this setting, it use should only be considered if (a) a patient had ingested up to 1 hour previously a potentially toxic amount of a poison known to be adsorbable to charcoal and (b) airway protection was assured since the charcoal can cause vomiting and aspiration. The dose in children up to 1 year of age is 1 g/kg, in children 1 to 12 years of age 25 to 50 g and in adolescents 25 to 100 g. It can be given orally or by nasogastric tube.

American Academy of Clinical Toxicology, European Association of Poisons Centres and Clinical Toxicologists: Position statement: Single-dose activated charcoal. J Toxicol Clin Toxicol 35:721-741, 1997.

103. In what settings is activated charcoal not advised?

Charcoal should not be given in poisonings involving:

- Caustics (charcoal can interfere with possible endoscopy)
- Drugs for which immediate oral antidotes are contemplated (e.g., late presentation of pure acetaminophen ingestion)
- Clinical presentation of ileus, hematemesis, or severe vomiting
- Household petroleum distillates (e.g., gasoline, kerosene) because of possible increased risk of aspiration
- Compounds for which it is ineffective, including acids, alcohols, alkalis, cyanide, iron, heavy metals, and lithium
- Via NG tube, when airway is not protected

104. In what setting would multi-dose activated charcoal be advised?

Multiple-dose activated charcoal therapy involves the repeated administration (more than 2 doses of 0.5 to 1.0 g/kg every 4 to 6 hours) of oral activated charcoal to enhance the elimination of drugs already absorbed into the body. The rationale behind its use is that drugs with a prolonged elimination half-life are more likely to have their elimination enhanced the longer an adsorptive agent is around in the GI tract. Potential complications include bowel obstruction, constipation, regurgitation and subsequent aspiration. Its use should be considered if a patient has ingested a life-threatening amount of *carbamazepine*, *dapsone*, *phenobarbital*, *quinine*, *benzodiazepines*, *phenytoin*, *tricyclic antidepressants*, or *theophylline*. Use in salicylate poisoning is controversial.

American Academy of Clinical Toxicology; European Association of Poisons Centres and Clinical Toxicologists: Position statement and practice guidelines on the use of multi-dose activated charcoal in the treatment of acute poisoning. Clin Toxicol 37: 731-751, 1999.

105. Should all children with ingestion be given a cathartic?

No. Cathartics may help to decrease absorption and lessen constipation caused by charcoal. Magnesium sulfate (250 mg/kg), magnesium citrate (4–8 ml/kg up to 300 ml), or sorbitol (70%, 1.5 gm/kg) are the usual choices. The contraindications are similar to those for activated charcoal. Care must be taken when cathartics are given to smaller children, as large volume loss may result. Repeated administration of magnesium-containing cathartics can cause hypermagnesemia, manifested by hypotonia, altered mental status, and in severe cases, respiratory failure. However, magnesium citrate is associated with less emesis than sorbitol.

Perry H, Shannon M: Emergency department gastrointestinal decontamination. Pediatr Ann 25:19–26, 1996.

106. How is the manipulation of urinary pH used in treating poisonings?

Acidification or *alkalinization* of the urine to enhance the excretion of weak acids and bases has been a traditional way to enhance the elimination of toxicologic agents. In recent years, its use has been limited because of the potential complications from fluid overload (e.g., pulmonary and cerebral edema), the risk of acidemia, and the use of other therapeutic advancements (e.g., hemodialysis). However, alkaline diuresis is still considered valuable in the management of acute overdoses of salicylates, barbiturates, or tricyclic antidepressants.

107. What ingestions and exposures have available antidotes?

Ingestion/Exposure	***Antidote***
Acetaminophen	N-acetylcysteine (Mucomyst)
Anticholinergics	Physostigmine
Benzodiazepines	Flumazenil
Beta-blockers	Glucagon
Carbon monoxide	Hyperbaric oxygen chamber
Calcium channel blocker	Calcium, glucagon
Cyanide	Sodium nitrite, sodium thiosulfate
Digoxin	Digibind (anti-digoxin antibody)
Ethylene glycol	Ethanol, fomepizole
Iron	Deferoxamine
Isoniazid	Pyridoxine
Lead	EDTA, DMSA
Mercury	Dimercaprol, DMSA
Methanol	Ethanol
Methemoglobinemic agents	Methylene blue
Opiates	Naloxone, nalmefene
Organophospates	Atropine, pralidoxime
Phenothiazines (dystonic reaction)	Diphenhydramine
Tricyclics	Bicarbonate
Warfarin (rat poison)	Vitamin K

108. Narcan is considered an antidote for which kinds of ingestions?

Narcan (naloxone) is an antidote for opioid drugs. It reverses the CNS and respiratory depression of morphine and heroin, as well as clear the depressed sensorium in overdoses due to many of the synthetic opioids, including propoxyphene, codeine, dextromethorphan, pentazocine and meperidine. It is a known antidote for clonidine, and its efficacy at reversal of the signs and symptoms of tetrahydrozoline (over-the-counter eye drop solutions and nasal decongestants) ingestion in children has been described.

The pediatric dose is 0.01-0.1 mg/kg. However, many authorities now recommend the following regimen for all suspected opioid, or opioid-like, acute poisonings:

Coma without respiratory depression—1.0 mg

Coma with respiratory depression—2.0 mg

These doses may be repeated every 2-10 minutes up to a total dose of 8-10 mg. If intravenous access is not available, the drug can be given intramuscularly, sublingually or endotracheally.

Holmes JF, Berman DA: Use of naloxone to reverse symptomatic tetrahydrozoline overdose in a child. Pediatr Emerg Care 15: 193-194, 1999.

109. Which ingestions are radiopaque on abdominal x-ray?

The mnemonic "CHIPS" indicates possible suspects.

C: **C**hloral hydrate

H: **H**eavy metals (arsenic, iron, lead)

I: **I**odides

P: **P**henothiazines, psychotropics (cyclic antidepressants)

S: **S**low-release capsules, enteric-coated tablets

The likelihood of radiopacity depends on numerous factors including weight of the patient, size of the ingestion, and composition of the pill matrix.

Barkin RM et al: Poisoning and overdose. In Barkin RM, Rosen P (eds): Emergency Pediatrics, 4th ed. St. Louis, Mosby, 1994, p 335.

110. What is a toxidrome?

A *toxidrome* is a clinical constellation of signs and symptoms that is very suggestive of a particular poisoning or category of intoxication. For example, patients with salicylate overdose commonly present with fever, hyperpnea and tachypnea, abnormal mental status (ranging from lethargy to coma), tinnitus, vomiting, and sometimes oil of wintergreen odor from methylsalicylate.

Shannon M: Ingestion of toxic substances by children. N Engl J Med 342:186-191, 2000

111. What breath odors may be associated with specific ingestions?

Characteristic odor	*Responsible toxin/drug*
Wintergreen	Methyl salicylate
Bitter almond	Cyanide
Carrots	Cicutoxin (of water hemlock)
Fruity	Ethanol, acetone (nail polish remover), isopropyl alcohol, chloroform
Fishy	Zinc or aluminum phosphide
Garlic	Organophosphate insecticide, arsenic, thallium
Glue	Toulene
Minty	Mouthwash, rubbing alcohol
Mothballs	Naphthalene, p-dichlorobenzene, camphor
Peanuts	Vacor rat poison (odor is from a flavoring agent)
Rotten eggs	Hydrogen sulfide, N-acetylcysteine, disulfuram
Rope (burned)	Marijuana, opium
Shoe polish	Nitrobenzene

Woolf AD: Poisoning in children and adolescents. Pediatr Rev 14:411–422, 1993.

112. What are the limitations of the routine toxicology screen?

Most toxicology screens are intended to detect drugs encountered in substance abuse. Even in larger pediatric hospitals, comprehensive toxicology screens generally include only a fraction of the drugs available to children. Most blood screens analyze for acetaminophen, salicylates and alcohols. Urine is often screened for substances of abuse and other common psychoactive drugs, including antidepressants, antipsychotics, benzodiazepines, sedative-hypnotics, and anticonvulsants. Other potential toxins which can cause mental status changes (carbon monoxide, chloral hydrate, cyanide, organophosphates) or circulatory depression (beta-blockers, calcium channel blockers, clonidine, digitalis) may not be included, but may be assayed via individual blood tests. In clinical studies, toxicology screens are most valuable in quantitative settings (i.e., assessing drug levels).

Belson MG et al: The utility of toxicologic analysis in children with suspected ingestions. Pediatr Emerg Care 15:383-387, 1999.

113. How do the types of alcohol ingestions vary?

All alcohols can cause CNS disturbances ranging from mild mentation and motor abnormalities to respiratory depression and coma. Each alcohol individually is associated with specific metabolic complications.

1. ***Ethanol***: (present in beverages, colognes and perfumes, aftershave lotion, mouthwash, topical antiseptic, rubbing alcohol)—in infants and toddlers, can cause the classic triad of coma, hypothermia and hypoglycemia and, in adolescents, can cause intoxication and mild neurologic findings. At levels > 500 mg/dl, it can be lethal.
2. ***Methanol***: (present in antifreeze and windshield washer fluid)—can cause severe, refractory metabolic acidosis and permanent retinal damage leading to blindness.
3. ***Isopropyl alcohol***: (present in jewelry cleaners, rubbing alcohol, windshield de-icers,

cements, paint removers)—can cause gastritis, abdominal pain, vomiting, hematemesis and CNS depression, moderate hyperglycemia, hypotension and acetonemia, without acidosis.

4. ***Ethylene glycol***: (present in antifreeze, brake fluid)—causes severe metabolic acidosis. In addition, it is metabolized to oxalic acid, which can cause renal damage by the precipitation of calcium oxalate crystals in the renal parenchyma and can lead to hypocalcemia.

114. Which alcohol is considered the most lethal?

Methanol. Deaths can arise from doses as little as 4 ml of pure methanol. Unique to methanol is that it becomes more toxic as it is metabolized. Methanol is broken down by alcohol dehydrogenase to formaldehyde and formic acid. It is the formic acid that causes the refractory metabolic acidosis and ocular symptoms.

115. Why may fomepixole replace ethanol as the primary antidote in methanol and ethylene glycol ingestions in children?

Both methanol and ethylene glycol require the enzyme alcohol dehydrogenase to create their toxic metabolites. Ethanol, given either intravenously or orally (the latter is more commonly used), competitively inhibits the formation of these metabolites by serving as a substrate for the enzyme. However, it is inebriating, may cause hypoglycemia and its kinetics are widely variable. Fomepixole is a safer and more effective blocker of alcohol dehydrogenase. Although significantly higher in cost, it may lower other costs by shorter and less intensive hospital stays.

Casavant MJ: Fomepizole in the treatment of poisoning. Pediatrics 107:170, 2001.

116. How is the osmolar gap helpful in diagnosing ingestions?

The *osmolar gap* is the difference between the measured osmolarity (obtained from freezing point depression) and the calculated osmolarity (calculated = 2 [serum Na] + BUN/2.8 + glucose/18). Normal osmolarity is about 290 mOsm/L. A significant osmolar gap suggests an alcohol poisoning, which typically produces exogenous osmoles.

117. What cautions should be observed regarding the use of physostigmine for an antihistamine overdose?

Antihistamine overdose can cause the *anticholinergic syndrome*. This is recalled by the mnemonic "mad as a hatter" (delirium), "red as a beet"(cutaneous vasodilation), "dry as a bone" (reduced salivation and sweating), "hot as a hare" (fever), and "blind as a bat" (loss of accommodation). It is the result of competitive antagonism of acetylcholine at muscarinic receptors. Physostigmine is an anticholinesterase that acts by maximizing muscarinic receptor stimulation by acetylcholine.

The use of physostigmine is controversial. In a patient with altered mental status and/or hallucinations, physostigmine may reverse the symptoms. However, if given too rapidly, it may stimulate seizure activity. It can also produce profound bradycardia, refractory asystole and death, particularly in patients with cardiac conduction abnormalities. Contraindications to its use include abnormal ECGs and concurrent tricyclic antidepressant overdose (with the higher likelihood of conduction abnormalities).

Shannon M: Toxicology reviews: Physostigmine. Pediatr Emerg Care 14: 224-226, 1998.

118. How can pupillary findings assist in the diagnosis of toxic ingestions?

***Miosis** (pinoint pupils):* Narcotics, organophosphates, phencyclidine, clonidine, phenothiazines, barbiturates (occasionally), ethanol (occasionally)

***Mydriasis** (dilated pupils):* Anticholinergics (atropine, antihistamines, cyclic antidepres-

	sants). sympathomimetics (amphetamines, caffeine, cocaine, LSD, Nicotine)
Nystagmus:	Barbiturates, ketamine, phencyclidine, phenytoin

119. If a child has ingested an acetaminophen-containing product, when should the first acetaminophen level be obtained?

A plasma level obtained ***four hours*** after ingestion is a good indicator of the potential for hepatic toxicity. Nomograms are available for determining risk. As a rule, doses under 150 mg/kg are unlikely to be harmful.

120. When should a "NAC attack" begin?

N-acetylcysteine (NAC) is a specific antidote for acetaminophen hepatotoxicity by serving as a glutathione-substitute in detoxifying the hepatotoxic metabolites. It should be used for any acetaminophen overdose with a toxic serum acetaminophen level within the first 24 hours after ingestion. It is especially effective if used in the first 8 hours after ingestion. If acetaminophen levels are not available on a rapid basis or the time since ingestion is not clear, it is preferable to initiate NAC(140 mg/kg orally and then 70 mg/kg orally every 4 hours for 17 doses) while awaiting consultation with a toxicologist or poison control center.

121. How does NAC prevent hepatotoxicity in acetaminophen overdose?

Normally 94% of acetaminophen is metabolized to glucuronide or sulfate form; 2% is excreted unchanged in urine and both of them are nontoxic. The remaining 4% is conjugated with glutathione (with the help of cytochrome P-450) to form mercaptopuric acid, which is also not hepatotoxic. When a significant acetaminophen overdose occurs, cytochrome P-450 becomes the major system for metabolizing the acetaminophen leading to depletion of hepatic stores of glutathione. When the glutathione is depleted to less than 70% of normal, a highly reactive intermediate metabolite binds to hepatic macromolecule causing hepatocellular necrosis. It is presumed that NAC replenishes the glutathione, thus helping the cytochrome P-450 in converting the excess acetaminophen into mercaptopuric acid.

122. What arterial blood gas is classic for salicylate poisoning?

Metabolic acidosis and ***respiratory alkalosis***. Salicylates directly stimulate the medullary respiratory drive center causing tachypnea with diminished PCO_2 (respiratory alkalosis) and cause lactic and ketoacidosis by inhibiting Krebs cycle enzymes, uncoupling oxidation phosphorylation and inhibiting amino acid metabolism (metabolic acidosis).

123. What is a quick way to confirm salicylate use by using a simple bedside test?

Several drops of 10% ferric chloride are added to 1 ml of a patient's urine. If the color changes to purple, it indicates the presence of salicylic acid (also positive with acetoacetic acid and phenylpyruvic acid).

124. What features suggest the possibility of lead toxicity in a child?

- Most children with elevated lead levels are asymptomatic. Plumbism, or lead intoxication, should be suspected if a child has:
- Pica: including a history of accidental ingestions or foreign body insertion in the nose or ear
- Vague or increasing abdominal complaints, such as anorexia, recurrent abdominal pain, constipation, and vomiting
- Vague behavioral effects, such as hyperactivity, irritability, malaise, or lethargy
- Progressive ataxia or afebrile seizure
- A history of unexplained or iron-deficiency anemia
- Basophilic stippling of peripheral RBCs

125. Should all children be screened for elevated lead levels?

Because of substantial regional and local variations in the prevalence of elevated lead levels, the recommendation to screen all children is controversial. Some states have adopted universal screening because increased lead levels have been associated with slowed mental growth and behavior disorders. In general, it is advisable to screen high-risk children, including those:

- Living in or visiting homes with peeling paint built before 1960 or undergoing renovation
- Having a sibling or playmate with elevated lead
- Living with an adult whose job or hobby involves lead
- Living near an industry likely to release lead (e.g., smelting plant, battery-recycling plant)

126. How do the signs and symptoms of acute and chronic lead intoxication differ?

Acute lead poisoning is rare in children and differs from chronic poisoning mainly in the occurrence of a reversible renal Fanconi-like syndrome. In *chronic* exposure, a glomerulonephritis with hypertension and renal failure may occur. The CNS effects are similar, however, and are the most feared consequences of pediatric plumbism. Lead encephalopathy may range from mild behavioral and cognitive dysfunction to severe, life-threatening coma, seizures, cerebral edema, and permanent neurologic sequelae in survivors.

127. Why is erythrocytic protoporphyrin (EP) no longer used as an initial screen for lead poisoning?

Elevated EP can be an indicator of abnormalities in heme biosynthesis, which can occur in lead poisoning. As the acceptable limit for blood lead has been progressively lowered (in 1991 to 10 µg/dl), the EP test is no longer considered sensitive. It identifies only a small percentage of children with blood levels of 10–25 µg/dl and misses > 50% of children with blood levels above 25 µg/dl. In addition, there is approximately a 2-week lag between significant lead accumulation and detectable rises in the EP level, therefore making it a poor indicator of recent lead exposure.

128. If elevated lead is discovered on a routine screen, what are the most likely sources of exposure?

The most common sources are:

- *Lead-based paint*: homes built before the 1960s (ban on residential use since 1977)
- *Home renovation*: releases lead-containing dust into environment
- *Soil*: contamination from nearby industries like smelting, soldering, battery-recycling, sandblasting and demolition
- *Drinking water:* older lead-containing pipes

Infrequent sources of exposure are cooking in ceramic or pewter cookware, lead-containing folk remedies, moonshine liquor made with lead vats or tubes, or parental occupation or hobbies (stained glass making, lead glazes for painting). In adolescents, inhaling leaded gasoline fumes can result in lead toxicity.

Campbell C, Osterhoudt KC: Prevention of childhood lead poisoning. Curr Opin Pediatr 12:428-437, 2000.

129. At what lead levels is chelation indicated?

< 25 µg/dl	Chelation not indicated
25–45 µg/dl	Chelation not routinely indicated, as no evidence exists that chelation avoids or reverses neurotoxicity. Some patients may benefit from (oral) chelation (e.g., succimer), especially if elevated levels persist

	despite aggressive environmental intervention and abatement.
45–70 μg/dl	Chelation indicated with either succimer or $CaNa_2EDTA$ (if no clinical symptoms suggestive of encephalopathy such as headache or persistent vomiting); if symptoms of encephalopathy, chelation with dimercaprol (BAL) and $CaNa_2EDTA$ indicated. Prior to chelation, an abdominal radiograph should be taken to evaluate for possible removable enteral lead.
> 70 μg/dl	Inpatient chelation therapy with dimercaprol and $CaNa_2EDTA$

Committee on Drugs: Treatment guidelines for lead exposure in children. Pediatrics 96:155–160, 1995.

130. Why are both British anti-Lewisite (BAL, or dimercaprol) and disodium EDTA ($CaNa_2EDTA$) used in the treatment of lead encephalopathy or levels greater than 70 μg/dL?

Chelation with $CaNa_2EDTA$ removes lead from the *extracellular* compartment and increases urinary excretion of lead by 20- to 50-fold. The lead-depleted extracellular compartment increases diffusion from the tissues into the blood. This process may initially aggravate symptoms of lead toxicity in encephalopathic or severe cases by increasing blood and CNS lead levels. BAL is given because it binds with both intracellular and extracellular lead. It must be administered prior to (about 4 hours) $CaNa_2EDTA$. An additional advantage is it can be used in renal impairment, as its excretion is primarily through the biliary tree.

131. How are children with tricyclic antidepressant (TCA) overdose managed?

TCA overdose is one of the most serious and potentially lethal ingestions in children. These children usually need to be closely monitored in a hospital setting. Not all TCA ingestions result in life-threatening toxicity, but patients should be observed for at least 6 hours in an emergency department for any clinical symptoms including evidence of anticholinergic effects (sinus tachycardia, dilated pupils, and hot, flushed, dry skin), seizures, and ECG abnormalities (ventricular ectopy, QRS prolongation, or evidence of frank dysrhythmias such as ventricular tachycardia). The latter are the most feared complication TCA overdose in children.

The complete management of TCA overdose in children is complex, but includes anticonvulsant therapy for seizures, sodium bicarbonate and occasionally magnesium sulfate to prevent and/or treat TCA-associated dysrhythmias, and fluids and vasopressors, including norepinephrine and dopamine, for hypotension.

132. What is the pathophysiologic basis for the toxicity in iron ingestions?

Iron is toxic in various ways. It has a direct caustic effect on the GI tract, and when absorbed in excess of the total iron-binding capacity, free iron causes shock due to vasodilation. Hepatotoxicity results from accumulation of free iron in hepatocytes.

133. Which clinical and lab features correlate with an acutely elevated serum iron?

Serum iron levels obtained 4-6 hours after ingestion correlate with severity of toxicity. Iron levels > 300 μg/dl are associated with mild toxicity of local GI symptoms, such as nausea, vomiting, diarrhea. A serum iron level of 500 μg/dl is associated with serious systemic toxicity, and a level of 1000 μg/dl is associated with death. Other laboratory tests that correlate with an elevated iron level include leukocytosis (>15,000/mm^3) and hyperglycemia (>150 mg/dl). Sometimes radiopaque tablets may be demonstrated on abdominal x-ray.

134. If a toddler may have swallowed some multivitamins, when can he go home?

The toxic compound in multivitamin overdose is iron. There are a large variety of children's chewable multivitamins that contain different amounts of elemental iron (none to 18 mg of elemental iron per tablet). The toxic dose of iron ingestion is at least 20 mg/kg of elemental iron, and the lethal dose of iron reported is in the range of 60–180 mg/kg of elemental iron. In a small child, a toxic dose is about 300 mg of elemental iron, which is the equivalent of 20 tablets of multivitamins containing 15 mg/tab of elemental iron. Frequently, the amount of ingestion is not known. Since iron can initially cause nausea, vomiting or abdominal pain, a child with suspected but unknown amount of iron poisoning can be observed. A child who has no complaints and has a normal physical exam after 4-6 hours of observation can be safely discharged home.

135. What are the classic four clinical stages of iron toxicity?

While the presence, duration and severity of these phases will vary considerably, the four phases (with time post-ingestion) are:

Stage 1: (0.5 – 6 hours)—direct mucosal GI toxicity causing nausea, vomiting, abdominal pain and/or GI hemorrhage

Stage 2: (6–24 hours)—latent period with resolution of symptoms

Stage 3: (4–40 hours)—systemic toxicity with shock, cyanosis, lethargy, coma or coagulopathy associated with hepatic necrosis and/or renal failure

Stage 4: (2–8 weeks)—stricture formation with gastric outlet or intestinal obstruction

136. What is the preferred method GI decontamination in iron overdose?

Whole bowel irrigation is effective and is the method of choice if patient has symptoms of iron toxicity. Syrup of ipecac is no longer recommended even in the first hour. Many adult strength iron containing pills are very large and are often too large for orogastric lavage. Activated charcoal is not effective since it does not adsorb iron.

137. How do the signs and symptoms of acute iron ingestion differ from those of other heavy metal poisonings?

Iron salt ingestion causes early GI symptoms and, in severe cases, hemorrhagic gastritis, shock, and coma. After 24–48 hours, evidence of hepatic damage ensues.

Lead poisoning may cause mild GI symptoms; however, encephalopathy with cerebral vasculitis, increased intracranial pressure and coma, seizures, and severe neurologic damage are the most feared complications.

Acute ***mercury salt*** poisoning causes both a hemorrhagic gastroenteritis and renal damage. The liver is generally not injured.

Arsenic poisoning affects multiple organs with marked skin and hair changes, neurologic effects (encephalopathy, peripheral neuropathy, tremor, coma, convulsions), fatty infiltration of the liver, renal tubular and glomerular damage, and cardiac involvement with conduction delays and dysrhythmias.

138. What is the value of a deferoxamine challenge?

Deferoxamine challenge occasionally may be useful as an additional screening test for mild to moderate iron poisoning if "stat" iron levels are not available. In the asymptomatic or mildly symptomatic patient, a dose of 15 mg/kg (up to 1 gm maximum) may be given intramuscularly. A positive test (orange or "vin rose" tint to the urine) signifies the excretion of feroxamine (deferoxamine–iron chelate). All patients with a positive challenge test should be admitted for continuing chelation therapy. A negative challenge test in a patient with *significant* symptoms does not rule out iron toxicity and should not be relied upon.

139. What is worse, drinking dishwashing detergent or toilet bowl cleaner?

You are better off with the toilet bowl cleaner, although both acid (toilet bowl cleaner) and alkali (dishwashing detergent) ingestions may cause severe esophageal burns. *Alkalis* cause injury by liquefaction necrosis, dissolving proteins and lipids, thereby allowing deeper penetration of the caustic substance and greater local tissue injury. With *acids*, coagulation necrosis of the tissue occurs. This results in the formation of an eschar which limits the penetration of the toxin into deeper tissues. Compared with acids, alkalis are more typically in solid and paste form which increases tissue contact time and tissue injury.

140. If a 4-year-old patient has a convincing history of drain pipe cleaner (i.e., sodium hydroxide or lye) ingestion but is asymptomatic without evidence of oral mucosal injury, when can he or she be discharged to home?

The presence or absence of local (facial and oro-pharyngeal) signs and symptoms may not predict injury to the remainder of the gastrointestinal tract. The need for endoscopy to evaluate esophageal injury (burns) in these patients is controversial. Some experts recommend endoscopy in any setting where a convincing history of caustic ingestion has occurred. However, other studies suggest that a child with a minor accidental ingestion who has no symptoms of vomiting, stridor, drooling or irritability and no evidence of facial or oro-pharyngeal burns on exam may be discharged to home after a period of observation and normal feeding.

Gorman, et al: Initial symptoms as predictors of esophageal injury in alkaline corrosive ingestions. Am J Med 10:189-194, 1992.

141. Are steroids helpful for caustic ingestion?

Steroids are controversial in the treatment of caustic ingestions. They are purported to reduce scar formation and strictures but may interfere with wound healing and predispose to perforation. Most authorities currently recommend steroids for all significant second-degree burns and advocate their omission for significant full-thickness burns (where their use might be hazardous as well as ineffectual) or first-degree burns (which are expected to heal without scarring regardless of treatment).

142. When does stricture formation occur in lye ingestion?

Although strictures may form as soon as 2–3 weeks after caustic ingestion, the development is somewhat variable. 80% manifest within 2 months and almost all within 1 year. In general, in the followup of patients exposed to caustics, esophagoscopy and barium swallow are performed 3 weeks after ingestion if a significant burn was noted at the time of initial presentation. Clinical follow-up should occur for 6 months, at which time a repeat barium swallow should be considered. Occasionally, a mild stricture that has been relatively asymptomatic will become problematic after an interval of years, particularly following growth spurts (e.g., at adolescence). Long-term follow-up is also important because of the increased risk of carcinoma of the esophagus following ingestion of lye.

143. Which hydrocarbons pose the greatest risk for chemical pneumonitis?

The household hydrocarbons with ***low viscosities*** pose the greatest aspiration hazard. These include furniture polishes, gasoline and kerosene, turpentine and other paint-thinners, and lighter fuels.

144. What are the indications for gastric emptying in a hydrocarbon ingestion?

- Only for those compounds that would cause systemic toxicity. They can be remembered using the mnemonic ***CHAMP***: ***C***amphor—seizures; ***H***alogenated—dysrhythmias and hepato-toxicity; ***A***romatic—bone marrow toxicity; ***M***etals—diverse heavy metal manifestations; and ***P***esticides.
- When the hydrocarbon was ingested in massive quantity
- There is co-ingestion of another toxic compound for which GI decontamination is indicated.

145. Which patients with hydrocarbon ingestions should be admitted?

All patients with significant clinical findings should be admitted. Children with a history of exposure are safe to discharge after 4-6 hours of observation if they have (1) no symptoms; (2) accidental ingestion; (3) very transient coughing or gagging; (4) a normal physical examination; (5) asymptomatic patient with abnormal chest x-ray with reliable follow-up.

146. What is the differential diagnosis in a 10-year-old boy who presents to the emergency department with delirium?

Delirium is defined as a transient and reversible dysfunction in cerebral metabolism manifested as decreased ability to maintain attention to external stimuli, disorganized thinking, reduced level of consciousness, perceptual disturbances, disorientation, and memory impairment. It can be the result of numerous causes, including toxins, as depicted by the foreboding mnemonic, "I WATCH DEATH":

I = **I**nfectious (encephalitis, meningitis, syphilis, AIDS)
W = **W**ithdrawal (alcohol, barbiturates, sedatives-hypnotics)
A = **A**cute metabolic (acidosis, alkalosis, electrolyte disturbance, hepatic failure, renal failure)
T = **T**rauma (heat stroke, postoperative, severe burns)
C = **C**NS pathology (abscesses, hemorrhage, normal pressure hydrocephalus, seizures, stroke, tumors, vasculitis)
H = **H**ypoxia (anemia, CO poisoning, hypotension, pulmonary/cardiac failure)
D = **D**eficiencies (B_{12}, niacin, thiamine)
E = **E**ndocrinopathies (hyper-/hypoadrenalcorticism, hyper-/hypoglycemia)
A = **A**cute vascular (hypertensive encephalopathy, shock, migraine)
T = **T**oxins/drugs (medications, pesticides, solvents)
H = **H**eavy metals (lead, manganese, mercury)

From Williams DT: Neuropsychiatric signs, symptoms, and syndromes. In Lewis M (ed): Child and Adolescent Psychiatry. Baltimore, Williams &Wilkins, 1991, p 343; with permission.

147. A patient receiving an antiemetic drug (e.g., promethazine) who develops involuntary, prolonged, twisting, writhing movements of the neck, trunk and arms likely has what condition?

Acute dystonia. This dystonic reaction is classically seen as an adverse side effect of antidopaminergic agents such as neuroleptics, antiemetics or metoclopramide. In children, phenothiazines are the most common culprit. Treatment includes administration of diphenhydramine (Benadryl) orally, intramuscularly or intravenously at 1 mg/kg/dose. Benztropine (Cogentin) is also used in adolescents.

148. What do "SLUDGE" and "DUMBELS" have in common?

Both are mnemonics used to remember the problems involved with organophospate poisoning, lipid-soluble insecticides used in agriculture and terrorism ("nerve gas"). Organophosphates inhibit cholinesterase and cause all the signs and symptoms of acetylcholine excess.

Muscarinic effects: increased oral and tracheal secretions, miosis, salivation, lacrimation, urination, vomiting, cramping, defecation, and bradycardia; may progress to frank pulmonary edema

CNS effects: agitation, delirium, seizures, and/or coma

Nicotinic effects: sweating, muscle fasciculation, and, ultimately, paralysis

The mnemonic ***SLUDGE*** is: **S**alivation, **L**acrimation, **U**rination, **D**efecation, **GI** cramps, **E**mesis.

The mnemonic **DUMBELS** is: **D**efecation, **U**rination, **M**iosis, **B**ronchorrhea/**B**radycardia, **E**mesis, **L**acrimation, **S**alivation.

149. A child is brought to the ED with a temperature of 105°, hypertension, and involuntary muscle contraction. What kinds of poisoning should be considered?

The combination of severe hyperthermia and increased muscle activity is common for a number of acute drug overdoses as well as withdrawal from alcohol and sedative hypnotic agents. The common acute overdoses that may present this way include cocaine, amphetamines and other sympathomimetic agents, monoamine oxidase inhibitors, lithium, phencyclidine, and some anticholinergic agents (including TCAs). Occasionally, the syndrome is seen as part of the so-called neuroleptic-malignant syndrome, which occurs with therapeutic dosing of antipsychotic agents.

150. What metal intoxication can mimic Kawasaki syndrome?

Mercury. *Acrodynia* is the term applied to one form of mercury salt intoxication that results in a constellation of signs and symptoms very similar to that currently recognized as Kawasaki syndrome. The classic presentation of acrodynia was described in children exposed to calomel, a substance used in teething powders, which was essentially mercurous chloride. The symptom complex included swelling and redness of the hands and feet, skin rashes, diaphoresis, tachycardia, hypertension, photophobia, and an intense irritability with anorexia and insomnia. Infants were often very limp, lying in a frog-like position, with impressive weakness of the hip and shoulder girdle muscles. Similar symptoms have been described in children exposed to other forms of mercury, including broken fluorescent light bulbs or diapers rinsed in mercuric chloride.

151. What causes Minamata disease?

Methylmercury exposure. The term derivatives from Minamata, Japan, where in the 1950s the local population was exposed to methylmercury through the ingestion of fish caught in the heavily contaminated Minamata Bay. Severe neurologic abnormalities developed in the older population, and 6% of children born from 1955–1959 had significant problems, including microencephaly and cerebral palsy.

Harada M: Minamata disease: Intrauterine and methylmercury poisoning. Teratology 18:285–288, 1978.

152. Where did the "mad hatter" get his name?

The ***encephalopathy*** of ***chronic elemental mercury poisoning*** was an occupational hazard of hat makers, who used mercury to produce felt.

153. How does the coma caused by barbiturates differ from that caused by psychotropic drugs?

Barbiturates are classic examples of the *sedative-hypnotic group* of drugs. Ingestions of these agents are manifested by a dose-dependent CNS depression with subsequent respiratory and cardiovascular depression. These patients usually have coma, occasionally with miotic pupils and depressed deep tendon reflexes; the coma is characterized by slowed vital signs and decreased muscle tone. This picture contrasts with that of the *psychotropic drugs* and *phenothiazines*, which often produce an anticholinergic effect, elevated vital signs, and increased muscle tone with progression to seizures.

154. Why is cyanide so toxic?

Cyanide ion binds to the heme-containing cytochrome a_3 enzyme in the electron transport chain of mitochondria, which is the final common pathway in oxidative metabolism. Thus, with a significant exposure, virtually every cell in the body becomes starved of oxygen at the mitochondrial level and is unable to function. The body does have minor routes of cyanide detoxification, including excretion by the lungs and liver via rhodanese, an hepatic enzyme that combines cyanide with thiosulfate to form the less toxic thiocyanate for renal excretion. However, these mechanisms are inadequate in the face of a significant cyanide exposure. As with carbon monoxide poisoning, symptoms tend to be most prominent among the metabolically active organ systems. In particular, the CNS is rapidly affected, causing headache and dizziness, which may progress to prostration, convulsions, coma, and death. Less severe ingestions may be noted initially by burning of the tongue and mucous membranes, with tachypnea and dyspnea due to cyanide stimulation of chemoreceptors.

155. In what settings should cyanide poisoning be suspected?

- *Suicidal ingestion*, often involving chemists who have access to cyanide salts as reagents
- *Fires* causing combustion of materials such as wool, silk, synthetic rubber, polyurethane and nitrocellulose, which resulting in the release of cyanide
- Patients who are on *nitroprusside continuous infusion*, an antihypertensive agent that contains five cyanide moieties per molecule

156. What kinds of plants account for the greatest percentage of deaths due to plant poisonings?

Mushrooms account for ≥ 50% of deaths due to plant poisoning. The most dreaded variety are the *Amanita* species, which initially cause intestinal symptoms by one toxin (phallotoxin) and then hepatic and renal failure by a separate toxin (amatoxin). Other mushrooms classes can cause a variety of early-onset (<6 hours) symptoms including muscarinic effects (e.g., sweating, salivation, colic), anticholinergic effects (e.g., drowsiness, mania, hallucinations), gastroenteritis and Antabuse-type effects if taken with alcohol.

157. After an enjoyable takeout meal of moo goo gai pan, an 8-year-old presents with facial burning and headache. What is the likely diagnosis?

The ***Chinese restaurant syndrome***. Several hours after ingestion of Chinese food, a patient may complain of burning and numbness of the face and neck, headache, and, occasionally, severe chest pain. Symptoms can persist up to 1–2 days. The pathophysiology remains unclear, but monosodium glutamate (MSG), a food additive, may be involved with glutamate acting as a neurotransmitter. Other studies suggest that the fermentation of typical ingredients in Chinese cooking (e.g., soy sauce, black beans, shrimp paste) may release histamines which account for the symptoms.

158. Is mistletoe toxic?

Mistletoe, the popular Christmas plant, is an evergreen with small white berries. Ingestions of small amounts of the berries, leaves, or stems may result in GI symptoms, including pain, nausea, vomiting, and diarrhea. Rarely, large ingestions have resulted in seizures, hypertension, and even cardiac arrest. In some countries, extracts of mistletoe have been used for illegal abortifacients, brewed in teas which are particularly toxic. In the United States, the typical call to a poison center concerns a child who eats one or two mistletoe berries, which in general, is unlikely to produce significant signs or symptoms. Kissing under the mistletoe may lead to greater hazards.

159. Should ingested disc batteries be removed?

Although the concern is that a disc battery may produce corrosive intestinal injury, most traverse the GI tract without incident. An initial x-ray for localization is indicated. If the disc battery is in the distal esophagus, removal is required. Otherwise, if the battery is in the stomach or beyond and the patient remains asymptomatic, watchful waiting is appropriate. If the battery is not seen in the stool by 5–7 days, a repeat x-ray should be obtained.

160. Would watchful waiting be appropriate management for a child with an x-ray revealing an open safety pin in the abdomen?

Even though an open safety pin is obviously a sharp object and may get stuck in the intestinal tract more easily than a round smooth object (e.g., coin, battery, marble), most pass without complications. If the patient develops no abdominal symptoms, watching waiting with follow-up x-rays is appropriate. If symptoms (e.g., pain, vomiting, distension) develop, surgical extraction is indicated.

161. What is the most common causes of aspirated foreign bodies resulting in respiratory symptoms and requiring bronchoscopic removal in children?

Peanuts. Easily the most common, causing nearly 40% of cases in some studies. Other causes include other nuts, other organic (food) materials, seeds (sunflower and watermelon), twigs, plastics, popcorn, pins and screws. Because the clinical picture of aspiration can mimic viral URI, the diagnosis is often delayed. Eliciting a thorough history involving possible aspiration (i.e., choking) is important, though not always present.

Black RE, et al: Bronchoscopic removal of aspirated foreign bodies in children. J Pediatr Surg 29:682-684, 1994.

162. What is the best way to remove a foreign body from the esophagus?

Three methods are used, and often local custom prevails regarding selection.

1. ***Esophagoscopy***, the most commonly used method, is done under general anesthesia.

2. A ***Foley catheter*** can be inserted beyond the foreign body, inflated, and then pulled back to remove the object. This extraction method is used by various centers, particularly for coins if the ingestion is < 24 hours old and no respiratory distress is present. Complications, such as airway obstruction by a displaced coin and esophageal perforation, are possible.

3. In ***bougienage***, the object is forced into the stomach.

TRAUMA

163. In a child with head trauma, is a skull x-ray a good screening study?

No. Use of skull films in the management of head trauma in children has been controversial. Skull films will reveal only bony abnormalities, not intracranial injuries (ICIs). While the presence of a skull fracture increases the relative risk for intracranial injury almost fourfold, the absence of a skull fracture on plain x-ray does not rule out an ICI. A normal skull film may be falsely reassuring. Plain x-rays are not considered sufficiently sensitive nor specific to be clinically useful in most settings.

Skull films may be considered in well-appearing children less than 3 months of age with a history of nontrivial head trauma without hematoma present or in children between 3 months and one year, who have a moderate to severe skull hematoma. Presence of a fracture would warrant CT evaluation. Also, many practitioners consider films for temporal injuries, given the proximity of the middle meningeal artery and increased epidural bleeding with a fracture at that site, even with a relatively minor injury.

Quayle SQ, Jaffe, DM, et al: Diagnostic testing for acute head injury in children: When are head computed tomographic scan and skull radiographs indicated? Pediatrics 99:11-17, 1997.

164. When should a CT scan be considered following head trauma?

- Glasgow coma scale < 15
- Focal neurologic abnormality
- Seizure (early, focal or prolonged)
- Skull fracture
- Full fontanel
- Loss of consciousness (especially if more than brief)

- Deteriorating or persistent altered level of consciousness, irritability or behavior
- Unremitting vomiting (especially if > 4-6 hrs) or progressive headache
- Signs of penetrating skull trauma or bony abnormality
- Age <3 months with nontrivial trauma
- Age less than two years with significant scalp hematoma

Adapted from Schutzman SA: Head injury. In Fleisher GR, Ludwig S (eds): Textbook of Pediatric Emergency Medicine, 4th ed. Baltimore, Lippincott Williams &Wilkins, 2000, p 272.

Greenes DS, Schutzman SA: Clinical indicators of intracranial injury in head-injured infants. Pediatrics 104:861-867, 1999.

165. What types of localized anatomic pathology can develop after acute head trauma?

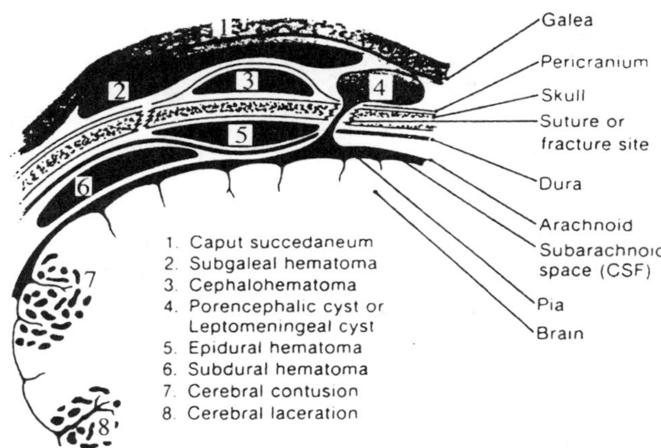

From Rosman NP, et al: Acute head trauma in infancy and childhood. Pediatr Clin North Am 26:708, 1979; with permission.

166. If a patient with head trauma has persistent hypotension and bradycardia despite resuscitative efforts, what should be considered?

Neurogenic shock. Trauma to the cervical or high thoracic spinal cord can often injure or ablate the descending sympathetic pathways, which results in the loss of vasomotor tone and sympathetic control of the heart. Treatment consists of cardiorespiratory support, atropine, fluid resuscitation, and sympathomimetics. The vast majority of patients respond to fluids alone.

167. How does hyperventilation lower increased intracranial pressure (ICP)?

Following severe head trauma, cerebral blood flow and cerebral blood volume increase and can result in an elevated ICP. Severely increased ICP may compromise cerebral perfusion pressure (defined as the mean arterial pressure minus ICP), contribute to ischemic injury and ultimately lead to herniation. Cerebral blood flow is influenced by $PaCO_2$. The hyperventilation of a patient to reduce the $PaCO_2$ from 40 mmHg to 25–30 mmHg reduces cerebral blood volume by approximately 50%, lowering ICP and thus improving cerebral perfusion pressure. However, lowering cerebral blood flow may have deleterious effects on outcome. There is debate on the exact role of hyperventilation (particularly prolonged) in head-injured children, and it is generally reserved for patients who have signs of acutely-increased intracranial pressure or herniation. It is not indicated as a preventative therapy.

Meyer P, et al: Critical care management of neurotrauma in children: New trends and perspectives. Childs Nerv Syst 15: 732-739, 1999.

168. What is the role of hypertonic saline solutions in the management of head trauma?

The use of 3% hypertonic saline is under study as an additional means of controlling cerebral edema and increased intracranial pressure following closed head injury. Its role is undetermined, but promising.

Peterson B, et al: Prolonged hypernatremia controls elevated intracranial pressure in head-injured pediatric patients. Crit Care Med 28:1136-1143, 2000.

169. When ICP is acutely elevated, how long before papilledema develops?

Generally, in **24–48 hours**.

170. What are the components of the Glasgow Coma Scale?

Developed in 1974 by the neurosurgical department at the University of Glasgow, the scale was an attempt to standardize the assessment of the depth and duration of impaired consciousness and coma, particularly in the setting of trauma. The scale is based on eye opening, verbal responses, and motor responses, with a total ranging from 3–15.

Glasgow Coma Scale

Best verbal response*	5	Oriented, appropriate conversation
	4	Confused conservation
	3	Inappropriate words
	2	Incomprehensible sounds
	1	No response
Best motor response	6	Obeys a verbal command
(to command or pain,	5	Localizes
such as rubbing	4	Withdraws
knuckles on sternum)	3	Abnormal flexion (decorticate posturing)
	2	Abnormal extension (decerebrate posturing)
	1	No response
Eye opening	4	Spontaneous
	3	In response to verbal command
	2	In response to pain
	1	No response

*Children < 2 years should receive full verbal scores for crying after stimulation.

171. How do the signs of CNS herniation differ?

- *Tentorial herniation* (unilateral herniation of temporal lobe from middle to posterior fossa through rigid tentorium)—ipsilateral third nerve findings (pupillary dilation, ptosis, loss of media gaze) and contralateral hemiparesis and decerebate posturing
- *Cerebellar tonsils through foramen magnum*—Abnormalities of tone, bradycardia, hypertension and progressive respiratory distress (Cushing's triad)
- *Subfalcine herniation* (herniation of one cerebral hemisphere beneath the falx cerebri to the opposite side): leg weakness and bladder abnormalities

Beware that these clinical findings tend to overlap, and an altered state of consciousness is often the initial symptom.

172. How, when, and where are car seats to be used?

All 50 states require that children riding in cars always be restrained in an approved safety seat based on weight or height as follows:

< 20 lbs	Rear-facing infant seat (also recommended by the AAP until *1 year of age*)
20–40 lbs	Forward-facing toddler seat
40–60 lbs	Booster seat with lap belt
> 60 lbs	Regular lap belt
> 48 in	Shoulder strap with belt

Bull MJ, Sheese J: Update for the pediatrician on child passenger safety: Five priniciples for safer travel. Pediatrics 106:1113-1116, 2000.

173. What are the most common problems found with seat belt use in children?

Safety seats are often installed or used incorrectly. The three most frequently found problems:

1. Seat not belted into vehicle tightly
2. Safety seat harness straps are not snug
3. Harness retainer clip not at armpit level

In various studies, these deficits have been identified in 34-88% of forward-facing or rear-facing seats.

Kohn M et al: Anticipatory guidance about child safety seat misuse: Lessons from safety seat "check-ups." Arch Pediatr Adolesc Med 154:606-609, 2000.

174. What are the dangers of air bags to children?

Children *under the age of 13 years* and *under 5 feet in height* should not be seated in the front seat of cars with air bags. Air bag deployment has been associated with such life-threatening injuries as cervical spine injuries and closed head trauma. Other, less serious injuries include facial, neck, and chest abrasions, facial and upper extremity burns and blunt and chemical ocular trauma.

McCaffrey M, et al: Air bags and children: A potentially lethal combination. J Pediatr Orthop 19:60-64, 1999.

175. What are the major signs of a blow-out fracture?

Traumatic force to the eye can result in a blow-out fracture affecting either the orbital floor or medial wall. The fracture may result from either a sudden increase in intraorbital pressure or from a direct concussive force to the bony walls. Symptoms and signs can include:

- Pain on upward gaze
- Diplopia on upward gaze
- Enophthalmos (i.e., posterior displacement of globe)
- Loss of sensation over upper lip and gums on injured side
- Inability to look upward on affected side due to entrapment of the inferior rectus muscle
- Crepitus over the inferior orbital ridge

176. How does the location of cervical spine fractures vary between younger children and older children/adults?

Younger children tend to have fractures of the *upper* cervical spine, whereas *older children and adults* have fractures more often involving the *lower* cervical spine, for the following reasons:

- Changing fulcrum of spine: In an infant, the fulcrum of the cervical spine is at approximately C2–3; in a child aged 5–6 years, C3–4; by age 8 to adulthood, C5–6. These changes are in large part due to the relatively large head size of a child compared to an adult.
- Younger children have relatively weak neck muscles.
- Younger children have poorer protective reflexes.

Woodward GA: Neck trauma. In Fleisher GR, Ludwig S (eds):Textbook of Pediatric Emergency Medicine, 4th ed. Baltimore, Williams &Wilkins, 2000, pp 1318.

177. What is a hangman fracture?

This fracture of the posterior elements of the C2 vertebra results from severe hyperextension of the neck. When the neck is placed in flexion, this may allow subluxation (spondylolisthesis) of C2 on C3, causing damage to the spinal cord.

178. Is there a set of clinical criteria that can limit the need for cervical spine films?

A recent study, including a subset of younger children, looked at five criteria as low probability for cervical injury: no midline cervical tenderness, no focal neurologic deficit, normal alertness, no intoxication, and no painful, distracting injury. In over 34,000 patients who underwent radiography for blunt trauma, the negative predictive value was 99.8% if the five criteria were met. More extensive studies in children will be needed to confirm its usefulness.

Hoffman JR et al: Validity of a set of clinical criteria to rule out injury to the cervical spine in patients with blunt trauma. N Engl J Med 343:94-99, 2000.

179. Which patients have SCIWORA?

Up to 60% of children with spinal cord injuries have **SCIWORA**, which is **S**pinal **C**ord **I**njury **W**ithout **R**adiographic **A**bnormality. Most are < 8 years of age with symptoms and signs consistent with spinal cord injury, but x-ray and CT studies reveal no bony abnormalities. It is postulated that the highly malleable pediatric spine allows the cord to sustain injury from flexion/extension forces without causing bony disruption. The more recent use of MRI in these children may help to clarify the cause(s).

Their initial neurological complaint should be taken seriously. Even with normal x-rays, a patient with an altered sensorium or neurologic abnormalities consistent with cervical cord injury (e.g., motor or sensory changes, bowel/bladder problems, vital sign instability) requires continued neck immobilization and more extensive evaluation.

180. In the evaluation of abdominal trauma in children, what are the indications for peritoneal lavage?

- Potential false-negative examination: head injury, altered sensorium due to medication, spinal cord trauma
- Potential false-positive examination: rib, pelvic, or spine fractures
- Unexplained hypovolemia
- Anesthetic need for unrelated injury
- Selected penetrating injury

Ziegler Mm, Gonzalez Del Rey JA: Major trauma. In Fleisher GR, Ludwig S (eds):Textbook of Pediatric Emergency Medicine, 4th ed. Baltimore, Williams &Wilkins, 2000, pp 1265.

181. Why is left shoulder pain after abdominal trauma a worrisome sign?

This may represent blood accumulating under the diaphragm resulting with pain referred to the left shoulder (*Kehr sign*). The sign can be elicited by LUQ palpation or by placing the patient in the Trendelenburg position. The finding is worrisome for possible solid organ abdominal injury, most commonly the spleen, and requires surgical consultation and radiographic studies, usually CT or ultrasound, to grade the extent of injury.

Powell M, et al: Management of blunt splenic trauma: significant differences between adults and children. Surgery 122:654-660, 1997.

182. What is the significance of a teardrop-shaped pupil noted in the evaluation of a child with eye trauma?

Ruptured globe. The misshapen pupil is the result of the contents of the iris coming forward and plugging the laceration or puncture. This is an ophthalmologic emergency with risk of permanent injury. Emergency management follows the mnemonic **SANTA**: **S**—

shield, **A**—antiemetics, **N**—NPO, **T**—tetanus, **A**—antibiotics. Most importantly, the eye must be immediately protected from further injury with a non-malleable shield which applies *no* pressure to the globe itself. The patient must be kept calm to prevent increases in intraocular pressure.

Rahman WM, O'Connor TJ: Facial Trauma. In Barkin RM (ed): Pediatric Emergency Medicine, Concepts and Clinical Practice. St. Louis, Mosby, 1997, pp 252-283.

183. How should the pupils be dilated?

Pupillary dilation is sometimes needed in the evaluation of eye trauma, in the search for retinal hemorrhages in suspected child abuse, in the ongoing examination of suspected increasing ICP (e.g., headaches, meningitis, head trauma), and in the ascertainment of papilledema prior to lumbar puncture. Pupillary control is dual—the pupillary dilator is sympathetically mediated; the pupillary sphincter is parasympathetically mediated (as is the ciliary muscle, which controls lens accommodation). Combinations of drops are often utilized involving sympathomimetics (e.g., phenylephrine 2.5%) and anticholinergics (e.g., tropicamide 0.5–1.0%, cyclopentolate 0.5%). All have rapid onsets (< 30 min) and short durations of action (e.g., phenylephrine, <3 hrs; tropicamide, < 6 hrs). Local custom will prevail, but one simple method of dilation is 1 drop of tropicamide 0.5%, repeated if necessary. Darker eyes are more difficult to dilate and may require repeat dosing.

Chiaviello CT, Bond GR: Dilating the pupil in the pediatric emergency department. Pediatr Emerg Care 4:216–218, 1994.

184. When are drops for pupillary dilation contraindicated?

These drops should not be used in patients requiring sequential neurologic exams (e.g., after severe head trauma) where increasing ICP with herniation is possible. They are also contraindicated in the setting of acute-angle glaucoma. The risk of inducing glaucoma is very low in children, but if symptoms of glaucoma (e.g., moderate eye pain, decreased vision, cloudy cornea, asymmetric pupil size, poor pupillary reaction) are present, dilation should be deferred. Of note, all drops can have side effects, and these can be minimized by pressure over the medial canthus to avoid systemic absorption.

185. When should an avulsed tooth be reimplanted?

Avulsion is the complete displacement of the tooth from its socket. Primary (i.e., baby) teeth should not be reimplanted, as nerve root damage or dental ankylosis may result. Secondary teeth should be repaired within 30 minutes (less than 10 minutes may be most optimal) to maximize the chance of tooth viability. Thus, early insertion after gently rinsing the tooth is preferable (even if not a perfect fit, reimplanation may prevent the root from drying). It is important to disturb the root as minimally as possible. If not reimplantable (e.g., uncooperative patient), a dislodged tooth should be gently rinsed, transported in milk or saliva or under a parent's tongue, and reimplanted temporarily until definitive dental care can be obtained.

Weiger R, Heuchert T. Management of an avulsed primary incisor. Endod Dental Traumatol 15:138-143, 1999.

186. What are the three most important considerations in evaluating nasal trauma?

1. ***Bleeding***. If persistent, bleeding should be controlled with pressure, topical vasoconstrictors, topical thrombin, cauterization, and anterior or posterior nasal packing.

2. ***Septal hematoma***. If the nasal septum is bulging into the nasal cavity, there is likely a hematoma which must be drained. If drainage is not done, abscess formation or pressure necrosis can result, leading to a saddle-nose deformity.

3. ***Watery rhinorrhea***. This may be a sign of cribriform plate, suborbital ethmoid, sphenoid sinus, or frontal sinus fracture with CSF leak. Radioisotope scans or CT scan with metrizamide dye can confirm the fracture. Hospitalization is warranted if positive.

More extensive facial trauma requires evaluation for many items, especially midface fractures and eye damage. Determining if the nose is fractured is a lower priority item because fracture reduction is done only if there is distortion of the nose. Furthermore, such distortion cannot be properly assessed acutely due to swelling.

187. How long before a broken nose in a child must be reduced?

If a nasal bone fracture causes asymmetry, which is noted as the swelling from acute trauma subsides, the fracture should be reduced within 4–5 days. A longer delay may result in malunion.

188. How does one distinguish nasal mucosal drainage from CSF leakage?

This often becomes an issue when children have nasal rhinorrhea following trauma. The simplest test is to check the glucose concentration. The CSF glucose is normally 40–80 mg/dl, whereas the glucose concentration of nasal mucus is normally near 0.

189. In a 7-year-old boy with an x-ray-proven pelvic fracture, what urologic procedure is needed and what procedure is relatively contraindicated?

The urethra as it passes through the prostate is very close to the pubic bone and is thus susceptible to injury by a pelvic fracture. Urethral damage should be suspected in all patients with pelvic fractures, even those without hematuria. The recommended diagnostic procedure is a ***retrograde urethrogram***. Of note, a boggy, high-riding prostate found on rectal exam and/or blood seen at the urethral meatus are clinical signs of possible urethral disruption. These two findings are contraindications for passing a ***Foley catheter***. A partial urethral disruption could potentially be made into a complete one with the passing of the catheter.

190. How is zipper entrapment remedied?

This situation most commonly occurs in boys with intact foreskins. Following use of a local anesthetic (1% lidocaine without epinephrine), release is accomplished by simple manipulation of the zipper, cutting the median bar of the zipper with a wire cutter or dividing the zipper transversely.

Strait RT: A novel method for removal of penile zipper entrapment. Pediatr Emerg Care 15:412-413, 1999.

191. Are single lateral cervical spine radiographs sufficient to "clear" a patient following neck injury?

No. In some studies, the sensitivity of a single view for fractures is only 80%. American College of Radiology guidelines recommend at least 3 views: *anteroposterior* (including C7-T1 junction, C1-C7), *lateral* and *open-mouth* (odontoid). The last view is often difficult to obtain in younger children. CT scan and MRI imaging are reserved for more extensive evaluation for spinal cord injury when the initial three views are negative in symptomatic patients. The use of oblique films is controversial.

Dalinka MK et al: Appropriateness criteria for imaging and treatment decisions. In: Cascade PN (ed), American College of Radiology Task Force on Appropriateness Criteria. Reston,VA, American College of Radiology, 1995.

192. What condition, if improperly treated, can result in a "saddle-nose" deformity?

Septal hematoma. Bleeding into the septum after nasal trauma compromises the blood supply to the nasal cartilage. Septal hematomas, recognizable by bulging of the septum into the nasal cavity, require prompt recognition to permit timely incision and drainage. If untreated, abscess (most common complication), necrosis, perforation, and nasal obstruction may occur. The saddle-nose deformity is the inward bowing of the nasal midline due to cartilaginous decay.

Canty PA, Berkowitz RG: Hematoma and abscess of the nasal septum in children. Arch Otolaryngology Head Neck Surg. 122:1373-1376, 1996.

The authors gratefully acknowledge the contributions of the following individuals:
Peter Dayan, M.D., Anju Wagh, M.D., Sharon Pan, M.D., Joan Bregstein, M.D.,
Stephen Gordon, M.D., Joel Berezow, M.D., Jonathan Bennett, M.D.,
Rob Best, M.D., Faez Ahmad, M.D., Mindy Stimell, M.D.

6. ENDOCRINOLOGY

Sharon Oberfield, M.D., *and Daniel* E. *Hale,* M.D.

ADRENAL DISORDERS

1. What is the differential diagnosis of primary adrenal insufficiency?

Inherited enzymatic defects: Congenital adrenal hyperplasia (multiple enzymatic defects)

Autoimmune: Isolated, autoimmune polyendocrine syndromes (APES I and II), Schmidt syndrome

Infectious: Tuberculosis, meningococcemia, disseminated fungal infections

Traumatic: Bilateral adrenal hemorrhage

2. What are the most common causes of secondary adrenal insufficiency?

Secondary causes can include failure of the hypothalamic and/or pituitary gland due to tumor, CNS trauma, irradiation, infection, or surgery. The most common cause, however, is ***prolonged glucocorticoid use*** for treatment of nonadrenal disease.

3. Can clinical clues suggest that adrenal insufficiency is a primary rather than secondary problem?

In *primary* adrenal insufficiency, ACTH levels rise due to disruption of the hormonal feedback loop. Hyperpigmentation can result from these elevated levels. In *secondary* adrenal insufficiency, ACTH levels are low, and no hyperpigmentation occurs. Furthermore, in secondary insufficiency, the zona glomerulosa of the adrenal gland (responsible for aldosterone secretion) remains intact. Therefore, hyperkalemia and/or volume depletion are distinctly uncommon, but hyponatremia may occur as a result of decreased capacity to excrete a water load. In contrast, primary deficiencies commonly lead to hyponatremia *and* hyperkalemia.

4. What is the optimal time for measuring serum cortisol levels?

The time depends on the question being addressed. If the question is whether the pituitary-adrenal axis is functioning normally, then cortisol should be measured at 8 AM and 11 PM. The response is also dependent on whether the patient is significantly stressed (e.g., serious illness) and has an established diurnal pattern. Morning values should be 8–19 μg/dl, and evening values should be 4–11 μg/dl. Hypofunction of the axis is likely to be demonstrated by a low AM cortisol, while hyperfunction is more likely to be shown by a high PM cortisol. More definitive evaluation of the axis can be obtained by using some combination of the cosyntropin stimulation test, corticotropin-releasing factor (CRF) test, and metyrapone test. If hyperfunction of the axis is suspected, 24-hour urinary free cortisol determination is more definitive, although multiple 24-hour urine collections may need to be obtained.

5. In newborns with congenital adrenal hyperplasia (CAH), why are girls more likely to be diagnosed earlier than boys?

The most obvious clinical feature of CAH in the newborn period is *ambiguous genitalia* due to androgen excess. In boys, androgen excess does not cause any clearly abnormal appearance of the external genitalia. In girls, however, ambiguous genitalia are common. CAH should always be considered in the differential diagnosis of ambiguous genitalia, particularly in genetic females.

6. Describe the clinical features of the various forms of congenital adrenal hyperplasia (CAH).

CAH refers to a group of autosomal recessive disorders that result from various enzymatic defects in the biosynthesis of cortisol. Depending on the enzyme involved, the blockade can result in excesses or deficiencies in the other steroid pathways (i.e., mineralocorticoids and androgens). 21-Hydroxylase deficiency accounts for > 90% of cases; the complete (salt-losing) and partial (simple virilizing) forms occur in about 1/12,000 births and have an equal sex distribution. A late-onset or attenuated form (mild deficiency) manifests in adolescent females with hirsutism and menstrual irregularities.

Clinical Features of Disorders of Adrenal Steroidogenesis

ENZYME DEFECT	SEXUAL AMBIGUITY		POSTNATAL VIRILIZATION	SALT WASTING	HYPERTENSION
	FEMALE	MALE			
21-Hydroxylase					
Salt-wasting	+	0	+	+	0
Simple virilizing	+	0	+	0	0
Late-onset	0	0	+	0	0
11-Hydroxylase	+	0	+	0	+
17-Hydroxylase	0	+	0	0	+
18-Hydroxylase	0	0	0	+	0
3β-Hydroxysteroid dehydrogenase	+	+	+	+	0
Desmolase	0	+	0	+	0

7. How do the major steroid preparations vary in potency?

Relative Potencies of Glucocorticoids

NAME	RELATIVE GLUCOCORTICOID POTENCY	RELATIVE DOSING (mg)	RELATIVE MINERALO-CORTICOID POTENCY
Cortisone	1	100	+
Hydrocortisone	1.25	80	++
Prednisone	5	20	+
Prednisolone	5	20	+
Methylprednisolone	6	16	0
9α-Fluorocortisol	20	5	+++++
Dexamethasone	50	1	0

Adapted from Donohoue PA: The adrenal cortex. In McMillan JA, et al (eds): Oski's Pediatrics, Principles and Practice, 3rd ed. Philadelphia, J.B. Lippincott, 1999, p 1814; with permission.

8. How do physiologic, stress, and pharmacologic doses of hydrocortisone differ?

Careful studies have shown that adrenal glucocorticoid production in the normal individual is about 7–8 mg/m^2/24 hr. Because 50–60% of oral hydrocortisone is absorbed, the recommended ***physiologic replacement*** orally is about 12–15 mg/m^2/24 hr.

Based on studies performed prior to the development of high-quality radioimmunoassays, a consensus developed that production of glucocorticoid increased about threefold when individuals were physiologically stressed. Hence, when the term ***stress dose*** is used, it generally means 50 mg of hydrocortisone/m^2/24 hr.

Glucocorticoids are extensively used in ***pharmacologic doses*** in the treatment of various inflammatory processes and in surgery or trauma to reduce or prevent swelling and inflammation. The doses are dependent on the underlying process and are often > 50 mg hydrocortisone/m^2/24 hr.

9. When does adrenal-pituitary axis suppression occur in prolonged glucocorticoid treatment?

As a general rule, the longer the duration of treatment and the higher the dose, the greater the risk of adrenal suppression. If pharmacologic doses of glucocorticoids are used for ***< 10 days***, there is a relatively small risk of permanent adrenal insufficiency, while daily use ***> 30 days*** carries a high risk of transient or permanent adrenal suppression.

10. How rapidly should prescribed doses of steroids be reduced?

No single rule can cover all possible circumstances. The rapidity of tapering depends on the duration of treatment, the amount and type of glucocorticoid used, and the disease process under treatment.

1. The reduction from pharmacologic to physiologic doses depends on the underlying disease. For example, a child with lupus who has been maintained on pharmacologic doses for weeks may need to be tapered very slowly (10% increments every 2 weeks) in order to avoid a rebound of disease.

2. If there is no obvious reason to taper slowly, then the dose can be reduced by 50% every 2 days until the patient is on the equivalent of physiologic dosing (12–15 mg hydrocortisone/m2/24 hr). The second phase, tapering from a physiologic dose, can then begin (see Question 11).

3. In cases of congenital adrenal hyperplasia or known hypopituitarism, reducing the dose below physiologic replacement amounts may be contraindicated.

11. A child has been on physiologic doses of prednisone (3–4 mg/m^2/day) for 4 months. What is the best way to discontinue the therapy safely?

1. Change to a hydrocortisone preparation with corresponding equivalency dose.

2. Reduce to ½ of physiologic dose for 2 weeks. If the child is stressed, the dose must be increased to an appropriate stress dose (50 mg/m^2/24 hr).

3. At the end of the second week, withhold the AM hydrocortisone dose and obtain an AM cortisol level.

   a. If AM cortisol is > 10 μg/dl, supplementation may be stopped. However, stress coverage is required until the adequacy of the adrenal-pituitary response to stress (ACTH stimulation test and/or metyrapone testing) can be determined.
   b. If AM cortisol is < 10 μg/dl, continue supplementation (6–8 mg/m2/24 hr). Repeat AM cortisol in 1 month. Stress coverage must be maintained.

CALCIUM METABOLISM AND DISORDERS

12. Is it the Chvostek or Trousseau sign that gets the tap?

Chvostek. Both are clinical manifestations of hypocalcemia or hypomagnesemia that occur because of neuromuscular irritability.

Chvostek sign: Tapping on the facial nerve in front of the ear results in movement of the upper lip.

Trousseau sign: Inflating a blood pressure cuff at pressures greater than systolic for 2 minutes results in carpopedal spasm.

13. What are the causes of hypercalcemia?

Remember the "high fives" (***H***igh 5-***I's***) rule: ***H*** (hyperparathyroidism) plus the 5 ***I's*** (idiopathic, infantile, infection, infiltrations, and ingestions) and ***S*** (skeletal disorders).

Hyperparathyroidism
- Familial
- Isolated
- Syndromic

Idiopathic
- Williams syndrome

Infantile
- Subcutaneous fat necrosis
- Secondary to maternal hypoparathyroidism

Infections
- Tuberculosis

Infiltrations
- Malignancy
- Sarcoidosis

Ingestions
- Milk-alkali syndrome
- Thiazide diuretics
- Vitamin A intoxication
- Vitamin D intoxication

Skeletal disorders
- Hypophosphatasia
- Immobilization
- Skeletal dysplasias

14. In what circumstances should hypoparathyroidism be suspected?

Historical
- May occur as part of the autoimmune polyendocrine syndrome (see Question 24)
- Associated with thymic aplasia and immunodeficiency (DiGeorge syndrome)
- Damage may occur as a complication of neck surgery or irradiation

Clinical
- Manifestations of hypocalcemia such as carpopedal spasm, bronchospasm, tetany, or seizures
- Lenticular cataracts (which can occur in other causes of long-standing hypocalcemia)
- Changing behaviors, ranging from depression to psychosis
- Mucocutaneous candidiasis (seen in familial form)
- Dry and scaly skin, psoriasis, and patchy alopecia
- Brittle hair and fingernails
- Enamel hypoplasia (if present during dental development)

Laboratory
- Low serum calcium with elevated phosphate
- Prolonged QT interval on ECG

15. An 8-year-old in a spica cast following hip surgery develops vomiting and a serum calcium of 15.3 mg/dl. What should be the level of concern?

A serum calcium concentration > ***15 mg/dl*** or the presence of ***significant symptoms*** (vomiting, hypertension) constitutes a ***medical emergency*** and requires immediate intervention to lower the calcium level. The initial mainstay of treatment is isotonic saline at 2–4 times maintenance rates and furosemide (1 mg/kg IV, every 6 hrs). Furosemide is a potent diuretic and calciuric agent. Meticulous monitoring of input and output and of serum and urinary electrolytes (including serum magnesium) is vital. ECG monitoring is mandatory because hypercalcemia can be associated with conduction disturbances, including premature ventricular contractions, ventricular tachycardia, prolonged PR interval, prolonged QRS duration, and atrioventricular block. Additional treatment with glucocorticoids and antihypercalcemic agents may also need to be employed.

16. If saline and furosemide fail as treatments for hypercalcemia, what other options are available?

The administration of glucocorticoids may decrease serum calcium levels by decreasing intestinal absorption of calcium. Bone antiresorptive agents, including mithramycin, calcitonin, and etidronate, have also been used successfully as therapies for hypercalcemia.

McKay C, Furman WL: Hypercalcemia complicating childhood malignancies. Cancer 72:256–260, 1993.

17. What are the main causes of hypocalcemia in children?

- ***Nutritional:*** inadequate intake of vitamin D and/or calcium
- ***Renal insufficiency:*** due to (a) increased serum phosphorus from decreased GFR with depressed serum calcium and secondary hyperparathyroidism or (b) decreased activity of renal α-hydroxylase, which is involved in converting the less-active 25-hydroxyvitamin D into the more active 1,25-$(OH)_2$ D.
- ***Nephrotic syndrome:*** with lowered serum albumin, total calcium levels are reduced. Additionally, intestinal absorption of calcium is decreased, urinary losses of cholecalciferol-binding globulin are increased, and urinary losses of calcium are increased with prednisone **therapy.**
- ***Hypoparathyroidism:*** (a) in infants, primary aplasia, hypoplasia, or DiGeorge syndrome or (b) in older children, autoimmune polyglandular disease or mitochondrial myopathy syndromes.
- ***Pseudohypoparathyroidism:*** a peripheral resistance syndrome with elevated parathyroid hormone and normal renal function.
- ***Disorders of calcium sensor genes.***

Fouser L: Disorders of calcium, phosphorus, and magnesium. Pediatr Ann 24:38–46, 1995.

CLINICAL SYNDROMES

18. How does the syndrome of inappropriate secretion of antidiuretic hormone (SIADH) develop?

Antidiuretic hormone (ADH) is released from the posterior pituitary gland and serves as a regulator of extracellular fluid volume. The secretion of ADH is regulated by changes in osmolality sensed by the hypothalamus and alterations in blood volume detected by carotid and left atrial stretch receptors. Intracranial pathology can increase the secretion of ADH directly by local CNS effects, and intrathoracic pathology can increase secretion by stimulating volume receptors. Medications (see Question 20) can directly promote ADH release as well as enhance its renal effects. SIADH is usually asymptomatic until symptoms of water intoxication and hyponatremia develop. Nausea, vomiting, irritability, personality changes, progressive obtundation, and seizures can result.

19. What are the 5 criteria for the diagnosis of SIADH?

1. Hyponatremia with reduced serum osmolality
2. Urine osmolality elevated compared with serum osmolality (a urine osmolality < 100 mOsm/dl usually excludes the diagnosis)
3. Urinary sodium concentration excessive for the extent of hyponatremia (usually > 20 mEq/L)
4. Normal renal, adrenal, and thyroid function
5. Absence of volume depletion

20. SIADH is associated with what conditions?

CNS abnormalities

- Infections (meningitis, encephalitis, abscess)
- Head trauma
- Postoperative (especially perinatal asphyxia)
- Hypoxic encephalopathy (especially pituitary manipulations)
- Tumor
- Hemorrhage (subarachnoid or intraventricular)
- Guillain-Barré syndrome

Intrathoracic disorders
- Infection (pneumonia, tuberculosis, empyema)
- Cystic fibrosis
- Positive-pressure ventilation
- Asthma
- Pneumothorax

Drug-related

Pituitary secretion enhanced
- Phenothiazines
- Vincristine
- Vinblastine
- Vidarabine
- Morphine

Renal effect enhanced
- Chlorpropamide
- Indomethacin

21. What clinical features suggest diabetes insipidus?

Because diabetes insipidus is caused by insufficiency of ADH, or the inability to respond to ADH, the signs and symptoms tend to be directly related to excessive fluid loss. The clinical spectrum may vary depending on the child's age. The infant may present with failure to thrive secondary to chronic dehydration or with a history of repeated episodes of hospitalizations for dehydration. There may also be a history of intermittent low-grade fever.

Often, caretakers report a large volume intake or an inability to keep a dry diaper on the infant. In the young child, diabetes insipidus may present as difficulty with toilet training. In the older child, the reappearance of enuresis, increasing frequency of urination, nocturia, or dramatic increases in fluid intake may herald the diagnosis. Frequent urination with large urinary volumes should lead to the suspicion of diabetes insipidus, and the absence of glucosuria is sufficient to rule out diabetes mellitus.

22. How is the diagnosis of diabetes insipidus (DI) made?

The child who sleeps for 8–12 hours without urinating or drinking fluids is unlikely to have DI. If the possibility of DI has been raised in such a child, measurement of the serum osmolality and urine osmolality shortly after awakening should be done. If the serum osmolality is normal (< 290 mOsm/L) and the urine is concentrated (> 800 mOsm/L), DI is unlikely.

In a child with a more compelling history (excessive thirst and urination, awakening at night to drink, water-craving behaviors), deprivation of water intake for a limited time accompanied by judicious monitoring of physical and biochemical parameters may be required. The *diagnosis* of DI rests on the demonstration of (a) an ***inappropriately dilute urine*** in the face of a rising or elevated serum osmolality; (b) ***urine output*** that remains ***high*** despite the lack of oral input; and (c) changes in physical parameters consistent with ***dehydration*** (weight loss, tachycardia, loss of skin turgor, dry mucous membranes). A child who, with water deprivation, appropriately concentrates urine and whose serum osmolality remains constant is unlikely to have DI.

If a child meets the criteria for the diagnosis of DI, the water-deprivation test is usually ended with the administration of some form of ADH, such as desmopressin (DDAVP) and the provision of fluids. If the urine subsequently becomes appropriately concentrated, this confirms the diagnosis of ADH deficiency (central DI). Failure to concentrate suggests renal resistance to ADH (nephrogenic DI).

Baylis PH, Cheetham T: Diabetes insipidus. Arch Dis Child 79:84-89, 1998.

23. Precocious puberty and café-au-lait spots are commonly seen in what syndrome?

McCune-Albright syndrome. This syndrome is the association of polyostotic fibrous dysplasia, precocious puberty, and café-au-lait pigmentation. These nevi classically have an irregular border ("coast of Maine"), while the lesions in neurofibromatosis have a more regular border ("coast of California"). McCune-Albright syndrome may occur in either an incomplete form (pigmented nevi and bony changes without precocious puberty) or expanded form (the hallmark features plus other findings such as gigantism, hyperthyroidism, Cushing syndrome, and ovarian cysts). It occurs most commonly in females. The syndrome is thought to be due to autonomous function of the involved gland (ovary, adrenal, thyroid).

24. What distinguishes MEN from APES?

Besides the occasional use of forks, the distinction involves the two groups of *polyendocrine disorders*. **MEN** (multiple endocrine neoplasia) involves the development of pluriglandular neoplasia. MEN type I (Werner syndrome) is characterized by adenomas of the pancreatic islet cells (with insulin and a gastrin production) and the pituitary gland (with prolactin secretion) and by hyperplasia or multiple adenomas of the parathyroids. MEN II (Sipple syndrome) is associated with medullary thyroid carcinoma, parathyroid adenomas, and, occasionally, pheochromocytomas. MEN III has features of MEN II plus multiple mucosal neuromas.

APES is autoimmune polyendocrine syndrome. APES I has its onset in childhood and is distinguished by hypoparathyroidism, adrenal insufficiency and mucocutaneous candidiasis. APES II occurs in adults and involves a variety of thyroid, adrenal, pancreatic, gonadal, and dermatologic abnormalities.

Hoff AO et al: Multiple endocrine neoplasias. Ann Rev Physiol 62:377-411, 2000.

DIABETES MELLITUS

25. What are the risks of developing insulin-dependent diabetes mellitus (type 1) if one sibling is affected?

Identical twins:	> 50%
HLA identical:	20%
HLA haploidentical:	5%
HLA nonidentical:	1%

Plotnick L: Insulin-dependent diabetes mellitus. Pediatr Rev 15:138, 1994.

26. Can the development of diabetes in other siblings be predicted?

In one series of 661 children who had a sibling with diabetes mellitus, 49 went on to develop type 1 diabetes. All but 6 cases were predicted on the basis of islet cell autoantibody formation or an abnormal glucose tolerance test. If a sibling develops such an antibody *and* an abnormal gluose tolerance test, the risk for the development of DM increases 1300-fold. Much research centers on ways of modulating the development of diabetes in those patients through the use of exogenous insulin or immunomodulators.

Mrena S et al: Staging of preclinical type 1 diabetes in siblings of affected children. Pediatrics 104:925-930, 1999.

27. Is the use of cow milk in infants a risk factor for the development of IDDM?

IDDM is believed most likely to result from an autoimmune destruction of pancreatic islet cells involving both a genetic predisposition and environmental insult. Multiple environmental factors, including viral infections and toxins, may serve as triggers. Early exposure to cow milk has been hypothesized as predisposing children to IDDM. However, early cow milk feeding has not been associated with the development of antibodies to islet cells and most experts do not believe its use is a risk factor.

Couper JJ et al: Lack of association between duration of breast-feeding or introduction of cow's milk and development of islet autoimmunity. Diabetes 48:2145-149, 1999.

28. How long does the "honeymoon" period last in newly diagnosed insulin-dependent diabetics?

The "honeymoon" usually begins within 1–2 weeks after the initiation of insulin treatment. It is a period of falling or minimal exogenous insulin requirements that reflects continued residual endogenous insulin production. The duration of the honeymoon in a particular individual may last for a few weeks or months but is not predictable. However, evidence is accumulating that it may be prolonged by the maintenance of excellent control. Cessation of the honeymoon is often heralded by elevated fasting blood glucose levels prior to breakfast or by an increasing insulin requirement.

29. How do the types of insulin vary in their timing and duration of action?

Kinetics of Action of Insulins

	ONSET OF ACTION (HRS)	PEAK OF ACTION (HRS)	DURATION OF ACTION (HRS)
Regular	0.5–1	2–4	5–7
Insulin zinc (prompt, Semilente)	1–3	2–8	12–16
Isophane (NPH)	3–4	6–8	18–24
Insulin zinc (Lente)	1–3	9–12	24–18
Protamine zinc	4–6	14–24	36
Insulin zinc (extended, Ultralente)	4–6	18–24	24–36
Humalog	.25	1–2	3–4

For most children with juvenile-onset diabetes, the mainstays of treatment are regular and NPH insulin. The most widely used forms of insulin are those derived from recombinant DNA technology. The other forms (beef/pork, pure pork, modified pork) are becoming increasingly hard to obtain, although some patients and physicians feel that these have superior qualities compared to the recombinant forms. Children and adolescents treated with recombinant NPH seem to be somewhat more likely to have hypoglycemia prior to lunch and hyperglycemia prior to supper. If that pattern is noted, use of a multi-dose regimen (3 or more injections/day) or switching to an animal insulin or Lente may alleviate both problems.

30. What are the typical insulin dosages given after the "honeymoon" period?

Prepubertal children generally require about 0.5 U/kg/day, while postpubertal individuals require 0.75–1.0 U/kg/day. Athletes or those with a low caloric intake may require less insulin.

31. When should the Somogyi phenomenon be suspected?

The *Somogyi phenomenon* is rebound hyperglycemia following an incident of hypoglycemia. This rebound is secondary to release of counter-regulatory hormones, which is the natural response to hypoglycemia. As tighter diabetic control is maintained, there is an increased likelihood of hypoglycemia and therefore the Somogyi phenomenon. If the hypoglycemia is recognized and treated promptly, rebound hyperglycemia is less likely to occur. Thus, the Somogyi is commonly reported more frequently at night because there is greater likelihood of unrecognized and untreated hypoglycemia when the child is asleep. The Somogyi phenomenon should be suspected when a child in excellent control begins to have

intermittent high blood glucoses in the morning. If that pattern is noted, blood glucose should be checked at 2–3 AM on several nights to determine if hypoglycemia is occurring. If hypoglycemia can be documented, the dose of bedtime insulin should be decreased and/or twice daily dosing changed to three times per day.

32. What causes the "dawn phenomenon"?

The term *dawn phenomenon* describes a rise in blood glucose that occurs in the early morning hours (5–8 AM), particularly in patients who have normal glucose levels throughout most of the night. The rise in glucose is thought to be due to several factors, including:

- The normal increase in the AM cortisol
- Cumulative effect of increased nocturnal growth hormone
- Insulinopenia, due to the length of time since the pre-supper injection

In some instances, the dawn phenomenon can be satisfactorily managed by shifting the NPH dose to a later time (pre-bedtime snack) and/or by using Lente.

33. How rapidly can renal disease develop after the onset of diabetes mellitus?

Microscopic changes in the glomerular basement membrane are present by 2 years after the diagnosis of diabetes. Microalbuminuria is often present by 10–15 years, followed by a proteinuric period (> 0.5 gm/24 hrs). Beyond this point, there is a relentless decline in glomerular function. An azotemic period begins on average by 17 years, and frank uremia occurs by 20 years. Retrospective studies suggest that as many as 50% of patients with IDDM diagnosed before age 30 will develop end-stage renal disease. Diabetic nephropathy accounts for 25% of patients receiving long-term renal dialysis in the United States.

34. When does retinopathy develop following the onset of diabetes mellitus?

Retinal disease in patients with diabetes is characterized by either background (simple) or proliferative retinopathy. By 25–30 years after the diagnosis of diabetes, 90% of patients have demonstrable retinal lesions. The onset of the proliferative form of retinopathy carries a high risk of blindness. Vitreous hemorrhage, scarring, and retinal hemorrhage occur frequently. Approximately 10% of patients develop proliferative retinopathy within 14 years. The disease will proceed to blindness in about 45% of patients within 5 years of the onset of proliferative changes. Diabetes is the leading cause of adult blindness in the United States. It is important to remember that knowledge concerning dietary management has expanded, the quality of the insulin has improved, and the ability to maintain better diabetic control has changed dramatically in the past 20 years. Therefore, the prognosis for both renal and retinal injury may be significantly better than the statistics outlined above. Studies have hown improved glycemic control delays the onset of microvascular damage.

35. Describe the three forms of diabetic neuropathy.

1. ***Mononeuropathy***. Involves a peripheral or cranial nerve. The usual presentation is the sudden appearance of foot drop, wrist drop, or paralysis of the III, IV, or VI cranial nerves. Generally, the abnormality subsides in several days.

2. ***Symmetrical peripheral polyneuropathy***. A symmetrical sensory loss occurs in the distal lower extremities. Upper extremity involvement and motor deficits are uncommon. Numbness, tingling, and burning of the affected extremities are common and generally are worse at night. The pain may be severe on occasion. Due to the loss of sensory input, injuries may occur that are asymptomatic. Increased surveillance for these injuries in affected patients is required.

3. ***Autonomic neuropathy***. This may result in orthostatic hypotension, sexual dysfunction, and motility disorders of the esophagus, stomach, gallbladder, small intestine, colon, and urinary bladder.

36. How is hemoglobin A_1C helpful in monitoring diabetic control?

Glycohemoglobin, also known as glycosolated hemoglobin or hemoglobin A_1C, is a hemoglobin-glucose combination formed nonenzymatically within the cell. Initially, an unstable bond is formed between glucose and the hemoglobin molecule. With time, this bond rearranges to form a more stable compound in which glucose is covalently bound to the hemoglobin molecule. The amount of the unstable form may rise rapidly in the presence of a high blood glucose level, while the stable form changes slowly and provides a time-average integral of the blood glucose concentration through the 120-day lifespan of the red blood cell. Thus, glycohemoglobin levels can provide an objective measurement of averaged diabetic control over time.

37. Is tight control of diabetes better than conventional control?

The Diabetes Control and Complications Trial (DCCT) followed over 1400 diabetics (nearly 200 of whom were adolescents). Study subjects were randomized to receive either standard diabetic therapy (e.g., twice daily insulin shots) or more intensive therapy (e.g., more frequent blood glucose monitoring and 3 or more shots daily). Intensive control reduced the risk of development of retinopathy by 53% and the occurrence of microalbuminuria by 55% compared with conventional control. The major adverse effect was a three-fold increase in the rate of severe hypoglycemia. Whether the benefits of tighter control outweigh the potential risks of hypoglycemia in younger pediatric patients remains unknown. Newer insulins (e.g., Humalog) can decrease the risk of hypoglycemia.

DCCT Research Group: Retinopathy and nephropathy in patients with type 1 diabetes four years after a trial of intensive therapy. N Engl J Med 342:381-389, 2000.

38. Why is a falling serum sodium concentration during the treatment of diabetic ketoacidosis (DKA) of concern?

Most patients with DKA have a significant sodium deficit of 8–10 mEq/kg which needs to be replaced. Following initial fluid boluses, fluids containing 0.5 normal saline or greater may be required. As a general rule, the serum [Na] is low at the outset and rises throughout the course of treatment. An initial [Na] > 145 mEq/L suggests severe dehydration or hyperosmolarity. An initial [Na] that is normal or low and begins to fall with treatment merits prompt attention since it indicates either inappropriate fluid management or the onset of inappropriate diuretic hormone secretion (SIADH) and can signal impending cerebral edema.

39. How should potassium deficits be replaced in children with DKA?

In almost all children, there is a potassium deficit of 6–10 mEq/kg, although the initial serum [K] value is often normal or high. If the initial [K] < 3.5 mEq/L, 60 mEq/L should be added to the infusion and close ECG monitoring should be instituted. If the initial [K] is 3.5–5.5, 40 mEq/L of potassium is used. When the initial [K] is > 5.5, only 20 mEq/L is recommended. If the initial K is >6, obtain an ECG and add K^+ only when the level falls to $\leq$ 5.5 and the patient has voided.

After the initial fluid bolus, the typical child in DKA will receive 0.5 normal saline containing 40 mEq/L of potassium. Half of the potassium may be given as potassium chloride and the other half as potassium phosphate if the serum calcium is normal. The initial rate will be about twice normal maintenance rates. It is strongly recommended that while the initial fluid bolus is being given, the physician carefully carefully calculate fluid and electrolyte replacement.

40. Why do potassium levels fall during management of DKA?

- Dilutional effects of rehydration
- Correction of acidosis (less K^+ exchanged out of cell for H^+ as pH rises)

• Insulin administration (increases cellular uptake of K^+)
• Ongoing urinary losses

Most patients are potassium-depleted, although the serum [K^+] is usually normal or elevated. A low [K^+] is particularly worrisome because it suggests severe potassium depletion.

41. How has the approach to fluid replacement in DKA changed over the past decade?

In an effort to prevent cerebral edema, recommendations for the initial fluid resuscitation in patients with DKA have undergone revision. Unless a patient is in shock, initial boluses should ideally not exceed 10 ml/kg and fluid replacement over 24-48 hours is recommended.

Rutledge J, Couch R: Am J Emerg Med 18:658-660, Oct. 2000.

42. Should bicarbonate be used in the treatment of children with DKA?

PRO	CON
Improved pH enhances myocardial contractility and response to catecholamines	Cardiac function problems are rare in children
Ventilatory response to acidosis blunted when pH < 7.0	Ventilatory response well maintained in children
No adverse effect of bicarbonate on oxygenation has been demonstrated clinically	May alter oxygen-binding of hemoglobin, potentially decreasing tissue oxygenation
Questionable relevance of CNS acidosis	Paradoxical CNS acidosis documented in humans
May be useful in the rare patient with hyperkalemia	Hypokalemia may result from uptake of K^+ as acidosis is corrected; low serum [K] is 6 times more common after bicarbonate treatment
	May be associated with increased hyperosmolarity and cerebral edema

The use of bicarbonate in the treatment of DKA in children has been both advocated and denounced. The establishment of an adequate intravascular volume and the provision of sufficient quantities of insulin are *far* more important in the treatment of DKA than bicarbonate. The decision to initiate bicarbonate therapy should be based on an arterial blood gas, *not* a venous blood gas. The three clear indications for bicarbonate therapy are:

1. ***Symptomatic hyperkalemia***
2. ***Cardiac instability***
3. ***Inadequate ventilatory compensation***

Each of these conditions requires admission to an intensive care unit where appropriate monitoring can be undertaken and ventilatory assistance provided if necessary.

43. When should glucose be added to the infusate in DKA?

When the ***glucose*** level ***approaches 300 mg/dl***. It is usually wise to order the appropriate glucose-containing fluid in advance. This is easy to do because the rate of fall of glucose is predictable when a child is on continuous intravenous insulin. After the glucose-containing infusate is introduced, the glucose-free infusate can be kept at the bedside in case the blood glucose begins to rise excessively, despite increased insulin rates.

44. Is continuous or bolus insulin better in the treatment of DKA?

The choice of route of administration depends in part on the particular situation. For example, hourly IM injections may be easier to manage while a child is being transported between institutions. However, continuous IV insulin is easier to titrate than IM injections. However, the differences may not be clinically significant. More importantly, injection of insulin subcutaneously is inappropriate until adequate hydration is established and the acidosis is resolving ([HCO_3–] > 15 mEq/L).

Continuous insulin is given initially at a rate of 0.1 U/kg/hr (after an initial bolus of 0.1 U/kg). This rate is adjusted to allow blood sugar to fall by about 100 mg/dl/hr. Alternatively, IM insulin can be used with an initial dose of 0.25 U/kg, followed by 0.1 U/kg/hr. Only regular insulin should be used. Intermediate or long-acting insulins are not appropriate in the treatment of DKA.

45. How is the transition made to intermittent insulin therapy as DKA is resolving?

The transition from insulin infusion to intermittent subcutaneous therapy is predicated on three factors:

1. *Normalization of biochemical parameters.* Insulin infusions should not be stopped until the blood sugar is < 300 mg/dl, pH is > 7.3, and HCO_3^- is > 15 mEq/L.

2. *Resumption of oral food intake.* As long as the patient is not eating and is receiving a constant supply of glucose by vein, it is easier to maintain a stable blood sugar using an insulin infusion rather than intermittent subcutaneous insulin. When oral intake is resumed, food is usually provided on an intermittent (bolus) basis. It is then reasonable to provide insulin in an intermittent fashion as well.

3. *Convenience/normal schedule.* Patients with diabetes generally are placed on a four-times-daily insulin regimen for the initial 24–36 hour period after an episode of ketoacidosis. Regular insulin is given prior to meals and the bedtime snack. For the first dose of insulin after an episode of DKA, the child can be allowed to eat with the insulin drip running. If food is retained for 30 minutes without problems, a dose of subcutaneous insulin (0.25 U/kg) can be administered and the insulin infusion shut off. Subsequent doses of insulin should be given prior to meals.

46. What signs and symptoms suggest worsening cerebral edema during the treatment of DKA?

Cerebral edema accounts for the majority of the 1–2% of case fatalities that occur in DKA. It is unpredictable, occurring often as biochemical abnormalities are improving. It may be sudden in onset or occur gradually. Those most susceptible are children < 5 years of age and newly-diagnosed diabetics. Signs and symptoms include:

- Decreasing sensorium
- Sudden and severe headache
- Incontinence
- Vomiting
- Change in vital signs
- Combativeness, disorientation, agitation
- Ophthalmoplegia
- Pupillary asymmetry or sluggish responses
- Papilledema
- Seizure

Early recognition is vital because intervention (e.g., IV mannitol, intubation, hyperventilation) can improve outcome in 50% of patients. The best methods to prevent its occurrence remain controversial.

Glaser N, et al: Risk factors for cerebral edema in children with diabetic ketoacidosis. N Engl J Med 344: 264-268, 2001.

Rosenbloom AL et al: Therapeutic controversy: prevention and treatment of diabetes in children. J Clin Endo Metab 85:494-522, 2000.

Maloney CP et al: Risk factors for developing brain herniation during diabetic ketoacidosis. Pediatr Neurol 21:721-727, 1999.

47. What pathophysiologic process characterizes type 2 diabetes?

Peripheral resistance to insulin action and insulin ***secretory defects***. This syndrome is most commonly associated with obesity, hypertension and cardiovascular disease. Previously rare in pediatrics, it has increased ten-fold in the 1990s in some centers in the U.S. and accounts for as high as 40% of new-onset diabetes cases. The reason for the increase is unclear, but is likely related to current trends of increasing childhood obesity, poor dietary habits and sedentary behavior.

Fagot-Campagna A et al: Type 2 diabetes among North American children and adolescents: An epidemiologic review and a public health perspective. J Pediatr 136:664-672, 2000.

48. What clinical and features suggest type 2 rather than type 1 diabetes?

Obesity is the hallmark of type 2 diabetes with up to 85% of affected children overweight or obese. Acanthosis nigricans (velvety hyperpigmented patches most prominent in intertriginous areas) is present in up to 95% of cases. Polycystic ovarian syndrome, another disorder associated with insulin resistance and obesity, is common. Unlike patients with type 1, most with type 2 present with glycosuria without ketonuria (although up to 33% can have ketonuria), absent or mild polyuria and polydipsia, and little or no weight loss. Family history is usually strongly positive for type 2 diabetes. Although classification can usually be made on the basis of clinical characteristics, measurement of levels of fasting insulin and C-peptide (low in type 1, normal or elevated in type 2) or islet cell autoantibodies (present in type 1, generally absent in type 2) can assist.

American Diabetes Association. Type 2 diabetes in children and adolescents. Pediatrics 105:671-680, 2000.

GROWTH DISTURBANCES

49. How do the growth rates of boys and girls differ?

In both both boys and girls, the rate or velocity of linear growth begins to decelerate at about 2 years of age. In girls, this deceleration continues until approximately age 11 years, at which time the adolescent growth spurt begins. For boys, the deceleration continues until about 13 years. The peak rate of increase in males occurs at age 14 years.

50. What is the best predictor of a child's eventual adult height?

Mid-parental height. This is an estimate of a child's expected genetic growth potential based on parental heights (preferably measured rather than by history).

For girls: ([father's height – 13 cm] + [mother's height])/2.

For boys: ([mother's height + 13 cm] + [father's height])/2.

This gives a rough range (± 5 cm) of expected adult height. The predicted height can be compared with the present height percentile, and any significant deviation can be a clue of an abnormal growth pattern in a child.

51. When have most children achieved the height percentiles consistent with parental height?

By age ***two***. Rough estimates of ultimate adult height can be obtained by taking a boy's length at age 2 and a girl's length at 18 months and doubling them.

52. Name the seven major categories of causes of short stature.

1. ***Genetic***
2. ***Constitutional delay*** ("late bloomer")
3. ***Chronic disease*** (e.g., inflammatory bowel disease, chronic renal failure, renal tubular acidosis, cyanotic congenital heart disease)
4. ***Chromosomal/syndromic*** (e.g., Turner [45, X], 18q–, Down, achondroplasia)
5. ***Endocrine*** (e.g., hypothyroidism, growth hormone deficiency, hypopituitarism, hypercortisolism [endogenous and exogenous])
6. ***Psychosocial*** (e.g., chaotic social situation, orphanage)
7. **Intrauterine** (e.g., small for gestational age)

Genetic patterns and constitutional delay account for the largest percentage of determined causes.

53. In a child with short stature, what rate of growth makes an endocrinologic cause unlikely?

Rates of growth are age-dependent. In general, a growth rate of ≥ ***6 cm/yr between ages 2–5 years*** or ≥ ***5 cm/yr in children between age 5 and*** the ***adolescent*** growth spurt makes an endocrinologic cause of short stature less likely. The importance of sequential measurements using standard growth charts cannot be underestimated. Growth rates below the 3rd percentile or crossing percentiles downward warrant further investigation.

54. In evaluating a short child, why should you ask about the time the parents reached puberty?

The age at which puberty occurred in other family members may help identify children with constitutional delay, since this entity tends to run in families. Most women will remember their age at menarche, and this age can be used as a reference for the age at which other pubertal events occurred. The strongest association for pubertal delay is between father and son. The most useful reference point for adult males is the age at which they reached adult height, since almost all normal males will have reached their adult height by 17 years of age (around high school graduation). Significant growth beyond this age suggests a history of pubertal delay.

55. When does the pubertal growth spurt occur?

For children with an average growth rate, pubertal growth begins earlier in girls mean age at take-off is 11 years for boys and 9 years for girls. Peak height velocity occurs at 13.5 years for boys, 11.5 years for girls. Peak velocity occurs at Tanner breast stage 2-3 for girls and Tanner testis stage 3-4 for boys. Of note, girls generally stop growing at an average of 14 years of age, but boys continue to grow until 17 years.

Abassi V: Growth and normal puberty. Pediatrics 102:507-511, 1998.

56. What other historical information is helpful in the diagnosis of short stature?

The gestational and birth history are often revealing. About one-third of small-for-date infants, while growing at normal rates, remain small throughout childhood and are unlikely to achieve a height consistent with their genetic potential. Girls with Turner syndrome are often short at birth, and many are noted to have edema of the hands and feet in the newborn period.

A ***review of systems*** should be undertaken with particular emphasis on systemic disease, intracranial pathology, and medication usage. Growth failure in inflammatory bowel disease may precede the onset of clinical disease by more than a year. Chronic headaches or visual difficulties may presage pituitary or hypothalamic pathology. Frequent use of steroidal hormones may suppress linear growth. Changes in the level of activity, sleeping patterns, or bowel habits can be an early indication of thyroid disease, while failure to change shoe size and excess abdominal obesity suggest a deficiency of growth hormone. An examination of photographs taken of the child and the child's siblings at various ages can be helpful in separating familial changes from clinical problems.

Access to ***previous growth records*** is absolutely essential since endocrine diseases affect the rate of linear growth. These records can often by obtained from the school, family physician, child's "baby book," or the door jam in the family home. If records are not available, it is useful to obtain heights every 3 months over a 6–12-month period prior to the initiation of extensive testing. Linear growth rate can be determined from accurate sequential height measurements. It is essential that this process be standardized and that the same observer obtain the measurement.

57. Are upper to lower body ratios helpful in the diagnosis of growth problems?

Disproportionate short stature generally refers to an inappropriate ratio between truncal length and limb length (upper to lower segment ratio). It is important that the ratio be compared to individuals of similar age and race, because there are both age-related and racial differences in the ratio. In the infant, the head and trunk are quite long relative to the limbs, so that the ratio of truncal length to limb length is about *1.7*.

Throughout childhood this ratio declines, so that by 7–10 years of age this ratio is about *1.0*. Variance from the normal ratio may occur in bony dysplasias (e.g., achondroplasia and hypochondroplasia), in certain syndromes (e.g., Marfan syndrome), and after specific types of therapy (e.g., spinal irradiation).

58. What laboratory studies should be obtained when evaluating short stature?

Extensive laboratory tests are generally not indicated unless the growth rate is abnormally low. Laboratory testing may include any or all of the following: complete blood count, urinalysis, chemistry panel, sedimentation rate, thyroxine, TSH, insulin-like growth factor-I (IGF-I), and IGF-binding protein-3 (IGFBP-3).

Random growth hormone levels are of little value because they are generally low in the daytime, even in children of average height. IGF-I (or somatomedin C) mediates the anabolic effects of growth hormone, and levels correlate well with growth hormone status. However, IGF-I can also be low in nonendocrine conditions, such as malnutrition and liver disease.

IGFBP-3, the major binding protein for IGF-I in serum, is also regulated by growth hormone. IGFBP-3 levels generally indicate growth hormone status and are less affected by nutritional factors than IGF-I. Many endocrinologists now use IGF-I and IGFBP-3 as their initial screening tests for GH deficiency.

Rosenfeld RG, et al: Diagnostic controversy: The diagnosis of childhood growth hormone deficiency revisited. J Clin Endocrinol Metab 80:1532–1540, 1995.

Evans AJ: Screening tests for growth hormone deficiency. J R Soc Med 88:161P–165P, 1995.

59. In a very obese child, how does height measurement help to determine whether an endocrinopathy might be the cause?

In children with simple obesity (e.g., familial), linear growth is enhanced, whereas in endocrinopathies it is usually impaired. If the height of a child is at or greater than mid-parental height percentile, an endocrine cause of the obesity is unlikely. An exception is Cushing syndrome, in which abnormal growth may not be a clue.

60. How does a growth chart help in the diagnosis of failure to thrive?

If an infant is demonstrating deceleration of a previously established growth pattern or growth consistently less than the 5th percentile, the pattern of growth of head circumference, height, and weight can help establish the likely cause. There are three main types of impaired growth: type I (retardation of weight with near-normal or slowly decelerating height and head circumference), type II (near-proportional retardation of weight and height with normal head circumference), and type III (concomitant retardation of weight, height, and head circumference). See charts on next page.

61. Why is a bone age determination so helpful in evaluating short stature?

The rate of bony maturation corresponds better with physical development than with chronologic age. Standards of normal skeletal radiographic maturation are available, and all children with possible pathologic short stature should have radiographs obtained for comparison. Generally, a radiograph of the left hand and wrist is obtained. A single bone age is of value in differentiating familial short stature and genetic diseases, in which bone age is normal, from other causes of short stature. A ***delayed bone age*** (> 2 SD below the mean) which correlates with the child's height age (age on growth chart at which child's height would be on the 50th percentile) is suggestive of *constitutional* delay, while a ***markedly delayed bone age*** is suggestive of *endocrinologic* disease. Serial bone ages each 6–12 months are often helpful, since in both the normal child and the child with constitutional delay, the bone age will

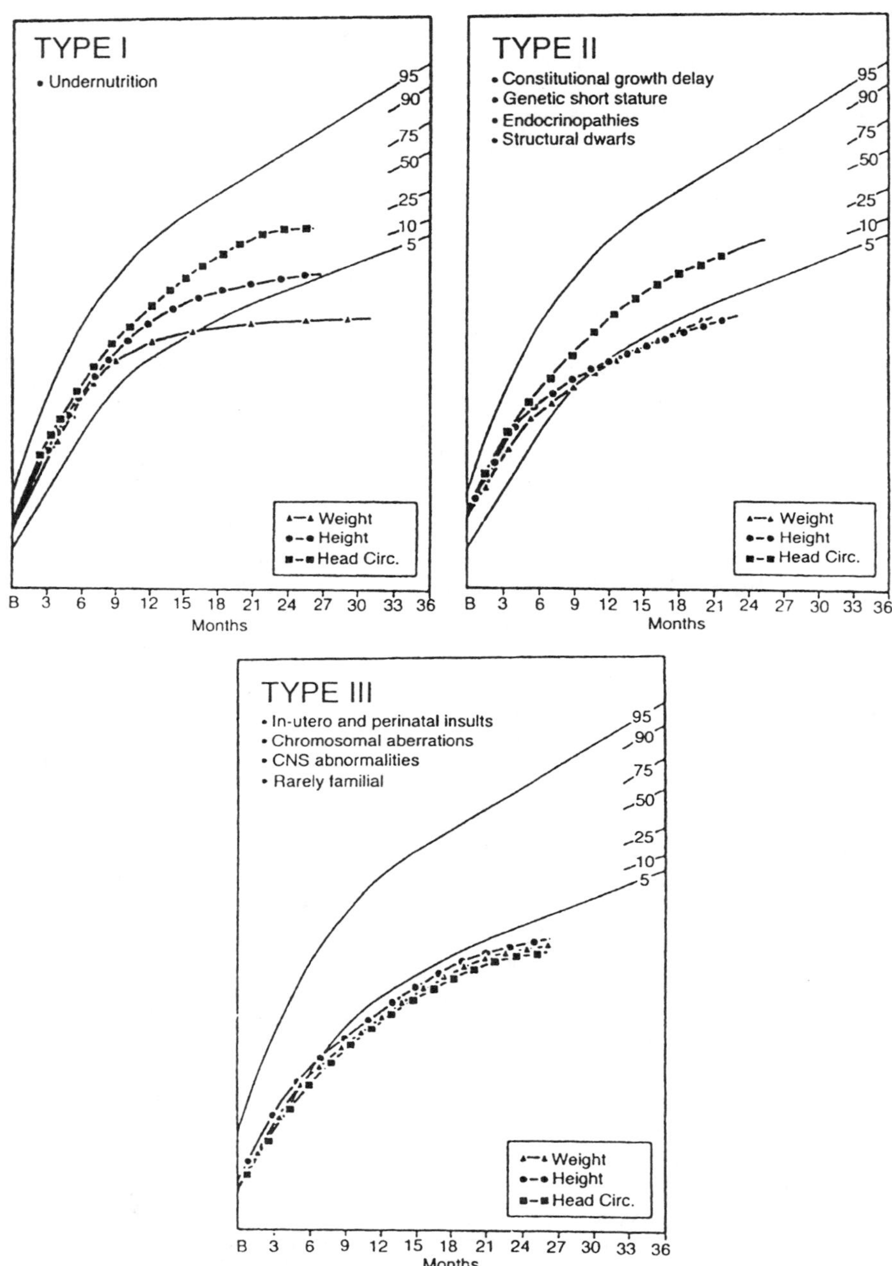

From Roy CC, Silverman A, Alagille DA: Pediatric Clinical Gastroenterology, 4th ed. St. Louis, Mosby-Year Book, 1995, pp 4–8; with permission.

advance in parallel with chronologic age. In endocrinologic disease, the bone age falls progressively further behind chronologic age. Bone age may be normal or delayed in chronic disease, dependent on the severity of disease, its duration, and type of treatment used.

62. What features suggest constitutional delay as a cause of short stature?

- No symptoms or signs of systemic disease
- Bone age delayed up to 2–4 years but consistent with height age
- Period of poorest growth occurring often from ages 18–30 months, with steady linear growth thereafter (normal rate of growth for bone age)
- Parental or sibling history of delayed development
- Height predictions consistent with family characteristics

63. How is constitutional delay managed?

If the results of history, physical examination, and clinical laboratory evaluation are unremarkable, the child is seen once every 3–6 months for accurate height measurements and determination of growth rate. A bone age may be done yearly to assess progression of bony maturation. In constitutional delay, the rate of bone maturation should keep pace with chronologic age. In children who are of mid-to-late pubertal ages (girls > 13, boys > 14 yrs) but showing minimal or no signs of puberty, selective use may be made of estrogen or testosterone supplementation to initiate puberty or additional assessment may be indicated.

64. What are the causes of growth hormone (GH) deficiency?

Growth hormone deficiency can result from isolated defects of GH biosynthesis and release or from a malignancy or structural abnormalities involving the pituitary and hypothalamus. In recent years, it has been increasingly recognized that both chemotherapy and craniospinal irradiation affect GH production. Trauma or disease involving the base of the skull (e.g., Wegener granulomatosis) may also affect its production.

65. How is growth hormone production tested?

GH production is extremely variable from day to day, even in normal children. Production by the pituitary is affected by a host of factors, including sleep and psychologic state, medications, and nutrition, as well as input from the hypothalamus and higher brain centers. These factors make testing for GH difficult. Furthermore, there is good evidence that specific subsets of children (e.g., those with Turner syndrome) make insufficient GH on a daily basis while they respond normally to pharmacologic stimuli.

Testing for GH can be divided into ***pharmacologic stimulation*** and ***physiologic evaluation***. *Stimulation tests* rely on specific agents known to cause the normal pituitary to release GH. Extensive protocols are available for this type of testing; the general protocol is to obtain a baseline blood level GH quantitation, followed by administration of the pharmacologic agent, and then repetitive blood specimens are drawn at various times afterward. The limitations of these tests are that (1) they only measure the acutely releasable pool and provide no information on how long the pool took to accumulate; (2) 5–10% of normal children will fail to respond to any single provocative agent; and (3) some children will give a normal response although they do not produce normal amounts of GH on a daily basis.

Physiologic testing potentially provides a more reliable indicator of how the hypothalamic-pituitary axis performs under the "usual" conditions. This testing requires either serial 24-hour urine collections for GH or the collection of blood every 20 minutes for a 12–24-hour period. These studies are problematic because of methodologic issues. For example, the act of withdrawing blood every 20 minutes may be stressful and painful or alter the normal sleep cycle, and these stimuli that may affect pituitary GH production or its regulation.

66. When did growth hormone become available by recombinant DNA technology?

Since ***1983***, all GH given in the U.S. has been made by recombinant techniques. Before that, U.S. GH was still extracted from collections of human pituitary glands. There were case reports of patients receiving the human-derived hormone who developed Creutzfeldt-Jakob disease, a neurodegenerative disorder caused by a slow virus or prion (proteinaceous infectious particle) with a long latency period. Many patients may still be at risk. Recombinant therapy has allowed more widespread use of GH in trials for short-stature syndromes (e.g., Turner, Noonan, Prader-Willi) and children with short stature due to chronic illness.

Vance ML, Mauras N: Growth hormone therapy in the adults and children. N Engl J Med 341:1206-1226, 1999.

67. Should growth hormone therapy be given to the normal short child?

One of the hotter areas of controversy in pediatric endocrinology. *Opponents* argue that short stature is not a disease, current height velocity may not be predictive and what constitutes growth hormone sufficiency and insufficiency is not clearly defined. Long-term safety remains under study, and some recent studies suggest impairment of testicular function in treated males. *Proponents* counter that the treatment is safe and does improve height in 50% of treated patients to at least 5 cm greater than pre-treatment predictions. Surveys have indicated that a majority of pediatric endocrinologists support growth hormone use in patients with short stature, normal growth hormone stimulation tests and subnormal growth velocity.

Voss LD: Growth hormone therapy for the normal short child: Who needs it and who wants it? The case against growth hormone therapy. J Pediatr 136:103-106, 2000.

Saenger PJ: The case in support of growth hormone therapy. J Pediatr 136:106-109, 2000.

Bertonelli S et al: Can growth hormone therapy in boys without growth hormone deficiency impair testicular function? J Pediatr 135:367-370, 1999.

Huntz RL et al: Effect of growth hormone treatment on adult height of children with idiopathic short stature. N Engl J Med 340:502-507, 1999.

68. What are the clinical manifestations of growth hormone excess?

Prior to puberty, the cardinal manifestations are an increase in growth velocity with minimal bone deformity and soft tissue swelling—a condition called ***pituitary gigantism***. Hypogonadotropic hypogonadism and delayed puberty often coexist with GH excess, and affected children exhibit eunuchoid body proportions. If the GH excess occurs after puberty (after epiphyseal closure), the more typical features of ***acromegaly*** occur, including coarsening of the facial features and soft tissue swelling of the feet and hands. GH excess is rare in children.

69. List the causes of tall stature.

Constitutional (familial)

Endocrine causes

Somatotropin excess (pituitary gigantism)

Androgen excess (tall as children, short as adults)

- True sexual precocity
- Pseudosexual precocity

Androgen deficiency (normal height as children, tall as adults)

- Klinefelter syndrome
- Anorchia (infection, trauma, idiopathic)

Hyperthyroidism

Genetic causes

- Klinefelter syndrome
- Syndromes of XYY, XXYY (tall as adults)

Miscellaneous syndromes and entities

- Marfan syndrome
- Cerebral gigantism (Soto syndrome)
- Total lipodystrophy
- Homocystinuria

From Gotlin RW, et al: Endocrine disorders. In Hay WW, et al (eds): Current Pediatric Diagnosis and Treatment, 12th ed. Norwalk, CT, Appleton & Lange, 1995, p 885; with permission.

HYPOGLYCEMIA

70. How is hypoglycemia defined?

A serum glucose of ***< 50 mg/100 ml*** is defined as hypoglycemia in childhood. Some argue for lower levels being used for term and preterm infants; however, these arguments are based on population sampling data rather than on physiology. Hypoglycemia is a laboratory finding, and its presence should lead to a diligent search for the underlying pathology.

71. Describe the clinical findings associated with hypoglycemia.

Neuroglycopenic symptoms include irritability, headache, confusion, unconsciousness, and seizure. *Adrenergic* signs include tachycardia, tremulousness, diaphoresis, and hunger. Any combination of the above signs and symptoms should lead to the measurement of the blood glucose level.

72. What are the causes of childhood hypoglycemia?

No single cause predominates in any age group. Therefore, the entire differential diagnosis must be considered in any child who presents with hypoglycemia.

Differential Diagnosis of Childhood Hypoglycemia

Increased glucose utilization
- Hyperinsulinism—islet-cell adenoma or hyperplasia (nesidioblastosis), oral hypoglycemic agents, exogenous insulin

Decreased glucose production
- Inadequate glycogen reserves—enzymatic defects in glycogen synthesis and glycogenolysis
- Ineffective gluconeogenesis—inadequate substrate (e.g., ketotic hypoglycemia), enzymatic defects

Diminished availability of fats
- Depleted fat stores
- Failure to mobilize fats (e.g., hyperinsulinism)
- Defective utilization of fats—enzymatic defects in fatty acid oxidation (e.g., medium-chain acyl CoA dehydrogenase deficiency)

Decreased fuels and fuel stores
- Fasting, malnutrition, prolonged illness, malabsorption

Increased fuel demand
- Fever, exercise

Inadequate counter-regulatory hormones
- Growth hormone or cortisol deficiency, hypopituitararism

73. An unconscious 3-year-old is brought to the emergency department with a serum glucose concentration of 26 mg/dl. What other laboratory tests should be done?

The principal laboratory evaluations should include the measurement of (1) the metabolic compounds associated with fasting adaptation, (2) the hormones that regulate these processes, and (3) drugs that can interfere with glucose regulation.

A 3-ml red-top tube of *blood* can be sent for measurement of:

- Markers of principal regulatory hormones: insulin, growth hormone, cortisol
- Markers of fatty acid metabolism: ketones (b-hydroxybutyrate and acetoacetate), free fatty acids, total and free carnitine
- Markers of gluconeogenic pathways: lactate, pyruvate, alanine

Urine can be tested for:

- Ketones
- Metabolic byproducts associated with known causes of hypoglycemia (e.g., organic acids, amino acids)
- Toxicology screen, especially for alcohol, salicylates

Taken together, these tests provide valuable clues as to the cause. For example, low levels of ketones and free fatty acids suggest that fat was not appropriately mobilized. As a consequence, ketones were not formed by the liver. Those biochemical abnormalities are seen in hyperinsulinemic states and can be confirmed by documenting a high level of circulating insulin. Low urinary ketones also suggest an enzymatic defect in fatty acid oxidation.

If appropriate studies are not obtained at the time of presentation and the cause remains unknown, a careful fasting study must be undertaken to evaluate fasting adaptation, since repeated profound hypoglycemic episodes are associated with significant morbidity and mortality.

Pershad J, et al: Childhood hypoglycemia in an urban emergency department: Epidemiology and diagnostic approach to the problem. Pediatr Emerg Care 14:268-271, 1998.

74. In patients with acute hypoglycemia, what are the treatment options?

The principal acute treatment is provision of ***glucose orally or intravenously***. If the patient is alert, orange juice or cola (4–8 oz) may be given. If the patient is obtunded, intravenous glucose (2–3 ml/kg of $D_{10}W$ or 1 ml/kg of $D_{25}W$) should be administered rapidly. If venous access cannot be achieved promptly, glucose can be provided via a nasogastric tube, as glucose is rapidly absorbed from the gut. The risk of prolonged hypoglycemia far outweighs the risk associated with passage of a nasogastric tube in an obtunded patient. Subsequently, the blood sugar should be monitored closely and, if necessary, maintained by the constant infusion of glucose (6–8 mg/kg/min). $D_{10}W$ given at about 1.5 times maintenance dose approximates that glucose rate. Larger quantities may be necessary, and the blood sugar should be closely followed.

Glucagon promotes glycogen breakdown. In settings where glycogen stores have not been depleted (e.g., insulin overdose), 1 mg of ***glucagon intramuscularly or subcutaneously*** will raise blood glucose levels.

Glucocorticoids should not be used routinely. Their only clear indication is in known primary or secondary adrenal insufficiency. In other settings, they have little acute value and may cloud the diagnostic process.

HYPOTHALAMIC/PITUITARY DISORDERS

75. What clinical signs or symptoms suggest hypothalamic dysfunction?

The signs and symptoms of hypothalamic dysfunction are as *variable* as the processes controlled by the hypothalamus, ranging from disorders of hormonal production to disturbances of thermoregulation. ***Precocious*** or ***delayed sexual maturation*** represent the most common presentations of hypothalamic endocrine abnormality in childhood. ***Diabetes insipidus***, ***psychic disturbances***, and ***excessive sleepiness*** are found in about one-third of all patients with hypothalamic dysfunction and may be the first manifestation of disease. Eating disorders (obesity, anorexia, bulimia) and convulsions are also reported. Dyshidrosis and disturbances of sphincteric control are occasionally seen.

76. List the intracranial or systemic processes that can interfere with hypothalamic-pituitary function.

Intracranial

- *Congenital:*
  - Inherited deficiencies of gonadotropin-releasing factor (GnRF), growth-hormone-releasing hormone (GHRH)
  - Syndromic—Laurence-Moon-Biedl, Prader-Labhart-Willi syndromes
  - Structural—craniopharyngioma, Rathke pouch cyst, hemangioma, hamartoma
- *Infectious*: meningitis, encephalitis

- *Tumors*: glioma, dysgerminoma, ependymoma
- *Trauma*: subarachnoid or intraventricular hemorrhage, surgical stalk section
- *Idiopathic*

Systemic

- *CNS abnormality demonstrable by scan or biopsy*:
  Kernicterus, congenital infection, sarcoidosis, Langerhans cell histiocytosis (eosinophilic granuloma), tuberculosis, neurofibromatosis, leukemia
- *CNS involvement is functional:*
  Anorexia nervosa, psychosocial dwarfism, chronic illness

77. What is the significance of an enlarged sella turcica on a skull film?

The sella turcica derives its name from the Latin words for *Turkish saddle*. The name reflects the anatomic shape of the saddle-like prominence on the upper surface of the sphenoid bone in the middle cranial fossa above which sits the pituitary gland. A variety of conditions can lead to sellar enlargement, including tumors of the pituitary or functional hypertrophy of the pituitary, which may occur in primary hypothyroidism or primary hypogonadism. Modern imaging techniques have supplanted the skull series as a tool for searching for pituitary or hypothalamic disease; however, an enlarged sella may be noted on children in whom skull series are obtained for other reasons (e.g., head trauma).

78. Which tests are useful in studying suspected hypothalamic and pituitary malfunction?

The choice of tests depends on the spectrum of historical features and clinical findings, but it is essential to rule out structural pathology prior to searching for functional abnormalities. Skull films are not adequate for this purpose; therefore, either an ***MRI*** or ***CT scan*** is required.

Studies of the pituitary-hypothalamus may include any or all of the following:

1. ***Prolactin.*** Random levels tend to be elevated in the presence of hypothalamic lesions. A normal level does not rule out structural abnormalities.

2. ***Thyrotropin-releasing hormone provocative test (TRH test).*** TRH normally promotes the rapid release of thyroid-stimulating hormone (TSH) by the pituitary. In the presence of pituitary or hypothalamic dysfunction, the release of TSH is often blunted and delayed. TRH also promotes release of prolactin. In hypothalamic dysfunction, the prolactin response is often altered as well.

3. ***Growth hormone production tests*** (see Question 64). These tests are generally indicated only if the child's growth rate is subnormal. Growth hormone releasing factor is now available for testing the pituitary responsiveness. It has proven useful, in some instances, in delineating pituitary causes of growth hormone underproduction from primary hypothalamic disease.

4. ***Gonadotropin-releasing hormone (GnRH) provocative test.*** Random levels of leuteinizing hormone and follicle-stimulating hormone are not generally helpful if one is searching for pituitary hypofunction. The results of the GnRH test must be correlated with the age of the child, since there are developmental changes in the response to GnRH.

5. Simultaneous ***urine and serum osmolalities.*** Anormal serum osmolality and a concentrated urine osmolality tend to rule out diabetes insipidus. If these results are equivocal, a water deprivation test may be required.

SEXUAL DIFFERENTIATION AND DEVELOPMENT

79. An infant is born with suspected ambiguous genitalia. What features of history and physical examination are key in the evaluation?

History: One should search for evidence of maternal androgen ingestion (rare now, but common in the 1960s with certain progestational agents), other hormonal use (e.g., for infertility or endometriosis), alcohol use, parental consanguinity, previous neonatal deaths, or a family history of previously affected children.

Physical examination: The presence of a *gonadal structure* in the labioscrotal fold strongly implies the presence of some Y chromosomal material. Gonads containing both ovarian and testicular components (ovotestes) have been found in the inguinal canal. However, it is rare to find an ovary in the inguinal canal. In the absence of a palpable gonad, no conclusions can be drawn regarding probable chromosomal sex. The size of the phallic structure and the location of the urethral meatus provide no information regarding genetic or chromosomal make-up. However, phallic size and function are important considerations when determining sex-of-rearing.

The presence of *midline abnormalities* (e.g., cleft palate) suggests hypothalamic or pituitary dysfunction, while congenital anomalies such as imperforate anus suggest structural derangements. Digital rectal exam will confirm the patency of the anus and may allow palpation of the uterus. Other anomalies should be noted since ambiguous genitalia can be a feature of numerous syndromes.

80. What is the most common cause of ambiguous genitalia?

There are numerous causes of ambiguous genitalia, and no particular cause appears to predominate. Nature is capable of endless variety; therefore, great caution must be exercised in assigning a diagnosis and gender to an affected child.

Undervirilized male (XY karyotype)

- *Androgen resistance*
  - Complete—testicular feminization
  - Partial
- *Defects in androgen synthesis*
  - 3β-Hydroxysteroid dehydrogenase deficiency
  - 5α-Reductase deficiency

Virilized female (XX karyotype)

- *Excess androgen*
  - Congenital adrenal hyperplasia
  - 21-Hydroxylase deficiency
  - 3β-Hydroxysteroid dehydrogenase deficiency

Maternal androgen exposure

- Medication
- Virilizing adrenal tumor

Intersex (mosaic karyotypes; e.g., XO/XY)

Structural abnormalities

81. Which studies are essential in the evaluation of ambiguous genitalia?

- ***Ultrasonography:*** This test is the most helpful in identifying internal structures, particularly the uterus and occasionally the ovaries. The absence of a uterus suggests that testes were present early in gestation and produced müllerian-inhibiting factor, causing regression of the müllerian-derived ducts (and thus the uterus). The injection of contrast medium into the urethrovaginal opening(s) will often demonstrate a pouch posterior to the fused labioscrotal folds. Occasionally, the cervix and cervical canal will be highlighted by this study as well.
- ***Chromosomal analysis:*** Obviously useful in predicting gonadal content. Of note, buccal smears searching for clumps of nuclear membrane chromatin (Barr bodies), representing the inactive X chromosome in girls, should not be used (even preliminarily) because of their high rates of inaccuracy.

- ***Measurement of adrenal steroids*** (17-hydroxyprogesterone, 11-deoxycortisol, 17-hydroxypregnenolone). 17-Hydroxyprogesterone is the precursor elevated in the most common variety of congenital adrenal hyperplasia associated with ambiguous genitalia (21-hydroxylase deficiency).
- ***Measurement of testosterone and dihydrotestosterone*** (DHT).

As important and useful as the testing is, it is also useful to have input from staff with expertise in this area, including a geneticist, pediatric endocrinologist, and pediatric urologist. It is also essential that information be synthesized by this group after all data are available and that it be communicated to the family by a single spokesperson.

American Academy of Pediatrics, Committee on Genetics, Section on Endocrinology and Section on Urology: Developmental anomalies of the external genitalia in the newborn. Pediatrics 106:138-142, 2000.

82. What major criteria are used to define a micropenis?

To be classified as a micropenis, the phallus must meet *two* major criteria:

1. The phallus must be ***normally formed***, with the urethral meatus located on the head of the penis and the penis positioned in an appropriate relationship to the scrotum and other pelvic structures. If these features are not present, then the term micropenis should be avoided.

2. The phallus must be > 2.5 SD below the appropriate mean for age. For a term newborn, this means that a penis ***< 2 cm in stretched length*** is classified as a micropenis.

It is essential that the phallus be measured appropriately. This entails the use of a rigid ruler pressed firmly against the pubic symphysis, depressing the suprapubic fat pad as much as possible. The phallus is grasped gently by its lateral margins and stretched. The measurement is taken along the dorsum of the penis. Note should also be made of the breadth of the phallic shaft. Micropenis must be recognized early in life so that appropriate diagnostic testing can be done.

Lee PA, et al: Micropenis. I. Criteria, etiologies and classification. Johns Hopkins Med J 146:156–163, 1980.

83. What causes a micropenis?

Regression of the müllerian system, fusion of the labioscrotal folds, and migration of the urethral meatus occur during the first trimester of gestation. Further growth of the phallus during the second and third trimester is dependent on the production of testosterone by the fetal testis in response to fetal pituitary luteinizing hormone (LH). Growth hormone also enhances penile growth *in utero*. Thus, the following disorders can result in micropenis:

- *Hypothalamic/pituitary dysfunction*: isolated, Kallmann syndrome, Prader-Willi syndrome, septo-optic dysplasia
- *Testicular dysfunction or failure*: intrauterine testicular torsion (vanishing testes syndrome), testicular dysplasia
- *Complex* (testicular and/or pituitary) or *idiopathic*: Robinow, Klinefelter, other X polysomies
- *Partial androgen resistance*

84. Outline the three main concerns in the initial evaluation of a 1-month-old with micropenis.

1. ***Is there a defect in the hypothalamic-pituitary-gonadal axis?*** Specific tests include measurement of testosterone, dihydrotestosterone, LH, and follicle-stimulating hormone (FSH). Because circulating levels of these hormones are normally quite high in the neonatal period, measurement of random levels during the first 2 months of life may be useful in identifying diseases of the testes and pituitary. Beyond 3 months of age, the tests are generally not useful because the entire axis becomes quiescent and remains so until late childhood. Depending on the patient's age, provocative tests may be necessary including: (a) repetitive

testosterone injection to evaluate the ability of the penis to respond to hormonal stimulation, (b) use of human chorionic gonadotropin (hCG) as a stimulus for testosterone production by the testes, and (c) GnRH administration to examine the responsiveness of the pituitary to stimulation. The trial of testosterone therapy is especially important because it indicates whether phallic growth is possible, and if not, gender reassignment becomes a consideration.

2. ***Does a possible pituitary deficiency involve other hormones?*** Isolated growth hormone deficiency, gonadotropin deficiency, and panhypopituitarism have been associated with micropenis. The presence of hypoglycemia, hypothermia, or hyperbilirubinemia (e.g., associated with hypothyroidism) in a child with micropenis should lead one to search for other pituitary hormone deficits and structural abnormalities of the CNS (e.g., septo-optic dysplasia).

3. ***Is there a renal abnormality?*** Because of the association of genital and renal abnormalities and nature's endless variations, it may be important in some cases to obtain an abdominal and pelvic ultrasound to better define the internal anatomy.

85. Review the spectrum of androgen resistance syndromes.

In males, the testis-determining factor (TDF, formerly "HY antigen") is encoded on the short arm of the Y chromosome. TDF induces the gonads to develop into testes. In the testes, Sertoli cells secrete müllerian inhibiting factor (MIF), and the müllerian ducts (responsible for the proximal vagina, uterus, and fallopian tubes) regress. Leydig cells secrete testosterone, which maintains the wolffian ducts (responsible for seminiferous tubules). Testosterone is converted by 5α-reductase to dihydrotestosterone (DHT), which virilizes the urogenital sinus and external genitalia. If there is no TDF, the cascade does not begin and the internal and external development is female.

Androgen resistance syndromes usually refer to peripheral defects, which can vary from a lack of receptors (androgen insensitivity) to a deficiency in 5α-reductase. In complete androgen insensitivity (testicular feminization), an XY male appears externally to be completely female. Because MIF production has also occurred, no internal female organs are present. Affected individuals often present at adolescence with primary amenorrhea. In 5α-reductase deficiency, external virilization of the genitalia is incomplete, and these children usually present at birth with ambiguous genitalia.

Griffin JE: Androgen resistance—the clinical and molecular spectrum. N Engl J Med 326:611, 1992.

86. If a second grade girl, age 7½ years, develops breast buds and pubic hair, is this normal or precocious?

Precocious puberty is the appearance of physical changes associated with sexual development earlier than normal. Traditionally, this has been the development of secondary sexual characteristics along female lines in girls who are < 8 years of age and along male lines in boys who are <9 years of age. In 1997, an office-based study of 17,000 healthy 3-12 year-old girls revealed that puberty was occurring on average 1 year earlier in white girls and 2 years earlier in black girls and suggested a revision of guidelines for the ages at which precocious puberty should be investigated. Many experts now recommend that an evaluation for precocious puberty of girls need not be undertaken for white girls >7 years or black girls >6 years with breast and/or pubic hair development. However, this remains controversial and a subject of ongoing debate and data collection. The recommendations for boys remain that investigations for pathologic etiologies be undertaken if pubertal changes begin before age 9 years.

Kaplowitz PB, et al: Reexamination of the age limit for defining when puberty is precocious in girls in the United States: Implications for evaluation and treatment. Pediatrics 104:936-941, 1999.

Herman-Giddens ME, et al: Secondary sexual characteristics and menses in young girls seen in office practice: A study from the pediatric research in office settings network. Pediatrics 99:505-512, 1997.

87. Breast buds are noted on a 2-year-old girl. Is this worrisome?

Premature thelarche, or the development of breast buds, is the most common variation of normal pubertal development. A form of mild estrogenization, it typically occurs between ages 1 and 3. It is usually benign and should not be associated with the onset of other pubertal events. Precocious puberty, rather than simple premature thelarche, should be suspected if:

- Breast, nipple, and areolar development reach Tanner III stage
- Androgenization with pubic and/or axillary hair begins
- Linear growth accelerates

Ongoing parental observation and periodic re-examination are all that are required if there are no signs of progression.

88. Which aspects of the physical exam are particularly important in evaluating a patient with precocious puberty?

- ***Evidence of CNS mass:*** examination of optic fundus for possible increased intracranial pressure; visual fields testing for evidence of optic nerve compression by a hypothalamic or pituitary mass
- ***Evidence of androgenic influence:*** presence of acne, facial and axillary hair; increased muscle bulk and definition; extent of other body/pubic hair; in boys, increased scrotal rugation accompanied by thinning and pigmentation, penile elongation
- ***Evidence of estrogenic influence:*** size of breast tissue and nipple/areolar contouring; vaginal mucosa color (increased estrogen causes cornification of vaginal epithelium with a color change from prepubertal shiny red to a more opalescent pink); labia minor (become more prominent and visible between the labia majora as puberty progresses)
- ***Evidence of gonadotropic stimulation:*** testicular enlargement > 2.5 cm in length or > 4 ml in volume (preferably measured using a Prader orchidometer of labeled volumetric beads). Of note, pubertal development without testicular enlargement usually suggests adrenal pathology.
- ***Evidence of other mass:*** asymmetric testicular enlargement; hepatomegaly; abdominal mass

89. Which radiologic and laboratory tests are indicated for evaluation of precocious puberty?

The evaluation may often be costly and complex, and in most cases, a specific cause will not be identified. As a general rule, the younger the child and the more rapid the onset of the condition, the greater the likelihood of detecting pathology. While precocious puberty occurs 80% of the time in girls, boys are more likely to have identifiable pathology.

Radiologic evaluation

- *Bone age:* This study helps to determine the duration of exposure to the elevated sex hormone. A significantly advanced bone age compared with chronologic age suggests long-term exposure.
- *Abdominal and pelvic ultrasound:* In boys, this test identifies possible adrenal masses, and in girls, adrenal masses, ovarian masses, or cysts. Increased uterine size and echogenicity suggest endometrial proliferation in response to circulating estrogen.

Laboratory

- *LH, FSH, estradiol, testosterone.*
- *Adrenal steroid levels* (17-hydroxyprogesterone, androstenedione, cortisol). More extensive testing may be needed in a virilized child if the initial studies are normal.
- *Provocative testing* of the hypothalamic-pituitary axis (using a synthetic GnRH) or of the adrenal gland using a synthetic ACTH, especially in the child presenting with slight but progressive pubertal changes.

90. Discuss the terms denoting aspects of precocious sexual development.

The terms used to describe precocious puberty reflect the fact that normal puberty is an orderly process by which female children are feminized and male children masculinized. The development of breast tissue without pubic hair is called *premature thelarche*. If pubic hair subsequently develops, the term *precocious puberty* is used. If pubic hair develops without breast tissue, it is *premature pubarche*. Since pubic hair development in the female is thought to be due to adrenal androgens, the term *premature adrenarche* is commonly used. If the pubertal changes are early and appear to proceed in the orderly fashion of breast budding, pubic hair development, growth spurt, and finally menstruation, the term *true precocious puberty* is used. When some of the changes of puberty are present but their appearance is isolated or out of normal sequence (e.g., menses without breast development), the term *pseudo-precocious puberty* is used. When the changes of puberty are consistent with the child's sex, they are called *isosexual;* when they are discordant with sex, they are *heterosexual*.

91. When along the pubertal spectrum does the male voice begin to crack?

Voice "breaking" has traditionally been regarded as one of the harbingers of puberty. However, sequential voice analysis reveals it is usually a *late* event in puberty, usually occurring between Tanner stage 3 and 4.

Harries MLL, et al: Changes in the male voice at puberty. Arch Dis Child 77:445-447, 1997.

THYROID DISORDERS

92. Which thyroid function tests are "standard"?

Diseases of the thyroid represent a heterogeneous group of disorders. As such, there are no "standard" thyroid function studies appropriate for all children with suspected thyroid disease. The choice of laboratory tests is based on the results of a careful history and physical examination.

Clinical findings suggesting *hyperthyroidism:* A ***thyroid-stimulating hormone (TSH)*** and ***thyroxine (T_4) level*** should be obtained. TSH suppression is probably the most sensitive indictor of hyperthyroid status. If the patient is symptomatic and has a suppressed TSH with a normal T_4, it will be necessary to obtain a triiodothyronine (T_3) radioimmunoassay, since cases of T_3-thyrotoxicosis do occur. If the patient is asymptomatic but has an elevated T_4, then some measure of binding capacity should be obtained, such as a T_3 uptake.

Clinical findings consistent with *hypothyroidism:* The laboratory evaluation consists of the ***quantitation of T_4*** and ***TSH***. A low T_4 and elevated TSH are diagnostic of hypothyroidism.

93. What is the significance of anti-thyroid antibodies in children?

In the pediatric population, ***chronic lymphocytic thyroiditis*** is the most common cause of hypothyroidism. The antibodies that are generally available as markers for this condition include *antimicrosomial*, *antithyroglobulin*, and *antithyroidal peroxidase* antibodies. Most laboratories will run at least 2 of these assays. A titer > 1:2000 on any assay provides strong evidence in favor of the diagnosis, but the absence of antibodies does not rule out chronic lymphocytic thyroiditis. High titers may be seen in Graves disease. Low titers may be present with a wide range of systemic diseases, particularly autoimmune processes.

94. Of what value is the T_3 resin uptake (T_3RU) test?

The *T_3RU test* is a measure of ***serum thyroid-binding capacity***. Because T_4 is primarily protein-bound, only a small amount exists in the unbound (free) state. Physiologically, the free T_4 is the metabolically active compound, but it is technically complex to assay directly. In most cases, it has proved simpler to measure T_3RU and total T_4 and to calculate the amount of T_4 that is unbound. In primary thyroidal disease, the T_3RU and the T_4 should go in the same direction (i.e., both increased or both decreased). If they go in opposite directions, it is probably a binding problem.

95. Which signs and symptoms in an infant suggest congenital hypothyroidism?

SYMPTOMS	SIGNS
Lethargy	Hypotonia, slow reflexes
Poor feeding	Poor weight gain
Prolonged jaundice	Jaundice
Constipation	Distended abdomen
Mottling	Acrocyanosis
Cold extremities	Coarse features
	Large fontanels/wide sutures
	Hoarse cry
	Goiter

96. What causes congenital hypothyroidism?

- *Primary*: agenesis/dysgenesis, ectopic, dyshormonogenesis
- *Secondary*: hypopituitarism, hypothalamic abnormality
- *Other*
    Transient
    Maternal factors—goitrogen ingestion, iodide deficiency

97. How common is goiter in newborns with congenital hypothyroidism?

Congenital goiter is seen in only **20%** of newborns with congenital hypothyroidism. Maternal ingestion of antithyroid medications, iodides, and goitrogens, congenital thyroid dyshormonogenic defects, and congenital hyperthyroidism are associated with palpable thyromegaly. Goiter in the newborn is difficult to recognize because of the infant's relatively short neck and increased subcutaneous fat. Palpation of the neck is often overlooked in newborn exams.

99. How effective are screening programs for congenital hypothyroidism?

Screening programs correctly identify ***90–95%*** of children affected with congenital hypothyroidism. Screening programs are most likely to miss infants with *large ectopic glands*, those with *partial defects* in thyroidal hormone biosynthesis, and individuals with *secondary (pituitary or hypothalamic) disease*. If an infant presents with a clinical picture of hypothyroidism and has had a normal newborn screen, it is important to realize that the false-negative rate of the screening is up to 10%.

99. Discuss the risks in delaying treatment for congenital hypothyroidism.

Therapy should begin as early as possible because outcome is related to the time treatment is started. Because < 20% of patients will have distinctive clinical signs at 3–4 weeks of age, screening is now performed on all newborns in the United States at 2–3 days of age, and most affected children are started on therapy prior to 1 months of age. The prognosis for intellectual development is directly related to the amount of time from birth to the initiation of therapy. Children begun on hormone replacement at < 30 days of age have a mean IQ of 106, but those whose treatment started at 3–6 months have a mean IQ of 70.

100. If a goiter is noted during a routine exam of an asymptomatic 7-year-old boy, what should be the next course of action?

The evaluation of a child with goiter is generally simple. In the absence of signs of thyroidal disease, history should be obtained regarding recent exposure to iodine or other halogens. A family history should be obtained regarding thyroidal disease since thyroiditis tends to run in families. The initial laboratory evaluation is typically T_4, TSH, and anti-thyroidal antibodies. If there is discrete nodularity within the thyroid or the gland is rock hard or tender, then further diagnostic evaluation (ultrasound, CT scan) may be indicated. Parathyroid enlargement or lymphoma may be misdiagnosed as a goiter.

101. What are the causes of acquired hypothyroidism in childhood?

The most common cause is ***chronic lymphocytic thyroiditis***.

102. What is the most common clinical presentation of Hashimoto thyroiditis?

Chronic lymphocytic thyroiditis (CLT), also called *Hashimoto disease* or *autoimmune thyroiditis*, is the most common thyroid problem in children and is thought to be caused by an autoimmune organ-specific process. Although symptoms of hypo- or hyperthyroidism may be present, the preponderance of pediatric patients are asymptomatic, and the condition is detected by the presence of a goiter. The diagnosis of CLT is primarily based on the demonstration of antithyroglobulin and/or antimicrosomal antibody in high titers (> 1:2000).

103. What should a parent be told about the prognosis of a child who has euthyroid goiter caused by chronic lymphocytic thyroiditis?

About ***50%*** of all children who present with euthyroid goiter will have resolution of the goiter over several years regardless of whether or not thyroxine replacement is given. However, it is not possible to predict which children will recover completely, which will remain euthyroid with goiter, and which will become hypothyroid. Any child identified with thyroid disease should have T_4 and TSH values monitored every 4-6 months.

104. What other autoimmune endocrine diseases are associated with chronic lymphocytic thyroiditis?

Adrenal insufficiency (Schmidt syndrome), diabetes mellitus, and autoimmune polyendocrine syndrome (type II).

105. What does a normal T_4 and an elevated TSH suggest?

The diagnosis of hypothyroidism is based on finding both a low T_4 and an elevated TSH. However, on occasion, the T_4 can be maintained in a normal range by increased stimulation of the thyroid gland by TSH. This combination of laboratory values is suggestive of a failing thyroid and is referred to as ***compensated hypothyroidism***. Since TSH is the most useful physiologic marker for the adequacy of a circulating level of thyroid hormone, an elevated TSH is an indication for thyroid replacement therapy. If the TSH is only minimally elevated and the child is asymptomatic, it is worthwhile to wait 4–6 weeks and repeat the T_4 and TSH levels before instituting therapy.

106. What is the most common cause of hyperthyroidism in children?

Graves disease is a multisystem disease characterized by hyperthyroidism, infiltrative ophthalmopathy, and, occasionally, an infiltrative dermopathy. The features of this disease may occur singly or in any combination. In the pediatric population, the ophthalmopathy seems to be less severe, and the dermopathy is rare. The full syndrome may never develop. There has been a tendency to use the terms Graves disease, thyrotoxicosis, and hyperthyroidism interchangeably, but there are many other causes of hyperthyroidism in childhood.

107. In addition to Graves disease, what conditions may cause hyperthyroidism?

Excess TSH: TSH-producing tumor

Abnormal thyroid stimulation: TSH receptor antibody
Thyroid autonomy: adenoma, multinodular goiter
Thyroid inflammation: subacute thyroiditis, Hashimoto thyroiditis
Exogenous hormone: ingestion, ectopic thyroid tissue

108. Describe the typical features of hyperthyroidism due to Graves disease.

History: The onset of symptoms is usually gradual, with increasing emotional lability and deteriorating school performance. Since the onset of Graves disease and puberty may coincide, many parents initially attribute the psychologic changes to adolescence. The younger child may simply be thought to be "hyperactive." Sleep disturbances, nervousness, and weight loss may be noted as well as easy fatigability and heat intolerance. Observation of the child's behavior while the history is being obtained from the parent is often instructive.

Physical examination: The oral temperature may be slightly increased (100°F). Weight may be low for height, and many children will be tall for age and genetic potential. Some children will have experienced an acceleration in growth rate at the same time that their behavior began to deteriorate. However, the onset of puberty may be delayed or accelerated. The pulse rate is usually inappropriately high for age. A widened pulse pressure or elevated blood pressure is often noted, although this is a more variable finding in children than in adults. A hyperactive precordium may accompany the changes in blood pressure, and a functional systolic murmur may be heard. Two- to fourfold thyroid enlargement is a consistent finding. The thyroid is usually firm, symmetrical, smooth, and nontender. The presence of a discrete node or area of tenderness warrants further investigation.

109. What causes Graves disease?

Graves disease is an autoimmune disorder in which TSH receptor antibodies bind to the TSH receptor, resulting in stimulation of thyroid hormone production and subsequent hyperthyroidism. Most thyroid receptor antibodies belong to the IgG class. The general name used for these antibodies is ***human thyroid-stimulating immunoglobulins***, formerly called long-acting thyroid stimulator.

110. How is the hyperthyroidism of Graves disease distinguished from that occasionally found in chronic lymphocytic thyroiditis?

Patients with hyperthyroidism due to CLT may be indistinguishable from those with Graves disease. The presence of ***ophthalmologic findings*** points toward the latter entity, but the absence of exophthalmos does not rule out Graves disease. The demonstration of ***human thyroid-stimulating antibodies*** is confirmatory of the Graves diagnosis, but these tests may not be readily available. The best way to distinguish between these two entities is by ***determining the uptake of radioactive iodine*** 6 and 24 hours after the administration of the isotope. Low or normal uptake supports the diagnosis of CLT, whereas elevated uptakes at 6 and 24 hours are more indicative of Graves disease.

111. In the child or adolescent with Graves disease, what other endocrine abnormalities can be observed?

A great number of endocrinologic functions are altered in Graves disease, but only a few of these changes are clinically relevant to children and adolescents.

- Hyperthyroidism may be associated with either ***delayed or early puberty***. The mechanisms for these alterations are not well understood.
- Postpubertal females often have ***menstrual irregularity*** prior to treatment. The intermenstrual interval may be either prolonged or shortened, and menstrual flow may be diminished. In rare circumstances, frank amenorrhea may occur.
- ***Hypercalcemia*** has been noted in patients with hyperthyroidism, and the serum *alkaline phosphatase* may also be elevated in affected children. These changes are simi-

lar to those found in hyperparathyroidism. However, parathyroid hormone levels are low or undetectable. True hyperparathyroidism and Graves disease may coexist and should be suspected if the hypercalcemia does not improve as the hyperthyroidism is controlled.

- The manifestation of ***thyroid hormone excess***—flushing, sweating, tachycardia, GI hypermotility—are similar to those seen in carcinoid syndrome. However, the plasma serotonin concentration, urinary 5-hydroxyindoleacetic acid excretion, and platelet monoamine oxidase activity are normal.

112. Why does exophthalmos occur in Graves disease?

The reason is unknown, but several facts suggest an autoimmune process:

- Histologic studies reveal lymphocytic infiltration of the retrobulbar muscles.
- Circulating lymphocytes are sensitized to an antigen unique to the retrobulbar tissues.
- The thyroglobulin—antithyroglobulin antibody complexes found in patients with Graves disease bind specifically to the extraorbital muscles.

113. What treatment options are available for children with Graves disease?

The three types of therapy are ***antithyroid medication***, ***radioactive (^{131}I) ablation***, and ***subtotal thyroidectomy***.

Cheetham TD, et al: Treatment of hyperthyroidism in young people. Arch Dis Child 78:207-209, 1998.

114. Describe the principal modes of actions and side effects of medications used to treat Graves disease.

The thionamide derivatives, propylthiouracil, and methimazole are the keystones of long-term management. However, their effective onset of action is slow since they block synthesis but not release of thyroid hormone. Propranolol is useful in treating many of the β-adrenergic effects of hyperthyroidism. It is used during the acute management of Graves disease but should be discontinued when the thyroid disease is controlled. Iodide, which can transiently block thyroid hormone release, and glucocorticoids are useful "stopgap" medications while awaiting the inhibitory effects of the thionamides. They are generally used only when the patient is acutely symptomatic (thyroid storm).

115. Has radioactive iodide fallen into disfavor as a treatment option for Graves disease?

On the contrary, radioactive iodide (^{131}I) is increasing in popularity. Concern had been voiced about the possible risk of thyroid carcinoma, leukemia, thyroid nodules, or genetic mutations, but as the individuals treated with ^{131}I during childhood have been followed for prolonged periods, experience suggests that children are *not* at a significantly increased risk.

Rivkees SA et al: The management of Graves' disease in children, with special emphasis on radioiodine treatment. J Clin Endo Metab 83:3767-3776, 1998.

116. During a routine physical exam, a solitary thyroid nodule is palpated on a asymptomatic 10-year-old. Can a "wait and see" approach be taken?

Absolutely not. In children with a solitary nodule, about 30–40% have a carcinoma, 20–30% have an adenoma, and the remainder will have thyroid abscess, thyroid cyst, multinodular goiter, Hashimoto thyroiditis, subacute thyroiditis, or nonthyroidal neck mass. Given the relatively high incidence of carcinoma, a thyroidal mass demands prompt evaluation. Previous irradiation to the head or neck is associated with a significantly increased incidence of thyroid carcinoma. A family history of thyroid disease increases the likelihood of chronic lymphocytic thyroiditis or Graves disease. The presence of tenderness or palpation or high titers of anti-thyroid antibodies points away from a malignant process. However, in all cases, radiologic studies should be undertaken, and in many cases, surgical exploration is required.

117. How should this solitary thyroid nodule be investigated?

The principal tools used in the investigation of a thyroid mass are ***^{123}I scanning*** and ***ultrasound***. *Ultrasound* is useful in delineating the size of the mass, its anatomic relationship to the rest of the thyroid, and the presence of cystic structures. ***^{123}I imaging*** that reveals a single nonfunctioning mass ("cold" nodule) suggests a carcinoma or adenoma and is a clear indication for surgery. Patchy uptake is more characteristic of chronic lymphocytic thyroiditis, while a poorly functioning lobe may be found in a subacute thyroiditis.

118. How is the euthyroid sick syndrome diagnosed?

This syndrome is an adaptive response to slow body metabolism. It is also called the *low T_3 syndrome* because the most consistent finding is a depression of serum T_3. Reverse T_3 (rT_3), a metabolically inactive metabolite, is increased, although this is rarely measured. T_4 and TBG levels may be low or normal. Free T_4 levels and TSH levels are normal. In sick preterm infants, the clinical picture is often confusing because levels of T_4, free T_4, and T_3 are naturally low. Infants and children with the euthyroid sick syndrome generally revert to normal as the primary illness resolves.

7. GASTROENTEROLOGY

Petar Mamula, M.D., Jonathan E. Markowitz, M.D., David A. Piccoli, M.D., and Chris A. Liacouras, M.D.

CLINICAL ISSUES

1. What constitutes the syndrome of cyclic vomiting?

As a clinical entity, *cyclic vomiting* is charactized by recurrent, stereotypical episodes of intense nausea and vomiting lasting hours to days, which punctuate periods of normal health. The frequency of episodes averages 12 per year (range, 1-70). Its etiology and pathogenesis remain unknown. In a study of 225 children with cyclic vomiting, 12% had identifiable conditions as a cause, including malrotation, acute hydronephrosis, CNS neoplasm, Addison disease, and disorders of fatty acid oxidation. Gastroesophageal reflux and sinusitis were noted in 41%, but not felt to be the primary cause of vomiting. Although 88% of patients with cyclic vomiting syndrome were felt to have idiopathic disease, a systematic search to look for underlying disorders should be undertaken. Cyclic vomiting syndrome shares features similar to vomiting episodes seen in migraine headaches and familial dysautonomia, and recent research on the idiopathic type is being directed toward alterations in the autonomic nervous system.

Rashed HR, et al: Autonomic function in cyclic vomiting syndrome and classic migraine. Dig Dis Sci 44:74S-78S, 1999.

Li BUK, et al: Heterogeneity of diagnoses presenting as cyclic vomiting. Pediatrics 102:583-587, 1998.

2. Which infants have dyschezia?

Those who strain and scream during prolonged attempts to defecate. The behavior can continue up to 20 minutes until a liquid or soft stool is passed. This can occur on multiple times daily for a few weeks until spontaneous resolution. It is presumed that the disorder is due to failure of coordination between increased intraabdominal pressure and relaxation of the pelvic floor. Physical examination should include rectal examination to exclude anorectal abnormalities. A normal physical exam and growth rate is reassuring to parents, who should be discouraged from maneuvers of rectal stimulation. The entity is commonly confused with colic and constipation.

Rasquin-Weber A, et al: Childhood functional gastrointestinal disorders. Gut 45:1160S-1168S, 1999.

3. What are the most frequent causes of pancreatitis in children?

Acute pancreatitis in children is relatively rare. Most cases are due to drugs, infections (primarily viral), systemic illness, or trauma. In up to 25% of cases, an etiology is not identified.

- *Drugs/toxins*: Alcohol, L-asparaginase, high-dose corticosteroids, sulfasalazine, thiazides, valproic acid
- *Infections*: Viral (mumps, coxsackie virus, Epstein-Barr virus, rubella, influenza A), *Mycoplasma pneumoniae*, *Salmonella*, ascariasis
- *Systemic disease*: Cystic fibrosis, diabetes mellitus, Henoch-Schönlein purpura, Kawasaki disease, renal failure, sarcoidosis, systemic lupus erythematosus
- *Trauma*
- *Anatomic abnormalities*: Biliary obstruction (stones, tumors), duodenal ulcer
- *Congenital abnormalities*: Annular pancreas, choledochal cyst, pancreas divisum

- *Metabolic*: Hypercalcemia, hypertriglyceridemia, Reye syndrome
- *Miscellaneous*: Familial, refeeding syndrome (following malnutrition)
- *Idiopathic*

Lerner A, et al: Pancreatic diseases in children. Pediatr Clin North Am 43:125–156, 1996.

4. In addition to serum amylase, what other tests are useful in the diagnosis of pancreatitis?

Multiple laboratory abnormalities can exist in pancreatitis, and although serum amylase is the most widely used test for diagnosis, it may not be the most sensitive or specific. It is usually elevated in the first 12 hours but then may return to normal within 24–72 hours. The serum lipase remains elevated for longer periods of time. Other tests have been advocated as being more useful for pancreatic injury than a simple serum amylase:

- Cationic trypsinogen
- Amylase:creatinine clearance ratio (> 5% suggests pancreatitis)
- Elevated hepatic transaminases, hyperglycemia, and hypocalcemia
- Abdominal x-rays showing pancreatic calcifications or abdominal ileus
- Abdominal ultrasonography revealing increased density, pancreatic enlargement, or pseudocyst formation

Of note, falsely elevated serum amylase can occur if amylase is released from other injured areas (e.g., salivary gland in mumps, intestine in Crohn disease, ovary and fallopian tube in salpingitis). Isoenzyme determinations can help to identify the source if the clinical picture is confusing.

5. What is hereditary pancreatitis?

Hereditary pancreatitis (HP) is a genetic disorder inherited in an autosomal dominant manner. It is caused by mutations in cationic trypsinogen, and it carries an approximate 80% life-time risk of developing symptoms of recurrent pancreatitis. HP is an uncommon cause of pancreatitis, accounting for about 1% of cases, with the majority of patients having their first episode within the first two decades of life. The treatment consists of symptomatic therapy, pancreatic enzyme supplementation, and avoidance of smoking and alcohol. Pancreatic duct stenting is being explored as an option. Prenatal testing is available.

Vaughan D, et al: Pancreatic duct stenting as a treatment for hereditary pancreatitis. Pediatrics 104:1129-1133, 1999.

6. How is ascites diagnosed by physical examination?

Severe ascites is commonly diagnosed by observation of the child in a supine and then upright position. Bulging flanks, umbilical protrusion, and scrotal edema (in males) are generally evident. Three main techniques are used when the diagnosis is not obvious:

1. ***Fluid wave*:** This sign can be elicited in a cooperative patient by tapping sharply on one flank while receiving the wave with the other hand. The transmission of the wave through fatty tissue should be blocked by a hand placed on the center of the abdomen.

2. ***Shifting dullness*:** With the patient supine, percussion of the abdomen will demonstrate a central area of tympany at the top surrounded by flank percussion dullness. This dullness shifts when the patient moves laterally or stands up.

3. ***"Puddle sign"*:** A cooperative and mobile patient may be examined in the knee-chest position. The pool of ascites is tapped while you listen for a sloshing sound or change in sound transmission with the stethoscope.

Small amounts of ascites can be extremely difficult to detect on physical exam in children. Although ascites can be demonstrated on radiographs, the most sensitive and specific test is an abdominal-pelvic ultrasound, which can detect as little as 150 ml of ascitic fluid.

7. How does the major cause of ascites in neonates differ from that in older children?

Older children: portal hypertension due to hepatic (e.g., chronic liver disease of multiple etiologies), prehepatic (e.g., portal vein thrombosis), or posthepatic (e.g., congestive heart failure, constrictive pericarditis) conditions

Infants: urinary ascites due most commonly to obstructive renal disease (e.g., posterior urethral valves)

8. Which features on plain radiographs are suspicious for ascites?

- Separation of bowel loops
- Abdominal haziness
- Indistinct psoas muscle shadow
- Increased pelvic density in the upright position
- *McCort sign*: increased distance (> 2 mm) between the properitoneal fat stripe and the right colon
- *Hellmen sign*: appearance of a radiolucent shadow between the lateral wall of the liver and the abdominal wall
- *Dog ear sign*: radiodensity superior and lateral to the bladder
- Obliteration of the lower lateral hepatic angle

Cochran WJ: Ascites. In McMillan JA, et al (eds). Oski's Pediatrics, Principles and Practice of Pediatrics, 3rd ed. Philadelphia, Lippincott Williams & Wilkins, 1994, p 1904.

9. In what clinical settings is rectal prolapse most commonly seen?

- Constipation
- Celiac disease
- Malnutrition
- Severe coughing (e.g., pertussis)
- Cystic fibrosis
- *Enterobius vermicularis* (pinworm) infestation
- Myelomeningocele
- Abnormalities of sacrum or coccyx
- Ehlers-Danlos syndrome

10. Which agents are known to cause food poisoning in children?

Food poisoning is best defined as a gastrointestinal upset resulting in nausea, vomiting, and diarrhea, with or without fever, and appearing within 72 hours of ingestion of food contaminated by microorganisms or toxins. The likely offending agents vary according to the nature and time of onset of symptoms after the ingestion.

Onset within 1–6 hrs, nausea and vomiting, no fever

- *Staphylococcus aureus* toxin
- *Bacillus cereus*

Abdominal cramps and diarrhea within 8–16 hrs

- *Clostridium perfringens*
- *Bacillus cereus*

Fever, abdominal cramps, diarrhea within 16–48 hrs

- Salmonella
- Shigella
- *Vibrio parahaemolyticus*
- Invasive *Escherichia coli*
- *Campylobacter jejuni*

Abdominal cramps, watery diarrhea within 16–72 hrs

- Enterotoxigenic *E. coli*

- *V. parahaemolyticus*
- *V. cholerae*, non-O1
- *V. cholerae*, O1 (endemic area)

Fever, abdominal cramps within 16–48 hrs

- *Yersinia enterocolitica*

Nausea, vomiting, paralysis within 18–36 hrs

- *Clostridium botulinum*

Tauxe RV, Hughes JM: Food-borne disease. In Mandell GL, Bennett JE, Dolin R (eds): Principles and Practice of Infectious Diseases, 4th ed. New York, Churchill Livingstone, 1995, pp 1012–1024.

11. How should the bowel be prepared prior to colonoscopy?

Children < 1 year of age

- Clear liquids for 24 hours
- Pediatric Fleet enemas the night before and the morning of the exam

Children > 1 year of age

- Clear liquids for 48 hours
- X-prep (senna extract) or magnesium citrate orally on 2 successive nights prior to exam
- Adult Fleet enema the night before and the morning of the exam; ***OR***
- GOLYTELY or CoLyte (2–4 liters over 3–4 hours) administered orally or via nasogastric tube the night before the procedure may be substituted in children over 5 years of age. It must be used with caution in younger children.

12. List the indications for lower GI colonoscopy or endoscopy in children.

- Hematochezia in absence of anal source
- Chronic diarrhea of unclear etiology
- Colitis of unclear etiology
- Diagnosis and management of inflammatory bowel disease
- Abnormality on barium enema
- History of familial polyposis
- Persistent severe unexplained lower abdominal pain
- Removal of foreign body
- Ureterosigmoidostomy, surveillance
- Dilation of a colonic stricture

13. When is colonoscopy contraindicated?

- Suspected perforation
- Recent abdominal surgery
- Inadequate bowel preparation
- Massive lower GI bleeding
- Toxic megacolon
- Unstable medical illness
- Coagulopathy

Fox VL: Colonoscopy. In Walker WA, et al (eds): Pediatric Gastrointestinal Disease, 2nd ed. St. Louis, Mosby, 1996, pp 1533–1541.

14. In children with recurrent abdominal pain, what historical features suggest a possible serious cause?

Recurrent abdominal pain is the most common chronic pain syndrome encountered in pediatrics. The vast majority have no identifiable organic basis. Features that suggest an identifiable cause include:

- Pain localizing away from the umbilicus
- Abnormalities in bowel function (constipation, diarrhea, incontinence)
- Vomiting
- Pain that awakens a child at night
- Pain with radiation to the back, shoulder, or lower extremities
- Dysuria
- Rectal bleeding
- Constitutional symptoms (fever, weight loss, altered rate of growth, rash, arthralgia)
- Presentation at age < 4 or > 15 years

- Family history of GI or systemic illness (peptic ulcer disease, inflammatory bowel disease, lactose intolerance)

Oberlander TF, Rappaport LA: Recurrent abdominal pain. Pediatr Rev 14:313–319, 1993.

15. How does the average volume of a swallow in a child compare with that of an adult?

Child (age 1¼–3½ yrs):	4.5 ml	*Adult male*:	21 ml
Adult female:	14 ml	*Average*:	0.27 ml/kg

Jones DV, Work CE: Volume of a swallow. Am J Dis Child 102:427, 1961.

16. What is intractable singultus?

Persistent hiccups.

17. How is the test for reducing substances in the urine performed?

Copper sulfate in a reagent tablet reacts with reducing substances in urine to convert cupric sulfate to cuprous oxide (the Benedict copper reduction reaction). The test provides useful information on carbohydrate metabolism by detecting reducing sugars: glucose, lactose, fructose, galactose, and pentose. Urine is collected in a clean container, and 5 drops are placed in a test tube and mixed with 10 drops of water. Fifteen seconds after the boiling reaction is stopped, the tube is gently shaken (but not stirred) and the color compared with the color chart. The test should be performed on a fresh or refrigerated specimen; otherwise, reducing sugars may be consumed by bacteria.

18. What are the causes of a false-positive result of testing for reducing substances in urine?

A number of substances in the urine can react positively with test tablets: ***salicylates, penicillin, ascorbic acid, nalidixic acid, cephalosporins,*** and ***probenicid*** (especially in large quantities).

19. What is the most commonly ingested foreign body?

Coins account for more than 20,000 visits yearly to emergency rooms in the U.S. Symptomatic patients are more likely to have the coin lodged in the esophagus, although a significant portion may be asymptomatic. Coins lodged in the esophagus should be removed endoscopically because of the risk of ulceration and perforation.

20. Which is potentially more dangerous after ingestion: a penny made in 1977 or 1987?

The penny from ***1987.*** In 1982, the composition of pennies changed. Coins minted after that date have higher concentrations of zinc, which is more corrosive and potentially more harmful after prolonged contact with stomach acid.

21. What is the difference radiographically between a coin in the esophagus and a coin in the trachea?

A coin in the esophagus appears *en face* in the anteroposterior view (sagittal plane), whereas a coin in the trachea appears *en face* on the lateral view (coronal plane). This occurs because the cartilaginous ring of the trachea is open posteriorly, but the opening of the esophagus is widest in the transverse position.

22. A teenage girl presents with symptoms of swallowing difficulties improved by positional head and neck changes, nocturnal regurgitation, and halitosis. What is the likely diagnosis?

Achalasia. The cardinal symptom of this motility disorder of the esophagus is dysphagia. The diagnosis is made by barium swallow and esophageal manometry. The manometric findings are diagnostic, including elevated basal lower esophageal sphincter pressure with failure to relax and the absence of peristalsis throughout the esophageal body during the swallow.

CONSTIPATION

23. When is the first stool normally passed?

Ninety-nine percent of infants will pass a stool within the first 24 hours, and 100% by 48 hours. Failure to pass a stool can be an indication of intestinal obstruction or anatomic abnormality. Approximately 95% of patients with Hirschsprung disease and 25% of patients with cystic fibrosis do not pass their first stool in the first 24 hours. The rule of early passage does not apply to premature babies, in whom delayed evacuation (> 24 hrs) is common, particularly with extreme prematurity.

24. What constitutes constipation in childhood?

Strictly speaking, constipation is defined as infrequent stooling, difficulty passing feces, or chronic fecal retention. Normal stool frequency varies from several times a day to 1 stool every 3 days. In children, constipation should be considered when the normal stooling pattern becomes more infrequent, when stools become hard or are difficult to expel, or when the child exhibits withholding patterns or behavioral changes toward moving his or her bowels. Soiling, or encopresis, can be a sign of constipation.

25. How should children with constipation be evaluated?

Any child suspected of having constipation should undergo a full history and physical examination. Common clinical features include a history of difficulty passing stools, withholding behavior, intermittent passage of extremely large stools, soiling, abdominal pain, rectal pain, or the development of anal fissures. An examination of the abdomen may reveal hard mobile masses which represent palpable stool. A rectal examination is extremely important. The presence of large amounts of stool in the rectal vault almost always indicates functional constipation. If no stool is present, Hirschsprung disease and abnormal anorectal anatomy should be considered. Failure to perform a rectal exam is a common omission in the evaluation of children, and impaction in chronic constipation often goes undetected. Abdominal radiographs can be used to show the degree of fecal retention and can be used to monitor treatment in children who have severe functional constipation.

Gold DM, et al: Frequency of digital rectal examination in children with chronic constipation. Arch Pediatr Adolesc Med 153:377-379, 1999.

26. Which clinical features differentiate chronic retentive constipation from Hirschsprung disease?

FUNCTIONAL CONSTIPATION	HIRSCHSPRUNG DISEASE
Meconium passes within 24 hrs	Meconium passes after 24 hrs
Vomiting unusual	Vomiting common
Begins during toilet training	Begins shortly after birth
Soiling (encopresis) occurs	Soiling very rare
No enterocolitis	Enterocolitis
Palpable stool in rectal vault	No stool in rectal vault
Dilated anal canal	Narrow anal canal
Normal growth	Failure to thrive

27. How is Hirschsprung disease diagnosed?

Hirschsprung disease results from the failure of normal migration of ganglion cell precursors to their location in the GI tract during gestation. The loss of ganglion cells always begins distally in the rectum, involves a contiguous portion of the colon, and can extend to variable lengths in the large and small intestine. Involvement can vary from total aganglionosis to short-segment disease. In Hirschsprung disease, a prone abdominal x-ray typically reveals a lack of air in the rectal vault. The diagnosis can be made by obtaining an unprepped *barium enema*, which will demonstrate a change in the caliber of the large intestine at the site where normal bowel meets aganglionic bowel (transition zone). An unprepped barium enema is required, since the use of cleansing enemas can dilate the abnormal portion of the colon and remove some of the distal impaction, thereby resulting in a false-negative result. Following the study, retention of barium for 24 or more hours is suggestive of Hirschsprung disease or a significant motility disorder. *Rectal suction biopsies or full-thickness surgical biopsies* will confirm the absence of ganglion cells. Anal manometry is less reliable in children and in small infants requires specialized equipment.

28. How is encopresis defined?

Encopresis, or fecal soiling, may be defined as the involuntary passage of fecal material in an otherwise healthy and normal child. Children with encopresis typically sense no urge to defecate. Fecal soiling is almost always associated with severe functional constipation.

29. How should children with chronic constipation and encopresis be managed?

Therapy for constipation and encopresis requires a multimodal approach.

- The rectosigmoid colon should be aggressively cleansed of fecal material. Commonly, multiple enemas over 2 or 3 days are needed. Adult enemas should be used in children over the age of 2.
- An oral lubricant, such as mineral oil or Kondremul, is necessary to promote continued passage of stool. In difficult cases, stimulant medications, such as milk of magnesia or Haley's MO, can be substituted. While fecal soiling typically improves rapidly, a maintenance dose of mineral oil may be required for a prolonged period of time.
- It is extremely important to educate patients and parents about the mechanics of the disorder. A high-fiber diet, possible limitation of cow milk, defined periods of toilet-sitting, and a behavior modification system rewarding normal bowel movements are essential for eventual success.

Felt B, et al: Guideline for the management of pediatric idiopathic constipation and soiling. Arch Pediatr Adolesc Med 153:380-385, 1999.

Iacono G, et al: Intolerance of cow's milk and chronic constipation in children. N Engl J Med 339:1100-1104, 1998.

30. How does the use of mineral oil affect the absorption of fat-soluble vitamins?

Mineral oil is extensively used for treatment of functional constipation. While several case reports have shown that the long-term use of mineral oil can potentially alter the absorption of fat-soluble vitamins (A, D, E, K), vitamin deficiencies rarely occur. However, when mineral oil is prescribed, a multivitamin supplement (given at a different time than the mineral oil) is commonly added to the child's diet.

DIARRHEA

31. Which is a better predictor of bacteria as a cause of diarrhea: blood in the stool or neutrophils (PMNs) in the stool?

Stool PMNs are more reliable as indicators of a bacterial etiology than a positive stool guaiac test for blood. While about 30–50% of patients with blood in the stool will have a bacterial etiology, up to 70% will not. Thus, the presence of blood has a fair specificity but poor sensitivity. Stool PMNs, on the other hand, have a specificity and sensitivity of around 85% with a positive predictive value of around 60%.

DeWitt T, et al: Clinical predictors of acute bacterial diarrhea in young children. Pediatrics 76:551–556, 1985.

32. How is the stool examined for white blood cells?

Unlike dipstick testing for urine white blood cells, you must find stool PMNs the old-fashioned way. A thin smear of fresh stool is placed on a slide and air-dried. The sample is covered with methylene blue for about 5 seconds, gently rinsed with tapwater, and air-dried again. The quantity of PMNs seen per high-power microscopic field can be classified as occasional, scattered, or diffuse.

33. Which historical questions are key in seeking the cause of diarrhea?

- Recent medications, especially antibiotics
- History of immunosuppression (e.g., recurrent major infections, history of malnutrition, AIDS, recent measles)
- Illnesses in other family members or close contacts
- Travel outside the United States
- Travel to rural or seacoast areas (e.g., with consumption of untreated water, raw milk, raw shellfish)
- Attendance in day care
- Recent foods
- Presence of family pets

34. How do patterns of acute diarrhea vary by the pathogen involved?

SECRETORY/ENTEROTOXIGENIC	INFLAMMATORY
Characterized by watery diarrhea and absence of fecal leukocytes	Characterized by dysentery (i.e., symptoms and bloody stools), fecal leukocytes, and erythrocytes
Food poisoning (toxigenic)	*Shigella*
Staphylococcus aureus	Invasive *E. coli*
Bacillus cereus	*Salmonella*
Clostridium perfringens	*Campylobacter*
Enterotoxigenic *Escherichia coli*	*Clostridium difficile*
Vibrio cholerae	*Entamoeba histolytica*
Giardia lamblia	
Cryptosporidium	
Rotavirus	
Norwalk-like virus	

From Northrup RS, Flanigan TP: Gastroenteritis. Pediatr Rev 15:463, 1994; with permission.

35. How quickly can the mucosa of the gut repair itself after a bout of viral gastroenteritis?

Acute viral gastroenteritis is usually a self-limited disease. Histologic recovery of the intestinal epithelium can be expected 7–10 days after virus excretion has ceased. Functional recovery of the bowel occurs shortly thereafter. Occasionally, in infants < 12 months of age, a severe postviral enteritis may occur for up to 6–12 weeks. Normally, the differentiated enteric epithelium replenishes itself every 3–5 days.

36. What is the best way to feed an outpatient infant who has an acute bout of diarrhea complicated by mild dehydration?

The AAP's Committee on Nutrition in 1985 recommended rapid rehydration over 4–6 hours with an oral glucose-electrolyte rehydration solution, followed by diluted formula or milk. Use of a lactose-free formula was not routinely recommended. For older infants or children, dietary supplementation with nonlactose, complex carbohydrate–rich foods, such as rice, cereal, bananas, or potatoes, was suggested within 24 hours after successful rehydration. This contrasted with the traditional approach of rehydration with clear fluids for 24–48 hours followed by a slowly advancing concentration of diluted milk or formula and the BRAT diet (bananas, rice, apples, toast and tea) or a regular diet for older children as the diarrhea resolved. Recent data indicate that earlier initiation of full-strength formula does not worsen and may decrease the duration of diarrhea, although data are conflicting regarding the use of full-strength lactose-free vs. lactose-containing formula. By one survey, two-thirds of practicing pediatricians recommend a lactose-free formula.

Provisional Committee on Quality Improvement: Practice parameter: The management of acute gastroenteritis in young children. Pediatrics 97:424–436, 1996.

37. How do the various oral electrolyte replacement solutions differ in composition from other liquids commonly used in rehydration?

Oral Replacement Solutions (ORS)

SOLUTION	CARBOHYDRATE* (g/L)	SODIUM (mEq/L)	POTASSIUM (mEq/L	BASE (mEq/L)	OSMOLALITY (mOsm/L)	CALORIES (cal/100 ml)
Diarrhea	—	50–100	25–35	25–40	250–300	—
WHO (recommended)	G: 20	60–90	20–30	25–35	< 300	8
WHO ORS	G: 20	90	20	30	300	8
Pedialyte	G: 25	45	20	30	260	10
Ricelyte	R: 30	50	25	34	210	12
Cereal-based ORS	St: 50	60–90	20	30	315	42
Gatorade	G: 50	20	3	3	330	10
Chicken broth	0	250	5	0	450	0
Cola	F/G: 50–150	2	0.1	13	550	12–16
Apple juice	F/G/S: 100–150	3	30	0	700	15–18
Tea	0	0–1	0–1	0	0–5	0

*G, glucose; F, fructose; R, rice syrup solids; S, sucrose; St, starch.

Each solution has some advantages and disadvantages. Many home remedies are either very deficient or very excessive in electrolytes or sugar. A main problem with recommended ORS solutions is their low caloric content, but development of cereal-based and polymer-based solutions, which increase calories without increasing osmolality, is in progress.

38. How can the WHO oral electrolyte (rehydration) solution be duplicated?

The WHO solution is 2% glucose, 20 mEq K^+/L, 90 mEq Na^+/L, 80 mEq Cl^-/L, and 30 mEq bicarbonate/L. This solution is approximated by adding $^3/_4$ tsp of salt, 1 tsp of baking soda, 1 cup of orange juice (for KCl), and 8 tsp of sugar to a liter of water. Of note, parental satisfaction in the U.S. with the WHO solution (reconstituted from packets) compares very favorably with more expensive, more readily-available commercial products.

Ladinsky M, et al: The World Health Organization oral rehydration solution in U.S. pediatric practice. Arch Pediatr Adolesc Med 154:700-705, 2000.

39. What is the role of probiotic organisms in the treament of antibiotic-associated diarrhea?

Probiotics (opposite of antibiotics) are living organisms which are felt to cause health benefits by replenishing some of the more than 500 species of intestinal bacteria that antibiotics can suppress and by inhibiting the growth of more pathogenic flora. In children receiving broad-spectrum antibiotics, about 20%-40% are likely to experience some degree of diarrhea. *Lactobacillus GG* has been shown to limit the degree of diarrhea.

Vanderhoof JA, et al: Lactobacillus GG in the prevention of antibiotic-associated diarrhea in children. J Pediatr 135:564-568, 1999.

Arvola T, et al: Prophylactic Lactobacillus GG reduces antibiotic-associated diarrhea in children with respiratory infections: A randomized study. Pediatrics 104:e64, 1999.

40. When is antidiarrheal pharmacologic treatment indicated in children?

Antidiarrheal agents include (1) anti-infective/antibiotic agents, (2) antimotility agents (e.g., opiates, diphenoxylate), (3) antisecretory agents (e.g., loperamide, somatostatin), and (4) binding agents (e.g., pectin, cholestyramine, charcoal, attapulgite). Antidiarrheal medications are seldom indicated in pediatrics. In most cases, treatment of diarrhea consists of fluid and electrolyte replacement by oral rehydration solutions. Antibiotics are useful in only a number of bacterial and parasitic diseases. Rarely, antidiarrheal agents are indicated in those children who have chronic diseases, such as cholestatic liver disease (cholestyramine), inflammatory bowel disease, short-gut syndrome, or other secretory diarrheas (loperamide). Opiates are almost never indicated.

Provisional Committee on Quality Improvement: Practice parameter: The management of acute gastroenteritis in young children. Pediatrics 97:424–436, 1996.

41. Is homeopathic treatment for diarrhea effective?

Homeopathic treatment utilizes naturally-occurring plant, animal and mineral substances to stimulate the immune system and other defense mechanisms of the body. The driving principle of homeopathy is that a substance which in large doses can cause symptoms in an healthy individual is useful in smaller amounts as a treatment when given to an ill person. Treatment is individualized and often involves very dilute medicines. Mechanisms of action remain unclear and positive results are often attributed to placebo effects. However, a number of studies have demonstrated positive benefits.

Jacobs J, et al: Homeopathic treatment of childhood diarrhea. Pediatrics 97:778-779, 1996.

42. Why is true diarrhea in the first few days of life especially concerning?

In addition to the greater potential for dehydration in a newborn, diarrhea in this age group more commonly is associated with major congenital intestinal defects involving electrolyte transport (e.g., congenital sodium- or chloride-losing diarrhea) or carbohydrate absorption (e.g., congenital lactase deficiency). While viral enteritis can occur in the nursery, any newborn with true diarrhea warrants thorough evaluation and possible referral to a tertiary center.

43. Why is *Salmonella* enteritis so concerning if present in a child less than 12 months of age?

In older children with *Salmonella* gastroenteritis, secondary bacteremia and dissemination of disease rarely occur. In infants, however, 5–40% may have positive blood cultures for *Salmonella*, and in 10% of these cases, *Salmonella* can cause meningitis, osteomyelitis, pericarditis, and pyelonephritis. Thus, in infants < 1 year old, outpatient management of diarrhea assumes even greater significance, particularly if *Salmonella* is suspected.

Management of Salmonella Enteritis in the First Year of Life

	MANAGEMENT
First Evaluation	
Colitis (dysentery, heme positive stool, fecal WBCs)	Stool culture Blood culture if < 3 mos of age or temperature > 39.5° C
Diarrhea (no colitis)	Consider viral or other causes first Stool culture if diarrhea prolonged (≥ 5 days) Stool and blood culture if < 3 mos and exposure to *Salmonella*

Management of Salmonella Enteritis in the First Year of Life (continued)

	MANAGEMENT
Follow-up	
Persistent diarrhea	Stool culture
Positive stool culture (blood culture +)	Admit, repeat cultures (including CSF)
	Systemic parenteral antibiotics (e.g., ceftriaxone, cefotaxime) regardless of appearance on repeat examination
Positive stool culture (blood culture –)	
Toxic, ill, or immunocompromised	As if blood culture-positive
Febrile, nontoxic	Admit, blood culture, systemic parenteral antibiotics if < 3 mos
Afebrile, improving	Home observation, periodic reexamination

Adapted from St. Geme JW III, et al: Consensus management of Salmonella infection in the first year of life. Pediatr Infect Dis J 7:615–618, 1988; with permission.

44. What are the etiologies of traveler's diarrhea?

The etiologies vary by location, but toxigenic *Escherichia coli* is clearly the most commonly identified cause.

MICROORGANISM	AVERAGE FREQUENCY (%)	RANGE (%)
Toxigenic *E. coli*	40–60	0–72
Invasive *E. coli*	< 5	0–5
Shigella	10	0–30
Salmonella	< 5	0–15
Campylobacter jejuni	< 5	0–15
Vibrio parahaemolyticus	< 5	0–30
Aeromonas	< 5	0–30
Giardia lamblia	< 5	0–6
Entamoeba histolytica	< 5	0–6
Rotavirus	5	0–36
No pathogen identified	40	20–85

From Gorbach SL, et al: Infectious diarrhea and bacterial food poisoning. In Sleisinger MH, Fordtran JS (eds): Gastrointestinal Disease, 5th ed. Philadelphia, W.B. Saunders, 1993, p 1153; with permission.

45. How can traveler's diarrhea be prevented?

Four strategies can be used to prevent traveler's diarrhea: (1) *anticipatory guidance* regarding food and beverage intake, (2) *bismuth subsalicylate,* (3) *anti-infective drugs*, and (4) *symptomatic control* and medications with direct action on the GI tract.

In high-risk areas in developing countries, avoid previously peeled raw fruits and vegetables and any foods or beverages prepared with tap water. Prophylactic bismuth subsalicylate (Pepto-Bismol) has been shown to minimize diarrheal illness in up to 75% of adults. While some authorities recommend its use in children, others argue against it because of the risk of salicylate intoxication. Prophylactic use of antimicrobial agents such as trimethoprim-sulfamethoxasole, neomycin, doxycycline, and ciprofloxacin can decrease the frequency of traveler's diarrhea in children and adults. However, routine use of antibiotics is not recommended because of potential risks of allergic drug reactions, antibiotic-associated colitis, and development of resistant organisms. If symptoms develop, empiric therapy is indicated, and the regimen of trimethoprim-sulfamethoxasole and Imodium (for children age > 2 years) is very effective. Immunization, while potentially an ideal solution, at present is not an alternative.

46. Which bacterial gastroenteritides may benefit from antimicrobial therapy?

ENTEROPATHOGEN	INDICATION OR EFFECT
Shigella	Shortens duration of diarrhea Eliminates organisms from feces
Campylobacter jejuni	Shortens duration Prevents relapse
Salonella	Indicated for Infants < 12 mos Bacteremia Metastatic foci (e.g., osteomyelitis) Enteric fever
Escherichia coli	
EPEC (enteropathogenic)	Use primarily in infants Intravenous use if invasive disease
ETEC (enterotoxigenic) EIEC (enteroinvasive)	Most illnesses brief and self-limited
Yersinia enterocolitica	None for gastroenteritis alone, but indicated if suspected septicemia or other localized infection
Clostridium difficile	10–20% relapse rate
Aeromonas hydrophila	Efficacy not clearly established

47. List the differential diagnosis of chronic diarrhea by age group.

NEWBORNS	INFANTS	TODDLERS	OLDER CHILDREN
Congenital short gut Congenital lactose intolerance Malrotation with intermittent volvulus Ischemia Defective Na^+/H^+ exchange Congenital chloride diarrhea Microvillus disease	Protein sensitization Infection Parenteral diarrhea (urinary or upper respiratory infection) Immunoglobulin deficiency Postgastroenteritis diarrhea Cystic fibrosis Celiac disease *Clostridium difficile*	Postgastroenteritis diarrhea Dietary (allergy, excess fruit juice ingestion) Toddler's diarrhea Hyperthyroidism Sucrase-isomaltase deficiency Constipation/impaction with overflow Teething (?)	Lactose intolerance Infection Inflammatory bowel disease Irrittable bowel Laxative abuse

From Gryboski J: The child with chronic diarrhea. Contemp Pediatr 10:73, 1993; with permission.

48. How does secretory diarrhea differ from osmotic diarrhea?

STOOLS	OSMOTIC DIARRHEA	SECRETORY DIARRHEA
Electrolytes	Na^+ < 70 mmol/L	Na^+ > 70 mmol/L
Osmotic gap*	> 100 mOsm	< 50 mOsm
pH	< 5	> 6
Reducing substance	Present	Absent
Volume	< 20 ml/kg/day	> 20 ml/kg/day
After fasting	< 10 ml/kg/day	> 20 ml/kg/day
Blood/pus/fat	Present or absent	Absent

*Osmotic gap = osmolality of the fecal fluid minus the sum of the concentrations of the fecal electrolytes. From Mehta DI, Lebenthal E: New developments in acute diarrhea. Curr Probl Pediatr 24:99, 1994; with permission.

49. How should children with secretory diarrhea be managed?

It is important to identify an etiology for secretory diarrhea. After the child is taken off feeds, a vigorous attempt must be initiated to maintain fluid and electrolyte balance. If this is successful, the child should be evaluated for proximal small bowel damage, enteric pathogens, and a baseline malabsorptive workup. If abnormalities of the mucosal integrity are suspected, a small bowel biopsy is performed, and if the findings are significantly abnormal, the patient may be given parenteral alimentation and gradual refeeding. Electron microscopy may reveal congenital abnormalities of the microvillus membrane and brush border.

If the evaluation is negative, hormonal causes of secretory diarrhea (such as a VIPoma, hypergastrinoma, or carcinoid syndrome) must be considered. The list of active GI hormones is rapidly expanding, and unusual tumors stimulating diarrhea have been identified. Bacterial overgrowth may cause a secretory process, although usually this diarrhea will abate somewhat with fasting. A number of congenital abnormalities have been identified and are classified under the diagnosis of intractable diarrhea of infancy. If no etiology is identified, severe protracted disease may occur, and central parenteral alimentation is initiated. Careful monitoring and maintenance of intravenous access are critical because of marked fluid shifts.

50. How common is asymptomatic *Clostridium difficile* carriage?

C. difficile is the agent most often implicated in antibiotic-associated colitis. Fever, abdominal pain, and bloody diarrhea begin as early as a few days after starting antibiotics (especially clindamycin, ampicillin, cephalosporins). The diagnosis in infancy is more difficult because the carriage rate for *C. difficile* is relatively high. Neonates have a colonization rate of about 20%, infants 30–40%, older children 10%, and adolescents 5%. Toxin assays are more indicative of *C. difficile*–associated disease than culture. However, the toxin may be present without any symptoms, especially in infants.

Kelley CP, et al: Clostridium difficile colitis. N Engl J Med 330:257–262, 1994.

51. Which antibiotics most commonly cause pseudomembranous colitis?

Pseudomembranous colitis is a severe condition seen in patients undergoing intensive antibiotic therapy. It is associated with profuse diarrhea, which may be watery or mucoid, and is usually green, foul-smelling, and often bloody, and is accompanied by abdominal cramps. Fever and leukocytosis are common, and stool smears frequently show leukocytes. Diagnosis is made by sigmoidoscopy, which reveals pseudomembranous plaques or nodules. The causative agent is toxin-producing *Clostridium difficile*. Pseudomembranous colitis has been reported most commonly with ampicillin, clindamycin, and cephalosporins, but most antibiotics may cause this condition.

52. What are the therapeutic alternatives for treatment of pseudomembranous colitis?

If the disease is not severe, children may be treated with withdrawal of antibiotics and good supportive care. More severely ill children should be treated with oral vancomycin or metronidazole. Some clinicians have advocated cholestyramine to bind *C. difficile* toxin.

53. How helpful is eosinophilia as a diagnostic sign of parasitic disease?

Normally, the total eosinophil count does not exceed $500/mm^3$. As a screening tool for suspected parasitic disease (e.g., in symptomatic patients returning from foreign travel), it has a very poor positive-predictive value (15–55%). Its negative-predictive value is better (73–96%), particularly if sequential eosinophil counts remain normal.

Mawhorter SD: Eosinophilia caused by parasites. Pediatr Ann 23:405–413, 1994.

54. Name the three most common presentations of giardiasis.

- Asymptomatic carrier state
- Chronic malabsorption with steatorrhea and failure to thrive

- Acute gastroenteritis with diarrhea, weight loss, abdominal cramps, abdominal distention, nausea, and vomiting

55. How reliable are the various diagnostic methods for detecting giardia?

- Single stool exam for trophozoites or cysts—50–75%
- Three stool exams (ideally 48 hours apart) for same—95%
- Single stool exam and stool ELISA test for giardia antigen—> 95%
- Duodenal aspirate or string test—> 95%
- Duodenal biopsy (gold standard)—closest to 100%

56. Which patients are particularly susceptible to giardiasis?

Those with ***cystic fibrosis, chronic pancreatitis, achlorhydria, agammaglobulinemia***, and ***hypogammaglobulinemia***.

57. What are the clinical features of cryptosporidial enteritis?

Most reported cases occur in immunocompromised patients, although limited outbreaks have occurred in normal hosts. Children infected with HIV are particularly susceptible. Acute infection typically has an incubation period of 1–7 days. The clinical features include fever, abdominal pain, nausea, vomiting, high-output diarrhea, and failure to thrive. The illness may resolve within a few days, or it may be prolonged for several weeks. Asymptomatic carriage has been reported.

58. What is the triad of findings in acrodermatitis enteropathica?

Diarrhea, hair loss, and ***dermatitis*** are the presenting signs of this rare autosomal recessive disorder. The name nicely describes the disorder. There is a classic *acral* distribution of the rash. It is usually eczematous, often with a vesiculobullous or pustular component, and involves skin around body orifices as well. As for *enteropathica*, serum zinc levels are extremely low, secondary to impaired GI absorption. Dietary insufficiency of zinc may give an identical clinical picture. This has been found in children on long-term total parenteral nutrition without sufficient zinc and in very premature infants due to decreased stores and increased requirement.

59. What features characterize "toddler's diarrhea"?

Toddler's diarrhea, also known as chronic nonspecific diarrhea and even irritable bowel syndrome, is a clinical entity of unclear etiology that occurs in infants between 6 and 40 months, often following a distinct identifiable enteritis and treatment with an antibiotic. Loose, nonbloody stools (at least two per day but usually more) occur without associated symptoms of fever, pain, or growth failure. Malabsorption is not a key feature.

Multiple causes may be present: overconsumption of fruit juices, relative intestinal hypermotility, increased secretion of bile acids and sodium, intestinal prostaglandin abnormalities. The diagnosis is one of exclusion, and toddlers should be evaluated for disaccharide intolerance, protein hypersensitivity, parasitic infestation, and inflammatory bowel disease. Treatment consists of reassurance, careful growth assessment, and psyllium bulking agents (as initial therapy). Other agents used with success have been cholestyramine and metronidazole.

60. In what settings can diarrhea be a severe life-threatening illness?

Severe diarrhea of any cause can lead to dehydration, which can cause significant morbidity and mortality. However, diarrhea can be a sign of a serious associated illness which in itself can be life-threatening:

- Intussusception
- Hemolytic-uremic syndrome
- Pseudomembranous colitis
- Salmonella gastroenteritis (neonatal or compromised host)
- Hirschsprung disease (with toxic megacolon)
- Inflammatory bowel disease (with toxic megacolon)

Fleisher GR: Diarrhea. In Fleisher GR, Ludwig S (eds): Textbook of Pediatric Emergency Medicine, 4th ed. Baltimore, Lippincott Williams & Wilkins, 2000, p 204.

61. How is the degree of dehydration estimated in a child?

Clinical Findings to Estimate the Degree of Dehydration

SIGNS AND SYMPTOMS	MILD	MODERATE	SEVERE
Body fluid lost (ml/kg)	< 50	50–100	> 100
Weight loss	< 5%	5–10%	> 10%
State of shock	Impending	Compensated	Uncompensated
General appearance	Thirsty, alert restless	Thirsty, restless or lethargic, irritable to touch, younger children more likely drowsy	Drowsy; limp, cold, sweaty; older may be apprehensive; infants may be comatose
Vital Signs			
Systolic BP	Normal	Normal (orthostatic)	Very low or absent
Heart rate	Normal	Slight elevation (orthostatic)	Very elevated
Respiration	Normal	Deep, may be rapid	Deep and rapid (hyperpnea)
Other Exam			
Radial pulse	Normal rate and strength	Rapid and weak	Feeble, rapid, may be impalpable
Capillary refill	< 2 sec	2–3 sec	> 3 sec
Skin elasticity	Retracts immediately	Retracts slowly	Retracts very slowly (> 3 sec)
Anterior fontanel	Flat	Depressed	Sunken
Mucous membranes	Normal/dry	Very dry	Very dry/cracked
Tears	Present	Absent	Absent
Skin color	Pale	Gray	Mottled
Lab Tests			
Urine			
Volume	Decreased (< 2–3 ml/kg/hr)	Oliguric (1 ml/kg/hr) (< 1 ml/kg/hr)	Anuric
Osmolarity (mOsm/L)	600	800	Maximal
Specific gravity	1.010	1.25	Maximal
Blood			
pH	7.40–7.22	7.30–6.92	7.10–6.80
BUN	Upper normal	Elevated	High
HCO_3	Lower normal	Decreased (16–19 mEq/L)	Very decreased (< 16 mEq/L)

Adapted from Shaw KN: Dehydration. In Fleisher GR, Ludwig S (eds): Textbook of Pediatric Emergency Medicine, ed. Baltimore, Lippincott Williams & Wilkins, 2000, p 198.

62. How accurate is blood urea nitrogen (BUN) as a means of assessing dehydration in children?

Notoriously unreliable. The BUN does not begin to rise until the glomerular filtration rate falls to approximately one-half of normal. It then rises about 1% each hour. It may rise even less in a fasting child with disease. In a prospective study, Bonadio et al. found that 80% of patients judged to be 5–10% dehydrated by common physical findings may have a normal BUN.

Bonadio WA, et al: Efficacy of measuring BUN in assessing children with dehydration due to gastroenteritis. Ann Emerg Med 18:755–757, 1989.

FOOD ALLERGIES

63. What are the most common food allergies in children?

Egg, cow milk, and ***peanut*** account for 75% of abnormal food challenges. Soy, wheat, fish, and chicken are also common allergens.

64. Are food allergies in infants more or less common than generally perceived?

As the saying goes, "It depends on where your bread is buttered." Nearly a third of parents report that their infant has an adverse food reaction, most equating this with allergy. In pediatric circles, the general perception is that true food allergies are relatively rare. The answer, as custom, lies somewhere between. A prospective study in Colorado of 489 infants followed from birth to age 3 showed 8% had allergies confirmed by food challenge. In Denmark, a prospective study of nearly 1800 infants showed a prevalence of cow's milk allergy of 2.2%. Of note, the natural history of food allergies in infants is disappearance in nearly 90% of cases by age 3.

Bock SA: Prospective appraisal of complaints of adverse reactions to foods in children during the first three years of life. Pediatrics 79:683–688, 1987.

Host A, Halken S: A prospective study of cow's milk allergy in Danish infants during the first three years of life. Allergy 45:587–596, 1990.

65. How are adverse food reactions characterized?

***Food allergy*:** Ingestion of food results in hypersensitivity reactions mediated most commonly by IgE.

***Food intolerance*:** Ingestion of food results in symptoms not immunologically mediated, and causes may include toxic contaminants (e.g., histamine in scromboid fish poisoning), pharmacologic properties of food (e.g., tyramine in aged cheeses), digestive and absorptive limitations of host (e.g., lactase deficiency), or idiosyncratic reactions.

66. What are the manifestations of milk protein allergy in childhood?

Milk protein allergy and milk intolerance have been blamed for nearly every symptom in infancy. It is important to distinguish between a milk protein allergy, a lactose intolerance, and the common side effects of significant milk ingestion.

Acute manifestations	**Subacute symptoms**
Angioedema	Chronic vomiting
Urticaria	Intestinal obstruction
Acute vomiting and diarrhea	Persistent diarrhea
Anaphylactic shock	Malabsorption
GI bleeding	Protein-losing enteropathy
	Hypoproteinemia with or without edema
	Upper GI bleeding
	Lower GI bleeding
	Hemoptysis
	Abdominal distention
	Failure to thrive
	Colic

Diarrhea of variable severity is the most common manifestation of a milk protein allergy. Histologic abnormalities of the small intestinal mucosa have been documented, with the most severe form seen as a flat villous lesion. Protein-losing enteropathy may result from disruption of the surface epithelium. The stools of children with primary milk protein intolerance often contain blood. At sigmoidoscopy there is an erythematous and friable mucosa, and biopsies demonstrate a cellular infiltration, often with eosinophils, and changes in the surface and glandular epithelium. *Heiner syndrome* is hematemesis and hemoptysis with failure to thrive associated with milk allergy.

67. Can laboratory tests confirm a diagnosis of milk allergy?

The laboratory tests available are *not* sensitive or specific enough to confirm the diagnosis fully. Tests of humoral or cellular immune function, RAST tests, intradermal skin testing, and IgE levels have not been diagnostic. Specific assays for serum immunoglobulins directed against individual proteins in milk formulas may be useful. The peroral small bowel biopsy may show signs of superficial damage, but postenteritis syndrome, celiac disease, and other diseases also present with this finding. The accurate diagnosis of milk protein allergy still relies on the clinical challenge test.

68. Why is the DBPCFC a must in diagnosing food allergy?

The *double-blind placebo-controlled food challenge* (DBPCFC), while in need of a catchier acronym, is the gold standard for evaluating food allergies. The initial choice of food to be tested is usually based on history, skin tests, or RAST testing. In a fasted patient without recent antihistamine use, small quantities of the chosen food (or placebo) are given in lypholized form (food rapidly frozen and dehydrated under high vacuum), capsules or liquid. The quantities are doubled every 30–60 minutes as the patient is observed for up to 8 hours, depending on the anticipated reaction. Observers must be capable of responding to possible anaphylaxis, which usually occurs in the first 2 hours. If no reaction has occurred, the observer should knowingly give the food being tested to ensure that a false-negative test has not occurred.

69. Why can children who are allergic to nuts usually eat peanuts without any problem?

Tree nuts (e.g., almonds, Brazil nuts, cashews, pecans, pistachios, and walnuts) are a relatively common cause of food allergy in adults and less commonly in children. *Peanuts* are a legume (like soy) and have no cross-reactivity with members of the nut family.

70. Does delaying the introduction of solid foods until 4–6 months reduce the risk of food allergies?

This remains unclear and relatively unstudied, but usually recommended. The theoretical reason for the delay is to allow intestinal mucosal maturation with less "leakiness" so that fewer antigens can penetrate and initiate an immunologic response. One setting in which delay appears to have proven benefit is in children with a strong family history of atopic dermatitis. Limiting solid foods in the first 4–6 months and also minimizing exposure to major allergenic foods (e.g., cow's milk, egg, peanut) diminish the prevalence and extent of atopic dermatitis.

Kajosaari M, Saarinen UM: Prophylaxis of atopic disease by six month's total solid food elimination. Arch Paediatr Scand 72:411–414, 1983.

GASTROESOPHAGEAL REFLUX

71. How rapidly do infants outgrow gastroesophageal reflux (GER)?

40% of healthy infants regurgitate more than once a day, and mild reflux does not represent disease. As a rule, in those infants who have more significant primary GER, 50% resolve by 6 months, 75% by 12 months, and 95% by 18 months. Of note, reflux in older children may be more widespread than appreciated. In a survey of parents of children and adolescents (3-17 years), frequent symptoms of heartburn regurgitation were relatively common (2-8% of patients).

Nelson SP, et al: Prevalence of symptoms of gastroesophageal reflux during childhood. Arch Pediatr Adolesc Med 154:150-154, 2000.

Orenstein SR: Gastroesophageal reflux. Pediatr Rev 20: 24-28, 1999.

72. What factors can contribute to the process of gastroesophageal reflux?

GER is defined as the egress of gastric contents proximal to the stomach. There are a variety of factors that contribute to GER in children. Anatomic abnormalities such as a hiatal hernia or defective diaphragmatic or crural musculature can cause GER. Anatomic abnormalities distal to the stomach, such as malrotation or duodenal webs, may cause intermittent partial obstruction or mechanical delayed gastric emptying. Functional abnormalities such as a decreased resting lower esophageal sphincter (LES) pressure, an increase in transient LES relaxations, delayed gastric emptying, increased intra-abdominal pressure, esophageal dysmotility, or abnormal esophageal acid clearance have also been implicated. The process can be exacerbated by medications that alter gastric acid production or diminish LES competence or by constant horizontal positioning, as occurs in some children with psychomotor disorders.

Holloway RH, Dent J: Pathophysiology of gastroesophageal reflux. Gastroenterol Clin North Am 19:517–535, 1990.

73. Which test is most reliable for the diagnosis of GER?

The diagnosis can be made either clinically or by diagnostic testing. Clinically, reflux should be suspected in any child who demonstrates frequent, effortless vomiting or regurgitation without evidence of GI obstruction. With regard to diagnostic testing, the upper GI barium study is not sensitive for identifying reflux, as it is seen in only 50% of affected patients. The "milk scan" is a more physiologic test, but it detects only postprandial reflux. Unfortunately, significant damage occurs during nocturnal reflux, which cannot be modeled by a "milk scan." Endoscopically, the presence of histologic esophagitis is suggestive but not diagnostic of reflux. Scintigraphy, a noninvasive test utilizing radiolabeled meal, is very specific but only moderately sensitive in predicting reflux. The ***24-hour pH probe*** continues to be the most reliable test for the diagnosis of GER.

74. How are the complications of GER treated?

Simple GER
- Counseling
- Thickened feeding
- Positional therapy

Esophagitis
- Antacids
- Cimetidine, ranitidine, or famotidine
- Sucralfate
- Prokinetic agents (bethanecol, metoclopramide)

Failure to thrive
- Nutritional rehabilitation
- Nasogastric feeding

Apnea
- Monitoring
- Fundoplication, if severe

Recurrent aspiration
- Fundoplication
- Jejunal feeding

Failure of medical and nutritional therapy
- Fundoplication

75. What are the endoscopic and pathologic findings in GER?

Simple reflux has no pathologic correlate. If reflux is complicated by esophagitis, there may be erythema, edema, friability, or frank ulceration of the distal esophagus. Histologically, the diseased portion of the esophagus may demonstrate neutrophilic or eosinophilic infiltration into the epithelium and occasionally ulceration.

76. An infant with known GER who periodically arches his or her back likely has what syndrome?

Sandifer syndrome is paroxysmal dystonic posturing with opisthotonus and unusual twisting of the head and neck (resembling torticollis) in association with GER. Typically, an esophageal hiatal hernia is also present.

77. How effective are milk-thickening agents as a treatment for GER?

While not as effective as once thought, thickened feedings do alleviate GER in 40–50% of infants, especially when the child is placed in the prone position with the head elevated approximately 30°.

78. Should antacids used in the treatment of GER be given before, during, or after feedings?

Antacids should be given 60–90 minutes following a meal and/or before bedtime. Antacids are used to buffer gastric acid, and the buffering capacity lasts up to 1 hour. Meals also buffer gastric acid, and thus antacids have minimal effect when given with meals.

79. What are common side effects of antacids?

Diarrhea, eructation, flatulence, nausea, vomiting, rash, and constipation. Rarely, antacids can cause hypophosphatemia, hypocalcemia, hypermagnesemia, gastric bezoars, abnormal gastric emptying, and fecaliths.

80. Does the use of theophylline worsen GER?

The effect of theophylline on the development of GER is controversial. While theophylline has been reported to inhibit lower esophageal sphincter tone, several studies have shown that the use of theophylline and/or bronchodilators causes no significant increase in the frequency or severity of GER.

81. What is the Nissen fundoplication?

The *Nissen fundoplication* is the most commonly performed anti-reflux surgical procedure. It involves wrapping a portion of the gastric fundus 360° around the distal esophagus in an effort to tighten the gastroesophageal junction.

82. Which infants are candidates for fundoplication?

The vast majority of infants with developmental reflux do not require fundoplication. It is indicated in patients with recurrent aspiration, refractory or Barrett esophagitis, reflux-associated apnea, and reflux-associated failure to thrive which is refractory to medical therapy. Patients with severe reflux and psychomotor retardation should be evaluated for a fundoplication if a feeding gastrostomy is contemplated.

83. What are the infectious causes of esophagitis?

Fungal
- *Candida albicans*
- *Aspergillus*
- *Torulopsis glabrata*

Viral
- Cytomegalovirus
- Varicella-zoster
- Herpes

Bacterial
- *Helicobacter pylori*

Protozoan
- *Trypanosoma cruzi*
- *Cryptosporidium*

GASTROINTESTINAL BLEEDING

84. What features on physical exam can help identify an unknown cause of GI bleeding?

Skin:
- Signs of chronic liver disease (e.g., spider angiomas, venous distension, caput medusae, jaundice)
- Signs of coagulopathy (e.g., petechiae, purpura)
- Signs of vascular dysplasias (e.g., telangiectasia, hemangiomas)
- Signs of vasculitis (e.g., palpable purpura on legs and buttocks suggests Henoch-Schönlein purpura)

Head and neck:	Signs of epistaxis (especially before placing nasogastric [NG] tube, which can induce bleeding)
	Hyperpigmented spots on lips and gums (suggests Peutz-Jeghers syndrome, which is associated with multiple intestinal polyps)
	Webbed neck (suggests Turner syndrome, which is associated with GI vascular malformations and inflammatory bowel disease)
Cardiac:	Murmur of aortic stenosis (in adults, associated with vascular Malformations of the ascending colon, although this association not certain in children)
Abdomen:	Splenomegaly or hepatomegaly (suggests portal hypertension and possible esophageal varices)
	Ascites (suggests chronic liver disease and possible varices)
Rectal:	Perianal ulcerations and skin tags (suggest inflammatory bowel disease)
	Presence of polyps, melena or hematochezia

Mezoff AG, Preud'homme DL: How serious is that GI bleed? Contemp Pediatr 11:60–92, 1994.

85. In acute GI bleeding, how may vital signs indicate the extent of volume depletion?

It is important to remember that in acute bleeding in children, it may take from 12–72 hours for full equilibration of a patient's hemoglobin to occur. Vital signs are much more useful in patient management in the acute setting.

VITAL SIGNS	BLOOD VOLUME LOSS
Tachycardia without orthostasis	5–10% loss
Orthostatic changes:	> 10% loss
Pulse increases by 20 bm	
BP decreases by 10 mmHg	
Hypotension and resting tachycardia	30% loss
Nonpalpable pulses	> 40% loss

From Mezoff AG, Preud'homme DL: How serious is that GI bleed? Contemp Pediatr 11:62, 1994; with permission.

86. What is the simplest way of differentiating upper GI from lower GI bleeding?

Nasogastric lavage. After insertion of a soft NG tube (12 Fr in small children, 14–16 Fr in older children), 3–5 ml/kg of room-temperature normal saline is instilled, and if bright red blood or coffee-ground material is aspirated, the test is positive. A pink-tinged effluent is not a positive test because it can simply denote dissolution of a clot and not active intestinal bleeding. By definition, upper GI bleeding occurs proximal to the ligament of Treitz. If the lavage is negative, it is unlikely that the bleeding is above this ligament and rules out gastric, esophageal, or nasal sources. However, bleeding from duodenal ulcers and duodenal duplications may sometimes be missed by these aspirates.

87. How does the type of bloody stool help pinpoint the location of a GI bleed?

- ***Hematochezia*** (bright red blood):
  Normal stool spotting on toilet tissue likely suggests distal bleeding, such as anal fissure, juvenile colonic polyp.
  Mucous or diarrheal stools (especially if painful) indicates left-sided or diffuse colitis.
- ***Melena*** (black, tarry stools) indicates blood denatured by acid and usually implies a lesion likely before the ligament of Treitz. However, melena can be seen in Meckel diverticulum (due to denaturation by anomalous gastric mucosa).
- ***Currant jelly*** (dark maroon) stools usually come from the distal ileum or colon and often are associated with ischemia, as with intussusception.

Since blood is a cathartic, intestinal transit time can be greatly accelerated and makes defining the site of bleeding by the magnitude and color of the blood difficult. This difficulty underscores the importance of the initial NG tube insertion.

88. What can cause false-negatives and false-positives in stool testing for blood?

Hemoglobin and its various derivatives (e.g., oxyhemoglobin, reduced hemoglobin, methemoglobin, carboxyhemoglobin) can serve as catalysts for the oxidation of guaiac (HemOccult) or benzidine (Hematest) when a hydrogen peroxide developer is added, producing a color change.

False negatives: Ingestion of large doses of ascorbic acid
Delayed transit time or bacterial overgrowth allowing bacteria to degrade the hemoglobin to porphyrin

False positives: Recent ingestion of red meat or peroxidase-containing fruits and vegetables (e.g., broccoli, radishes, cauliflower, cantaloupes, turnips)

89. How do the causes of *lower* GI bleeding vary by age group?

NEWBORNS	INFANTS	CHILDREN
Anal fissure	Anal fissure	Anal fissure
Allergic proctocolitis	Infectious diarrhea	Polyp
Infectious diarrhea	Allergic proctocolitis	Infectious diarrhea
Hirschsprung disease	Meckel's diverticulum	Lymphonodular hyperplasia
Necrotizing enterocolitis	Intussusception	Inflammatory bowel disease
Volvulus	GI duplication	Henoch-Schönlein purpura
Stress ulcer	Peptic ulcer	Meckel's diverticulum
Vascular malformation	Foreign body	Peptic ulcer
GI duplication		Hemolytic uremic syndrome
		Vascular malformations

*In order of frequency.

From Mezoff AG, Preud'homme DL: How serious is that GI bleed? Contemp Pediatr 11:82, 1994; with permission.

90. A previously asymptomatic 18-month-old presents with large amounts of painless rectal bleeding (red but mixed with darker clots). What is the likely diagnosis?

Meckel diverticulum. This outpouching occurs from the failure of the intestinal end of the omphalomesenteric duct to obliterate. Up to 2% of the population may have a Meckel diverticulum, and about half contain gastric mucosa. Most are usually silent throughout life. Meckel is twice as common in males and usually presents in the first 2 years of life as massive painless bleeding, red or maroon in color. Tarry stools are observed in about 10% of cases. A history of previous minor episodes may be obtained. The presentation can range from shock to intussusception with obstruction, volvulus, or torsion. Meckel diverticulitis, which occurs in 10–20% of cases, may be indistinguishable from appendicitis.

91. What percentage of patients with Meckel diverticulum will have a falsely negative technetium-99m scintiscan?

Up to ***45%***. If clinical suspicion remains high, a nuclear medicine study with tagged RBCs or surgical or laparoscopic exploration is indicated.

Teitelbaum DH, et al: Laparoscopic diagnosis and excision of Meckel's diverticulum. J Pediatr Surg 29:495–497, 1994.

92. How can the reliability of the Meckel scintiscan be improved?

This radionuclide study employs ^{99m}Tc pertechnetate, which is taken up by the heterotopic gastric muscosa. Both pentagastrin (an HCl-stimulating hormone) or H_2 antagonists (e.g., cimetidine) may improve sensitivity. False-positives can occur in other anomalies containing ectopic gastric mucosa (e.g., duplication cysts) or inflammatory bowel disease. False-negative studies also occur, and angiography may be needed (especially with brisk bleeding). In rare instances, the diagnosis is made only at the time of laparotomy.

93. In a child with a juvenile polyp, how common are polyposis syndromes?

Juvenile polyps are the most common type of intestinal tumor in children, usually presenting with hematochezia. Up to 1/3 can have chronic blood loss with microcytic anemia. Juvenile polyposis is common (up to 12%) in patients with symptomatic polyps, especially with right-colonic polyps, anemia and adenomas. The importance of establishing a diagnosis of a polyposis syndrome is that some (Peutz-Jeghers and juvenile polyposis coli) are associated with a risk of developing adenocarcinoma as high as 30% in as early as 10 years.

Hoffenberg EJ, et al: Symptomatic colonic polyps in childhood: Not so benign. J Pediatr Gastroenterol Nutr 28:175-181, 1999.

94. Describe the management for massive upper GI bleeding.

Massive upper GI hemorrhage is a life-threatening emergency, and initial therapy precedes the specific diagnostic evaluation. Management includes:

- Brief history and character of bleeding, previous episodes, bleeding disorders
- Vital signs
- Intravascular access and serologic studies (CBC, LFTs, coagulation profile, crossmatch)
- Nasogastric tube insertion
- Full history and physical examination
- Transfusion and intravascular support
- Determination of probable etiology

1. *Peptic disease*
   Diagnostic endoscopy
   Therapeutic endoscopy
   H_2-blockers, antacids, sucralfate
   If no resolution,
   Surgical repair of ulcer
   Partial resection
2. *Variceal bleeding*
   Diagnostic endoscopy
   Therapeutic endoscopy
   Vasopressin, octreotide
   If no resolution,
   Sengstaken-Blakemore tube
   Emergency portosystemic shunt
   Esophageal devascularization
3. *Mallory-Weiss tear*
4. *Superficial vascular anomaly*
   Endoscopic ablation

95. How do the causes of *upper* GI bleeding vary by age group?

NEWBORNS	INFANTS	CHILDREN
Swallowed maternal blood	Epistaxis	Epistaxis
Hemorrhagic gastritis	Gastritis	Tonsillitis/sinusitis
Stress ulcer	Esophagitis	Gastritis
Idiopathic	Stress ulcer	Gastric/duodenal ulcer
Coagulopathy	Gastric/duodenal ulcer	Medications
Gastric outlet obstruction	Foreign bodies	Mallory-Weiss tears
Gastric volvulus	Gastric volvulus	Tumors
Pyloric stenosis	Esophageal varices	Hematologic disorders
Antral or pyloric webs		Esophageal varices
		Münchausen/Münchausen-by-proxy syndrome

*In order of frequency.

From Mezoff AG, Preud'homme DL: How serious is that GI bleed? Contemp Pediatr 11:82, 1994; with permission.

96. Why is the buffering of gastric acid important in controlling upper GI bleeding?

- Acid is ulcerogenic and can cause and propagate erosions.
- Coagulation is better in a neutral or alkaline environment than in an acidic one.
- Platelet plugs are disrupted by gastric pepsins, but these pepsins function less well in a neutral or alkaline environment.

Mezoff AG, Preud'Homme DL: How serious is that GI bleed? Contemp Pediatr 11:79, 1994.

97. Name the six most common causes of massive GI bleeding in children.

- Esophageal varices
- Hemorrhagic gastritis
- Peptic ulcer (mainly duodenal)
- Meckel diverticulum
- Crohn disease with ileal ulcer
- Arteriovenous malformation

Treem WR: Gastrointestinal bleeding in children. Gastrointest Endosc Clin North Am 5;78, 1994.

HEPATIC/BILIARY DISEASE

98. What are the most sensitive indicators of hepatic function?

The most sensitive indicator of hepatic disease is the ***fasting serum bile salt assay***. Bile salts are synthesized and excreted by the liver to promote fat absorption and conserved by ileal reabsorption into the enterohepatic circulation. While highly sensitive, this assay is of no use in hepatic failure. Since hepatic failure denotes the impairment of hepatic function, the most clinically useful assays monitor the processes of synthesis, detoxification, excretion, and metabolic regulation. Synthesis of serum proteins, such as albumin, and clotting factors are important indicators of hepatic function, but interpretation can be complicated by infection, disseminated intravascular coagulation, and third-space fluid shifts. Other measures of true hepatic function include transamination and urea synthesis and drug detoxification and elimination. Tests of aminopyrine, methacetin, caffeine, and galactose metabolism have all been recently used in an attempt to quantify hepatic function in a meaningful way.

99. How should a normal child with isolated hepatomegaly be evaluated?

All children with isolated hepatomegaly should have a careful history and physical examination. Family history of liver disease, previous exposure to hepatitis, foreign travel, blood transfusions, and drugs or toxins should be determined. One should verify that the liver is indeed large and not displaced by adjacent structures or hyperinflation. The consistency, character, and tenderness of the liver will provide information about possible etiologies. The spleen should be carefully palpated. Cutaneous signs of chronic liver disease and portal hypertension, lymphadenopathy, retinal pathology, cardiac lesions, and abdominal venous hums may indicate a particular etiology. Isolated hepatomegaly without splenomegaly or CNS involvement should be evaluated systematically to conserve resources.

100. What is the differential diagnosis for hepatomegaly?

Hepatocytic inflammation

Infectious (bacterial, viral, mycobacterial, fungal, abscess, parasitic)

Noninfectious (toxic, drug-induced, autoimmune, postobstructive)

Kupffer cell (septicemia/systemic infection, malignancy, granulomatous hepatitis, vitamin A toxicity)

Congestion (congestive heart failure, Budd-Chiari, sickle cell, vascular tumors)

Infiltration

Nonneoplastic (extramedullary hematopoiesis, cysts, benign tumors)

Neoplastic (Langerhans cell histiocytosis, leukemia, lymphoma, metastatic tumors, hepatoblastoma, hepatocellular carcinoma)

Storage (glycogen storage disease, mucopolysaccharidoses, lipidoses, gangliosidoses)

Metabolic (α_1-antitrypsin disease, galactosemia, hereditary fructose intolerance, hereditary tyrosinemia, Wilson disease, hemochromatosis, Reye syndrome, fatty-acyl-CoA dehydrogenase deficiency)
Steatosis (malnutrition, hyperalimentation, acute refeeding, steroids)
Portal tract (congenital hepatic fibrosis, idiopathic cirrhosis)
Bile duct abnormalities (arteriohepatic dysplasia, obstruction, biliary atresia, sclerosing cholangitis)
Miscellaneous (juvenile rheumatoid arthritis, systemic lupus erythematosus, cerebrohepatorenal syndrome, cystic fibrosis, endocrine [hypopituitarism, hypothyroidism, hypocorticolism])

101. A 3-year-old who experiences mild fluctuating jaundice in times of illness "just like his Uncle Kevin" is likely to have what condition?

***Gilbert syndrome*,** which is due primarily to a decrease in hepatic glucuronyl transferase activity. Normally, bilirubin is diconjugated to glucuronic acid. In Gilbert, the defective total conjugation results in increased production of monoglucuronides in bile and mild elevation in serum unconjugated (indirect) bilirubin. The syndrome is inherited in an autosomal dominant fashion with incomplete penetrance (boys outnumber girls by 4:1). Frequency of this gene in the population is estimated at 2–6%. Elevations of bilirubin are noted during times of medical and physical stress, particularly fasting.

102. What is the animal model for Gilbert syndrome?

***The Bolivian squirrel monkey*.**

103. Is there a treatment for Crigler-Najjar syndrome?

Crigler-Najjar syndrome is a genetic disorder characterized by either almost complete (type I) or partial (type II) deficiency of the enzyme bilirubin-UGT (bilirubin-uridinephosphoglucuronate glucuronosyltransferase), which is critical in bilirubin conjugation. The hallmark of the disease is high levels of unconjugated bilirubin, which commonly leads to kernicterus around the time of puberty. Currently available palliative treatments, including chronic phototherapy and intermittent plasmapheresis, have significantly improved survival rates. The current definitive treatment is liver transplantation, but advances are being made in hepatocyte transplantation and gene therapy.

Fox IJ, et al: Treatment of the Crigler-Najjar syndrome type 1 with hepatocyte transplantation. N Engl J Med 338:1422-1426, 1998.

104. List the most common causes of direct hyperbilirubinemia in an infant.

Biliary atresia, α_1-***antitrypsin deficiency, arteriohepatic dysplasia***, and cholestasis secondary to ***total parenteral nutrition*** or sepsis in the premature infant.

105. What types of liver injury are associated with various drugs?

TYPE OF LIVER INJURY	DRUG
Zonal liver necrosis	Acetaminophen Phenytoin Isoniazid Ketoconazole
Cholestasis	
Canalicular	Sex hormones Cyclosporine
Hepatocanalicular	Erythromycin Chlorpromazine

	Azathioprine Cimetidine
Microvesicular steatosis	Valproic acid Tetracycline
Granulomatous hepatitis	Sulfonamides Carbamazepine
Biliary cirrhosis	Methotrexate

From Mews C, Sinatra F: Chronic liver disease in children. Pediatr Rev 14:429, 1993; with permission.

106. What are the causes of chronic hepatitis in children?

Viral hepatitis	**Metabolic/genetic disorders**
Hepatitis B	Wilson disease
Hepatitis C	α_1-antitrypsin deficiency
Delta hepatitis	Cystic fibrosis
Cytomegalovirus	Steatohepatitis
Autoimmune hepatitis	**Toxic hepatitis**
Anti-smooth muscle antibody-positive	Drugs
Anti-liver-kidney microsomal antibody-positive	Hepatotoxins
	Radiation

From Mews C, Sinatra F: Chronic liver disease in children. Pediatr Rev 14:427, 1993; with permission.

107. In children with α_1-antitrypsin deficiency, which organ system is initially involved, lung or liver?

α_1-Antitrypsin is a major inhibitor of several proteolytic enzymes, primarily leukocyte elastase. It was first described in adults with chronic obstructive pulmonary disease. Since leukocyte elastase functions relatively unchecked, elastic fibers in the lung are digested with resultant destruction of alveolar walls and eventual panacinar emphysema. However, since the pulmonary effects take years to evolve, this condition rarely presents with pulmonary disease in children. More common presentations are neonatal cholestasis, hepatomegaly, chronic hepatitis, or, rarely, cirrhosis with liver failure. The pathophysiology of the liver disease is less clear. α_1-antitrypsin is synthesized in the liver, and in affected children, variants of the protein may be blocked from release from the hepatocyte. Some studies suggest that the buildup of these variants may be toxic and lead to chronic liver injury.

108. How is Pi typing useful in the evaluation of α_1-antitrypsin deficiency?

Pi typing (short for protease inhibitor typing) takes advantage of the fact that there are over 70 variants of the α_1-antitrypsin protein, each with a different electrophoretic mobility. Alleles are inherited in a codominant fashion, and thus a gene from each parent is expressed in one individual. MM is the normal phenotype and has the highest activity. ZZ has the lowest activity and most common association with liver disease. PiMM is the most common Pi type, with a distribution of about 87%, PiMS represents 8% and PiMZ 2%. The incidence of PiZZ ranges between 1:2000–5000.

109. An infant with cholestasis, triangular facies, and a pulmonic stenosis murmur is likely to have what syndrome?

One of the most common etiologies of neonatal cholestasis and hepatitis is arteriohepatic dysplasia, or ***Alagille syndrome***. Now called ***syndromic bile duct paucity***, it consists of a constellation of conjugated hyperbilirubinemia and cholestasis, typical triangular facies, cardiac lesions of pulmonic stenosis, peripheral pulmonic stenosis, or occasionally more significant lesions, butterfly vertebrae, and eye findings of posterior embryotoxon and Axenfeld anomaly, or iris processes. The patient may have extreme cholestasis, with pruritus and marked hypercholesterolemia. Although some patients have developmental delay, most develop appropriately. The usual mode of inheritance of Alagille syndrome is autosomal dominant.

110. Describe the clinical findings in portal hypertension.

Obstruction to portal flow is manifested by two physical signs: ***splenomegaly*** and ***increased collateral venous circulations***. Collaterals are evident on physical examination in the anus and abdominal wall and by special studies in the esophagus. Hemorrhoids may suggest collaterals, but in older patients these are present in high frequency without liver disease, and thus their presence has no predictive value. Dilation of the paraumbilical veins produces a rosette around the umbilicus (the caput medusae), and the dilated superficial veins of the abdominal wall are visible. A venous hum may be present in the subxiphoid region from varices in the falciform ligament.

111. How do the clinical presentations of acute and chronic liver failure vary?

Hepatic failure may be acute and fulminant, or it may follow a prolonged chronic course. In *fulminant hepatic failure*, there is a worsening of the hyperbilirubinemia and a decreased synthetic capacity which is evidenced by a worsening coagulation profile (vitamin-K resistant) and decreasing concentrations of fibrinogen, urea, and serum albumin. Encephalopathy, with concomitant increases in serum ammonia, may develop. As the liver mass shrinks, hepatic transaminases (a marker of liver damage) may paradoxically fall toward normal. These patients are at high risk for hypoglycemia.

Chronic hepatic failure, caused by a wide variety of infectious, toxic, and metabolic abnormalities, is characterized by jaundice and cutaneous manifestations (spider angiomas, caput medusae, palmar erythema). Fluid retention, development of ascites, renal hypoperfusion, and metabolic acidosis may occur. Mental status alterations and tremulous asterixis are chronic neurologic features. Ominous signs are GI bleeding, renal failure, cerebral edema, and coma.

112. A patient with liver failure develops confusion. Why worry?

Hepatic encephalopathy can present as either a rapid progression to coma or as mild fluctuations in mental status over extended times. A single underlying cause has not been established, but suspected toxins include ammonia, other neurotoxins, and a relatively increased GABA activity. Management is as follows:

- Treat any precipitating factors (e.g., infection, hemorrhage)
- Limit protein to 0.5–2.0 gm/kg/day
- Use modified amino acid preparations
- Administer lactulose, 1 ml/kg every 6 hrs, until diarrhea begins and then titrate to achieve mild diarrhea
- Antibiotics (Neomycin) to reduce the ammonia production
- Peritoneal dialysis may be indicated in severe coma and prior to liver transplantation
- Intracranial pressure monitoring in advanced cases

113. In children with liver failure, how should GI hemorrhage be managed?

- Pass an NG tube to monitor upper GI hemorrhage in patients with portal hypertension
- Daily vitamin K IV(0.2 mg/kg) for 3 days, and continue if response is seen
- Judicious administration of fresh frozen plasma for clinical bleeding
- Have blood cross-matched at all times; for children with variceal bleeding, have 40 ml/kg whole blood and 0.2 U/kg platelets available
- For gastritis or peptic ulceration, treat with ranitidine (2–6 ml/kg/day) and maintain gastric pH > 5

114. What is the most common indication for pediatric liver transplantation?

The most common indication is ***extrahepatic biliary atresia*** with chronic liver failure after a Kasai hepatoportoenterostomy. Other common indications include inborn errors of metabolism (e.g., α_1 antitrypsin deficiency, hereditary tyrosinemia, Wilson disease) and idiopathic fulminant hepatic failure.

115. Liver transplantation in children: what is the long-term outcome?

In the past two decades, since the introduction of cyclosporine, the long-term outcome for patients with liver transplantation has improved markedly. Initially, the one-year survival rate was less than 50% for children. Current one-year survival rates for infants are > 80% with very little mortality from the first to the fifth year after transplant. The greatest improvement in the mortality rate has occurred in the pretransplantation waiting period. Initially, > 50% of infants died while on the transplantation list because of inadequate organ supply. Although regional centers for allotment and fair priority scoring systems have helped in part, the most significant advancement has been the development of technology allowing reduced size "split-livers" from adults to be used in infants. The use of living-related donors in the future may also help the organ supply for livers.

116. Which patients are at risk for cholelithiasis?

	PIGMENT STONE	CHOLESTEROL STONE
Demography		
Race	—	Native American
Sex	—	Females
Age	—	Adolescence
Diet	—	Obesity
Total parenteral nutrition	+++	—
Hemolytic disease (esp. sickle cell disease, thalassemia, hereditary spherocytosis	+++	—
Cystic fibrosis	—	+++
Ileal disease	—	+++
Defects in bile salt synthesis	—	+++
Hypertriglyceridemia	—	+++
Diabetes mellitus	—	+++

Adapted from Shaffer EA: Gallbladder disease. In Walker WA, Watkins JB (eds): Pediatric Gastrointestinal Disease. Philadephia, B.C. Decker, 1991, p 1154; with permission.

117. Are there predisposing factors for cholecystitis in children and adolescents?

Most are conditions that predispose to the formation of gallstones. Acalculous cholecystitis occurs in only about 15% of cases. In addition to the risk factors for gallstones (see Question 107), other predisposing factors include pregnancy, obesity, and family history of biliary disease.

INFLAMMATORY BOWEL DISEASE

118. How do ulcerative colitis and Crohn disease vary in their intestinal distribution?

Ulcerative colitis is limited to the superficial mucosa of the colon. It always involves the rectum and extends proximally to a variable extent. Limited distal ulcerative colitis has been termed ulcerative proctitis and in children may have a better prognosis. Regional enteritis, or *Crohn disease*, is a transmural inflammation of the bowel that may affect the entire tract from the mouth to the anus. The syndrome of limited Crohn colitis may be difficult to differentiate from ulcerative colitis.

119. What features differentiate ulcerative colitis from Crohn disease?

	ULCERATIVE COLITIS	CROHN DISEASE
Incidence (10–19-year olds)	2/100,000	3.5/100,000
Onset during childhood	15–20%	20–25%
Clinical presentation	Diarrhea—50% Rectal bleeding—> 90% Weight loss—65% Growth failure—10% Pain with defecation	Diarrhea—80% Rectal bleeding—50% Weight loss—85% Growth faiure—35% Anorexia, postprandial pain; extraintestinal signs may predominate
Site of disease at presentation	Rectal involvement—100% Left-sided colitis—50–60% Severe pancolitis—10%	Ileum± colon—50–70% Colon alone—10–20% Proximal small bowel—10–15% Gastroduodenal—< 5%
Endoscopic findings	Continuous inflammation 100% rectal involvement Erythema, edema, friability, ulceration on abnormal mucosa	Focal or segmental inflammation Rectal sparing Aphthous or linear ulcerations on normal-appearing mucosa Cobblestoning Abnormal terminal ileum—> 50%
Histologic findings	Mucin depletion Villous mucosal surface pattern Crypt abscesses Epithelial atypia Continuous disease	Epithelioid granulomas Histiocytic infiltrates Pericrypitis Submucosal extension of inflammation Discontinuous disease

From Hofley PM, Piccoli DA: Inflammatory bowel disease in children. Med Clin North Am 78:1283, 1994; with permission.

120. As the severity of ulcerative colitis increases, how does the treatment vary?

Treatment varies according to the age of the patient and the duration and severity of disease. Mesalamine (5-aminosalicylic acid) is the usual first therapy in all cases of ulcerative colitis. Steroid or 5-aminosalicylic acid enemas may control distal-limited disease. In more severe cases, prednisone (or any of the steroid group) is used to induce remission. When outpatient therapy is unsuccessful, elemental diets or parenteral alimentation are instituted. Long courses of intake restriction and aggressive intravenous nutritional therapy are likely to be efficacious. Immunosuppressive therapy (6-mercaptopurine or azathioprine) has a role in the maintenance of remission. When medical therapy fails or when toxic megacolon is present, surgical therapy is necessary.

Hanauer SB: Drug therapy: Inflammatory bowel disease. N Engl J Med 334:841–848, 1996.

121. What are the potential toxicities of intravenous cyclosporine?

Renal dysfunction, hepatic dysfunction, neurologic complications (from paresthesias to seizures), and immunosuppression.

122. What laboratory testing should be done before initiating cyclosporine therapy?

Baseline ***electrolytes, BUN, creatinine,*** and ***liver function tests*** should be done. Preexisting abnormalities should cause the clinician to strongly consider whether cyclosporine should be used. Stool studies document the absence of infectious colitis, including **bacterial culture** and ***Clostridium difficile*** **toxin assays** for toxins A and B. In patients on longstanding steroid therapy, **CMV colitis** should be excluded. Low **serum magnesium** or **cho-**

lesterol levels predispose to seizures and should be considered a relative contraindication to intravenous cyclosporine therapy.

123. What is infliximab?

Infliximab (Remicade) is a chimeric, monoclonal IgG antibody against tumor necrosis factor-α (TNF-α). TNF-α is a proinflammatory cytokine present in high levels in the blood and tissues of patients with Crohn disease. Infliximab has been shown to be effective in inducing remission in a subset of patients with severe disease.

124. In a child diagnosed with inflammatory bowel disease (IBD), what are the potential long-term complications?

The complications and presentations of IBD have considerable overlap.

- *Severe perianal disease* can be a debilitating complication. More prevalent in Crohn disease, it may range from simple skin tags to total devastation of the perineum. Deep perianal abscesses can interfere with the ability to sit and walk, and open drainage is often necessary. More extensive surgical removal may result in damage to the sphincter and subsequent incontinence. Fistulization to the vagina, bladder, or skin may occur.
- In Crohn disease, *enteroenteral fistulae* may occur and "short-circuit" the absorptive process. The thickened bowel may obstruct or perforate, requiring operation. The recurrence rate is high after surgery, repeated operations are often necessary, and short bowel syndrome may result. In many cases a permanent ostomy is placed, although pouch construction and continent ileostomies have become more common.
- In ulcerative colitis, the patient may require *surgery* because of the severity or duration of disease. In the past, most patients had total colectomy and ileostomy, but the current recommended procedure is a subtotal colectomy and an endorectal pullthrough with rectal mucosal stripping. This procedure maintains intestinal continuity, and the patient develops normal rectal continence, although with increased stool frequency.
- *Toxic megacolon* may occur with either form of IBD but is much more common with ulcerative colitis. After a progressive course, fever and a decrease in diarrhea usually herald a distended, tender, and tympanitic abdomen. The profound dilation of the bowel may be segmental or total, and massive hemorrhage or perforation may ensue. Mortality is high if toxic megacolon is not identified and treated aggressively.
- *Growth retardation and delayed puberty* are seen in both diseases but are more common in Crohn disease. The insidious onset may result in several years of linear growth failure before the correct diagnosis is made. With epiphyseal closure, linear growth is terminated, and short adult stature will be permanent.
- *Hepatic complications* of IBD include chronic active hepatitis and sclerosing cholangitis, which may require liver transplantation.
- *Nephrolithiasis* may occur in patients with resections or steatorrhea due to increased intestinal absorption of oxalate.
- Chronic reactive and restrictive *pulmonary disease* has been noted.
- Arthralgias are common, but destructive *joint disease* is uncommon.

125. What relatively rare liver disease is more common in patients with inflammatory bowel disease?

Primary sclerosing cholangitis. Between 1% and 3% of patients with IBD (more common in ulcerative colitis than Crohn disease) may develop this condition, which is characterized by fibrosis and inflammation of extra- and intrahepatic bile ducts and elevation of liver enzymes including gamma-glutamyl transferase (GGT). The etiology is unknown, although immune mechanisms are likely. The diagnosis is based on the characteristic findings on liver biopsy and endoscopic retrograde cholangiopancreatography or magnetic resonance cholangiogram.

126. Are children with IBD at increased risk for malignancy?

The risk of malignancy has not been studied systematically in pediatric populations with IBD. The risk in adults depends both on the disease and its duration. After 10 years of ulcerative colitis, the risk rises dramatically (1–2% increased incidence of malignancy per year). The risk is felt to be higher in patients with pancolitis compared to those with limited left-sided disease. The carcinomas associated with ulcerative colitis are often poorly differentiated and metastasize early. They have a poorer prognosis and are more difficult to identify by radiographic and colonoscopic examinations. Most authors indicate that carcinoma of the bowel is much less common in Crohn disease, although this has been disputed. The risk of lymphoma is increased in patients with Crohn disease. Immunosuppressive therapy such as azathioprine may also increase the risk of neoplasia.

127. When is surgery indicated in IBD in children?

Crohn disease	**Ulcerative colitis**	
Perforation with abscess formation	*Urgent:*	Hemorrhage
Obstruction with or without stenosis		Perforation
Uncontrolled massive bleeding		Toxic megacolon
Draining fistulas and sinuses		Acute fulminant colitis unresponsive to maximal medical therapy
Toxic megacolon	*Elective:*	Chronic disease with recurrent severe exacerbations
Growth failure in patients with localized areas of resectable disease		Continuous incapacitating disease despite adequate medical treatment
		Growth retardation with pubertal delay
		Disease of > 10 years' duration with evidence of epithelial dysplasia

From Hofley PM, Piccoli DA: Inflammatory bowel disease in children. Med Clin North Am 78:1293–1295, 1994; with permission.

128. Which has a better prognosis, Crohn disease or ulcerative colitis?

The outcome for patients with ulcerative colitis is better unless toxic megacolon or carcinoma develops. In these patients, surgery is curative, and the chronic morbidity depends on the type of surgery employed. Patients with Crohn disease can be expected to lead a functional and productive life. However, as many as three-fourths require surgery within 5 years, and only half of those with growth failure achieve significant catch-up growth.

MALDIGESTION/MALABSORPTION

129. How does late-onset lactase deficiency vary by ethnicity?

Approximate Percentage of Low Lactase Activity by Ethnic Group

United States		Worldwide	
White	20%	Dutch	0%
Hispanic	50%	French	32%
Black	75%	Filipino	55%
Native American	90%	Vietnamese	100%

After high levels in infancy, lactase levels decline progressively; after age 5 years, most people have lactase levels of about 10% of infancy. Since it is statistically more common to have these lower levels, the term *deficiency* may be a misnomer. Lactose intolerance may develop if excessive lactose loads are ingested.

130. What conditions produce secondary lactose deficiency?

Any disorder that alters the mucosa of the proximal small intestine may result in secondary lactose intolerance. For this reason, the lactose tolerance test is commonly used as a screening test for intestinal integrity, although this has the disadvantage of concomitantly identifying all primary lactose malabsorbers. Although a combination of factors is present in many disease processes, secondary lactose intolerance can be organized into lesions of the microsurface, total surface, transit time, and site of bacterial colonization in the small bowel.

At microvillus/brush border
- Postenteritis
- Bacterial overgrowth
- Inflammatory lesions (Crohn disease)

At level of the villus
- Celiac disease
- Allergic enteropathy
- Eosinophilic gastroenteropathy

Bulk intestinal surface area
- Short bowel syndrome

Altered transit with early lactose entry into colon
- Hyperthyroidism
- Dumping syndromes
- Enteroenteral fistulas

131. Which disorders of carbohydrate absorption are inherited?

Monosaccharides
- Glucose-galactose malabsorption

Disaccharides
- Congenital alactasia (lactase deficiency)
- Congenital sucrase-isomaltase deficiency
- Trehalase deficiency

Polysaccharides
- Congenital amylase deficiency
- Pancreatic insufficiency syndromes
- Schwachman syndrome
- Cystic fibrosis

Glucose-galactose malabsorption is an autosomal recessive disorder of carrier-mediated transport; patients have a normal ability to absorb fructose. Sucrase-isomaltase deficiency is the most common of the congenital abnormalities of carbohydrate absorption; the combined defect always coexists, and incidence is as high as 10% in some populations. By contrast, congenital lactase deficiency is extremely rare. Trehalase is a brush border enzyme whose only function is to digest trehalose. The source of trehalose is mushrooms, and occasionally gas and diarrhea attributed to rich or spicy foods may be due to this deficiency. Obviously, this disease is of little clinical importance (except to mushroom farmers). Additionally, all humans lack enzymes to digest stachyose and raffinose, two sugars in high concentration in beans. This explains the "beans syndrome," which for most people is clinically similar to lactose intolerance.

132. What is gluten?

After starch has been extracted from wheat flour, *gluten* is the residue that is left. This residue is made up of multiple proteins that are distinguished by their solubility and extraction properties. For example, the alcohol-soluble fraction of wheat gluten is wheat gliadin. It is this protein component that is primarily responsible for the mucosal injury that occurs in the small bowel in patients with celiac sprue.

133. Why does the flat villous lesion in the small intestine develop in celiac disease?

The relationship of the small intestinal flat villous lesion to celiac disease is well established, but the pathogenesis is still unclear. One theory is that an intestinal enzyme that normally digests gluten is absent, resulting in a toxic reaction that produces changes in the intestinal epithelium. This enzyme has been actively sought but never conclusively proven. A number of immunologic abnormalities have been suggested in celiac patients. Children with celiac disease have circulating antigliadin antibodies, and there is an increase in IgA- and IgM-containing plasma cells in the lamina propria. The number of intraepithelial lymphocytes is also increased. Each of these phenomena may disappear on a prolonged gluten-free diet. Celiac disease is associated with HLA B8, DR3, and DR7. The lectin hypothesis is based on the theory that a cell surface membrane defect may allow gluten to act as a lectin, and the subsequent reaction cause cell toxicity. Other hypotheses have focused on an increased permeability of the mucosal barrier or precipitation by viral infections.

134. What clinical features suggest celiac disease?

Gluten-sensitive enteropathy (celiac disease) is a relatively common cause of severe diarrhea and malabsorption in infants and children. Children with celiac disease commonly present between ages 9 and 24 months with failure to thrive, diarrhea, abdominal distention, muscle wasting, and hypotonia. After several months of diarrhea, growth slows. Weight typically decreases before height. Often, these children become irritable and depressed and display poor intake and symptoms of carbohydrate malabsorption. Vomiting is less common. On examination, the growth defect and distention are commonly striking. There may be a generalized lack of subcutaneous fat, with wasting of the buttocks, shoulder girdle, and thighs. Edema, rickets, and clubbing may also be seen.

135. How is the diagnosis of celiac disease confirmed?

To diagnose celiac disease, ***multiple small bowel biopsies*** must be obtained. In a typical sequence, the first biopsy on gluten should show villous atrophy, with increased crypt mitoses and disorganization and flattening of the columnar epithelium. This should resolve fully on the second biopsy after a strict gluten-free diet. To confirm the diagnosis and eliminate the possibility of a coincidental recovery after an infectious enteritis, a third biopsy must be obtained after the patient has again been challenged with gluten. This biopsy again must show the manifestations of the disease. While biopsy remains the gold standard, two main ***antibody tests***—antiendomysial and antitissue transglutaminase (tTG)—may shorten the expense and invasiveness of this sequence. In many patients, the titer falls dramatically with treatment and increases again with challenge.

Russo PA, et al: Comparative analysis of serologic screening tests for the initial diagnosis of celiac disease. Pediatrics 104:75-78, 1999.

136. Why might a 2-year-old with typical clinical features of celiac disease, including classic small-bowel biopsy findings, have negative antibody studies?

Antibodies found in patients with celiac disease—anti-gliadin IgA (AGA), anti-endomysial (EMA), antireticulin (ARA) and antitissue transglutaminase (tTG)—are IgA antibodies. Selective IgA deficiency is the most common primary immunodeficiency in Western countries with a prevalence of 1.5–2.5 per thousand. Celiac disease is 10–20 times more common in individuals with selective IgA deficiency than in the general population. Therefore, in highly suspicious cases with negative antibody panels, a quantitative IgA level can be helpful to rule out IgA deficiency. Alternatively, one could measure antigliadin IgG antibodies, but these have the lowest specificity of the celiac antibodies.

Catassi C, Fabiani E: The spectrum of coeliac disease in children. Bailliere Clin Gastroenterol 11:485-507, 1997.

137. Is a lifelong gluten-free diet necessary in celiac disease?

With some anecdotal reports of patients doing well with normalized duodenal biopsies after the reinstitution of a gluten-containing diet, the question has been raised if celiac disease is truly a lifelong disorder. On the basis of long-term follow-up studies of patients after the discontinuation of the diet, the risks of complications even in the absence of symptoms require that the only recommended approach is "zero-gluten" for a lifetime.

Chartrand LJ, Seidman EG: Celiac is a lifelong disorder. Clin Invest Med 19:357-361, 1996.

138. In addition to celiac disease, what disorders are associated with a flat villous lesion?

Acute enteritis
- Bacterial disease
- Viral disease
- Protozoal (*Giardia*)
- Radiation enteritis

Allergic enteropathy
- Milk-soy protein allergy
- Celiac disease
- Eosinophilic gastroenteritis

Immunoregulatory abnormalities
- Immunodeficiency
- Graft vs. host disease

Chronic enteritis
- Tropical sprue, Whipple disease
- Intractable enterocolitis
- Lymphoma

Malnutrition
- Protein calorie
- Folate deficiency
- Iron deficiency

Congenital
- Congenital villous atrophy

139. How is fat malabsorption determined?

72-hour fecal fat collections, measuring both the dietary fat intake and fecal fat excretion, remain the gold standard. This quantative method can be difficult in younger infants. Other tests include Sudan staining of stool for fat globules (a qualitative test, if positive, indicating gross steatorrhea), the steatocrit, and monitoring absorbed lipids after a standardized meal. Future methods may include breath testing (similar to carbohydrate testing). In an animal model, radioactively-labeled mixed triglyceride (^{13}C-MTG) has been given by mouth and exhaled air measured. With normal lipolytic activity in the GI tract, $^{13}CO_2$ is split off and can be sampled in exhaled air.

Kalivianakis M, et al: Validation in an animal model of the carbon 13-labeled mixed triglyceride breath test for the detection of intestinal fat malabsorption. J Pediatr 135:444-450, 1999.

140. How is the steatocrit measured?

The *steatocrit* is a rapid measurement of the percentage of fat in a spot sample of stool. It is done by homogenizing stool with sand and water. From this slurry, a microhematocrit tube is filled and spun in a centrifuge. The lipid portion rises to the top and the percentage of fat layer calculated (much like a spun hematocrit). Newborns normally excrete up to 15% fat, and this percentage falls with age. A value above 5% is abnormal for any child over age 3. It can be a crude estimate of fat malabsortion, but experts differ on its value.

Addison GM: Acid steatocrit. J Pediatr Gastroenterol Nutr 22:227, 1996.

Columbo C, et al: The steatocrit: A simple method for monitoring fat malabsorption in patients with cystic fibrois. J Pediatr Gastroenterol Nutr 6:926-930, 1987.

NUTRITION

141. In the world of ideal pediatric nutrition, what are the various requirements for protein, fat, and carbohydrates?

Protein should account for 7–15% of caloric intake and should include a balance of the 11 essential amino acids. Protein requirements range from 0.7–2.5 gm/kg/day. Fats should provide 30–50% of caloric intake. While most of these calories are derived from long-chain triglycerides, sterols, medium-chain triglycerides, and fatty acids may be important in certain diets. Linoleic acid and arachidonic acid are essential for tissue membrane synthesis, and approximately 3% of intake must be composed of these triglycerides. The remaining 50–60% of calories should come from carbohydrates. About half of these are contributed by mono- and disaccharides, such as sucrose and lactose, and the remainder as starch.

142. Which fatty acid is the most essential?

Linoleic acid. It is converted to longer chain fatty acids with multiple double bonds, which are essential components of membranes. Arachidonic acid is also a component of membranes, but it can be synthesized from linoleic acid. A dietary intake of linoleic acid at a level of 1–2% of dietary calories will prevent both the biochemical and clinical manifestations of essential fatty acid deficiency. Oral fats high in linoleic acid include safflower oil (72%), sunflower oil (61%), and corn oil (54%).

143. If recommended caloric intakes are maintained, what is normal daily weight gain in young children?

AGE	WEIGHT GAIN (GRAMS)	RECOMMENDED CALORIC INTAKE (KCAL/KG/DAY)
0–3 mos	26–31	100–120
3–6 mos	17–18	105–115
6–9 mos	12–13	100–105
9–12 mos	9	100–105
1–3 yrs	7–9	100
4–6 yrs	6	90

It should be noted that when babies are primarily breastfed, growth during months 3–18 is less than that indicated in the table. On average, breastfed babies gain 0.65 kg less than formula-fed infants in the first year of life.

Dewey KG, et al: Growth of breast-fed and formula-fed infants from 0 to 18 months: The DARLING Study. Pediatrics 89:1035–1041, 1992.

National Research Council, Food and Nutrition Board: Recommended Daily Allowances. Washington, D.C., National Academy of Sciences, 1989.

144. What is the calorie-nitrogen ratio?

The relationship between energy and protein intake. Usually a ratio of 150:1 or more is required, but this ratio is modified in states of increased protein utilization or decreased protein metabolism.

145. What are the recommended bottle feedings by age?

AGE	NO. OF FEEDINGS	OZ PER FEEDING
Birth–1 wk	6–10	1–3
1 week–1 mo	7–8	2–4
1 mo–3 mos	5–7	4–6
3 mos–6 mos	4–5	6–7
6 mos–9 mos	3–4	7–8
10 mos–12 mos	3	7–8

146. Why is honey not recommended for infants in the first year of life?

Honey, as well as some commercial corn syrups, has been associated with infantile botulism. *Clostridium botulinum* spores contaminate the honey and are ingested. In infants, intestinal colonization and multiplication of the organism may result in toxin production and lead to symptoms of constipation, listlessness, and weakness.

147 How is nutritional status objectively assessed in children?

• The most easily obtainable information comes from a carefully plotted ***growth chart***. Anthropometric data give an estimate of the height, weight, and head circumference of a child, compared to a population standard. Growth curves also provide a plot of weight for height (or stature). At any single point in time, this is a more accurate representation of the current nutritional status of the child. A change in the child's percentile after the first 6–12 months may signify the presence of a nutritional problem or systemic disease.

• ***Compare actual with ideal body weight*** (average weight for height age). The ideal body weight is determined by plotting the child's height on the 50th percentile and recording the corresponding age. The 50th percentile weight for that age is obtained, and this ideal body weight is divided by the actual weight. The result is expressed as a percentage, the percent ideal body weight, which gives a better stratification of patients with significant malnutrition. A %IBW of > 120 is obese, 110–120 is overweight, 90–110 normal, 80–90 mild wasting, 70–80 moderate wasting, and < 70 severe wasting.

• ***Measurement of midarm circumference*** provides information about the subcutaneous fat stores, and the midarm-muscle circumference (calculated from the triceps skinfold thickness) estimates the somatic protein or muscle mass. Subscapular skinfold thickness measurements may be preferable in infants. These values can be used to calculate the percent body fat in children. Potential errors in calculation arise when there is overhydration or underhydration, extreme obesity, musculoskeletal disorders, and profound mental-motor retardation.

• ***Laboratory assessment*** of nutritional status can provide objective data about the patient. Vitamin and mineral status can be directly assayed. Measurements of albumin (half-life 14–20 days), transferrin (half-life 8–10 days), and prealbumin (half-life 2–3 days) can provide information about protein synthesis, but each may be affected by certain diseases. The ratio of albumin to globulin may decrease in protein malnutrition. The creatinine height index is a measure of lean body mass, which decreases as muscle protein is used as an energy source. Specific measurements of nitrogen balance may be obtained to determine the degree of protein anabolism or catabolism.

148. What are the medical consequences of obesity in children and adolescents?

- Increased height
- Early menarche
- Advanced bone age
- Increased blood pressure
- Increased incidence of sleep apnea
- Increased incidence of cholelithiasis
- Increased long-term cardiovascular risks

149. How can examination of the head alone suggest problems of malnutrition?

CLINICAL SIGN	NUTRIENT DEFICIENCY
Epithelial	
Skin	
Xerosis, dry scaling	Essential fatty acids
Hyperkeratosis, plaques around hair follicles	Vitamin A
Ecchymoses, petechiae	Vitamin K
Hair	
Easily plucked, dyspigmented, lackluster	Protein-calorie
Mucosal	
Mouth, lips, and tongue	B vitamins
Angular stomatisis (inflammation at corners of mouth)	B_2 (riboflavin)
Cheilosis (reddened lips with fissures at angles)	B_2, B_6 (pyridoxine)
Glossitis (inflammation of tongue)	B_6, B_3 (niacin), B_2
Magenta tongue	B_2
Edema of tongue, tongue fissures	B_3
Spongy, bleeding gums	Vitamin C

CLINICAL SIGN	NUTRIENT DEFICIENCY
Ocular	
Conjunctival pallor due to anemia	Vitamin E (premature infants), iron, folic acid, vitamin B_{12}, copper
Bitot's spots (grayish, yellow, or white foamy spots on the whites of the eye)	Vitamin A
Conjunctival or corneal xerosis, keratomalacia	Vitamin A
Periorbital edema	Protein

150. What causes Harrison grooves?

Harrison grooves are horizontal depressions extending from the lower end of the sternum to the midaxillary line along the 6th and 7th costal cartilages. This corresponds to the sites of attachment of the anterior portion of the diaphragm. The grooves can be congenital, a sign of rickets, or rarely, associated with atrial septal defects.

151. How do marasmus and kwashiorkor differ clinically?

Although both disorders are due to a deficiency in energy intake, the syndromes differ dramatically because of the available protein sources. *Kwashiorkor* is edematous malnutrition due to low serum oncotic pressure. The low serum proteins result from a disproportionately low protein intake compared to the overall caloric intake. These children appear replete or fat, but have dependent edema, hyperkeratosis, and atrophic hair and skin. They generally have severe anorexia, diarrhea, and frequent infections and may have cardiac failure. *Marasmus* is severe nonedematous malnutrition caused by a mixed deficiency of both protein and calories. Serum protein and albumin levels are usually normal, but there is a marked decrease in muscle mass and adipose tissue. Signs are similar to those noted in hypothyroid children, with cold intolerance, listlessness, thin sparse hair, dry skin with decreased turgor, and hypotonia. Diarrhea, anorexia, vomiting, and recurrent infections may be noted.

152. With what laboratory tests should a patient on hyperalimentation be monitored?

- *Daily until stable, then twice per week*
  Serum glucose, sodium, potassium, chloride, bicarbonate
  BUN and creatinine
  Calcium, phosphate, magnesium
- *Weekly*
  Complete blood count with platelets
  Bilirubin and LFTs
  Cholesterol and triglycerides
  Albumin, total protein, total iron-binding capacity
- *As indicated by disease state*
  Serum B_{12}, iron, trace elements, serum amino acids

153. What are the major complications of intravenous hyperalimentation?

Mechanical, infectious, and metabolic.

1. ***Mechanical complications*** vary with the type of infusion and the delivery system, and include local or distant site thrombosis, perforation of the vasculature or heart, and accidental breakage or infiltration of the infusate into the subcutaneous, pleural, or pericardial space. Unfortunately, accidental dislodgment or disconnection is all too common in pediatric patients, and an emergency clamp should always be accessible.

2. Line-associated ***sepsis*** is a life-threatening complication that is associated with poor line aseptic technique. Any patient with fever and a central line should have an immediate set of peripheral and "line" cultures obtained and be started on antibiotics pending the

results. Because sepsis can be seeded by contaminated IV solutions, all equipment should be cultured in suspected line sepsis.

3. The ***metabolic complications*** of hyperalimentation may be limited by close monitoring but potentially span an enormous range including:

- Congestive heart failure and pulmonary edema from excessive infusate
- Hyper- and hypoglycemia
- Electrolyte, mineral, and vitamin disorders
- Hyperlipidemia
- Metabolic acidosis
- Hyperammonemia
- Anemia
- Demineralization of bone (i.e., rickets)
- Hepatic disorders (e.g., cholestasis, cholelithiasis, hepatitis)
- Eosinophilia (of unknown cause)

154. Who can develop the refeeding syndrome?

Chronically malnourished patients. The refeeding syndrome can occur in these individuals when a sudden exposure to excessive calories may begin a metabolic cascade due to the sudden surge of anabolic hormones in a nutritionally depleted host. Sudden hyperglycemia followed by increased insulin levels may lead to the rapid intracellular movement of glucose, potassium, magnesium, and phosphorus. Hypoglycemia, hypo-kalemia, and hypophosphatemia may then result in cardiac dysfunction. Atrophied skeletal and cardiac muscle may become more susceptible to the rapid decrease in available ATP and may result in weakness or heart failure.

PEPTIC ULCER DISEASE

155. What are the signs and symptoms of primary peptic ulcer (PUD) in childhood?:

Abdominal pain is the most common symptom of primary PUD. It is present in 90% of patients. While the quality and character of the pain can be variable, it is usually localized to the epigastric region. Classically, ulcer pain is temporally related to meals, but in children, this association occurs only about half the time. ***Nocturnal pain*** occurs in about 60% of patients and is a key feature in distinguishing organic from nonorganic pain. ***Melena*** is a feature in about a third of cases. Vomiting, hematemesis, and perforation are uncommon features.

156. How does the presentation of secondary ulcer disease differ from primary PUD?

Secondary ulcers, in association with other conditions, are often silent until very acute symptomatology develops. ***Pain*** occurs only in about 25% of patients, but 80% develop ***melena***, 60% have ***hematemesis***, and 30% have ***perforation***, often with severe bleeding and shock. The secondary ulcers have much higher mortality, morbidity, and need for surgical intervention. In primary PUD, symptoms are often recurrent and protracted. Delays in diagnosis can last for up to 2–4 years.

157. What conditions are associated with secondary ulcers in children?

- *Systemic diseases:* sepsis, acidosis, sickle cell anemia, cystic fibrosis, systemic lupus erythematosus, renal failure, severe hypoglycemia
- *Traumatic injury:* head trauma, burns, major surgery
- *Drugs/toxins:* corticosteroids, nonsteroidal anti-inflammatory drugs, theophylline, tolazoline, aspirin

158. What treatments are available for PUD in children?

Acid-neutralizing antacids

- Effective in promoting ulcer healing
- Used more commonly for symptomatic pain relief because of poor compliance due to large volumes (0.5 ml/kg/dose) required for therapy and potential side effects (e.g., diarrhea and constipation)
- Side effects (e.g., diarrhea and constipation)

H_2-receptor antagonists

- Include cimetidine, ranitidine, famotidine
- Well-tolerated in children with few side effects
- Also effective as prophylaxis in setting of systemic illness, head trauma, or surgery

"Proton pump" inhibitors

- Prototype is omeprazole, a substituted benzimidazole, which irreversibly binds to the gastric parietal cell, inhibiting H^+–K^+ exchange

Sucralfate

- Chemical complex of sucrose actasulfate and aluminum hydroxide which binds to the ulcer base and acts as a barrier; adsorbs pepsin and neutralizes hydrogen ions

Anticholinergics

- Decrease acid secretion
- At effective doses, side effects (e.g., dry mouth and blurred vision) may be significant

Antibiotics

- As treatment for *Helicobacter pylori* infection
- Most effective treatment remains unclear, but combination therapy with amoxicillin, bismuth subsalicylate (Pepto-Bismol), and metronidazole has an eradication rate of 60–90%

159. What is the relationship of *Helicobacter pylori* infection with antral gastritis, peptic ulcer disease, and recurrent abdominal pain in children?

An area of considerable interest, debate, and research. In adults, *H. pylori* has been associated with duodenal ulceration in over 90% of patients and with gastric ulceration in 70% of patients. However, asymptomatic colonization complicates the picture. In asymptomatic adult volunteers, 20–25% of patients have *H. pylori* colonization, as contrasted with only 4% of asymptomatic children. Studies seem to indicate that in children, there is a strong relationship between *H. pylori* and antral gastritis and primary duodenal ulcer disease, but a weak relationship between *H. pylori* and gastric ulcers and recurrent abdominal pain.

Hassall E: Peptic ulcer disease and current approaches to *Helicobacter pylori*. J Pediatr 138:462-468, 2001.

MacArthur C et al: Helicobacter pylori and childhood recurrent abdominal pain: Lack of evidence for a cause and effect relationship Can J Gastroenterol 13:607-610, 1999.

160. What methods are available for detecting the presence of *Helicobacter pylori* in the stomach or duodenum?

Non-invasive tests

- Stable isotope ^{13}C-urea breath test
- Serology (serum ELISA IgG and IgA titers)
- Stool antigen test

Invasive tests

- Culture of biopsy specimen
- PCR testing of biopsy specimen
- Identification of histologic gastritis
- Special stains for *H. pylori*

H. pylori produces urease, which can metabolize urea and produce CO_2, which is then exhaled by the patient. ^{13}C-labeled urea, given orally to the patient, exploits this peculiar metabolic step. If *H. pylori* is present in the proximal GI tract, labeled CO_2 is released. This is a reliable test, but requires (nonradioactive) labeled substrate and a mass-spectroscopy center for the assay. The ELISA assay detects the presence of antibody but is not as reliable for differentiating active disease from asymptomatic colonization. Levels of antibody titer may have a role in monitoring therapeutic response. Stool antigen testing is a newer modality and shows great promise as a screening tool.

The definitive diagnosis of *H. pylori*–associated gastritis requires endoscopic mucosal biopsies of the gastric antrum. The biopsy is cultured for *H. pylori* by direct inoculation of fresh minced tissue onto special media in the endoscopy lab or evaluated by polymerase chain reaction testing. Multiple specimens are also sent for histologic evaluation. Convincing evidence of *H. pylori* disease occurs when there is gastritis, and special stains (silver stain or acridine orange) identify the organism in the overlying mucus. When *H. pylori* occurs in the absence of gastritis or ulcer disease, as commonly happens in adults, the bacterial presence may indicate colonization rather than infection. In a recent study, all tests except serology were highly accurate in establishing the diagnosis in children.

Ni Y-H, et al: Accurate diagnosis of Helicobacter pylori infection by stool antigen test and 6 other currently available tests in children. J Pediatr 136:823-827, 2000.

161. Which patients should be evaluated for Zollinger-Ellison syndrome (ZES)?

ZES, a rare diagnosis in children, is ulcer disease caused by a gastrin-secreting tumor (gastrinoma). Patients usually present with symptoms secondary to peptic ulcer disease, and nearly all patients with ZES develop ulcers at some time in the course of the disease. In general, these ulcers are more persistent and progressive and commonly less responsive to treatment. Although the duodenal bulb is the most common location for both ZES and non-ZES associated ulcers, atypical ulcers in the distal duodenum or jejunum are more common in ZES. In children, any ulcer that does not heal after the first course of therapy should be investigated, as should patients with gastric acid hypersecretion and prominent gastric rugae.

162. How is the diagnosis of Zollinger-Ellison syndrome confirmed?

A simple screening test is the ***fasting serum gastrin level***, which should be obtained when the patient is not receiving acid blockade (H_2 blockers) or antacids. An elevated level requires prompt further investigation. Usually, the gastrin level is at least threefold elevated in patients with ZES. Unfortunately, many patients with an elevated gastrin level do not have ZES. Furthermore, some patients with a normal gastrin level may have a hormone-secreting tumor. When the diagnosis is strongly suspected but the serum gastrin concentration is low, a ***gastric acid secretion test*** is useful. Arteriography and CT scanning may be useful in locating a tumor, but in a large number of cases, even exploratory laparotomy may not identify the lesion.

SURGICAL ISSUES

163. What is the natural history of an umbilical hernia?

Most umbilical hernias < 0.5 cm spontaneously close before a patient is 2 years old. Those between 0.5 cm and 1.5 cm take up to 4 years to close. If the umbilical hernia is > 2 cm, it may still close spontaneously but may take up to 6 years or more. Unlike an inguinal hernia, incarceration and strangulation are very rare in an umbilical hernia.

Yazbeck S: Abdominal wall developmental defects and omphalomesenteric remnants. In Roy CC, et al (eds): Pediatric Clinical Gastroenterology, 4th ed. St. Louis, Mosby–Year Book, 1995, pp 134–135.

163. Which umbilical hernias warrant surgical repair?

Because of the high probability of self-resolution, indications for surgery are controversial. Some authorities argue that a hernia > 1.5 cm at age 2 years warrants closure due to its likely persistence for years. Others argue that since the likelihood of incarceration is small for umbilical hernias, surgical closure is warranted prior to puberty only for persistent pain, history of incarceration, or associated psychologic disturbances.

165. When should an infant with inguinal hernia have it electively repaired?

Once the diagnosis of inguinal hernia is made, it should be repaired as soon as possible. In a large study of children with incarcerated hernia, 40% of patients had a known inguinal hernia prior to incarceration and 80% were awaiting elective repair. Eighty percent of the children with incarceration of a hernia were infants under age 1 year, and especially in this age group, delay of repair should be minimized.

Stylianos S, et al: Incarceration of inguinal hernia in infants prior to elective repair. J Pediatr Surg 18:582–583, 1993.

166. Does surgical repair of one hernia warrant intraoperative exploration for another?

A controversial topic. Surveys have shown that during the repair of a clinical unilateral inguinal hernia, 65–90% of pediatric surgeons routinely explore the contralateral side in boys and 84–90% report they do so routinely in girls. Proponents of bilateral exploration argue that there is a high incidence of later contralateral hernia, particularly in children under age 2 years and in those in whom the initial presentation is on the left. 548 children with unilateral hernia repair without contralateral exploration were followed prospectively. 28% with incarcerated hernia later developed a contralateral hernia. 9% overall developed a contraleral hernia at a median interval of 6 months. Whether or not this 10% recurrence rate mandates contralateral exploration forms much of the basis of the controversy.

Tackett LD, et al: Incidence of contralateral inguinal hernia: A prospective analysis. J Pediatr Surg 34:684-688, 1999.

167. How are incarcerated inguinal hernias reduced?

Incarceration occurs most commonly in the first year of life. Because the infant will likely need to be admitted, nothing should be given to eat or drink. Reduction is most easily accomplished if the infant is calm (preferably asleep), warm, and, if possible, in a slightly reverse Trendelenburg position. Analgesia, such as 0.1 mg/kg of IV morphine, may facilitate the relaxed state. With one hand, the examiner stabilizes the base of the hernia by the internal inguinal ring and, with the other hand, milks the sac distally to progressively force fluids and/or gas through the ring to eventually allow complete reduction. If unsuccessful, immediate surgery is indicated.

168. Under what clinical settings should manual reduction of an inguinal hernia not be attempted?

When the patient has clinical findings of shock, perforation, peritonitis, GI bleeding or obstruction, or evidence of gangrenous bowel (bluish discoloration of the abdominal wall).

169. How do causes of intestinal obstruction vary by age?

Infant/young child

- Pyloric stenosis
- Inguinal hernia
- Malrotation
- Intestinal atresia or stenosis
- Intraluminal web
- Adhesions
- Intussusception
- Appendicitis
- Intestinal duplication
- Omphalomesenteric remnants
- Hirschsprung disease

Older child

- Appendicitis (perforated)
- Adhesions
- Inguinal hernia
- Inflammatory bowel disease
- Intussusception (lead-point)
- Malrotation
- Omphalomesenteric remnants

From Caty MG, Azizhan RG: Acute surgical conditions of the abdomen. Pediatr Ann 23:194, 1994; with permission.

170. What is the significance of green vomiting in the first 72 hours of life?

In the neonatal period, green vomiting should always be interpreted as a sign of potential intestinal obstruction requiring surgical intervention. In one study of 45 infants with green vomiting, 20% had surgical conditions (e.g., malrotation, jejunal atresia, jejunal stenosis), 10% had nonsurgical obstruction (e.g., meconium plug and microcolon), and 70% had idiopathic vomiting which self-resolved. If plain radiographs are equivocal or abnormal, upper or lower GI contrast studies should be done.

Lilien LD, et al: Green vomiting in the first 72 hours in normal infants. Am J Dis Child 140:662–664, 1986.

171. How is the volumetric method helpful in determining the need for imaging studies in vomiting infants?

In infants <4 months with *nonbilious vomiting*, aspiration of gastric contents after a period of NPO for 3-4 hours can be helpful. If the volume is less than 5 ml, a nonobstructive etiology is unlikely.

Mandell GA, et al: Cost-effective imaging approach to the nonbilious vomiting infant. Pediatrics 103:1198-1202, 1999.

172. What are the clinical findings of malrotation of the intestine?

Malrotation of the intestine is due to the abnormal rotation of the intestine around the superior mesenteric artery during embryologic development. Arrest of this counterclockwise rotation may occur at any degree of rotation. The lesion may present with *in utero* volvulus or may be asymptomatic throughout life. Infants may present with intermittent vomiting or complete obstruction. Any infant with bilious vomiting should be considered emergent and requires careful evaluation for volvulus and other high-grade surgical obstructions. Recurrent abdominal pain, distention, or lower GI bleeding may result from intermittent volvulus. Full volvulus with arterial compromise results in intestinal necrosis, peritonitis, perforation, and an extremely high incidence of mortality. Because of the extensive nature of the lesion, postoperative short gut syndrome is present in many patients who require resection.

173. Describe the x-ray findings associated with malrotation.

The upper GI series will show malposition and malfixation of the ligament of Treitz. The proximal small bowel may be located in the right upper quadrant, but this is not always true. The cecum viewed from either the upper GI series or barium enema may be unfixed or malpositioned. In both malrotation and volvulus, the plain films may be entirely normal. There may be proximal obstruction with gastroduodenal distention. In volvulus, the barium studies may show an obstruction near the gastroduodenal junction, often with a twisted appearance.

174. In an asymptomatic child with an incidental finding of malrotation, is surgery indicated?

Because of the persistent possibility of acute volvulus and intestinal obstruction, surgery is *always* indicated when intestinal malrotation is diagnosed.

175. In what settings should intussusception be suspected?

Ileocolic intussusception is twice as common in boys and usually occurs before the second year of life. Half of all cases occur between 3 and 9 months. Most cases do not have any identifiable etiology, but there is a seasonal clustering in the spring and fall which may be related to the increase in respiratory and enteric infections during those times, with resultant reactive intestinal lymphoid tissue. Colicky pain is seen in over 80% of cases but may be absent. It typically lasts 15–30 minutes, and the baby usually sleeps between attacks. In about two-thirds of cases, there is blood in the stool (currant jelly stools). Other presentations include massive lower GI bleeding or blood streaking on the stools. The infant may appear quite toxic, dehydrated, or in shock. Fever and tachycardia are common. A right lower quadrant mass may be palpable, or the area may feel surprisingly empty. Distention may accompany decreased bowel sounds. Radiographs typically demonstrate a small bowel obstruction pattern, but the diagnostic study of choice is a barium enema, which should be performed in all children with symptoms < 48 hours in duration. In 80% of cases, the barium enema under fixed hydrostatic pressure will reduce the intussusception. If this is unsuccessful, surgical reduction is necessary.

176. How commonly does intussusception present with the classic findings?

The classic triad of symptoms of intussusception consists of ***colicky pain, vomiting,*** and passage of ***bloody mucous*** stool. Unfortunately, this classic presentation is the exception. In studies of patients with intussusception, 80% of patients did not have this triad of symptoms, about 30% had blood in the stool, and this percentage dropped to about 15% if the abdominal pain was present for < 12 hours. Palpation of a mass can suggest the diagnosis, but a high degree of suspicion is key.

177. What causes intussusception?

Intussusception is caused by one proximal segment of the bowel being invaginated and progressively drawn caudad and encased by the lumen of distal bowel. This causes obstruction and may occlude the vascular supply of the bowel segment. There is commonly a lead point on the proximal bowel which initiates the process. Lead points have included juvenile polyps, lymphoid hyperplasia, hypertrophied Peyer patches, eosinophilic granuloma of the ileum, lymphoma, lymphosarcoma, leiomyosarcoma, leukemic infiltrate, duplication cysts, ectopic pancreas, Meckel diverticulum, hematoma, Henoch-Schönlein syndrome, worms, foreign bodies, and appendicitis.

Navarro O, et al: Lead points of intussusception. Pediatr Radiol 30:594-603, 2000.

178. What is the most common type of intussusception?

Ileocolic intussusception. It is also the most common cause of intestinal obstruction in infancy). Cecocecal and colocolic intussusceptions are less common. Gastroduodenal intussusception is rare and is usually associated with a gastric mass lesion such as a polyp or a leiomyoma. Enteroenteral intussusception is seen after surgery and in patients with Henoch-Schönlein syndrome.

179. How frequently does intussusception recur?

Idiopathic ileocolic intussusception recurs in about **3–9%** of all cases. Intussusceptions in older children tend to recur at a higher frequency if the causative lesion is not removed. It is important to investigate cases of recurrent intussusception for an underlying lesion.

Daneman A, et al: Patterns of recurrence of intussusception in children: A 17-year review. Pediatr Radiol 28:913-919, 1998.

180. Rotavirus vaccine and intussusception: how are they intertwined?

The oral rotavirus vaccine, licensed in the U.S. in 1998, was suspended from use when increased rates of intussusception were noted.

Murphy TV, et al: Intussusception among infants given an oral rotavirus vaccine. N Engl J Med 344:564-572, 2001.

181. Duodenal or jejunoileal atresia—which is associated with other embryonic abnormalities?

Duodenal atresia is caused by a persistence of the proliferative stage of gut development and a lack of secondary vacuolization and recanalization. It is associated with a high incidence of other early embryonic abnormalities. Extraintestinal anomalies occur in two-thirds of patients. In jejunoileal atresia, the lesion occurs after the establishment of continuity and patency, as evidenced by distal meconium seen in these patients. The etiology is postulated to be a vascular accident, volvulus, or mechanical perforation. Jejunoileal atresias are usually not associated with any other systemic abnormality.

182. How does the infant with biliary atresia classically present?

In classic cases, a term infant develops a recognizable jaundice by the third week of life, with increasingly dark urine and acholic stools. Usually the child appears well, with acceptable growth. The skin color sometimes appears somewhat greenish yellow. The spleen becomes palpable after the third or fourth week, at which time the liver is usually hard and enlarged. In other cases, the jaundice is clearly present in the conjugated form during the first week of life. There is also a strong association between the polysplenia syndrome and biliary atresia.

183. What are the complications of the Kasai procedure?

The *Kasai procedure* is a hepatic portoenterostomy performed for biliary atresia. The remnants of the extrahepatic biliary tree are identified, and a cholangiogram is performed to verify the diagnosis. Dissection and resection of the remaining extrahepatic ducts and the fibrous plate present at the porta are then performed. A Roux-en-Y jejunal limb is constructed to drain bile from the porta, and in some cases, this limb is temporarily exteriorized at a double-barrel ostomy. Postoperative complications include intestinal obstruction, early and late ascending cholangitis, peristomal breakdown, and stomal varices. In nearly half the cases, the procedure does not establish bile flow, and in most patients, there is ongoing inflammation and the development of portal hypertension.

184. When should a Kasai procedure be performed?

As soon as possible. Earlier operation results in a dramatically improved outcome. Patients operated before 70 days of age have increased likelihood of a successful procedure, although exceptions at both ends of this spectrum are common. Some surgeons now suggest that infants diagnosed late in the course should have a primary liver transplant rather than a hepatic portoenterostomy.

185. Why is distinguishing between a high and low imperforate anus so important?

The distinction is based on whether the blind end of the terminal bowel or rectum ends above (high-type) or below (low-type) the level of the pelvic levator musculature. The patients with high-type imperforations will have ectopic fistulae (rectourinary, rectovaginal), urologic anomalies (hydronephrosis or double collecting system), and lumbosacral spine defects (sacral agenesis, hemivertebrae). The surgical repair in these patients is much more extensive, and future problems of incontinence, fecal impaction, and strictures are much more likely.

186. What is the classic presentation of pyloric stenosis?

An infant 3–6 weeks of age presents with progressive nonbilious projectile vomiting leading to dehydration with hypochloremic, hypokalemic, metabolic alkalosis. On physical exam, a pyloric "olive" is palpable and peristaltic waves are visible.

187. How is pyloric stenosis diagnosed?

If the classic signs and symptoms are present in association with the typical blood chemistry findings (hypochloremia, hypokalemia, metabolic alkalosis), the diagnosis can be made on clinical grounds. If the diagnosis is in doubt, ultrasound can be used to visualize the hypertrophic pyloric musculature. Upper GI contrast studies demonstrate pyloric obstruction with the characteristic "string sign" and enlarged "shoulders" bordering the elongated and obstructed pyloric channel.

188. What is the mechanism of hyperbilirubinemia in babies with pyloric stenosis?

Unconjugated hyperbilirubinemia has been noted in 10–25% of babies with pyloric stenosis. While an enhanced enterohepatic circulation for bilirubin probably plays a role in the pathogenesis of the hyperbilirubinemia, hepatic glucoronyl transferase activity is markedly depressed in these jaundiced infants. The mechanism of diminished glucoronyl transferase activity is not known, although inhibition of the enzyme by intestinal hormones has been suggested.

189. In a patient with suspected pyloric stenosis, why is an acidic urine very worrisome?

As vomiting progresses in infants with pyloric stenosis, a worsening hypochloremic metabolic alkalosis develops. Multiple factors (e.g., volume depletion, elevated aldosterone levels) result in maximal renal efforts to reabsorb sodium. In the distal tubule, this is typically achieved by exchanging sodium for potassium and hydrogen. When total body potassium levels are very low, hydrogen is preferentially exchanged, and a paradoxic aciduria develops (in the setting of an alkaline plasma). This acidic urine is an indication that intravascular volume expansion and electrolyte replenishment (especially chloride and potassium) are urgently needed.

190. What is the connection between pyloric stenosis and erythromycin?

In studies of infants who have received erythromycin, primarily as prophylaxis after exposure to pertussis, the incidence of pyloric stenosis is significantly increased.

Honein MA, et al: Infantile hypertrophic pyloric stenosis after pertussis prophylaxis with erythromycin: A case review and cohort study. Lancet 354:2102-2105, 1999.

191. What syndromes are associated with pyloric stenosis?

- Trisomy 18
- Long-arm deletion 21
- Turner syndrome
- Smith-Lemli-Opitz syndrome
- Cornelia de Lange syndrome

192. What is the short bowel syndrome?

The *short bowel syndrome* results from extensive resection of the small intestine. Normally, the majority of carbohydrates, proteins, fats, and vitamins are absorbed in the jejunum and proximal ileum. The terminal ileum is responsible for the uptake of bile acids and vitamin B_{12}. Short bowel syndrome results in failure to thrive, malabsorption, diarrhea, vitamin deficiency, bacterial contamination, and gastric hypersecretion.

193. Why are infants with short bowel syndrome prone to renal calculi?

Chronic intestinal malabsorption results in an increase of intraluminal fatty acids, which saponify with dietary calcium. Thus, nonabsorbable calcium oxalate does not form, excessive oxalate is absorbed, and hyperoxaluria with crystal formation results.

194. In extensive small bowel resection, how much is "too much"?

Infants who retain 20 cm of small bowel as measured from the ligament of Treitz can survive *if the ileocecal valve is intact*. If the ileocecal valve has been removed, the infant usually requires a minimum of 40 cm of bowel to survive. The importance of the ileocecal valve appears to relate to its ability to retard transit time and minimize bacterial contamination of the small intestine.

195. What conditions may mimic appendicitis?

- Gastroenteritis
- Mesenteric adenitis
- Constipation
- Pelvic inflammatory disease
- Pyelonephritis
- Right lower lobe pneumonia
- Ruptured ovarian follicle/ovarian torsion
- Inflammatory bowel disease
- Henoch-Schönlein purpura
- Primary peritonitis
- Perforated peptic ulcer
- Pancreatitis

From Caty MG, Azizhan RG: Acute surgical conditions of the abdomen. Pediatr Ann 23:193, 1994; with permission.

196. Appendicitis in children: clinical, laboratory or radiologic diagnosis?

The diagnosis of appendicitis has traditionally been a clinical one. The classic picture in children is a period of *anorexia* followed by *pain, nausea,* and *vomiting*. Abdominal pain begins periumbilically and then shifts after 4–6 hours to the right lower quadrant. Fever is low grade. Peritoneal signs are detected on exam. In unequivocal cases, experienced surgeons would argue that no lab tests are needed.

Laboratory studies have limited value in equivocal cases. *WBC count* > 18,000/mm^3 or a marked left shift is unusual in uncomplicated cases and suggests perforation or another diagnosis. A *urinalysis* with many wbcs suggests a urinary tract infection as the primary pathology.

Limited CT with rectal contrast (CTRC) is emerging as a powerful tool in diagnosis with sensitivities and specificities between 98%-100% in children. 3% diatrizoate meglumine saline solution is instilled into the colon in a slow controlled drip. Oral and IV contrast are not needed. Diagnosis is based on the visualization of an abnormal appendix or pericecal inflammation or abscess with or without the presence of an appendicolith. CRTC can supplement or supplant abdominal ultrasound studies. Plain abdominal films are of limited value.

Garcia Pena BM, et al: Cost and effectiveness of ultrasonography and limited computed tomography for diagnosing appendicitis in children. Pediatrics 106:672-676, 2000.

Karakas SP, et al: Acute appendicitis in children: comparison of clinical diagnosis with ultrasound and CT imaging. PediatrRadiol 30:94-98, 2000.

Garcia Pena BM, et al: Ultrasonography and limited computed tomography in the diagnosis and management of appendicitis in children. JAMA 1041-1046, 1999.

197. How specific is the diagnosis of appendicitis if an appendicolith is noted on x-ray?

Although an appendicolith (or fecalith) on x-ray studies (plain film or CT) is significantly associated with appendicitis, it is not sufficiently specific to be the sole basis for the diagnosis. On CT studies, they can be noted in 65% of patients with appendicitis and in up to 15% of patients without appendicitis. The positive predictive value of finding an appendicolith is about 75% and in its absence a negative predictive value of only 26%.

Lowe LH, et al: Appendicolith revealed on CT in children with suspected appendicitis: How specific is it in the diagnosis of appendicitis? Am J Roentgenol 175:981-984, 2000 .

198. Should a digital rectal exam be performed on all children with possible appendicitis?

Tradition says yes, but reviews of studies of the practice indicate that in children it can be emotionally and physically traumatic and associated with a high false-positive interpretation. It may be most helpful in equivocal cases involving pelvic or retrocecal appendicitis (about a third of cases), suspected abscess formation or for attempted palpation of adnexal/cervical tissues when vaginal examination is not indicated. Thus, many clinicians now view it as "investigatory" rather than "routine" and only when results will change management.

Brewster GS, Herbert ME: Medical myth: a digital rectal examination should be performed on all individuals with possible appendicitis. West J Med 173:207-208, 2000.

199. In children taken to surgery for suspected appendicitis, how often is perforation of the appendix present?

It depends to a large extent on the age of the child (and, of course, on the skill of the clinician). Unfortunately, due to the variable location of the appendix, the clinical presentation of pain in appendicitis is often very different from the classical case. The younger the child, the more difficult the diagnosis. In infants < 1 year of age, nearly 100% of patients who come to surgery have a perforation. Fortunately, appendicitis is rare in this age group because the appendiceal opening at the cecum is much larger than the tip and obstruction is unusual. In children < 2 years, 70–80% are perforated, and in those up to 5 years, 50% are perforated. Particularly in younger children, a high index of suspicion is necessary and rapid diagnosis is critical. If the onset of symptoms can be pinpointed (usually anorexia related to a meal), 10% of patients will have perforation in the first 24 hours, but over 50% will perforate by 48 hours.

8. GENETICS

Elaine H. Zackai, M.D., Kwame Anyane-Yeboa, M.D., JoAnn Bergoffen, M.D., Alan E. Donnenfeld, M.D., and Jeffrey E. Ming, M.D., Ph.D.

AUTOSOMAL TRISOMIES

1. Excluding chromosomal analysis, what laboratory tests suggest that a woman is carrying a fetus with trisomy 21?

The combination of low levels of ***maternal serum alpha-fetoprotein*** and ***unconjugated estriol*** and elevated levels of ***human chorionic gonadotropin*** (the so-called *triple screen*) can identify 60% of fetuses with Down syndrome with a false-positive rate of 5–7%. Abnormal screening tests can prompt definitive studies of chromosomal analysis.

2. What is the main advantage of chorionic villus sampling (CVS) over amniocentesis?

CVS is the aspiration of chorionic villi via a transcervical catheter or transabdominal needle using ultrasound guidance. The main advantage of CVS is that it can be done between 10–12 weeks of gestation compared with the usual 16-week timing of amniocentesis.

3. Describe the features of the three most common autosomal trisomies.

Common Autosomal Trisomies

FEATURE	TRISOMY 21	TRISOMY 18	TRISOMY 13
Eponym	Down syndrome	Edward syndrome	Patau syndrome
Liveborn incidence	1/800	1/8000	1/15,000
Tone	Hypotonia	Hypertonia	Hypo- or hypertonia
Cranium/brain	Mild microcephaly, flat occiput, 3 fontanels	Microcephaly, prominent occiput	Microcephaly, sloping forehead, occipital scalp defects, holoprosencephaly
Eyes	Upslanting, epicanthal folds, speckled iris (Brushfield spots)	Small palpebral fissures, corneal opacity	Micro-ophthalmia, hypotelorism, iris coloboma, retinal dysplasia
Ears	Small, low-set, overfolded upper helix	Low-set, malformed	Low-set, malformed
Facial features	Protruding tongue, large cheeks, low flat nasal bridge	Small mouth, micrognathia	Cleft lip and palate
Skeletal	Clinodactyly 5th digit, gap between toes 1 and 2, excess nuchal skin, short stature	Clenched hand, absent 5th finger distal crease, hypoplastic nails, short	Postaxial polydactyly, hypoconvex fingernails, clenched hand
Cardiac defect	40%	60%	80%
Survival	Long-term	90% die within first year	80% die within first year
Other features	(see below)	Rocker bottom feet, polycystic kidneys, dermatoglyphic arch pattern	Genital anomalies, polycystic kidneys, increased nuclear projections in neutrophils

4. Are Brushfield spots pathognomonic for Down syndrome?

No. Brushfield spots are speckled areas that occur in the periphery of the iris. They are seen in about 75% of patients with Down syndrome but also in up to 10% of normal newborns.

5. What clinical findings occur most frequently in Down syndrome infants?

Frequency of Positive Phenotypic Findings in Infants with Down Syndrome

Sagittal suture separated	98%	Muscle weakness	81%
Oblique palpabral fissure	98	Hypotonia	77
Wide space between first and second toes	96	Brushfield spots	75
False fontanel	95	Mouth kept open	65
Plantar crease between first and second toes	94	Protruding tongue	58
Hyperflexibility	91	Epicanthal folds	57
Increased neck tissue	87	Single palmar crease	50–55
Abnormally shaped palate	85	Brachyclinodactyly	50–51
Hypoplastic nose	83		

Modified from Pueschel SM: The child with Down syndrome. In Levine et al: Developmental-Behavioral Pediatrics. Philadelphia, W.B. Saunders, 1983, p 356; with permission.

6. What is the chance that a newborn with a simian crease has Down syndrome?

A single transverse palmar crease is present in 4% of normal newborns. Bilateral palmar creases are found in 1%. These features occur twice as commonly in males than females. However, 50–55% of newborn infants with Down syndrome have a single transverse crease. Since Down syndrome occurs in 1/800 live births, the chance that a newborn with a simian crease has Down syndrome is only ***1 in 60***.

7. What is the expected intelligence and personality of a child with Down syndrome?

The IQ range is generally 35–65, with a mean reported IQ of 54. Occasionally, the IQ may be higher. Intelligence deteriorates in adulthood, with clinical and pathologic findings consistent with advanced Alzheimer disease. Autopsy results from brains of deceased adults with Down syndrome reveal both neurofibrillary tangles and senile plaques, as found in Alzheimer disease. By age 40, the mean IQ is 24. Children with Down syndrome are generally affectionate and docile. They tend toward mimicry and are noted usually to enjoy music, having a good sense of rhythm. However, 13% have serious emotional problems, and coordination is usually poor.

8. What causes the dementia of Down syndrome?

athologic evidence of senile dementia or Alzheimer disease (i.e., senile plaques, neurofibrillary tangles, and granulovascuolar degeneration) was reported in individuals with Down syndrome for the first time in 1929. Currently, it is believed that overexpression of a gene for the amyloid precursor (PreA4) located on the long arm of chromosome 21 may lead to amyloid deposition in Down syndrome patients.

Rumble B, et al: Amyloid A4 protein and its precursors in Down syndrome and Alzheimer's disease. N Engl J Med 320:1446–1452, 1989.

9. Why do older individuals with Down syndrome rarely develop atherosclerotic heart disease?

The enzyme cystathionine β-synthase (CBS) is needed to form cystathione from homocysteine and serine. Deficiency of this enzyme results in homocystinuria, which is characterized by precocious atherosclerosis and plasma accumulation of methionine and homocysteine. The gene for CBS is found on chromosome 21, and its activity is increased in cultured fibroblasts of Down syndrome patients. The plasma level of homocysteine has also been shown to be lower in Down syndrome patients after an overnight fast and a methionine load. It has been suggested that the higher enzymatic activity could be related to the lower incidence of atherosclerosis in individuals with Down syndrome.

10. Why is maternal age of 35 at delivery chosen as the cutoff for recommending amniocentesis for chromosome analysis?

There is a well-known association between advanced maternal age and trisomies (including XXY, XXX, trisomy 13, 18, and 21).

Maternal Age	Approximate Risk of Down Syndrome
30	1:1000
35	1:365
40	1:100
45	1:50

Most cases of Down syndrome involve nondisjunction at meiosis I in the mother. This may be related to the lengthy stage of meiotic arrest between oocyte development in the fetus until ovulation, which may occur as much as 40 years later.

11. What percentage of all babies with Down syndrome are born to women over the age of 35?

Only 20%. While their individual risk is higher, women in this age bracket account for only 5% of all pregnancies in the United States.

Haddow JE, et al: Prenatal screening for Down syndrome with use of maternal serum markers. N Engl J Med 327:588–593, 1992.

12. What percentage of cases of Down syndrome are due to translocations?

3.3% of all cases of Down syndrome are due to unbalanced robertsonian translocations in which a third copy of chromosome 21 is present, attached to an acrocentric chromosome. The chance of translocation Down syndrome is two to three times greater in children of younger mothers (6–8% of mothers under 30). One of three infants with translocation Down syndrome will have a parent with a robertsonian translocation. Two-thirds of the time, translocation Down syndrome occurs as a de novo event in the infant.

13. What is the overall recurrence risk of Down syndrome?

In chromosomally normal women ***under age 40***, the recurrence risk for Down syndrome is ***1%*** (assuming the father's chromosomes are also normal). Above age 40, the risk of having a child with Down syndrome increases, primarily as a function of maternal age. If the mother carries a translocation, the recurrence risk is 10%. If the father carries a translocation, the recurrence risk is 3–5%. One theory for this observed discrepancy between maternal and paternal rates of translocation Down syndrome is hindered motility of chromosomally abnormal sperm.

14. Does advanced paternal age increase the risk of having a child with trisomy 21?

There does not appear to be an increased risk of Down syndrome associated with paternal age until after age 55. Some studies have noted an increased risk of Down syndrome after this age, although others have not. The reports are controversial, and the statistical analysis needed to perform such a study is cumbersome. It is known that approximately 10% of all trisomy 21 cases derive the extra chromosome 21 from the father.

15. Why has the incidence of Down syndrome decreased from 1.6/1000 live births to 1.0–1.2/1000 live births over the past 25 years?

The decrease in incidence is a result of the reduction of births in older women and prenatal diagnosis. The risk for older women has not changed, but at the present time only 20%of children with Down syndrome are born to mothers over 35 years of age, whereas 25 years ago 50 % of the children with Down syndrome were born to older mothers.

16. Which is technically correct: Down's syndrome or Down syndrome?

In 1866, John Langdon Down, physician at the Earlswood Asylum in Surrey, England, described the phenotype of a syndrome which now bears his name. However, it was not until 1959 that it was determined that this disorder is caused by an extra chromosome 21. The correct designation is ***Down syndrome***.

CLINICAL ISSUES

17. What genetically inherited disease has the highest known mutation rate per gamete per generation?

Neurofibromatosis. The estimated mutation rate for this disorder is 1×10^{-4} per haploid genome. The clinical features are café-au-lait spots and axillary freckling in childhood followed by development of neurofibromas in later years. There is approximately a 10% risk of malignancy with this condition, and mental deficiency is common.

18. Which disorders with ethnic and racial predilections most commonly warrant maternal screening for carrier status?

DISORDER	ETHNIC OR RACIAL GROUP	SCREENING MARKER
Tay-Sachs disease	Ashkenazi Jewish, French, French Canadian	Decreased serum hexosaminidase A concentration
Sickle cell anemia	Black, African, Mediterranean, Arab, Indian, Pakistani	Presence of sickling in hemolysate followed by confirmatory hemoglobin electrophoresis
Alpha- and beta-thalassemia	Mediterranean, Southern and Southeast Asian, Chinese	Mean corpuscular volume < 80μm³, followed by confirmatory hemoglobin electrophoresis

From D'Alton ME, DeCherney AH: Prenatal diagnosis. N Engl J Med 328:115, 1993; with permission

19. Why are mitochondrial disorders transmitted from generation to generation by the mother and not the father?

Mitochondrial DNA abnormalities (e.g., many cases of ragged red fiber myopathies) are passed on from the mother because mitochondria are present in the cytoplasm of the egg and not the sperm. Transmission to males or females is equally likely; however, expression is variable because mosaicism with normal and abnormal mitochondria in varying proportions is very common.

Johns DR: Mitochondrial DNA and disease. N Engl J Med 333:638–644, 1995.

20. Which syndromes are associated with advanced paternal age?

Advanced paternal age is well documented to be associated with new dominant mutations. The assumption is that the increased mutation rate is due to accumulation of new mutations from many cell divisions. The more cell divisions, the more likely an error (mutation) will occur. The mutation rate in fathers > 50 is five times higher than the mutation rate in fathers < 20 years of age. Autosomal dominant new mutations that have been mapped and identified including ***achondroplasia***, ***Apert syndrome***, and ***Marfan syndrome***.

21. What is the most common genetic-lethal disease?

Cystic fibrosis (CF). A genetic-lethal disease is one that interferes with a person's ability to reproduce due to early death (before childbearing age) or impaired sexual function. CF is the most common autosomal recessive disorder in whites, occurring in 1/1600 (1 of every 20 individuals is a carrier for this condition). CF is characterized by widespread dysfunction of exocrine glands, chronic pulmonary disease, pancreatic insufficiency, and intestinal obstructions. Males are azospermic. The median survival is approximately 29 years.

22. Assuming that the husband is healthy and that no one in the wife's family has cystic fibrosis, what is the risk that a couple will have a child with cystic fibrosis if the husband's brother has the disease?

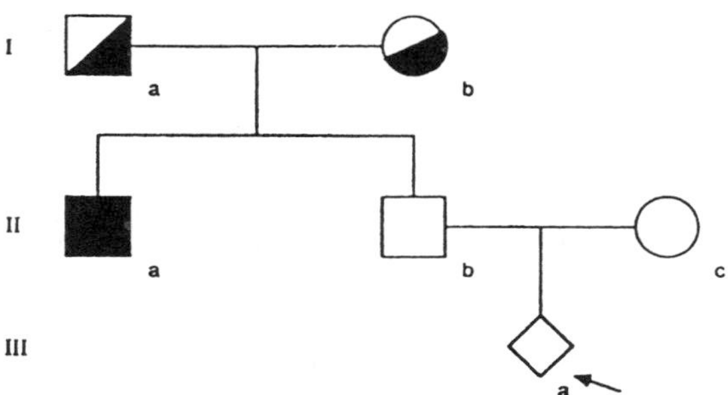

1. Since IIa is affected with CF, both his parents must be carriers.
2. The chance of IIb being a carrier is 2/3, since we know he is not affected by CF.
3. The risk of IIc being a carrier is 1/20 (the population risk).
4. The chance of IIIa being affected is: father's carrier risk × mother's carrier risk × the chnce that both will pass on their recessive CF gene to their child; 2/3 × 1/20 × 1/4 = **1/120**.

23. What are the "fat baby" syndromes?

- ***Prader-Willi*** (obesity, hypotonia, small hands and feet)
- ***Beckwith-Wiedemann*** (macrosomia, omphalocele, macroglossia, ear creases)
- ***Sotos*** (macrosomia, macrocephaly, large hands and feet)
- ***Weaver*** (macrosomia, accelerated skeletal maturation, camptodactyly)
- ***Bardet-Biedl*** (obesity, retinal pigmentation, polydactyly)
- ***Infants of diabetic mothers***

24. What is the H_3O of Prader-Willi syndrome?

Hyperphagia, hypotonia, hypopigmentation, and ***obesity***. Up to 50% of patients, most with mental retardation, have a deletion on the long arm of chromosome 15. The gene(s) responsible for Prader-Willi syndrome are subject to *parental imprinting*. Imprinting refers to the process by which expression of a gene depends on whether it has been inherited from the mother or the father. The gene(s) associated with Prader-Willi syndrome are paternally imprinted, meaning that loss of the paternal copy will result in the phenotype of Prader-Willi. A closely related area of the long arm of chromosome 15 is maternally imprinted, and loss of the maternal copy leads to Angelman syndrome. Angelman syndrome is characterized by severe developmental delay, abnormal gait, inappropriate laughter, and excessive movements, especially of the arms.

Deal CL: Parental genomic imprinting. Curr Opin Pediatr 7:445–458, 1995.

25. Name the two most common forms of dwarfism recognizable at birth.

There are 21 different skeletal dysplasia syndromes that were classified at the International Nomenclature of Constitutional Diseases of Bone meeting as "recognizable at birth." The most common is ***thanatophoric dwarfism***, a *lethal* chondrodysplasia characterized by flattened, Ushaped vertebral bodies, telephone-receiver-shaped femurs, macrocephaly, and redundant skinfolds causing a pug-like appearance. Thanatophoric means death-loving (an apt description). The incidence is 1 in 6400 births.

Achondroplasia is the most common *viable* skeletal dysplasia, occurring 1 in 26,000 live births. Its features are small stature (mean adult height 4¢2_), macrocephaly, depressed nasal bridge, lordosis, and a trident hand. Some patients develop hydrocephalus due to a small foramen magnum. X-ray findings include narrowing of the interpedicular distance as one proceeds caudally. Both achondroplasia and thanatophoric dysplasia are due to mutations in fibroblast growth factor receptor 3. In achondroplasia the mutation is in the transmembrance domain, while the mutation in thanatophoric dysplasia is either in the intracellular domain (type II) or the extracellular domain (type I).

Tavormina PL, Shiang R, Thompson LM, et al: Thanatophoric dysplasia (types I and II) caused by mutations in fibroblast growth factor receptor 3. Nature Genetics 9:321–328, 1995.

26. What are the risks of having a second child with autism?

The prevalence of autism in the siblings of autistic children has been estimated to be about ***2–3%,*** which is 50–100 times greater than the expected rate of autism in the population (4–5/10,000). However, many families choose to limit further child bearing, and therefore, this estimate may be low. The genetics of autism are still unclear.

27. What chromosomal abnormality is found in cri du chat syndrome?

Cri du chat syndrome is due to a ***deletion*** of material from the ***short arm of chromosome 5*** (i.e., 5p–) which causes many problems including growth retardation, microcephaly, and severe mental retardation. Patients have a characteristic *cat-like cry* in infancy from which the syndrome derives its name. In 85%of cases, the deletion is a de novo event. In 15%, it is due to malsegregation from a balanced parental translocation.

28. Which syndromes are characterized by a senile-like appearance?

- ***Progeria*** (alopecia, atrophy of subcutaneous fat, skeletal dysplasia, early death)
- ***Werner syndrome*** (cataract, thick skin, sparse, gray hair)
- ***Cockayne syndrome*** (growth deficiency, retinal degeneration, impaired hearing, thick skin)
- ***Rothmund-Thomson syndrome*** (poikiloderma, cataract, ectodermal dysplasia)

29. List the syndromes and malformations associated with congenital limb hemihypertrophy.

- Russell-Silver syndrome
- Conradi-Hünermann syndrome
- Klippel-Trenaunay-Weber syndrome
- Beckwith-Wiedemann syndrome
- Wilms tumor
- Hypomelanosis of Ito
- CHILD syndrome (**C**ongenital **H**emidysplasia, **I**chtyosiform erythroderma, **L**imb **D**efects)
- Neurofibromatosis

One of every 32 patients with isolated hemihypertrophy is at risk for developing Wilms tumor. For this reason, renal and abdominal ultrasound should be offered periodically in childhood as a screening device for patients with hemihypertrophy.

30. Which genetic disorders are associated with hypoplastic left heart syndrome?

While most newborns with hypoplastic left heart syndrome have this defect as an isolated abnormality, several syndromes in which this congenital heart malformation is a component have been identified: Down syndrome, Turner syndrome, Smith-Lemli-Opitz syndrome, trisomy 13, trisomy 18, and Ivemark syndrome. Before extensive reconstructive surgery is attempted, it may be prudent to obtain a chromosomal analysis in cases where malformations are noted.

31. In the evaluation of a stillborn infant, how does the general appearance of the fetus suggest a likely etiology?

A *fresh embryo* or fetus implies a rapid expulsion after intrauterine or intrapartum death. These fetuses are usually without major anomalies and have normal karyotypes. Causes of death commonly are placental abruption, cord accidents, and ascending infection. A *macerated embryo* or fetus indicates prolonged retention in utero. In this circumstance, structural anomalies or chromosomal abnormalities are more frequent.

32. In which fetal and infant deaths are autopsies strongly advised?

- Infants with external or suspected internal structural abnormalities
- Infants with intrauterine growth retardation
- Infants with nonimmune hydrops
- Families with a previous unexplained loss
- Infants with no obvious cause of death
- Macerated fetuses

In addition to an autopsy, other studies that should be considered include chromosomal analysis, skeletal radiographs, placental and cord histologic studies, titers for congenital infection, and, if hydropic, evaluation for a hemoglobinopathy (e.g., alpha thalassemia), or possible metabolic storage disease.

33. How should women with recurrent pregnancy loss be evaluated?

ouples with *recurrent pregnancy loss*, variably defined as either two or three losses, should be considered for the following evaluations:

- *Cytogenetic analysis* of both parents to rule out mosaicism or a balanced translocation.
- *Hysterosalpingogram* to rule out malformations of the uterine cavity (congenital, DES-induced, myomas, and intrauterine synechiae)
- *Infectious evalution* for Mycoplasma, *Chlamydia,* and other pathogens
- *Immunologic evaluation* for antiphospholipid antibody, anticardiolipin antibody, and antinuclear antibody (e.g., systemic lupus erythematosus)
- *Endometrial biopsy* or *progesterone level* analysis to rule out a luteal phase defect
- *Thyroid function tests*
- *Evaluation* of any suspected *systemic illnesses*

34. Give 8 reasons why a disease might be genetically determined but the family history be negative.

1. Autosomal recessive inheritance
2. X-linked recessive inheritance
3. Genetic heterogeneity (e.g., retinitis pigmentosa may be transmitted as AR, AD, or X-linked recessive)
4. Spontaneous mutation
5. Nonpenetrance
6. Expressivity (i.e., variable expression)
7. Extramarital paternity
8. Phenocopy (i.e., an environmentally determined copy of a genetic disorder)

Juberg RC: ...but the family history was negative. J Pediatr 91:693–694, 1977.

DYSMORPHOLOGY

35. How are structural dysmorphisms categorized?

• ***Malformation:*** a problem of poor formation (likely genetically based) in which the abnormality is present at the onset of development (e.g., hypoplastic thumbs of Fanconi syndrome)

• ***Disruption:*** an extrinsic destructive process interferes with previously normal development (e.g., thalidomide causing limb abnormalities)

• ***Deformation:*** an extrinsic mechanical force causes abnormalities, which are usually asymmetrical (e.g,. breech position causing tibial bowing and positional club feet)

• ***Dysplasia:*** an abnormal cellular organization or function that generally affects only a single tissue type (e.g., cartilage abnormalities that result in achondroplasia)

36. What are the principal kinds of morphologic defects in infants with multiple anomalies?

• ***Developmental or polytopic field defect:*** a pattern of anomalies derived from the disturbance of a single region or part of an embryo which responds as a coordinated unit to extrinsic or intrinsic influences. Field defects are believed to be derivatives of a single malformative or disruptive process. For example, if the rostral mesoderm is disturbed early in development, multiple anomalies of the head and face can occur.

• ***Sequence:*** a pattern of multiple anomalies derived from a single known (or presumed) prior anomaly or mechanical factor. For example, the entity of micrognathia, glossoptosis, and cleft soft palate is more properly called the Pierre Robin sequence (rather than syndrome) because the small mandible likely causes the developing tongue to be pushed posteriorly, which does not allow the posterior palatal shelves to close properly.

• ***Syndrome:*** the nonrandom occurrence of multiple anomalies, with such an increased frequency that a pathogenetically causal relationship (often of unknown cause) is felt to be involved. For example, chromosomal syndromes (e.g., Down) have characteristic clinical features.

• ***Association:*** the nonrandom occurrence of multiple anomalies without a known field defect, sequence initiator, or causal relationship, but with such a frequency that the malformations have a statistical connection.

37. How common are major and a minor malformations in newborns?

Major malformations are unusual morphologic features that cause medical, cosmetic, or developmental consequences to the patient. *Minor anomalies* are features that do not cause medical or cosmetic problems. Approximately ***14%*** of newborn babies will have a minor malformation, whereas only ***2–3%*** of newborns will have a major anomaly.

38. Identify the most common major congenital anomalies in the U.S.

Anencephaly and ***spina bifida***. The combined prevalence is 0.5–2.0/1000 live births.

39. What is the clinical significance of a minor malformation?

Recognition of minor malformations in a newborn may serve as an *indicator* of altered morphogenesis or as a valuable clue to the diagnosis of a specific disorder. The presence of several minor malformations is unusual and often indicates a serious problem in morphogenesis. For example, when three or more minor malformations are discovered in a child, there is a > 90% risk of a major malformation also being present. The most common minor malformations involve the face, ears, hands, and feet. Almost any minor defect may occasionally be found as an unusual familial trait.

40. How common are minor anomalies in newborns?

Common Minor Anomalies

PHYSICAL FEATURE	BLACK INFANTS (%)	WHITE INFANTS (%)
Palpable metopic suture	42	64
Third sagittal fontanel	10	3

Double hair whorl	6	7
Overfolded ear helix	51	38
Preauricular sinus	5	0.8
Preauricular tag	0.7	0.3
Epicanthal folds, bilateral	1	1.4
Brushfield spots, bilateral	0.2	7
Anteverted nostrils	2	2.6
Supernumerary nipple	2.2	0.2
Umbilical hernia	6	0.7
Sacral dimple	0.6	4.8
Clinodactyly of both 5th fingers	4.5	5.2
Syndactyly, 2nd–3rd toes	0.5	0.6

Adapted from Holmes LB: Congenital malformations. In Behrman BE (ed): Nelson Textbook of Pediatrics, 14th ed. Philadelphia, W.B. Saunders, 1992, p 295, with permission.

41. What are the 3 principal types of sequences?

1. ***Malformation*** sequences (resulting from poor formation of tissues)
2. ***Deformation*** sequences (resulting from mechanical factors)
3. ***Disruptive*** sequences (initiated by a disruptive process)

Examples include:

- DiGeorge sequence
- Early urethral obstruction sequence
- Extrophy of cloaca sequence
- Oligohydramnios sequence
- Caudal dysplasia sequence
- Pierre Robin sequence
- Extrophy of bladder sequence
- Rokitansky sequence
- Sirenomelia sequence
- Early amnion rupture sequence
- Jugular lymphatic obstruction sequence

42. Describe the most common associations.

CHARGE: **C**oloboma of the eye, **H**eart defects, **A**tresia of the choanae, **R**etardation (mental and growth), **G**enital anomalies (in males), **E**ar anomalies

MURCS: **M**üllerian duct aplasia, **R**enal aplasia, **C**ervicothoracic **S**omite dysplasia

VATER: **V**ertebral, **A**nal, **T**racheo-**E**sophageal, **R**enal or **R**adial anomalies

VACTERL: VATER anomalies plus **C**ardiac and **L**imb anomalies

43. What are the major vascular disruption sequences?

• ***Poland anomaly***: unilateral defect of the pectoralis muscle and syndactyly of the hand. This is thought to be due to an early deficit of blood flow through the subclavian artery to the distal limb and pectoral region.

• ***Hydranencephaly***: congenital absence of the cerebral hemispheres. Although the cause of this devastating defect can be varied, bilateral internal carotid artery occlusion has been commonly postulated.

• ***Proximal focal femoral hypoplasia***: unilateral dysgenesis of the proximal femur. Etiologies for this defect include familial genetic disorders, teratogenic influences, viral agents, maternal diabetes, trauma, and ischemia caused by vascular disruption.

• ***Oromandibular-limb hypogenesis spectrum***: craniofacial, limb, and often brain defects. This spectrum of anomalies suggests a diffuse disruptive vascular occlusion or hemorrhagic etiology.

44. What malformations are associated with oligohydramnios and polyhydramnios?

In early pregnancy (< 4 mos), the majority of amniotic fluid is produced by transudation through the placental membranes and fetal skin. Later in pregnancy, the bulk of amniotic fluid arises as a product of fetal urination. At term, the fetus swallows approximately 500 ml of amniotic fluid per day and urinates an equivalent amount. Fetal urine production increases rapidly from 3.5 ml/hr at 25 weeks to 25 ml/hr at term. Any malformation that leads to impaired urine production will cause *oligohydramnios*, including renal dysplasia, renal agenesis, and bladder outlet obstruction. When uteroplacental insufficiency occurs, the fetus is often faced with poor nutritive and volume support. The fetus becomes intravascularly depleted, leading to increased fluid conservation and decreased urine output, causing oligohydramnios. Oligohydramnios is often associated with intrauterine growth retardation.

The etiology of *polyhydramnios* may be broken down into maternal causes (30%), fetal causes (30%), and idiopathic causes (40%). Maternal disorders, such as diabetes, erythroblastosis fetalis, and preeclampsia, are often associated with excess amniotic fluid. Fetal disorders that commonly predispose to polyhydramnios are CNS anomalies (anencephaly, hydrocephaly, neurologic disorders, etc.), GI disorders (tracheoesophageal fistula, duodenal atresia), fetal circulatory disorders, and multiple gestation. The etiology for polyhydramnios in fetuses with CNS and upper GI anomalies is presumed to be impaired fetal swallowing ability.

45. What causes Potter syndrome?

Potter syndrome has come to be synonymous with fetal malformations caused by extreme oligohydramnios. Lack of amniotic fluid leads to fetal compression, a squashed, flat face, clubbing of the feet, pulmonary hypoplasia, and, commonly, breech presentation. Normal fetal lung development is dependent on *in utero* "breathing" and inhalation of amniotic fluid. In the absence of amniotic fluid, pulmonary hypoplasia occurs and is the cause of death for most fetuses with Potter syndrome. The underlying mechanism in Potter syndrome was initially reported to be renal agenesis or renal dysplasia. However, bladder outlet obstruction and prolonged premature rupture of the membranes may also cause this sequence. Some prefer that Potter syndrome be defined solely as renal agenesis.

46. If an infant is born with Potter syndrome, why should the parents undergo a renal ultrasound?

Renal agenesis is thought to be a sporadic or multifactorial condition, although autosomal dominant inheritance with variable expression (i.e., unilateral renal agenesis in a parent) has also been postulated. For this reason, obtaining a renal ultrasound on parents of a child with renal agenesis is advised. If the parents have normal renal evaluations, the empirically determined recurrence risk is approximately 3%. If one of the parents has unilateral renal agenesis, the recurrence risk may be as high as 50% due to a presumed autosomal dominant gene.

47. How do clinodactyly, syndactyly, and camptodactyly differ?

- *Clinodactyly:* curvature of a toe or finger (usually the fifth) due to hypoplasia of the middle phalanx, which is the last fetal bone to develop in the hands and feet. Normal curvature can consist of up to 8° of in-turning. Curvature beyond this is considered a minor anomaly.
- *Syndactyly:* an incomplete separation of fingers (usually 3rd and 4th) or toes (usually 2nd or 3rd)
- *Camptodactyly:* abnormal persistent flexion of fingers or toes

48. Name the three major types of dermal ridge patterns.

Dermal ridge patterns are formed early in embryogenesis. Their pattern is influenced by genetic inheritance, the influence of teratogens, congenital infections, and chromosomal abnormalities. The distal phalanges have a variety of dermal ridge patterns that can be classified in three major types: ***arches***, ***whorls***, and ***loops***. Infants with trisomy 18 commonly have a high frequency of arches,.an unusual finding in chromosomally normal individuals. In the foot, there is a pattern at the base of the great toe. In 50%of patients with trisomy 21, a simple arch pattern (called an open field) will be found. This occurs in < 1%of controls.

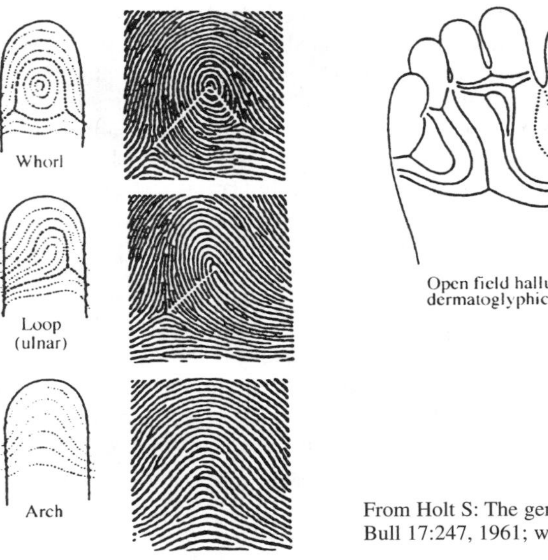

From Holt S: The genetics of dermal ridges. Br Med Bull 17:247, 1961; with permission.

49. Are preauricular ear tags a significant finding?

Preauricular pits and *tags* are minor anomalies that occur in about 0.3–1.0% of individuals, with a wide variance in frequency among racial groups. They are twice as common in females as in males and can be inherited as an autosomal dominant trait. They are believed to represent remnants of early embryonic branchial cleft or arch structures. As isolated findings, they do not warrant additional evaluations.

50. What is the proper way to test for low-set ears?

This designation is made when the upper portion of the ear (helix) meets the head at a level below a horizontal line drawn from the lateral aspect of the palpebral fissure. The best way to measure is to align a straight edge between the two inner canthi and determine whether the ears lie completely below this plane. In normal individuals, approximately 10% of the ear is above this plane.

From Feingold M, Bossert WH: Normal values for selected physical parameters: An aid to syndrome delineation. In Bergsma D (ed): The National Foundation-March of Dimes Birth Defects Series 10:9, 1974.

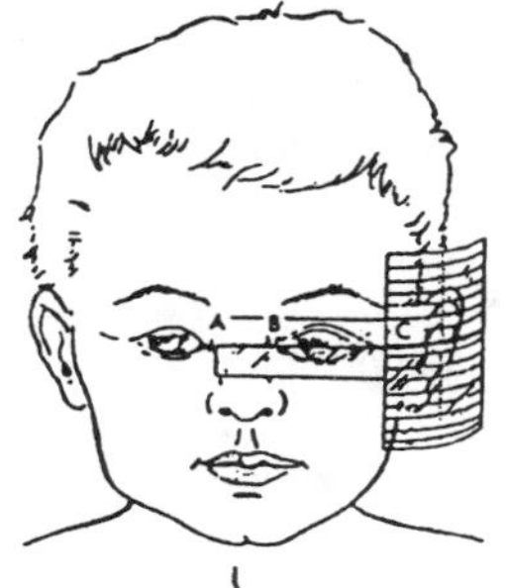

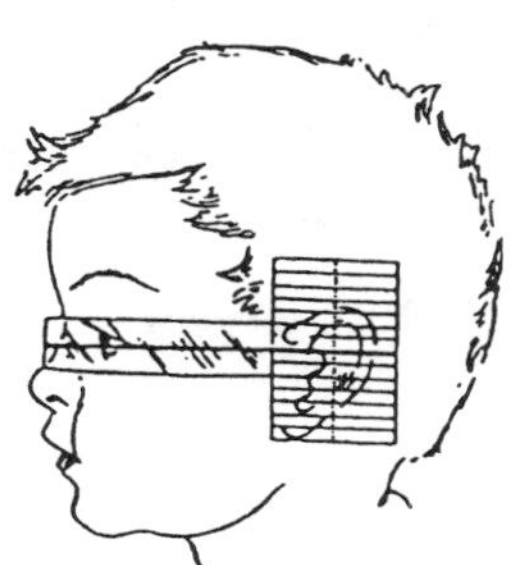

51. Where is the Darwinian tubercle located?

Also called the *auricular tubercle*, this is a cartilaginous bump on the ***upper part of the outer ear*** below and posterior to the helix. It is a minor variant that should not be considered an anomaly.

52. Why do the sclerae of patients with osteogenesis imperfecta appear blue?

Phylogenetically, the sclerae are closely related to the skeleton. In many animals, the sclera contains cartilage and osseous material. The primary component of sclera in humans is collagen. It is not surprising that in osteogenesis imperfecta and many other connective tissue diseases, the sclerae are abnormally thin and transparent, since abnormal collagen formation is the underlying defect in many of these disorders. The bluish color of the sclera in patients with connective tissue (especially collagen) diseases is thought to be due to visualization of the bluish-colored uvea (the eye layer behind the retina) as seen through a more transparent sclera. Uvea literally means grape, the name being derived from the similarity in their colors.

53. What is the significance of lip pits?

Lip pits derive from small, accessory salivary glands that fistulize on either side of the midline lower lip. This finding is most characteristic of Van der Woude syndrome, whose other features are cleft lip and/or palate and missing second premolars. Inheritance is autosomal dominant, yet variable expression often occurs, and in some cases only the lip pits will be present without the associated cleft lip and/or palate. Lip pits are seen less commonly in the rare popliteal pterygium syndrome.

54. What is the inheritance pattern of cleft lip and palate?

Most cases of cleft lip and palate are inherited in a ***polygenic*** or ***multifactorial pattern***. The male to female ratio is 3:2, and the incidence in the general population is approximately 1/1000. Recurrence risk after one affected child is 3–4%; after two affected children, 8–9%.

55. How can hypertelorism be rapidly assessed?

If an imaginary third eye would fit between the eyes, hypertelorism is possible. Precise measurement involves measuring the distance between the center of each eye's pupil. This is a difficult measurement in newborns and uncooperative patients because of eye movement. In practice, the best way to determine hypotelorism or hypertelorism is to measure the inner and outer canthal distances, then plot these measurements on standardized tables of norms.

56. Which syndromes are associated with iris colobomas?

Colobomas of the iris are due to abnormal ocular development and embryogenesis. They are frequently associated with chromosomal syndromes, most commonly trisomy 13, 4p–, 13q–, and triploidy. In addition, they may be commonly found in the CHARGE association, Goltz syndrome, and Rieger syndrome. Whenever iris colobomas are noted, chromosome analysis is recommended. The special case of complete absence of the iris (aniridia) is associated with the development of Wilms tumor and may be caused by an interstitial deletion of the short arm of chromosome 11.

57. How large is the posterior fontanel in the healthy term infant?

In 97% of full-term infants, the posterior fontanel is normally ***fingertip size or smaller***. Large posterior fontanels can be seen in infants with congenital hypothyroidism, skeletal dysplasias, or increased intracranial pressure.

58. On which side does the newborn "crown" usually sit?

In the fetus, hair follicles on the skin surface grow downward during weeks 10–16. During this time, the brain and scalp expand outward in a dome-like fashion, pulling the follicles in different directions, and at 18 weeks, when the hair erupts, patterns are set. The "crown," or parietal hair whorl, is the focal point of this outgrowth. At birth, it is usually a few centimeters anterior to the posterior fontanel. 55% of single parietal scalp whorls are left of midline (presumably secondary to the larger size of the left brain), 30% are right-sided, and 15% are midline. 5% of normal individuals have bilateral hair whorls. Abnormal positioning of the hair whorl (particularly a posterior location) can be seen in microcephaly.

GENETIC PRINCIPLES

59. Why is chromosomal banding such a valuable asset?

Chromosome banding was introduced in the early 1970s and has revolutionized cytogenetics. Prior to banding, all chromosomes appeared as solid, dark figures and could not be individually identified. Stains such as Giemsa and quinacrine can now be used to differentially stain certain chromosome regions, producing a characteristic striped pattern that can accurately identify each chromosome. Even small chromosome fragments can often be identified on the basis of their banding patterns. Contiguous gene disorders are syndromes due to a microdeletion of specific chromosomal regions. Examples of microdeletion syndromes include Prader-Willi syndrome, Angelman syndrome, Miller-Dieker syndrome, and DiGeorge/velocardiofacial syndrome. While the deletions are sometimes detectable on a karyotype, submicroscopic deletions cannot be visualized even on high-resolution chromosome banding. These deletions can be detected by fluorescent in situ hybridization (FISH). In this technique, a DNA probe specific for the chromosomal region of interest is hybridized to the chromosomes. A fluorescent signal is attached to the probe so that the number of copies of the DNA corresponding to the probe can be determined for each cell. Normally, two copies of each region, one on each chromosome, should be present. If a deletion has occurred, only one of the copies will be seen. This technique has aided in the diagnosis of microdeletion syndromes that were formerly difficult to detect because of their small size.

Gopal Rao VVN, Roop H, Carpenter NJ: Diagnosis of microdeletion syndromes: high-resolution chromosome analysis versus fluorescence in situ hybridization. Am J Med Sci 309:208–212, 1995.

60. Why has the polymerase chain reaction (PCR) revolutionized molecular genetics?

Most DNA techniques require a microgram of DNA, and this amount is often difficult to obtain. PCR is a technique that allows a millionfold amplification of a specific DNA fragment from a sample as small as a billionth of a microgram. The DNA to be amplified is denatured by heating the sample. In the presence of DNA polymerase and excess deoxynucleotide triphosphates, oligonucleotides that hybridize specifically to the target sequence prime new DNA synthesis. The first cycle is characterized by a product of indeterminate length. However, the second cycle produces the discrete short product which accumulates exponentially with each successive round of amplification. This leads to the millionfold amplification of the discrete fragment over the course of 20–30 cycles. PCR and other recently developed molecular techniques have led to a boom in the identification of genes associated with clinical disorders.

Muenke M: Finding genes involved in human developmental disorders. Curr Opin Genet Dev 5:354–361, 1995.

61. How are restriction enzymes used in the diagnosis of genetic disorders?

Restriction enzymes (restriction endonucleases) are enzymes purified from bacteria which cut double-stranded DNA at precise nucleotide sequences. Each enzyme is named for the organism from which it was obtained (e.g., *Eco*RI from *Escherichia coli*), and each has its own specific recognition sequence of 4–8 bases (e.g., GAATTC). If there is an alteration at this recognition site, the sequence becomes unrecognizable to the restriction enzyme, and the DNA will not be cut. Restriction enzyme analysis is one approach for direct detection of some mutant genes. For example, the sickle cell mutation (adenine changes to thymine at codon 6) alters the recognition site for the restriction enzyme *Mst*II. Cleavage at the normal location does not occur in the DNA molecules that contain the mutation, and a longer fragment is created. Techniques are available to size the resulting enzyme fragments to see if a normal or variant fragment (i.e., gene) exists.

62. Why is RFLP an MVP in genetic analysis?

The lengths of DNA digested by restriction enzymes result in fragments of various sizes. If a patient has a mutation, the size of the fragments may vary because the DNA sequence at the restriction site has been altered. These *restriction fragment length polymorphisms* (RFLP) may be inherited with certain diseases and differ from the general population when certain restriction enzymes and identifying DNA probes are used. Comparative analysis can identify carriers.

63. What is a linkage map?

Linkage is the coinheritance of two or more nonallelic genes because their loci are in close proximity on the same chromosome. A *linkage map* is a chromosome map showing the relative positions of genetic markers of a given species, as determined by linkage analysis.

64. How does mosaicism develop?

Mosaicism is the possession of multiple chromosomally different cell lines in a single individual. Most mosaicism involves the sex chromosomes and occurs because of defects in mitosis in an early embryo. Normally, chromosomes duplicate and separate equally in mitotic division. Mosaicism occurs when the chromosomes fail to separate (mitotic nondisjunction) or fail to migrate (anaphase lag). In general, the greater the proportion of abnormal cell lines, the more abnormal the phenotype. The earlier in embryonic development an abnormal cell line is established, the higher the percentage of abnormal cells in that individual.

65. What causes chimerism in infants?

The term *chimera* is derived from the Greek mythological monster which, according to Homer, had the head of a lion, body of a goat, and tail of a dragon. In cytogenetic parlance, chimerism is the presence of two or more cell lines in an individual which are derived from two separate zygotes. The most common cause of chimerism is the mixing of blood from unlike-sexed twins, resulting in a karyotype of 46,XX/46,XY. Chimerism can also result from the admixture of cells from a nonviable twin into a surviving fetus or, most rarely, from incorporation of two zygotes into a single embryo.

66. What is the risk of having a child with a recessive disorder when the parents are first or second cousins?

First cousins may share more than one deleterious recessive gene. They have $\frac{1}{8}$ of their genes in common, and their progeny are homozygous at $\frac{1}{16}$ of their gene loci. Second cousins have only $\frac{1}{32}$ genes in common. The risk that consanguineous parents will produce a child with a severe or lethal abnormality is ***6%*** for first-cousin marriages and ***1%*** for second-cousin marriages.

67. Identify the common symbols used in the construction of a pedigree chart.

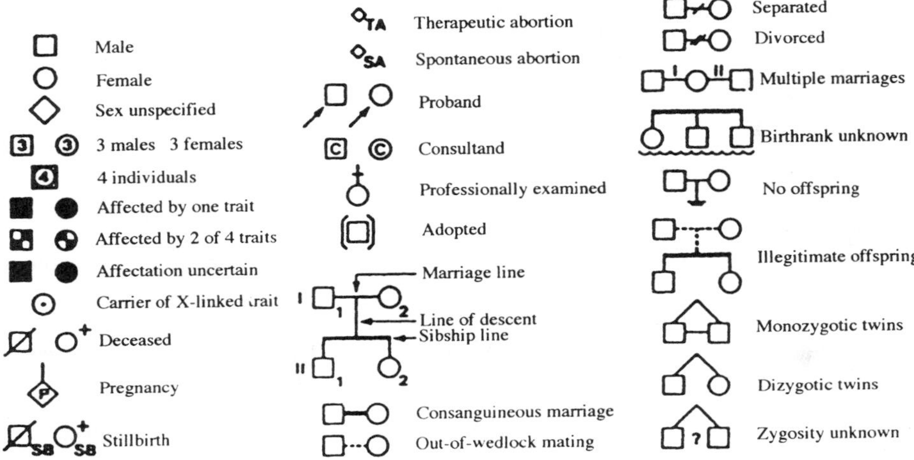

68. How does a reciprocal translocation differ from a robertsonian translocation?

A *chromosome translocation* is a transfer of chromosomal material between two (or more) nonhomologous chromosomes. The exchange is usually *reciprocal* (the two segments trading places). The genetic content of the individual is therefore complete but rearranged. *Robertsonian* translocation represents a special variety of chromosome translocation in which the long arms of two acrocentric chromosomes (#13, 14, 15, 21, or 22) fuse at their centromeres. The breaks may occur within, above, or below the centromeres. The short arms are usually lost, but this does not produce an abnormality since the genetic material on the short arms of acrocentric chromosomes occurs in multiple copies throughout the genome. A phenotypically normal individual with a robertsonian translocation has only 45 chromosomes inasmuch as the long arms of two acrocentric chromosomes are fused into one.

69. Why is a parent with a 14;21 robertsonian translocation at risk for having multiple miscarriages and/or children with birth defects?

When a parent with a translocation undergoes gametogenesis, six chromosomally different types of gametes can be formed due to unequal segregation of chromosomes during meiosis. The possible outcomes are trisomy 14 (which will abort), monosomy 14 (which will abort), monosomy 21 (which will abort), normal, trisomy 21 (Down syndrome), and a balanced robertsonian translocation (just like the parent).

70. How can an autosomal recessive disease occur when only one parent is a carrier?

Uniparental disomy is an inheritance pattern in which a child receives two identical chromosomes from one parent and none from the other. The most likely explanation is an abnormality in meiosis whereby one gamete receives an extra copy of a homologous chromosome due to an error in separation. This gamete with two copies from one parent then unites with the gamete of the other parent. If the second gamete lacks that particular chromosome (i.e., nullisomic gamete), a normal karyotype results. If the second gamete contains that particular chromosome, a trisomic zygote results. During embryonic development, this trisomy may be lost, resulting in a normal karyotype. Uniparental disomy has been reported in some patients with Prader-Willi, Angelman, and Beckwith-Weidemann syndromes as well as cystic fibrosis and hemophilia A.

71. How can the same genotype lead to different phenotypes?

In ***parental imprinting*** (an area of the regulation of gene expression that is incompletely understood), the expression of an identical gene is dependent on whether the gene is inherited from the mother or father. For example, in Huntington disease, the clinical manifestations occur much earlier if the gene is inherited from the father rather than the mother. Modification of the genes by methylation of the DNA during development has been hypothesized as one explanation of the variability.

72. 46,XY,t(4:8)(p21;q22)—what does it all mean?

46	Normal number of chromosomes
XY	Genetic male
t(4:8)	The first set of parentheses refers to the chromosomes. The symbol in front indicates the change: **t** stands for reciprocal translocation, **del** for deletion, **dup** for duplication, and **inv** for inversion.
(p21;q22)	The second set of parentheses refers to the bands on the chromosomes. The short arm symbol is **p**; the long arm symbol is **q**.

In this case, a genetic male with a normal number of chromosomes has a reciprocal translocation between the short arm of chromosome 4 at band 21 and the long arm of chromosome 8 at band 22.

SEX CHROMOSOME ABNORMALITIES

73. What are the features of the four most common sex chromosome abnormalities?

Most Common Sex Chromosome Disorders

	47,XXY (KLINEFELTER)	47,XYY	47,XXX	45,X (TURNER)
Frequency of live births	1/2000	1/2000	1/2000	1/8000
Maternal age association	+	–	+	–
Phenotype	Tall, eunuchoid habitus, underdeveloped secondary sexual characteristics, gynecomastia	Tall, severe acne, indistinguishable from normal males	Tall, indistinguishable from normal females	Short stature, web neck shield chest, pedal edema at birth, coarctation of the aorta
IQ and behavior	80–100; behavioral problems	90–110; behavioral problems; aggressive behavior	90–110; behavioral problems	Mildly deficient to normal intelligence spatial-perceptual difficulties
Reproductive function	Extremely rare	Comon	Common	Extremely
Gonad	Hypoplastic testes, Ledig cell hyperplasia, Sertoli cell hypoplasia, seminiferous tubule dysgenesis, few spermatogenic precursors	Normal size testes, normal testicular histology	Normal size ovaries, normal ovarian histology	Streak ovaries with deficient follicles

From Donnenfeld AE, Dunn LK: Common chromosome disorders detected prenatally. Postgrad Obstet Gynecol 6:5, 1986; with permission.

74. What did Lyon hypothesize?

The Lyon hypothesis is that in any cell, only one X chromosome will be functional. Any other X chromosomes present in that cell will be condensed, late replicating, and inactive (called the Barr body). The inactive X may be either paternal or maternal in origin, but all descendants of a particular cell will have the same parentally derived chromosome inactive. Inactivation is initially random, occurring at the 16-day (blastocyst) stage of embryonic development. For example, in normal females (46,XX), one X chromosome is inactive. In normal males (46,XY), the X is always active, since it is the only one present. In 48,XXXY individuals, there will be two inactive X chromosomes per cell. The process of X inactivation allows for gene dosage compensation in females and poly-X males.

75. Is it possible to get identical twins of different sexes?

Yes. If anaphase lag (loss) of a Ychromosome occurs at the time of cell separation into twin embryos, a female fetus with karyotype 45,X (Turner syndrome) and a normal male fetus (46,XY) results.

76. How commonly does mosaicism occur in Turner syndrome?

At least ***35%*** of chromosome abnormalities in individuals with Turner syndrome are mosaics. The most common are 45,X/46,XX, and 45,X/46,XX/47,XXX, and 45,X/46,XY. Whenever a cell line with a Y chromosome is identified in a phenotypic female, gonadectomy is recommended due to a high risk of malignancy in the gonads of these individuals.

77. Of the four most common types of sex chromosomal abnormalities, which is identifiable at birth?

Only infants with ***Turner syndrome*** have physical features easily identifiable at birth. Features include:

- Dorsal hand and pedal edema
- Web neck (pterygium colli)
- Broad chest with wide-spaced nipples
- Prominent ears
- Low posterior hairline
- Congenital elbow flexion (cubitus valgus)
- Narrow, hyperconvex nails
- Short fourth metacarpal and/or metatarsal

78. What causes the webbing of the neck in Turner syndrome?

Failure of canalization between the cervical and jugular lymphatic vessels causes trapped lymphatic fluid to accumulate progressively and to form large posterior nuchal cysts called cystic hygromas. Occasionally, resolution of fluid accumulation may occur during gestation with regression of the cystic hygroma, formation of nuchal webbing (called pterygium colli), nuchal skin redundancy, alteration in the zone of hair growth, protrusion of the lower auricles, and morphologic alterations of the fetal face. This is known as the *jugular lymphatic obstruction sequence*. It is hypothesized that if only a partial or temporary obstruction occurs, egress of lymphatic fluid may be possible, and the cystic hygroma will resolve with only redundant nuchal skinfolds remaining. Therefore, the entire obstruction sequence will not develop. However, others believe that the pathogenesis of the web neck is not related to lymphatic obstruction but occurs as a primary developmental defect due to the chromosomal abnormality.

79. Describe the similarities and differences between Noonan syndrome and Turner syndrome.

Similarities: short stature, web neck, cardiac defects, low posterior hairline, broad chest, wide-spaced nipples, edema of the dorsum of the hands and feet, cubitus valgus

Differences:

Turner syndrome	***Noonan syndrome***
Affects females only	Affects both males and females
Chromosome disorder (45,X)	Normal chromosomes, autosomal dominant disorder
Near-normal intelligence	Mental deficiency
Coarctation of aorta is most common cardiac defect	Pulmonary stenosis is most common cardiac defect

Amenorrhea and sterility due to ovarian dysgenesis	Normal menstrual cycle in females

80. What is the most common inherited form of mental retardation?

Fragile X syndrome. It affects an estimated 1 in 1000 males and 1 in 2000 females. Approximately 2%-6% of male subjects and 2%-4% of female subjects with unexplained mental retardation will carry the full fragile X mutation.

81. What is the nature of the mutation in fragile X syndrome?

When the lymphocytes of an affected male are grown in a folate-deficient medium and the chromosomes examined, a substantial fraction of X chromosomes demonstrate a break near the distal end of the long arm. This site, the fragile X mental retardation-1 gene (FMR-1), was identified and sequenced in 1991. At the center of the gene is a repeating trinucleotide sequence (CGG) which, in normal individuals, repeats 6–45 times. However, in carriers, the sequence expands to 50–200 times (called a premutation), and in fully affected individuals, it expands to 200–600 copies. These longer sequences cause malfunctioning of the gene. Expansion of trinucleotide repeat sequences are responsible for several other diseases, including the neurodegenerative disorders myotonic dystrophy, spinocerebellar ataxia type 1, Kennedy disease, and Huntington disease.

82. What are the associated medical problems in fragile X syndrome in males?

Flat feet (80%), macro-orchidism (80% after puberty), mitral valve prolapse (50 – 80% in adulthood), recurrent otitis media (60%), strabismus (30%), refractive errors (20%), seizures (15%), scoliosis (< 20%).

Lachiewicz AM et al: Physical characteristics of young boys with fragile X syndrome. Am J Med Genet 92:229-236, 2000.

83. What is the outcome for girls with fragile X?

Heterozygous females who carry the fragile X chromosome have more behavioral and developmental problems (including attention deficit hyperactivity disorder), cognitive difficulties (50% with an IQ in the mentally retarded or borderline range), and physical differences (prominent ears, long and narrow face). Cytogenetic testing is recommended for all sisters of fragile X males.

Hagerman RJ, et al: Girls with fragile X syndrome: Physical and neurocognitive status and outcome. Pediatrics 89:395–400, 1992.

84. How common are subtle chromosomal rearrangements in children with unexplained mental retardation (MR)?

In cases of moderate to severe MR, chromosomal and genetic disorders account for 30%-40% and environmental factors for 10%-30%, but no explanation exists in 40%. In mild mental retardation, 70% of cases have unknown causes. Using fluourescence in-situ hybrization (FISH) techniques, subtle rearrangements were discovered in 7.4% of moderate-to-severe MR and 0.5% of mild MR. Most common were abnormalities (balanced translocation and submicroscopic subtelomeric rearrangements) in chromosomal ends (terminal bands called subtelomeric regions). Subtelomeric probes should be considered in screening all individuals with unexplained MR.

Knight SJL et al: Subtle chromosomal rearrangements in children with unexplained mental retardation. Lancet 354:1676-1681, 1999.

85. What is the name of the name of the condition associated with facial capillary hemangioma, developmental delay and seizures in some affected individuals?

Sturge-Weber syndrome.

In this condition, there is a facial capillary hemangioma, which is usually unilateral, but may be bilateral and in most cases is within the area innervated by the trigeminal nerve. There may be glaucoma or bupthalmos and angioma of the leptomeninges present as well.

The condition is due to lack of regression of an embryonic vascular plexus. Seizures, hemipariesis and developmental delay may occur. Developmental delay is more likely if seizures occur in the first year of life. Calcifications of the cerebral cortex with a typical "tramline" appearance appear after 2 years of age. CT scan and MRI are the best modalities for demonstrating the intracranial lesions. Sturge-Weber syndrome is almost always sporadic.

86. What genetic disorder is associated with polyostosis fibrous dysplasia, café-au-lait spots with "coast of Maine" borders and sexual precocity?

The ***McCune-Albright syndrome***.

This sporadic disorder is associated with café-au-lait patches, which tend to be large and terminate abruptly at the midline. The majority of reported cases are females.
Polyostosis fibrous dysplasia and sexual precocity are present in the syndrome. There may also be hyperfunction of multiple endocrine tissues. somatic mutations in Exon 8 of the Gsα gene have been documented. The mutations are postzygotic and mosaic in distribution. The mutations result in increase cyclic AMP formation and hyperfunction of multiple endocrine tissues.

87. What is an "ash-leaf spot?"

This is a hypopigmented skin lesion, which has a lance-ovate shape and resembles the shape of a mountain ash tree. This and other hypomelanotic macules are seen in about 80% of individuals with tuberous sclerosis (TSC). Other skin lesions of TSC are so called (1) adenoma sebaceum, which are better called facial angiofibromas because histologically they are made up of connective tissue and blood vessels, (2) shagreen patch, a raised orange-skin like patch in the thoracolumbar region (3) forehead plaques are raised patches which appear in childhood. (4) ungual and subungual fibromas appear in adulthood and grow under or around the toenails. Seizures occur in about 60% of patients and mental retardation about an equal number. Renal angiomyolipomas are seen in up to 80% of individuals and may lead to renal failure in adults.

Congenital rhabdomyosarcomas are almost always associated with tuberous sclerosis. TSC is an autosomal dominant disorder. There are two genes, TSC1 is on chromosome 9q34 and TSC2 on 16p13. Both genes have been cloned and a variety of mutations have been identified in different TSC patients.

88. What is the single most frequent manifestation of Turner syndrome at birth?

Lymphedema of the feet and/or hands may be the only manifestation of Turner syndrome in the newborn period. Other features, which may be present at that age, are short neck with excess nuchal folds, wide-spaced nipples and coarctation of the aorta.

89. What syndrome is associated with CATCH22?

This acronym has been used to describe the salient features of ***DiGeorge/Velo-cardio-facial syndrome***.

C : **C**ongenital heart disease
A : **A**bnormal face
T : **T**hymic aplasia/hypoplasia
C : **C**left palate
H : **H**ypocalcemia
22: microdeletion of chromosome **22**q11

The cardiovascular lesions frequently encountered are tetralogy of Fallot, truncus arteriosis, interrupted aortic arch, right-sided aortic arch and double outlet right ventricle. Any infant with any of the above cardiovascular lesions should be screened for DiGeorge/Velo-cardio-facial syndrome.

90. "Go FISH" usually means what in genetic parlance?

Fluorescence In Situ Hybridization (FISH). This is a molecular cytogenetic method of combining DNA probes and fluorescence methods in identifying whole chromosomes or specific regions of a chromosome. It is most often used in pediatric patients for the detection of microdeletions in conditions such as Prader-Willi syndrome, Angelman syndrome, DiGeorge syndrome, and unusual chromosome translocations. It is also used widely in cancer cytogenetics.

American Academy of Pediatrics, Committee on Genetics: Molecular genetic testing in pediatric practice: A subject review. Pediatrics 106:1494-1497, 2000.

91. What is a "triplet" expansion disorder?

These are a group of genetic disorders, which are caused by abnormal expansion of trinucleotide repeat sequences.

Examples of such disorders are fragile "X" syndrome, myotonic dystrophy, Huntington Disease, the spinocerebellar ataxias, Friedrich ataxia and Kennedy disease.

In each of these disorders, the normal copy of the gene is made up of trinucleotide repeats (triplets), which vary in number from person to person but may not exceed a predetermined size. When the number of trinucleotide repeat exceeds the threshold, the repeats may become exceedingly large and impair the function of the gene leading to an abnormal phenotype.

For example, in fragile "X" syndrome, the normal gene is made up of CGG trinucleotide repeats of up to about 50. Affected individuals, mostly males but also females, have repeating CGG-units, which exceed 230. Carrier females and males that have a premutation state carry a CGG-repeat size of 50-230. It is expected that over time, many other disorders belonging to this class of genetic disorders will be described.

In myotonic dystrophy, the normal gene has 5-35 CTG repeats but in affected individuals repeat size may range from 100 to 2000. There is a tendency for the repeat number to increase from one generation to the next. This explains the phenomenon of "anticipation" in which the age of onset of myotonic dystrophy is earlier and more severe in younger generations.

TERATOLOGY

92. Which drugs are known to be teratogenic?

Most teratogenic drugs exert a deleterious effect in a minority of exposed fetuses. Exact malformation rates are unavailable due to the inability to perform a statistical evaluation on a randomized, controlled population. Known teratogens include:

DRUG	MAJOR TERATOGENIC EFFECT	DRUG	MAJOR TERATOGENIC EFFECT
Thalidomide	Limb defects	Androgens	Virilization
Lithium	Ebstein tricuspid valve anomaly	Tetracycline	Teeth and bone maldevelopment
Aminopterin	Craniofacial and limb anomalies	Streptomycin	Ototoxicity
Methotrexate	Craniofacial and limb anomalies	Warfarin	Nasal hypoplasia, bone maldevelopment
Phenytoin	Facial dysmorphism, dysplastic nails	Penicillamine	Cutis laxa
Trimethadione	Craniofacial dysmorphism, growth retardation	Accutane retinoic acid)	Craniofacial and cardiac
Valproic acid	Neural tube defects	Propylhiouracil	Goiter
Diethylstilbestrol (DES)	Müllerian anomalies, clear cell adenocarcinoma	Radioactive iodine	Hypothyroidism

93. Describe the characteristic features of the fetal hydantoin syndrome.

***Craniofacial*:** Broad nasal bridge, wide fontanel, low-set hairline, broad alveolar ridge, metopic ridging, short neck, ocular hypertelorism, microcephaly, cleft lip/palate, abnormal or low-set ears, epicanthal folds, ptosis of eyelids, coloboma, and coarse scalp hair

***Limbs*:** Small or absent nails, hypoplasia of distal phalanges, altered palmar crease, digital thumb, and dislocated hip

Approximately 10% of infants whose mothers took phenytoin (Dilantin) during pregnancy have a major malformation; 30% have minor abnormalities.

94. Does cocaine cause fetal malformations?

***Yes*.** Several malformations are associated with maternal cocaine use. All are believed to be due to a disruption in normal organ growth and development as a result of vascular insufficiency. Intestinal atresias due to mesenteric artery vasoconstriction or thrombosis and urinary tract anomalies, including urethral obstruction, hydronephrosis, and hypospadias, are most commonly reported. Limb reduction defects, often described as transverse terminal defects of the forearm or amputation of the digits of the hands and feet, have also been identified. The type of disruption will depend on the timing of cocaine exposure during pregnancy, the dosage and frequency of cocaine administration, and susceptibility of the embryo or fetus. The teratogenic influences of cocaine are not limited to the first trimester. Vasoconstriction may lead to infarction in a wide variety of organs; however, it is most common in the fetal brain. Additionally, uteroplacental insufficiency due to vasculopathy, chronic abruption, thrombosis, or a combination of these problems is a well-known cause of intrauterine growth retardation in cocaine-exposed fetuses.

95. What amount of alcohol is safe to ingest during pregnancy?

This is unknown. The full dysmorphologic manifestations of fetal alcohol syndrome are associated with heavy intake. However, most infants will not display the full syndrome. For infants born to women with lesser degrees of alcohol intake during pregnancy who demonstrate more subtle abnormalities (e.g., cognitive and behavioral problems), it is more difficult to ascribe risk because of confounding variables (e.g., maternal illness, pregnancy weight gain, other drug use, especially marijuana). Furthermore, it appears that infants prenatally exposed to similar amounts of alcohol are likely to have different consequences for reasons that are unclear. Because current data do not support the concept that any amount of alcohol is safe during pregnancy, the AAP recommends abstinence from alcohol for women who are pregnant or planning to become pregnant.

Committee on Substance Abuse and Committee on Children with Disabilities: Fetal alcohol syndrome and fetal alcohol effects. Pediatrics 91:1004–1006, 1993.

96. What are the frequent features of the fetal alcohol syndrome?

Skull	Microcephaly, mid-face hypoplasia
Eyes	Short palpebral fissures, epicanthal folds, ptosis, strabismus
Mouth	Hypoplastic philtrum, thin upper lip, prominent lateral palatine ridges, retrognathia in infancy, micrognathia or relative prognathia in adolescence
Nose	Flat nasal bridge, short and upturned nose
Cardiac	Ventricular septal and atrial septal defects
Skeletal	Pectus excavatum, altered palmar crease patterns, small fifth fingernails
Skin	Hemangiomas
CNS	Mild to moderate mental retardation, poor coordination, fine motor impairment, hypotonia, irritability in infancy, hyperactivity in childhood
Growth	Prenatal: small for gestational age Postnatal: < 2 SD for length and weight, disproportionately diminished adipose tissue

97. What happens to children with fetal alcohol syndrome when they grow up?

A follow-up study of 61 adolescents and adults revealed that relative short stature and microcephaly persisted, but facial anomalies became more subtle. Academic functioning, particularly in arithmetic, was delayed to the early grade-school level. Intermediate or significant maladaptive behavior was present in 100% of patients. Severely unstable family environments were common.

Streissguth AP, et al: Fetal alcohol syndrome in adolescents and adults. JAMA 265:1961–1967, 1991.

9. HEMATOLOGY

Anne F. Reilly, M.D., and Steven E. McKenzie, M.D., Ph.D.

BONE MARROW FAILURE

1. What are the types of bone marrow failure?

Bone marrow failure is manifested by *pancytopenia* or, at times, by *cytopenia* of a *single cell type*. It can be *acquired* (acquired aplastic anemia) or *inherited/genetic* (e.g., Fanconi anemia, Kostmann syndrome, Diamond-Blackfan anemia, amegakaryocytic thrombocytopenia, thrombocytopenia-absent radius).

2. What are the causes of acquired aplastic anemia?

After careful exclusion of the known causes listed below, over 80% of cases remain classified as *idiopathic*. A variety of associated conditions include:

Radiation

Drugs and *chemicals*
- Regular: cytotoxic, benzene
- Idiosyncratic: chloramphenicol, anti-inflammatory drugs, antiepileptics, gold

Viruses
- Epstein-Barr virus
- Hepatitis (primarily B)
- Parvovirus (in immunocompromised hosts)
- HIV

Immune diseases
- Eosinophilic fasciitis
- Hypogammaglobulinemia

Thymoma

Pregnancy

Paroxysmal nocturnal hemoglobinuria

Preleukemia

Adapted from Alter BP, Young NS: The bone marrow failure syndromes. In: Nathan DG, Orkin SH (eds): Nathan and Oski's Hematology of Infancy and Childhood, 5th ed. Philadelphia, W.B. Saunders, 1998, p 238.

3. What is the definition of severe aplastic anemia?

Severe disease includes a ***hypocellular bone marrow biopsy*** (< 30% of the normal hematopoietic cell density for age) and ***decreases in at least two of three peripheral blood counts***: neutrophil count < 500 cells/mm^3, platelet count < 20,000/ mm^3, or reticulocyte count < 1% after correction for the hematocrit. Categorization has important prognostic and therapeutic implications.

4. What are the treatments and prognosis for children with aplastic anemia?

In the absence of definitive treatment, fewer than 20% of children with severe acquired aplastic anemia survive for > 2 years. When bone marrow transplantation is performed using an HLA-identical sibling donor, the 2-year survival rate exceeds 85%. The usual approach to the newly diagnosed child with severe acquired aplastic anemia is to perform bone marrow transplantation if there is a HLA-identical sibling to serve as the donor.

Approximately 80% of children with severe aplastic anemia do not have a sibling donor for bone marrow transplantation. These children receive medical therapy, usually the combination of anti-thymocyte (ATG), cyclosporine, and hematopoietic growth factors, such as granulocyte–macrophage colony-stimulating factor (GM-CSF) or granulocyte colony-stimulating factor (G-CSF). Two year response and survival rates for combination medical therapy now exceed 80% in children.

5. What is the probable diagnosis in a 6-year-old with pancytopenia, short stature, abnormal thumbs, and areas of hyperpigmentation?

Fanconi anemia, or constitutional aplastic anemia, is a genetic disorder in which numerous physical abnormalities are often present at birth, and aplastic anemia occurs around age 5 years. The more common physical abnormalities include hyperpigmentation, anomalies of the thumb and radius, small size, microcephaly, and renal anomalies, such as absent, duplicated, or pelvic horseshoe kidneys. When patients are recognized early in life on the basis of the physical abnormalities, the early signs of bone marrow failure, including elevated mean corpuscular volume (MCV), may be detected before clinical problems related to pancytopenia occur. Mild thrombocytopenia may occur in infancy or early childhood, but the platelet count may remain only slightly depressed for 4 or 5 years until the usual picture of bone marrow failure occurs. *Chromosomal breakage analysis* can be used to make the diagnosis, and *molecular diagnosis* can confirm the diagnosis and be used to test relatives. On studies of peripheral blood lymphocytes, a high percentage of patients with Fanconi anemia will have chromosomal breaks, gaps, or rearrangements, especially in the face of treatment with double-stranded DNA crosslinking agents e.g., diepoxybutane (DEB) and mitomycin C. The genes responsible for Fanconi anemia groups A, C, and G have been identified, and molecular analysis for causative mutations is available.

6. Do aplastic anemia and Fanconi anemia lead to leukemia?

For *aplastic anemia*, late clonal hematological disease includes PNH (paroxysmal nocturnal hemoglobinuria), myelodysplasia, and acute myeloid leukemia. The actuarial incidence after 5 to 10 years from diagnosis and treatment of aplastic anemia is on the order of *20%* for these complications in aggregate. The natural history of *Fanconi anemia*, as a chromosome breakage syndrome, is one of elevated risk for hematologic and non-hematologic malignancies in the 2nd to 4th decades of life.

7. How is transient erythroblastopenia of childhood (TEC) distinguished from Diamond-Blackfan anemia?

Both are disorders of red cell production that occur in early childhood. It is extremely important to distinguish TEC from Diamond-Blackfan syndrome—TEC is a self-limited disorder, whereas Diamond-Blackfan syndrome usually requires life-long treatment. While there is an overlap in the age of presentation, Diamond-Blackfan syndrome commonly causes anemia in the first 6 months of life, whereas TEC occurs more frequently after age 1 year. Both disorders are characterized by a low hemoglobin level and an inappropriately low reticulocyte count. The bone marrows may be indistinguishable, showing reduced or absent erythroid activity in both cases. The red cells in patients with Diamond-Blackfan syndrome have fetal characteristics that are useful in distinguishing this disorder from TEC, including increased mean cell volume, elevated level of hemoglobin F, and presence of i antigen. The level of adenine deaminase may be elevated in patients with Diamond-Blackfan syndrome but normal in children with TEC. 25% of Caucasian patients with Diamond-Blackfan anemia have been found to have mutations in the gene for ribosomal protein S19 (RP S19), and molecular diagnosis for RP S19 gene mutations is very helpful when positive.

Draptchinskaia N, et al: The gene encoding ribosomal protein S19 is mutated in Diamond-Blackfan anaemia. Nature Genetics. 21(2):169-75, 1999.

Willig T-N, et al: Identification of new prognosis factors from the clinical and epidemiologic analysis of a registry of 229 Diamond-Blackfan anemia patients. Pediatr Res 46:553-561, 1999.

8. What is Kostmann syndrome?

Kostmann syndrome is ***severe congenital neutropenia***. At birth or shortly thereafter, very severe neutropenia (absolute neutrophil count of 0–200/mm^3) is noted, often at the time of significant bacterial infection, such as deep skin abscess, pneumonia, or sepsis. Even with antibiotic treatment, there is a high mortality in infancy unless G-CSF therapy is used to elevate the neutrophil count. An alternative treatment is bone marrow transplantation from an HLA-identical sibling donor.

CLINICAL ISSUES

9. What is the hemoglobin value (lower limit of normal) below which children are considered to be anemic?

Newborn (full term)	13.0 gm/dl	*4–8 years*	11.5
3 months	9.5	*8–12 years*	11.5
1–3 years	11.0	*12–16 years*	12.0

Dallman P, Siimes MA: Percentile curves for hemoglobin and red cell volume in infancy and childhood. J Pediatr 94:27, 1979.

10. In patients with severe chronic anemia, how rapidly can transfusions be given?

When anemia is chronic, there has been cardiovascular adaptation and a relatively normal blood volume. Excessively rapid transfusions can lead to congestive heart failure. For patients with a hemoglobin < 5 gm/dl who exhibit no signs of cardiac failure, a safe regimen is to transfuse packed red blood cells at a rate of *1–2 ml/kg/hr* by continuous infusion until the desired target is reached. One ml/kg will raise the hematocrit by 1% in most patients. Judicious use of a diuretic like furosemide or automated erythrocytapheresis in larger children can be considered.

Jayabose S, et al: Transfusion therapy for severe anemia. Am J Pediatr Hematol Oncol 15:324–327, 1993.

11. When does the physiologic anemia of infancy occur?

Physiologic anemia occurs at 8–12 weeks in full-term infants and 6–8 weeks in premature infants. Full-term infants may exhibit hemoglobin levels as low as 9 gm/dl at this time and very premature infants as low as 7 gm/dl.

12. Why does the physiologic anemia of infancy occur?

The mechanism(s) responsible for physiologic anemia is not completely understood. Red blood cell (RBC) survival time is decreased in both premature and full-term infants. Furthermore, the ability to increase erythropoietin production in response to ongoing tissue hypoxia is somewhat blunted, even though the response to exogenous erythropoietin is normal. The precise signals that tell infants to increase RBC production are not clear. However, factors that control the infant's ability to deliver oxygen to tissues (e.g., oxygen saturation, hemoglobin-oxygen dissociation curve, cardiac output, red cell mass) as well as the metabolic demands of these tissues appear to be important.

13. In what settings of shortened RBC survival can the reticulocyte count be normal or decreased?

As a rule, the reticulocyte count is elevated in conditions of shortened RBC survival (e.g., hemoglobinopathies, membrane disorders, immune hemolysis) and decreased in anemias characterized by impaired RBC production (e.g., iron deficiency, aplastic anemia). The reticulocyte count may be unexpectedly low in setting of shortened RBC survival if an aplastic or hypoplastic crisis is occurring at the same time, such as is seen with parvovirus infection. In addition, in immune-mediated hemolysis the autoantibody may react with antigens present on reticulocytes, leading to increased clearance of these cells. In chronic states of hemolysis, the marrow may become unresponsive secondary to micronutrient deficiency (e.g., iron, folate) or a reduction in erythropoietin production as seen in chronic renal failure.

14. How does the pathophysiology of anemia differ in acute and chronic infection?

Chronic infection and other inflammatory states impair the release of iron from reticuloendothelial cells, thereby decreasing the amount of this necessary ingredient available for RBC production. The lack of mobilizable iron may be due to the action of proinflammatory cytokines such as IL-1 and TNFα. Giving additional iron under these circumstances further increases reticuloendothelial iron stores and does little to help the anemia. *Acute infection* may cause anemia through a variety of mechanisms, including bone marrow suppression, shortened RBC lifespan, red cell fragmentation, and immune-mediated RBC destruction.

15. Describe the differential diagnosis for children presenting with splenomegaly and anemia.

The main question is whether the anemia is the cause of the splenomegaly or the splenomegaly is the cause of the anemia. Examples of anemia causing splenomegaly include hemolytic anemias in which the spleen plays an active role, such as membrane disorders, sickling disorders, and thalassemia syndromes. The major example of splenomegaly causing anemia is hypersplenism due to chronic liver disease and portal hypertension. In this instance, the anemia results from sequestration of RBCs in the enlarged spleen. Accompanying features usually include mild leukopenia and thrombocytopenia.

Anemia causing splenomegaly	***Splenomegaly causing anemia***
• Membrane disorders	• Cirrhotic liver disease
• Hemoglobinopathies	• Cavernous transformation of portal vessels
• Enzyme abnormalities	• Storage diseases
• Immune hemolytic anemia	• Persistent viral infections

16. A 14-month-old presents with marked cyanosis, lethargy, and normal oxygen saturation by pulse oximetry after drinking from a neighbor's well. What is the likely diagnosis?

Methemoglobinemia should always be considered when a patient presents with cyanosis without demonstrable respiratory or cardiac disease. The most common causes are oxidant toxins, such as antimalarial drugs or nitrates in food or well water. Congenital methemoglobinemia is due to inherited abnormalities of the enzymes that lead to reduction of methemoglobin, or presence of the abnormal M hemoglobins that seem to stabilize hemoglobin in the ferric form. Recently the use of inhaled nitric oxide as therapy for persistent pulmonary hypertension has led to neonatal cases of methemoglobinemia.

Symptoms can range from simple cyanosis (methemoglobin < 30%) to headache, lethargy, and altered consciousness (30–70%). Levels above 70% can be fatal. In an acute situation when levels are > 30%, treatment consists of 1–2 mg/kg of 1% methylene blue administered intravenously over 5 minutes and repeated in 1 hour if levels have not fallen to normal. Failure to respond to therapy should raise the possibility of G6PD deficiency, which prevents the conversion of methylene blue to the metabolite that is active in the treatment of methemoglobinemia. In these cases, hyperbaric oxygen therapy or exchange transfusion may be necessary. Chronic methemoglobinemia, as observed with inherited enzyme abnormalities or M hemoglobinopathies, may result in chronic cyanosis without symptoms. In these patients, oral ascorbic acid may occasionally be useful. Of note, patients with cyanosis due to methemoglobinemia can have normal oxygen saturation as measured by pulse oximetry since the oximeter operates by measuring only hemoglobin that is available for saturation.

17. How can the diagnosis of methemoglobinemia be made at the bedside?

In methemoglobinemia, the inability of the red cell to maintain hemoglobin iron in the ferrous (Fe^{2+}) state leads to a loss of oxygen-carrying capacity. When a drop of blood from a patient with methemoglobinemia is placed on a piece of filter paper, it generally has a brownish color. When the filter paper is waved in the air, the color of the blood remains brown because the hemoglobin is unable to bind oxygen. In contrast, blood from a normal individual turns from brown to red when the filter paper is waved in the air.

18. Why are infants at greater risk for the development of methemoglobinemia?

- *Anti-oxidant defense mechanisms* (e.g., soluble cytochrome b_5 and NADH-dependent cytochrome b_5 reductase) are 40% lower in infants than teenagers.
- Infants' *intestinal pH* is relatively alkaline compared with older children's. If nitrates are ingested (as in fertilizer-contaminated well water), this higher pH more readily allows bacterial conversion of nitrate to nitrite, which is a potent oxidant.
- They are more susceptible to various *oxidant exposures:* nitrate reductase from foods such as undercooked spinach, menadione (vitamin K_3) for prevention of neonatal hemorrhage, over-the-counter teething preparations with benzocaine, or metoclopramide for gastroesophageal reflux.

Bunn HF: Human hemoglobins: Normal and abnormal. In: Nathan DG, Orkin SH (eds): Nathan and Oski's Hematology of Infancy and Childhood, 5th ed. Philadelphia, W.B. Saunders, 1998, pp 729-751.

19. Which organs produce erythropoietin?

The ***kidney*** is the primary manufacturing site, but the cell of origin is unclear. The fetal **liver** and, to a lesser extent, adult liver are also capable of production. The role of macrophages in synthesis is disputed.

20. What are indications for erythropoietin (EPO) therapy in the pediatric population?

The most clearly proven indication is therapy for the ***anemia*** associated with *end-stage renal disease*. Other indications include anemia induced by *chemotherapy*, anemia for *HIV-positive* patients on antiretroviral therapy, and anemia of *chronic inflammation*. The use of EPO in the neonatal setting as prophylaxis or treatment for various types of anemia (e.g., anemia associated with prematurity, fetal isoimmune hemolytic anemia) remains under study. Frequently, supplemental iron is needed for full efficacy of erythropoietin, even when the iron stores are full but cannot be mobilized, as in anemia of chronic inflammation. The most common general side effects include an influenza-like syndrome, development of iron deficiency in the absence of iron supplementation, and neutropenia (rarely). Side effects such as hypertension, clotting of vascular access devices, and seizures are much more prevalent in adults being treated for end-stage renal disease.

21. What are the indications for the use of leukoreduced red blood cells?

When packed red cells are prepared from whole blood and then filtered, most of the remaining white cells are removed from the product. Since febrile transfusion reactions are usually due to leukocytes, filtered products should be used for patients who have experienced such reactions to previous blood transfusions. Filtered red cells are also effective in reducing the transmission of cytomegalovirus in at risk individuals. In addition, use of filtered blood components reduce the risk of HLA alloimmunization, desirable in repeatedly transfused patients and those who may need stem cell or solid organ transplants.

22. What is the most common genetic disease among persons of northern European descent?

Hemochromatosis has a prevalence of 1:200 to 1:250 for homozygosity and a carrier rate of 1:8 to 1:12. Screening has traditionally been done by measuring serum transferrin, iron saturation and ferritin levels. Transferrin saturation may be elevated by age 10 and in almost all homozygous individuals by age 40. Early diagnosis is key as measures can be undertaken to delay cirrhosis. A recently identified novel MHC class I gene called HFE has been identified and testing for this gene will likely replace iron studies as the main screening tool. In most cases of hereditary hemochromatosis, the gene is mutated. In the U.S., it is estimated that 80%-90% of patients with hemochromatosis have the abnormality.

El-Serag HB et al: Screening for hereditary hemochromatosis in siblings and children of affected patients: A cost-effective analysis. Ann Intern Med 132:261-269, 2000.

COAGULATION DISORDERS

23. What features on history or physical exam help pinpoint the cause of a bleeding problem?

The history sought should be that of both the patient and the patient's extended family. While there can be considerable overlap, in general, *platelet* problems result in petechiae, especially on dependent parts of the body and mucosal surfaces. Additional manifestations of platelet disorders include epistaxis, hematuria, menorrhagia, and gastrointestinal hemorrhages. Ecchymoses are suspicious for *coagulation factor deficiencies* or *platelet* problems when they occur in unusual areas, are out of proportion to the extent of described trauma (also seen in child abuse), or are present in different stages of healing. Delayed bleeding from old wounds and extensive hemorrhage (particularly into joint spaces or following immunizations) are also suggestive of coagulation protein disorders. Bleeding from multiple sites in an ill patient is worrisome for *disseminated intravascular coagulation*. Of note, if a patient has tolerated tonsillectomy and/or adenoidectomy or extraction of multiple wisdom teeth without major hemorrhage, a significant inherited bleeding disorder is unlikely.

24. What are the inheritance patterns of the common bleeding disorders?

The inheritance of von Willebrand disease, the most common coagulopathy, is autosomal dominant in the majority of cases. Factor VIII deficiency (hemophilia A) and factor IX deficiency (hemophilia B) are inherited in an X-linked pattern so that females are carriers and males are affected. Inquiry about affected maternal male first cousins or uncles is appropriate. In general, heterozygotes for clotting factor deficiencies are not clinically affected. However, evidence indicates that some heterozygotes for deficiencies or dysfunction of anticoagulant proteins, such as Factor V Leiden, protein C and antithrombin III, may have problems related to hypercoagulation such as venous thrombosis.

25. Why is the lack of a family history of bleeding problems only moderate evidence against the likelihood of hemophilia A in a patient?

The abnormal Factor VIII gene responsible for hemophilia A exhibits marked heterogeneity, and up to a third of cases (either the immediate carrier mother or the son himself) may have developed a spontaneous mutation. Molecular diagnosis of the most common mutation in severe Factor VIII deficiency, a gene inversion in the distal portion of the gene, in the affected male, the mother and maternal relatives may help in understanding the family history.

26. Which is more common, factor VIII or factor IX deficiency?

Factor VIII deficiency (hemophilia A) is more common, affecting 80–85% of all patients with clinically diagnosed factor deficiency.

27. How are the doses of replacement factor calculated for a hemophiliac with or without life-threatening hemorrhage?

For moderate (1–5% of normal factor levels) to severe (< 1% of normal) hemophilia, recombinant Factor VIII or Factor IX concentrates are the treatments of choice. For minor hemorrhages, such as knee and elbow bleeds, factor levels should be increased to 20–30% of normal. For major bleeding episodes, such as hip bleeds, intracranial hemorrhage, or bleeding around the airway, factor levels should be raised to 70–100% and repeat dosing strongly considered under close medical supervision. Each unit of Factor VIII or Factor IX is equivalent to the activity in 1 ml of normal plasma. With the recombinant products, a dose of one unit/kg should increase the Factor VIII level by 1.5 to 2% and the Factor IX level by 1%.

Lee C: Recombinant clotting factors in the treatment of hemophilia. Thromb Haemostas 82: 516-524, 1999.

Kelly K et al: Superior in vivo response of recombinant factor VIII concentrate in children with hemophilia A. J Pediatr 13: 507-509, 1997.

28. Why do hemophiliacs bleed if there are two pathways of coagulation, intrinsic and extrinsic?

The concept of the intrinsic and extrinsic pathways of coagulation has been useful in identifying the basis for abnormalities in the PT (prothrombin time) and aPTT (activated partial thromboplastin time) screening tests. The ***extrinsic pathway*** initiates clotting through factor VII and tissue factor (TF) and together with the common pathway is measured by the PT. The ***intrinsic pathway*** is activated via Factor XII, and together with the common pathway is measured by the aPTT. A newer understanding of the clotting process has emerged in recent years, emphasizing the central role of thrombin and the role of membrane-associated coagulation protein complexes, as depicted in the figure. Clotting is closely regulated in space and time. While Factor VII/TF initiates most clotting in the body, the complex is rapidly inactivated by TFPI (tissue pathway factor inhibitor). The thrombin generated activates Factor XI, and further activation from there to activation of Factor X requires physiological levels of Factor VIII and IX. If functional levels of one of these (Factor VIII or Factor IX) is too low, efficient clotting cannot proceed and bleeding results.

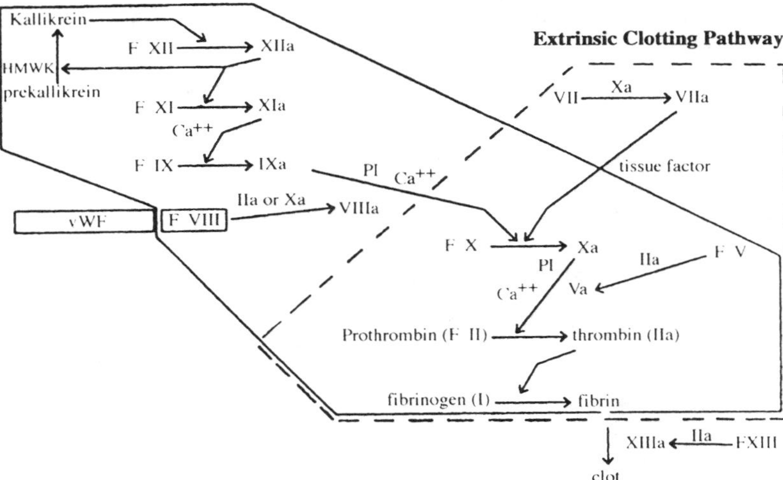

Adapted from Montgomery RR, et al: Newborn haemostasis. Clin Haematol 14:443, 1985; with permission.

29. Can someone with isolated Factor XII deficiency causing an elevated aPTT undergo surgery?

The aPTT test requires functional Factor XII in the test tube to activate Factor XI, and in Factor XII deficiency the aPTT is prolonged. However, because there is an alternative for activation of Factor XI in the body via FVII/TF leading to generation of thrombin, the risk of perioperative bleeding with isolated Factor XII deficiency is considered to be that of the average patient. It is prudent to know the personal and family bleeding histories in an individual with a prolonged aPTT, to rule out Factor XI, IX, VIII and von Willebrand factor deficiencies, and to rule out the presence of an inhibitor of coagulation, before the diagnosis of isolated Factor XII deficiency can be made.

30. What can cause an elevation of the PT with other coagulation testing being normal?

Factor VII deficiency. As noted above, PT measures the function of the common pathway factors (including X, V, II, fibrinogen) as well as the extrinsic pathway (tissue factor and Factor VII). The aPTT measures the common pathway plus the function of the intrinsic pathway (including Factors XII, XI, IX, VIII). Isolated Factor VII deficiency selectively elevates the PT. Other causes of elevated PT, liver disease, Vitamin K deficiency, or warfarin toxicity, are not selective in lowering Factor VII activity.

31. What are the half-lives of exogenously administered factors VIII and IX?

The half-lives for the *first* doses of Factors VIII and IX are 6–8 hours and 4–6 hours, respectively. With *subsequent* doses, Factor VIII has a half-life of 8–12 hours, while factor IX has a half-life of 18–24 hours. Thus, for serious bleeding, the second dose of Factor VIII should be given 6–8 hours after the first, while the second dose of Factor IX should be given 4–6 hours after the first. Subsequent doses are usually given every 12 hours for factor VIII replacement and every 24 hours for Factor IX, but measurement of actual factor levels may be necessary to guide therapy in life-threatening situations.

Gill JC: Transfusion principles for congenital coagulation disorders. In Hematology: Basic Principles and Practice, 3rd ed. R. Hoffman, et al (eds). New York, Churchill Livingstone, 2000, pp 2282-2290.

32. In hemophiliacs who develop inhibitors to factor infusions, what differentiates "low responders" from "high responders"?

About 25% of patients with hemophilia A (but < 5% with hemophilia B) develop IgG antibodies to Factor VIII following infusion. Depending on the extent of response, the development of inhibitors can greatly complicate management. *Low responders* do not exhibit significant increases in titers with repeated transfusions and can be treated with increased amounts of factor VIII. *High responders* have an anamnestic response to factor replacement, and repeated treatments can result in substantial elevations in inhibitor titers. A variety of approaches may be tried including:

- Recombinant Factor VIIa infusion
- Activated and nonactivated prothrombin complex concentrates (to bypass the block)
- Porcine factor VIII (which has little cross-reactivity with human Factor VIII)
- In emergent situations, administration of large quantities of Factor VIII, perhaps by continuous infusion and/or after plasmapheresis to lower inhibitor levels. This treatment, however, will lead to even higher inhibitor titers in a matter of days.

Hedner U: Treatment of patients with Factor VIII and Factor IX inhibitors with special focus on the use of recombinant Factor VIIa. Thrombo Haemostas 82: 531-539, 1999.

33. What is the role of desmopressin (DDAVP) in the treatment of hemophilia and von Willebrand disease?

DDAVP, a synthetic analog of vasopressin, increases levels of factor VIII and von Willebrand factor by allowing release from storage sites. It can be used for patients with mild hemophilia or von Willebrand disease. It is contraindicated in Type IIB von Willebrand disease, as it has been associated with more severe thrombocytopenia in those patients. A dose of 0.3 μg/kg given intravenously will raise baseline levels by 300–400% in many individuals. More recently, unit dose intranasal DDAVP formulated specifically for bleeding disorders (Stimate) has become available. Its use requires documentation of efficacy for the specific patient and reduction in free water intake for approximately 8 hours following intranasal use to avoid hyponatremia.

34. Can hemophilia be cured?

Gene therapy offers hope of this. A phase I trial of gene therapy for Factor IX deficiency in adults has encouraging early results with respect to safety and possible efficacy, but much more work remains to be done. The gene encoding Factor VIII is much larger, and this has complicated its use in gene therapy.

Kay M, et al: Evidence for gene transfer and expression of Factor IX in haemophilia B patients treated with an AAV vector. Nature Genetics 24: 257-261, 2000.

35. Who gets "hemophilia C"?

More commonly called *Factor XI deficiency*, this is an uncommon cause of hemophilia (<5% of total patients). Unlike the X-linked nature of hemophilia A and B, it is an autosomal recessive disease that occurs most frequently in ***Ashkenazi Jews***.

Asadai R, et al: Factor XI deficiency in Ashkenazi Jews in Israel. N Engl J Med 325:153–158, 1991.

36. Why is factor IX deficiency also called "Christmas disease"?

In 1952, investigators in England noted that when blood from one group of hemophiliacs was added to the blood of another group of hemophiliacs, the clotting time was shortened. This provided the basis for the discovery of plasma substances in addition to what was then called antihemophilic globulin (and now called Factor VIII) responsible for normal clotting. The name was derived because the first patient examined in detail with the unusual clotting deficiency (later designated as Factor IX) was a boy named Christmas. The publication of the landmark article in fact occurred in the last week in December 1952.

Biggs R, et al: Christmas disease: A condition previously mistaken for haemophilia. BMJ 262: 1378–1382, 1952.

37. What causes the coagulation abnormalities in von Willebrand disease?

von Willebrand disease is actually a group of disorders that involves the von Willebrand factor (vWF), which is a multimeric glycoprotein complexed to factor VIII in the plasma. The common variants are listed below. vWF serves as a bridge between damaged endothelium and adhering platelets and facilitates platelet attachment. von Willebrand disease is a heterogenous disorder caused by qualitative or quantitative abnormalities in vWF. Either variety of abnormality can result in improper formation of a platelet plug and reduction in Factor VIII quantities (due to the importance of vWF in minimizing the clearance of Factor VIII from plasma and in accelerating its cellular synthesis). Coagulation abnormalities in children with severe disease can include a prolonged bleeding time, prolonged PTT, decreased Factor VIII coagulant activity, decreased factor VIII antigen, and decreased ability of patient plasma to induce aggregation of normal platelets in the presence of ristocetin, the so-called ristocetin cofactor activity.

Common Variants of von Willebrand Disease

	TYPE 1	TYPE IIA	TYPE IIB
Frequency	70–80%	10–12%	3–5%
Genetic transmission	Autosomal dominant	Autosomal dominant	Autosomal dominant
Ristocetin cofactor activity	↓	↓↓↓	±↓
Low-dose ristocetin-induced platelet aggregation	Normal	Normal	Increased
Multimeric electrophoretic pattern	Normal mixture (various sizes)	Large and intermediate forms absent	Large multimers absent

Adapted from Montgomery RR, Scott JP: Hemostasis: Diseases of the fluid phase. In Nathan DG, Oski FA (eds): Hematology of Infancy and Childhood, 4th ed. Philadelphia, W.B. Saunders, 1993, p 1622; with permission.

38. What are the best screening diagnostic tests for suspected von Willebrand disease?

The diagnosis can be difficult because test results can vary widely among patients. Stress, pregnancy, or medications (e.g., oral contraceptives) can cause variation even in an individual patient. Although the bleeding time and PTT are often abnormal, in milder disease, they are frequently normal. Thus, they are insensitive alone as screening tests. However, if in addition to the bleeding time and PTT, the vWF activity (i.e., ristocetin cofactor activity) is measured, over 90% of patients with von Willebrand disease will demonstrate at least one abnormality. More extensive (and expensive) testing, including vWF antigen, factor VIII clotting activity, ristocetin-induced platelet aggregation, and multimer analysis, can be done to determine subtype or to eliminate false-negatives if clinical suspicion remains high.

39. In what settings outside the newborn period can vitamin K abnormalities contribute to a bleeding diathesis?

Vitamin K is essential for gamma-carboxylation of both procoagulants (including Factors II, VII, IX, X) and anticoagulants (proteins C and S). Gamma-carboxylation occurs in the liver and converts the proteins to their functional forms. Vitamin K is obtained in three ways: (1) as dietary fat-soluble K_1 (phytonadione) from leafy vegetables and fruits, (2) as K_2 (menaquinone) from synthesis by intestinal bacteria, and (3) as water-soluble K_3 (menadione) from commercial synthesis. *Malabsorptive intestinal disorders* (e.g., cystic fibrosis, Crohn disease, short bowel syndrome), *prolonged antibiotic therapy* (which diminishes intestinal bacteria), *prolonged hyperalimentation without supplementation*, and *malnutrition* can result in diminished stores. *Chronic hepatic disorders* (e.g., hepatitis, α_1-antitrypsin deficiency) can diminish both absorption of fat-soluble vitamin K (secondary to diminished bile salt production) and utilization of vitamin K in factor conversion. *Drugs* that can disrupt vitamin K include phenobarbital, phenytoin, rifampin, and warfarin.

40. What is the best test for distinguishing between coagulation disturbances secondary to hepatic disease, disseminated intravascular coagulation (DIC), and vitamin K deficiency?

Factors II, V, VII, IX, and X are made in the liver, and all of these factors except Factor V are vitamin K-dependent. Therefore, measurement of ***Factor V*** is a useful test to distinguish liver disease from vitamin K deficiency, since this factor is reduced in the former and normal in the latter disorder. Factor VIII is reduced in patients with DIC because of the consumptive process, but this factor is normal or increased in liver disease and vitamin K deficiency. Therefore, the ***Factor VIII*** level is a good test to distinguish DIC from the other two disorders.

Coagulation Abnormalities in Liver Disease, Vitamin K Deficiency, and DIC

	FACTOR V	FACTOR VII	FACTOR VIII
Liver disease	Low	Low	Normal or increased
Vitamin K deficiency	Normal	Low	Normal
DIC	Low	Low	Low

41. What is the treatment of choice for DIC?

DIC occurs most commonly in the context of bacterial sepsis and hypotension. The best treatment is reversal of the underlying cause through treatment of the infection and appropriate fluid and pressor management. If bleeding is severe or if hemorrhage is occurring in a life-threatening location, platelets and fresh frozen plasma should be given to make up for the loss of these elements which are occurring from consumption. Heparin has not been proved to be effective in increasing survival in patients with sepsis and DIC. The replenishment of depleted antithrombin III levels with antithrombin III concentrate may decrease the risk of new thromboses.

42. How is anticoagulant therapy monitored in children?

The goal of therapy with *unfractionated heparin* therapy is to raise the ***PTT*** to 1.5–2 times the normal level. However, the relationship between heparin level and prolongation of the PTT depends on the particular reagents that are used in the coagulation laboratory. Therefore, it is useful to check with the coagulation laboratory to see if they have established a range for the PTT at therapeutic heparin levels. *Low molecular weight heparin* (LMWH), which is usually administered subcutaneously, does not require monitoring of the aPTT under normal circumstances because the dose-response with this form of heparin is much more predictable. The reduction in laboratory costs partially offsets the higher cost of the drug itself, and it is often the drug of choice for home use. In neonates and small children, laboratory monitoring of the anti-Factor Xa activity is recommended in LMWH therapy. Also, the dosing of LMWH frequently needs to be adjusted upward in infants due to differences in metabolism in comparison with older children and adults.

Changes in the ***PT*** are used to monitor *warfarin (coumadin)* therapy. In the past, the prolongation of the PT by 1.5 times normal was the usual therapeutic goal. However, differences in reagents used in different laboratories made it difficult to monitor individual patients tested in different laboratories or to compare patients enrolled in multicenter clinical trials. The INR (international normalized ratio) provides a measure of prolongation of the PT that is standardized against a common reagent. Thus, a therapeutic INR of 2–3.5 means the same thing no matter where the test is performed.

Andrew M, et al: Thromboembolic Complications during Infancy and Childhood. Hamilton, Ontario, BC Decker, 2000.

43. What are the common hereditary disorders that predispose a child to thrombosis?

- ***Factor V Leiden:*** An abnormal Factor V protein that is resistant to the normal antithrombotic effect of activated protein C. (Heterozygote for Factor V mutation present in 3-6% of children.)
- ***Protein C deficiency:*** Protein C inactivates Factors V and VIII and stimulates fibrinolysis. Homozygous individuals can present in the newborn period with purpura fulminans.
- ***Protein S deficiency:***Protein S serves as a cofactor for the activity of protein C.
- ***Antithrombin III deficiency:*** Antithrombin III is involved in the inhibition of thrombin, Factor X, and to a lesser extent, Factor IX.

Other thrombophilic disorders include a ***variation in prothrombin*** (gene position 20210 AT) and ***hyperhomocysteinemia***, often due to mutation in the MTHFR gene. Acquired prothrombotic states in neonates can be due to ***antiphospholipid antibodies*** from an affected mother.

Male C, et al: Clinical significance of lupus anticoagulants in children. J Pediatr 134:1999-205, 1999.

Hagstron JN, et al: Prevalence of factor V Leiden mutation in children and neonates with thromboembolic disease. J Pediatr 133:777-781, 1998.

HEMATOLOGY LABORATORY

44. Of the seven red cell parameters given by a Coulter counter, which are measured and which are calculated?

The Coulter counter, the most commonly used automated electronic cell counter, utilizes the impedance principle. A precise volume of blood passes through an narrow aperture and impedes an electrically charged field, and each "blip" is counted as a cell. The larger the red cell, the greater the electric displacement. In a separate chamber, the same volume is hemolyzed and colorimetrically analyzed to determine the hemoglobin concentration.

Measured values
- Red blood cell (RBC) count
- Mean corpuscular volume (MCV)
- Hemoglobin (Hb)

Calculated values
- Mean corpuscular hemoglobin (MCH, in pg/cell) = (10 × [Hb/RBC])
- Mean corpuscular hemoglobin concentration (MCHC, in gm/dl) = (100 × [Hb/Hct])
- Hematocrit (Hct, in %) = (RBC × [MCV/10])
- Red cell distribution width (RDW) = coefficient of variation in RBC size

45. What factors can interfere with electronically derived red cell indices?
- ***Hyperleukocytosis:*** Overestimates the hemoglobin determination because of increased turbidity during measurement. Similarly, the MCV and RBC count can be artifactually elevated (usually when WBC count > 50,000/mm^3) because WBCs are counted as RBCs.
- ***Cold agglutinins:*** May lower the RBC count, as aggregated collections are counted as a single cell. MCV may thus be artifactually high.
- ***Hyperglycemia:*** When hyperglycemia is prolonged, RBCs become hyperosmolar and expand when placed in diluent. This results in an artifactually high MCV and hematocrit.
- ***Hypernatremia:*** Similar to hyperglycemia.
- ***Hypertriglyceridemia:*** If very elevated, can increase turbidity and result in an artifactually high hemoglobin concentration.

Stockman J: Using electronic RBC counts to diagnose anemia. Contemp Pediatr 6:99, 1989.

46. How does the mean corpuscular volume help provide a quick screen of the possible causes of anemia?

Microcytic: iron deficiency, thalassemias, sideroblastic anemia

Normocytic: autoimmune hemolytic anemia, hemoglobinopathies, enzyme deficiencies, membrane disorders, anemia of chronic inflammation

Macrocytic: disorders of B_{12} and folic acid metabolism, bone marrow failure

47. What is a quick rule of thumb for approximating MCV?

70 + (age in years). This number (in mm^3) approximates the lower limit of MCV in children less than the age of 10 years, below which microcytosis is present.

48. In addition to an elevated reticulocyte count, what laboratory studies suggest increased destruction (rather than decreased production) of RBCs as a cause of anemia?
- ***Increased serum erythrocyte lactate dehydrogenase (LDH):*** More commonly seen in hemolytic diseases, it can be greatly elevated in ineffective erythropoiesis (e.g., megaloblastic anemia).
- ***Decreased serum haptoglobin:*** When RBCs lyse, serum haptoglobin binds the released hemoglobin and is excreted. However, up to 2% of the population has congenitally absent haptoglobin.
- ***Hyperbilirubinemia (indirect):*** Usually increased with RBC lysis. However, it may also be elevated in ineffective erythropoiesis (e.g., megaloblastic anemia). Additionally, 2% of the population have Gilbert disease. In these patients, acute infection can cause a transient elevation of bilirubin secondary to liver enzymatic dysfunction rather than hemolysis.

49. What is the difference between the direct and indirect Coombs test?

Coombs serum is rabbit anti-human Ig. In the *direct* test, the Coombs serum is added directly to a patient's washed RBCs. The occurrence of agglutination means that the patient's RBCs have been sensitized *in vivo* by antibody. The *indirect* test involves incubating a patient's serum with RBCs of a known type and adding Coombs serum. If *in vitro* sensitization occurs, agglutination will result, indicating antibodies are present against the known blood type. Direct Coombs testing is vital in diagnosing autoimmune hemolytic anemias, while indirect testing is key in blood crossmatching.

50. How is the corrected reticulocyte count calculated?

Because the reticulocyte count is expressed as a percentage of total RBCs, it must be corrected according to the extent of anemia with the following formula: *reticulocyte % × (patient Hct/normal Hct) = corrected reticulocyte count*. For example, a very anemic 10-year-old patient with a hematocrit of 7% (contrasted with an expected normal hematocrit of 36%) and a reticulocyte count of 5% has a corrected reticulocyte count of 1.0% (5% × 7%/36% = 1%), which is not appropriately elevated as might be seen in severe iron deficiency. The key concept is the appropriateness of the reticulocyte response to anemia: the corrected "retic count" should be elevated if the bone marrow is working properly and has all the right nutrients for making RBCs, including iron, folate and vitamin B_{12}.

51. What is the significance of targeting on an RBC smear?

Red cell targets on a peripheral smear are caused by excessive membrane relative to the amount of hemoglobin. Therefore, *target cells* are found when the membrane is increased, as in patients with liver disease, or when the intracellular hemoglobin is diminished, as in patients with iron deficiency or thalassemia trait. Target cells may also be found in patients with certain hemoglobinopathies, such as hemoglobin C and hemoglobin SC. In these instances, the target cells are caused by aggregation of the abnormal hemoglobin.

52. In what conditions are Howell-Jolly bodies found?

Howell-Jolly bodies are nuclear remnants found in red cells of patients with ***reduced or absent splenic function*** and in patients with ***megaloblastic anemias***. They are occasionally present in the red cells of premature infants. Howell-Jolly bodies are dense, dark, and perfectly round, and their characteristic appearance makes them easily distinguishable from other red cell inclusions and from platelets overlying red cells.

53. What is the cause of Heinz bodies?

Heinz bodies represent ***precipitated denatured hemoglobin*** in the red cell. Heinz bodies occur when the hemoglobin is intrinsically unstable, as in hemoglobin Koln, or when the enzymes that normally protect hemoglobin from oxidative denaturation are abnormal or deficient, as in G6PD deficiency. These inclusions are not visible with a routine Wright-Giemsa stain but can be seen readily with methyl violet or brilliant cresyl blue stains.

54. Of what clinical value is the sedimentation rate?

An elevated erythrocyte sedimentation rate (ESR) is a nonspecific marker for inflammatory disease. The rate of sedimentation increases when inflammatory paraproteins bind to the RBC surface. The test may be of some value in suggesting the presence of deep-seated infection or collagen vascular disease, particularly in patients with fever of unknown origin. Unfortunately, there are few data to define the predictive value of the ESR in this setting. A better use of the ESR may be the monitoring of the response to therapy in particular infections, such as bacterial endocarditis and osteomyelitis. In these conditions, a falling ESR is considered to be a reliable indicator of the resolution of the inflammatory process.

55. What conditions give a low sedimentation rate?

Low ESRs may be due to a ***reduction in the concentration of large proteins*** (nephrosis, liver disease, congestive heart failure), **abnor*mal red cell membrane*** (sickle cell disease), or ***polycythemia*** (cyanotic congenital heart disease). A low ESR, however, has little diagnostic value. In fact, it may create confusion by masking the normally increased ESR that is expected during infection in, for example, a patient with nephrotic syndrome and peritonitis or a patient with sickle cell anemia and osteomyelitis.

56. For which hematology disorders is molecular diagnsosis available and useful?

This is an ever-growing list, including:

Hemoglobin disorders: sickle cell disease; α-thalassemia syndromes; β-thalassemia syndromes; δ-thalassemia syndromes

RBC enzyme disorders: G6PD (A- and other variants), PK deficiency

RBC membrane disorders: hereditary spherocytosis (α spectrin, β spectrin, band 3, ankyrin)

Neutrophil disorders: Leukocyte adhesion deficiency (LAD) type I, LAD II, chronic granulomatous disease, cyclic neutropenia

Platelet disorders: Glanzmann thrombasthenia; Bernard-Soulier syndrome; Wiskott-Aldrich syndrome and X-linked thrombocytopenia

Procoagulant protein deficiencies: Factor VIII; Factor IX; Factor XI among others

Prothrombotic disorders: Factor V Leiden; prothrombin; MTHFR

Bone marrow failure disorders: Fanconi anemia; Diamond Blackfan anemia

Iron overload: hereditary hemochromatosis

HEMOLYTIC ANEMIA

57. What two types of RBC forms are commonly seen on the peripheral smear in patients with hemolytic anemia?

1. ***Spherocytes or microspherocytes***. These forms can be seen in any hemolytic anemia that results from a loss of RBC membrane surface area (e.g., Coombs positive hemolytic anemia, DIC, or hereditary spherocytosis).

2. ***Schistocytes***. These various forms of fragmented RBCs can be seen in microangiopathic hemolytic anemia, a form of intravascular hemolysis from mechanical disruption (e.g., prosthetic heart valves, hemolytic-uremic syndrome, cavernous hemangioma).

58. Which disorder is most commonly associated with an elevated mean cell hemoglobin concentration (MCHC)?

Hereditary spherocytosis. The hyperchromic appearance of spherocytes and microspherocytes is due to loss of surface membrane, an excess of hemoglobin, and mild cellular dehydration. In other hemolytic anemias associated with spherocytosis, the percentage of spherocytes is usually insufficient to raise the MCHC.

59. Name the two most common inherited disorders of red cell membranes.

Hereditary spherocytosis and hereditary elliptocytosis. *Hereditary spherocytosis* is characterized by hemolysis (anemia, reticulocytosis, jaundice, splenomegaly), spherocytosis, and, in most cases, a family history of hemolytic anemia. The diagnosis can be made by establishing presence of the clinical findings, and by the finding of increased osmotic fragility of the red blood cells. HS is inherited as an autosomal dominant disorder about 75% of the time. *Hereditary elliptocytosis* is characterized by variable hemolysis, with predominance of elliptocytes on the blood smear. HE is usually inherited in an autosomal dominant pattern.

60. How are disorders of red cell membranes diagnosed?

Most membrane disorders can be identified by careful analysis of red cell morphology on the peripheral smear. The characteristic spherocytes, elliptocytes, ovalocytes, or stomatocytes are usually readily apparent. The osmotic fragility test is used frequently to confirm the diagnosis of spherocytosis, since spherocytes are more sensitive to osmotic lysis than normal red cells because of their reduced surface to volume ratio. Most membrane disorders are associated with an abnormality in cation and/or water transport across the red cell membrane. Specific studies of intracellular ion and water content may be useful in diagnosing the more unusual varieties of membrane disorders. Additional studies include analysis of membrane proteins or the genes associated with these proteins.

61. Why can hereditary spherocytosis (HS) present at multiple ages?

The time of presentation of hereditary spherocytosis is largely dependent on the severity of the disease. HS is caused by abnormalities of red cell membrane skeletal proteins; there are multiple known molecular defects which result in varying degrees of hemolysis in HS. When hemolysis is brisk, the initial presentation may be jaundice in the neonatal period or anemia during early infancy. Some children first present with an aplastic crisis, for example in response to a parvovirus infection, in which the hemoglobin level and reticulocyte count are both low. The latter finding may initially obscure the diagnosis since an elevated reticulocyte count is expected in a hemolytic disorder. Children with less severe hereditary spherocytosis may not be recognized until a routine blood count reveals a low hemoglobin level or until an enlarged spleen is found on examination. Some persons with mild disease will escape detection until they are adults, and they develop gallstones or have a child who is diagnosed with the disorder.

62. Why is splenectomy usually curative for hereditary spherocytosis?

In hereditary spherocytosis, an abnormality in the skeletal structure of the red cell membrane allows sodium influx into the RBC followed by water, which swells the cell and decreases its deformability. This problem is accentuated when the RBC reaches the spleen, where conditions are ideal for the destruction of metabolically incompetent red cells. In this case, the increased rate of glycolysis which is needed to compensate partially for the sodium leak is compromised by the low pH and the small amount of available glucose in the spleen. In addition, the poor deformability of the swollen RBC may lead to trapping of the cell in the cords of the spleen and loss of membrane to the surrounding macrophages. This results in a further reduction in the surface to volume ratio of the RBC, leaving the cell even less deformable and more vulnerable to a metabolic or mechanical death in its next trip through the spleen. This prominent role of the spleen in the pathophysiology of the hemolytic anemia in hereditary spherocytosis explains why splenectomy is usually curative.

63. In which settings do isoimmune and autoimmune hemolytic anemia most commonly appear?

Isoimmune: Red cell antigen incompatibility between mother and fetus
Transfusion of incompatible blood

Autoimmune: Idiopathic (most common)
Infectious (including *Mycoplasma pneumoniae*, infectious mononucleosis, varicella, viral hepatitis)
Drugs (antimalarials, penicillin, tetracycline)
Hematologic disorders (Evans syndrome)
Systemic autoimmune disorders (including systemic lupus erythematosus, dermatomyositis)

Tabbara IA: Hemolytic anemias: Diagnosis and management. Med Clin North Am 76:649–668, 1992.

64. How should children with a suspected immune-mediated hemolytic anemia be evaluated?

Quickly and carefully, as this may be a life-threatening disease. History and physcial examination are key. Typical findings may include rapid onset of pallor, jaundice, dark urine, abdominal pain, splenomegaly, and fever. The laboratory evaluation should include a CBC, reticulocyte count (elevated), evaluation of the peripheral blood smear (possible red cell fragments, spherocytes, polychromasia, and occasionally nucleated rbcs), a direct Coombs test, indirect bilirubin, and if suggested by history, a cold agglutinin titer. Approximately 10% of patients with autoimmune hemolytic anemia are Coombs negative. Thus, patients should be treated for autoimmune hemolytic anemia if the disease is strongly suspected, even if the direct Coombs test is negative.

In children older than 10 years of age, immune hemolytic anemia is more likely to be secondary to an underlying disease rather than the idiopathic or autoimmune IgG-mediated type seen in younger children. Cold agglutinin (IgM) disease is uncommon in pediatric patients, except in the setting of mycoplasmal infection.

65. What are the differences between autoimmune hemolytic anemias caused by "warm" and "cold" antibodies?

Warm: These are usually IgG antibodies with maximum activity at 37°C. They are directed most commonly against the Rh antigens, and generally do not require complement for *in vivo* hemolysis. Hemolysis is predominantly *extravascular* with consumption primarily in the spleen. Warm antibody-mediated hemolytic anemia is more likely to be associated with underlying disease (especially SLE in females) and to become chronic. Splenectomy and/or immunosuppression (such as with steroids) are often effective therapies.

Cold: These are IgM antibodies with maximum activity between 0°–30°C; they are directed most commonly against I or i antigen. Hemolysis is most commonly *intravascular*, via complement activation; extravascular hemolysis which does occur involves primarily hepatic consumption. Cold antibody-mediated hemolytic anemia is more commonly associated with acute infection (e.g., *Mycoplasma pneumoniae*, cytomegalovirus). Patients are less likely to develop chronic hemolysis, and therapy such as splenectomy and immunosuppression are often ineffective.

66. An 8-year-old black male developed jaundice and very dark urine 24–48 hours after beginning nitrofurantoin for a urinary tract infection. What is the likely diagnosis?

Glucose-6-phosphate dehydrogenase (G6PD) deficiency is the most common hemolytic anemia caused by an RBC enzymatic defect. The enzyme G6PD is a key component of the pentose phosphate pathway, which ordinarily generates sufficient NADPH to maintain glutathione in a reduced state (and available for combating oxidant stresses). The deficiency is inherited in an X-linked recessive fashion. In patients who are deficient (most commonly those of African, Mediterranean or Asian ancestry), oxidant stresses (particularly certain drugs) can result in hemolysis.

67. In a patient with G6PD deficiency, why is the initial diagnosis often difficult in the acute setting?

The amount of G6PD enzymatic activity is dependent on the age of the RBC. Older RBCs have the least, reticulocytes the most. In an acute hemolytic episode, the older cells are destroyed first, younger ones may remain, and reticulocytes increase. If erythrocytic G6PD levels are measured at this point, the result may be misleadingly near or above the normal range. If clinical suspicions remain, repeating the test when the reticulocyte count is reduced will give a more accurate measurement.

68. What are the clinical manifestations of G6PD deficiency?

Children with the GdA– or the GdMediterranean variants of G6PD deficiency are usually hematologically normal unless exposed to an oxidant stress. Acute intravascular hemolysis may occur with drugs such as the antimalarial agent chloroquine, toxins such as naphthalene found in some mothballs, or viral infections. These hemolytic episodes are characterized by an abrupt fall in hemoglobin level and a rise in reticulocyte count. Hemoglobinuria may be manifested as a positive test for blood by dipstick in the absence of red cells on microscopic analysis. Jaundice may accompany the hemolysis. The red cells have a characteristic appearance during acute hemolytic episodes. The peripheral smear shows blister cells in which the hemoglobin is pushed to one side of the cell, leaving a clear area beneath the membrane on the opposite side. In the GdA– variant, the hemolytic episode is usually self-limited since the reticulocytes have a normal complement of enzyme activity and are therefore resistant to the oxidant stress of the drug, toxin, or infection. Recovery usually occurs within 48–72 hours. In the GdMediterranean variant, acute hemolysis is more common and more severe due to the lower overall level of enzyme activity.

69. Why do children with pyruvate kinase (PK) deficiency tolerate anemia better than children with other anemias?

PK deficiency is an RBC glycolytic enzyme deficiency that most commonly affects those of northern European ancestry. Levels of 2,3-diphosphoglycerate (a glycolytic intermediate) are increased in patients with PK deficiency, and this compound shifts the oxygen dissociation curve to the right. As a result of this shift, oxygen is more readily delivered from the red cells to the tissue. This rightward shift is much greater than is ordinarily found in patients with similar degrees of anemia due to other causes. Thus, some symptoms typically associated with anemia may be less severe or even absent in patients with PK deficiency.

IRON-DEFICIENCY ANEMIA

70. At what age do exclusively breastfed infants become at risk for iron deficiency?

Healthy *term* infants who are exclusively breastfed are at risk for iron deficiency ***after 6 months*** of age. The age of risk for exclusively breastfed *premature* infants can be more complicated, particularly for the smaller and sicker infants, and recommendations vary. The lower iron stores of premature infants are more rapidly depleted compared to term babies. As a rule, the smaller the baby, the earlier and greater the amount of iron-supplementation needed. Very low-birth-weight babies (1000–1500 gm) should have supplementation (2–3 mg/kg/day) by 1 month of age, and extremely low-birth-weight babies (< 1000 gm) even sooner (2–4weeks). Of note, multiple transfusions can decrease or delay the need for supplementation because they are a source of iron (1 mg/ml) once the cells have completed their lifespan.

71. Why are infants who begin cow milk at an early age susceptible to iron-deficiency anemia?

Although breast milk and cow milk contain about the same amount of iron (0.5–1.0 mg/l), nonheme iron is absorbed at 50% efficiency from breast milk but only at 10% from cow milk. In addition, cow milk may cause microscopic gastrointestinal bleeding in younger infants due to mucosal injury, possibly from sensitivity to bovine albumin. In older infants, cow milk may interfere with iron absorption from other sources.

Fuchs G, et al: Gastrointestinal blood loss in older infants: Impact of cow milk versus formula. J Pediatr Gastroenterol Nutr 16:4–9, 1993.

Sullivan P: Cow's milk induced intestinal bleeding in infancy. Arch Dis Child 68:240–245, 1993.

72. In which pediatric groups should screening for iron-deficiency anemia be considered?

- Low birth weight
- Consumption of whole cow milk before 7 months of age
- Use of formula not fortified with iron

- Low socioeconomic status
- Exclusive breastfeeding (without solid or formula supplementation) beyond 6 months of age
- Perinatal blood loss
- Teenage females (if menstruation is heavy or with pregnancy)

Oski F: Iron deficiency in infancy and childhood. N Engl J Med 329:190–193, 1993.

73. How common is anemia in teenage athletes?

Frank anemia is uncommon. However, nonanemic iron deficiency may be found in approximately one-half of adolescent female athletes and up to one-eighth of male athletes, particularly long-distance runners. However, an adverse effect of this iron deficiency on athletic performance in the absence of anemia has never been conclusively demonstrated. On the other hand, iron depletion (with or without anemia) may be associated with lassitude, decreased concentration ability, and mood swings.

Ballin A, et al: Iron state in female adolescents. Am J Dis Child 146:803–805, 1992.

Rowland TW: Iron deficiency in the young athlete. Pediatr Clin North Am 37:1153–1162, 1990.

74. As iron becomes depleted from the body, what is the progression at which lab tests change?

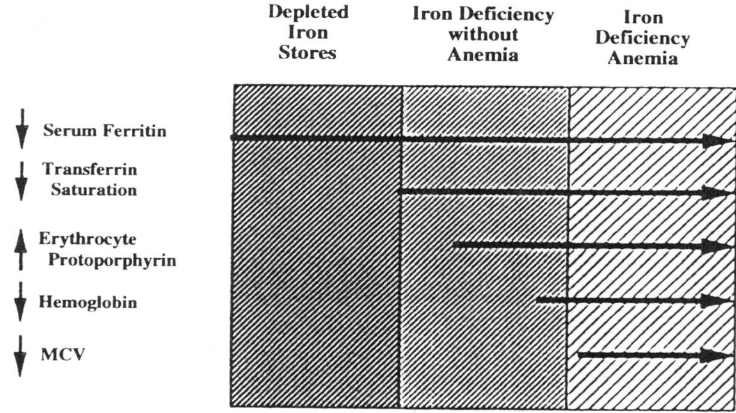

The left end of the line for each test indicates the point at which the result deviates from its baseline. As shown in this diagram, in general, depletion of marrow, liver, and spleen reserves (as represented by ferritin) occurs first, followed by a decrease in transport iron (as represented by transferrin saturation), and finally a fall in hemoglobin and mean cell volume (MCV). The diagram illustrates that absence of anemia does not exclude the possibility of iron deficiency and that iron depletion is relatively advanced before anemia develops. Tests of soluble transferrin receptor have become of interest in iron deficiency anemia, because the elevated levels are very sensitive indicators.

From Dallman PR, et al: Iron deficiency and related nutritional anemias. In: Nathan DG, Oski FA (eds): Hematology of Infancy and Childhood, 4th ed. Philadelphia, W.B. Saunders, 1993, p 427; with permission.

75. How might the reticulocyte hemoglobin content be helpful in the diagnosis of iron deficiency?

Because the reticulocyte is the most recently produced red blood cell in circulation, the earliest sign of iron deficiency many be a fall in the concentration of hemoglobin in reticulocytes (CHr). This number can be calculated from automated counting equipment and may be a reliable and inexpensive alternative to ferritin. Studies have indicated that patients with a CHr ≥ 30 pg have virtually no chance of iron deficiency.

Brugnara C, et al: Reticulocyte hemoglobin content to diagnose iron deficiency in children. JAMA 281:2225-2230, 1999.

Cohen AR: Choosing the best strategy to prevent childhood iron deficiency. JAMA 281:2247-2248, 1999.

76. How do acute inflammatory states affect tests for iron deficiency?

The *ferritin* level, used to monitor body iron stores, is exquisitely sensitive to inflammation, increasing even with mild upper respiratory infections. Elevations of ferritin may persist for some time. In contrast, *serum iron*, *transferrin* level, and percent *transferrin saturation* may decrease with infection or inflammation. *Free erythrocyte protoporphyrin* should not be affected by acute inflammation but may increase in chronic inflammatory states. All of these changes increase the difficulty of evaluating iron stores in the patient with acute or chronic inflammation.

77. How is the red cell distribution width (RDW) helpful in diagnosing microcytic anemia?

The *RDW* is a quantification of *anisocytosis* or *variation in red cell size*. It is derived from the RBC size histogram measured by automated cell counters and is reported as a percentage. In children, normal values range from about 11.5–14.5% but can vary between instruments. Statistically, it is the coefficient of variation of red cell volume distribution. Practically, when elevated in a patient with microcytosis, it suggests that iron deficiency is a more likely cause of anemia than thalassemia trait. Children with thalassemia trait tends to have values that overlap with normal RDW values. Of note, the combination of an RDW above the normal range with free erythrocyte protoporphyrin > 35 μg/dl is sensitive and specific for iron-deficiency anemia.

Cesana BM, et al: Relevance of red cell distribution width (RDW) in the differential diagnosis of microcytic anaemias. Clin Lab Haematol 13:141–151, 1991.

78. In a child with suspected iron-deficiency anemia, is a therapeutic trial with iron an acceptable diagnostic approach?

If an infant or child is otherwise well, a therapeutic trial of 4–6 mg/kg/day of elemental iron can substitute for additional diagnostic testing (e.g., ferritin, transferrin saturation, free erythrocyte protoporphyrin) since dietary iron deficiency is the most likely cause of microcytic anemia. If the child is iron-deficient, compliant with therapy, and there is not ongoing undetected blood loss, the hemoglobin should rise in about 2 weeks by > 1 gm/dl. If the hemoglobin does rise, therapy should be continued for an additional 2 months to replenish iron stores.

79. After iron therapy is initiated, how early can a response be detected?

2–5 days: Increase in reticulocyte count

7–10 days: Increase in hemoglobin level

For patients with mild iron-deficiency anemia, the hemoglobin level should be checked after several weeks of therapy. For patients with more severe anemia, it may be useful to check the hemoglobin and reticulocyte levels after a few days to make certain that the hemoglobin has not declined to dangerous levels and that the reticulocyte response is beginning.

80. What foods affect the bioavailability of nonheme iron?

Decreased by: Phosphates, tannates, polyphenols and oxalates found in cereal, eggs, milk, cheese, tea, and complex carbohydrates.

Increased by: Fructose, citrate, and especially ascorbic acid found in red kidney beans, cauliflower, and bananas. In children with iron deficiency, administration of replacement iron with a vitamin C-fortified fruit juice 30 minutes before a meal makes physiologic sense.

81. What are the indications for parenteral iron therapy?

Parenteral iron is appropriate for patients in whom oral iron is not tolerated, when rapid restoration of iron stores is necessary (for example, when ongoing losses make oral iron therapy ineffective), or for those situations in which oral iron is poorly absorbed (such as inflammatory bowel disease or severe malabsorption). Newer forms of iron for intravenous use make this the preferred route over intramuscular use, but monitoring for adverse reactions is still prudent.

82. What are the differences between pica, geophagia, and pagophagia?

All are clinical markers that suggest the diagnosis of iron deficiency. *Pica* is a more general term indicating a hunger for material not normally consumed as food. *Geophagia* refers to the consumption of dirt or clay, and *pagophagia*, to excessive consumption of ice. These are distinguished from *cissa*, which is the physiologic craving of pregnancy for unusual food items or combinations.

83. Discuss the relationship between iron deficiency and development in infants and toddlers.

Multiple studies have shown an association between iron deficiency in infants aged 9–24 months and lower motor and cognitive scores and increased behavioral problems when compared with nonanemic controls. Some longer-term studies suggest that the developmental impairments may be long-lasting. Debate remains on whether this relationship is causal and, if so, whether the correction of anemia leads to a reversal of the problems.

Buchanan GR: The tragedy of iron deficiency during infancy and childhood. J Pediatr 135:413-415, 1999.

84. Why are iron-deficient children at increased risk for lead poisoning?

- Pica associated with iron deficiency increases likelihood of ingestion of lead-contaminated items.
- GI absorption of lead may be increased in patients who consume less iron-containing nutrients.

Watson WS, et al: Food iron and lead absorption in humans. Am J Clin Nutr 44:248–256, 1986.

MEGALOBLASTIC ANEMIA

85. What is megaloblastic anemia?

Megaloblastic anemia refers to a macrocytic anemia accompanied by a characteristic hyperplastic bone marrow with changes in the erythropoietic precursors, in addition to changes in the white cell and platelet precursors. There is erythroid hyperplasia with increased number of young erythroid precursors, and erythroid maturation is abnormal (ineffective erythropoiesis). Megaloblastic anemia is most often caused by nutritional deficiency of folates, or by deficiency of vitamin B_{12} secondary to poor nutrition or malabsorption in the gastrointestinal tract.

86. Is megaloblastic anemia responsible for most macrocytic anemias in children?

No. Macrocytic anemia can be found in conditions associated with a high reticulocyte count (e.g., hemolytic anemia or hemorrhage), bone marrow failure (e.g., Fanconi anemia, aplastic anemia, Diamond-Blackfan syndrome), liver disease, Down syndrome, and hypothyroidism.

87. What findings on a complete blood count are suggestive of megaloblastic anemia?

Red cells: Elevated mean corpuscular hemoglobin (MCH) and mean cell volume (MCV, often 106 fl or more) with normal mean corpuscular hemoglobin concentration (MCHC); marked variability in cell size (anisocytosis) and cell shape (poikilocytosis)

Neutrophils: Hypersegmentation (more than 5% of neutrophils with 5 lobes, or a single neutrophil with 6 lobes)

Platelets: Usually normal, thrombocytopenia in more severe anemia

88. What are the causes of vitamin B_{12} (cobalamin) deficiency in children?

Decreased intake	***Decreased absorption***
May occur in vegetarians who consume no animal products	Ileal mucosal abnormalities (e.g., Crohn disease)
Seen in exclusively breastfed infants of B_{12}-deficient mothers	Surgical resection of terminal ileum
General malnutrition	Competition for cobalamin in bacterial overgrowth syndromes or infection with fish tapeworm *Diphyllobothrium latum*)
	Congenital abnormalities of the receptor for vitamin B_{12}–intrinsic factor complex
	Gastric mucosal defects that interfere with secretion of intrinsic factor

89. How does the pathophysiology of juvenile pernicious anemia differ from that of adult pernicious anemia?

Intrinsic factor (a glycoprotein) is released from gastric parietal cells and binds vitamin B_{12} to form a complex that is ultimately absorbed in the terminal ileum. Pernicious anemia is due to lack of intrinsic factor. *Juvenile pernicious anemia* is due most commonly to a congenital inability to secrete intrinsic factor. Since transplacental vitamin B_{12} stores (from nonvegetarian mothers) can last for years, symptoms can be delayed for up to 5 years in children. Gastric acidity and histology are normal, and the cause is unknown. In *adult pernicious anemia*, autoantibodies are produced against gastric parietal cells (resulting in achlorhydria); in addition, there is decreased production of intrinsic factor and, in many cases, antibodies to intrinsic factor are also found. These antibodies are not typically found in children. However, they can cross the placenta and impair cobalamin absorption during the first few weeks of life.

90. How is the Schilling test done?

This is a test to identify the cause of vitamin B_{12} deficiency. Administration of radiolabeled B_{12} by mouth is followed by an intramuscular (IM) dose of unlabeled B_{12}. Urine is collected for 24 hours and assayed for percent excretion of the oral dose (normal, 10–35%). The IM B_{12} is given to saturate tissue B_{12}-binding sites to facilitate excretion of the oral dose. Normal results depend on both the availability of intrinsic factor and undisturbed intestinal absorption. Oral intrinsic factor may also be given if results are abnormal. In pernicious anemia, excretion will normalize with administration of exogenous intrinsic factor, while in disorders of the terminal ileum, urinary excretion remains low even with intrinsic factor since absorption is defective.

91. What are the best dietary sources of folate and B_{12}?

Folate: Rich foods include liver, kidney, and yeast. Good sources include green vegetables (particularly spinach) and nuts. Moderate sources include fruits, bread, cereals, fish, eggs, and cheese. Rice, milk, meat, and poultry are poor sources of folate. Pasteurization or boiling destroys folate.

Vitamin B_{12}: Humans do not manufacture B_{12}; bacteria and fungi do. Animals require it, while plants do not. Consequently, our major dietary source of vitamin B_{12} is consumption of animal tissue, milk, or eggs. Seafood, which live on bacterial diets, are also a good dietary source. Of note, B_{12} is required for normal folate metabolism.

92. A 10-month-old fed exclusively goat milk is likely to develop what anemia?

Megaloblastic anemia due to folic acid deficiency. Goat milk contains very little folic acid compared with cow milk. Infants consuming large amounts, especially if not receiving significant supplemental solid foods, are susceptible. In addition, the diagnosis can be complicated by the higher risk of coexistent iron-deficiency anemia in this age group.

PLATELET DISORDERS

93. How can a platelet count be estimated from a peripheral smear?

As a rule, each platelet visible on a high-power microscopic field (100x) represents 15,000–20,000 platelets/mm^3. If platelet clumps are observed, the count is usually > 100,000/mm^3.

94. What factors can interfere with the automated platelet count?

Since automated cell counters utilize only size to identify platelets, small objects such as red cell fragments, white cell fragments, or leukemic blast fragments may be counted as platelets, falsely elevating the automated count. Conversely, the automated count may be depressed if large or giant platelets are counted as red cells. Inadequate anticoagulation of the sample may also cause a falsely low platelet count. Platelets may also agglutinate in vitro in some patients by EDTA (anticoagulant)-dependent antibodies. In this disorder, the cause of platelet clumping is an IgG or IgM antibody directed against a platelet antigen that is present only in the presence of EDTA. This has been referrred to a pseudothrombocytopenia, and is usually benign. Diagnosis is suspected by examination of the smear and confirmed by drawing the blood into an alternative anticoagulant, such as sodium citrate.

95. How much does a platelet transfusion raise the platelet count?

0.1–0.2 unit/kg of transfused platelets should raise the platelet count by 40,000/mm^3, or 1.0 unit/m^2 should raise the count by 10,000/mm^3. In normal patients, platelet survival time is 7–10 days but is often considerably shorter in thrombocytopenic patients due to a variety of causes.

96. A previously healthy 3-year-old develops mucosal petechiae, multiple ecchymoses, and a platelet count of 20,000/mm^3 2 weeks after a bout of chickenpox. What is the most likely diagnosis?

Acute idiopathic (immune) thrombocytopenic purpura (ITP). ITP is one of the most common bleeding disorders of childhood, and the presentation is postinfectious in about 50% of cases.

97. What is the natural history of acute childhood ITP?

With or without medical treatment, 50–60% of patients with acute ITP will have normal platelet counts within 1–3 months of diagnosis and 75% are well after 6 months. By 1 year, only 10% of children with ITP remain thrombocytopenic, and some of the children with chronic ITP still improve as long as 5–10 years after diagnosis. Because of this predominantly benign natural course of ITP, careful consideration is necessary before instituting treatment that is hazardous or irreversible.

98. In a toddler with suspected ITP, what is the significance of a palpable spleen on exam?

Although patients with ITP may rarely have a palpable spleen tip, the presence of splenomegaly in a patient with thrombocytopenia warrants more aggressive evaluation for an associated problem (e.g., collagen-vascular disease, hypersplenism).

99. In patients with suspected ITP, should a bone marrow evaluation be done?

A topic of much debate. A major concern is that without a bone marrow aspiration, the diagnosis of leukemia may be delayed or the course of illness worsened by treatment (typically corticosteroids) that is begun for presumed ITP. However, it is very rare that patients with leukemia present with isolated thrombocytopenia. Local custom will likely prevail regarding the need for bone marrow examination in the setting of "classic" acute ITP, but heightened consideration should be given if: (1) other cell lines are involved, (2) history and physical examination have atypical features (e.g., weight loss, hepatosplenomegaly), and (3) steroid therapy is to be used. In survey studies, most pediatric hematologists in the U.S. will manage ITP without active bleeding by not performing a bone marrow examination and by administering IVIG, if available, to raise a platelet count.

Vesely S, et al: Self-reported diagnostic and management strategies in childhood idiopathic thrombocytopenic purpura: Results of a survey of practicing pediatric hematology/oncology specialists. J Pediatr Hematol Oncol 22: 55-61, 2000.

100. When should medical treatment be given for acute ITP without active bleeding?

Because the long-term prognosis of ITP does not appear to be influenced by medical treatment, the management of a newly diagnosed child with ITP and no serious bleeding remains controversial. The principal concern is susceptibility to intracranial bleeding, which occurs in < 1% of affected patients (but can have 30–50% mortality), almost always when the platelet count is <10,000/mm^3. Local custom will prevail, but some authorities will treat medically when the platelet count is <10,000/mm^3 and/or there is active mucous membrane hemorrhage, to minimize the chance of intracranial catastrophe and to avoid excessive limitations of physical activity that might otherwise be imposed on a child with ITP.

101. If a child with ITP requires treatment, how does the response to different treatments compare?

IVIG: Intravenous immune globulin (IVIG), 0.8–1.0 gm/kg/day, raises the platelet count in approximately 85% of patients. The response usually occurs within 48 hours and persists for 3–4 weeks. Up to 75% of patients will have some degree of limited adverse reaction (e.g., nausea, vomiting, headaches, fever). IVIG is more expensive than steroids.

Corticosteroids: Corticosteroids are similarly effective, but oral steroids take about twice as long (4 days) to raise the platelet count significantly. The steroid effect may be multifactorial because signs of hemorrhage tend to decrease before the increase in platelets occurs. Side effects of long-term frequent steroid use are multiple.

Anti-D immunoglobulin: Anti-D can be given intravenously to individuals with adequate hemoglobin count, (Rh)D-positive RBCs, and intact splenic function. It is more rapidly given than IVIG, with a slightly smaller proportion of responders.

102. Are platelet transfusions of any value in ITP?

ITP is a disorder of increased platelet destruction rather than decreased production. In some severe cases, the platelet half-life might be as little as 10 minutes (normal 7–10 days). Because the antiplatelet antibody produced by the patient is as "effective" against donor platelets as it is against the patient's own platelets, transfusions usually do not increase the peripheral platelet count. Nonetheless, patients with ITP and life-threatening bleeding may benefit from platelet transfusion, since there may be a local hemostatic effect even in the absence of a demonstrable effect on the peripheral blood platelet count.

103. Which children with ITP are candidates for splenectomy?

Splenectomy improves the platelet count in up to 90% of patients. Since spontaneous remission is common in acute ITP, splenectomy is usually limited to bleeding that is life-threatening and unresponsive to medical therapies. Patients with ITP lasting > 1 year with continued bleeding, severe thrombocytopenia, or with unacceptable restrictions may be reasonable candidates for splenectomy. If possible, splenectomy should be deferred until a child is at least 5 years old to minimize the risk of overwhelming sepsis that can occur in younger splenectomized patients. Preoperative immunization against Hib, pneumococcus, and meningococcus (if available) is advisable.

104. How does the age of presentation of ITP influence the long-term outcome?

Children with the onset of ITP after age 10 years are more likely to develop chronic ITP, which by definition is persistence > 6–12 months. Chronic ITP is more commonly associated with other underlying problems (e.g., systemic lupus erythematosus, autoimmune thyroid disease, HIV infection), and the likelihood of spontaneous remission is significantly diminished.

105. A 6-month-old boy has an eczema, recurrent pneumonia, and a platelet count of 25,000/mm^3 with small platelets noted on the blood smear. What condition is likely?

Wiskott-Aldrich syndrome. This X-linked recessive syndrome is characterized by multiple immunologic defects (especially poor B-cell response to polysaccharide antigens and diminished T-cell function), eczema, and persistent thrombocytopenia. The *small platelet size* is a particularly important diagnostic clue.

106. What are other inherited disorders of platelet function?

Membrane glycoprotein abnormalities	***Granule defects***	***Metabolic abnormalities***
Bernard-Soulier syndrome	Hermansky-Pudlak syndrome	Impaired arachidonic acid release
Glanzmann thrombasthenia	Chédiak-Higashi syndrome	Cyclo-oxygenase deficiency
	Gray platelet syndrome	

Several rare, inherited disorders of platelet function involve membrane receptors or metabolic processes important for platelet aggregation and the formation of a primary platelet plug. In more severe disorders, such as Glanzmann thrombasthenia, bleeding usually occurs early in life. Hemorrhagic manifestations include prolonged bleeding from circumcision, sustained GI bleeding, and oral mucosal bleeding. Platelet transfusions are effective initially, but over time, there is a high risk of alloimmunization to donor platelets.

107. In what conditions in children is thrombocytosis most commonly seen?

- Acute infections (e.g., upper and lower respiratory tract infections)
- Chronic infections (e.g., tuberculosis)
- Iron deficiency anemia
- Hemolytic anemia
- Blood loss
- Medications (including vinca alkaloids, epinephrine, corticosteroids)
- Trauma (with tissue damage)
- Inflammatory disease (e.g., Kawasaki disease)
- Malignancy (including chronic myelogenous or megakaryocytic leukemia)
- Chronic renal disease

Yohannan MD, et al: Thrombocytosis: Etiologic analysis of 663 patients. Clin Pediatr 33:340–343, 1994.

108. What level of thrombocytosis requires treatment?

It depends primarily on etiology, duration and any comorbid conditions. A high platelet count in most children does not appear to be a cause of significant morbidity, as it is often transient In some centers, aspirin in doses of 81 mg daily is administered when the platelet count exceeds $1.5 \times 10^6/mm^3$. Early introduction of aspirin therapy may be more important if the patient has other problems that might contribute to hyperviscosity, such as a high WBC count or hemoglobin level. Essential thrombocythemia is more common in adults, but persistently very high platelet counts with these abnormal platelets can be associated with thrombosis. Recently anegrilide has been of use in such patients.

SICKLE CELL DISEASE

109. Why screen for sickle cell disease during the neonatal period?

It is a proven lifesaver. Sickle cell disease is often asymptomatic in the first months of life. In the neonatal period, the presence of large amounts of fetal hemoglobin reduces the rate of polymerization of HbS and the sickling of red cells containing this abnormal hemoglobin. As the amount of fetal hemoglobin decreases after age 3–6 months, patients with sickle cell disease are increasingly likely to experience their first clinical manifestations. These can include pneumococcal sepsis and splenic sequestration, which are associated with significant morbidity and mortality. If a neonate is identified with sickle cell disease, parental education can be given, and early daily prophylactic penicillin initiated.

Vinchinsky E, et al: Newborn screening for sickle cell disease: Effect on mortality. Pediatrics 81:749–755, 1988.

110. When does functional asplenia occur in children with sickle cell disease?

It may begin ***as early as 5 or 6 months*** of age and may precede the presence of Howell-Jolly bodies in the peripheral smear. Most children with HbSS over 5 years of age have functional asplenia, with a small, atrophied spleen. Clinical experience indicates that the period of increased risk for serious bacterial infection parallels the development of functional asplenia. Loss of splenic function usually occurs later in patients with HbSC or HbS β^+-thalassemia.

111. What clinical and laboratory factors detectable in infancy may be associated with poor prognosis in sickle cell disease?

When poor outcome is defined as death, stroke, frequent acute chest syndrome and/or frequent painful episodes, occurrence of dactylitis (hand-foot pain and swelling), elevated leukocyte count, and hemoglobin level less than 7 gm/dl are specific markers for increased risk of severe disease. An elevated pitted RBC count may also be predictive.

Miller ST et al., Prediction of adverse outcomes in children with sickle cell disease. N Engl J Med 342: 83-89, 2000.

112. Is the finding of a palpable spleen during the exam of a 13-year-old with a sickling disorder unusual?

It is a strong clue to the presence of HbSC or HbS β^+-thalassemia. In HbSS, the spleen is rarely palpable after 5 or 6 years of age.

113. What are the two major pathophysiologic mechanisms in sickle cell anemia which cause the morbidities associated with the disease?

***Hemolysis*:** Sickle red blood cells undergo both intra- and extravascular hemolysis, leading to anemia, reticulocytosis, jaundice, gallstones, and occasional aplastic crisis.

***Vasoocclusion*:** intermittent and chronic vasoocclusion results in both acute exacerbations such as painful crisis and stroke, and chronic disease manifestations such as retinopathy and renal disease. Adhesion of sickled erythrocytes to activated vascular endothelium is a principal pathologic component.

114. List the morbidities associated with sickle cell disease.

Acute
- Infection
- Vaso-occlusive (painful) crisis
- Splenic sequestration
- Severe anemia secondary to aplastic crisis or hemolytic crisis
- Acute chest syndrome
- Cerebral infarction or hemorrhage
- Priapism

Long-term
- Chronic lung disease
- Renal failure
- Congestive heart failure
- Retinal damage
- Leg ulcers
- Aseptic necrosis of the hip or shoulder
- Poor growth

115. A 6-month-old black male has painful swelling of both hands. What is the most likely diagnosis?

Hand-foot syndrome, or ***dactylitis***. This common early manifestation of sickling disorders in infants and young children is characterized by painful swelling of the hands, feet, and proximal fingers and toes caused by symmetric infarction in metacarpals, metatarsals, and phalanges. Lack of systemic signs, presence of symmetric involvement, and young patient age help distinguish hand-foot syndrome from the much less common osteomyelitis which may also complicate sickle cell disease.

116. How should a child with a painful crisis be managed?

A painful (or vaso-occlusive) crisis is one of the most difficult and challenging problems in the treatment of sickle cell disease. The mainstays of treatment are fluid therapy to prevent dehydration and analgesia. Approaches to pain control are notoriously varied and untested. The guiding principles are adequate relief of pain, awareness of drug side effects, and close familiarity with a particular drug, including its usual dose and route of administration. Treatment is considerably easier when the physician is familiar with or inquires of an individual patient's particular pattern of painful episodes and analgesic response.

For outpatients with an acute painful crisis, ibuprofen or acetaminophen and codeine are reasonable choices. Patients with intensely painful crises require hospitalization for opioid (including morphine and meperidine) analgesics, ideally given intravenously. Patient-controlled analgesia (PCA) offers the dual benefit of a constant infusion and intermittent boluses of an analgesic. Within parameters set by the physician, the patient determines the frequency of bolus doses. Other supplementary agents, including nonsteroidal analgesics (e.g., ketorolac), vasodilators/membrane active agents (e.g., cetiedil citrate), and high-dose methylprednisone, are presently under study. For severe crises unresponsive to standard measures, blood transfusions to reduce the amount of sickle cells to < 40% may be beneficial. Of note, the reasons for the enormous variability in occurrences among sickle cell patients remain unclear. Forty percent never experienced a painful crisis in a 10-year study.

Yaster M, et al: The management of pain in sickle cell disease. Pediatr Clin North Am 47:699-710, 2000.

117. How should children with sequestration crisis be managed?

Acute sequestration crisis represents a true emergency in sickle cell disease and is the second leading cause of death in young children with sickle cell disease. The clinical problem is primarily one of hypovolemic shock due to pooling of blood in the acutely enlarged spleen. The hemoglobin level may drop as low as 1 or 2 gm/dl. The major therapeutic effort should be directed toward ***volume replacement*** with whatever fluid is handy. In most instances, normal saline or colloid solutions will be adequate until properly cross-matched blood is available. Acute sequestration crisis is one of the few instances in sickle cell disease in which ***transfusion*** with whole blood is appropriate, since the problem is one of hypovolemia and anemia rather than anemia alone. If whole blood is not available, packed RBCs alone or packed RBCs plus plasma may be an alternative therapy.

118. How is abdominal pain due to a sickle cell crisis distinguished from a surgical abdomen?

Patiently and carefully. Children with this clinical scenario should be treated as if they may have a surgical abdomen, including omission of high dose analgesics, cessation of oral intake, and early surgical consultation. Clinical clues to suggest sickle cell crisis include the presence of bowel sounds, concomitant vaso-occlusive pain elsewhere, and a report by the patient that the pain is typical for his or her previous vaso-occlusive crises. Plain films are indicated to rule out perforation of a viscus in severe cases, and ultrasound may help to identify a localizing source such as cholecystitis or appendicitis. If clinical deterioration occurs with adequate hydration and moderate analgesia, surgical exploration should be strongly considered. Although simple or exchange transfusion preoperatively is recommended to help prevent the development of acute chest syndrome postoperatively, truly emergent surgery should *never* be delayed.

119. What causes "acute chest syndrome" in sickle cell patients?

Acute chest syndrome refers to the constellation of findings (e.g., fever, cough, chest pain, pulmonary infiltrates) that can resemble pneumonia or pulmonary infarction. The exact mechanism is unknown, and the cause is likely multifactorial. Various infections (e.g., viral, chlamydial, or mycoplasmal) may initiate respiratory inflammation which ultimately causes localized hypoxia. Increased pulmonary sickling may then result. Rib and other bone infarcts can also occur, and hypoventilation may result from chest splinting. Pulmonary fat embolism has been seen to occur, particularly in the setting of a preceding bony painful crisis (such as thigh). Overly vigorous hydration can lead to pulmonary edema.

Stuart MJ, Setty BNY: Sickle acute chest syndrome: Pathogenesis and rationale for treatment. Blood 94:1555-1560, 1999.

120. How should the acute chest syndrome in sickle cell patients be treated?

Acute chest syndrome should be managed aggressively, as it may progress very rapidly to severe disease with respiratory failure in some cases. Optimization of ventilation is vital, including supplemental oxygen, pain relief adequate to minimize splinting, and incentive spirometry, with additional measures as needed. Judicious hydration, analgesics, and antibiotics should be given. Blood transfusion, including erythrocytapheresis (automated RBC exchange transfusion) has been shown to improve the status of patients with acute chest, and should be considered for patients with severe or worsening disease.

121. How common is priapism a problem in children with sickle cell disease?

Priapism is an unwanted, painful erection usually unrelated to sexual activity. It is an underappreciated morbidity in adolescents, usually occurring at least once by age 20 and typically by age 12. Most patients are unaware of the term and the consequences. Early intervention may prevent irreversible penile fibrosis and impotence.

Mantadakis E, et al: Prevalence of priapism in children and adolescents with sickle cell anemia. J Pediatr Hematol Oncol 21:518-522, 1999.

122. Why is hydroxyurea beneficial in some patients with sickle cell disease?

Hydroxyurea, a chemotherapeutic agent used in some forms of leukemia, has as one of its side effects the ability to increase fetal hemoglobin production. Cells with higher concentrations of fetal hemoglobin are less prone to sickle. In addition, hydroxyurea decreases red cell–endothelial cell adhesion thought to contribute to vasoocclusion in sickle cell disease. Adult patients treated with hydroxyurea report fewer and less intense painful crises, and have fewer episodes of the acute chest syndrome. The hemoglobin usually rises 1–1.5 g/dl with therapy.

Koren A, et al: Effect of hydroxyurea in sickle cell anemia: A clinical trial in children and teenagers with severe sickle cell anemia and sickle cell beta-thalassemia. Pediatr Hematol Onc 16:221-232, 1999.

123. How common is sickle cell trait in the United States?

Heterozygosity for the sickle gene occurs in about 8% of blacks in the U.S., 3% of Hispanics in the eastern U.S., and a much smaller percentage of individuals of Italian, Greek, Arabic, and Veddah Indian heritage. Of note, 2% of blacks in the U.S. have hemoglobin C trait.

124. Does sickle cell trait have any morbidity?

Under normal physiologic conditions, RBCs in individuals with sickle cell trait contain only 30–40% sickle hemoglobin, which is insufficient to cause sickling. However, in hypoxic settings, sickling may occur. At high altitudes (such as mountain climbing or unpressurized aircraft), splenic infarction is possible. In addition, portions of the kidney may have physiologically low oxygen concentrations which can interfere with function and lead to hyposthenuria and hematuria (usually microscopic and asymptomatic). Higher rates of sudden unexplained death in military recruits have raised questions about the danger of severe, prolonged exertion in patients with sickle trait. However, most authorities place no restriction on activity. Life expectancy is not altered by sickle cell trait.

125. Do patients with sickle cell disease require special preparation for surgery?

Yes. Patients with sickle cell are at increased risk of surgical complications and sickle cell problems when undergoing general anesthesia and surgery. The most common morbidities are *acute chest syndrome* and *painful crisis*. Patients should, in most cases, receive blood transfusions pre-operatively; simple transfusion to a hemoglobin of 10-11g/dl, is sufficient in many cases. Adequate hydration should be ensured, which often requires intravenous hydration in patients unable to take fluids by mouth. Post-operatively, meticulous attention to ventilation and oxygenation includes supplemental oxygen when needed, use of frequent incentive spirometry, and adequate pain relief to prevent splinting.

126. What is the second most common worldwide hemoglobin variant?

Hemoglobin E. This variant is particularly high in the southeast Asian population (especially those of Laotian, Thai, and Cambodian heritage). Heterozygotes are asymptomatic; homozygotes can have a mild microcytic anemia. The most common abnormal findings on a peripheral smear are microcytosis and target cells.

THALASSEMIA

127. What accounts for the variability in clinical expression of the thalassemias?

The thalassemias are a heterogeneous group of disorders due to diminished or absent normal globin chain production. Normally, 4 α-globin genes and 2 β-globin genes are expressed to make the tetrameric globin protein, which then combines with a heme moiety to make the predominant hemoglobin in red cells, HbA (subunits $\alpha_2\beta_2$). Depending on the number of genes that are deleted, the production of polypeptide chains is diminished. In α-thalassemia, deletions of the α-globin gene(s) occur, and in β-thalassemia, mutations of β-globin gene(s) occur. When one class of polypeptide chains is diminished, this leads to a relative excess of the other chain. The result is ineffective erythropoiesis, precipitation of unstable hemoglobins, and hemolysis due to intramedullary RBC destruction.

Clinical heterogeneity results from variability in the number of gene deletions (particularly in α-thalassemia). However, as a rule, the greater the number of deletions, the more severe the symptoms. A large number of point mutations have been identified in various populations which can contribute to the phenotypic diversity. In addition, the inheritance of other thalassemia genes, such as δ or the persistence of fetal hemoglobin, can modify the clinical course.

128. How is the diagnosis of thalassemia made in most clinical laboratories?

Homozygous β-thalassemia is detected by the absence (β^0) or reduction (β^+) relative to HbF ($\alpha_2\gamma_2$ or fetal hemoglobin) in the amount of HbA ($\alpha_2\beta_2$) on *hemoglobin electrophoresis*. The carrier state for β-thalassemia is characterized by a low mean cell volume (MCV) and, in most instances, an increased level of HbA_2 ($\alpha_2\delta_2$) or HbF. The levels of these two hemoglobins are most accurately measured by column chromatography. Estimation or quantitation from electrophoretic patterns is frequently misleading. Alpha thalassemia trait remains a diagnosis of exclusion (low MCV in the absence of an identifiable cause) in the clinical laboratory, although the enumeration of missing alpha genes is easily accomplished by molecular techniques. Newer PCR-based DNA tests for the common variants has become very useful recently, and can be quite useful in genetic counseling.

129. Why is splenomegaly common in thalassemia?

The excess α-globin chains in the red cells of patients with β-thalassemia and the excess β-globin chains in the red cells of patients with α-thalassemia form inclusion bodies on the red cell membranes. These cells are cleared by the spleen because of their diminished flexibility, and the spleen enlarges as a result. The spleen may also enlarge as it attempts to make red cells to compensate for the severe anemia and as it stores iron that accumulates from repeated red cell transfusions.

130. Describe the clinical features of the α-thalassemia syndromes.

When all 4 alpha globin genes are missing or nonfunctional, this results in severe intrauterine anemia and hydrops fetalis. Extraordinary therapy such as *in utero* transfusion may result in survival. Absence of 3 functional alpha globin genes results in Hb H disease, a chronic moderate to severe anemia, with jaundice and splenomegaly, which may necessitate RBC transfusion therapy. Absence of 2 alpha globin genes is associated with mild microcytic anemia. Absence of one alpha globin gene is clinically silent.

Clinical Features in α-Thalassemia

SYNDROME	USUAL GENOTYPE	α GENE NUMBER	CLINICAL FEATURES
Normal	α α/α α	4	Normal
Silent carrier	α –/α α	3	Normal
α-Thalassemia trait	α –/α – α α/– –	2	Mild microcytic anemia
HbH disease	– –/α α	1	Moderate microcytic anemia Splenomegaly Jaundice
Homozygous α-thalassemia	– –/– –	0	Fetal hydrops due to severe anemia

131. What are the clinical features of the β-thalassemia syndromes?

Thalassemia minor: minimal or no anemia (hemoglobin 9–12 gm/dl); microcytosis; elevated rbc count

Thalassemia intermedia: microcytic anemia with hemoglobin usually > 7 gm/dl;

growth failure; hepatosplenomegaly; hyperbilirubinemia; and thalassemic facies (i.e., frontal bossing, mandibular malocclusion, prominent malar eminences due to extramedullary hematopoiesis) develop between ages 2–5 years

Thalassemia major (Cooley anemia): severe anemia (hemoglobin 1-6 gm/dl) usually in the first year of life; hepatosplenomegaly; growth failure

Olivieri NF: The beta-thalassemias. N Engl J Med 341:99-109, 1999.

131. How can coexistent iron deficiency increase the difficulty of diagnosing β-thalassemia?

β-thalassemia trait is usually diagnosed by hemoglobin electrophoresis, with quantitative hemoglobins revealing elevated HbA_2 and/or HbF levels. Iron deficiency can cause a lowering of HbA_2, masking the diagnosis. With iron replacement, the hemoglobin A_2 will rise to the expected elevated levels in β-thalassemia trait.

132. What are the adverse effects of chronic iron overload in children with thalassemia?

The major cause of morbidity and mortality from transfusional iron overload is related to iron accumulation in the *heart*, manifested as congestive heart failure, dysrhythmias, and, less frequently, pericarditis. Common iron-induced *endocrine* abnormalities include delay in growth and sexual development, hypoparathyroidism, and hypothyroidism. Diabetes due to iron overload is irreversible, even with intensive chelation. Excessive *hepatic* iron storage causes progressive liver fibrosis and cirrhosis, although death from cardiac disease occurs before most patients develop major problems related to liver dysfunction.

133. How do you reduce iron accumulation in children requiring repeated transfusions?

The two most common diseases associated with transfusion-related iron overload are thalassemia major and sickle cell disease. Strategies for reducing iron accumulation include:

- ***Chelation therapy:*** Subcutaneous or intravenous deferoxamine has been the standard therapy for transfusional overload. Effective oral iron chelators are under development.
- ***Splenectomy:*** Used primarily in thalassemia (and a small subgroup of sickle cell patients) with hypersplenism which results in premature destruction of RBCs.
- ***Diet:*** Drinking tea with meals reduces dietary iron absorption and may be most helpful in diseases such as thalassemia intermedia, in which the bulk of excessive iron is dietary in origin.
- ***Erythrocytapheresis:*** Automated erythrocytapheresis rather than repeated simple transfusions may markedly reduce transfusional iron loading in sickle cell disease.

We would like to acknowledge input and support from Elias Schwartz, M.D., and Margaret Keller, Ph.D., and our appreciation of (and reliance on) the prior chapter on Hematology and Immunology in *Pediatric Secrets, 2nd edition,* by Drs. Bruce P. Himelstein, Steven D. Douglas and Alan R. Cohen.

10. IMMUNOLOGY

Georg A. Holländer, M.D., and Anders Fasth, M.D., PhD.

CLINICAL ISSUES

1. Which immunologic factors account for the increased incidence of sepsis in preterm infants during the first months of life?

Inadequate concentrations of IgG antibodies, diminished neutrophil storage pool in the bone marrow, impaired phagocytic and intracellular killing capacity, and decreased activity of the alternate and classical complement pathway contribute to the higher incidence of morbidity and mortality among preterm infants with sepsis.

2. What is the significance of IgG subclass deficiencies?

IgG can be classified according to structural, chemical and biologic differences into four subclasses: IgG_1, IgG_2, IgG_3, IgG_4. The relative contribution of each to total IgG is 70%, 20%, 7% and 3%, respectively. In response to protein antigens, IgG_1 and IgG_3 subclasses predominate, while IgG_2 and IgG_4 are typically noted with polysaccharide antigens. In the mid-1970s, reports began to appear describing children with recurrent infections (primarily sinopulmonary) who had selective subclass deficiencies. Most common was IgG_2, but multiple other combinations have since been described. Patients with selective deficiency and recurrent infection may benefit from polysaccharide–protein conjugate vaccines, prophylactic antibiotics, and, if the infections are severe, intravenous immunoglobulin.

Considerable debate exists regarding the treatment and clinical importance of subclass deficiencies because:

- IgG values have a very wide and age-dependent range.
- Methodologic variability among laboratories is widespread.
- Specific antibody responses may be more important than absolute subclass quantities.
- Coexistent immunologic problems (e.g., IgA deficiency) may be present.
- Subclass deficiencies can be the presenting abnormality in more serious immunologic disorders (e.g., ataxia-telangiectasia, common variable immunodeficiency, chronic mucocutaneous candidiasis, adenosine deaminase deficiency).
- Some younger patients with subclass deficiencies have immunoglobulin levels that return to normal with maturation.

Shackelford PG: IgG subclasses: Importance in pediatric practice. Pediatr Rev 14:291–296, 1993.

3. What are the immunologic risks for asplenic patients?

Overwhelming bacterial infections have been noted in children and adults with anatomical or functional asplenia. The incidence of mortality from septicemia is increased by 50-fold in individuals after traumatic loss of splenic function. The risk of bacteremia is higher in younger than in older children and may be greater during the first few years following splenectomy. *S. pneumoniae, H. influenzae* type B and *N. meningitidis* are the most frequent pathogens observed in asplenic children.

4. How is neutropenia defined?

Neutropenia is arbitrarily defined as an absolute neutrophil count (ANC) of < $1500/mm^3$. The ANC is determined by multiplying the percentage of bands and neutrophils by the total white blood cell count. An ANC of < 500/mm^3 is severe neutropenia. As a rule, the lower the ANC, the greater the risk of infectious complications. In the first 2 years of life (outside the neonatal period) when normal white blood counts are generally lower, an ANC < 1000/mm^3 is considered neutropenic.

5. What is the most common cause of transient neutropenia in children?

Viral infections, including influenza, adenovirus, coxsackie virus, respiratory syncytial virus (RSV), hepatitis A and B, measles, rubella, Epstein-Barr virus, cytomegalovirus, and varicella. The neutropenia usually develops in the first 2 days of illness and may persist for up to a week. Multiple factors likely contribute to the neutropenia, including a redistribution of neutrophils (increased margination rather than circulation), sequestration in reticuloendothelial tissue, increased utilization in injured tissues, and marrow suppression. In general, otherwise healthy children with transient neutropenia due to viral infections are at low risk for serious infectious complications.

6. Excluding intrinsic defects in myeloid stem cells, what conditions are associated with neutropenia in children?

- ***Bone marrow replacement:*** leukemia, myelofibrosis
- ***Drugs:*** sulfonamides, penicillin, antithyroid drugs, phenothiazines, benzodiazepines, aspirin, gold salts, acetaminophen
- ***Immunologic:*** neonatal alloimmune (secondary to maternal IgG directed against fetal neutrophils), autoimmune (e.g., antineutrophil antibodies in systemic lupus erythematosus)
- ***Metabolic:*** hyperglycinemia, isovaleric acidemia, propionic acidemia, methylmalonic acidemia, glycogen storage disease type IB
- ***Nutritional:*** anorexia nervosa, marasmus, B_{12}/folate deficiency, copper deficiency
- ***Sequestration:*** splenic enlargement

Curnutte JT: Disorders of granulocyte function and granulopoiesis. In Nathan DG, Oski FA (eds): Hematology of Infancy and Childhood, 4th ed. Philadelphia, W.B. Saunders, 1993, pp 945–949.

7. How should an infant or child with neutropenia be evaluated?

The evaluation of the patient with neutropenia should begin with a good history, focusing on prior illness or infection, toxin or drug exposure, growth and development, and family history. If the data are available, prior blood counts should be reviewed to determine if the neutropenia is newly acquired, longstanding, or congenital. Physical examination should focus on a search for mucosal or skin infection and phenotypic abnormalities, which may suggest another primary disorder such as Fanconi anemia, cartilage-hair hypoplasia, or Shwachman-Diamond syndrome. Delayed growth may be a clue to repeated infections or accompanying abnormalities such as malabsorption in Shwachman-Diamond syndrome.
If other cytopenias are present, a bone marrow examination is indicated immediately to rule out infiltrative disease or one of the bone marrow failure syndromes. If the neutropenia is isolated, any drugs which may be causative should be discontinued and all underlying infections or systemic illnesses treated. If the neutropenia persists, one should obtain serial blood counts to determine whether the low neutrophil count reoccurs in a predictable sequence, which would suggest the diagnosis of cyclic neutropenia.

Other diagnostic tests depend upon historical elements and available laboratory findings which might suggest an etiology. Relevant diagnostic tests might include viral serology, pancreatic function testing for babies with a history of diarrhea or growth failure to rule out Shwachman-Diamond syndrome, folate and vitamin B_{12} levels if dietary history or blood cell morphology suggests a megaloblastic anemia, blood counts on family members if the family history is positive for repeated infections or early death, and evaluation for autoimmune or metabolic causes in the patient with multi-system disease.

8. What should top your diagnostic list in a 5-year-old with short stature, steatorrhea, neutropenia, and metaphyseal dysostosis on x-ray?

Schwachman-Diamond syndrome comprises a constellation of findings, including pancreatic insufficiency (resulting in malabsorption and failure to thrive), bone marrow failure, short stature, and characteristic bony changes. A unifying cause has not been identified.

Cipolli M, et al: Schwachman's syndrome: Pathomorphosis and long-term outcome. J Pediatr Gastroenterol Nutr 29:265-272, 1999.

9. What is the significance of a leukemoid reaction?

A *leukemoid reaction* usually refers to a white cell count > 50,000/mm^3 and an accompanying shift to the left. Causes include bacterial sepsis, tuberculosis, congenital syphilis, congenital or acquired toxoplasmosis, and erythroblastosis fetalis. Infants with Down syndrome may also have a leukemoid reaction that is often confused with acute leukemia during the first year of life.

10. Name the three most common causes of eosinophilia in children in the U.S.

Eosinophilia, usually defined as > 10% eosinophils or an absolute eosinophil count of ≥1000/mm^3, is most commonly seen in three atopic conditions: ***atopic dermatitis, allergic rhinitis,*** and ***asthma***.

11. What conditions are associated with extreme elevations of eosinophils in children?

- Visceral larval migrans (toxocariasis)
- Other parasitic disease (trichinosis, hookworm, ascariasis, strongyloidiasis)
- Eosinophilic leukemia
- Hodgkin disease
- Drug hypersensitivity
- Idiopathic hypereosinophilic syndrome

Lukens JN: Eosinophilia in children. Pediatr Clin North Am 19:969–981, 1972.

12. When is the best time to draw blood for evaluation of eosinophilia?

Midnight. Circulating blood eosinophils have a diurnal variation, with the highest values occurring near midnight and the lowest around noontime. This pattern may be a reflection of the diurnal nature of cortisol secretion, which is lower in the evening. Exogenous steroid administration is known to lower peripheral eosinophil counts. However, the small clinical significance (and large family repercussions) do not warrant midnight phlebotomy.

13. Which disorders are associated with basophilia?

- *Hypersensitivity reactions:* drug or food hypersensitivity, urticaria
- *Inflammation/infection:* ulcerative colitis, rheumatoid arthritis, influenza, chickenpox, tuberculosis
- *Myeloproliferative diseases:* chronic myelogenous leukemia, myeloid metaplasia

Dinauer MC: The phagocytic system and disorders of granulopoiesis and granulocyte function. In Nathan DG, Orkin SH (eds): Nathan and Oski's Hematology of Infancy and Childhood, 5th ed. Philadelphia, W.B. Saunders, 1998, p. 924.

14. How do children with neutrophil disorders present?

Neutrophil disorders include those affecting quantity (e.g., various neutropenias) and function (e.g., chemotaxis, phagocytosis, bactericidal activity). These defects should be considered part of the differential diagnosis in patients with *delayed separation of the umbilical cord, recurrent infections with bacteria or fungi* of low virulence (but minimal problems with recurrent viral or protozoal infections), *poor wound healing*, and *specific locales of infection* (e.g., recurrent furunculosis, perirectal abscesses, gingivitis).

15. Since infections are a clinical warning sign for primary immunodeficiencies, which frequencies are suspicious for a decreased host defense?

- Eight or more ear infections within a year
- Two or more serious sinus infections or pneumonias within a year
- Two or more serious infections such as meningitis, osteomyelitis, sepsis, etc.

16. How common are primary immunodeficiencies?

Primary immunodeficiencies: ***1:10,000*** (excluding asymptomatic IgA deficiency).

- B cell defects: 50%
- Combined cellular and antibody deficiencies: 20%
- T cell-restricted deficiencies:10%
- Phagocytic disorders: 18% and
- Complement component disorders: 2%

17. What are the typical clinical findings of the various primary immunodeficiencies?

	PREDOMINANT B-CELL DEFICIENCY	PREDOINANT T-CELL DEFICIENCY	PHAGOCYTIC DEFECTS	COMPLEMENT DEFECTS
Age of onset	After maternal antibodies have disappeared (usually > 6 mos)	Early infancy	Early infancy	Any age
Type of infection	Gram$^+$, gram$^-$ (encapsulated) bacteria *Mycoplasma* *Giardia* *Cryptosporidium* *Campylobacter* Enteroviruses	Viruses, in particular CMV_1, CBV Systemic BCG postvaccination Fungal *Pneumocystis carinii*	Gram$^+$, gram$^-$ bacteria Catalase$^+$ organisms in CGD, especially *Aspergillus*	*Streptococcus* *Neisseria*
Clinical findings	Recurrent respiratory tract infections Diarrhea Malabsorption Ileitis, colitis Cholangitis Arthritis Dermatomyositis Meningoencephalitis	Poor growth and failure to thrive Oral candidates Skin rashes Sparse hair Opportunistic infections Graft-versus host disease Bony abnormalities Hepatosplenomegaly	Poor wound healing Skin diseases, e.g., seborrheic dermatitis, impetigo, abcess Cellulitis without pus Suppurative adenitis Periodontitis Liver abcess Crohn disease Osteomyelitis Bladder outlet obstruction	Rheumatoid disorders Angioedema Increased susceptibility to infections

18. How likely is it that a patient with a primary immunodeficiency is diagnosed within the first year of life?

Approximately ***40%*** of all cases are diagnosed within the first 12 months of life, an equal percentage are detected, in addition, by 5 years of age, and another 15% before the age of 16. Only 5% of all primary immunodeficiency disorders are diagnosed in adulthood.

19. Why are male children more likely to suffer from a primary immunodeficiency?

Several primary immunodeficiency disorders are linked to the X-chromosome: agammaglobulinemia, hyper-IgM syndrome, severe combined immunodeficiency (the common cytokine receptor gamma chain deficiency), lympho-proliferative syndrome, Wiskott-Aldrich syndrome, one form of chronic granulomatous disease, properidin deficiency. This fact accounts for the observation that the male:female ratio is 4:1 among patients with a primary immunodeficiency that are younger than 16 years of age.

20. Which is the most common type of primary immunodeficiency?

Selective IgA deficiency is the most common primary immunodeficiency. The prevalence of selective IgA deficiency has been calculated to range from 1:220 to 1:3,000 depending on the population studied. However, most IgA deficient subjects remain healthy, which has been attributed to a compensatory increase of IgM in bodily secretions. A minority of these patients demonstrate normal levels of secretory IgA and normal numbers of IgA-bearing mucosal plasma cells. Although IgA represents < 15% of total immunoglobulin, it is predominant on mucosal surfaces. Therefore, most patients with symptoms have recurrent diseases involving mucosal surfaces, including otitis media, sinopulmonary infections, and chronic diarrhea. Systemic infections are rare.

21. What are the diagnostic criteria for IgA deficiency?

Serum concentrations of IgA ***below 0.05 g/L*** are diagnostic and almost invariably associated with a concomitant lack of secretory IgA. Serum levels for IgM are normal and concentrations for IgG (in particular IgG_1 and IgG_3) may be increased in one-third of all IgA deficiency patients.

22. What is the association of autoimmune disorders and IgA deficiency?

Autoimmune disorders have been described in up to 40% of patients with selective IgA deficiency including systemic lupus erythematosus, rheumatoid arthritis, thyroiditis, celiac disease, pernicious anemia, Addison disease, idiopathic thrombocytopenic purpura and autoimmune hemolytic anemia.

23. How common are anti-IgA antibodies in patients with IgA deficiency?

At the time of diagnosis, approximately 20–40% of patients have detectable anti-IgA antibodies (IgG_1, IgG_4, occasionally IgM and, rarely, IgE). The etiology of this immune response is invariably unknown but could include an IgA epitope mimicking food products. Anti-IgA antibodies (in particular IgE) may cause anaphylaxis upon injection of IgA-containing blood products.

24. Why is immunoglobulin therapy not utilized as a treatment for selective IgA deficiency?

Unless a patient has a concurrent IgG subclass deficiency (and even in this setting, therapy is controversial), gamma globulin therapy is not indicated and relatively contraindicated because:

- The short half-life of IgA makes frequent replacement therapy impractical.
- Gamma globulin preparations have insufficient IgA quantities to restore mucosal surfaces.
- Patients can develop anti-IgA antibodies with the potential for hypersensitivity complications, including anaphylaxis.

25. In an infant with panhypogammaglobulinemia, how can quantitation of B and T lymphocytes in peripheral blood help distinguish the diagnostic possibilities?

- *Normal numbers of T lymphocytes, no detectable B lymphocytes*: X-linked agammaglobulinemia (Bruton's disease)
- *Normal numbers of T and B lymphocytes*: transient hypogammaglobulinemia of infancy, common variable immunodeficiency

- *Decreased numbers of T lymphocytes, normal or decreased numbers of B lymphocytes*: severe combined immunodeficiency
- *Decreased CD4 lymphocytes*: HIV infection

Lederman HM: Disorders of humoral immunity. In Oski FA, et al (eds): Principles and Practice of Pediatrics, 2nd ed. Philadelphia, J.B. Lippincott, 1994, p 185.

26. What are the criteria for the diagnosis of X-linked agammaglobulinemia?

X-linked agammaglobulinemia (XLA) is typically characterized by four findings: Onset of recurrent bacterial infections before the age of five; serum immunoglobulin values for IgG, IgM and IgA well below 2 standard deviations (SD) of the normal for age; absent isohaemagglutinins; a poor to absent response to vaccines; and less than 2% peripheral B cells ($CD19^+$).

27. What are the typical laboratory findings and clinical features of common variable immunodeficiency (CVID)?

Laboratory evaluations in CVID typically demonstrate low IgG levels and low to absent IgA and IgM serum concentrations. Similarly, specific antibodies to previously encountered pathogens and vaccines and isohaemagglutinins are low to absent. A large proportion of CVID patients exhibit a depressed switch from IgM to IgG. Although lymphocyte subsets are normal in the majority of CVID patients, standard T cell function tests (e.g. in vitro proliferation in response to mitogenes, nominal antigens and allogeneic cells) are subnormal in approximately half of all patients.

Symptoms of CVID may first occur during childhood or, more often, after puberty and include increased infections, particularly in the respiratory tract, involvement of the gastrointestinal tract (chronic malabsorption, nodular lymphoid hyperplasia, gastric atrophy with achlorhydria) and autoimmune disorders (e.g., rheumatoid arthritis, autoimmune hemolytic anemia, pernicious anemia, neutropenia, thrombocytopenia, chronic active hepatitis, vertiligo, parotitis).

28. What are the typical clinical manifestations of X-linked agammaglobulinemia (XLA)?

Newborns with XLA have normal serum levels of IgG at birth and few, if any, symptoms. Typically, symptoms begin at the age of 4–12 months, although as many as 20% of XLA patients present clinical symptoms as late as 3–5 years of age. Infections are the most common clinical manifestation and frequently occur due to encapsulated bacteria, *Staphylococcus aureus*, *Salmonella, Campylobacter, Mycoplasma*, and *Giardia lamblia*. Infections may be localized to the respiratory tract (e.g., otitis media, sinusitis, pneumonia), skin (e.g., pyoderma), GI tract (e.g., diarrhea), or spread hematogenously (e.g., sepsis, meningitis, septic arthritis). Patients with XLA are at an increased risk for chronic entroviral infections and viral hepatitis.

29. How are immunoglobulins prepared for intravenous use?

Commercially available human serum immunoglobulins for intravenous use (IVIG) are prepared from large pools of donors (3000 to more than 6000 individuals). These products differ mainly in (i) their content of IgA, which may be relevant for patients with complete IgA deficiency, and (ii) the composition of stabilizers (glucose, sucrose, sorbitol)

30. For which clinical conditions are immunoglobulins approved?

Initially used to treat agammaglobulinemia, indications for IVIG include:

- Primary humoral immunodeficiencies of the humoral immunity
- Kawasaki disease
- Chronic lymphocytic leukemia with hypogammaglobulinemia and recurrent infections

- Bone marrow transplant recipients with recurrent infections
- Idiopathic thromaocytopenic purpura (ITP)
- HIV infection
- Autoimmune and inflammatory diseases, including Guillain-Barré syndrome, multifocal motor neuropathy, chronic demyelinating polyneuropathy, dermatomyositis and polymyositis.

31. What are the adverse reactions to IVIG?

Approximately 10% of patients receiving IVIG treatment experience mild side effects including headaches, myalgias, nausea, vomiting, and facial flushing. The majority of these side effects are related to the presence of acute or chronic infections, the rate of infusion and/or the temperature of the IVIG solution. Uncommon reactions are chest tightness and bronchospasm. Aseptic meningitis with rapid onset of severe headaches and photophobia has been noted, especially in patients with a history of migraines. Anaphylaxis due to anti-IgA antibodies is a rare side effect. Acute and chronic renal failure may occur in patients with preexisting renal diseases and in those receiving sucrose containing IVIG solutions.

32. What is the underlying disorder in an 8-year old girl with atypical eczema, pneumatoceles and bouts of severe furunculosis?

Hyper-IgE syndrome is the most likely diagnosis. This disease is clinically characterized by:

- *Recurrent infections* (almost invariably caused by *Staphylococcus aureus*) of skin, lung (causing frequently persistent pneumatoceles), ears, sinuses, eyes, joints and viscera
- *Atypical eczema* with lichenified skin
- *Coarse facial features*
- *Osteopenia* of unknown cause
- *Delayed tooth exfoliation* (i.e., prolonged retention of primary teeth)

The laboratory evaluation of the hyper-IgE syndrome reveals massively elevated IgE levels associated with IgG subclass and specific antibody deficiencies, variable dysfunctions of neutrophils and an imbalance of cytokine production due to a Th2 predominance (IL-4, IL-5).

Grimbacher B, et al: Hyper-IgE syndrome with recurrent infections—an autosomal dominant multisystem disorder. N Engl J Med 340:697-702, 1999.

33. What is the likely diagnosis of a 5-year-old girl presenting with recurrent sinopulmonary infections, progressive anomalies in station and gate, and vascular malformations in both conjunctivae?

This patient suffers from ***ataxia-telangiectasia*** (A-T, also known as Louis-Bar syndrome). This autosomal recessive disorder has fairly constant neurological features (early onset of cerebellar ataxia, choreoathetosis, dysartric speech), and telangiectasia which are typically confined to the skin of the face, the ears and the conjunctivae. These vascular malformations are usually apparent after the onset of neurological manifestations. Increased infections become evident by the age of three and primarily affect the upper and lower airways. A-T patients are particularly susceptible to bacterial and viral pathogens but not to generalized opportunist fungal or protozoan infections. Recurrent pneumonias progressively lead to respiratory insufficiency. The clinical features of A-T and the family history provide the best clues for diagnosis. Laboratory evaluations reveal variable immunoglobulin concentrations (but often reduced IgA, IgE and occasionally IgG2 levels), possibly due to a defect in B-cell differentiation or T-cell helper cells. T-cell numbers (CD4 >CD8) and function are usually reduced.

34. What is the classic triad of Wiskott-Aldrich syndrome?

Thrombocytopenia with small platelet volume, ***eczema*** and ***immunodeficiency.*** An X-linked disorder, the initial manifestations are often present at birth and consist of petechiae, bruises and bloody diarrhea due to thrombocytopenia. The eczema is similar in presentation to classical atopic eczema (antecubital and popliteal fossa). Infections are common and include (in decreasing frequency): otitis media, pneumonia, sinusitis, sepsis and meningitis. The severity of immunodeficiency may vary but usually affects both T and B cell functions. Importantly, this immunodeficiency is progressive and associated with a high risk of developing cancer. A teenager has a statistical risk of 10–20% risk of a lymphoid neoplasm. Of note, only about a third of Wiskott-Aldrich patients present with this classic triad.

Sullivan KE, et al: A multi-insitutional survey of the Wiskott-Aldrich syndrome. J Pediatr 125:876, 1995.

35. Where are WASPs found?

WASP is the acronym for the ***W***iskott-***A***ldrich ***s***yndrome ***p***rotein which is encoded by the gene defective in this disorder. The WASP-family members associate with numerous signaling molecules known to alter the actin cytoskeleton. The lack of cell surface microvilli, a unique cytoskeletal abnormality, has been noted on lymphocytes defective in WASP.

Snapper SB, Rosen FS: The Wiskott-Aldrich Syndrome Protein (WASP): Roles in signaling and cytoskeletal organization. Ann Rev Immunol 17: 905-929, 1999.

36. What is the CATCH 22?

The acronym stands for ***c***ardiac anomalies, ***a***bnormal facies, ***t***hymic hypoplasia, ***c***left palate and ***h***ypocalcemia associated with chromosomal deletions within ***22***q11. *CATCH 22* represents a field defect affecting the normal development of branchial arch-derived structures and thus accounts for a number of heterogeneous disorders, including the DiGeorge syndrome.

37. Which is the most important single laboratory test if severe combined immunodeficiency (SCID) is suspected?

A full blood count to document ***lymphopenia*** (2000/mm^3) is the single most important laboratory test in the initial evaluation of SCID. However, a minority of SCID patients (approximately 20%) may have a normal absolute lymphocyte count.

38. What are the typical clinical features of SCID?

- Recurrent bacterial infections (typically pneumonia, otitis media, sepsis)
- Persistent viral infections (RSV, enterovirus, parainfluenza, CMV)
- Opportunistic infections (*Pneumocystitis carinii,* fungi).
- Failure to thrive
- Diarrhea (enterovirus, rotavirus)
- Other features may include skin rash (due to maternal-fetal engraftment with graft-versus-host disease, Omenn syndrome (associated with RAG-deficiency) and hepatosplenomegaly (due to materno-fetal engraftment, transfusion of non-irradiated blood, or following generalized BCG infection after immunization).

39. Which are the four subtypes of severe combined immunodeficiency (SCID), and what is their relative frequency?

Classification of Subtypes of SCID

SUBTYPE	T CELL	B CELL	NK CELL	RELATIVE FREQUENCY	EXAMPLE	MODE OF INHERITANCE
I	–	–	–	20 %	Adenosine deaminase deficiency	AR
II	–	–	+	20 %	RAG deficiency	AR
III	-	+	–	55 %	Receptor common-γ-chain deficiency	XL
					Jak 3 deficiency	AR
IV	–	+	+	<5 %	CD3 deficiency	AR
					IL-7 Rα deficiency	AR

AR = autosomal recessive; XL = X-linked.

40. In children with severe combined immunodeficiency (SCID), how often is a family history positive for affected relatives?

50–60%. SCID can be inherited in both an autosomal recessive and an X-linked form.

Stephan JL, et al: Severe combined immunodeficiency: A retrospective single-center study of clinical presentation and outcome in 117 patients. J Pediatr 123:564–572, 1993.

41. What disease did the "bubble boy" have?

Adenosine deaminase (ADA) ***deficiency***. In this form of severe combined immunodeficiency, the lack of ADA results in abnormalities of B-cell and T-cell function and increased susceptibility to infection. The bubble served as a means of minimizing contagion but also promoted social isolation. While bone marrow transplantation has been curative as a treatment, ADA deficiency is the first disease (by initial reports) to be treated by gene therapy (i.e., insertion of functional ADA genes into the patient's autologous cells and followed by infusion).

42. What are the clinical phenotypes of adenosine deaminase deficiency?

Neonatal/infantile onset (80–90%): Clinically and immunologically virtually indistinguishable from all forms of classical SCID: lymphopenia with absent humoral and cellular immune functions, failure to thrive, severe infections with fungal, viral and opportunistic pathogens. 50% of the patients have skeletal abnormalities at the costochondral junction (flared ribs).

Delayed onset (15–20%): Recurrent infections, in particular sino-pulmonary infections and septicemia with a frequent failure to generate specific antibodies. Increased IgE levels, IgG subclass deficiencies and automimmunity (hypoparathyroidism, type 1 diabetes, hemolytic anemia, and idiopathic thrombocytopenia) provide evidence of immune dysregulation.

Shovlin CL, et al: Adult onset immunodeficiency caused by inherited adenosine deaminase deficiency. J Immunol 153:2331, 1994.

43. Which is the molecular defect of chronic granulomatous disease ?

Chronic granulomatous disease (CGD) is characterized by a profound defect in the oxygen metabolic burst in myeloid cells following the phagocytosis of microbes. The molecular mechanisms responsible for this disease are heterogenous, as any defect of the four subunits which constitute the NADPH-oxidase can cause CGD. In consequence, superoxide, oxygen radicals and peroxide production are lacking, and patients with CGD cannot kill catalase-positive pathogenic bacteria and fungi (e.g. *Staphylococcus aureus, Nocardia, Seratia, Aspergillus,* and others).

44. What types of infections are commonly seen in children with CGD?

Superficial staphylococcal skin infections, particularly around the nose, eyes, and anus, are common. Severe adenitis, recurrent pneumonia, indolent osteomyelitis, and chronic diarrhea are frequent. Of note, a male child with a liver abscess should be considered to have chronic granulomatous disease until proven otherwise.

45. What are the cornerstones of CGD treatment?

- Prevention of infections through immunization, prophylactic antibiotic and anti-*Aspergillus* treatment and avoidance of certain sources of pathogens
- Use of prophylactic recombinant human interferon-γ
- Early and aggressive use of parenteral antibiotics
- Surgical treatment of recalcitrant infections

Bemiller LS, et al: Safety and effectiveness of long-term interferon-γ therapy in patients with chronic granulomatous disease. Blood Cells Mol Dis 21:239, 1995.

46. Which disorder has to be considered in a newborn patient with delayed separation of the umbilical cord?

Patients with ***leucocyte adhesion deficiency*** type I (LAD I) suffer from a profound impairment of leucocyte mobilization into extravascular sites. The hallmark of this disorder is the complete absence of neutrophils at the site of infection and inflammation (e.g. wound healing).

47. What is the basis for leukocyte adhesion deficiency (LAD I)?

Leukocytes express a functionally related glycoprotein complex on the cell surface with a common β subunit and a cell-specific family of α subunits. LAD is a deficiency of various members of subfamilies of surface proteins due to mutations in the common integrin subunit (CD18). Affected cells do not migrate properly because they are unable to adhere to endothelial or connective tissue surfaces. In addition to delayed umbilical cord separation, clinically affected children can present with, skin infections with little pus formation, impaired wound healing, severe periodontal disease and persistent leukocytosis.

48. An 8-month-old with oculocutaneous albinism and recurrent pyogenic skin and respiratory tract infections likely has what syndrome?

Chédiak-Higashi syndrome is an autosomal recessive disorder characterized by leukocytes containing giant lysosomal granules, abnormal phagocytosis (due to deficient degranulation), and abnormal chemotaxis.

49. An infant with hypocalcemic tetany, a loud cardiac murmur, and dysmorphic facies likely has what syndrome?

DiGeorge syndrome (also called DiGeorge sequence or anomaly). The clinical pattern results from maldevelopment of the third and fourth pharyngeal pouches during embryogenesis, resulting in a spectrum of malformations including:

- *Cardiac defects*: aortic arch anomalies, and conotruncal anomalies, especially truncus arteriosus
- *Parathyroid absence* or *hypoplasia* with abnormal calcium homeostasis
- *Abnormal facies*, including low-set ears, short philtrum, hypertelorism, notched ear pinna, micrognathia, and downslanting palpebral fissures
- *Thymic hypoplasia*

The thymic maldevelopment is variable in degree and usually results in diminished numbers of T cells. However, clinically significant immunologic abnormalities are often absent.

50. What makes the lymphocyte bare in the bare lymphocyte syndrome?

The *bare lymphocyte syndrome* is characterized by absence of class I and/or class II MHC-HLA antigens. Lack of MHC antigens interferes with processes of recognition and cytotoxic defense. The immunologic features are similar to those noted with combined immunodeficiency diseases. There is severe lymphopenia and increased susceptibility to infection, particularly viral.

51. What are the two main phenotypes associated with complement component deficiencies?

Generally, deficiencies of the *early* complement components (C1, C4, C2, or C3 and Factor I and Factor H deficiencies) are associated with autoimmune diseases (glomerulonephritis, systemic lupus erythematosus, dermatomyocytis, scleroderma and vasculitis) or with a predisposition to infections with encapsulated organisms. Deficiencies of the *terminal* components (C5, C6, C7, C8, and possibly C9) are associated with recurrent neisserial diseases.

52. Which potential life-threatening disorder of the complement system is associated with non-pruritic swelling and occasional recurrent abdominal pain?

Angioedema of any part of the body including the airway and the intestine occurs as a consequence of ***hereditary C1 inhibitor deficiency*** and the failure to inactivate the complement and kinin systems. The condition has also been called hereditary angioneurotic edema (HANE). Infections, oral contraceptives, pregnancy, minor trauma, stress and others have been noted to precipitate this autosomal dominant disease. Diagnosis is confirmed by direct assay of the inhibitor level. Clinical presentations include:

- *Recurrent facial and extremity swelling*—acute, circumscribed edema that is not painful, red, or pruritic, clearly distinguishing it from urticaria. Usually self-resolves in 72 hours.
- *Abdominal pain*—recurrent, often severe, colicky pain, due to interstitial wall edema with vomiting and/or diarrhea; may be misdiagnosed as an acute abdomen.
- *Hoarseness, stridor*—a true emergency, as death by asphyxiation may occur due to laryngeal edema. Epinephrine, hydrocortisone, and antihistamines are often of only limited benefit, and tracheostomy is needed if there is progression of symptoms.

53. What are the indications for interferon therapy?

It is a growing list. Recombinant **IFN** α has been used as adjuvant treatment in multiple conditions including various malignancies (including hairy-cell leukemia), condyloma acuminata, hepatitis (C and D), and large or diffuse hemangiomas. **IFN** β is used experimentally to treat selected tumors. **IFN** γ has a role in a number of infectious (e.g., chronic granulomatous disease, chronic active hepatitis, leishmaniasis), fibrotic (e.g., scleroderma, keloids), and IgE-mediated diseases (e.g., atopic dermatitis, hyper-IgE syndrome).

DEVELOPMENTAL PHYSIOLOGY

54. How do immunoglobulin levels change during the first years of life?

- ***IgG*** levels in a full-term baby are equal or higher (5-10%) than maternal levels due to active placental transport. With an IgG half-life of 21 days, this transported maternal IgG reaches a nadir after 3–5 months. As the infant begins to make IgG, the level begins to rise slowly, is 60% of adult level at 1 year and achieves adult level by 6–10 years of age.
- ***IgM*** concentrations are normally very low at birth and 75% of normal adult concentrations are usually achieved by about 1 year of age.
- ***IgA*** is the last immunoglobulin produced and approaches 20% of adult value by one year, but full adult levels are not reached until adolescence. Because delays in production of IgA are not unusual, the diagnosis of IgA deficiency is difficult to make with certainty in a child < age 2 years.
- ***IgD*** and ***IgE***, both of which are present in low concentrations in the newborn, reach 10–40% of adult concentrations by 1 year of age.

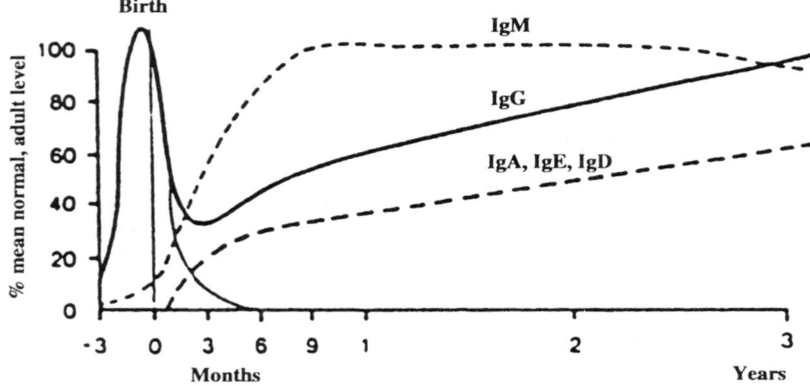

Normal development of serum immunoglobulin levels. (From Hobbs JR: Primary immune paresis. In Adinolfi M (ed): Immunology and development. Clinics in Developmental Medicine, no. 34. London, Spastics Int Medical Publ./William Heinemann Medical Books Ltd., 1969, pp 114–158; with permission.)

55. What determines immunoglobulin levels in infancy?

Immunoglobulin serum concentrations are determined by the amount of maternal IgG transported across the placenta, by catabolism of maternal IgG, and by the rate of synthesis of the infant's own IgM, IgG and IgA. The development of specific antibodies is dependent on antigen exposure, antigen presentation, and the availability of T cell help and T cell maturation. Newborns readily produce antibodies against (vaccine) proteins while polysaccharides fail to induce an adequate response during the first two years of life.

56. At what point in the development of the embryo can phenotypically mature B and T cells be detected?

Surface IgM-positive B cells are detected by the 9th week of gestation in the fetal liver. These cells are detected in the bone marrow, peripheral blood and the spleen by 12 weeks. IgG- and IgA-positive B cells appear between 10 and 12 weeks' gestation. $CD4^+$ and $CD8^+$ T cells can be detected in the fetal liver and the spleen by 14 weeks of gestation. Thus, lymphocytes with a mature phenotype are already present by the second trimester of fetal development.

57. Why aren't antibodies produced by the fetus in appreciable quantities?

- The fetus is in a sterile environment and is not exposed to foreign antigens.
- The active transport of maternal IgG across the placenta may suppress fetal antibody synthesis.
- Fetal and neonatal monocyte/macrophages may not process foreign antigens normally.

58. What is the role of the thymus?

The thymus is the primary lymphoid organ for the production and generation of T cells bearing the αβT cell receptor. Importantly, the thymus is responsible for the central selection of the T cell repertoire which allows the establishment of tolerance towards self-antigens and responsiveness to non-self (i.e., foreign) antigens.

59. At what age does thymic function cease?

At birth, the thymus is at two thirds of its mature weight and reaches its peak mass at around 10 years of life. Subsequently, thymic size declines but substantial function (as measured by the output of new T cells) persists into the very late adulthood (70-80 years of age).

Douek DC, et al: Changes in thymic function with age and during the treatment of HIV infection. Nature 396: 690-5, 1998.

60. What are the advantages of breast milk to the immune system of infants?

Several studies have reported that human milk enhances the development of the immune system, especially when measuring antibody formation. For example, antibody levels in response to immunization with conjugate *Haemophilous influenzae type B* vaccine are significantly higher in breast fed babies than in formula fed babies, suggesting that breast feeding enhances the active immune response in the first year of life.

Pabst HF, Spady DW: Effect of breast-feeding on antibody-response to conjugate vaccine. Lancet 336: 269, 1990.

61. What is the role of the receptor common γ-chain for the development and function of T cells and natural killer (NK) cells?

On the cell surface, the receptor common γ-chain associates with different transmembrane proteins to form the specific cytokine receptors for IL-2, IL-4, IL-7, IL-9 and IL-15, respectively. These cytokines are important for T and NK cell proliferation, and differentiation. In particular, IL-2 is important for peripheral T cell homeostasis; IL-4 for the polarization of Th2 cells; IL-7 for lymphoid precursor survival/expansion; and IL-15 for NK cell development and homeostasis.

IMMUNOLOGIC PRINCIPLES

62. What is the normal lymphocytic makeup of the peripheral blood?

Approximately 55–80% of the lymphocytes are T cells, 5–20% are B cells, and 5–20% are natural killer (NK) cells. There are usually a small number of cells that cannot be accounted for using the routine typing reagents.

63. Describe the life cycle of a polymorphonuclear (PMN) leukocyte.

It takes about 14 days for an immature myeloblast to develop into a mature PMN. After departing the bone marrow, the PMN circulates in the blood for up to 20 hours and then migrates to tissue where it resides for 1–2 days.

64. How do natural killer (NK) cells differ from other lymphocytes?

NK cells are large granular lymphocytes that lyse tumor or viral-infected target cells. This type of immunity does not require antibody and is not MHC restricted.

65. What are CD antigens?

CD, or cluster designated, antigens are one or more cell-surface molecules, detectable by monoclonal antibodies, that define a particular cell line or state of cellular differentiation.

66. What is the immunological importance of the major histocompatibility complex (MHC) antigens?

The MHC molecules are part of the immunoglobulin-gene super-family. MHC molecules are responsible for the rejection of unrelated tissues following transplantation. Every antigen, both non-self and self, is recognized by T cells in conjunction with MHC molecules. *Class I MHC gene products* (human leukocyte antigens [HLA] A, B, and C) are expressed on every living cell. *Class II MHC antigens* (HLA-D/DR) are expressed in large quantities only on B cells, dendritic cells, monocyte, macrophages, and activated T cells. CD4 (helper T cells) recognize foreign antigens in conjunction with Class II molecules, whereas CD8 (cytotoxic T cells) recognize foreign antigens in association with Class I MHC antigens.

67. What are the four types of hypersensitivity reactions?

Type I	IgE-mediated; immediate or anaphylactic (e.g., urticaria, allergic rhinitis)
Type II	Antibody-dependent cytotoxicity (e.g., Goodpasture syndrome, erythroblastosis fetalis)
Type III	Immune complex or Arthus reaction (e.g., poststreptoccal glomerulonephritis, serum sickness)
Type IV	Delayed hypersensitivity (e.g., contact dermatitis, tuberculin skin testing)

68. What are the activation pathways of the complement system?

The complement system can be activated via the ***classical pathway***, ***the lectin activation pathway*** and the ***alternative pathway***. The *classical pathway* (C1q, C1r, C1s, C4, C2) is usually activated when C1 binds to an antigen-antibody complex or to LPS, C-reactive protein or some types of viruses (including HIV). The *lectin pathway* is activated by direct recognition of microorganisms and their products (e.g. LPS), or by the recognition of hypoglycosylated IgG as mediated by the C-type MBLectin (previously known as mannose binding protein) recognizing certain sugar residues. The *alternative activation pathway* (C3, Factor D, P, and B) is directly activated by carbohydrate moieties of microorganisms.

Sumiya M, et al: Molecular basis of opsonic defect in immunodeficient children. Lancet 337: 1569, 1991.

69. What are the functions of the various interferons (IFN)?

Interferons are glycoproteins that were initially discovered as factors produced by cells during the course of viral infections. Three major types (α, β, γ) have been identified. IFNs α and β are produced by leukocytes and fibroblasts in response to viral infections, and γ is produced by T cells in response to an antigen or mitogen. The effects of interferons on cellular functions are widespread including:

Inhibit	Enhance	Mixed effects
Cell proliferation	Promyelocytic and monoblastic leukemic cell differentiation	Erythroleukemic cell differentiation
Tumor growth	Phagocytosis by macrophages	Production of antibodies
Fibroblast-adipocyte differentiation	Accessory cell functions of macrophages (IFN γ > IFN α, β)	Cell-mediated immune phenomena
	Endotoxin-induced interleukin-1 secretion by macrophages (IFN γ, α, β)	
	Generation of cytotoxic T lymphocytes	
	Activity of NK cells	
	Expression of class I and II MHC antigens and Fc receptors	

From Stites DP, Terr AI, Parslow TG: Medical Immunology, 9th ed. Norwalk, CT, Appleton & Lange, 1997; with permission.

LABORATORY ISSUES

70. **Which laboratory tests allow a broader evaluation of the humoral immune system?**

- ***Serum immunoglobulin levels, quantitative***: IgM, IgG, IgA and IgE . A combined IgG, IgA, and IgM level <400 mg/dL suggests immunoglobulin deficiency; >5000 IU/ml for IgE suggests hyper-IgE syndrome.
- ***IgG-subclasses:*** These immunglobulins generally should be measured primarily in patients older than six years of age and in certain circumstances, such as in patients with selective IgA deficiency, and normal to low IgG concentrations but demonstrated

functional antibody deficiency; and in patients with recurrent sino-pulmonary infections.

Specific antibody titers: in response to documented infections and vaccinations.

- Isohemagglutin titer (anti-A, anti-B): ≤1:4 after age 1 suggests specific IgM deficiency
- Tetanus/diphtheria (IgG_1)
- Pneumococcal polysaccharide antigens (IgG_2)
- Viral respiratory agents (IgG_3)

Determination of B cell numbers: in the peripheral blood by use of flow cytometry (CD19, CD20).

B cell proliferation and immunoglobulin production: by *in vitro* assays.

71. What is flow cytometry?

Flow cytometry is a diagnostic tool of cellular immunology to assess the cell surface and intracytoplasmic expression of proteins (antigens) by use of specific antibodies or substrates. Applicable only to single cell suspensions, this technique analyzes the size and granularity of cells as well as the (usually three) different wave lengths of light emitted from dyes excited by a laser beam. The dyes are conjugated to specific antibodies and thus determine antigen specificity (usually CD determinants).

72. Which diagnostic tests allow the specific evaluation of T cell functions?

- ***Total lymphocyte count:*** Although most T-cell immunodeficiencies are not associated with a decreased lymphocyte count, a total count < 1500/mm³ suggests a deficiency.
- ***T cell subpopulations:*** total T cells with < 60% mononuclear cells, helper (CD4) cells < 200/µl, or CD4/CD8 < 1.0 suggest T-cell deficiency.
- ***Delayed-type hypersensitivity skin testing.***
- ***Proliferative responses*** to mitogens, antigens and allogeneic cells.
- Acquisition of ***activation markers*** on T cells (using flow cytometry).
- ***Cytotoxic assay.***
- ***Cytokine synthesis.***
- ***Adenosine deaminase*** and ***purine nucleoside phosphorylase*** determination in RBCs.
- ***Molecular biological studies*** (including karyotyping and fluorescent *in situ* hybridizations).
- ***Histology*** of *thymic* and *lymph node biopsies.*

73. What is the value of skin testing for the diagnosis of T cell deficiencies?

Skin tests for the assessment of delayed-type hypersensitivity are difficult to evaluate. A positive test is useful in eliminating the diagnosis of severe T cell deficiency, while a negative test may either reflect a T cell defect or may result from the lack of an anamnestic response to the antigens used. Seventy-five percent of normal children aged 12–36 months will respond to *Candida* skin testing at 1:10 dilution; by 18 months, approximately 90% of normal children will respond to one of a panel of recall antigens (tetanus toxoid, trichophyton, and *Candida*); the younger the child, the less likely the reactivity. The cell-mediated reaction may be obscured by a humoral (Arthus) reaction due to previous priming.

74. What is the importance of the CD4/CD8 ratio?

The *CD4/CD8 ratio* is an index of helper to suppressor cells and may be significantly altered in a variety of immundeficiencies. In normal individuals, the ratio ranges from 1.4-1.8/1.0. In viral infections (particularly HIV), the ratio can be reduced, and in bacterial infections it can be increased.

75. How is white cell function evaluated in children with suspected disorders?

Neutrophils and monocyte/macrophages are enumerated and examined morphologically after histochemical staining. Monoclonal antibodies directed against CD14 (a surface antigen on monocytes) are used in conjunction with flow cytometry to quantify the number of monocytes/macrophages. Suspected abnormalities in hexose monophosphate activity (as seen in children with chronic granulomatous disease) can be investigated with either nitroblue tetrazolium dye reduction or a dichlorofluorescein assay. Chemotaxis is commonly assayed in agarose, and *in vitro* quantitative microbicidal assays can be used to assess the bactericidal capacity of isolated neutrophils and monocytes.

76. What are the principal tests used for the diagnosis of chronic granulomatous disease (CGD)?

The ***nitroblue tetrazolium (NBT) test*** and the ***chemiluminescence test***. Both rely on documenting the absence or greatly diminished respiratory burst seen in the stimulated neutrophils of CGD. The *NBT test* is a dye-reduction assay in which neutrophils are stimulated in the presence of yellow NBT. Ordinarily, NBT is reduced intracellularly to an insoluble blue compound (formazan) by the activation of the oxygen machinery of neutrophils. In CGD, these insoluble crystals do not form in normal numbers. *Chemiluminescence* is an alternative method to measure the metabolic burst of activated neutrophils. Numerous oxygen radicals react with substrates on microbes to form unstable intermediates which, in turn, emit light energy on their return to ground state. This energy can be measured as chemiluminescence (amplified by luminol) using flow cytometry. Decreased emissions are seen in CGD.

77. How is the classic complement cascade evaluated?

The primary screening test is the $\boldsymbol{CH_{50}}$. It assesses the ability of an individual's serum (in varying dilutions) to lyse sheep RBCs after those cells are sensitized with rabbit IgM anti-sheep antibody. The CH_{50} is an arbitrary unit indicating the quantity of complement necessary for 50% lysis of the RBCs in a standardized setting. Test results are usually expressed as a derived reciprocal of the test dilution needed for 50% lysis. The test is relatively insensitive, as major reductions in individual complement components are necessary before the CH_{50} is altered. Therefore, determination ***C3*** and ***C4 levels*** are often included in the initial screening of a child with a suspected complement deficiency.

11. INFECTIOUS DISEASES

Alexis M. *Elward,* M.D., *David* A. *Hunstad,* M.D., *and*
Joseph W. *St. Geme,* III, M.D.

ANTI-INFECTIVE THERAPY

1. In prescribing antibiotics for obese children, should the dosage be based on the actual or ideal weight of the child?

As a rule, most antibiotics distribute poorly into fat, and fat cells do not metabolize the drug. Therefore, ideal body weight (for height) is a better determinant of total daily dosage than actual weight.

2. Which antibiotics are contraindicated in hepatic failure?

Antibiotics that are primarily excreted or detoxified in the liver should be avoided or used with extreme caution in patients with impaired hepatic function. Examples of such drugs include chloramphenicol, tetracycline, erythromycin, clindamycin, rifampin, and isoniazid. If these agents are used, their dosage should be modified to account for the diminished excretion. Other drugs that should be used with caution or for which serum levels should be monitored in patients with severe liver disease include metronidazole, antifungal azoles, nitrofurantoin, and pyrazinamide.

3. How common are rashes related to ampicillin?

Minor reactions to ampicillin are manifested by a morbilliform, erythematous, papular rash that appears about 3 days after initiation of therapy. These rashes are common (7% of ampicillin courses) and are thought to be due to IgM complexes formed with penicilloyl antigens. They resolve spontaneously as IgG-blocking antibodies are formed. Clinical resolution occurs even though ampicillin therapy is continued. Ampicillin rashes should be distinguished from immediate (type I), IgE-mediated hypersensitivity reactions. The latter are rare (1 in every 20,000 courses of ampicillin) and occasionally life-threatening, with manifestations including an urticarial rash, shock, bronchospasm, and laryngeal edema. Usually, this allergic reaction follows immediately upon exposure to the drug, but a milder form may be delayed from a few hours to a few days.

Boguniewicz M, Leung DYM: Hypersensitivity reactions to antibiotics commonly used in children. Pediatr Infect Dis J 14:221–231, 1995.

4. How are children with allergy to penicillin managed?

Only about 10% of children with a history of adverse reactions to penicillin have an IgE-mediated sensitivity to the drug as demonstrated by a positive skin test. However, it is imperative that a thorough history be elicited in children with a history of an adverse reaction to penicillin.

Some experts have advocated skin testing in children with such histories to determine whether a reported adverse reaction to the drug is, in fact, IgE-mediated. There is an approximate 95% sensitivity in skin testing when both Prepen (penicilloyl-polylysine, a major antigenic determinant) and penicillin G are used. The sensitivity of skin testing is improved when minor determinants of penicillin are included in the skin testing panel. Other authorities advocate providing alternative antibiotic therapy in patients with a previous adverse reaction to penicillin. According to this approach, if for some reason alternative drug therapy is not possible, then penicillin skin testing can then be performed.

Skin testing itself poses a risk, including the possibility of anaphylaxis, and should be performed by an individual experienced in such procedures and in an appropriate clinical setting. In situations in which penicillin-specific IgE has been demonstrated and in which it is imperative that the patient receive a penicillin drug, desensitization can be performed by experienced medical personnel in a clinical setting capable of handling emergency situations.

Boguniewicz M, Leung DYM: Management of the patient with allergic reactions to antibiotics. Pediatr Pulmonol 12:113–122, 1992.

5. What is the advantage of Augmentin over amoxicillin?

Augmentin is a combination antibiotic that contains amoxicillin and clavulanic acid. Clavulanic acid is a β-lactamase inhibitor and adds activity against many β-lactamase producing organisms, including *Haemophilus influenzae, Moraxella catarrhalis, Staphylococcus aureus*, and the majority of penicillin-resistant anaerobes.

6. What are the different classes of penicillins?

Penicillins are divided into 5 categories based on structure and antibacterial activity. The categories are as follows:

Class	***Examples***	***Spectrum of activity***
Natural penicillins	Penicillin G Penicillin V	Non-β-lactamase producing gram positive bacteria and anaerobes
Aminopenicillins	Ampicillin Amoxicillin	Same as natural penicillins, plus gram-negative cocci and some *Enterobacteriaceae*
Penicillinase-resistant penicillins	Methicillin Nafcillin Oxacillin	*Staphylococcus aureus,* some coagulase-negative staphylococci, streptococci
Carboxy- and indanyl penicillins	Carbenicillin Ticarcillin	Gram-negative aerobic rods resistant to ampicillin, including *P. aeruginosa*
Extended-spectrum Ureidopenicillins	Azlocillin Mezlocillin Piperacillin	Like carboxy- and indanyl penicillins, but with more activity against streptococci and *Haemophilus* spp.

7. What are the differences among first-, second-, third-, and fourth-generation cephalosporins?

First-generation cephalosporins (e.g., cefazolin, cephalexin, cefadroxil)

- Alternative drugs for patients allergic to penicillins, although there is a 5–10% risk of cross-reactivity
- Prophylaxis in orthopedic and cardiovascular surgery
- Better *Staphylococcus aureus* coverage compared to second- and third-generation cephalosporins
- Lack of efficacy against *Haemophilus influenzae*

Second-generation cephalosporins (e.g., cefaclor, cefuroxime, cefprozil, cefpodoxime)

- Increased spectrum of activity, including many gram-negative organisms
- Prophylaxis for intra-abdominal and pelvic surgery (e.g., cefoxitin)
- Improved compliance with oral medications (most with twice-daily dosing)
- Poor penetration into CSF
- No anti-pseudomonal activity

Third-generation cephalosporins (e.g., ceftriaxone, cefotaxime, cefixime)

- Broadest spectrum, including excellent activity against gram-negative bacteria

- Generally less activity against gram-positive organisms than earlier generations
- Very high blood and CSF levels achievable in relation to MIC for bacterial strains
- Wide therapeutic index with generally minimal toxicity (similar to previous generations)
- Some offer single-daily dosing
- Most expensive

Fourth-generation cephalosporins (e.g., ceftazidime, cefepine)

- Spectrum similar to third-generation agents, with the addition of anti-pseudomonal activity

Darville T, Yamauchi T: The cephalosporin antibiotics. Pediatr Rev 15:54–62, 1994.

8. What is the mechanism of resistance to β-lactam antibiotics by *Streptococcus pneumoniae*?

Penicillin and related β-lactams inhibit the replication of *Streptococcus pneumoniae* by binding to one or more of the enzymes involved in synthesis of peptidoglycan, an important component of the cell wall. These enzymes include higher molecular weight transpeptidases and a lower molecular weight carboxypeptidase and are referred to as penicillin-binding proteins (PBPs). Resistant isolates of *S. pneumoniae* have mutations in one or more PBPs, resulting in decreased affinity for β-lactams. Of note, since resistance is independent of β-lactamase, β-lactamase inhibitors offer no benefit in treating resistant *S. pneumoniae*.

9. Are antibiotic-resistant pneumococci more virulent than sensitive strains?

The occurrence of infection due to antibiotic-resistant *Streptococcus pneumoniae* is a growing problem in both children and adults. Resistance has been documented to penicillins, cephalosporins, erythromycin, tetracycline, and trimethoprim-sulfamethoxazole. Up to 50% of pneumococcal isolates from sterile body sites are non-susceptible to penicillin (MIC ≥ 0.1 μg/ml), and of these, 50% are also non-susceptible to cefotaxime and ceftriaxone (MIC ≥ 1 μg/ml). The strongest risk factors for infection due to non-susceptible strains include day care attendance and recent treatment with antibiotics. It does not appear that the non-susceptible strains are more virulent or present with a different clinical picture than susceptible strains. For CNS infection, treatment requires the use of cefotaxime or ceftriaxone plus vancomycin. In some cases, rifampin may be necessary as well.

American Academy of Pediatrics. Pneumococcal infections. In: Pickering LK (ed): 2000 Red Book: Report of the Committee on Infectious Diseases, 25th ed. Elk Grove Village, IL, American Academy of Pediatrics, 2000, p. 454.

Friedland IR, McCracken GH Jr: Management of infections caused by antibiotic-resistant Streptococcus pneumoniae. N Engl J Med 331:377–382, 1994.

10. What are the uses and side effects of chloramphenicol?

Chloramphenicol has activity against many gram-positive and gram-negative bacteria, but its use is limited because newer alternatives with less serious side effects are available. Rickettsial infections (e.g., Rocky Mountain spotted fever) and some other zoonoses can still be treated with chloramphenicol, but tetracycline or doxycycline is preferred in most cases.

In neonates, chloramphenicol toxicity manifested by circulatory collapse (gray baby syndrome) occurs because hepatic metabolism of the drug is poor. It is necessary to determine serum levels frequently (daily to every other day) to anticipate this complication; the serum chloramphenicol level should be maintained between 10 μg/ml and 25 μg/ml. In older children, this syndrome is not seen, and the only common side effect is reversible bone marrow suppression. One in 20,000-40,000 courses of the drug will lead to an idiosyncratic, non-dose-dependent fatal aplastic anemia.

11. In which patients should trimethoprim-sulfamethoxazole be avoided or used with caution?

Trimethoprim-sulfamethoxazole (TMP-SMX) acts by inhibiting the folic acid pathway of bacteria. Disruption of human folate metabolism may occur, affecting rapidly replicating cells, especially in the bone marrow and skin. Avoidance or cautious use is suggested in the following settings:

1. Patients who have not received folate supplementation and who are known or expected to be deficient in folate, because of:
   a. Phenytoin use
   b. Therapy with another folate antagonist
   c. Protein-calorie malnutrition
   d. Prematurity
2. Pregnancy
3. Fragile X syndrome
4. Known sensitivity to any sulfonamide
5. Age ≤ 2 months
6. History of skin rash while receiving TMP-SMX
7. G6PD deficiency

From Gutman LT: The use of trimethoprim-sulfamethoxazole in children: A review of adverse reactions and indications. Pediatr Infect Dis J 3:355, 1984; with permission.

12. Which antibiotic is associated with the "red man syndrome"?

The red man syndrome is a frequent occurrence with the rapid infusion of ***vancomycin*** and is characterized by flushing of the neck, face, and thorax. The histamine release underlying this reaction is directly caused by vancomycin. It is not mediated by IgE and therefore does not represent a true hypersensitivity reaction. Generally the reaction can be avoided by slowing the rate of drug infusion. Administration of an H_1-receptor antagonist (e.g., diphenhydramine) before vancomycin is given is also effective in preventing this reaction.

13. How should infections with vancomycin-resistant organisms be managed?

Resistance to vancomycin was first observed in *Enterococcus faecium* and has now been seen in *E. faecalis*. Many patients have succumbed to bacteremia or other invasive infections with vancomycin-resistant enterococci (VRE). Most of these infections are acquired nosocomially. Basic tenets of therapy apply: foreign bodies should be removed, infected fluid collections should be drained, and the patient should be isolated to prevent spread. Antimicrobial agents with activity against some VRE strains exist, but these agents are not bactericidal. The newly licensed streptogramin agent quinupristin-dalfopristin (Synercid) and the oxazolidinone antibiotic linezolid (Zyvox) have shown promise in early use.

Several cases of infection due to *Staphylococcus aureus* with intermediate susceptibility to vancomycin (VISA) have been reported. Treatment of these infections is similar to that described above for VRE. Some VISA isolates show reduced expression of PBP2a, a protein that is critical to the phenotype of methicillin resistance. This change in expression of PBP2a may permit the use of semisynthetic penicillins against some vancomycin-resistant strains.

14. What is the mechanism of action of linezolid?

Linezolid is the first licensed antibiotic belonging to a class referred to as oxazolidinones. These antibiotics are ***inhibitors of protein synthesis*** and are bacteriostatic against a variety of bacteria. Linezolid may be especially useful in treating infections due to vancomycin-resistant enterococci, methicillin-resistant *Staphylococcus aureus*, and β-lactam-resistant *Streptococcus pneumoniae*.

15. What is Synercid?

Synercid is a combination antibiotic that includes quinupristin and dalfopristin, which belong to the streptogramin family. These agents inhibit bacterial protein synthesis by irreversibly binding to the 50S bacterial ribosomal subunit. Quinupristin and dalfopristin bind to different sites on the 50S subunit, and quinupristin acts by inhibiting peptide chain elongation, while dalfopristin directly interferes with peptidyl transferase.

16. How can the emergence of antibiotic-resistant pathogens be minimized?

- Appropriate handwashing to reduce transmission of resistant organisms to other patients.
- Use of the most potent, narrow-spectrum antibiotic possible for an appropriate length of time.
- Minimization of empiric use of broad-spectrum antibiotics.
- Avoidance of antibiotic treatment of illnesses that are likely viral.
- Awareness of local antibiotic resistance patterns.

Woodin KA, Morrison SH: Antibiotics: Mechanisms of action. Pediatr Rev 15:440–447, 1994.

17. Are any antiviral agents effective in eradicating cytomegalovirus (CMV) infection?

Both ***ganciclovir*** and ***foscarnet*** have activity against CMV. Ganciclovir has been studied more thoroughly and has efficacy in HIV-infected patients who have CMV retinitis and in some transplant patients with local or systemic CMV infection. Foscarnet has been used primarily when an isolate develops resistance to ganciclovir.

18. What are the advantages of valacyclovir and famciclovir over acyclovir?

Valacylovir is the L-valyl ester prodrug of acyclovir and following oral administration is rapidly and almost completely converted to acyclovir. The bioavailability of valacyclovir is considerably higher than that of acyclovir, allowing less frequent dosing.

Famciclovir is the diacetyl ester of penciclovir, which is an acyclic guanosine analog similar to acyclovir in spectrum of activity and potency against herpesviruses. Famciclovir is a prodrug that is well absorbed orally and rapidly converted to penciclovir. Again, compared with acyclovir, the bioavailability of famciclovir allows less frequent dosing.

19. Why is chicken soup so helpful for URIs?

The benefits of chicken soup have been of lore for hundreds of years, beginning in the 12th century when physician and philosopher Maimonades extolled its virtue. The precise mechanisms of its anecdotal therapeutic benefits remain elusive. One recent study at the University of Nebraska found that the non-particulate component of chicken soup *in vitro* inhibited neutrophil migration in a concentration-dependent manner. This anti-inflammatory effect may be one mechanism by which chicken soup mitigates the symptoms of URIs.

Rennard BO, et al: Chicken soup inhibits neutrophil chemotaxis in vitro. Chest 118: 1150-1157, 2000.

CLINICAL ISSUES

20. Name the three stages of pertussis infection (whooping cough).

1. ***Catarrhal*** (1–2 wks): low grade fever, upper respiratory infection symptoms
2. ***Paroxysmal*** (2–4 wks): severe cough occurring in paroxysms, onset of inspiratory "whoop"
3. ***Convalescent*** (1–2 wks): resolution of symptoms

21. What is the most common cause of death in children with whooping cough?

Ninety percent of deaths are attributable to ***pneumonia***, which most often develops as a secondary bacterial infection. These cases can be easily missed in the paroxysmal phase, when respiratory symptoms are so prominent and usually attributed solely to pertussis. A new spiking fever should prompt a careful search for an evolving pneumonia.

22. Is erythromycin of value in pertussis infection?

If used in the first 14 days of illness or before the paroxysmal stage, erythromycin can decrease the severity of symptoms during the paroxysmal stage. If the diagnosis is established later in the course, erythromycin should still be administered, as it eliminates nasopharyngeal carriage of *B. pertussis* and limits the spread of disease. The dose is 50 mg/kg/day (divided QID) for 14 days, maximum total daily dose of 1 gm. Recent evidence suggests that treatment with azithromycin (10-12 mg/kg/day in one dose) or clarithromycin (15-20 mg/kg/day divided BID) for 5-7 days is also effective in eradicating carriage and preventing transmission.

23. Do antibiotics prevent the development of pneumonia after an upper respiratory tract infection (URI)?

Over 90% of URIs are caused by viruses, and children younger than age 5 (especially those in day care environments) can experience 6–8 URI episodes per year. Multiple studies have shown that antibiotic treatment of URIs does *not* shorten their course or prevent the development of pneumonia.

Gadomski AM: Potential interventions for preventing pneumonia among young children: Lack of effect of antibiotic treatment for upper respiratory infections. Pediatr Infect Dis J 12:115–120, 1993.

24. What is the treatment of choice for *Listeria monocytogenes* infection?

In most cases, treatment should include ampicillin or penicillin. Based on synergy in vitro and in animal models, most experts advise adding gentamicin in cases of meningitis and for patients with bacteremia and severe immunodeficiency.

Vancomycin has been used with success in some penicillin-allergic patients with bacteremia, but others have developed *Listeria* meningitis during therapy with this agent. Cephalosporins lack activity against *Listeria monocytogenes* and should not be used.

25. Sternal edema is classically the sign of what infection?

Mumps.

26. How does the Hatchcock sign help distinguish swelling due to mumps from swelling caused by adenitis?

Upward pressure applied to the angle of the mandible produces tenderness with mumps (*Hatchcock sign*). This maneuver produces no tenderness with adenitis.

27. What clinical criteria are used to diagnose staphylococcal toxic shock syndrome?

Temperature > 38.9°C

***Rash*:** diffuse macular erythroderma

***Desquamation*:** particularly of palms and soles 1–2 weeks after onset of illness

***Hypotension*:** systolic BP < 90 mm Hg (adults), <5th percentile (children), or orthostatic changes

Multisystem involvement—*3 or more of the following*:

Gastrointestinal: vomiting or diarrhea at the onset of the illness

Musculoskeletal: severe myalgia or elevated creatine kinase level

Mucous membrane: conjunctival, vaginal, or oropharyngeal hyperemia

Renal: elevated blood urea or creatinine, or pyuria without urinary tract infection

Hepatic: elevated alanine or aspartate aminotransferase level

CNS: disorientation or other alteration of consciousness

Hematologic: platelet count < 100 x 10^9/L

Negative results on:

Cultures of blood, throat, and CSF (except blood cultures growing *Staphylococcus aureus*)

Serologic or other tests for Rocky Mountain spotted fever, leptospirosis, and measles

Wharton M, et al: Case definitions for public health surveillance. MMWR 39(RR13):1-43, 1990.

28. What clinical criteria are used to diagnose streptococcal toxic shock syndrome?

Isolation of group A streptococci from a normally sterile site (blood, CSF, pleural fluid) or nonsterile site (throat, vagina)

***Hypotension*:** systolic BP < 90 mm Hg (adults) or < 5th percentile (children)

***Multisystem involvement*—*2 or more of the following*:**

Renal: creatinine level more than twice the upper limit of normal for age

Hematologic: platelet count < 100 × 10^9/L or evidence of DIC

Hepatic: elevated alanine or aspartate aminotransferase level

Respiratory: Adult respiratory distress syndrome

Dermatologic: Generalized erythematous macular *rash* that may desquamate; soft tissue necrosis, including necrotizing fasciitis, myositis, or gangrene

The Working Group on Severe Streptococcal Infections: Defining the group A streptococcal toxic shock syndrome. JAMA 269:390-1, 1993.

29. Discuss the distinguishing features of staphylococcal scalded skin syndrome, staphylococcal toxic shock syndrome, and streptococcal toxic shock syndrome.

Distinguishing Features of Stapylococcal Scalded Skin Syndrome, Staphyloccal Toxic Shock Syndrome, and Streptococcal Toxic Shock Syndrome

CLINICAL FEATURES	STAPHYLOCOCCAL SCALDED SKIN SYNDROME	STAPHYLOCCAL TOXIC SHOCK SYNDROME	GROUP A STREPTOCOCCAL TOXIC SHOCK-LIKE SYNDROME
Organism	*Staphylococcus aureus* Usually phage group 11, type 71	*Staphylococcus aureus* Usually phage group 1, type 29	Group A streptococci Usually type 1, 3, or 18 Exotoxin A production
Site of infection	Usually focal Mucocutaneous border: nose, mouth, diaper area Sometimes inapparent	Mucous membranes Infected wound or furuncle Sometimes inapparent	Blood, abscess, pneumonia, empyema, cellulitis, necrotizing fasciitis Sometimes inapparent
Skin rash	Tender erythroderma: face, neck, generalized Bullae, no petechiae	Tender erythroderma: trunk, hands, feet Edema of hands, feet	Erythroderma: trunk, extremities
Desquamation	Early, first 1–2 days, generalized	Late, 7–10 days, mostly hands and feet Hyperemia of oral and vaginal mucosa	Late, 7–10 days, mostly hands and feet Hyperemia of oral and vaginal mucosa
Mucous membranes	Normal	Hypertrophy of tongue papillae	Hypertrophy of tongue papillae
Conjunctivae	Normal	Markedly injected	Injected
Course	Insidious, 4–7 days benign, < 1% mortality	Fulminant, shock with secondary multiple organ failure, 10% mortality	Fulminant, shock with early primary multiple organ failure, 30–50% mortality

From Bass JW: Treatment of skin and skin structure infections. Pediatr Infect Dis J 11:154, 1992; with permission.

30. What percentage of cases of staphylococcal toxic shock syndrome are nonmenstrual?

Over the past two decades, the epidemiology of toxic shock syndrome has changed, reflecting changes in tampon composition and a decrease in absorbency. In 1996, over 50% of repoted cases were nonmenstrual. The syndrome occurs in the setting of focal staphylococcal colonization or focal infections, including empyema, osteomyelitis, soft tissue abscess, surgical infections, and burns.

31. What are the biphasic features of leptospiral infection?

Both anicteric and icteric cases of leptospirosis have two phases:

First phase: fever, headache, conjunctivitis, myalgia, abdominal pain; leptospires found in CSF and blood; lasts 4–7 days.

Second phase: phase of immunologic response; leptospires found in urine; lasts 4–30 days

Anicteric type (90%): rash, meningitis, uveitis

Icteric type (10%): jaundice, myocarditis, hemorrhage, renal dysfunction

32. In a recovering patient, where in the body do leptospires persist the longest?

The ***aqueous humor***. Regions of the eye serve as an immunologic barrier, allowing chronic carriage for months. Some affected patients have recurrent uveitis.

33. Which diseases are transmitted by ticks?

Disease	***Agent***
Lyme disease	*Borrelia burgdorferi*
Relapsing fever	*Borrelia* species
Tularemia	*Francisella tularensis*
Rocky Mountain spotted fever	*Rickettsia rickettsii*
Queensland tick typhus	*R. australis*
Boutonneuse fever	*R. conorii*
Asian tick typhus	*R. sibirica*
Colorado tick fever	Arbovirus
Tick-borne encephalitis	Arbovirus
Ehrlichiosis	*Ehrlichia chaffeensis, E. equi, E. phagocytophila, E. ewingii*
Babesiosis	*Babesia microti, B. divergens, B. bovis*

Kaplan SL: Arthropods. In: Feigin RD, Cherry JD (eds): Textbook of Pediatric Infectious Diseases, 4th ed. Philadelphia, W.B. Saunders, 1998, p. 2537.

34. What are the two primary types of human ehrlichiosis?

Human monocytic ehrlichiosis *(HME)* and ***human granulocytic ehrlichiosis*** *(HGE).*

Both are febrile illnesses caused by different agents but with similar clinical pictures of significant systemic symptoms (e.g., intense headache, chills, myalgia) and occasional rash. The presentation can mimic Rocky Mountain spotted fever. Particular features include anemia, lymphopenia, leukopenia, thrombocyopenia, hyponatremia, elevated liver function tests and CSF abnormalities (e.g., lymphocytic pleocytosis, elevated total protein).

Jacobs RF, Schultze GE: Ehrlichiosis in children. J Pediatr 131:184-192, 1997.

35. Which ticks are associated with transmission of human ehrlichiosis?

The Lone Star tick, *Amblyomma americanum*, appears to be responsible for transmission of most cases of human monocytic ehrlichiosis, caused by *Ehrlichia chaffeensis*. In some geographic areas, the American dog tick, *Dermacentor variabilis*, may also transmit *E. chaffeensis*.

The deer tick *Ixodes scapularis* is involved in transmission of most cases of human granulocytic ehrlichiosis, caused by the HGE agent (highly homologous to *E. phagocytophila* and *E. equi*). A minority of cases are transmitted by the Lone Star tick, which is the vector for *E. ewingii*, a dog pathogen recently implicated as an occasional cause of human granulocytic ehrlichiosis.

36. What is the preferred treatment for human ehrlichiosis?

Doxycycline is the drug of choice to treat human ehrlichiosis. Early clinical experience suggested that chloramphenicol may also be effective, but *in vitro* susceptibility testing of

E. chaffeensis and the HGE agent revealed resistance to chloramphenicol. Although tetracyclines are generally contraindicated in children younger than 8 years old because of associated dental staining, short courses of treatment with these agents, especially doxycycline, are unlikely to cause dental abnormalities.

37. What are the six forms of tularemia?

Tularemia is caused by *Francisella tularensis*, a gram-negative coccobacillus. Blood-feeding arthropods and flies are the most important vectors of tularemia in the U.S. In addition, animal contact is an important mode of acquiring tularemia, typically related to skinning, dressing, or eating infected rabbits, muskrats, beavers, or squirrels.

The classic forms of tularemia include the following: ***glandular, ulceroglandular, oculoglandular*** (Parinaud syndrome), ***pharyngeal, pneumonic***, and ***typhoidal*** (disseminated).

38. What is the preferred treatment for tularemia?

The drug of choice for tularemia is *streptomycin*, although gentamicin is a suitable and common alternative. Tetracycline and chloramphenicol have been used but are associated with a high rate of relapse, presumably because they are bacteriostatic for *F. tularensis*.

39. What the heck are the HACEKs?

The *HACEK* organisms include *Haemophilus aphrophilus, Haemophilus paraphrophilus, Actinobacillus actinomycetemcomitans, Cardiobacterium hominis, Eikenella corrodens*, and *Kingella kingae*. These organisms share the property of slow growth in culture and have a predilection for producing endocarditis. They should be considered in cases of apparently culture-negative endocarditis.

40. In the setting of clinical signs and symptoms of encephalitis, what EEG pattern is suggestive of herpes simplex virus disease?

Periodic lateralized epileptiform discharges (PLEDs). PLEDs may be seen in other, rarer forms of encephalitis, such as Epstein-Barr virus encephalitis, Creutzfeldt-Jakob disease, and subacute sclerosing panencephalitis.

41. What is the best approach to diagnosing herpes simplex virus (HSV) encephalitis in children?

Encephalitis due to HSV is a devastating disease with significant mortality and morbidity. Antiviral therapy (e.g., with acyclovir) is successful only if the diagnosis is made early. In the past, no single noninvasive method could simply and reproducibly diagnose HSV encephalitis; definitive diagnosis relied on brain biopsy. In recent years, a number of studies have demonstrated that analysis of CSF using the polymerase chain reaction (PCR) allows rapid and accurate diagnosis. According to Lakeman et al., PCR detects over 98% of cases and may be more sensitive than brain biopsy. When performed with the proper precautions and controls, PCR is also highly specific. With this information in mind, the need for brain biopsy has diminished considerably. Nowadays, brain biopsy should be considered only when (1) PCR is negative and the diagnosis remains obscure; or (2) PCR is positive, but the clinical course is atypical for HSV encephalitis and the response to antiviral therapy is slow.

Lakeman FD, et al: Diagnosis of herpes simplex encephalitis: Application of polymerase chain reaction to cerebrospinal fluid from brain-biopsied patients and correlation with disease. J Infect Dis 171:857–863, 1995.

DeVincenzo JP, Thorne G: Mild herpes simplex encephalitis diagnosed by polymerase chain reaction: A case report and review. Pediatr Infect Dis J 13:662–664, 1994.

42. Can acyclovir be used to prevent or treat oral HSV infections?

In immunocompetent hosts, oral acyclovir offers significant therapeutic benefit in primary HSV gingivostomatitis but has limited efficacy in the treatment of recurrent herpes labialis. Topical acyclovir has not shown consistent benefit in either of these settings. Prophylaxis with oral acyclovir can reduce the number of recurrences in adults with herpes labialis but has not been studied in children.

43. How long should animals be observed in confinement when rabies is a concern?

When animals are shedding the virus and are thus capable of being contagious, they are usually sick within 5 days after the onset of shedding. In some experimental settings, this asymptomatic period can last up to 14 days. The standard in the United States is to confine dogs and cats for 10 days following a suspicious human contact. There has not been a report of a case of rabies transmission by an animal that remained healthy during that time period.

44. What causes visceral larva migrans?

Toxocara canis (a dog helminth) and *T. cati* (a cat helminth) cause this infiltrative granulomatous disease. Clinical features include fever, hepatomegaly, myocardial involvement, retinal disease, and pneumonitis.

45. Other than definitive serologic tests, which two laboratory tests are most suggestive of *Toxocara* infections?

1. ***Marked eosinophilia*** (20–90% of peripheral white blood cells)
2. ***Markedly elevated isohemagglutinin titers*** (i.e., anti-A and/or anti-B titers in individuals who are not blood type A or B)

46. What is the difference between a paronychia and a felon?

A *paronychia* is an inflammation or infection in the soft tissue adjacent to the nail (*onyx* = *nail*, Greek). A *felon* is an infection (often an abscess) in the fat pad spaces (also known as volar pulp) of the distal phalanx.

47. How quickly do central lines become colonized?

The timing and rate of central line colonization depend on a number of factors. Manipulation of the catheter (e.g., for blood drawing, medication administration, or flushing) and poor hand-washing by health care providers are probably most important in increasing the risk of colonization. In general, the likelihood of colonization increases with the length of time the catheter has been in place. Colonization rates have been reported to be <10% for catheters less than 3 days old, approximately 15% for catheters 3–7 days old, and about 20% for catheters in place over 7 days.

48. What is the most proper medical term for oral thrush?

Acute pseudomembranous candidiasis. Quite a mouthful. Although thrush is sometimes confused with residual formula in the mouth, formula is more easily removed with a tongue blade. When thrush is scraped, small bleeding points often occur on the underlying mucosa.

CONGENITAL INFECTIONS

49. Which congenital infections cause cerebral calcifications?

Cerebral calcifications are most frequently observed in congenital ***Toxoplasma*** and ***cytomegalovirus*** (CMV) infections. Toxoplasmosis often produces dense round calcifications scattered diffusely throughout the white matter of the brain, although it may also present as curvilinear streaks in the basal ganglia. Calcification in CMV-infected infants is typically periventricular, but there is considerable overlap between the presentations of these two diseases. Herpes simplex virus has also been reported to cause massive bilateral calcifications of the cerebral hemispheres, as has congenital rubella infection (rarely).

50. What are the late sequelae of congenital infections?

The late sequelae of chronic intrauterine infections are relatively common and may occur in infants who are asymptomatic at birth. Most sequelae present later in childhood rather than infancy.

Late Sequelae of Chronic Intrauterine Infection

CMV	Hearing loss,* minimal to severe brain dysfunction* (motor, learning, language, and behavioral disorders)
Rubella	Hearing loss,* minimal to severe brain dysfunction* (motor, learning, language and behavioral disorders), autism,* juvenile diabetes, thyroid dysfunction, precocious puberty, progressive degenerative brain disorder*
Toxoplasmosis	Chorioretinitis,* minimal to severe brain dysfunction,* hearing loss, precocious puberty
Neonatal herpes	Recurrent eye and skin infection, minimal to severe brain dysfunction
Hepatitis B virus	Chronic subclinical hepatitis, rarely fulminant hepatitis

*Seen with infections that are subclinical in early infancy.
From Plotkin SA, Alpert G: Pediatr Clin North Am 33:465, 1986; with permission.

51. What is the most common congenital infection?

Congenital ***CMV*** infection, which in some large screening studies occurs in up to 1.3% of newborns. However, 90–95% of infected neonates are asymptomatic.

52. How is CMV transmitted from mother to infant?

CMV can be transmitted by the ***transplacental route*** or through contact with ***cervical secretions*** or ***breast milk***. On occasion, transmission may occur by contact with saliva or urine.

53. How do complications vary between newborns with CMV infection who are symptomatic versus asymptomatic at birth?

Complications in Symptomatic versus Asymptomatic Newborns with CMV

	% OCCURRENCE	
COMPLICATION	SYMPTOMATIC	ASYMPTOMATIC
Death	5.8	0.3
Microcephaly	37.5	1.8
Sensorineural hearing loss	58	7.4
Bilateral hearing loss	37	2.7
Moderate to profound hearing loss (60-90 dB)	27	1.7
Chorioretinitis	20.4	2.5
IQ <70	55	3.7
Seizures	23.1	0.9
Paresis/paralysis	12.5	0

From Remington JS, Klein JO: Infections of the Fetus and Newborn Infant, 4th ed. Philadelphia, W.B. Saunders, 1995, p. 335, with permission.

54. Which infants with CMV infection have the worst prognosis?

- Neonates born to mothers with primary CMV infection during pregnancy

- Infants with symptoms at birth (particularly those with CNS signs)
- Infants with microcephaly and/or intracranial calcifications
- Neonates with CMV-specific IgM

Overall JC Jr: Viral infections of the fetus and neonate. In: Feigin RD, Cherry JD (eds): Pediatric Infectious Diseases, 4th ed. Philadelphia, W.B. Saunders, 1998, p. 868.

55. What is the risk to the fetus if the mother is infected with parvovirus B19 during pregnancy?

The risk of fetal loss is ***between 2% and 10%*** and is greatest when maternal infection occurs during the first half of pregnancy. Fetal loss occurs as a consequence of hydrops, which develops as a result of parvovirus-induced anemia. An elevated maternal serum alpha-fetoprotein level may be a marker for an adverse outcome. The signs of parvovirus infection in adults are not very distinctive but may include fever, a maculopapular or lace-like rash, and joint pain.

56. What are the consequences of primary varicella infection in the first trimester?

The ***congenital varicella syndrome*** consists of a constellation of features, the most typical of which is atrophy of a limb, usually associated with a cicatricial lesion involving the affected limb. Other features include neurologic and sensory defects, as well as eye abnormalities (chorioretinitis, cataracts, microphthalmia, Horner syndrome). The congenital varicella syndrome usually follows maternal infection in the first trimester, though it may be seen following infection up to 20 weeks into gestation. The largest prospective study reported to date found 4 cases of fetal varicella syndrome in 141 pregnancies, yielding an incidence of < 3%.

57. When should varicella zoster immune globulin be given to a newborn?

Varicella-zoster immune globulin (VZIG) should be given as soon as possible to a newborn whose mother developed varicella from 5 days before to 2 days after delivery. During this period of high risk, the fetus is exposed to high circulating titers of virus without benefit of maternal antibody synthesis. In contrast, if the child's mother develops primary infection more than 5 days before delivery, maternal antibody is synthesized and provides passive protection for the fetus. Similarly, if symptoms develop in the child's mother more than 48 hours after delivery, it is assumed that the fetus was not exposed to maternal viremia.

Premature neonates exposed to varicella in the neonatal period are also candidates for VZIG:

1. If the infant is ≥ 28 weeks gestation and the mother has no history of chickenpox.
2. If the infant is < 28 weeks gestation or ≤ 1,000 g, regardless of maternal history, because little maternal antibody crosses the placenta prior to the third trimester of pregnancy.

58. Do urogenital mycoplasmas have a role in neonatal disease?

Ureaplasma urealyticum has been associated with low birth weight and bronchopulmonary dysplasia; it has been recovered from neonates with respiratory distress, pneumonia, and meningitis. Its causative role in these diseases has not been proven. In one study, *Mycoplasma hominis* was recovered from the CSF in 23 (5.9%) of 387 neonates evaluated for bacterial sepsis, but only one infant had a CSF profile suggestive of meningitis. Several other reports of apparent *M. hominis* meningitis have been published. This organism has also been reported to cause neonatal eye infection.

59. If a mother is culture-positive for *Ureaplasma urealyticum* or *Mycoplasma hominis*, what is the likelihood of transmission to the newborn infant?

Vertical transmission occurs in ***up to 60%*** of exposed newborns. Risk of transmission is higher in preterm and low-birthweight infants and correlates with prolonged rupture of membranes and maternal fever. Infants delivered by cesarean section over intact membranes have a very low rate of colonization compared to those delivered vaginally.

60. What are the features of the congenital rubella syndrome?

Rubella virus is a teratogenic agent that induces a number of characteristic congenital abnormalities. Some of these abnormalities are present only in the neonatal period, while others persist through life. The features of congenital rubella syndrome can be divided into three broad categories:

1. ***Transient***—including low birthweight, hepatosplenomegaly, thrombocytopenia, hepatitis, pneumonitis, and radiolucent bone lesions.
2. ***Permanent*** —including deafness, cataracts, and congenital heart lesions (patent ductus arteriosus > pulmonary artery stenosis > aortic stenosis > ventricular septal defects).
3. ***Developmental***—including psychomotor delay, behavioral disorders, and endocrine dysfunction.

The *most characteristic* features of congenital rubella syndrome are congenital heart disease, cataracts, microphthalmia, corneal opacities, glaucoma, and radiolucent bone lesions.

61. Should all pregnant women be screened for herpes simplex virus (HSV) infection during pregnancy?

Neonatal HSV disease is usually contracted at delivery from contact with genital secretions that contain infectious virus. In most cases, the mother is asymptomatic and has no history of clinical herpes genitalis (i.e., she has unrecognized primary infection). Existing data indicate that antepartum cultures of the maternal genital tract fail to predict viral shedding at the time of delivery. As a consequence, routine antepartum cultures are not recommended.

62. What are risk factors for the development of neonatal HSV disease?

Among infants born vaginally to mothers with primary herpes genitalis, 30–50% will develop HSV disease. Only 3–5% of infants born to mothers with active recurrent disease become infected. Of note, distinguishing between primary and recurrent herpes infections by history and clinical exam is often difficult. Low birthweight is an independent risk factor. Fetal scalp monitoring may result in direct inoculation of the virus into the baby's scalp. Cesarean section is advocated by many authors for women who are in labor at term and have visual evidence of active genital HSV lesions, especially if membranes have been ruptured for less than 6 hours. Operative delivery after 6 hours of rupture is less effective in reducing the risk of neonatal infection.

63. What are the three forms of neonatal HSV disease?

Occurring with approximately equal frequency, the three patterns of neonatal HSV disease are:

1. ***Mucocutaneous disease*** (localized to the skin, eye, or mouth)
2. ***Encephalitis***
3. ***Disseminated disease*** (± *CNS involvement*) with a picture resembling bacterial sepsis

It is important to note that only one third of infants with either localized encephalitis or disseminated disease will present with visible skin lesions.

64. How should the neonate with suspected HSV disease be treated?

In infants with mucocutaneous disease, the diagnosis can be established with viral cultures of skin lesions, eye, rectum, or nasopharynx. In patients with systemic disease, the diagnosis can be made with viral cultures or PCR studies of blood and CSF.

Both acyclovir and vidarabine have activity against HSV. Acyclovir is the preferred drug and is administered in a dose of 20 mg/kg IV every 8 hours for 14-21 days.

65. How often does relapse occur after an infant is "successfully" treated for an HSV infection?

In one study, 8% of patients with encephalitis or disseminated disease developed recurrent disease within one month of completing a 10 day course of treatment. In all cases, recurrence presented with encephalitis. In the same study, among patients with skin lesions, 19-35% developed recurrent skin lesions within one month of completing therapy and 46% developed recurrent skin involvement by 6 months.

Whitley R, et al: A controlled trial comparing vidarabine with acyclovir in neonatal herpes simplex virus infection. N Engl J Med 324:444-449, 1991.

66. In which groups of women is prenatal hepatitis B surface antigen (HBsAg) screening recommended?

In the past, women were screened for HBsAg if they fell into a high-risk group based on ethnic origin, immunization status, or history of exposure to blood products, intravenous drugs, or high-risk partner(s). However, historical information only reveals a portion of HBsAg carriers, and it is recommended that *all* pregnant women be screened for HBsAg.

67. What is the relationship between age of acquisition of hepatitis B virus and the likelihood of chronic hepatitis B infection?

Chronic hepatitis B virus infection with persistence of hepatitis B surface antigen (HBsAg) occurs in as many as 90% of infants infected by perinatal transmission, in an average of 30% of children 1-5 years old when infected, and in 2-6% of older children, adolescents, and adults who become infected.

Schiff ER: Update in hepatology. Ann Intern Med 130:52-57, 1999.

68. How should infants born to mothers with hepatitis A, B, or C infection be managed?

Immunization with hepatitis B vaccine is recommended for all infants, regardless of maternal history. The first dose should be given by age 2 months. The second dose should follow the first by at least one month, and the third dose should be given at age 6-18 months. For infants born to women who are HBsAg-positive, hepatitis B immune globulin (HBIG, 0.5 mL IM) and the first dose of hepatitis B vaccine should be administered *within 12 hours of delivery* to reduce the risk of infection. Though breast milk is capable of transmitting hepatitis B virus, the risk of transmission in HBsAg-positive mothers whose infants have received timely HBIG and hepatitis B vaccine is *not* increased by breastfeeding.

Neonates born to mothers with active hepatitis A infection are unlikely to contract the virus, and efficacy of postnatal prophylaxis with hepatitis A immune globulin (0.02 mL/kg IM) has not been proven. With this information in mind, no prophylaxis is recommended.

The risk of vertical transmission of hepatitis C virus is approximately 5%, and no preventive therapy exists. Mothers with hepatitis C infection should be advised that transmission of hepatitis C by breastfeeding has not been documented. Accordingly, maternal hepatitis C infection is not a contraindication to breastfeeding, although mothers with cracked or bleeding nipples should consider abstaining.

69. How do the clinical features of early and late congenital syphilis differ?

The manifestations of congenital syphilis are protean and may be divided into early and late findings. Early manifestations occur during the first 2 years of life; late manifestations occur after 2 years of age.

Early and Late Manifestations of Congenital Syphilis

EARLY CONGENITAL SYPHILIS (310 PATIENTS)		LATE CONGENITAL SYPHILIS (271 PATIENTS)	
Hepatomegaly	32%	Frontal boss of Parrot	87%
Skeletal abnormalities	29	Short maxilla	84
Splenomegaly	18	High palatal arch	76
Birthweight < 2500 gm	16	Hutchinson triad	75
Pneumonia	16	Hutchinson teeth	63
Severe anemia, hydrops, edema	16	Interstitial keratitis	9
Skin lesions	15	VIII nerve deafness	3
Hyperbilirubinemia	13	Saddle nose	73
Snuffles, nasal discharge	9	Mulberry molars	65
Painful limbs	7	Higouménakis sign	39
CSF abnormalities	7	Relative protuberance of mandible	26
Pancreatitis	5	Rhagades	7
Nephritis	4	Saber shin	4
Failure to thrive	3	Scaphoid scapulae	0.7
Testicular mass	0.3	Clutton joint	0.3
Chorioretinitis	0.3		
Hypoglobulinemia	0.3		

Adapted from Gutman LT: Syphilis. In Feigin RD, Cherry JE (eds): Pediatric Infectious Diseases, 3rd ed. Philadelphia, W.B. Saunders, 1992, pp. 556–557; with permission.

70. How is the diagnosis of congenital syphilis made?

The diagnosis of early congenital syphilis is often difficult and is based on clinical, serologic, and epidemiologic considerations. Nontreponemal serologic tests should be performed on all pregnant women and are often used to screen newborn infants for possible congenital infection with *T. pallidum.* Such tests include the rapid plasma reagin (RPR) card test and the Venereal Disease Reference Laboratory (VDRL) slide test. Serum from the infant is preferred to cord blood, since cord specimens can produce false-positive results. A mother who has been treated adequately for syphilis during pregnancy can still passively transfer antibodies to the neonate, resulting in a positive titer in the infant in the absence of infection. In this circumstance, the infant's titer is usually less than the mother's and reverts to negative over several months.

If blood from mother or infant yields a positive nontreponemal serologic test, a specific treponemal test is performed on the infant's blood. Examples currently in use include the fluorescent treponemal antibody absorption (FTA-ABS) test and the microhemagglutination test for *T. pallidum* (MHA-TP). Evaluation of infants with suspected congenital syphilis should also include a complete blood count, analysis of the cerebrospinal fluid (including a CSF VDRL), and long-bone radiographs (unless the diagnosis has been otherwise established).

In infants with suspected or confirmed infection, aqueous crystalline penicillin G is the drug of choice.

71. What is the prozone phenomenon?

Agglutination of an antigen by an antibody requires that the antigen and antibody be present in appropriate relative concentrations. When the antibody concentration is far greater than the amount of antigen, agglutination will not occur. This is considered the "prozone" of the dilution range of the antibody. In some infants with congenital syphilis, serum antibody levels are so high that undiluted serum fails to agglutinate the nontreponemal antigens used to diagnose syphilis (i.e., the VDRL and RPR are nonreactive). To account for the possibility of the prozone phenomenon in infants being evaluated for congenital syphilis, VDRL or RPR titer should be determined with *and* without dilution of the serum.

72. If a pregnant woman is found to have *Chlamydia trachomatis* in her birth canal, what is the most appropriate course of action?

A pregnant woman with a known chlamydial infection should be treated with oral erythromycin to reduce the risk of neonatal chlamydial pneumonia and conjunctivitis. Simultaneous treatment of the male partner(s) with doxycycline (100 mg PO bid) or azithromycin (1 gm PO as a single dose) should also be undertaken.

73. What is the risk to a fetus following primary maternal *Toxoplasma* infection?

The risk depends on the time during pregnancy that the mother becomes infected. Assuming the mother is untreated, first-trimester infection is associated with a fetal infection rate of approximately 25%, second-trimester infection with a rate > 50%, and third-trimester infection with a rate of roughly 65%. The severity of clinical disease in congenitally infected infants is inversely related to gestational age at the time of primary maternal infection.

74. If a mother acquires *Toxoplasma* during pregnancy, can transmission to the fetus be prevented?

Treatment with spiramycin before 17 weeks gestation or with pyrimethamine plus sulfadiazine after 17 weeks gestation can prevent transmission of the parasite to the fetus. Data from several studies suggest that the risk of congenital toxoplasmosis can be reduced by 50–60%, although other studies do not show benefit. The rationale for such treatment is based on the observation that there may be a significant lag period between the onset of maternal infection and infection in the fetus. There is no maternal therapy that will prevent sequelae once congenital toxoplasmosis has developed.

Wallon M, et al: Congenital toxoplasmosis: Systematic review of evidence of efficacy during pregnancy. BMJ 318:1511-1514, 1999.

75. What is the typical presentation of congenital toxoplasmosis?

As with other congenital infections, the presentations are varied. Presentations range from severe disease (in about 10%) with fever, hepatosplenomegaly, chorioretinitis, and/or neurologic features (seizures, hydrocephalus, microcephaly) to apparent lack of signs or symptoms. In the latter group, which constitutes about two-thirds of cases, intracranial calcifications are often present, and long-term risks include impaired vision, learning disabilities, mental retardation, and seizures.

76. How can a woman minimize the chance of acquiring a *Toxoplasma* infection during pregnancy?

Measures relate to personal hygiene, food preparation, and exposure to cats.

- Prepare meat by cooking to > 150°F, smoking it, or curing it in brine.
- Wash fruits and vegetables before consumption.
- Wash hands and kitchen surfaces thoroughly after contact with raw meat or unwashed fruits or vegetables and after gardening.
- Avoid changing cat litter boxes, or wear gloves while changing the litter and wash hands thoroughly afterward. Changing the litter every 1-2 days will also reduce risk.

THE FEBRILE CHILD

77. Fever in children—is it friend or foe?

In certain situations, fever is beneficial, and in others it is detrimental. Gonococci and some treponemes are killed at temperatures ≥ 40°C (104°F), and benefits from fever therapy have been reported in cases of gonococcal urethritis and neurosyphilis. In addition, fever appears to hamper growth of some types of pneumococci and some viruses. Fever also is associated with a decrease in the amount of free serum iron, an essential nutrient for many pathogenic bacteria. Modest fever can accelerate a variety of immunologic responses, including phagocytosis, leukocyte chemotaxis, lymphocyte transformation, and interferon production.

On the other hand, other data indicate that high fever can impair the immune response. In addition, while the metabolic effects of fever are well-tolerated by most children, in some situations these effects can be dangerous. Examples include patients at risk for cardiac or respiratory failure and those with neurologic disease or with septic shock. Fever can precipitate febrile seizures in the susceptible population, children between 6 months and 5–6 years of age.

78. At what temperature does a child have fever?

A simple question without a simple answer. Because body temperatures vary among individuals and age groups and vary over the course of the day in a given individual (lowest around 4–5 AM and highest in late afternoon and early evening), a precise cutoff point is difficult to determine. In children age 2–6 years, diurnal variation can range up to 0.9°C (1.6°F). Infants tend to have a higher baseline temperature pattern, with 50% having daily rectal temperatures > 37.8°C (100.0°F); after age 2 years, this elevated baseline falls. In addition, activity and exercise (within 30 min), feeding or meals (within 1 hr), and hot foods (within 1 hr) can cause body temperature elevations. Most authorities agree that in a child age < 3 months, a rectal temperature > 38°C (100.4°F) constitutes fever. In infants age 3–24 months, who tend to have a higher baseline, a temperature ≥ 38.3°C (101°F) likely constitutes fever. In those age > 2 years, as the baseline falls, fever more commonly is defined as a rectal temperature > 38°C (100.4°F).

79. Where did the popular notion of a normal temperature being 98.6°F originate?

98.6°F was established as the mean healthy temperature in 1868 after >1 million temperatures from 25,000 patients were analyzed. Ironically, these were axillary temperatures, and the waters of what constitutes normal have been muddied since.

Mackowiak PA, et al: A critical appraisal of 98.6°F, the upper limit of the normal body temperature, and other legacies of Carl Reinhold August Wunderlich. JAMA 268:1578–1580, 1992.

80. How does temperature vary among different body sites?

Rectal	Standard
Oral	0.5–0.6°C (1°F) lower
Axillary	0.8–1.0°C (1.5–2.0°F) lower
Tympanic	0.5–0.6°C (1°F) lower

81. If a tympanic thermometer is used, does the presence of otitis media increase the reading?

Tympanic thermometers work by measuring naturally occurring infrared emissions from the eardrum and surrounding structures. Otitis media causes only a very minor (approximately 0.1°C) difference in the reading. Mastoiditis and otitis externa may cause greater differences because of increased local blood flow. Cerumen, which is translucent to infrared emissions, does not affect readings.

82. How should the temperature of young infants be taken?

In infants < 3 months of age, when fever can be more significant clinically, a rectal temperature is the preferred method. Tympanic recordings are much less sensitive in this age group because the narrow, tortuous external canal can collapse, resulting in readings obtained from the cooler canal rather than the warmer tympanic membrane. Axillary temperatures often underestimate fever. The oral route is usually not used until a child is 5–6 years old.

83. Can excessive bundling raise an infant's temperature?

Prospective studies have found mixed results. One study of newborns in a warm environment of 80°F found that rectal temperatures in bundled infants could be elevated above 38°C, the "febrile range." Another study of infants up to age 3 months found that in room temperatures of 72–75°F, the bundling of infants up to 65 minutes did not produce any rectal temperatures > 38°C. A clinical method that can distinguish disease-related fevers from possible environmental overheating is the "abdomen-toe" temperature differential. A foot as warm as the abdomen suggests an overly warm environment, while a foot that is cooler suggests fever with peripheral vasoconstriction.

Grover C, et al: The effects of bundling on infant temperature. Pediatrics 94:669–673, 1994.

Cheng TL, Partridge JC: Effect of bundling and high environmental temperatures on neonatal body temperature. Pediatrics 92:238–240, 1993.

84. Does teething cause fever?

Long a doctrine of grandmothers, the suggested association between teething and temperature elevation may have some basis in fact. In one study of 46 healthy infants with rectal temperatures recorded for 20 days prior to the eruption of their first tooth, nearly half had a new temperature elevation above 37.5° on the day of the eruption. Other studies have shown some statistical association with slight temperature increase. In any event, significantly elevated fever should never be ascribed simply to teething. Listen to the grandmothers, but verify.

Macknin ML, et al: Symptoms associated with infant teething. Pediatrics 105:747-752, 2000.

Jaber L, et al: Fever associated with teething. Arch Dis Child 67:233–234, 1992.

85. Do sponge baths reduce fever?

Because fever is the result of an elevated set-point of the thermoregulatory center in the hypothalamus, a critical intervention to reduce temperature is to return the set-point to normal. This effect can be achieved by treatment with any of several drugs, including acetaminophen, ibuprofen, and other nonsteroidal antiinflammatory agents. While aspirin has the same effect, it is no longer recommended for routine treatment of fever in children due to its association with Reye syndrome. Provided the set-point has been normalized, external cooling (by sponging with cold, cool, or tepid water) can be effective in reducing fever. Sponging with ice water is most effective but is very uncomfortable. Water in the range of 29.4–32°C (85–90°F) is preferred. Alcohol sponge baths are not recommended because of the potential for significant absorption of alcohol through the skin.

86. Can viral infections and bacterial infections be distinguished based on response to antipyretic therapy?

The traditional theory was that a viral illness responds better to antipyretics than does a bacterial infection. However, there is little evidence to support this contention, and response to antipyretic therapy should not be used as a diagnostic aid.

87. What is occult bacteremia?

Occult bacteremia refers to the finding of bacteria in the blood of patients, usually aged 3–36 months, who are febrile without an apparent focus of infection. This term should be distinguished from *septicemia*, which refers to the growth of bacteria in the blood from a child with the clinical picture of toxicity and shock.

88. Is there an association between the degree of fever and the incidence of bacteremia?

In children the relationship between fever and likelihood of bacteremia has been examined most thoroughly in patients who are febrile yet have no localizing signs on physical examination. In general, the risk of bacteremia in this population increases with the magnitude of fever. In a classic study involving febrile children < 2 years of age who were seen in an ambulatory clinic, bacteremia was present only if the rectal temperature was ≥ 38.9°C (102°F). In another series of febrile children seen in a pediatric emergency room, among patients with temperatures > 41.1°C (106°F), the incidence of bacteremia was 13%.

McCarthy PL, Dolan TF: Hyperpyrexia in children: Eight-year emergency room experience. Am J Dis Child 130:849–851, 1976.

Teele DW, et al: Bacteremia in febrile children under 2 years of age: Results of cultures of blood of 600 consecutive febrile children in a "walk-in" clinic. J Pediatr 87:227–230, 1975.

89. What constitutes the Yale Observation Scales?

This set of 6 items of observation and physical signs was designed at Yale to assist in detecting serious illness in febrile children < 24 months of age. Normal (1 point), moderate impairment (3 points), and severe impairment (5 points) scores are given for ***quality of cry, reaction to parental stimulation, state of alertness, color, hydration,*** and ***response to social overtures***. Scores of ≤ 10 correlate with a low likelihood of serious illness, primarily in infants > 2 months old.

McCarthy PL, et al: Observation scales to identify serious illness in febrile children. Pediatrics 70:802–809, 1982.

90. What is the proper way to evaluate and manage febrile illness in infants <60 days of age?

A very contentious area. On average, about 10% of febrile infants < 2 months of age have serious bacterial infections (bacteremia, meningitis, osteomyelitis, septic arthritis, urinary tract infection, or pneumonia). One third to one half of these infections are associated with bacteremia. In the past, the approach to the evaluation and management of febrile young infants has varied. Many studies have attempted to identify criteria for a "low-risk" group of infants with a very small risk of serious bacterial infection. Clinical algorithms have ranged from routine lumbar punctures and empiric antibiotic use to neither lumbar punctures nor empiric antibiotics for well-appearing infants. One approach to the outpatient management of the febrile infant (29-60 days, temp ≥ 38°C) is that of the Children's Hospital of Philadelphia. Patients are categorized as "low-risk" and followed as outpatients without antibiotic therapy if the following criteria are met:

- Well-appearing infant
- No evidence of focal infection on physical exam
- Total peripheral blood WBC count 5,000 - 15,000/mm^3
- CSF WBC < 8/mm^3 and Gram stain negative
- Urinalysis: < 10 WBC high-power field (hpf) and ≤ 3 bacteria on spun specimen
- No pulmonary infiltrate on chest radiograph, if performed

Of infants who meet these criteria and were observed without antibiotics, the risk of serious infection is exceedingly low. The CHOP experience and others suggest that infants who meet low-risk criteria may not require antibiotic therapy and/or hospitalization, provided the social setting is suitable and close outpatient follow-up is possible.

Currently, infants < 28 days of age are generally hospitalized for empiric therapy, but some authors advocate outpatient management of selected "low-risk" neonates.

Baker MD, et al: The efficacy of routine outpatient management without antibiotics of fever in selected infants. Pediatrics 103:627-631, 1999.

Baker MD, Bell LM: Unpredictability of serious bacterial illness in febrile infants from birth to 1 month of age. Arch Pediatr Adolesc Med 153:508-511, 1999.

Baker MD, et al: Outpatient management without antibiotics of fever in selected infants. N Engl J Med 329:1437-1441, 1993.

91. How should older infants and toddlers (2–36 months of age) with fever and no apparent source be managed?

As with infants < 2 months of age, the management of older children with fever and no identifiable source remains controversial. The basis for this controversy relates to the difficulty in distinguishing viral illness from occult bacteremia and the fear of occult bacteremia leading to more serious infection, especially meningitis. In recent years, consideration of this issue has been influenced by the remarkable success of the *Haemophilus influenzae* vaccination program. In the past, *H. influenzae* occult bacteremia was relatively common and, in ~ 10% of cases, was associated with progression to meningitis. *Streptococcus pneumoniae* now accounts for > 90% of all episodes of occult bacteremia, but *S. pneumoniae* occult bacteremia seldom progresses to meningitis.

Strategies for management of febrile young children aged 2–36 months vary. For patients with temperatures ≥ 39°C, some experts advocate use of a protocol involving:

1. Urine culture for males < 6 months of age and females < 2 years of age
2. Stool culture if stool has blood or mucus or > 5 WBCs/hpf
3. Blood culture

Empiric antibiotics (e.g., oral amoxicillin or intramuscular ceftriaxone) are then prescribed pending culture results. Other specialists consider the degree of fever and height of the WBC count or absolute neutrophil count (ANC) to assess the likelihood of bacteremia and the need for empiric antibiotic therapy (WBC count ≥ 15,000/mm^3 and ANC ≥10,000/mm^3 are associated with a greater risk of occult bacteremia). Still others advise no testing and no empiric therapy and emphasize that parents be provided with specific information about signs and symptoms that should prompt reevaluation.

It should be noted that the introduction of the heptavalent pneumococcal vaccine, which is 90% efficacious in preventing invasive disease, will likely make obsolete the use of wbc counts, blood cultures and expectant empiric antibiotic therapy in those patients who have received the vaccine.

Baraff LJ: Management of fever without source in infants and children. Ann Emerg Med 36:602-614, 2000.

92. How helpful is the band count in distinguishing the likelihood of viral versus bacterial infections in young infants?

Alas, the song from the band has no lyrics. A study looking at the value of the band count in the peripheral blood smear in young febrile infants (3-24 months) was not of value in distinguishing bacterial from viral infections. Band counts may be more helpful in infants less than 3 months of age.

Kupperman N, et al: Immature neutrophils in the blood smears of young febrile children. Arch Pediatr Adolesc Med 153:261-266, 1999.

93. When is a chest radiograph indicated in a febrile young infant?

While some clinicians believe that chest x-rays should be performed in all febrile infants < 2–3 months of age, others reserve this study for infants who have respiratory symptoms or signs, including cough, tachypnea, irregular breathing, retractions, rales, wheezing, or decreased breath sounds. In a study of infants < 8 weeks of age who were admitted with fever, 31% of patients with respiratory manifestations had an abnormal chest x-ray compared with only 1% of asymptomatic infants.

Crain EF, et al: Is a chest radiograph necessary in the evaluation of every febrile infant less than 8 weeks of age? Pediatrics 88:821–824, 1991.

94. Which children with "seizure and fever" need to have a lumbar puncture?

Consultation of pediatric textbooks, physicians in practice, and residency program directors reveals no consensus on this question. The concern is that the seizure might be a manifestation of meningitis. Specific signs of meningitis, such as stiff neck and bulging fontanel, are often lacking in affected patients who are younger than 12–18 months of age. Many authorities mandate LPs for children < 18 months who have had a seizure with fever, regardless of clinical appearance. It is a difficult issue to resolve, but unless a child is alert and completely well-appearing at the time of examination, a lumbar puncture should be seriously considered.

The occurrence of a simple febrile seizure as the sole manifestation of meningitis in a child is very unusual. In one retrospective study of 503 children with meningitis, none with bacterial meningitis presented solely with a seizure. Other studies have shown that bacterial meningitis, even in younger children, is nearly always accompanied by some abnormal sign or symptom, particularly lethargy or a toxic appearance.

Green SM, et al: Can seizures be the sole manifestations of meningitis in febrile children? Pediatrics 92:527–534, 1993.

95. Is there a risk in performing a lumbar puncture in a bacteremic infant?

A definitive estimate of this risk in humans is not available. Such an estimate would require a systematic study, taking into account such variables as magnitude of the bacteremia, amount of blood introduced into the CSF, and the patient's immune status. It is unlikely that such a study could ever be performed, and even if it were, its application to individual cases would be impossible. Suffice it to say that the risk is small and would never outweigh the risk of not doing a lumbar puncture.

96. Does changing needles during the collection of blood cultures reduce contamination?

No. In one study of 303 children, replacing the needle used for venipuncture with a fresh, sterile needle before inoculating the blood into a culture medium resulted in no change in the contamination rate. As a side note, if the incubation of a blood culture is delayed ≥ 2 hours, the likelihood of positivity may be significantly decreased, especially for *Streptococcus pneumoniae* and *Neisseria meningitidis*.

Roback MG, et al: Delayed incubation of blood culture bottles: Effect on recovery rate of Streptococcus pneumoniae and Haemophilus influenzae type b. Pediatr Emerg Care 10:268–272, 1994.

Isaacman DJ: Lack of effect of changing needles on contamination of blood cultures. Pediatr Infect Dis J 9:274–278, 1990.

97. In what clinical settings are blood cultures for anaerobic bacteria indicated?

While it is commonplace to inoculate both aerobic and anaerobic blood culture bottles when blood cultures are obtained from pediatric patients, the yield of anaerobic cultures is very low. As part of a diagnostic evaluation for sepsis, patients who satisfy the following criteria are more likely to have a positive anaerobic blood culture:

- Abdominal signs and symptoms
- Debilitation with sacral decubitus ulcers or cellulitis
- Poor dentition, oral mucositis, or chronic sinusitis
- Underlying neutropenia, especially in the setting of high-dose steroids
- Underlying sickle cell disease
- Pharyngitis and possible septic thrombophlebitis
- Human bite wounds or crushing trauma

Zaida AK, et al: Value of routine anaerobic blood cultures for pediatric patients. J Pediatr 127:263-268, 1995.

98. How long should one wait before a blood culture is designated negative?

Bacterial growth is evident in the vast majority of cultures of infected blood within 48 hours. With the use of conventional culture techniques and subculture at 4 and 14 hours, Pichichero and Todd found that 101 of 105 positive cultures yielded growth within 48 hours. Using a radiometric technique, Rowley and Wald reported that 40 of 41 cultures positive for group B streptococcus and 15 of 16 cultures growing *Escherichia coli* were identified within 24 hours. Use of continuous monitoring culture techniques at Children's Hospital of Philadelphia allowed detection of 95% of critical pathogens in less than 24 hours.

While 48-72 hours is generally sufficient time to isolate common bacteria present in the bloodstream, fastidious organisms may take longer to grow. Therefore, when one suspects anaerobes, fungi, or other organisms with special growth requirements, a longer time should be allowed before concluding that a culture is negative.

PCR technology, with the potential ability to detect bacterial DNA in blood in minutes, may revolutionize the practice of expectant antibiotic therapy.

McGowan K, et al: Outpatient pediatric blood cultures: Time to positivity. Pediatrics 106:251-255, 2000.

Belgrader P, et al: PCR detection of bacteria in seven minutes. Science 284:449-450, 1999.

Rowley AH, Wald ER: Incubation period necessary to detect bacteremia in neonates. Pediatr Infect Dis J 5:540, 1986.

Pichichero MD, Todd JK: Detection of neonatal bacteremia. J Pediatr 94:958, 1979.

99. How should a child with fever and petechiae be evaluated?

In a patient with fever and petechiae, the most significant concern is serious systemic bacterial infection. Fortunately, when prospectively evaluated, the incidence of bacteremia or clinical sepsis in this setting is low (<2%) and 0/357 well-appearing children had meningococcemia when evaluated.

History: Elicit information about exposures, travel, animal contacts, and immunizations.

Physical exam: Assess vital signs, general appearance, signs of toxicity, evidence of nuchal rigidity, presence of purpura and distribution of petechiae (patients with systemic bacterial infection rarely have petechiae confined to the head and neck).

Laboratory: Obtain blood culture, complete blood count with differential, and prothrombin and partial thromboplastin times; consider examination of cerebrospinal fluid.

Mandl KD, et al: Incidence of bacteremia in infants and children with fever and petechiae. J Pediatr 131:398-404, 1997.

100. What infections can be associated with fever and petechiae?

Bacterial

- Meningococcemia
- *Streptococcus pneumoniae* sepsis
- *Staphylococcus aureus* sepsis
- *Haemophilus influenzae* sepsis
- Listeriosis
- Disseminated gonococcal infection
- Group A streptococcal sepsis

Rickettsial

- Rocky Mountain spotted fever
- Ehrlichiosis

Viral

- Enterovirus (especially coxsackie A9, echovirus 9)
- Epstein-Barr virus
- Cytomegalovirus
- Atypical measles

Parasitic

- Malaria

101. To which infection do the Stiehm and Damrosch criteria apply?

The presence of 3 or more of the Stiehm and Damrosch criteria define a poor prognosis for patients with meningococcemia:

1. Presence of petechiae for < 12 hours prior to admission
2. Shock
3. Absence of meningitis (< 20 WBCs in CSF)

4. Normal or low peripheral WBC count
5. Low or normal erythrocyte sedimentation rate

Stiehm ER, Damrosch DS: Factors in the prognosis of meningococcal infection. J Pediatr 68:457–467, 1966.

102. When is fever considered a fever of unknown origin (FUO)?

FUO is defined as the presence of persistent fever (temperature > 38°C or > 100.4°F) in a patient in whom a careful history, a thorough physical examination, and preliminary laboratory data fail to reveal the probable cause. For study purposes, in adults the duration of fever that constitutes an FUO is ≥ 3 weeks, while in children the duration varies from ≥ 8 days to ≥ 2–3 weeks.

103. What is the eventual etiology of fever in children with FUO?

In a summary of 446 cases, the following causes were identified:

	No. of cases	*% of cases*
Infection	198	44.4%
Respiratory	102	22.9
Other	97	21.7
Collagen disease	57	12.8
Inflammatory bowel disease	7	1.6
Neoplasm	25	5.6
No diagnosis	48	10.7
Resolved	56	12.6
Miscellaneous	54	12.1

Gartner JC Jr: Fever of unknown origin. Adv Pediatr Infect Dis 7:6, 1992; with permission.

104. How should a child with FUO be evaluated?

FUO is more likely to be an unusual presentation of a common disorder than a common presentation of a rare disorder. After obtaining a complete and detailed history and performing a thorough physical examination, one should avoid indiscriminately ordering a large battery of tests. The erythrocyte sedimentation rate (ESR) may be a helpful screening test, with an elevated value suggesting more serious illness. Additional laboratory studies should be directed as much as possible toward the most likely diagnostic possibilities.

105. In children with FUO, how helpful are CT scans and nuclear medicine studies in determining the diagnosis?

Minimally. In a prospective study of 109 patients with FUO, scanning procedures (e.g., abdominal CT scan, gallium or indium scanning, technetium bone scanning) had very low utility in the absence of clinical findings suggesting a localized process. Similarly, bone marrow examination had little value when hematologic abnormalities were lacking.

Steele RW, et al: Usefulness of scanning procedures for diagnosis of fever of unknown origin in children. J Pediatr 119:526–530, 1991.

106. What is PFAPA?

PFAPA is the acronym for the syndrome of ***p**eriodic* ***f**ever,* ***a**phthous stomatitis,* ***p**haryngitis* and cervical ***a**denitis*. A clinical syndrome of unclear etiology responsive to corticosteroids, this is perhaps the most common cause of regular, recurrent fevers in children.

Feder HM Jr: Periodic fever, aphthous stomatitis, pharyngitis, adenitis: A clinical review of a new syndrome. Curr Opin Pediatr 253-256, 2000.

Long S: Syndrome of periodic fever, aphthous stomatitis, pharyngitis, and adenitis (PFAPA): What it isn't. What is it? J Pediatr 135:1-5, 1999.

107. In addition to PFAPA, which syndromes are associated with periodic fevers?

Predictable periodic fever is a cardinal feature of a small number of diseases and is uncommon in infectious diseases and malignancies.

Characteristic of PFAPA versus Other Intermittent Fever Syndromes

	PFAPA	FAMILIAL MEDITERRANEAN FEVER	HYPER IgD	SYSTEMIC ONSET JUVENILE RHEUMATOID ARTHRITIS
Onset at <5 years of age	Common	Unusual	Common	Common
Length of fever episode	4 days	2 days	4 days	> 30 days
Interval between fever episodes	2–8 weeks	Not periodic	Not periodic	Hectic quotidian
Associated symptoms	Aphthous stomatitis, pharyngitis, adenitis	Painful pleuritis, peritonitis	Arthralgias abdominal pain diarrhea splenomegaly rashes	Rash, generalized lymphadenopathy, hepatosplenomegaly, arthritis
Ethnic/geographic	None	Mediterranean	Dutch	None
Special laboratory test results	None	Gene analysis	Elevated serum IgD concentration	None
Sequelae	None	Amyloidosis	None	Symmetric polyarthritis

From Thomas KT, et al: Periodic fever syndrome in children. J Pediatr 135:15-21,1999, p. 19; with permission.

HIV INFECTION

108. When did HIV testing begin on blood intended for transfusion?

Spring of 1985. Patients at greatest risk for transfusion-acquired AIDS are those transfused from 1978 to spring 1985.

109. How is a "Western blot" test done?

Western blot is the most sensitive and specific test currently available for detection of antibodies against HIV. It is more accurate than enzyme immunoassay, which occasionally yields false-positive reactions. On the other hand, Western blot is expensive, lacks standardization among laboratories, and may be difficult to interpret.

Western blot for HIV is performed as follows. Purified HIV is separated into protein components by polyacrylamide gel electrophoresis. These components are transferred from the gel to a nitrocellulose membrane. Serum is placed over the membrane and incubated. If specific antibodies are present against one or more HIV antigen, they will bind to the relevant antigen. The antibodies are then illuminated by the addition of an enzyme–anti-IgG complex, which binds to the HIV antibody. A substrate is added and is converted to a colored compound in the presence of bound enzyme. The amount of color produced can be quantified.

110. How common is maternal to infant transmission of HIV?

Virtually all infants born to HIV-seropositive mothers will acquire antibody to the virus transplacentally. However, at most only 15–40% of these infants will ultimately develop active HIV infection. Approximately 70% of maternal–infant HIV transmission occurs during late gestation or labor and delivery, and 30% of transmission occurs intrapartum.

In a landmark study published in 1994, treatment with AZT administered antepartum and intrapartum to the mother and postnatally to the infant reduced transmission by approximately two-thirds. In a more recent study conducted in Africa, treatment with nevirapine administered intrapartum to the mother (200 mg at the onset of labor) and postnatally to the infant (2 mg/kg at 72 hours of life or time of discharge) resulted in a 47% decrease in the rate of transmission.

Currently HIV-infected pregnant women in the U.S. are treated the same as nonpregnant adults, generally with comination antiretroviral therapy. Treatment with AZT alone is reserved for the rare pregnant woman with a normal CD4 count and a low or undetectable viral load who otherwise would not require therapy. All HIV-exposed newborn infants should receive AZT at 2 mg/kg/dose every 6 hours for the first 6 weeks of life.

Guay LA, et al: Intrapartum and neonatal single dose nevirapine compared with zidovudine for prevention of mother to child transmission of HIV-1 in Kampala, Uganda. Lancet 354:795-802, 1999.

Connor EM, et al: Reduction of maternal-infant transmission of human immunodeficiency virus type I with zidovudine treatment. N Engl J Med 331:1173–1180, 1994.

111. What are the risk factors for perinatal transmission of HIV?

Higher maternal viral load is associated with a higher risk of vertical transmission. Women who receive AZT monotherapy have higher transmission rates than women receiving combination antiretroviral therapy. Other risk factors for transmission include rupture of membranes greater than 4 hours, fetal instrumentation with scalp electrodes and forceps, and breastfeeding.

In a recent meta-analysis of 16 prospective cohort studies including more than 8000 mother-child pairs comparing vertical transmission rates among women who delivered via instrumental vaginal delivery, non-instrumental vaginal delivery, elective C-section, or non elective C-section, the rates of vertical transmission were shown to be highest among women who delivered vaginally, with no antiretroviral therapy (19%, range 17.9-20%). Rates were lowest in women who underwent elective C-section with antiretroviral treatment (2%, range 0.1-4%). There are no recommendations from the American College of Obstetrics and Gynecology (ACOG) to routinely perform elective C-sections on HIV infected women. Instead, the decision should be made by individual obstetricians and their patients.

Nduati R, et al: Effect of breastfeeding and formula feeding on transmission of HIV-1: A randomized clinical trial. JAMA 283:1167-1174, 2000.

The International Perinatal HIV Group: The Mode of Delivery and the Risk of Vertical Transmission of Human Immunodeficiency Virus Type 1. N Engl J Med 340: 977-987,1999.

112. How is a newborn infant whose mother is infected with HIV confirmed to be HIV-infected?

The standard methods used to diagnose HIV infection in older children and adults rely on detection of antibody to HIV by ELISA or Western blot. Since maternal antibody may persist in the infant well into the second year of life, these techniques are unreliable until approximately 18 months of age. The diagnosis of HIV infection in the newborn therefore usually relies on direct detection of the virus or viral components in the infant's blood or body fluids. Three methods are currently available:

1. ***Detection of HIV nucleic acid:*** PCR of DNA extracted from peripheral blood mononuclear cells is the preferred test for diagnosis of HIV infection in infants. In the first 48 hours of life, the sensitivity of PCR for HIV DNA is approximately 30%. By 2 weeks of age PCR will detect approximately 93% of infected infants, and at 1 month of age PCR will be positive in nearly all infected infants.

2. ***Culture:*** A positive culture for HIV from an infant's blood is diagnostic of infection. Sensitivity and specificity exceed 90% in infants > 1 month of age. However, sensitivity can be as low as 50% in the immediate newborn period, probably because of very low levels of

viremia in some newborn infants. Culturing of HIV is labor-intensive and expensive and is currently available only in specialized centers.

3. ***Antigen detection:*** An HIV core protein, designated p24 antigen, can be detected in blood using an ELISA. Antigen detection is significantly less sensitive than culture and PCR, and false positive results occur in infants younger than 1 month of age.

Infants born to HIV-infected women should be tested by HIV DNA PCR during the first 48 hours of life, then between 2 weeks and 2 months of age, and then at 3 to 6 months of age. Any time a positive result is obtained, testing should be repeated on a second blood sample as soon as possible. The diagnosis of HIV infection is established if 2 separate samples are positive by PCR. The diagnosis can be excluded when results from 2 samples at or beyond 1 month of age are negative, with at least 1 sample at or beyond 4 months of age.

113. What are the earliest and most common manifestations of AIDS in HIV-infected infants?

The vast majority of infants with congenital HIV infection are asymptomatic at birth, although occasional patients have diffuse lymphadenopathy and hepatosplenomegaly. Early reports of an "HIV embryopathy," with characteristic dysmorphic features, have not been confirmed in prospective trials. Hence, congenital HIV infection cannot be diagnosed reliably on the basis of clinical manifestations in the newborn period.

The progression from asymptomatic HIV infection to AIDS follows a much more fulminant course in infants who acquire the infection congenitally as compared to those who are infected through other routes. In the United States, most vertically infected infants become ill prior to 1 year of age, with the average age of onset of severe immunodeficiency occurring between 5 and 10 months of age.

Infants with HIV commonly present with failure to thrive, mucocutaneous candidiasis, hepatosplenomegaly, interstitial pneumonitis, or a combination of these features. Toddlers and older children may present with generalized lymphadenopathy, recurrent bacterial infections, parotitis, or neurologic disease.

Pneumonia due to *Pneumocystis carinii* eventually develops in greater than one-third of patients and may be the presenting symptom in 10% of HIV-infected children. All infants between 6 weeks and 4 months of age who are at risk for HIV infection should receive chemoprophylaxis against *Pneumocystis* until the diagnosis is clarified. Another common feature of pediatric AIDS is lymphoid interstitial pneumonitis, a chronic progressive interstitial lung disease that is often associated with EBV infection. Neurologic dysfunction develops in 90% of children with HIV infection.

Pizzo PA, Wilfert CM: Preventing Pneumocystis carinii pneumonia in human immunodeficiency virus-infected children: New guidelines for prophylaxis. Pediatr Infect Dis J 15:165–168, 1996.

1994 Revised classification system for human immunodeficiency virus infection in children less than 13 years of age. MMWR 43(RR12):1–10, 1995.

114. What are the common pulmonary diseases in children with AIDS?

Both infectious and noninfectious pulmonary diseases are common presenting complaints in children with AIDS. These include:

- *Pneumocystis carinii* pneumonia
- Cytomegalovirus pneumonia
- Lymphocytic interstitial pneumonitis
- Infection with *Mycobacterium avium* complex

115. How is lymphocytic interstitial pneumonitis (LIP) distinguished from *Pneumocystis carinii* pneumonia (PCP)?

LIP is a chronic pulmonary interstitial disease of unknown cause that occurs in about 50% of pediatric AIDS patients and is characterized by infiltration of the lungs with lymphocytes and plasma cells. Occasionally, concomitant hilar adenopathy is present. The chest x-ray frequently reveals a reticulonodular pattern. The onset of symptoms is gradual, and tachypnea and hypoxia are late findings. LIP typically develops in patients in whom the risk for opportunistic infection is low (i.e., the CD4+ lymphocyte count is not severely decreased). PCP usually occurs when CD4+ counts are low and has a relatively rapid onset with early development of tachypnea and hypoxia. The chest x-ray usually reveals a diffuse alveolar-interstitial process. LIP may respond to steroids, while PCP is treated with trimethoprim-sulfamethoxazole (or alternatively pentamidine) with the addition of steroids for severe hypoxemia. Patients with LIP have considerably longer periods of survival than those with PCP.

116. When should PCP prophylaxis begin and end for an HIV-exposed infant?

The peak incidence of PCP in HIV-infected infants occurs at age 3 months, with a range of 4 weeks to 6 months. Given that vertical transmission of HIV cannot be excluded until the patient has two negative PCRs at least one month apart, both of which must be at age ≥ 1 month and one of which must be at age ≥ 4 months, PCP prophylaxis should be initiated at age 4-6 weeks and continued until at least 4 months of age. If the HIV status of the child is indeterminate or confirmed positive, PCP prophylaxis should be continued until 12 months of age.

Recommended regimens include:

1. TMP/SMX 150 mg/m^2/day po divided BID 3 days/week
2. Dapsone 2 mg/kg po qd
3. Pentamidine (aerosolized, in children older than 5 years) 300 mg monthly

117. What immunologic abnormalities are seen in children with HIV infection?

Most patients have elevated serum immunoglobulins, and about 10% have hypogammaglobulinemia. Failure to make antibodies to specific antigens (e.g., tetanus toxoid, pneumococcal polysaccharides) is common. In more advanced infection, the ratio of helper-suppressor (CD4/CD8) T cells is decreased, absolute lymphopenia is present, and in vitro mitogenic responses are diminished.

118. Among infants with HIV infection, how does the CD4 count influence classification?

According to the 1994 revised Pediatric HIV Classification System, for children ≤ 12 months of age, CD4 counts ≥ 1,500/ml and ≥ 25% of total lymphocytes are considered normal and correspond to Category 1 (no immunosuppression). CD4 counts ranging from 750-1499/ml or 15-24% of total lymphocytes correspond to Category 2 (moderate suppression). CD4 counts < 750/ml or <15% of total lymphocytes correspond to Category 3 (severe suppression).

119. Describe the major hematologic manifestations of pediatric HIV infection.

The hematologic manifestations of pediatric HIV infection are due to several factors, including: (1) direct cytopathic effects of HIV on blood cell precursors; (2) autoantibody production; (3) drug toxicity; and (4) opportunistic infections that involve the bone marrow. Anemia is very common and may be due to bone marrow suppression, immune hemolysis, or chronic disease. Neutropenia and neutrophil dysfunction may be caused by HIV, drugs (zidovudine, didanosine, TMP-SMX), or intercurrent infection. Thrombocytopenia may be a presenting finding of HIV infection, emphasizing the importance of HIV testing in patients thought to have idiopathic thrombocytopenic purpura (ITP). Thrombotic thrombocytopenic purpura is more common in adults but rarely has been seen in children with HIV infection. Coagulopathy may be secondary to HIV-induced hepatitis, lupus-like anticoagulants, autoantibodies to clotting factors, or disseminated intravascular coagulation accompanying systemic infection.

Hilgartner M: Hematologic manifestations in HIV-infected children. J Pediatr 119: S47–S49, 1991.

120. What special recommendations regarding vaccination should be made for the child infected with HIV?

- OPV is no longer recommended for routine use in children in the US, and is specifically contraindicated in HIV-infected children and members of their households.
- BCG vaccine should not be administered to children with HIV infection who live in the US. On the other hand, BCG is recommended for children who are aymptomatic and live in areas of the world with a high incidence of tuberculosis.
- MMR is recommended for all children with HIV infection *except* those with severe immunosuppression. Of note, there is at least one report of a child with AIDS who developed fatal pneumonia attributable to vaccine-type measles virus. Furthermore, a protective immune response to MMR rarely develops in severely immunocompromised HIV-infected patients.
- Pneumococcal and influenza vaccines are indicated for both symptomatic and asymptomatic patients with HIV infection.
- Varicella vaccine should be considered for HIV-infected children who have no evidence of immunosuppression and at most have mild signs and symptoms. Limited data indicate that the vaccine is safe, immunogenic, and effective in these children.
- Passive immunization with intravenous gammaglobulin has been demonstrated to decrease the incidence of opportunistic infections in HIV-infected children with CD4 counts > 200.

Committee on Infectious Diseases and Committee on Pediatric AIDS, American Academy of Pediatrics. Measles immunization in HIV-infected children. Pediatrics 103:1057-60, 1999.

121. How common is the transmission of HIV from infected children to household contacts?

Extremely rare. Only two case reports clearly implicate an infected sibling as the source of HIV infection. Nevertheless, children with HIV infection should be instructed regarding good hygiene and appropriate behavior, and their families should be counseled about HIV and its transmission.

122. Should a classroom teacher be told that a child is HIV-positive?

There is no absolute requirement to inform a classroom teacher, a school principal, or any other school official about a child's HIV status. It is not necessary for anyone except the child's physician to be aware of the diagnosis. Nevertheless, in certain circumstances it may be advisable for a family to communicate with a teacher or a principal.

American Academy of Pediatrics. Human immunodeficiency virus. In: Pickering, LK (ed): 2000 Red Book: Report of the Committee on Infectious Diseases, 25th ed. Elk Grove Park, IL, American Academy of Pediatrics, 2000, p. 345.

123. What is the relationship between viral load and prognosis?

In several large, prospective cohort studies of adult patients, HIV-1 viral load (RNA copies/mL) both independently and in combination with CD4 count predicted progression to AIDS and death from an infectious disease (AIDS-defining diagnosis). Of patients with high HIV RNA levels (≥ 30,000 copies/mL) and CD4 counts less than 200, 83% developed AIDS within 5 years and 76.4% died from an AIDS-defining infectious disease. No patients with undetectable viral loads (<500 copies/mL) and high CD4 counts (>500) developed AIDS or succumbed to death from an infectious disease.

The relationship between viral load and prognosis is less clear in children. However, high HIV-1 RNA levels at birth and during primary viremia have been shown to be associated with rapid progression to AIDS and death in children infected perinatally.

Delta coordinating Committee and Virology Group: An evaluation of HIV RNA and CD4 cell count as surrogates for clinical outcome. AIDS 13:565-73, 1999.

Dickover RE: Early prognostic indicators in primary perinatal human immunodeficiency Virus type I Infection: Importance of viral RNA and the timing of transmission on long-term outcome. J Infect Dis 178: 375-87, 1998.

124. In what part of the population is HIV increasing most rapidly?

Female adolescents. The most recent data from the CDC indicate that of 1,384 female adolescents and adults with AIDS, 708 (54%) acquired HIV via heterosexual contact. Vertical transmission of HIV has decreased dramatically since the introduction of prepartum and intrapartum AZT in pregnant HIV-infected women together with postnatal AZT in their HIV-exposed infants.

125. What are the risk factors for HIV transmission following a needlestick injury?

- High viral inoculum (patient with advanced disease or acute retroviral disease)
- Large volume of blood (from a large diameter needle)
- Deep puncture wound

Overall, the risk of transmission from needles contaminated with the blood of an HIV-infected patient is roughly 0.3%. The above risk factors were identified in a case-control study that involved 33 healthcare workers and 665 controls.

Cardo DM, et al: A Case-Control Study of HIV Seroconversion in Health Care Workers After Percutaneous Exposure. N Engl J Med 337:1485-90, 1997.

126. When should postexposure prophylaxis be given following a needlestick injury?

Postexposure prophylaxis has been shown to reduce transmission of HIV in healthcare workers by approximately 81%. Data from health care workers suggest that prophylaxis is most effective when given within 1-2 hours of exposure, and data from animal studies suggest that prophylaxis is not effective if initiated more than 24 hours after exposure. It is recommended postexposure prophylaxis be continued for 4 weeks.

There are currently no guidelines for postexposure prophylaxis in children. Many experts recommend application of the CDC guidelines for healthcare workers to children injured by needles potentially contaminated by patients. Needlestick injuries occurring in parks/playgrounds where no source person can be identified require the healthcare provider to weigh the risks and benefits of postexposure prophylaxis. Some experts recommend prophylaxis for injuries that occur in an area where HIV and/or intravenous drug use is prevalent, if blood can be seen on or in the needle, or if the needle is large diameter.

Public Health Service Guidelines for the Management of Health-Care Worker Exposures to HIV and Recommendations for Postexposure Prophylaxis. MMWR 47:1-28, 1998.

127. What are the major classes of antiretroviral agents used to treat HIV, and what are their mechanisms of action?

There are three major classes of antiretroviral drugs: ***nucleoside reverse transcriptase inhibitors*** (NRTIs), ***non-nucleoside reverse transcriptase inhibitors*** (NNRTIs), and ***protease inhibitors*** (PI).

NRTIs competitively inhibit the HIV reverse transcriptase (which converts HIV RNA into DNA) and terminate the elongation of viral DNA. They require intracellular phosphorylation for activation. NRTIs have little to no effect on chronically infected cells, as their site of action is before incorporation of viral DNA into host DNA. This class of drugs includes zidovudine (AZT), lamivudine (3TC), stavudine (d4T), zalcitabine (ddC), didanosine (ddI), and abacavir.

NNRTIs also inhibit the HIV reverse transcriptase, although at a different site than do NRTIs. They bind directly to the active site of HIV reverse transcriptase and do not require activation. This class of drugs includes delavirdine, efavirenz and nevirapine.

PIs inhibit the HIV protease, which cuts HIV RNA prior to viral budding. This class of drugs includes amprenavir, nelfinavir, ritonavir, indinavir, saquinavir, and lopinavir.

128. What are the principles behind the initiation of antiretroviral therapy?

Early treatment is associated with virologic, immunologic, and clinical benefits. According to the International AIDS Society-USA panel, antiretroviral therapy is recommended for any *adult* patient who has a plasma HIV-1 RNA level greater than 5000 to 10,000 copies/mL and who is committed to long-term complex therapy.

The first regimen is likely to be the most effective in achieving a sustained clinical and virologic response and is thus the most important. Viral resistance develops quickly, particularly under pressure from drugs administered intermittently or as single agents. Initial regimens should generally include at least two different classes of antiretrovirals. Regimens under study include the following: two NRTIs and a PI, 1 NRTI and 2 NNRTIs, 2 PIs with or without 1 or 2 NRTIs, 1 PI and 1 NNRTI with or without 2 NRTIs, and 3 NRTIs.

Antiretroviral therapy is recommended for HIV-infected *children* in the following circumstances:

1. Age less than 12 months (infants are at high risk for disease progression, and immunologic and virologic parameters have poorer predictive value in these patients than in older children and adults)
2. HIV RNA levels > 100,000 copies/mL, regardless of clinical or immune status of the child
3. Evidence of immune suppression (immune category 2 or 3) or clinical symptoms of HIV infection, regardless of the age of the child or the viral load
4. Substantially increasing viral loads on repeated testing (more than a five-fold increase for children younger than age 2 years and more than a three-fold increase for children 2 years of age or older)

Antiretroviral therapy should be considered for asymptomatic patients 30 months of age or older with HIV RNA levels of 10,000 to 20,000 copies/mL.

Antiretroviral Therapy and Medical Management of Pediatric HIV Infection. Pediatrics 102: 1005-1062, 1998.

Carpenter CJ, et al: Updated Recommendations of the International AIDS Society-USA Panel. JAMA 280:78-86, 1998.

129. What are the common bone marrow toxicities associated with antiretroviral therapy?

Anemia is common, occurring in up to 9.4% of children receiving AZT (v. 4-5% of those on other regimens). Typically HIV infected children with anemia respond to erythropoeitin and do not require cessation of therapy.

Neutropenia is very common, occurring in 6-27% of children receiving antiretroviral therapy, particularly those taking AZT and ddI. HIV-infected children typically tolerate neutropenia well, without serious infectious complications unless the neutropenia is severe and prolonged (absolute neutrophil count < 250 cells/mm^3). Before changing antiretroviral therapy, a trial of G-CSF is warranted. Other common causes of neutropenia include HIV infection itself and other drug toxicity (TMP-SMX is a common culprit).

Thrombocytopenia occurs in 30% of untreated children with HIV infection and is more commonly an initial presentation of HIV infection rather than a complication of antiretroviral therapy. In initial trials severe thrombocytopenia was seen in 2% of children receiving either ddI and AZT or 3TC and AZT. IVIG is used to treat severe thrombocytopenia; if this intervention fails, corticosteroids can be attempted.

130. Which antiretroviral is associated with a severe, potentially fatal hypersensitivity reaction?

3–5% of patients treated with ***abacavir*** (Ziagen) experience a hypersensitivity reaction characterized by fever, nausea, vomiting, diarrhea, abdominal pain, fatigue, respiratory symptoms (occurring in 20% of patients and including cough, dyspnea, and pharyngitis) and rash. The drug should be discontinued and not restarted, as restarting can result in more severe symptoms within hours, including life-threatening hypotension and sudden death.

131. Which antiretroviral agent is commonly associated with CNS symptoms, including nightmares and hallucinations?

Efavirenz (also known as Sustiva). In controlled trials 53% of patients receiving efavirenz compared with 25% patients receiving control regimens experienced CNS symptoms, including dizziness, insomnia, impaired concentration, somnoloence, abnormal dreams, and hallucinations. Symptoms usually occur within the first two days of treatment and resolve within 2-4 weeks. Bedtime dosing minimizes the impact of these side effects.

132. Which class of antiretrovirals is associated with abnormal glucose metabolism, lipodystrophy, and dyslipidemias?

All PIs can cause hyperglycemia, new-onset diabetes mellitus, spontaneous bleeding, lipodystrophy and dyslipidemias.

133. What adjustments are necessary when co-administering ddI and antifungal agents?

Ketoconazole and itraconazole should be administered at least two hours before or after dosing with ddI because they are better absorbed at an acidic gastric pH. Other antimicrobials that require gastric acidity and should be administered roughly two hours before or after ddI include dapsone, doxycycline, and fluoroquinolones.

134. Which drug combinations used to treat HIV can produce life-threatening arrythmias?

Astemizole, terfenadine, cisapride, triazolam, or midazolam used in combination with macrolides, azoles, or protease inhibitors can cause life-threatening arrythmias.

IMMUNIZATIONS

135. Why is the buttocks a poor location for intramuscular injections in infants?

The gluteus maximus is not a good choice for injections because:

- The gluteus muscles are incompletely developed in some infants.
- There is potential for injury to the sciatic nerve or superior gluteal artery if the injection is misdirected.
- Some vaccinations, particularly those for rabies, influenza and hepatitis B, may be less effective if injected into fat.

If injections into the buttocks are given to older children, the proper site is the gluteus medius in the upper outer quadrant, rather than the gluteus maximus, which is more medial.

Zuckerman JN: The importance of injecting vaccines into muscle. BMJ 321:1237-1238, 2000.

Lawton EL, Hayden GF: Immunization, medication and tuberculin skin test administration procedures. In: Lohr JA (ed): Pediatric Outpatient Procedures. Philadelphia, J.B. Lippincott, 1991, pp 25–26.

136. Is there any risk associated with administering multiple vaccines simultaneously?

Immune responses to one vaccine generally do not interfere with those to other vaccines, and thus most vaccines can be administered simultaneously (at separate sites) without concern regarding effectiveness. Exceptions include interference among the 3 oral poliovirus serotypes in OPV vaccine and simultaneous administration of cholera and yellow fever vaccines.

137. Should premature babies receive immunization based on postconceptional age or chronologic age?

In most cases, premature babies should be immunized based on postnatal *chronologic* age. If a premature infant is still in the hospital at 2 months of age, the vaccines routinely scheduled at that age should be administered, including diphtheria, tetanus, acellular pertussis, *Haemophilus influenzae* type b, and inactivated poliovirus vaccines.

For premature infants who weigh less than 2 kg at birth and whose mothers are hepatitis B vaccine surface antigen (HBsAg) negative, the optimal time to initiate immunization against hepatitis B remains unclear. Based on the finding that seroconversion rates are relatively low in these infants when immunization is initiated shortly after birth, it is recommended that immunization be delayed until just before hospital discharge or until 2 months of age.

Premature infants who weigh less than 2 kg at birth and whose mothers are HBsAg-positive should receive hepatitis B immune globulin (HBIG) and the first dose of hepatitis B vaccine within 12 hours of birth. If the maternal HBsAg status is unknown, hepatitis B vaccine should be administered at birth; maternal HBsAg status should then be determined, and HBIG should be administered if the mother is HBsAg-negative.

138. Should there by any change in the immunization schedule for children with cerebral palsy?

No. In particular, patients with static cerebral palsy should receive immunization against pertussis at the normally recommended times. If cerebral palsy is associated with a neurologic disorder that is evolving, then vaccination with pertussis vaccine should be withheld until the condition is in a stable phase. The decision to proceed with pertussis vaccination in these instances may often require discussion with a pediatric neurologist.

139. Which vaccines are egg-embryo-based vaccines?

Of the more common immunizations administered to children, measles and mumps vaccine preparations are grown in chick embryo fibroblast culture. Recent studies indicate that children with egg allergy are at low risk for anaphylaxis to MMR and do not require skin testing prior to administration of this vaccine. Influenza vaccine also contains egg protein and on rare occasions induces immediate hypersensitivity reactions, including anaphylaxis. In children who have a history of severe anaphylactic reactions to eggs and who are scheduled to receive influenza vaccine, skin testing is recommended. However, in most cases these children should not receive influenza vaccine because of the risk of reaction, the likely need for yearly immunization, and the availability of chemoprophylaxis against influenza infection.

140. Discuss the relative merits of OPV and IPV.

Both the live oral poliovirus (OPV or Sabin) vaccine and the inactivated poliovirus (IPV or Salk) vaccine are effective in preventing poliomyelitis. OPV induces intestinal immunity, is simple to administer, and results in immunization of some contacts of vaccinated persons (a phenomenon referred to as herd immunity). On the other hand, on rare occasions OPV can produce paralytic polio. IPV results in seroconversion in 95% or more of recipients to each of the 3 serotypes after 2 doses and in 99-100% of recipients after 3 doses. Enhanced potency IPV induces mucosal immunity, although to a lesser extent than does OPV. Finally, IPV has no risk of producing paralytic polio.

The American Academy of Pediatrics now recommends a 4-dose all-IPV vaccine schedule for routine immunization of all infants and children in the US. OPV is contraindicated in the US except in the following circumstances:

- Mass vaccination campaigns to control outbreaks of paralytic polio
- Unimmunized children who will be traveling in the next 4 weeks to an area where polio is endemic
- Children whose parents refuse the recommended number of injections to complete the schedule of routine immunizations

141. What is the difference between whole cell and acellular pertussis vaccines?

Whole cell pertussis vaccines consist of whole bacteria that have been inactivated and are nonviable. These vaccines contain lipooligosaccharide and other cell wall components that result in a high incidence of adverse effects. Acellular pertussis vaccines contain one or more *B. pertussis* proteins that serve as immunogens. All contain at least detoxified pertussis toxin, and some contain other antigens as well, including filamentous hemagglutinin (FHA), fimbrial proteins, and pertactin. The acellular vaccines are associated with a much lower incidence of side effects and thus are preferred for all doses in the US.

142. Given the number of licensed acellular pertussis vaccines, what are the recommendations regarding interchangeability?

When feasible, the same DTaP product should be used for the first 3 doses of the pertussis immunization series. However, when information about the type of DTaP vaccine received previously is unavailable, any of the DTaP vaccines licensed for use in the primary series can be used. For the fourth and fifth doses, any of the licensed products is acceptable, without consideration of the prior vaccines received.

143. What are the absolute contraindications to pertussis immunization?

The adverse events after pertussis immunization that represent absolute contraindications to further administration of pertussis vaccine include the following:

- Immediate anaphylactic reaction
- Encephalopathy within 7 days of vaccination

The adverse events that represent precautions for further administration of pertussis vaccine include the following:

- A seizure, with or without fever, within 3 days of immunization
- Persistent, severe, inconsolable screaming or crying for ≥ 3 hours within 2 days of immunization
- Collapse or shock-like state within 2 days of vaccination
- Fever ≥ 40.5°C (104.9°F), unexplained by another cause, within 2 days of immunization

When a contraindication to pertussis immunization exists, DT vaccine should be administered instead.

144. How often do major neurologic complications or death occur from pertussis vaccine?

The only case-controlled study addressing this issue was the National Childhood Encephalopathy Study (NCES), which was conducted in England from 1976–1979. This study reported that DTP immunization (using whole cell pertussis vaccine) was temporally related to the development of acute encephalopathy in approximately 1 in 110,000 doses. About one-third of these children had permanent brain damage. This figure formed the basis for previous estimates of a 1 in 310,000 incidence of permanent neurologic deficits following DTP immunization. However, an expert panel reevaluated these data and concluded that limitations of the study design and the small number of cases precluded valid interpretation regarding the incidence of permanent brain damage following DTP immunization. Additional studies have not provided evidence to support a causal association between DTP immunization and permanent neurologic injury.

The American Academy of Pediatrics Committee on Infectious Diseases concluded that according to current data, the DTP vaccine has not been proved to be a cause of brain damage. The Committee also stated that while the data do not disprove the association, if brain damage does result from DTP immunization, the occurrence must be exceedingly rare.

Committee on Infectious Diseases: The relationship between pertussis vaccine and central nervous system sequelae: Continuing assessment. Pediatrics 97:279–281, 1996.

146. How long does protection against pertussis last after infection versus immunization?

Vaccine-induced immunity is of relatively short duration. Based on studies of patients immunized against pertussis and exposed to a sibling with pertussis, protection against infection is approximately 80% for the first 3 years after immunization, dropping to 50% at 4–7 years and to near zero at 11 years. It is hypothesized that subclinical infection during the period of waning immunity may be a factor in prolonging protection following immunization in some instances.

Protective immunity following natural infection with *Bordetella pertussis* is long-lasting. In addition, the immunity induced by natural infection appears to provide better protection than that induced by vaccination, even in the first 3 years following vaccination.

Wardlaw AC, Parton R (eds): Pathogenesis and Immunity in Pertussis. New York, John Wiley & Sons, 1988, p 284.

147. What are the age restrictions regarding pertussis vaccination?

Based on current recommendations, generally pertussis vaccines should not be given to children over 7 years of age. At least with whole cell pertussis vaccine, there is an increased incidence of localized reactions to the vaccine in older children and adults, and pertussis is usually a mild illness when it occurs past early childhood. In general, postexposure antimicrobial prophylaxis is preferred to vaccination in this setting. However, in rare instances, it may be advisable to immunize certain older individuals. For example, during an epidemic when unknown exposures may occur with increased frequency, patients with chronic lung disease should be immunized.

148. What is the difference between the pediatric (DT) and adult (dT) types of diphtheria and tetanus toxoid vaccines?

The *DT vaccine* contains standard doses of diphtheria and tetanus toxoids and should be used to immunize all children younger than 7 years of age when pertussis immunization is not required or is contraindicated. The *dT vaccine* contains a much smaller dose of diphtheria toxoid compared with the standard tetanus toxoid dose. It should be used to immunize children over 7 years old and adults and is less likely to produce the severe reactions seen in older individuals given the higher dose. dT can be used when tetanus toxoid is required for wound management, as a booster against both tetanus and diphtheria is required every 10 years to ensure continuing tetanus and diphtheria immunity in adulthood.

149. If a pregnant woman is given the rubella vaccine in her first trimester, what is the risk to the fetus?

There is a theoretical risk that congenital rubella infection will occur. The Centers for Disease Control and Prevention has collected information from 226 susceptible women who received the present rubella vaccine during the first trimester and found that 2% of the infants born to these women had subclinical infection but none had congenital defects. Based on these data, the maximum risk of congenital rubella associated with first-trimester vaccination is estimated to be 1.6%. Receipt of rubella vaccine during pregnancy is not an indication for interruption of the pregnancy.

150. What are the contraindications to immunization with MMR?

• ***Intercurrent illness***. In general, in an otherwise well child, low-grade fever and upper respiratory tract symptoms are not considered contraindications to immunization with MMR. However, more serious illness should prompt a delay in immunization until the child recovers.

• ***Immunosuppression***. Examples include primary disorders of the immune system and immunodeficiency secondary to malignancies, treatment with immunosuppressive drugs, and treatment with radiation. Among patients with HIV infection, MMR is contraindicated if severe immunosuppression is present.

• ***Allergies***. Because the MMR vaccine contains trace amounts of neomycin, a previous anaphylactic reaction to neomycin is a contraindication to the use of this vaccine. While the mumps and measles components of MMR are derived from chick embryo fibroblast tissue cultures, these components do not contain significant amounts of egg proteins. Furthermore, recent studies indicate that children with egg allergy are at low risk for anaphylactic reactions with MMR. As a consequence, children with egg allergy can receive MMR routinely.

• ***Passive immunity***. Administration of immune globulin, whole blood, or other antibody-containing blood products may interfere with response to MMR for variable periods of time, depending on the dose administered. In general, MMR should be delayed at least 3 months and sometimes longer (up to 11 months after the dose of immune globulin for Kawasaki disease).

• ***Pregnancy***. There is no evidence that MMR vaccine administered during pregnancy injurs the developing fetus, but due to theoretical concerns, the vaccine should not be administered to women who are pregnant or contemplating pregnancy within 3 months.

• ***Personal** or **family history of convulsions***. Children with a personal or immediate-family history of seizures have a slightly increased risk of seizures after measles vaccination. However, such history is not a contraindication to vaccination but rather should serve to alert the family and physician of the possibility

150. When was inactivated (killed) measles vaccine used?

1963–1968. About 1.8 million doses were given.

151. What is the relationship between the MMR vaccine, autism and inflammatory bowel disease?

In the late 1990s, reports from Great Britain suggested that increased immunization rates with the MMR vaccine might be a cause of apparent increasing rates of autism and in addition constituted a risk factor for the development of Crohn disease and ulcerative colitis. However, subsequent published studies have not supported any such association.

Dales L, et al: Time trends in autism and in MMR immunization coverage in California. JAMA 285:1183-1185, 2001.

Davis RL, et al: Measles-mumps-rubella and other measles-containing vaccines do not increase the risk for inflammatory bowel disease. Arch Pediatr Adolesc Med 155:354-359, 2001.

152. What are the differences between the licensed hepatitis B vaccines?

Two highly effective and safe hepatitis B vaccines have been licensed for use in the US. Both are produced by recombinant DNA technology. The original plasma-derived vaccine is no longer produced in this country, but plasma-derived products are available in other countries. Recombivax HB contains 10 μg of HBsAg protein per ml, while Engerix-B contains 20 μg of HBsAg protein per ml, in both cases adsorbed to aluminum hydroxide. Despite the difference in the concentration of HBsAg protein, the two vaccines achieve equal rates of seroconversion in infants, children, adolescents, and young adults.

153. Under what circumstances should hepatitis A vaccine be used?

Currently, two inactivated hepatitis A vaccines (Havrix and Vaqta) are available in the US. Both vaccines are approved for individuals older than 2 years and are administered in a 2-dose schedule. Recommendations for the use of hepatitis A vaccine include the following:

- As preexposure prophylaxis for susceptible people traveling to countries with intermediate or high endemic rates of hepatitis A infection. In this circumstance, vaccine is preferable, but immunoglobulin is an acceptable alternative.
- For children living in communities with consistently elevated hepatitis A rates, defined as twice the national average
- For people with chronic liver disease
- For homosexual and bisexual men
- For patients with clotting factor disorders
- For people at risk of occupational exposure to hepatitis A (e.g. handlers of nonhuman primates and individuals working with hepatitis A virus in a laboratory setting)

Hepatitis A vaccine should also be considered for staff at day care centers, staff at custodial care institutions, hospital personnel, and food handlers.

154. Can immunization prevent disease caused by pneumococci?

In the past, the 23-valent plain polysaccharide pneumococcal vaccine was able to prevent most invasive disease (bacteremia, meningitis, and pneumonia) in children over 2 years of age; immunogenicity in those under 2 years of age was limited. A recently licensed 7-valent pneumococcal conjugate vaccine uses a mutant diphtheria toxin (CRM_{197}) as a carrier protein to increase immunogenicity in infants and toddlers. The serotypes contained in this vaccine represent 75-80% of those causing invasive disease in the United States. Early studies indicate that the vaccine can prevent over 90% of invasive disease in infants and young children caused by these serotypes.

Black S, et al: Efficacy, safety, and immunogenicity of heptavalent pneumococcal conjugate vaccine in children. Pediatr Infect Dis J 19:187-95, 2000.

155. Who should receive the pneumococcal vaccine?

According to recommendations from the American Academy of Pediatrics Committee on Infectious Diseases, the 7-valent conjugate vaccine should be administered to all children 23 months and younger at 2, 4, 6, and 12-15 months of age. In addition, the 7-valent vaccine is recommended for all children 24-59 months who are at high risk for invasive pneumococcal disease, including children with sickle cell disease, other causes of functional or anatomic asplenia, HIV infection, chronic cardiac disease, chronic pulmonary disease, chronic renal insufficiency, diabetes mellitus, CSF leak, primary immunodeficiency, or a condition associated with immunosuppression (e.g., organ or bone marrow transplantation, drug therapy, or radiation therapy). In order to provide protection against a broader range of serotypes, these high-risk children should also a dose of the 23-valent plain polysaccharide vaccine at least 6-8 weeks after the last dose of the conjugate vaccine. When elective splenectomy is performed for any reason, scheduled immunization with either the 7-valent or the 23-valent vaccine should be performed at least 2 weeks before the splenectomy. Similarly, when possible, patients anticipating cancer chemotherapy or immunosuppression should be immunized at least 2 weeks before the initiation of therapy.

156. What are the pediatric indications for the influenza vaccine?

Two types of killed influenza vaccine are available: the split vaccine is used for children < 13 years of age, and the whole virus vaccine is used for older children and adults. Each year in the autumn, a new preparation is made, aimed to cover the expected antigenic types for the winter season. Vaccination should be undertaken each year as soon as possible after the vaccine becomes available. When the vaccine is given for the first time, two doses are given, 1 month apart; in subsequent years, the same patient should be given only one dose. The vaccine is not recommended for children < 6 months of age.

Children at high risk for severe influenza infection who should be vaccinated include those with:

- Chronic lung diseases, e.g., asthma, bronchopulmonary dysplasia, cystic fibrosis
- Congenital heart disease causing significant hemodynamic disturbance
- Sickle cell anemia and other hemoglobinopathies
- Immunosuppressive disorders or therapy
- Chronic renal dysfunction
- Chronic metabolic disease, including diabetes mellitus
- Diseases requiring long-term aspirin therapy (which may increase the risk for developing Reye syndrome following influenza)

In addition, children who are close contacts of high risk patients should be vaccinated. There is controversy regarding whether the clinical course of influenza is severe enough to warrant routine vaccination for all children.

Neuzil KM, et al: The effect of influenza on hospitalizations, outpatient visits, and courses of antibiotics in children. N Engl J Med 342:225-231, 2000.

McIntosh K, Lieu T: Is it time to give the influenza vaccine to healthy infants? N Engl J Med 342: 275-276, 2000.

Cox NJ, Subbarao K: Influenza. Lancet 354:1277-1282, 1999.

157. Under what circumstances should meningococcal vaccine be given?

A quadrivalent meningococcal vaccine containing capsular polysaccharide from serogroups A, C, Y, and W135 is available in the U.S. and is approved for use in children ≥ 2 years of age. Of note, serogroup B isolates account for approximately one-third of cases of meningococcal disease, and serogroup B polysaccharide is absent from the vaccine.

Routine vaccination against meningococcal disease is not recommended in children because in this population the rate of disease is low and the immune response is poor and relatively short-lived. However, vaccination is considered advisable for children ≥ 2 years of age in high-risk groups, including those with functional or anatomic asplenia or complement deficiency.

According to recent recommendations from the U.S. Public Health Service Advisory Committee on Immunization Practices (ACIP), college freshmen living in dormitories should be offerred the meningococcal vaccine. In 1998-1999, the rate of meningococcal disease for college freshmen living in dormitories was 4.6/100,000, compared to 0.7/100,000 for undergraduates in general and 1.5/100,000 for people 18-23 years old who were not in college. A study of university freshmen in England found that 7% of entering freshmen were carriers for *N. meningitidis* and this rate rose to almost 35% by the end of one month.

Meningococcal vaccine is given to all military recruits in the U.S. and should be considered for individuals traveling to areas of epidemic or hyperendemic disease. In addition, the current vaccine may be useful as an adjunct to chemoprophylaxis in the control of outbreaks caused by a vaccine serogroup.

Neal KR, et al: First year university and N. meningitidis carriage rates. BMJ 320:846-849, 2000.

158. Who should receive post-exposure prophylaxis against rabies?

Children bitten by dogs, cats, or ferrets known or suspected to be rabid should receive immediate immunization and rabies immune globulin (RIG). If the animal escapes, public health authorities should be consulted. Bats, skunks, raccoons, foxes and most other carnivores should be regarded as rabid unless they are caught, euthanized and proven to be free of rabies. Bites of squirrels, rabbits, hamsters, gerbils, guinea pigs, chipmunks, rats, and mice usually do not require antirabies treatment.

Prophylaxis includes one-time administration of RIG in a total dose of 20 units per kg of body weight. As much of this dose as possible is infiltrated around the wound, and the remainder is given intramuscularly at a separate site. At-risk children should also receive five doses of rabies vaccine. Four formulations of three different rabies vaccines are currently licensed for use in the United States.

159. Beyond candidates for post-exposure prophylaxis, who should receive rabies human diploid cell vaccine (HDCV)?

Pre-exposure vaccination is recommended for individuals at high risk for contact with rabies, such as veterinarians, animal handlers, cave explorers, certain laboratory workers, and individuals living in or visiting areas where the risk of rabies exposure is high.

160. What are the most common adverse reactions to intravenous immunoglobulin?

The incidence of adverse reactions associated with intravenous immunoglobulin (IVIG) is less than 5%. In most cases, the reactions are mild and self-limited. Severe reactions occur infrequently and do not generally contraindicate further use of IVIG. Adverse events include the following:

- Pyrogenic reactions (fever, chills)
- Minor systemic reactions marked by headache, myalgia, anxiety, nausea, or vomiting
- Vasomotor manifestations, with flushing, tachycardia, and blood pressure lability
- Aseptic meningitis
- Hypersensitivity reactions, including anaphylaxis, which generally occurs in patients who are absolutely deficient in IgA and have IgG antibodies directed against IgA.

161. What are the recommendations for storage of varicella vaccine?

Varicella vaccine (Varivax) comes lyophilized and should be stored in a frost-free freezer at an average temperature of –15°C or colder. It can be stored at refrigerator temperature (2°-8°C) for up to 72 continuous hours before administration. The diluent used for reconstitution should be stored either at room temperature or in a refrigerator. Following reconstitution, the vaccine should be injected within 30 minutes.

162. How effective is the varicella vaccine if given following exposure to the illness?

Highly effective (95% for prevention of any disease, 100% for prevention of moderate to severe disease) when used within 36 hours after exposure in an environment involving close contract. The reason may be that natural varicella infection may require 5-7 days for the wild virus to propogate in the respiratory tract before primary viremia and dissemination occur, while the vaccine virus may elicit humoral and cellular immunity in significantly less time.

Watson B, et al: Postexposure effectiveness of varicella vaccine. Pediatrics 105:84-88, 2000.

163. Of the vaccines included in the routine schedule, which ones contain live viruses?

MMR and ***varicella***. OPV is a live attenuated virus vaccine but is no longer recommended for routine use. Other live virus vaccines include adenovirus and yellow fever virus.

164. What are the recommendations for interchangeability of *H. influenzae* type b (Hib) vaccines?

In the US there are four Hib conjugate vaccines, including HbOC, PRP-OMP, PRP-T, and PRP-D. In all cases, these vaccines consist of the type b capsular polysaccharide (polyribosylribitol phosphate or PRP) covalently linked to an immunogenic carrier protein. HbOC, PRP-OMP, and PRP-T are recommended for infants beginning at 2 months of age, while PRP-D is recommended only for children 12 months of age or older. Except for the age constraint regarding PRP-D, all of the Hib vaccines are considered interchangeable for primary and booster immunization. Of note, HbOC and PRP-T are administered at 2, 4, 6, and 12-15 months of age, and PRP-OMP is administered at 2, 4, and 12-15 months. If PRP-OMP is administered in a primary series, the recommended number of doses to complete the series is determined by the other Hib conjugate vaccine.

165. What are the 3 general circumstances for passive administration of preformed antibody?

1. When an individual is deficient in antibody synthesis as a result of a congenital or acquired B-lymphocyte defect
2. When an individual susceptible to a specific infection is exposed to that infection, especially when the person has a high risk of complications from the infection (e.g., a child with leukemia exposed to varicella), or when time does not permit protection by active immunization alone (e.g., exposure to rabies or hepatitis B)
3. When an individual has a toxin- or immune-mediated disease where antibody may suppress the effects of the toxin (e.g., botulism or tetanus) or suppress the immune response (e.g., Kawasaki disease)

166. What are the indications for palivizumab?

Palivizumab is a humanized mouse monoclonal antibody directed against an RSV protein and approved for prevention of RSV disease in selected children. According to the American Academy of Pediatrics, recommendations for *consideration* of palivizumab include the following:

- Infants and children younger than 2 years of age with chronic lung disease who have required medical therapy for their lung disease within 6 months of the expected RSV season
- Infants born at ≤ 32 weeks gestation within 6 months of the expected RSV season
- Children with severe immunodeficiencies (e.g. severe combined immunodeficiency or advanced AIDS)

167. What are the recommendations regarding administration of live-virus vaccines to patients on corticosteroid therapy?

Children on corticosteroid treatment can become immunosuppressed. Although some uncertainty exists, there is adequate experience to make recommendations regarding administration of live-virus vaccines to previously healthy children receiving steroid treatment. In general, live-virus vaccines should *not* be administered to children who have received prednisone or its equivalent in a dose of ≥ 2 mg/kg/day (or ≥ 20 mg per day for individuals whose weight is > 10 kg) for 14 days or more. Treatment for briefer periods, with lower doses, or with topical preparations or local injections should not contraindicate the use of these vaccines.

168. What is thimerosal?

Thimerosal is a mercury-containing preservative that has been used as an additive to vaccines for decades because of its effectiveness in preventing contamination, especially in open multidose containers. In an effort to reduce exposure to mercury, vaccine manufacturers, the FDA, the AAP, and other groups are working to remove thimerosal from vaccines that contain this compound.

169. What is the National Childhood Vaccine Injury Act?

This Act went into effect in 1986 and requires physicians and other health care professionals who administer vaccines to maintain permanent immunization records and to report specific adverse events via the Vaccine Adverse Event Reporting System (VAERS).

The vaccines to which these requirements apply include measles, mumps, rubella, varicella, polio, hepatitis B, pertussis, diphtheria, tetanus, and *H. influenzae* type b.

170. What is the National Vaccine Injury Compensation Program?

This program is a no-fault system that allows people who believe they have suffered an injury or death as a result of administration of a covered vaccine to seek financial compensation. Claims related to the covered vaccines must be evaluated through the program before civil litigation can be pursued. This program has been in place since 1988 and has resulted in a marked reduction in the number of lawsuits against health care professionals and manufacturers and has helped to maintain a stable vaccine supply.

INFECTIONS WITH RASH

171. What is the traditional numbering of the "original" six exanthemas of childhood and when were they first described?

First disease	Measles (rubeola), 1627
Second disease	Scarlet fever, 1627
Third disease	Rubella, 1881
Fourth disease	Filatov-Dukes disease (described in 1900 and felt to be a distinct scarlatiniform type of rubella or attributed more recently to exotoxin-producing *Staph aureus*; term is no longer used)
Fifth disease	Erythema infectiosum, 1905
Sixth disease	Roseola infantum (exanthem subitum), 1910

Weisse ME: The fourth disease: 1900-2000. Lancet 357:299-301, 2001.

172. What is "atypical" about atypical measles?

- It occurs primarily in patients who have received inactivated measles vaccine.
- Koplik spots are unusual.
- The rash begins on distal extremities and spreads toward the head (in typical measles, the exanthem spreads from the head to the feet).
- Conjunctivitis and coryza are not part of the prodrome.
- Hepatosplenomegaly is common.

Cherry JD: Measles. In: Feigin RD, Cherry JD (eds): Textbook of Pediatric Infectious Diseases, 4th ed. Philadelphia, W.B. Saunders, 1998, pp 2063-2064.

173. What are the circumstances associated with measles cases in the US?

From 1989 to 1991, the incidence of measles in the US increased as a consequence primarily of low immunization rates in preschool children. Since 1992, the incidence of measles in the US has been low, with fewer than 1000 reported cases per year. Cases continue to occur from importation of the virus from other countries. In addition, vaccine failure occurs in approximately 5% of vaccine receipients after a single dose of vaccine and is responsible for some cases. Waning immunity after immunization may be a factor in occasional cases. Of note, vaccine failure after 2 doses of measles vaccine administered after 12 months of age is uncommon.

Global Measles Control and Regional Elimination, 1998-1999. MMWR 48 (49):1124-1130, 1999.

National Vaccine Advisory Committee: The measles epidemic: The problems, barriers, and recommendations. JAMA 266:1547–1552, 1991.

174. Why is post-measles blindness so common in underdeveloped countries?

As many as 1% of all patients with measles in underdeveloped regions experience progression of keratitis to blindness. In contrast, measles keratitis in developed countries is usually self-limited and benign. There are two principal reasons for the progression to blindness among patients with measles in underdeveloped countries:

1. Vitamin A deficiency—Vitamin A is needed for corneal stromal repair, and a deficiency allows epithelial damage to persist or worsen. Many malnourished children have accompanying vitamin A deficiency, and vitamin A supplements may be of benefit during active illness.
2. Malnutrition—Malnutrition may predispose to corneal superinfection with herpes simplex virus.

175. How common is human herpesvirus type-6 (HHV-6) infection in children?

Infection with HHV-6 is ubiquitous and occurs with high frequency in infants, 65% of whom have serologic evidence of primary infection by their first birthday. HHV-6 infection results in typical cases of roseola and is also associated with a number of other common pediatric problems, including "fever without localizing findings," nonspecific rash, and EBV-negative mononucleosis. In a study by Hall and coworkers, up to one-third of all febrile seizures in children age < 2 years were due to HHV-6 infections. On rare occasions, the virus has been associated with fulminant hepatitis, encephalitis, and a syndrome of massive lymphadenopathy called Rosai-Dorfman disease.

Hall CB, et al: Human herpesvirus-6 infection in children. N Engl J Med 331:432–438, 1994.

176. What are the etiologic agents of exanthem subitum (roseola).

Multiple agents are likely. HHV-6 was discovered in 1986, and in 1988, Japanese investigators isolated it from four children with exanthem subitum. In 1994, human herpesvirus type 7 (HHV-7) was also isolated from children with the clinical features of roseola.

177. What are the typical features of roseola?

Most children have an abrupt onset of high fever (> 39°C) with no prodrome. Fever usually lasts 3–4 days but can range from 1–8 days. Within 24 hours of defervescence, a discrete erythematous macular or maculopapular rash appears on the face, neck, and/or trunk. Erythematous papules (Nagayama spots) may be noted on the soft palate and uvula in two-thirds of patients. Other common findings on exam include mild cervical lymph node enlargement, edematous eyelids, and a bulging anterior fontanel in infants. A variety of symptoms can accompany the fever, including diarrhea, cough, coryza, and headache.

Caserta MT, et al: Primary human herpesvirus 7 infection: a comparison of human herpesvirus 7 and human herpesvirus 6 infections in children. J Pediatr 133:386-389, 1998.

178. What is the spectrum of disease caused by parvovirus B19?

- Erythema infectiosum (most common; a childhood exanthem, also called fifth disease or slapped cheek disease because of the classic appearance of the rash)
- Arthritis and arthralgia (most common in adults)
- Intrauterine infection with hydrops fetalis
- Transient aplastic crisis in patients with underlying hemolytic disease
- Persistent infection with chronic anemia in patients with immunodeficiencies
- No symptoms

179. Describe the characteristic rash of Rocky Mountain spotted fever.

- Usually seen by third day of illness (5–11 days after tick bite)
- Initially blanching red macules which become petechial
- Begins on wrists and ankles and spreads to extremities and trunk within hours
- Involves palms and soles

180. Describe the characteristic rash of ehrlichiosis.

Among patients with ehrlichiosis, rash occurs variably. Approximately 30% of adults and 60% of children develop a rash, which typically begins on the trunk and then spreads to the extremities. The rash can be maculopapular or petechial.

181. What is the Weil-Felix test?

The Weil-Felix test was used in the past to diagnose Rocky Mountain spotted fever (RMSF). This test was based on the fact that rickettsiae share antigens that cross-react with the *Proteus vulgaris* OX-19 and OX-2 antigens. However, only a fraction of patients with RMSF have elevated titers to the *P. vulgaris* OX-19 and OX-2 antigens, and titers can be elevated in patients with leptospirosis, brucellosis, *Borrelia* infections, typhoid fever, and serious liver disease as well. Accordingly, the Weil-Felix test has little value in the diagnosis of RMSF.

In most cases, the diagnosis of RMSF is established by measuring acute and convalescent titers against *Rickettsia rickettsiae*, including indirect immunofluorescence antibody (IFA), enzyme immunoassay (EIA), or complement fixation (CF) titers. During the acute phase of the illness, RMSF can be diagnosed by PCR on the blood in some cases.

182. How long after exposure to chickenpox (varicella) do symptoms develop?

99% of patients develop symptoms between 11–20 days following exposure.

183. Should "well" children with varicella be treated with acyclovir?

Studies have shown that oral acyclovir therapy (20 mg/kg, up to 800 mg) four times daily for 5 days, initiated within 24 hours after the onset of rash, decreases the maximum number of lesions by 15–30%, shortens the duration of the development of new lesions, and shortens the duration of fever by 1 day. The American Academy of Pediatrics Committee on Infectious Diseases opted not to recommend acyclovir for routine use in uncomplicated varicella for otherwise healthy children under age 13 because of "marginal therapeutic effect, the cost of the drug, feasibility of drug delivery in the first 24 hours of illness, and the currently unknown and unforeseen possible dangers of treating as many as 4 million children each year." Of note, the varicella vaccine is now recommended for routine use in children.

American Academy of Pediatrics: Varicella-zoster infections. In: Pickering LK (ed): 2000 Red Book, Report of the Committee on Infectious Diseases, 25th ed. Elk Grove Village, IL, American Academy of Pediatrics, 2000, p. 626.

Committee on Infectious Diseases: Use of oral acyclovir in otherwise healthy children with varicella. Pediatrics 91:674–676, 1993.

184. What is the risk of varicella-associated complications in normal children 1–14 years old?

More than 3.5 million cases of chickenpox occur in the United States each year, with the great majority occurring in children < 14 years of age. The most common complications include secondary bacterial skin infections (generally due to streptococci or staphylococci), neurologic syndromes (cerebellitis, encephalitis, transverse myelitis, and Guillain-Barré syndrome), and pneumonia. Thrombocytopenia, arthritis, hepatitis, glomerulonephritis, and Reye syndrome occur less commonly. Myocarditis, pericarditis, pancreatitis, and orchitis are described but are rare.

The frequency of these complications in normal children is not known precisely, but it is estimated to be low on the basis of hospitalization and mortality data. In particular, approximately 4500 otherwise normal children are hospitalized in the U.S. each year because of chickenpox. In normal children, the death rate due to varicella averages about 1 in 50,000 cases.

Arvin AM : Varicella-zoster zirus. Clin Microbiol Rev 9: 361-381, 1996.

Preblud SR: Varicella: Complications and costs. Pediatrics 78:728–735, 1986.

185. How common are second episodes of varicella?

Approximately ***1 in 500*** cases. They are more likely to occur in children who develop their first episode during infancy or whose first episode is subclinical or very mild.

Gershon A: Second episodes of varicella: Degree and duration of immunity. Pediatr Infect Dis J 9:306, 1990.

186. In children with herpes zoster, what is the distribution of the rash?

Compared with adults, who most commonly have lesions in the lower thoracic and upper lumbar regions, children may have more cervical and sacral involvement with resultant extremity and inguinal lesions.

50% *Thoracic*
20% *Cervical*
20% *Lumbosacral*
10% *Cranial nerve*

If there are lesions on the tip of the nose, herpes zoster keratitis is more likely because of possible involvement of the nasociliary nerve. When the geniculate ganglion is involved, there is risk of developing the Ramsay Hunt syndrome, which consists of ear pain with auricular and periauricular vesicles and facial nerve palsy.

187. Should children with zoster be treated with antiviral agents?

Routine antiviral therapy is not indicated. In general, the prognosis for children with herpes zoster is very good with extremely low probabilities of postherpetic neuralgia or of associations with undiagnosed malignancy.

Petursson G, et al: Herpes zoster in children and adolescents. Pediatr Infect Dis J 17:905-908, 1998.

188. Who gets herpes gladiatorum?

Herpes gladiatorum is a term used for ocular and cutaneous infection with herpes simplex virus type 1 occurring in wrestlers and rugby players. The infection is transmitted primarily by direct skin-to-skin contact and is endemic among high school and college wrestlers.

189. When did the World Health Organization certify that smallpox had been globally eradicated?

1980.

LYMPHADENITIS/LYMPHADENOPATHY

190. What are the most common causes of lymphadenitis in normal, otherwise healthy children?

In order of frequency:

1. *Staphylococcus aureus*
2. Group A β-hemolytic streptococcus
3. *Bartonella henselae* (cat scratch disease)
4. *Mycobacterium tuberculosis*
5. Nontuberculous mycobacteria

191. An intensely erythematous but nontender submandibular or tonsillar node is most suggestive of what infectious process?

Nontuberculous mycobacterial infection.

192. How is the diagnosis of nontuberculous mycobacterial disease made?

In children, infection with nontuberculous mycobacteria (NTM) most commonly takes the form of localized lymphadenitis. The submandibular or preauricular glands are most often affected. Suggestive clinical features include adenopathy with minimal warmth and tenderness together with induration in response to PPD skin testing and a negative chest x-ray. Skin test antigens specific for NTM are of limited usefulness due to cross-reactivity with antigens of *M. tuberculosis*. Definitive diagnosis of NTM infection depends on culture of the organism from infected tissue. Histopathologic examination of the tissue cannot adequately differentiate NTM from *M. tuberculosis*.

Less common forms of disease due to NTM include pulmonary and disseminated infection. These occur almost exclusively in debilitated patients, particularly patients with AIDS, in whom *M. avium* complex infections have become prevalent. On occasion, children with cystic fibrosis can develop symptomatic pulmonary disease due to NTM. In these forms of infection, the diagnosis relies on culture of the organism from the relevant body site, such as sputum or blood.

193. Swollen, tender pectoral nodes are most suggestive of what infection?
Cat scratch disease.

194. What is the etiologic agent of cat scratch disease?

Based on serologic studies and testing of infected tissues with PCR and culture, it appears that most, if not all, cases of cat scratch disease are caused by *Bartonella henselae*. This organism was first isolated in 1991 and has also been associated with bacillary angiomatosis and peliosis hepatis, which occur primarily in adults with HIV infection.

195. What is the typical course of the lymphadenitis in cat scratch disease?

Cat scratch disease (CSD) is characterized by *chronic* regional lymphadenitis. Typically, an otherwise healthy child or adolescent presents with regional lymphadenopathy of several weeks duration. A history of exposure to cats, particularly kittens, is obtained in up to 90% of patients. In most cases fever is absent or low grade. Other symptoms can include malaise, arthralgia, headache, anorexia, myalgia, and abdominal, extremity, neck, or back pain. In many patients, a round nontender red papule several millimeters in diameter develops near the scratch after 3 to 10 days and can persist for a few days to three weeks. One to two weeks after the scratch, regional lymph nodes draining the area gradually enlarge, peaking in size after 2-3 weeks. The nodes remain unchanged for the next 2-3 weeks and then gradually shrink over another 2-3 weeks. They are usually moderately tender and are associated with overlying erythema and fluctuance. The lymph nodes most commonly involved are axillary, epitrochlear, cervical, submandibular, inguinal, and preauricular. Enlarged pectoral nodes are highly suggestive of CSD.

196. How common is disseminated infection in cat scratch disease?

5-25% . This form of the disease is characterized by severe, prolonged systemic symptoms, including fever, malaise, fatigue, myalgia, arthralgia, and abdominal pain. Granulomatous lesions may be detected by ultrasound in the liver and spleen.

Parinaud oculoglandular syndrome is an occasional presentation of CSD. This syndrome is characterized by granulomatous lesions on the palpebral conjunctiva associated with swelling of ipsilateral preauricular nodes. Direct eye rubbing after contact with a cat is the presumed mode of inoculation.

Among the most disturbing presentations of CSD is *encephalitis*, which is associated with convulsions in 46-80% of patients. In one series of 76 patients with neurologic complications of cat scratch disease, 61 had encephalopathy. The average age was 10.6 years. Nearly twice as many males as females were affected. 50% of patients with encephalopathy did not have fever; 26% had fever > 39°C. Combative behavior was common, occurring in nearly 40% of patients. Other common signs and symptoms included headache and malaise.

Four of the 61 patients had ataxia lasting 1- 8 weeks after presentation with encephalopathy. Other rare findings in this series included bilateral sixth nerve palsy, transient aphasia, transient hemiplegia, and temporary hearing loss. CSF parameters are typically normal or reveal a mild elevation in protein. CT scans and MRI scans are usually normal. Fortunately, the prognosis for full neurologic recovery is excellent.

Other neurologic presentations include polyneuritis, myelitis, and neuroretinitis. Rarely, CSD manifests as osteomyelitis, atypical pneumonia, thrombocytopenic purpura, or nonthrombocytopenic purpura.

Grando D et al: Bartonella henselae associated with Parinaud's oculoglandular syndrome. Clin Infect Dis 38:1156-1158, 1999.

Bass JW, et al: The expanding spectrum of Bartonella infections: II. Cat-scratch disease. Pediatr Infect Dis J 16: 163-79, 1997.

197. Are antibiotics indicated for CSD?

In nearly all cases, lymphadenitis due to CSD resolves within several weeks to months from its onset. On occasion, the nodes suppurate, necessitating excision to prevent spontaneous drainage. Incision and drainage is generally not recommended, as this therapy may be associated with a higher incidence of chronic drainage and fistula formation.

The use of antibiotics in uncomplicated CSD is controversial, as commonly used antibiotics are ineffective and most patients recover spontaneously. In a small series of patients (n=35) with cervical lymphadenitis, azithromycin was shown to reduce the size of cervical lymph nodes to 20% of the original lymph node volume by 4 weeks after therapy.

Based on *in vitro* antibiotic susceptibility testing and uncontrolled clinical studies, several antibiotics appear to offer benefit in patients with more severe forms of *Bartonella* infection. Examples include azithromycin, doxycycline, trimethoprim-sulfamethoxasole, ciprofloxacin, gentamicin, and rifampin.

Arisoy E,S et al: Hepatosplenic cat-scratch disease in children: Selected clinical features and treatment. Clin Infect Dis 28: 778-84, 1999.

Bass JW et al: Prospective randomized double blind placebo-controlled evaluation of azithromycin for treatment of cat-scratch disease. Pediatr Infect Dis J 17 : 447-52, 1998.

198. How is the diagnosis of cat scratch disease made?

In most clinical microbiology laboratories, *Bartonella henselae* is difficult to culture. Experienced laboratories have reported success with chocolate or blood agar plates incubated for at least 30 days.

Currently the gold standard for diagnosis is serologic testing with an IFA assay performed at the Centers for Disease Control and Prevention. An antibody titer of greater than 1:64 is considered a positive result. Cross reactivity exists between *Bartonella henselae* and *Bartonella quintana,* so high positive antibody titers to *B. henselae* are sometimes associated with low positive titers to *B. quintana.*

Warthin-Starry silver staining of infected tissues is sometimes helpful in establishing a diagnosis. However, in one series only 4 of 32 patients with serologically confirmed cat scratch disease had a positive Warthin-Starry stain. Thus, silver staining is considered unreliable for excluding the diagnosis of cat scratch disease.

PCR is not yet available commercially but is performed at the CDC and in some clinical microbiology laboratories and appears to be very sensitive.

199. What are the common presentations for Epstein-Barr virus (EBV) infections?

EBV infection is frequently asymptomatic in young children. In adolescents and young adults, infection typically results in infectious mononucleosis, which is characterized as follows:

Clinical: Fever, pharyngitis, lymphadenopathy (75–95%), splenomegaly (50%)
Hematologic: > 50% mononuclear cells, > 10% atypical lymphocytes

Serologic: Transient appearance of heterophile antibodies; emergence of persistent antibodies to EBV

A wide variety of symptoms (e.g., malaise, headache, anorexia, myalgias, chills, nausea) can occur. Neurologic presentations are rare but can include encephalitis, meningitis, myelitis, Guillain-Barré syndrome, and cranial or peripheral neuropathies.

200. How was the monospot test developed?

In 1932, Paul and Bunnell observed that patients with infectious mononucleosis make antibodies that agglutinate sheep RBCs. These antibodies are referrred to as heterophile antibodies and serve as the basis for the monospot test, which is a rapid slide agglutination test. Nowadays usually horse or beef RBCs are used because they are more sensitive to agglutination than are sheep RBCs. Heterophile antibodies can also occur in serum sickness and as a normal variant. If there is clinical confusion, differential absorption can pinpoint the cause. Heterophile antibodies in infectious mononucleosis do not react with guinea pig kidney cells, whereas those of serum sickness do. Normal variant heterophile antibodies do not react with beef RBCs.

Durbin WA, Sullivan JL: Epstein-Barr virus infections. Pediatr Rev 15:63–68, 1994.

201. How common are heterophile antibodies in infectious mononucleosis?

In typical infectious mononucleosis with fever, tonsillopharyngitis, and lymphadenopathy, 75% of older children and adolescents have heterophile antibodies by the end of the first week of illness and 85–90% by the third week. These percentages are much lower in infants and children younger than 4 years of age, and false-negative screening with the monospot test is common in these groups as well as in patients without classic infectious mononucleosis.

202. What is the natural course of serologic responses to EBV infection?

A variety of distinct EBV antigens, including viral capsid antigen (VCA), early antigen (EA), and nuclear antigen (EBNA), can elicit antibody responses. Acute infection is best characterized by the presence of anti-VCA IgM.

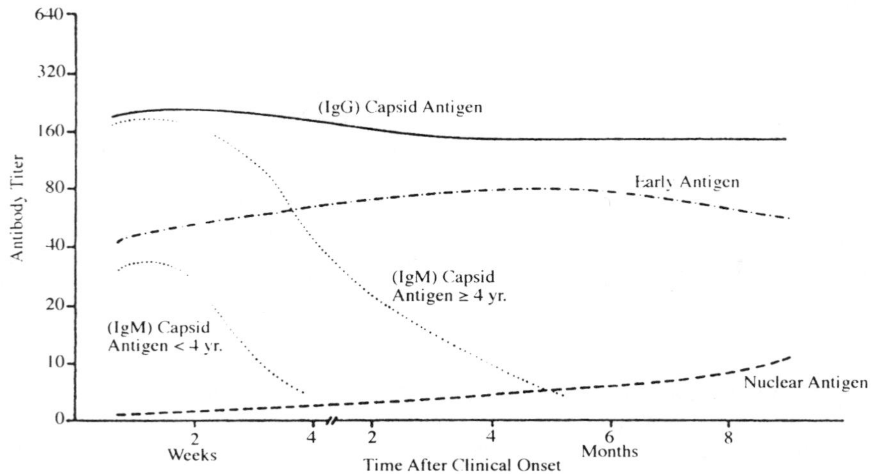

From Sumaya CV: Infectious mononucleosis. In: Oski FA, et al (eds): Principles and Practice of Pediatrics, 2nd ed. Philadelphia, J.B. Lippincott, 1994, p. 1316; with permission.

203. When are steroids indicated in children with EBV infection?

For the relief of respiratory obstruction due to enlarged tonsils. Some authorities have also advocated their use for severe autoimmune hemolytic anemia, aplastic anemia, neurologic disease, and severe life-threatening infection, such as liver failure.

204. Which other organisms can cause an infectious mononucleosis-like picture?

Cytomegalovirus, *Toxoplasma gondii*, human herpesvirus-6, adenovirus, HIV, and rubella.

205. What are the clinical presentations of acquired cytomegalovirus (CMV) infection?

When acquired cytomegalovirus infection is symptomatic, in normal hosts it produces fever, malaise, and nonspecific aches and pains. The peripheral blood smear reveals an absolute lymphocytosis and many atypical lymphocytes. In contrast to EBV-infectious mononucleosis, lymphadenopathy and tonsillitis are not prominent. Liver involvement is very common and liver function tests are commonly abnormal. Like EBV disease, CMV mononucleosis can persist for several weeks.

MENINGITIS

206. What are the most common signs and symptoms of meningitis in infants aged < 2 months?

In general, the findings in neonates and young infants with meningitis are minimal and often subtle. Temperature instability (fever or hypothermia) occurs in approximately 60% of infected infants, increasing irritability in about 60%, poor feeding or vomiting in roughly 50%, and seizures in about 40%. Lethargy, respiratory distress, and diarrhea are frequent nonspecific manifestations of meningitis in this patient group. On physical exam, approximately 25% of newborns and young infants have a bulging fontanelle, and only 13% have nuchal rigidity. The diagnosis of meningitis cannot be excluded based on the absence of these physical findings in infants.

Pong A, Bradley JS: Bacterial meningitis and the newborn infant. Infect Dis Clin North Am 13: 711-733, 1999.

207. What percentage of neonates with bacterial sepsis and positive blood cultures have meningitis?

Up to 25% of infants less than 28 days old with bacterial sepsis and positive blood cultures will have culture-confirmed meningitis.

208. Which occurs more commonly, aseptic or bacterial meningitis?

Aseptic meningitis. Prior to the availability of the *Haemophilus influenzae* type b conjugate vaccines, one-third of all cases of meningitis were bacterial and two-thirds were aseptic. Now the percentage of cases that are aseptic is even higher.

209. What is the most common cause of aseptic meningitis?

Aseptic meningitis consists of clinical and laboratory indications of inflammation of the meninges (e.g., CSF pleocytosis and increased protein) without evidence of bacterial infection on Gram stain or culture. Over 80% of cases are caused by *enteroviruses* (i.e., coxsackievirus, enterovirus, echovirus, and, rarely, poliovirus).

210. Is intracranial pressure elevated in patients with meningitis?

In acute bacterial meningitis, pressure is elevated in up to 95% of cases. Elevations are also commonly seen in tuberculous and fungal meningitis. The extent of elevation in viral meningitis is less well studied.

211. Should CT scans be performed prior to a lumbar puncture (LP) in the evaluation of possible meningitis?

CT scans are not routinely indicated prior to an LP unless any of the following are present:

- Signs of herniation (rapid alteration in consciousness, abnormalities of pupillary size and reaction, absence of oculocephalic response, fixed oculomotor deviation of eyes)
- Papilledema
- Abnormalities in posture or respiration
- Generalized seizures (especially tonic), which are often associated with impending cerebral herniation
- Overwhelming shock or sepsis
- Concern about a condition mimicking bacterial meningitis (e.g., intracranial mass, leadintoxication, tuberculous meningitis, Reye syndrome)

Haslam RH: Role of CT in the early management of bacterial meningitis. J Pediatr 119:157–159, 1991.

212. What is the range of values found in CSF of infants and children who do not have meningitis?

CSF Values Found in Infants and Children without Meningitis

	WBCs/mm^3	PROTEIN (MG/DL)	CSF/BLOOD GLUCOSE (%)
Newborn infants			
Preterm	0–29	65–150	55–105
Term	0–32	20–170	44–248
Infants and children	0–6	15–45	60–90

From McCracken GH: Current management of bacterial meningitis in infants and children. Pediatr Infect Dis J 11:170, 1992; with permission.

213. If bloody CSF is collected during a lumbar puncture, how is CNS hemorrhage distinguished from a traumatic artifact?

Most often, the blood is due to traumatic rupture of small venous plexes that surround the subarachnoid space, but pathologic bloody fluid can be seen in multiple settings (e.g., subarachnoid hemorrhage, herpes simplex encephalitis). Distinguishing features that suggest pathologic bleeding include:

- Bleeding that does not lessen during collection of multiple tubes
- Xanthochromia of the CNS supernatant
- Crenated RBCs noted microscopically

214. How do the CSF findings vary in bacterial, viral, fungal, and tuberculous meningitis in children beyond the neonatal period?

Although a large overlap is possible (e.g., bacterial meningitis can be associated with a low WBC count early in the illness, or viral meningitis often can be associated with a predominance of neutrophils early or even persistently in the illness), the usual findings are:

Typical Findings in Bacterial, Viral, Fungal, and Tuberculous Meningitis

CSF FINDINGS	BACTERIAL	VIRAL	FUNGAL/TUBERCULOUS
WBC/mm^3	> 500	< 500	< 500
PMNs	> 80%	< 50%	< 50%
Glucose (mg/dl)	< 40	> 40	< 40
CSF/blood ratio	< 30%	> 50%	< 30%
Protein (mg/dl)	> 100	< 100	> 100

Adapted from Powell KR: Meningitis. In: Hoeckelman RA, et al: (eds). Primary Pediatric Care, 2nd ed. St. Louis, Mosby, 1992, p 1354; with permission.

215. How is a traumatic lumbar puncture interpreted?

To interpret the number of WBCs in the CSF following a traumatic lumbar puncture, a correction factor is needed:

$$\text{True WBCs (CSF)} = \text{Actual WBCs (CSF)} - \frac{[\text{WBCs (blood)} \times \text{RBCs (CSF)}]}{\text{RBCs (blood)}}$$

Ashwal S, et al: Bacterial meningitis in children: Current concepts of neurologic management. Curr Probl Pediatr 24:267–284, 1994.

216. When is the best time to obtain a serum glucose level in an infant with suspected meningitis?

Because the stress of a lumbar puncture can elevate serum glucose, the serum sample is ideally obtained just before the lumbar puncture. When the blood glucose level is elevated acutely, it can take at least 30 minutes before there is equilibration with the CSF.

217. How often does bacterial meningitis present in younger patients with normal findings on the initial CSF examination?

In ***up to 3%*** of cases in children aged 3 weeks to 18 months with positive bacterial cultures of the CSF, the initial CSF evaluation (i.e., cell count, protein and glucose concentrations, and Gram stain) can be normal. Of note, in almost all of these cases, physical examination reveals evidence of meningitis or suggests serious illness and the need for empiric antibiotics.

Polk DB, Steele RW: Bacterial meningitis presenting with normal cerebrospinal fluid. Pediatr Infect Dis J 6:1040–1042, 1987.

218. Does antibiotic therapy prior to lumbar puncture affect CSF indices?

In most cases of bacterial meningitis, a few doses of antibiotic will not markedly alter the CSF. Gram stain usually still demonstrates bacteria with typical staining properties, and chemistry values and cell counts are abnormal. Even when children have received appropriate antibiotic therapy for 44–68 hours, chemical and cytologic analysis of the CSF generally still reflects a bacterial process. In earlier studies of patients with *Haemophilus influenzae* meningitis who received oral antibiotic therapy prior to lumbar puncture, CSF cultures often grew the organism. In contrast, there is a tendency for oral therapy to sterilize the CSF of children with meningococcal disease or with meningitis due to sensitive *Streptococcus pneumoniae*.

219. What are the most common organisms responsible for bacterial meningitis in the US?

0–1 month

- Group B streptococci
- *Escherichia coli*
- *Listeria monocytogenes*
- *Streptococcus pneumoniae*
- Miscellaneous Enterobacteriaceae
- *Haemophilus influenzae* (nontypable and type b)
- Coagulase-negative staphylococci (in hospitalized preterm infants)

1–23 months

- *Streptococcus pneumoniae*
- *Neisseria meningitidis*
- Group B streptococci
- *Haemophilus influenzae*

2–18 years

- *Neisseria meningitidis*
- *Streptococcus pneumoniae*
- *Haemophilus influenzae*

The incidence of *H. influenzae* meningitis has fallen dramatically with the introduction of effective vaccines.

Schuchat A, et al: Bacterial meningitis in the United States in 1995. N Engl J Med 337: 970-976, 1997.

220. Why is *Haemophilus influenzae* type b more virulent than nontypable *Haemophilus* strains?

H. influenzae type b expresses the type b polysaccharide capsule, which is a polymer of ribose and ribitol-5 phosphate. In the absence of type-specific antibody, the type b capsule promotes intravascular survival by preventing phagocytosis and complement-mediated bactericidal activity. It is likely that other factors also contribute to the unique virulence of *H. influenzae* type b.

221. What are the drugs of choice for empiric treatment of bacterial meningitis in children older than 1 month?

In cases of suspected bacterial meningitis, both vancomycin and a third-generation cephalosporin are recommended for empiric therapy, as resistance to penicillin and cephalosporins is present in 10-30% of *Streptococcus pneumoniae* isolates. The exception would be when the gram stain suggests another etiology (e.g. gram-negative diplococci). Following determination of antibiotic susceptibility, antibiotics can be tailored accordingly. Animal experiments and studies of patients with meningitis reveal that vancomycin penetrates into the CSF relatively well in the setting of inflamed meninges. Treatment failures have been reported when the dosage of vancomycin is less than 60 mg/kg/day. Vancomycin should not be used alone to treat *S. pneumoniae* meningitis, as data in animal models indicate that bactericidal levels may be difficult to maintain. The combination of vancomycin plus cefotaxime or ceftriaxone has been shown to produce a synergistic effect in vitro, in animal models, and in the CSF of children with meningitis.

Ahmed A: A critical evaluation of vancomycin for treatment of bacterial meningitis. Pediatr Infect Dis J 16: 895-903, 1997.

American Academy of Pediatrics, Committee on Infectious Diseases: Therapy for children with invasive penumococcal infections. Pediatrics 99: 289-299, 1997.

222. How quickly is the CSF sterilized in children with meningitis?

In successful therapy, the CSF is usually sterile ***within 36–48 hours*** of initiation of antibiotics.

223. How long after treatment has been initiated must individuals with meningitis remain in respiratory isolation?

24 hours. Respiratory isolation is recommended for patients with suspected *Haemophilus influenzae* type b or meningococcal meningitis but can be discontinued after 24 hours of therapy.

224. What is the accepted duration of treatment for bacterial meningitis?

The duration of antibiotic treatment is based on the causative agent and clinical course. In general, a minimum of 5 days of therapy is required for meningococcal meningitis, 7–10 days for *Haemophilus influenzae* meningitis, and 10 days for pneumococcal meningitis. Disease due to group B streptococci or *Listeria monocytogenes* should be treated for 14–21 days, and meningitis caused by gram-negative enteric bacilli should be treated for a minimum of 21 days after the CSF has become sterile. Among patients with complications such as brain abscess, subdural empyema, delayed CSF sterilization, persistence of meningeal signs, or prolonged fever, the duration of therapy may need to be extended and should be individualized.

225. What is the role of corticosteroids in the treatment of bacterial meningitis?

The inflammatory response plays a critical role in producing the CNS pathology and resultant sequelae of bacterial meningitis. A series of studies have demonstrated that treatment with dexamethasone reduces the incidence of hearing loss and other neurologic sequelae in infants and children with *Haemophilus influenzae* meningitis. According to these studies, dexamethasone therapy should be started before initiation of antibiotic therapy and should be administered intravenously in a dose of 0.15 mg/kg. In the original studies, doses were repeated every 6 hours to complete 16 doses over 4 days. More recent data suggest that a regimen consisting of 8 doses given every 6 hours over 2 days is equally efficacious. For cases of meningitis caused by pathogens other than *Haemophilus influenzae*, the current recommendations by the American Academy of Pediatrics are to *consider* the use of dexamethasone. The role of steroids in meningitis due to other bacterial pathogens, particularly *S. pnuemoniae*, remains controversial.

Arditi M, et al: Three-year multicenter surveillance of pneumococcal meningitis in children: clinical characteristics, and outcome related to penicillin susceptibility and dexamethasone use. Pediatrics 102: 1087-1097, 1998.

McIntyre, et al: Dexamethasone as adjunctive therapy in bacterial meningitis. A meta-analysis of randomized clinical trials since 1988. JAMA 278: 925-31, 1997.

226. Should children receiving therapy for bacterial meningitis be retapped?

It is widely agreed that a repeat lumbar puncture is advisable in patients with meningitis due to penicillin-resistant *Streptococcus pneumoniae* or gram-negative enteric bacilli and in children who show no clinical response to therapy in 24–36 hours. Repeat lumbar puncture is also recommended for patients with prolonged or recurrent fever, for those with recurrent meningitis, and for immunocompromised hosts. Repeat CSF examination is unnecessary for patients whose course of illness is uncomplicated. An exception is neonatal meningitis, in which retapping to confirm sterilization is recommended because of the greater difficulty in tracking the infant's clinical course and because of the variable response of the immature neonatal immune system. Furthermore, in neonatal meningitis time to sterilization correlates inversely with prognosis.

Wubbel L, McCracken GH: Management of bacterial meningitis. Pediatr Rev 19: 78-84, 1998.

227. In a patient with meningitis, what are the indications for a CT scan or MRI?

CT scan and MRI are especially useful in identifying intracranial complications of bacterial meningitis, such as subdural collections of fluid (including subdural empyema), brain abscess, cerebrovascular thrombosis, and hydrocephalus. The following suggest the presence of an intracranial complication and should prompt a neuroimaging study: (1) prolonged obtundation, (2) prolonged irritability, (3) seizures developing after the third day of therapy, (4) focal seizures, (5) focal neurologic deficits, (6) increasing head circumference, (7) persistent elevation of CSF protein or neutrophil count, and (8) recurrence of disease. In cases of neonatal meningitis caused by *Citrobacter diversus* (also called *Citrobacter koseri*), brain abscess should be anticipated, and a CT scan or MRI should performed early in the course. In these patients, repeat scans are useful to monitor the response to antibiotic therapy and determine the need for surgical intervention.

Wubbel L, McCracken GH: Management of bacterial meningitis. Pediatr Rev 19: 78-84, 1998.

228. How common is persistent or recurrent fever in meningitis?

In the absence of dexamethasone treatment, fever persists for at least 5 days after initiation of antibiotics in most children with meningitis. It lasts for 5–9 days in 10–15% of cases and for 10 or more days in another 10–15% of patients. Fever that returns after a minimum of 24 hours of normal temperatures is considered recurrent fever and occurs in approximately 15% of patients.

Lin T-Y, et al: Fever during treatment for bacterial meningitis. Pediatr Infect Dis J 3:319–332, 1984.

229. What are the most common causes of prolonged fever in meningitis?

- Disease at other foci (e.g., arthritis)
- Nosocomial infection
- Thrombophlebitis (related to intravenous catheters and infusates)
- Sterile or infected abscesses from intramuscular injections
- Drug fever

Subdural effusions have also been associated with prolonged fever, but these occur commonly among children with meningitis and are probably not a cause of fever.

230. How should prolonged fever during treatment for meningitis be managed?

Patients who remain febrile for > 5 days and who are irritable or have persistent neck stiffness should undergo a repeat lumbar puncture. Similarly, children who appear well yet have fever for ≥ 10 days should also undergo repeat lumbar puncture. If the CSF examination reveals a protein concentration > 100 mg/dl, a glucose concentration < 30 mg/dl, or > 25% neutrophils, persistent infection is a possibility. Studies should be obtained to exclude an abscess or resistant isolate. If the CSF values are approaching normal, antibiotic therapy can usually be discontinued at the usual time. In this situation, nosocomial viral infection or drug fever would be likely.

Nelson JD: Management problems in bacterial meningitis. Pediatr Infect Dis J 4:S41-44, 1985.

231. How commonly are subdural effusions noted in bacterial meningitis?

Subdural effusions are common in bacterial meningitis and should be considered part of the disease rather than a complication. Estimates of their incidence vary from 10–50%. The incidence is highest in young infants and in patients with *Haemophilus influenzae* meningitis. Most authorities now agree that routine tapping of subdural effusions is unnecessary. Removal of fluid is reserved for patients showing signs of increased intracranial pressure or focal neurologic signs. Approximately 1% of patients with meningitis will have a subdural empyema; the typical presentation is fever, irritability, and meningeal signs. Subdural empyema can be diagnosed by CT and requires drainage and prolonged antibiotic therapy.

232. If a child develops bacterial meningitis, what should the parents be told about long-term outcomes?

In children beyond the newborn period, sequelae such as spasticity, paralysis, ataxia, seizures, school problems, and visual and hearing disorders can persist. Hydrocephalus is very rare. In a meta-analysis evaluating the three main bacterial causes of meningitis, disease due to *Streptococcus pneumoniae* was associated with considerably more mortality and morbidity than was infection caused by *Neisseria meningitidis* or *Haemophilus influenzae*. Among patients with pneumococcal meningitis, 17% had mental retardation, 12% had spasticity, 14% had a seizure disorder, and 15% had profound deafness. Mortality was as high as 15%. A more recent three-year multicenter surveillance study of invasive pneumococcal infections examined outcomes of meningitis due to *Streptococcus pneumoniae* in 180 children. The case fatality rate was 7.7%. 25% of children had evidence of neurologic sequelae at the time of hospital discharge, and 32% had unilateral or bilateral deafness. There were no differences in outcomes between patients with and without penicillin- or cephalosporin-resistant organisms. Predictors of mortality included coma on admission, requirement for mechanical ventilation, and shock.

Arditi M, et al: Three-year multicenter surveillance of pneumococcal meningitis in children: clinical characteristics and outcome related to penicillin susceptibility and dexamethasone use. Pediatrics 102 :1087-1097, 1998.

Baraff LJ, et al: Outcomes of bacterial meningitis in children: A meta-analysis. Pediatr Infect Dis J 12:389–394, 1993.

233. How should contacts of children with *Neisseria meningitidis* disease be managed?

Antibiotic prophylaxis is indicated for household and daycare or nursery school contacts of patients with invasive meningococcal disease. Only those medical personnel who have had intimate contact with the patient (e.g., through intubation or mouth-to-mouth resuscitation) require antibiotic prophylaxis. Surveillance cultures of contacts should not be performed to determine the need for prophylaxis. In most instances, options for chemoprophylaxis include rifampin, ceftriaxone, and ciprofloxacin (for those $\geq$ 18 years of age).

A quadrivalent plain polysaccharide vaccine containing capsular polysaccharide from serogroups A, C, Y, and W135 is approved in the U.S. for use in children 2 years of age and older. Because secondary cases can occur several weeks after onset of disease in an index case, meningococcal vaccine should be considered as an adjunct to chemoprophylaxis when an outbreak is caused by a serogroup A, C, Y, or W135 strain.

American Academy of Pediatrics. Meningococcal infections. In: Pickering LK (ed): 2000 Red Book, Report of the Committee on Infectious Diseases, 25th ed. Elk Grove Village, IL, American Academy of Pediatrics, 2000, p. 398-401.

Committee on Infectious Diseases: Meningococcal disease prevention and control strategies for practice-based physicians. Pediatrics 97:404–412, 1996.

OCULAR INFECTIONS

234. Among neonates with conjunctivitis, what is the timing for the various etiologies?

Cause	*Time of Onset*
Chemical	< 2 days
Neisseria gonorrhoeae	2-7 days
Chlamydia trachomatis	5-14 days
Herpes simplex virus	6-14 days

235. In children with conjunctivitis and otitis media, what is the most likely etiologic agent?

Nontypeable *Haemophilus influenzae* is the most common cause of the so-called conjunctivitis-otitis syndrome, which is characterized by concurrent conjunctivitis and otitis media.

236. Can bacterial conjunctivitis be distinguished from viral conjunctivitis on clinical grounds alone?

Classically, bacterial conjunctivitis is more common in infants and young children, with the discharge being purulent or mucopurulent. Viral conjunctivitis presents with a serous exudate in children of all ages. Bacterial infections are commonly associated with otitis media, and otoscopy should be performed on all patients. However, clinical findings can overlap. Both bacteria and viruses can cause unilateral or bilateral symptoms.

Common bacterial etiologies of conjunctivitis include nontypable *Haemophilus influenzae*, *Streptococcus pneumoniae* and *Moraxella catarrhalis*. Staphylococcal species frequently grow in cultures but usually are not a primary cause of the pathology. Aside from culture, the best way to distinguish the culprit is by Giemsa stain of a conjunctival scraping. Neutrophils predominate in bacterial infections, lymphocytes in viral infections, and eosinophils in allergic conjunctivitis.

Weiss A: Acute conjunctivitis in childhood. Curr Probl Pediatr 24:4–11, 1994.

237. What is keratoconjunctivitis?

Keratoconjunctivitis is an inflammatory process that involves both the conjunctiva and cornea. Superficial inflammation of the cornea occurs commonly in association with viral and bacterial conjunctivitis, particularly in adults. Hence, many cases of conjunctivitis are more correctly termed keratoconjunctivitis.

Epidemic keratoconjunctivitis is caused by adenovirus serotypes 8, 19, and 37. Some organisms, including *Pseudomonas aeruginosa*, *Neisseria gonorrhoeae*, and herpes simplex virus, have a propensity to cause more severe infection of the cornea. Infection due to these pathogens must be recognized early in order to prevent corneal scarring with subsequent vision loss.

238. When are topical antibiotics not sufficient in treating acute conjunctivitis?

Topical therapy for chlamydial conjunctivitis is generally ineffective in teenagers and should never be used as sole therapy in the neonate because of the high likelihood of concomitant respiratory tract colonization (which can eventually progress to pneumonia). Viral conjunctivitis, of course, does not respond to topical antibiotics. Finally, infections due to *Neisseria gonorrhoeae*, *Pseudomonas aeruginosa*, *Haemophilus influenzae* type b, and *N. meningitidis* require systemic therapy to prevent the serious complications seen with these organisms.

239. What is the best method of prophylaxis for ophthalmia neonatorum?

Previously, *Neisseria gonorrhoeae* was the most common cause of neonatal conjunctivitis (generally referred to as ophthalmia neonatorum). With the use of 1.0% silver nitrate drops, the rate of this disease dropped to 0.03% among liveborn infants. However, silver nitrate drops frequently cause a chemical conjunctivitis and are not completely effective against *Chlamydia*, which is now the predominant etiology of neonatal conjunctivitis. Erythromycin 0.5% ophthalmic ointment and tetracycline 1.0% ophthalmic ointment are now used in most nurseries the US, although their efficacy in preventing chlamydial disease remains unclear. Worldwide, other methods are utilized. In one large study of > 3000 infants in Kenya, 2.5% povidone-iodine ophthalmic solution was a more effective prophylaxis against neonatal conjunctivitis than silver nitrate drops or erythromycin ointment. Providone-iodine solution was also considerably cheaper than the alternatives.

Isenberg SJ: A controlled trial of povidone-iodine as prophylaxis against ophthalmia neonatorum. N Engl J Med 332:562–566, 1995.

240. What is the recommended therapy for gonococcal ophthalmia neonatorum?

Gonococcal ophthalmia neonatorum is a serious disease with the potential for blindness and should be treated with a parenteral antibiotic. Therapy should include a single dose of ceftriaxone (25–50 mg/kg IV or IM, not to exceed 125 mg) or cefotaxime (100 mg/kg IV or IM). Eye irrigation with buffered saline should be instilled until the discharge resolves. The diagnosis of gonococcal ophthalmia should prompt a thorough search for disseminated gonococcal infection. Careful physical examination should be performed, and blood and CSF cultures should be obtained. In infants who fail to respond adequately to therapy, simultaneous infection with *Chlamydia trachomatis* should be considered.

241. Can newborns with chlamydial conjunctivitis be treated with topical therapy alone?

Newborns diagnosed with chlamydial conjunctivitis should receive systemic therapy with oral erythromycin (50 mg/kg/day in 4 divided doses) for 14 days. Topical therapy will not eradicate the organism from the upper respiratory tract and fails to prevent development of chlamydia pneumonia. Close follow-up is indicated to ensure the absence of relapse.

242. Are ophthalmic solutions better than ophthalmic ointments in eradicating conjunctivitis?

Ophthalmic ointments are usually preferred in infants and young children because they can be instilled more reliably and remain in the eye for a longer time. In older children, ophthalmic solutions may be preferred to prevent the blurring of vision that occurs with ointments. In general, the efficacy of ophthalmic ointments is presumed to be superior to that of solutions. However, several antibiotics are available in high concentration solutions. These "fortified" formulations have not been compared prospectively to other preparations but are widely used because of their presumed enhanced efficacy.

243. What are the side effects of neomycin in eye ointment preparations?

Neomycin eye ointment can cause a localized contact dermatitis. Less commonly the medication can sensitize individuals and lead to rash or other systemic reactions upon reexposure to neomycin. Anaphylactic reactions are rare, but if they occur, the subsequent use of MMR vaccine is contraindicated, as it contains this antibiotic.

244. What is the most common cause of the Parinaud oculoglandular syndrome?

Parinaud syndrome is characterized by granulomatous or ulcerating conjunctivitis and prominent preauricular or submandibular adenopathy. The most common cause is ***cat scratch disease***, but other causes include tularemia, sporotrichosis, tuberculosis, syphilis, and infectious mononucleosis.

245. How is orbital cellulitis distinguished from periorbital (or preseptal) cellulitis?

Periorbital cellulitis involves the tissues anterior to the eyelid septum, while *orbital cellulitis* involves the orbit and is sometimes associated with abscess formation and cavernous sinus thrombosis. Distinction between these processes requires assessment of ocular mobility, pupillary reflex, visual acuity, and globe position, which are normal in periorbital cellulitis but may be abnormal in orbital cellulitis. An abnormality in any of these four areas mandates radiologic evaluation (usually CT scan of the orbit) and possible surgical drainage. Significant eyelid swelling can occur with both periorbital and orbital cellulitis, making visualization of the globe difficult. However, by using eyelid retractors, usually an adequate exam can be obtained.

246. What is the difference between a hordeolum, a stye, and a chalazion?

A *hordeolum* is a purulent infection of any one of the sebaceous or apocrine sweat glands of the eyelid, including the glands of Moll and Zeis, which drain near the eyelash follicle, and the meibomian glands, which drain nearer the conjunctiva. Clinically, a hordeolum is recognized as a red, tender swelling. It is usually due to *S. aureus*.

A *stye* is an external hordeolum, on the skin side of the eyelid.

A *chalazion* is an internal hordeolum, on the conjunctival side of the eyelid.

In all cases, these lesions are treated with warm compresses and topical antibiotic drops and usually resolve within 7 days. A chalazion is more likely to become chronic and to require surgical excision.

OTITIS MEDIA

247. How commonly does cerumen obscure the diagnosis of otitis media?

Cerumen is secreted by sebaceous and apocrine glands at the base of hair follicles in the outer third of the ear and comes in all forms—wet and brown in African-Americans and whites, and dry and flaky in Orientals. Surprisingly, as many as 50% of white children have no obvious cerumen seen on inspection. When otitis media is part of a differential diagnosis (as in unexplained fever), cerumen must be removed to allow visualization of the tympanic membrane. As many as 30% of cases of otitis media are obscured by this waxy roadblock. Unfortunately, lack of pain is not a helpful clue in diagnosis in that 15–20% of children with otitis media do not have ear pain. The old tale of otitis media being associated with soft wax (from melting by the "hot ear") is unfounded, with that finding occurring in only 10% of cases.

Schwartz RH et al: Cerumen removal: How necessary is it to diagnose acute otitis media? Am J Dis Child 137:1065–1068, 1983.

248. What is the best way to remove cerumen?

A variety of methods and folklore are tried. Removal by curretage via direct visualization (preferably through an otoscope) is commonly used, but it can be uncomfortable and difficult if immobilization of the child is incomplete. When time permits, ceruminolytic agents can be installed to soften the wax followed by gentle irrigation. A recent study comparing docusate sodium (Colace) with trimethanolamine polypeptide (Cerumenex) found the former more effective. Water jet irrigation devices are used, but at higher pressures there is a risk of perforation.

Singer AJ, et al: Ceruminolytic effects of docusate sodium: A randomized, controlled trial. Ann Emerg Med 36:228-232, 2000.

249. Is ear pulling a reliable sign of infection?

In the absence of other signs or symptoms (e.g., fever, upper respiratory infection symptoms), ear pulling alone is a very poor indicator of acute otitis media.

Baker RB: Is ear pulling associated with ear infection [letter]? Pediatrics 90:1006–1007, 1992.

250. How often will acute otitis media resolve spontaneously without antibiotics?

In 60% or more. It is this high rate of spontaneous improvement that confounds the comparison of drug treatments. Of note, the likelihood of spontaneous resolution depends on the microbiologic etiology and is estimated at 20% with *Streptococcus pneumoniae*, 50% with *H. influenzae*, 80% with *M. catarrhalis*, and 100% with respiratory viruses.

251. Should all children with acute otitis media be treated with antibiotics?

Because of the high rate of spontaneous improvement, some suggest that children may not require antibiotic therapy for uncomplicated otitis media, especially children over 2 years of age. However, placebo-controlled trials have demonstrated that treatment with an antimicrobial agent shortens the duration of symptoms and reduces the likelihood of persistent infection. The argument for routine use of antimicrobial agents in otitis media is strengthened by the rare but potentially fatal complications of untreated otitis media. In the preantibiotic era, approximately 3% of cases of otitis media were associated with intracranial complications, including mastoiditis, meningitis, brain abscess, and lateral sinus thrombosis. Since the availability of antimicrobial therapy, the incidence of intracranial complications has decreased to approximately 0.15%. Because of the potential for complications, in the U.S. watchful waiting is not generally recommended. In Europe, the use of therapeutic tympanocentesis as an alternative to antibiotics is more commonly practiced.

Blumer JL: Fundamental basis for rational therapies in acute otitis media. Pediatr Infect Dis J 18:1130-1140, 1999.

252. How should infants with otitis media be managed?

With infants 0-8 weeks, the main concern is whether a localized infection (i.e., otitis media) has disseminated and become systemic. Controversial issues include the extent of work-up (e.g., lumbar puncture) and need for hospitalization. Serious bacterial infection is infrequently associated with isolated otitis media in non-toxic appearing infants between the ages of 2-8 weeks. Some experts argue that outpatient management is appropriate. Febrile infants should have a more extensive laboratory evaluation. Clinical practice varies regarding the inpatient versus outpatient management of those infants with essentially normal blood, urine and CSF tests. This variation is in large part due to the decreased reliability of clinical observation in infants less than two months of age.

Nozicka CA, et al: Otitis media in infants aged 0-8 weeks: Frequency of associated serious bacterial disease. Pediatr Emerg Care 15:252-254, 1999.

253. Following an acute episode of otitis media, how long does the middle ear effusion persist?

Approximately 70% of patients will continue to have an effusion at 2 weeks, 40% at 1 month, 20% at 2 months, and 5–10% at 3 months.

254. What are the most common viral and bacterial agents that cause otitis media?

Tympanocentesis yields positive bacterial cultures in 65–90% of cases of acute otitis media. Virus or viral antigen is detected from middle ear fluid in 10–25% of cases. The significance of virus in middle ear fluid is debated, though it seems clear that antecedent viral infection is an important factor in the pathogenesis of otitis media and that concomitant viral infection may prolong the course of bacterial otitis media and lead to treatment failures.

Common Bacteria and Viruses Identified in Middle Ear Fluid

BACTERIAL ISOLATES		VIRAL ISOLATES	
Streptococcus pneumoniae	43%	Respiratory syncytial virus	7%
Moraxella catarrhalis	21%	Rhinovirus	3%
Haemophilus influenzae	18%	Influenza virus	2%
Streptococcus pyogenes	4%	Adenovirus	2%
Other	4%	Parainfluenza virus	2%

Viruses are the percent of total aspirates.

Adapted from Ruuskanen O, et al: Viruses in acute otitis media: Increasing evidence for clinical significance. Pediatr Infect Dis J 10:425–427, 1991.

Heikkinen T, et al: Increasing importance of viruses in acute otitis media. Ann Med 32:157-163, 2000.

255. What percentage of otitis media is caused by penicillin-resistant organisms?

In some areas, up to 40% of *S. pneumoniae* has some degree of ampicillin resistance because of alterations in penicillin-binding proteins. In addition, approximately 30% of *Haemophilus influenzae* isolates and over 80% of *Moraxella catarrhalis* isolates produce β-lactamase. Given the prevalence of *H. influenzae* and *M. catarrhalis* as additional causes of otitis media, roughly 20%-30% of all cases will have relative resistant to amoxicillin. Many authorities have recommended that amoxicillin be given at higher doses (70-90 mg/kg/day), particularly in children who have received antibiotic therapy in the previous three months.

McCracken GH: Prescribing antimicrobial agents for treatment of otitis media. Pediatr Infect Dis J 18:1141-1146, 1999.

Bradley JS: Oral versus intramuscular antibiotic therapy for acute otitis media: Which is best? Pediatr Infect Dis J 18:1147-1151, 1999.

256. Among patients with otitis media, what are the indications for tympanocentesis?

- A "toxic" appearing child
- An unsatisfactory response to antibiotics
- A suppurative complication
- Underlying immunosuppression
- Some experts would consider tympanocentesis in newborn infants with otitis media because the spectrum of potential pathogens may be broader than in an older child.

257. When is operative intervention indicated in children with mastoiditis?

Most children with mastoiditis will need a conduit to facilitate drainage of pus. The surgical approach to establishing such a conduit may be as simple as a tympanostomy tube. Posterior auricular fluctuance should be drained by incision and drainage, which should be undertaken urgently if signs of neurologic involvement are detected.

258. What are the immediate and long-term complications of otitis media?

The most dangerous immediate complications of acute otitis media involve local suppurative spread to structures within the temporal bone and beyond into other compartments of the cranial vault. Examples of such complications include mastoiditis, labyrinthitis, facial nerve paralysis, osteomyelitis, epidural abscess, lateral sinus thrombosis, otic hydrocephalus, meningitis, and brain abscess. Fortunately, in the antibiotic era, these complications have become rare. Other complications include perforation of the tympanic membrane, tympanosclerosis, fixation of the ossicles, cholesteatoma, chronic otitis media, and hearing loss. There is evidence that repeated bouts of otitis media may have adverse effects on speech development, language acquisition, and cognitive abilities.

259. When should prophylactic antibiotics be considered in children with recurrent otitis media?

Several studies have demonstrated that chronic use of an oral antimicrobial agent can marginally decrease the incidence of recurrent otitis media. Amoxicillin (20 mg/kg once daily) and sulfisoxazole have been studied most thoroughly, though trimethoprim-sulfamethoxasole and erythromycin have also been found to be effective.

In an effort to control the use of antibiotics and minimize selection for resistant organisms, antibiotic prophylaxis should be reserved for patients with 3 or more distinct and well-documented episodes per 6 months or 4 or more episodes per 12 months. When initiated, the duration of prophylactic therapy should be no more than 6 months.

Dowell SF, et al.: Otitis media—principles of judicious use of antimicrobial agents. Pediatrics 101:165-171, 1998.

260. What are the indications for tympanostomy tubes?

Tympanostomy tubes are most commonly inserted for the treatment of otitis media with effusion (OME) or for prophylaxis against recurrent otitis media. OME, also known as serous otitis media, secretory otitis media, or "glue ear," is defined as the presence of fluid in the middle ear in the absence of acute inflammation. It is felt to be a sequela of acute otitis media and is the most common cause of hearing deficit in children. A child with fluid persisting in both middle ears ≥ 3 months should undergo hearing evaluation. If significant hearing impairment is detected, placement of tympanostomy tubes should be considered, although prompt placement does not appear to improve developmental outcome at age 3 years. Tympanostomy tubes have been shown to improve hearing during the initial 6 months after the procedure. On the other hand, benefits are less marked beyond 6 months, partially due to extrusion of the tubes.

For patients with recurrent otitis media, the benefit of tube placement is modest and must be weighed against the risk of complications, which include sclerosis, retraction, and atrophy of the eardrum. Therefore, in the child with recurrent otitis media or secretory otitis media, a trial of long-term antimicrobial therapy appears justified. If this therapy is ineffective, then tympanostomy tube placement is a reasonable option.

Paradise JL, et al.: Effect of early or delayed insertion of tympanostomy tubes for persistent otitis media on developmental outcomes at the age of three years. N Engl J Med 344:1179-1187, 2001.

Otitis Media Guideline Panel: Managing otitis media with effusion in young children. Pediatrics 94:766–772, 1994.

261. Should a child with tympanostomy tubes be allowed to swim?

Otolaryngologists differ widely in their guidance to parents about issues of swimming and bathing. Controlled studies have shown that the rate of otorrhea is similar between non-swimmers (15%) and surface swimmers without earplugs (20%). If diving or underwater swimming is planned, fitted earplugs are recommended. Bath water with shampooing can cause inflammatory changes in the middle ear, and thus earplugs should be used if head dunking is anticipated during bathing. An *in vitro* study (using a head model) found water entry greatest with submersion in soapy water and with deeper swimming.

Hebert RL II, et al: Tympanostomy tubes and water exposure: A practical model. Arch Otolaryngol Head Neck Surg 124:1118-1121, 1998.

Isaacson G, Rosenfeld RM: Care of the child with tympanostomy tubes: A visual guide for the pediatrician. Pediatrics 93:924–929, 1994.

262. Is the pneumococcal vaccine useful for prevention of otitis media?

As *Streptococcus pneumoniae* is the most common bacterial cause of OM, the introduction of the heptavalent vaccine for younger children had been hoped to substantially decrease the incidence of otitis media. Studies have shown positive, but small benefits, including a 7% overall decrease in the number of episodes of acute otitis media (including pneumococcal and non-pneumococcal), a 9% decrease in the incidence of frequent otitis media, and a 20% decrease in the placement of tympanostomy tubes.

Black S, et al: Efficacy, safety, and immunogenicity of heptavalent pneumococcal conjugate vaccine in children. Pediatr Infect Dis J 1:187-95, 2000.

263. A child with the acute onset of ear pain and double vision likely has what condition?

Gradenigo syndrome is an acquired paralysis of the abducens muscle with pain in the area served by the ipsilateral trigeminal nerve. It is caused by inflammation of the sixth cranial nerve in the petrous portion with involvement of the gasserian ganglion. The inflammation is usually due to infection from otitis media or mastoiditis. Symptoms may include weakness of lateral gaze on the affected side, double vision, pain, photophobia, tearing, and hyperesthesia.

PHARYNGEAL/LARYNGEAL INFECTIONS

264. Can group A streptococcal pharyngitis be diagnosed clinically?

Streptococcal pharyngitis is a disease with variable clinical manifestations. Clues suggesting streptococcal disease include the abrupt onset of headache, fever, and sore throat with subsequent development of tender cervical lymphadenopathy, tonsillar exudate, and palatal petechiae. The presence of concurrent conjunctivitis, rhinitis, or cough suggests a viral process. The physical findings are by no means diagnostic. Even the most skilled clinician cannot exceed an accuracy rate of about 75%. A throat culture or a rapid antigen test is essential for confirming streptococcal infection.

265. What is the rationale for treatment of group A streptococcal pharyngitis?

- To prevent acute rheumatic fever. Even with the low incidence of acute rheumatic fever in the United States, it is still prevalent in much of the world.
- To shorten the course of the illness, including headache, sore throat, and lymph node tenderness.
- To reduce the spread of infection and prevent suppurative complications.
- Some cases of acute glomerulonephritis may also be prevented.

266. Should patients with group A streptococcal pharyngitis have a post-treatment throat culture?

In general, repeated courses of antibiotics are not indicated for patients who become asymptomatic but whose throat cultures remain positive for group A streptococci after appropriate antibiotic therapy. Accordingly, post-treatment throat cultures are of little value. Exceptions include individuals with a history of rheumatic fever and patients who have family members with rheumatic heart disease.

Dajani A, et al: Treatment of acute streptococcal pharyngitis and prevention of rheumatic fever: A statement for health professionals. Pediatrics 96:758–764, 1995.

267. How does one differentiate a patient with a sore throat who is a streptococcal carrier with an intercurrent viral pharyngitis from one who is having repeated episodes of group A streptococcal pharyngitis?

Streptococcal carrier:

- Signs and symptoms of viral infection (rhinorrhea, cough, conjunctivitis, diarrhea)
- Little clinical response to antibiotics (sometimes difficult to assess because of self-resolving nature of viral infections)
- Group A streptococcus present on cultures between episodes
- No serologic response to infection (i.e., anti-streptolysin O, anti-DNase B)
- Same serotype of group A streptococcus in sequential cultures

Recurrent group A streptococcal pharyngitis:

- Signs and symptoms consistent with group A streptococcal infection
- Marked clinical response to antibiotics
- No group A streptococcus on cultures between episodes
- Positive serologic response to infection
- Different serotypes of group A streptococcus on sequential cultures

Pichichero ME, et al: Incidence of streptococcal carriers in private practice medicine. Arch Pediatr Adolesc Med 153:624-628, 1999.

Gerber MA: Treatment failures and carriers: Perception or problems? Pediatr Infect Dis J 13:576–579, 1994.

268. What are the acceptable alternative therapies for group A streptococcal pharyngitis?

Penicillin V is the drug of choice for group A streptococcal pharyngitis, except in penicillin-allergic individuals. Of note, there are no documented reports of group A streptococci that are resistant to penicillin. The dose is 250 mg 2 to 3 times per day for 10 days for children and 500 mg 2 to 3 times per day for 10 days for adolescents and adults. Intramuscular benzathine penicillin or Bicillin (a mixture of benzathine penicillin and procaine penicillin) is an alternative and has the advantage of guaranteed compliance but the disadvantage of associated pain. A single daily dose of amoxicillin for 10 days is also effective. For patients with allergy to pencillin, erythromycin has been used most widely, but clarithromycin for 10 days and azithromycin for 5 days are appropriate as well. Narrow spectrum cephalosporins and clindamycin represent additional options. Tetracyclines, sulfasoxizole, and trimethoprim-sulfamethoxazole should not be used, as many strains of group A sreptococcus are resistant to tetracyclines, and sulfonamides fail to eradicate group A streptococci from the pharynx.

269. When can children treated for positive streptococcal throat cultures return to school or daycare?

Although clinical improvement often occurs promptly, most patients remain culture-positive at 14 hours after initiating antibiotics. However, by 24 hours nearly all patients are culture-negative. To minimize contagion, children should receive a full 24 hours of antibiotic therapy.

Snellman LW, et al: Throat cultures for group A streptococci. Pediatrics 91:1166–1170, 1993.

270. Do toddlers less than age 2 years get strep pharyngitis?

Traditonal teaching has been that toddlers rarely develop strep pharyngitis. Recent studies indicate that the incidence of infection and prevalence of carriage is greater than previously thought. In studies of patients less than 2 years with fever and clinical pharyngitis, the range of GABHS positivity was 4-6%. In well children, the carrier rate about 6%. Of note, the rate of rheumatic fever is exceedingly low in children less than age 3 years.

Nussinovitch M, et al: Group A beta-hemolytic streptococcal pharyngitis in preschool children aged 3 months to 5 years. Clin Pediatr 38:357-360, 1999.

Berkovitch M, et al: Group A streptococcal pharyngotonsillitis in children less than 2 years of age—more common than is thought. Clin Pediatr 38:365-366, 1999.

271. How long after the development of streptococcal pharyngitis can treatment be initiated and still effectively prevent rheumatic fever?

Treatment should be started as soon as possible, but little is lost in waiting for throat culture results to establish the diagnosis. Antibiotic treatment prevents acute rheumatic fever even when therapy is initiated as long as 9 days after the onset of the acute illness.

272. What is the difference between herpangina and Ludwig angina?

Herpangina is a common viral infection during the summer and fall and is characterized by posterior pharyngeal, buccal, and palatal vesicles and ulcers. Coxsackieviruses A and B and echoviruses are the most common causative agents. In young children, it is often accompanied by a high fever (103–104°F). Herpangina is distinguished from herpes simplex infections of the mouth, which are more anterior and involve the lips, tongue and gingiva.

Ludwig angina is an acute diffuse infection (usually bacterial) of the submandibular and sublingual spaces with brawny induration of the floor of the mouth and tongue. Airway obstruction can occur. The infections usually follow oral cavity injuries or dental complications (e.g., extractions, impactions).

273. What is quinsy?

Peritonsillar abscess (from Lower Latin for an inflammation of the throat).

274. How is a peritonsillar abscess distinguished from peritonsillar cellulitis?

A peritonsillar abscess is diagnosed when a discrete mass is palpated. The bulging abscess causes displacement of the uvula. Trismus occurs more commonly in the setting of abscess than simple cellulitis, which is characterized by signs of diffuse inflammation only.

275. What x-ray features suggest the diagnosis of a retropharyngeal abscess?

When a patient's neck is extended, a measurement of the prevertebral space exceeding two times the diameter of the C2 vertebra suggests an abscess. Pockets of air in the prevertebral space also suggest abscess. The retropharynx extends to T1 in the superior mediastinum, so empyema or mediastinitis is also possible whenever a retropharyngeal abscess is identified.

276. Which age group is most susceptible to retropharyngeal abscess?

This disease is most common between the ages of 1 and 6 years. There are several small lymph nodes in the retropharynx which usually disappear by age 4 or 5. These lymph nodes drain the posterior nasal passages and nasopharynx, and they may become involved if those sites are infected.

277. What are the indications for removing the tonsils and adenoid?

Paradise and colleagues have written extensively on this subject and divide indications into definite and relative.

Definite

- Tonsillar or adenoidal hypertrophy, causing obstructive apnea, cor pulmonale, or interference with swallowing
- Persistent or recurrent tonsillar hemorrhage
- Malignancy

Relative

- Peritonsillar abscess
- Recurrent documented tonsillitis
- Muffled, "hot potato" vocalizations caused by marked tonsillar hypertrophy
- Halitosis, caused by tonsillar crypt debris unresponsive to gargling
- Chronic otitis media with effusion

Paradise JL: Tonsillectomy and adenoidectomy. In Burg FD, et al (eds): Current Pediatric Therapy, 16th ed. Philadelphia, W.B. Saunders, 1999, pp. 510-512.

278. What is Lemierre disease?

Lemierre disease is another name for post-anginal sepsis, which is caused by *Fusobacterium necrophorum* and is characterized by jugular vein septic thrombophlebitis with metastatic dissemination to the lung and other sites. This disease is most common in adolescents and young adults. It usually begins with exudative pharyngitis, followed by extension to the jugular vein. Typical symptoms and signs include fever and dysphagia along with neck pain, swelling, and stiffness.

279. What is the typical presentation of pharyngitis due to *Arcanobacterium haemolyticum*?

Arcanobacterium haemolyticum has been identified increasingly as a cause of exudative pharyngitis, particularly in adolescents. Classically the infection is associated with an erythematous maculopapular rash on the extremities and trunk. Many isolates are resistant to penicillin, and thus first-line treatment is usually erythromycin or a related macrolide.

280. How should children with epiglottitis be managed?

Acute epiglottitis is a medical emergency, and all children should be assumed to have a critical airway, i.e., capable of imminent occlusion. Because of the risk of airway obstruction upon agitation, the patient should be allowed to remain with parents, free from restraint. Examination should be performed as cautiously as possible. Continuous observation regardless of the setting (e.g., radiology suite), avoidance of supine positioning, and arrangements for admission to an intensive care unit are mandatory. Ideally, the epiglottis is visualized directly in an operating room, and the child is intubated immediately afterward.

Previously, > 90% of cases were caused by *Haemophilus influenzae* type b. However, because of the routine use of Hib vaccines in infants, the incidence of epiglottitis has decreased dramatically, and pneumococci, staphylococci, and streptococci now account for a relatively large percentage of cases.

281. How is epiglottitis distinguished clinically from croup?

Clinical Distinctions Between Group and Epiglottitis

GROUP	EPIGLOTTITIS
Age	
Younger (6 mos–3 yrs)	Older (3–7 yrs)
Onset of stridor	
Gradual (24–72 hrs)	Rapid (8–12 hrs)
Symptoms	
Prodromal URI	Minimal rhinitis
Harsh, brassy cough	Little coughing
Hoarseness	Muffled voice
Slightly sore throat	Pain in throat
Signs	
Mild fever	High fever (> 39° C)
Not toxic	Toxic appearance

Variable distress	Severe distress; sits upright; may drool
Harsh inspiratory stridor	Low-pitched inspiratory stridor
Expiratory sounds uncommon	May have a low-pitched expiratory sound
Radiology	
Subglottic narrowing	Edema of epiglottis and aryepiglottic folds (positive "thumb" sign)

282. What are the criteria for admission of a child with viral croup?

- *Clinical signs of impending respiratory failure*: marked retractions, depressed level of consciousness, cyanosis, hypotonicity, and diminished or absent inspiratory breath sounds
- *Laboratory signs of impending respiratory failure*: $PCO_2 > 45$ mm Hg, $PaO_2 < 70$ mmHg in room air
- *Clinical signs of dehydration*
- *Social considerations*: unreliable parents, excessive distance from hospital
- *Historic considerations*: high-risk infant with history of subglottic stenosis, prior intubations

283. Are steroids efficacious in croup?

The use of corticosteroids (including oral and intramuscular dexamethasone and nebulized budesonide) has been shown to be beneficial in patients hospitalized for croup. In particular, corticosteroid treatment reduces the incidence of intubation and results in more rapid respiratory improvement. In addition, among patients with mild or moderate croup, corticosteroids appear to reduce the use of nebulized racemic epinephrine and the need for hospitalization. At present the most common dose of dexamethasone is 0.6 mg/kg, but lower doses are under study. The dose of budesonide is 2-4 mg.

Ausejo M, et al: The effectiveness of glucocorticoids in treating croup: Meta-analysis. BMJ 319:595-600, 1999.

Johnson DW, et al: A comparison of nebulized budesonide, intramuscular dexamethasone, and placebo for moderately severe croup. N Engl J Med 339:498-503, 1998.

284. If a child has received racemic epinephrine as a treatment for croup, is hospitalization required?

In earlier days, children treated with racemic epinephrine were routinely hospitalized to observe for potential rebound mucosal edema and airway obstruction, regardless of how they appeared clinically. However, a number of recent studies have shown that children who are free of significant stridor or retractions at rest 2-3 hours after the administration of racemic epinephrine can be safely discharged, provided adequate follow-up is assured. Of note, in most of these studies oral or IM dexamethasone (0.6 mg/kg) was also administered.

Rizos JD, et al: The disposition of children with croup treated with racemic epinephrine and dexamethasone in the emergency department. J Emerg Med 16:535-539, 1998.

Ledwith CA, et al: Safety and efficacy of nebulized racemic epinephrine in conjunction with oral dexamethasone and mist in the outpatient treatment of croup. Ann Emerg Med 25:331–337, 1995.

285. Is a cool mist vaporizer truly of benefit in croup?

The usual advice for home management of croup includes the use of a cool mist vaporizer. The theory is that the coolness serves as a vasoconstrictor and that the mist serves to thin respiratory secretions. Interestingly, this therapy remains time-honored but is largely unproven. One small study found no differences between control and mist-treated infants. The calming effects of being held by a parent during the mist treatment may have greater impact.

Bourchier D, et al: Humidification in viral croup: A controlled trial. Aust Paediatr J 20:289, 1984.

286. What is meant by pseudomembranous croup?

"Pseudomembranous croup" is an old term that was used for what is now referred to as bacterial tracheitis. (Of note, "membranous croup" is the historical term for diphtheria.)

Bacterial tracheitis is usually caused by *Staphylococcus aureus* and occurs following trauma to the neck or trachea or after a viral respiratory tract infection such as croup. The presentation is similar to that of severe croup or epiglottitis. As a consequence, a lateral neck film is often obtained to rule out epiglottitis and sometimes reveals narrowing of the trachea due to a thick, purulent exudate which can extend into both mainstem bronchi.

287. What is spasmodic croup?

Spasmodic croup is a poorly understood cause of recurrent stridor in young children (usually 1–3 years old) and resembles acute infectious laryngotracheobronchitis in many respects. However, unlike infectious croup, a prodrome of upper respiratory symptoms is usually absent, and the patient is usually afebrile. The onset is sudden, typically at night, with inspiratory stridor and a brassy cough that responds to therapies used for infectious croup (e.g., cool mist, racemic epinephrine, corticosteroids). Recurrence is common. The pathogenesis is unclear, but an allergic and hypersensitivity component is suspected. In the rare patient who requires intubation, the typical finding is the pale and boggy mucosa of allergy and not the inflamed swelling of a primary infection.

SINUSITIS

288. When do the sinuses develop during childhood?

The maxillary and ethmoid sinuses are present at birth. Pneumatization of the sphenoid sinuses begins at approximately 2–3 years of age and is usually complete by about age 6. Frontal sinus pneumatization varies considerably, beginning around 3–7 years of age and finishing by age 12.

289. What percentage of teenagers do not have frontal sinuses when x-rays are obtained?

Frontal sinus pneumatization is absent in approximately ***10%*** of the normal population.

290. List the predisposing factors for development of chronic sinusitis.

Allergic rhinitis, *anatomic abnormalities* (e.g., polyps, enlarged adenoids), *impairment of mucociliary clearance* (e.g., cystic fibrosis, primary ciliary dyskinesia), *foreign bodies* (e.g., nasogastric tube), and *abnormalities in immune defense* all predispose to chronic sinusitis.

291. Does a thick, green nasal discharge on day two of a respiratory illness indicate a bacterial sinus infection?

Absolutely not. The character of nasal secretions (e.g., purulent, discolored, tenacious) does not distinguish viral from bacterial. Treatment of early (<7–10 days) of purulent nasal discharge is a common cause of antibiotic overuse.

O'Brien KL, et al: Acute sinusitis—Principles of judicious use of antimicrobial agents. Pediatrics 101:14-17, 1998.

292. Is transillumination helpful in diagnosing sinusitis in children?

In general, transillumination of the sinuses is of very limited value in the diagnosis of acute sinusitis in young children.

293. What is the role of plain radiographs in the diagnosis of sinusitis?

Acute sinusitis usually presents in one of two ways, either with acute onset of fever >39° C and purulent nasal discharge or with prolonged nasal discharge and cough continuing without improvement for longer than 10 days. Most clinicians treat suspected acute sinusitis empirically, without performing imaging studies. Although plain radiographs are easy to obtain and are relatively inexpensive, they lack sensitivity in diagnosing sinusitis. In addition, they lack specificity, especially in children without clinical symptoms of sinusitis.

294. Which radiographic views are potentially useful in evaluating sinusitis?

In children younger than age 6, only the maxillary and ethmoid sinuses are clinically important, and 80% of children in this age group with acute sinusitis will have both sets of sinuses involved. Caldwell (anteroposterior) and Waters (occipitomental) views are necessary to assess these sinuses. To evaluate the frontal and sphenoid sinuses in older children, a lateral view is most informative.

295. What constitutes an abnormal sinus x-ray?

- Complete opacification of a sinus cavity
- Mucosal thickening of at least 4 mm
- Presence of an air-fluid level

While these findings are not specific for sinusitis, they are helpful in confirming a diagnosis of acute sinusitis in patients with suggestive signs and symptoms (i.e., nasal discharge and cough persisting for > 10 days without improvement or high fever and purulent nasal discharge for > 3 days).

296. When should CT scans be considered in diagnosing sinusitis?

In most cases, a sinus CT scan is unnecessary. CT scans are more sensitive than sinus x-rays but also suffer from a lack of specificity. Scenarios that might warrant use of CT include:

- Complicated sinus disease with either orbital or CNS abnormalities
- Multiple recurrences
- Prolonged symptoms unresponsive to treatment, suggesting possible anatomic abnormalities and raising sinus surgery as a consideration

Wald ER: Sinusitis. Ped Annal 27:811-818, 1998.

297. Which organisms are responsible for acute and chronic sinusitis in the pediatric age group?

In acute, uncomplicated sinusitis, the etiologic organisms closely parallel those associated with acute otitis media: *Streptococcus pneumoniae*, *Haemophilus influenzae*, and *Moraxella catarrhalis*. In patients with chronic sinusitis, the most common pathogens remain *S. pneumoniae*, *H. influenzae*, and *M. catarrhalis*, along with *S. aureus* and anaerobes. Mucormycosis is an important concern in immunosuppressed patients, and *Pseudomonas* must always be considered in patients with cystic fibrosis.

298. For how long should sinus infections be treated?

The duration of therapy for acute sinusitis in children has not been studied systematically. However, for patients whose symptoms improve dramatically within 3-4 days of initiating treatment, a 10-day course of therapy is usually effective. For patients who respond more slowly to antibiotics, treatment until symptoms resolve plus another 7 days is reasonable.

TUBERCULOSIS

299. Who should be screened for tuberculosis?

Previously, routine periodic screening with multiple puncture tests (tine tests) was a norm for the entire population of children. However, routine screening of low-risk children in low-prevalence areas is no longer advised. Current recommendations are as follows:

Children who should be tested immediately:

- Contacts of persons with confirmed or suspected infectious TB
- Children with radiographic or clinical findings suggestive of TB

- Children immigrating from endemic countries
- Children with a history of travel to endemic countries

Children who should be tested annually:

- Children with HIV or living in a household with an HIV-infected person
- Incarcerated adolescents

Children who should be tested every 2-3 years:

- Children exposed to the following groups: HIV-infected, homeless, nursing home residents, institutionalized adolescents or adults, illicit drug users, migrant farm workers

Children who should be considered for testing at 4-6 and 11-16 years of age:

- Children whose parents immigrated from endemic regions of the world
- Children residing in high-prevalence areas

American Academy of Pediatrics. Tuberculosis. In: Pickering LK (ed): 2000 Red Book: Report of the Committee on Infectious Diseases. Elk Grove Village, IL: American Academy of Pediatrics, 2000, p. 597.

300. When are the various strengths of PPD used?

The standard strength PPD (Mantoux test) contains 5 tuberculin units (TU) of purified protein derivative and is designated intermediate strength. This preparation is used for routine skin test screening. PPD is also available in 1-TU and 250-TU strengths, but these preparations are not generally recommended.

301. How is the Mantoux (PPD) test interpreted in children?

The Mantoux test is interpreted in the context of clinical signs and symptoms and epidemiologic risk factors (e.g., known exposure). Positive tests are defined as follows:

Reaction ≥ 5 mm:

- Children in close contact with confirmed or suspected cases of TB
- Children with radiographic or clinical evidence of TB disease
- Children receiving immunosuppressive therapy
- Children with immunodeficiency disorders, including HIV infection

Reaction ≥ 10 mm:

- Children younger than 4 years of age
- Children with diabetes mellitus, chronic renal failure, malnutrition, or other chronic conditions
- Children born in high-prevalence regions of the world, whose parents were born in such areas, or who have traveled to such areas
- Children frequently exposed to adults who are HIV-infected, homeless, incarcerated, illicit drug users, or migrant farm workers

Reaction ≥ 15 mm:

- Children over 4 years of age with no risk factors

American Academy of Pediatrics. Tuberculosis. In: Pickering LK (ed): 2000 Red Book, 25th ed. Elk Grove Village, IL, American Academy of Pediatrics, 2000, p. 594.

302. What are the reasons for false-negative skin testing with PPD?

- Testing during incubation period (2–10 weeks)
- Problems with administration technique
- Severe systemic TB infection (miliary or meningitis)
- Immunosuppression, malnutrition, or immunodeficiency
- Concurrent infection: measles, varicella, HIV, Epstein-Barr virus, *Mycoplasma*, mumps, rubella
- Recent measles immunization

From Callahan CW: Tuberculosis. In: Schidlow DV, Smith DS (eds): A Practical Guide to Pediatric Respiratory Diseases. Philadelphia, Hanley & Belfus, 1994, p 107; with permission.

303. Why is a multiple puncture test (tine test) not considered an ideal test for tuberculosis?

- The exact dose of antigen (either PPD or old tuberculin) cannot be standardized, and thus interpretation is difficult. As a result, any positive test must be confirmed with a Mantoux test.
- In a patient with a positive tine test, the need for follow-up Mantoux test can lead to a booster phenomenon if the patient has had a previous BCG vaccine or infection with nontuberculous mycobacteria, again making interpretation difficult.
- Significant variability exists in false-negative and especially false-positive rates.
- The use of tine tests has a tendency to result in parental reporting, which can be very unreliable.

Starke JR, Correa AG: Management of mycobacterial infection and disease. Pediatr Infect Dis J 14:455–470, 1995.

304. How should patients with a positive tuberculin test be evaluated?

History should search for clues suggestive of active infection, such as recurrent fevers, weight loss, adenopathy, or cough. A history of recurrent infections, either in the patient or a family member, may be suggestive of HIV infection, a risk factor for infection with *Mycobacterium tuberculosis*. Information from previous tuberculin skin testing is invaluable. Epidemiologic information includes an evaluation of possible exposure to TB. A family history is obtained, including questions pertaining to chronic cough or weight loss in a family member or other contact. Travel history and current living arrangements should be elucidated. If the patient has immigrated to North America, a history of BCG vaccination should be ascertained.

Physical exam should focus on pulmonary, lymphatic, and abdominal systems. Examination should corroborate a history of BCG vaccination.

Laboratory evaluation, including a chest x-ray with a lateral film, is the next stage. Family members and close contacts should undergo skin testing. In certain circumstances, chest x-rays should be performed on the child's contacts.

If there are no clinical or radiographic features suggestive of active TB, then no further evaluation is warranted, and the child is treated as having asymptomatic infection with *M. tuberculosis*. A single antituberculous agent (e.g., isoniazid) is prescribed for 9 months duration. If any of the preceding evaluation suggests active infection, sputum, gastric aspirates, urine, and other appropriate specimens (such as lymph node tissue) should be obtained for mycobacterial culture and Ziehl-Neelsen or auramine-rhodamine staining. The child should be treated with combined antituberculous medications while awaiting culture results, and an aggressive search for the source of the child's infection should be initiated.

305. In a younger child suspected of having tuberculosis, how should gastric aspirates be obtained?

Because younger children rarely produce sputum, gastric aspirates are a better source for culture of mycobacteria. They yield the organism in up to 40% of cases. The aspirate should be obtained early in the morning as the child awakens to sample overnight accumulation of respiratory secretions. The sample should be collected in a saline-free fluid, and the pH should be neutralized if any delay in processing is anticipated.

306. How are children with active tuberculosis treated?

Recommendations for the treatment of active TB in children have evolved over the past several years. Previously, at least 9 months of therapy were suggested for uncomplicated pulmonary disease. Studies in adults and children have demonstrated that 6 months of combined antituberculous therapy (short-course therapy) is as effective as 9-month therapy.

To date, the combined results of nine studies in pediatric patients have demonstrated the efficacy of 6-month therapy to be > 95%.

The current standard regimen for active pulmonary TB in children consists of 2 months of daily isoniazid, rifampin, and pyrazinamide, followed by 4 months of isoniazid and rifampin (daily or twice weekly). If drug resistance is a concern, either ethambutol or streptomycin is added to the initial 3-drug regimen until drug susceptibilities are determined. Meningitis, disseminated disease, and bone or joint infections are treated for 2 months with isoniazid, rifampin, pyrazinamide, and streptomycin once daily, followed by 7-10 months of isoniazid and rifampin (daily or twice weekly).

307. Why are multiple antibiotics used in treating tuberculosis?

Two features of *Mycobacterium tuberculosis* make the organism difficult to eradicate once infection has been established. First, mycobacteria replicate slowly and may remain dormant for prolonged periods, but are susceptible to drugs only during active replication. Second, drug-resistant organisms exist naturally within a large population, even prior to the initiation of therapy. These features render the organism, when present in significant numbers, extremely difficult to eradicate with a single agent. Indeed, the ability to cure patients with asymptomatic infection with a single agent is based on the presence of a small number of organisms that are exposed to a bactericidal antibiotic for an extended period of time.

308. What are the side effects of rifampin?

Rifampin commonly causes an orange discoloration of tears and urine. Contact lenses may be permanently discolored or destroyed. Less common adverse effects include allergic or hypersensitivity reactions, hepatotoxicity, and a flu-like syndrome that occurs particularly with intermittent administration. Hepatotoxicity is unusual in previously healthy children. Adolescent and adult patients should be warned that rifampin may decrease the efficacy of oral contraceptives and may antagonize the effects of oral anticoagulants.

309. Why is pyridoxine supplementation given to patients who are receiving isoniazid?

Isoniazid interferes with pyridoxine metabolism and may result in peripheral neuritis or convulsions. Administration of pyridoxine is generally not necessary for children who have a normal diet, as they have adequate stores of this vitamin. Children and adolescents with diets deficient in milk or meat, breast-fed infants, and pregnant women should receive pyridoxine supplementation during isoniazid therapy.

310. How effective is BCG vaccination?

The bacille Calmette-Guérin (BCG) vaccines are among the most widely used in the world at present and are also perhaps the most controversial. The difficulties stem from the marked variation in reported efficacy of BCG against *Mycobacterium tuberculosis* and *M. leprae* infections. Depending on the population studied, efficacy against tuberculosis has ranged from 0–80%. Similarly, the efficacy against leprosy has ranged from 20–60% in prospective trials.

The vaccines were derived from a strain of *M. bovis* in 1906 and were subsequently dispersed to several laboratories around the world, where they were propagated under non-standardized conditions. Hence, the vaccines in use today cannot be considered homogeneous. This may explain the observed variation in efficacy.

311. Is there any indication for BCG use in the United States?

BCG is rarely used in the United States. It is given primarily to tuberculin-negative individuals who are in close contact with active cases of untreated or ineffectively-treated pulmonary tuberculosis. It may be considered for groups with an excessive rate of new infections or when the usual methods of treatment have failed or are not feasible. BCG is a live vaccine and should not be used in individuals with abnormal immunity (e.g., those with HIV, with primary immunodeficiency, or undergoing chemotherapy).

312. How do you tell the difference between the scar from smallpox vaccination and the scar of BCG vaccination?

The scar due to BCG vaccination is a round, slightly depressed area with irregular edges, 4–7 mm in diameter. Occasionally it is raised. The scar resulting from smallpox vaccination is often irregular in shape, larger, and less likely to be associated with keloid formation.

Fine PEM, et al: The distribution and implications of BCG scars in northern Malawi. Bull WHO 67:35–42, 1989.

313. How does BCG immunization influence tuberculosis skin testing?

Generally, interpretation of PPD tests is the same in BCG recipients as it is in nonvaccinated children. If positive, consideration should be given to several factors in deciding who should receive antituberculous therapy. These factors include time since BCG immunization, number of doses received, prevalence of TB in the country of origin, contacts in the United States, and radiographic findings.

314. Why do children with tuberculosis rarely infect other children?

TB is transmitted via infected droplets of mucus that become airborne when an individual coughs or sneezes. Compared with adults, children with TB have several factors that minimize their contagiousness:

- Low density of organisms in sputum
- Lack of cavitation or extensive infiltrates on chest x-ray
- Lower frequency of cough
- Lower volume and higher viscosity of sputum
- Shorter duration of respiratory symptoms

Starke JR: Childhood tuberculosis during the 1990s. Pediatr Rev 13:343–353, 1992.

315. In addition to tuberculosis, what other airborne microbes can cause respiratory disease?

Airborne Microbial Diseases

DISEASE	AIRBORNE SOURCE
Aspergillosis	Conidiaspores from decaying vegetation and soil
Brucellosis	Aerosolized from carcasses of domestic and wild animals
Chickenpox	Aerosolized from respiratory secretions
Coccidioidomycosis	Arthroconidia from soil and dust
Cryptococcosis	Aerosolized from bird droppings
Histoplasmosis	Conidiaspores from bat or bird droppings
Legionnaire disease	Aerosolized contaminated water, especially air-conditioning cooling towers
Measles	Aerosolized respiratory secretions
Mucormycosis	Spores from soil
Psittacosis	*Chlamydia psittaci* from birds
Q fever	*Coxiella burnetii* from a variety of farm and other animals
Tularemia	Aerosolized from multiple wild animals, especially rabbits
Viral Nasopharyngitis, bronchiolitis, pneumonia	Aerosolized respiratory secretions

12. METABOLISM

Gerard T. Berry, M.D., and Mark Yudkoff, M.D.

AMINO ACID DISORDERS

1. What is the risk to the fetus of a mother known to have phenylketonuria (PKU)?

Hyperphenylalaninemia during pregnancy can result in a variety of fetal malformations and long-term sequelae, including microcephaly, mental retardation, growth retardation, cardiac defects, and skeletal malformations. The risk of injury to a fetus increases with the maternal phenylalanine level. For mothers with classic PKU who are not on a phenylalanine-restricted diet, the risk of significant fetal injury is essentially 100%. For untreated mothers with milder variants of PKU (blood phenylalanine levels of 10–20 mg/dl), the risk is 10–20%.

2. Why is vitamin C given to newborn premature infants with a positive PKU test?

The most common cause of an abnormal PKU blood screening test in premature infants is hyperphenylalaninemia secondary to transient tyrosinemia of the newborn. Transient tyrosinemia appears to be caused by inadequate activity of *p*-hydroxyphenylpyruvic acid dioxygenase, a vitamin-C-dependent enzyme in the tyrosine degradative pathway. Administration of vitamin C increases the activity of the enzyme and facilitates metabolism of both tyrosine and its precursor, phenylalanine.

3. What are the varieties of hyperphenylalaninemia?

Types of Hyperphenylalaninemia

DISORDER	BLOOD PHENYLALANINE LEVEL (MG/DL)	ENZYME DEFECT	THERAPY
Classic phenylketonuria	> 20	Phenylalanine hydroxylase	Diet
Atypical phenylketonuria	12-20	Phenylalanine hydroxylase	Diet
Persistent mild hyperphenylketonuria	2-12	Phenylalanine hydroxylase	Diet
Transient hyperphenylalaninemia	2-20	4α- carbinolamine dehydratase + unknown	None
Transient tyrosinemia	2-12	? *p*-OH-phenylpyruvic acid dioxygenase deficiency ? Secondary to low vitamin C	Vitamin C, low-protein formula
Dihydropteridine reductase deficiency	12-20	Dihydropteridine reductase	Dopa, OH-tryptophan, tetrahydrobiopterin
Biopterin synthesis defects	12-20	Dihydrobiopterin synthetase, GTP-cyclohydrase, 6-pyruvoyl tetrahydrobiopterin synthetase	Dopa, OH-tryptophan, tetrahydrobiopterin

4. Which children with PKU require treatment?

In addition to classic PKU, for which blood phenylalanine levels typically are > 20 mg/dl with unrestricted protein intake, several variant forms of PKU also have blood levels of phenylalanine that are persistently elevated above the normal range (< 2 mg/dl). Long-term follow-up studies indicate that phenylalanine levels > 10 mg/dl require some limitation of dietary phenylalanine intake. Diet therapy probably must be maintained throughout life.

5. What is the outcome for children with PKU treated in early infancy?

Theoretically, all complications of classical PKU can be prevented by (1) limitation of dietary phenylalanine to only the amount required for growth and (2) provision of adequate dietary tyrosine, which cannot be synthesized from phenylalanine by phenylalanine hydroxylase. The mean IQ of children who are treated from birth is only slightly lower than those of their unaffected siblings. Increasingly severe cerebral injury occurs when institution of dietary treatment is delayed after birth or if the diet is poorly managed after diagnosis.

6. What is the clinical significance of transient tyrosinemia in the newborn infant?

Neonates (especially premature infants) with transient tyrosinemia may be more lethargic than normal infants and may feed poorly. Controversy remains about the long-term significance of transient tyrosinemia and whether treatment with vitamin C and/or protein restriction is required. Two reports suggest that these infants are at increased risk for mild neurologic and developmental abnormalities during later childhood, but a definitive study has yet to be performed. A bias of ascertainment (i.e., sick premature infants) may explain these findings. Nevertheless, when hypertyrosinemia is found in an infant, a reasonable attempt should be made to restore the tyrosine and phenylalanine levels to normal with vitamin C and/or protein restriction.

7. Describe the characteristic clinical signs of alkaptonuria.

In alkaptonuria, incomplete metabolism of tyrosine and phenylalanine results in an increased concentration of homogentisic acid in blood and urine. Features include:

- Dark urine on exposure to air (e.g., in a diaper)
- Ochronosis (grayish discoloration of connective tissue)
- Degenerative arthritis
- Valvulitis and aortic degeneration

8. What physical findings help differentiate homocystinuria from Marfan syndrome?

CHARACTERISTIC	MARFAN SYNDROME	HOMOCYSTINURIA
Lens dislocation	Upward usually	Downward usually
Cornea, sclera	Flattened, bluish sclera	Normal
Body habitus and skeleton	Tall, arachnodactyly, pectus deformity	Same
Joints	Markedly hyperextensible	Normal or mildly contracted; ankle eversion
Skin	Hyperextensible, striae	Eczema; malar flush; livedo reticularis
Hair	Normal	Thin, dry, reddish
Heart/major vessels	Mitral valve prolapse; regurgitant aortic murmurs; aneurysms and sudden death	Mitral valve prolapse in some cases; aneurysms not typical; strokes frequent
Peripheral vasculature	Varicosities can occur	Diabetic-like peripheral vascular disease
Intelligence	Normal	Mental retardation common (50%); psychiatric disturbances frequent
Inheritance	Autosomal dominant; sibs and one parent often affected	Autosomal recessive; parents unaffected but may be consanguineous
Other	Emphysema, pneumothorax	Hepatomegaly; osteoporosis

9. Why are patients with homocystinuria at risk for thrombotic disease?

Most evidence points to homocysteine-mediated endothelial damage, thereby exposing surfaces that activate platelet aggregation and thrombus formation. By forming disulfide adducts with free cysteine, homocysteine interferes with the formation of essential cysteine–cysteine disulfide bonds in the proteins that are found in the vascular wall and in the suspensory connective tissue of the lens. The functions of many other proteins, such as protein C and coagulation factor VII, are also affected and may contribute to the vascular lesions that often develop in this disease.

10. Explain the difference between cystinuria and cystinosis.

Cystinuria is a defect of renal tubular and (in some cases) intestinal transport of dibasic amino acids (cystine, lysine, arginine, ornithine). The relative insolubility of cystine gives rises to renal stones. Clinical symptoms are limited to those caused by chronic renal lithiasis—recurrent infection, obstruction, renal colic, hypertension, and renal failure. Abnormal growth or other complications attributable to low body cystine or other dibasic amino acid occur rarely, if ever.

Cystinosis is a lysosomal storage disease caused by defective lysosomal transport of cystine. In classic infantile nephropathic cystinosis, most clinical abnormalities are attributable to the renal Fanconi syndrome that is present in almost all affected individuals. The biochemical characteristics are hyperchloremic metabolic acidosis from excessive bicarbonaturia, hypophosphatemia, glucosuria, and generalized aminoaciduria. The presenting clinical problems are growth failure, rickets, photophobia, and pigmentary retinopathy. As the infants grows into childhood, there appears glomerular dysfunction that progresses to renal failure, usually by age 10. Milder "adolescent" and "adult" forms of cystinosis are also known.

11. What entity classically causes the "blue diaper syndrome"?

Blue discoloration of the diaper is caused by ***intestinal malabsorption*** of the ***amino acid tryptophan*** as an apparently isolated defect of intestinal amino acid transport. Malabsorbed tryptophan is converted by colonic bacteria to indican, which causes blue staining of the diaper on exposure to air. Patients with tryptophan malabsorption may develop hypercalciuria, nephrocalcinosis, and failure to thrive. Curiously, patients with Hartnup disease, an inborn error of intestinal and renal transport of all neutral amino acids including tryptophan, do not develop the blue diaper syndrome despite intestinal malabsorption of tryptophan and conversion to indican and other indoles. Blue discoloration of diapers also has several nonmetabolic causes—methylene blue administration, food colorings, amitriptyline or triamterene ingestion, copper poisoning, and *Pseudomonas* urinary tract infections (bluish green).

CARBOHYDRATE DISORDERS

12. Name the three types of galactosemia.

- Galactose-1-phosphate uridyltransferase deficiency (classic galactosemia)
- Galactokinase deficiency
- Uridine diphosphogalactose epimerase deficiency

13. List the most common clinical findings in children with classic galactosemia.

Acute

- Poor feeding and vomiting
- Poor growth
- Jaundice, severe or prolonged; early in course of neonatal-onset disease, unconjugated bilirubin predominates
- Liver dysfunction—coagulopathy and elevated serum transaminases
- Cataracts

- Irritability and lethargy
- *Escherichia coli* sepsis

Chronic

- Developmental disability that may be progressive (below), especially affecting language and intelligence
- Gastrointestinal symptoms following lactose ingestion
- Primary ovarian failure

14. What are the pathogenic mechanisms responsible for the clinical manifestations of galactosemia?

Increased levels of several metabolites of galactose are believed (but, in most cases, not proved) to cause injury:

Galactose-1-phosphate	Renal Fanconi syndrome
	Hepatocellular disease
	Decreased RBC survival leading to indirect hyperbilirubinemia
Galactitol (dulcitol)	Cataracts
	? Pseudotumor cerebri
Unknown	Hypergonadotropic hypogonadism
	Mental retardation or cognitive deficits

15. What is the long-term outcome for children with classic galactosemia treated early in infancy?

Children with classic galactosemia who are treated from birth with galactose-free diets are spared the acute complications of galactosemia. However, ovarian insufficiency, which occurs in most affected females, may be caused by prenatal influences on ovarian development. In a few individuals, significant CNS disease (ataxia, dystonia, tremor) may develop late in childhood and progress despite excellent dietary management. In addition, minor neurologic problems, such as learning disabilities and speech disorders, occur in most patients despite strict observance of a galactose-free diet.

16. What is the earliest metabolic derangement seen in hereditary fructose intolerance?

Hypophosphatemia is the most characteristic metabolic derangement in hereditary fructose intolerance (hepatic aldolase B deficiency). Hypophosphatemia can occur within a few minutes of ingestion of fructose and before clinical symptoms appear and is usually followed by hypertransaminasemia. Somewhat slower in evolution are ***hypoglycemia*** and severe ***gastrointestinal distress***. Rapid hepatic uptake of inorganic phosphate for phosphorylation of fructose is probably the major factor causing the hypophosphatemia, but other factors, such as hyperphosphaturia, may contribute.

17. Does fructose produce any adverse effects?

Ingestion of excessive amounts of fructose in a normal individual can lead to lactic acidosis, hyperuricemia, and dental caries. Individuals with hereditary fructose intolerance who avoid all sources of fructose have a notable lack of dental caries.

18. What is the long-term outcome for children with hereditary fructose intolerance treated in infancy?

Most individuals with hereditary fructose intolerance (many of whom have self-selected a sucrose- and fructose-free diet) have normal health, growth, and intelligence. However, a few individuals under apparently good dietary management develop growth retardation because of sensitivity to very small amounts of fructose in the diet. Others on "fructose-free" diets develop seizures and deafness, but the relationship of these abnormalities to abnormal fructose metabolism or to possible unidentified dietary sources of fructose is uncertain.

19. Name the major natural sources of fructose ("fruit sugar") in the human diet.

- Most fruits and vegetables
- Sucrose (beet or cane sugar) = glucose-fructose disaccharide
- Molasses and many other natural sweeteners
- Processed corn sugar ("high-fructose" corn syrup)
- D-Sorbitol (artificial sweetener, oxidized to fructose in the liver)
- Some medications, especially liquid preparations (from sucrose)

20. What are the characteristic EKG findings in Pompe disease (type II glycogen storage disease)?

Gigantic QRS complexes in all leads coupled with an abnormally short P-R interval.

21. Why do patients with von Gierke (type I glycogen storage) disease develop bleeding tendencies?

A platelet defect, presumably secondary, occurs in many patients with type I glycogen storage disease (glucose-6-phosphatase deficiency). Platelets from these patients show impaired release of ADP in response to collagen and epinephrine. The cause is unknown.

22. In addition to Pompe disease, which glycogen storage diseases affect primarily muscle?

McArdle disease (type V with deficient muscle phosphorylase) and ***Tarui disease*** (type VII with deficient muscle phosphofructokinase). Clinically, they are similar, with increasing fatigue and cramps after exercise. Myoglobinuria may be noted. Since both enzyme deficiencies result in blockage of the glycolytic pathway, lactate will not rise after exercise as is normal. Definitive diagnosis is made by muscle biopsy with direct enzyme measurement.

CLINICAL ISSUES

23. Which metabolic diseases can present as sudden infant death syndrome (SIDS) or an acute life-threatening event (ALTE)?

- Fatty acid oxidation defects
- Some organic acidemias
- Defects of aldosterone and glucocorticoid metabolism
- McArdle syndrome (myophosphorylase deficiency) (rare)
- Mitochondrial defects, e.g., Leigh syndrome (rare)

Although early reports suggested that medium-chain acyl-CoA dehydrogenase deficiency may be especially common among SIDS deaths, this claim has not been supported by several large population studies that used strict diagnostic criteria for SIDS.

24. What causes neonatal hyperammonemia?

- Congenital urea cycle defects
- Organic acidemias (particularly methylmalonic aciduria, propionic acidemia, isovaleric acidemia)
- Fatty acid oxidation defects
- Other causes: idiopathic transient hyperammonemia (THAN), hypercatabolic states, excessive dietary protein, severe hepatocellular disease, neonatal hemochromatosis, urinary tract infection with urea-splitting organisms (e.g., *Proteus*) and patent ductus venosus

25. How do patients with urea-cycle defects present?

1. ***Neonatal catastrophe***—symptomatology similar to that of sepsis neonatorum
   - Seizures, hypertonicity, vomiting, coma, death
   - Extreme elevations of NH_3: > 1000 μg/dl (588 (μmoles/L)
2. ***Subacute presentation in infancy***
   - Recurrent vomiting and growth failure
   - Intermittent ataxia
   - Seizures, mental retardation, developmental regression
3. ***Presentation later in childhood***
   - Psychomotor retardation
   - Intermittent ataxia
   - Vomiting, protein intolerance—history of poor feeding during infancy
   - Overt symptoms after mild illness
4. ***Asymptomatic variant***
   - Usually shows amino acid abnormality without hyperammonemia

From Cohn RM, Roth KS (eds): Metabolic Disease: A Guide to Early Recognition. Philadelphia, W.B. Saunders, 1983, p 138; with permission.

26. What are the treatments of choice for urea-cycle disorders?

Acute

- Continuous arteriovenous hemofiltration or hemodialysis
- High-concentration glucose infusions ± insulin in order to favor tissue anabolism
- Aggressive treatment of fevers
- Correction of amino acid deficiencies to prevent secondary catabolism
- Sodium benzoate and sodium phenylbutyrate to increase ammonia excretion via alternate pathways
- Arginine for excretion of ammonia as argininosuccinic acid in argininosuccinic aciduria and as citrulline in patients with citrullinemia

Maintenance

- Low-protein diet with supplemental essential amino acids
- Avoidance of fasting or other catabolic stress
- Sodium benzoate, sodium phenylbutyrate
- Supplementation with specific urea-cycle amino acids to prevent a deficiency state (and subsequent catabolism) or to enhance ammonia excretion (e.g., arginine in argininosuccinic aciduria)

27. What is the source of the organic acids in children with organic acidemias?

Most organic acidemias are actually due to defects in amino acid metabolism, but the enzymatic defects occur far down the catabolic pathway, after amino groups have been removed (e.g., methylmalonic acidemia is a downstream abnormality in metabolism of valine and isoleucine). Organic acidemias due to primary abnormalities in organic acid metabolism, such as lactic acidemia and dicarboxylic aciduria, also occur.

28. Why do organic acidemias cause neonatal illness?

The mitochondrion is the cell's powerhouse. Body tissues that demand a major expenditure of energy are especially vulnerable to an interruption of their energy supply secondary to disturbed mitochondrial function. As such, brain, muscle, heart, liver, and the GI and renal transport systems fail due to clinical disorders of the mitochondrion. A variety of conditions can abruptly embarrass mitochondrial function and result in multisystem dysfunction. In the newborn, an organic acidemia may produce an acute form of encephalopathy manifested initially as feeding intolerance, vomiting, and lethargy, which progresses rapidly to coma, seizures, flaccid paralysis, respiratory depression, reduced gag reflex, and ultimately death. These signs are not specific for mitochondrial failure but suggest overwhelming, widespread CNS dysfunction. Their differential diagnosis includes sepsis, meningitis, intracranial hemorrhage, stroke and any catastrophic neurologic illness. Neonates with hyperammonemia due to urea-cycle enzyme defects manifest comparable signs; cerebral edema is often present and may contribute to a fatal outcome.

29. How are the organic acidemias diagnosed?

Gas chromatography of a urine specimen can identify the abnormality in 80–90% of cases. However, combined gas chromatographic–mass spectrometric analysis should be performed to confirm the identity. The renal tubule does not effectively reabsorb organic acids, and consequently urine has been preferred to blood for evaluation. For screening purposes, though, the relatively new technique of dual-tandem mass spectrometric analysis of carnitine-esters in blood may indirectly enhance the capability to diagnose organic acidemias (see question 30).

30. Why does secondary carnitine deficiency develop in the organic acidemias?

In most organic acidemias, the deficient enzyme resides in the mitochondrion, where the enzyme substrate is the CoA derivative of the organic acid, e.g., propionyl-CoA in propionic acidemia. The CoA derivative can react with free mitochondrial carnitine to form the cognate carnitine ester, e.g., propionylcarnitine. Excess formation of the carnitine ester, which is detectable in blood and urine, leads to free carnitine deficiency.

31. A 19-month-old boy with developmental delay, failure to thrive, spasticity, choreoathetosis, and compulsive self-mutilating behavior probably has what metabolic abnormality?

The child has ***Lesch-Nyhan syndrome*,** an X-linked recessive trait, due to complete deficiency of hypoxanthine-guanine phosphoribosyl transferase (HGPRT). This enzyme is involved in the reutilization of purine bases following degradation of their corresponding nucleotides. If the purine bases are not recycled they are oxidized to uric acid, which is then formed to excess. Mothers often report the yellow-red, sand-like urate crystals in the diapers during the newborn period.

Although affected infants (always male) may appear normal at birth, hypotonia, frequent vomiting, and delayed motor development are usually recognized in the first few months. Evidence of extrapyramidal dysfunction—dystonia, chorea, and athetosis—usually appears in the second 6 months of life. Between the first and second year, the evolution of spasticity and dysarthria often suggests the diagnosis of cerebral palsy. After 18 months, the compulsive self-destructive behavior usually develops; common manifestations include lip mutilation, finger-biting, and head-banging. A very high renal clearance of uric acid occasionally results in normal serum levels in infancy. However, the urine uric acid/creatinine ratio is pathologically elevated. Milder deficiencies of the enzyme may present as only spasticity and/or extrapyramidal disease without self-mutilation.

32. What is the etiology of Reye syndrome?

The cause remains unknown. Pathologically, the disease was characterized by widespread mitochondrial failure, which leads to the characteristic findings of acidosis, hyperammonemia, and hypoglycemia without significant ketosis (hypoketotic). Liver biopsy reveals fatty infiltration, minimal inflammation, and ultrastructural changes in mitochondria. These acquired metabolic abnormalities were usually associated with life-threatening brain edema.

33. Describe the biphasic course of Reye syndrome.

***Prodrome*:** mild upper respiratory illness or various viral illnesses (including influenza A and B, varicella, adenovirus, Epstein-Barr virus, herpes zoster, rubeola, mumps)

***Acute*:** pernicious vomiting, afebrile; progression in some to encephalopathy with delirium, stupor, seizures, coma

34. Why has Reye syndrome virtually disappeared?

The dramatic reduction in the use of aspirin is the key factor in the United States. Several case-control studies have identified a statistical association between aspirin use during an antecedent viral illness and the development of Reye syndrome. Both aspirin use and the incidence of Reye syndrome in young children started to decrease during the 1980s. By 1984, the median age of patients with this diagnosis had increased, a change that reflected less aspirin use in young children. Almost all patients who now present with a Reye syndrome–like illness suffer from a metabolic disease such as a urea-cycle defect (ornithine transcarbamylase deficiency), organic acidemia (isovaleric acidemia) and fatty acid oxidation defect (medium chain acyl-CoA dehydrogenase deficiency).

Belay ED et al: Reye's syndrome in the United States from 1981 through 1997. N Engl J Med 340:1377-1382, 1999.

35. When visiting the Caribbean, should you accept a gift of unripe fruit from the ackee tree?

Don't eat it. The fruit contains hypoglycin A, the toxin responsible for Jamaican vomiting sickness. The disease can be fatal and begins with vomiting and hypoglycemia that can progress to hepatic steatosis and coma. The disease may resemble Reye syndrome.

36. Which metabolic diseases are responsive to pyridoxine (vitamin B_6)?

- Homocystinuria
- Oxaluria
- Cystathioninuria
- Pyridoxine-dependent seizures (putative deficiency of glutamate decarboxylase)
- β-Alaninemia

37. What are the causes of hyperuricemia?

Overproduction

- Hypoxanthine-guanine phosphoribosyl transferase (HGPRT) deficiency (Lesch-Nyhan syndrome)
- Hypercatabolic states (e.g., severe anoxia, leukemia, tumor lysis)
- Fatty-acid β-oxidation defects
- Hereditary fructose intolerance
- Glycogen storage diseases
- Reye syndrome

Toxin or drug-induced

- Ethanol poisoning
- Lead intoxication
- Diuretics (most)
- Aspirin
- Nicotinic acid
- Radiocontrast agents
- Chronic ingestion of acids

Other

- Cystinosis, Fabry disease, oxalosis due to renal insufficiency
- Hypo- or hyperparathyroidism
- Hypothyroidism
- High meat or fructose diets

38. List the inherited disorders of neurotransmitter metabolism.

- Pyridoxine-responsive seizures (putative glutamate decarboxylase deficiency)
- Dopamine-β-hydroxylase deficiency (hypotension; autonomic dysfunction)
- Tyrosine hydroxylase deficiency (hypotonia; developmental retardation)
- Gaba transaminase deficiency (hypotonia; developmental retardation)
- Succinic-semialdehyde dehydrogenase deficiency (4-OH-butyric aciduria) (hypotonia; developmental retardation)
- L-Aromatic amino acid decarboxylase deficiency (hypotonia, hypokinesia, athetosis, oculogyric crisis, ptosis, diaphoresis)

39. What is the metabolic defect in Wilson disease?

Wilson disease is an autosomal recessive defect of copper metabolism that is caused by a congenital deficiency of the copper transporter/ATPase, ATP7B. The defective gene resides on the long arm of chromosome 13. The major biochemical abnormalities include low serum ceruloplasmin, decreased incorporation of copper into ceruloplasmin, increased urinary copper excretion, and markedly increased levels of copper in many tissues, notably the liver, basal ganglia, and cornea (Kayser-Fleischer rings). A cardinal feature is the high amount of free copper circulating in plasma unbound to ceruloplasmin.

40. What are the common clinical presentations of Wilson disease?

Hepatic/hematologic	**Neurologic**
• Jaundice and hepatitis	• Psychiatric disturbance
• Cirrhosis	• Tremor, extrapyramidal movement disorder
• Fulminant hepatic failure	• Intellectual and behavioral deterioration
• Hemolytic anemia	• Convulsions

Sanchez-Albisua I et al: A high index of suspicion: The key to an early diagnosis of Wilson's disease in childhood. J Pediatr Gastroenterol Nutr 28:186-190, 1999.

41. How is the diagnosis of Wilson disease confirmed?

The combination of markedly increased copper levels in a liver biopsy specimen (> 400 μg/gm wet weight), low serum ceruloplasmin, and increased urinary copper excretion strongly suggests classic Wilson disease but is not absolutely diagnostic. The additional finding of Kayser-Fleischer rings is nearly pathognomonic of Wilson disease; however, their absence, especially in children, does not rule out the disease, and copper deposits in the cornea may also rarely be seen in other severe liver diseases, such as Indian biliary cirrhosis. The most specific diagnostic test is the demonstration of the slow rate of disappearance of radiolabeled copper from the bloodstream. Newer methods include measurement of radioactive copper uptake and retention by cultured fibroblasts, which is increased in Wilson disease.

42. Is there a treatment of choice for Wilson disease?

D-Penicillamine, a copper-chelating agent, is the drug of choice. Another copper-chelating drug, trientine, has been used successfully in patients who have discontinued penicillamine because of hypersensitivity reactions. Zinc sulfate, which inhibits intestinal copper absorption, has also been used.

43. Describe the two main clinical features of the porphyrias.

The porphyrias are inborn errors in heme biosynthesis with overproduction of heme precursors. About 15% of heme is synthesized in the liver and the remainder in bone marrow. The precursors vary in their solubility, tissue depositions, and photosensitivity. Two main categories of presentations predominate:

Neurovisceral Symptoms
- Abdominal pain and vomiting
- Constipation or diarrhea
- Muscle weakness
- Mental status changes
- Peripheral nerve disease
- Hypertension and/or tachycardia
- Convulsions
- Bulbar paralysis
- Fever

Photosensitivity Skin Lesions
Acute
- Edematous skin plaques
- Bullae and vesicle formation
- Urticaria
- Purpura

Chronic
- Scarring, erosions, thickening
- Hypertrichosis
- Sensitivity to trauma
- Hyperpigmentation

44. How are the porphyrias broadly classified?

The ***acute porphyrias*** (acute intermittent porphyria, variegate porphyria and hereditary coproporphyria) present with severe pain, confusion, autonomic changes and paralysis. The ***cutaneous porphyrias*** (erythropoietic porphyria, porphyria cutanea tarda and congenital erythropoietic porphyria) present with blistering, severe photosensitivity, hirsutism and discoloration. Mixed presentations are possible with variegate porphyria and hereditary coproporphyria.

45. Link the various types of porphyrias with the phenotype including enzyme deficiency and the inheritance pattern.

DISEASE	ENZYME DEFICIENCY	NEURO-VISCERAL ATTACKS	PHOTO-SENSITIVITY	HEPATIC DISEASE	HEMO-LYTIC ANEMIA	AGE OF ONSET	INHERITANCE
Erythropoietic porphyrias							
Erythropoietic porphyria	Uroporphyringen III cosynthase	—	++++	—	++	Childhood	AR
Erythropoietic protoporphyria	Ferrochelatase	—	++	±	—	Childhood	AD
Hepatic porphyrias							
Acute intermittent porphyria	PGB deaminase	++++	—	+	—	Postpubertal	AD
ALA dehydratase deficiency Porphyria	ALA dehydratase	++++	—	—	—	Postpubertal	AR
Porphyria variegata	Protoporphyrinogen Oxidase	++	++	—	—	Postpubertal	AD
Hereditary copro-porphyria	Coproporphyrinogen oxidase	++	+	±	—	Postpubertal	AD
Porphyria cutanea tarda*	Uroporphyrinogen decarboxylase	—	—	++†	—	Adult	Sporadic, Some AD

AR = autosomal recessive; AD = autosomal dominant; ALA = δ-aminolevulinic acid.
*AR form is hepatoerythropoietic porphyria and is characterized by childhood onset of severe photosensitivity.
†Probable contributing cause (e.g., alcoholic liver disease) rather than primary manifestation of porphyria.

46. Why are females more commonly affected by clinical problems of porphyria than males?

In the biosynthesis of heme, the rate-limiting step involves the first enzyme, ALA-synthase. When this enzyme is stimulated, additional precursors accumulate downstream at the point of specific enzyme blocks. Estrogen is an important inducer of ALA-synthase, and this appears to be the key reason for the greater problems encountered by females. For example, symptoms of acute intermittent porphyria are rare before puberty and oral contraceptives often cause exacerbations.

47. What accounts for the varying clinical features of the mucopolysaccharidoses?

Mucopolysaccharidoses are examples of storage disorders of lysosomes, which are intracellular organelles that degrade structural macromolecules. If enzymes are deficient, metabolites predominantly accumulate in the tissues that are primarily responsible for their degradation.

Mucopolysaccharide	*Site of Accumulation*
Heparan sulfate	CNS
Dermatan sulfate	Bone, viscera (esp. liver)
Keratan sulfate	Bone
Chondroitin sulfate	Cartilage

48. Describe the radiographic features that characterize the mucopolysaccharidoses.

A constellation of x-ray findings, termed ***dysostosis multiplex***, is found:

- *Skull*: enlarged and elongated with a thickened calvaria
- *Sella turcica*: shaped like a wooden-shoe or boot
- *Vertebral bodies* (especially lower thoracic and upper lumbar): hypoplasia of antero-superior areas resulting in "beaked" appearance; in Morquio syndrome, platyspondylisis (flattening of vertebral bodies with surface irregularities)
- *Ribs*: thickened (except at spinal insertion), "oar shaped"
- *Metacarpals*: "baby-bottle" appearance with proximal narrowing and distal widening
- *Humerus, ulna*: distal angulation
- *Pelvis*: flaring of iliac bones, shallow acetabulum, progressive coxa valga
- *Long bones*: shortened, thickened

49. Can a metabolic disease in the fetus have an adverse effect on the mother?

Long-chain 3-hydroxyacyl-CoA dehydrogenase deficiency, a fatty-acid oxidation defect in the fetus, can cause acute fatty liver of pregnancy in the mother.

50. An 8-month-old presents with vomiting, lethargy, hypoglycemia, and no ketones on urinalysis. What condition is likely?

Medium-chain acyl-CoA dehydrogenase deficiency (MCAD). Disorders of fatty-acid oxidation and/or a deficiency of carnitine (the principal transporter of fatty acids into mitochondria) can result in maladaptation to the fasting stress that often accompanies an intercurrent illness. Hypoketotic hypoglycemia results from the inability to utilize fatty acids, which are the primary source of ketones. MCAD affects 1:5000–1:10,000 live births in families of Northern European ancestry. The clinical presentation varies from asymptomatic children who are detected with a screening test to those with severe vomiting, encephalopathy, coma, and death. This latter picture occurs in 25% of patients with their first episode and may be confused with Reye syndrome or SIDS.

51. What common laboratory abnormalities are found in disorders of mitochondrial fatty-acid oxidation?

- Hypoketotic hypoglycemia
- Abnormal urinary dicarboxylic aciduria (metabolites of fatty acids)
- Hypocarnitinemia

- Abnormally increased urinary acylglycines (e.g., suberylglycine)
- Increased plasma or urinary acylcarnitines (e.g., octanoylcarnitine)
- Abnormal plasma free fatty acid levels
- Specific mutations on DNA analysis

52. How are fatty acid oxidation disorders treated?

- Avoidance of prolonged fasting.
- If oral intake is limited, provide adequate IV glucose in excess of basal hepatic glucose production (6 mg/kg/min for newborns, 2 mg/kg/min for adults).
- If the defect affects only long-chain fatty-acid metabolism, limit dietary fat and/or provide only medium-chain fatty acids (C6–C10) in addition to minimal amounts of essential fatty acids.
- If carnitine levels are low, oral L-carnitine can be used to restore levels to normal (but the benefits are questionable).

53. A 3-month-old has hypotonia, hepatomegaly, a high forehead with flat facies, and increased serum very-long-chain fatty acids. What condition is likely?

Zellweger syndrome (cerebrohepatorenal syndrome) is caused by a defect in assembly of the peroxisome, an intracellular organelle involved in various metabolic functions, including lipid metabolism and oxidation of very-long-chain fatty acids.

54. In what disease is "Lorenzo's oil" used as attempted therapy?

Adrenoleukodystrophy is an X-linked peroxisomal disease that is characterized by progressive demyelination beginning around 6 years of age in the classical form. A more aggressive, infantile form also exists. A key to diagnosis is the presence of high blood levels of very-long-chain fatty acids, which are not oxidized normally because of abnormal peroxisomal function. Lorenzo's oil refers to a mixture of oleic and erucic acids has been used to treat adrenoleukodystrophy. Lorenzo's oil, popularized in a Hollywood movie, can normalize plasma fatty-acid levels, but does not alter the clinical course.

van Geel BM, et al: Progression of abnormalities in adrenomyeloneuropathy and neurologically asymptomatic x-linked adrenoleukodystrophy despite treatment with "Lorenzo's oil." J Neurol Neurosurg Psych 67:290-299, 1999.

55. Is the Smith-Lemli-Opitz syndrome, a congenital disorder with multiple malformations, an example of an inborn error of metabolism?

Yes. The disease, inherited as an autosomal recessive trait, is caused by a defect in cholesterol biosynthesis which leads to organ dysgenesis in the fetus. As a consequence of an enzyme deficiency, 7-dehydrocholesterol cannot be converted to cholesterol.

56. Do all patients with mutations of mitochondrial DNA show a persistent lactic acidosis?

No, but many do, because impaired electron transport chain function is usually the result of these mutations. Because more than one copy of mitochondrial DNA, inherited solely from the mother, is contained in a mitochondrion, and there may be thousands of mitochondria per cell, the systemic nature of the disease process in a particular patient depends on the number of cells in a tissue with a critical number of diseased mitochondria, the metabolic demands of the tissue, its replicative capacity, and probably other unknown factors. If the burden of mutated mitochondrial DNA is high in muscle, brain, or liver, whole body oxidative metabolism will be impaired, and the patient will manifest a lactic acidosis. However, the expression of severe disease in the absence of a lactic acidosis may occur because of limited regional involvement in an organ such as the brain.

57. Are the diseases due to mitochondrial DNA mutations limited to familial inheritance patterns with transmission from mother to all children?

No. There are sporadic cases, and while in the familial forms transmission of mutated mitochondrial DNA to offspring must be 100%, the expression of disease may be < 100%. Examples of sporadic disease include Kearns-Sayre syndrome, Pearson syndrome, and acquired zidovudine-induced mitochondrial myopathy. They are usually associated with DNA deletions. The MELAS (mitochondrial encephalopathy with lactic acidosis and strokes) syndrome is associated with a maternal inheritance pattern and, like most of these familial disorders, is secondary to a single base mutation in mitochondrial DNA.

GENERAL CONCEPTS

58. How are inborn errors of metabolism diagnosed prenatally?

Virtually all can be diagnosed prenatally using a number of different techniques.

- The most common procedure is enzyme analysis of cultured fibroblasts (obtained by chorionic villus sampling or amniocentesis) for the metabolic defect in question. An example is the measurement of hexosaminidase A activity from cultured amniotic fluid cells in a fetus at risk for Tay-Sachs disease.
- Measuring the concentration of a substrate which accumulates in excess due to a specific metabolic block (e.g., measure 17-hydroxyprogesterone in amniotic fluid from a fetus at risk for 21-hydroxylase deficiency, or congenital adrenal hyperplasia).
- Molecular genetic investigation for direct gene analysis or familial linkage studies (e.g., linkage studies in a fetus at risk for ornithine transcarbamylase deficiency, a lethal X-linked urea-cycle defect).

59. Which inborn errors of metabolism can cause rickets?

Any condition that causes a phosphaturic state:

- Cystinosis
- Galactosemia
- Wilson disease
- Hereditary fructose intolerance
- Hereditary tyrosinemia
- Fanconi-Bickel syndrome

60. In what settings should inborn errors of metabolism be suspected?

- Onset of symptoms correlating with dietary changes
- Loss or leveling of developmental milestones
- Patient with strong food preferences or aversions
- Parental consanguinity
- Unexplained sibling death, mental retardation, or seizures
- Unexplained failure to thrive
- Unusual odor
- Hair abnormalities, especially alopecia
- Microcephaly or macrocephaly
- Abnormalities of muscle tone
- Organomegaly
- Coarsened facial features, thick skin, limited joint mobility, hirsutism

61. What are the characteristic features of the Fanconi-Bickel syndrome?

This extremely rare autosomal recessive disease due to a deficiency of the facilitated glucose (galactose) transporter GLUT2 causes liver enlargement with glycogen accumulation, renal Fanconi syndrome and galactose intolerance.

62. A deficiency of what facilitated glucose transporter expressed in brain causes seizures because of hypoglycorrhexia but with normal blood glucose levels?

GLUT1.

63. What inborn errors of metabolism commonly cause acidosis during the neonatal period?

Severe metabolic acidosis in the neonatal period is more often caused by sepsis or cardiac defects than inborn errors of metabolism, but the latter do occur. Disorders of pyruvate metabolism, gluconeogenesis, and branched-chain amino acid catabolism are the most common inherited metabolic diseases causing metabolic acidosis in the newborn. In addition, metabolic acidosis with a normal anion gap occurs in disorders that impair renal uptake of bicarbonate or secretion of hydrogen ion. *Ketonuria with acidosis* in the newborn period is an especially important sign of an inborn error of metabolism and should be assumed to be caused by a metabolic disease until proved otherwise.

64. How do inborn errors of metabolism vary in clinical and laboratory features?

Inborn errors of metabolism can affect any organ system. The range of clinical presentation would extend to the full gamut of disease. A useful conceptual framework divides this group of disorders into those that involve a disruption of intermediary metabolism like most aminoacidurias and urea cycle defects. These diseases typically involve a sudden decompensation of clinical status. In contrast, the inborn errors of metabolism that involve structural molecules, like the many forms of lysosomal storage disease, usually involve a course of progressive degeneration rather than an episodic illness.

Clinical Findings in Inborn Errors of Metabolism

CLINICAL MANIFESTATIONS	GENERAL TYPE OF DISORDER TO CONSIDER								
LABORATORY FINDINGS	A	B	C	D	E	F	G	H	I
Episodic nature	++	++	++	++	+	+	—	—	—
Poor feeding	++	+	++	+	+	+	+	—	—
Abnormal odor	+	+	—	+	—	—	—	—	—
Lethargy, coma	+	+	+	+	+	+	—	—	—
Seizures	+	+	+	—	+	+	+	—	+
Developmental regression	+	+	+	—	+	—	+	++	+
Hepatomegaly	+	+	+	+	+	+	+	+	+
Hepatosplenomegaly	—	—	—	—	—	—	—	+	+
Splenomegaly	—	—	—	—	—	—	—	—	+
Hypotonia	+	+	+	+	+	+	+	—	+
Cardiomyopathy	—	+	—	+	+	+	—	+	—
Coarse facies	—	—	—	—	—	—	—	++	—
Birth defects	—	+	—	—	+	—	+	—	—
Hypoglycemia	+	+	—	+	+	+	—	—	—
Acidosis	+	++	—	+	+	+	—	—	—
Hyperammonemia	+	+	++	+	+	—	—	—	—
Ketosis	+	+	+	—	—	+	—	—	—
Hypoketosis	—	—	—	+	—	—	—	—	—

A–amino acidopathies; B–organic acidopathies; C–urea-cycle defects; D–fatty-acid oxidation defects; E–mitochondrial disorders; F–carbohydrate disorders; G–peroxisomal disorders; H–mucopolysaccharidoses; I–sphingolipidoses. ++ = usually present; + = may be present; — = usually not present.

From Wappner RS: Biochemical diagnosis of genetic disease. Pediatr Ann 22:284, 1993; with permission.

65. What key urine odors are associated with inborn errors of metabolism?

Cabbage Tyrosinemia, type I

Cat urine 3-Methylcrotonyl-CoA carboxylase deficiency

Fish	Trimethylaminuria
Hops	Oasthouse urine disease
Maple syrup	Maple syrup urine disease
"Mousy" or musty	Phenylketonuria
Sweaty feet or cheesy	Isovaleric acidemia; glutaric aciduria, type II

66. Which inherited metabolic disorders are commonly associated with hypoglycemia?

- Primary errors of glucose synthesis and release, i.e., gluconeogenesis and glycogenolysis
- Defects of fatty-acid oxidation and ketogenesis, the main sources of fuel for gluconeogenesis
- Hyperinsulinism
- Defects causing "metabolic poisoning" of glucose metabolism, principally the organic acidurias

67. What is the differential diagnosis for ketotic and nonketotic hypoglycemia?

Ketotic hypoglycemia

- 3-Ketoacyl-CoA thiolase deficiency (short chain)
- Acetoacetyl-CoA thiolase deficiency
- Succinyl-3-ketoacyl CoA transferase deficiency
- Glycogen storage diseases I, III, VI
- Hereditary fructose intolerance
- Respiratory chain defects and related mitochondrial defects
- Growth hormone deficiency
- Hypopituitarism
- Accelerated starvation syndrome

Nonketotic or hypoketotic hypoglycemia

- Hyperinsulinism
- Hypopituitarism
- Fatty-acid β oxidation defects and systemic carnitine deficiency
- 3-Hydroxy, 3-methyl glutaric acidemia
- Defective Ketostix or Dextrostix

68. In an acutely ill child with suspected metabolic disease, how does the liver size provide a clue to the possible diagnosis?

Generally, in patients with inborn errors of metabolism, hepatomegaly in association with acute illness is more typical of disorders of carbohydrate or fatty-acid metabolism. Less commonly, patients with urea-cycle enzyme defects or organic acidemias, such as methylmalonic acidemia, may manifest hepatomegaly. In patients without hepatomegaly, a disorder of amino acid metabolism, such as maple syrup urine disease or nonketotic hyperglycemia, is more likely. It should be noted mild elevations of the serum transaminases can occur in many metabolic diseases, even in the absence of frank hepatomegaly.

69. What strategies are used in the chronic management of inborn errors of metabolism?

- ***Dietary manipulation*** to avoid the substrate for deficient enzymes and precursor accumulation (e.g., give a low-phenylalanine diet in patients with phenylketonuria)
- ***Augment the excretion*** of toxic metabolites (e.g., glycine treatment of isovaleric acidemia)
- ***Supplement*** with an inadequately produced enzyme product (e.g., arginine therapy for urea-cycle disorders)
- ***Administer additional coenzyme*** to increase the activity of an abnormal enzyme (e.g., vitamin B_{12} in methylmalonic acidemia)
- ***Provide deficient enzyme*** (e.g., enzyme infusion in Gaucher disease, liver transplantation in hereditary tyrosinemia, gene replacement therapy)

Goodman SI, Greene CL: Metabolic disorders of the newborn. Pediatr Rev 15:359–365, 1994.

LIPID DISORDERS

70. How are lipoproteins categorized?

The three major lipoprotein groups are classified by their density or electrophoretic properties: very-low-density lipoproteins (VLDL or pre-β), low-density lipoproteins (LDL or β), and high-density lipoproteins (HDL or α_1). In addition, chylomicrons and an intermediate-density lipoprotein (IDL or "floating β") can be found in plasma, although their quantities are typically much less, except in children with disorders of lipid metabolism.

71. What are normal cholesterol levels for children and adolescents?

	Total Cholesterol (mg/dl)	LDL-Cholesterol (mg/dl)
Acceptable	< 170	< 110
Borderline	170-199	110-129
High	> 200	> 130

72. How is LDL cholesterol calculated?

LDL cholesterol = total cholesterol – [HDL cholesterol + (total triglyceride/5)]

73. Which children should have their cholesterol measured?

This is a controversial issue with proponents and opponents of universal screening. Current recommendations, developed by the National Cholesterol Education Committee and the American Academy of Pediatrics, adopt a middle ground—to screen all children aged ≥ 2 years if there is:

1. Family history of parents or grandparents aged 55 or younger with documented premature cardiovascular disease
2. History of a parent with elevated total cholesterol (> 240 mg/dl)
3. Parental and/or family history is unobtainable (e.g., adoption)

Proponents of universal screening have since argued that the guidelines are not sufficiently sensitive and may miss up to 50% of children with elevated lipids.

American Academy of Pediatrics, Committee on Nutrition: Cholesterol in childhood. Pediatrics 101:141-147, 1998.

74. Outline the six arguments against universal screening for elevated cholesterol.

1. Instrumentation for cholesterol measurement is not standardized, and some children will be mislabeled.
2. If pediatric dietary recommendations (e.g., total fat < 30% of calories) are routinely followed, many children with hypercholesterolemia will achieve normal levels.
3. Serum cholesterol may not be the most sensitive indicator of future atherosclerotic heart disease.
4. Tracking (persistence of high or low levels over time) is not precise for serum cholesterol.
5. Although fatty arterial plaques occur in children, atherosclerotic events are rare before the third decade, and present evidence suggests reversibility at that age with treatment.
6. Cost of universal screening is large compared to benefits.

Newman TB, Garber AM: Cholesterol screening in children and adolescents. Pediatrics 105:637-638, 2000.

Newman TB, et al: Problems with the report of the Expert Panel on blood cholesterol levels in children and adolescents. Arch Pediatr Adolesc Med 149:241–247, 1996.

75. How is the primary genetic hyperlipidemias classified?

FREDERICKSON TYPE	LIPIDS INCREASED	LIPOPROTEINS INCREASED	PREVALENCE	CLINICAL FINDINGS
I	Triglyceride	Chylomicrons	Very rare	Eruptive xanthomas, pancreatitis, recurrent abdominal pain, lipemia retinalis, hepatosplenomegaly
IIa	Cholesterol	LDL	Common	Tendon xanthomas, PVD
IIb	Cholesterol, triglyceride	LDL + VLDL	Common	PVD, no xanthomas
III	Cholesterol, triglyceride	VLDL remnants (IDL)	Rare	PVD, yellow palm creases
IV	Triglyceride	VLDL	Uncommon	PVD, xanthomas, hyperglycemia
V	Triglyceride, cholesterol	VLDL + chylomicrons	Very rare	Pancreatitis, lipemia retinalis, xanthomas, hyperglycemia

PVD = premature vascular disease.

76. What is the most common hyperlipidemia in childhood?

Type IIa, familial hypercholesterolemia with elevated cholesterol and LDL. This condition results from a lack of functional LDL receptors on cell membranes due to various mutations. When LDL cannot attach and release cholesterol to the cell, feedback suppression of HMG-CoA reductase (the rate-limiting enzyme in cholesterol synthesis) does not occur, and cholesterol synthesis continues excessively. In the homozygous form of Type IIa, xanthomas may appear before age 10 and vascular disease before age 20. However, the homozygous form is very rare, with an incidence of 1 in 1 million births. The heterozygous variety has a much higher incidence of 1 in 500 but is less likely to produce clinical manifestations in children.

The type most likely to present in childhood is type I hyperlipoproteinemia. This disorder is characterized by an excess of chylomicron triglycerides, which typically causes recurrent abdominal pain and hepatosplenomegaly in the first 5 years of life. Although rare, it is more common than homozygous familial hypercholesterolemia (type IIa). As a rule, most of the common familial hyperlipidemias are not associated with clinical disease during childhood, but usually manifest as atherosclerotic heart disease or xanthomata in the third or later decades.

77. What are the treatments of choice for familial hypercholesterolemia?

Dietary restriction of cholesterol and fat, plus a lipid-lowering resin such as cholestyramine. Cholestyramine and the related resin, colestipol, lower plasma cholesterol by trapping bile acids in the gut and thereby causing more cholesterol to be shunted to bile acid synthesis. Other therapies include direct removal of lipoproteins by plasmapheresis, pharmacologic doses of the vitamin niacin (nicotinic acid), and orthotopic liver transplantation. Inhibitors (the "statins") of the rate-limiting enzyme of cholesterol synthesis, HMG-CoA reductase, are also available and undergoing clinical testing in children. *Ex vivo* gene therapy using liver cells and retroviral vectors is currently under study in adults.

Stein EA et al: Efficacy and safety of lovastatin in adolescent males with heterozygous familial hypercholesterolemia: A randomized controlled trial. JAMA 281:137-144, 1999

Knopp RH: Drug treatment of lipid disorders. N Engl J Med 341:498-511, 1999

78. What are the causes of secondary hyperlipidemia in childhood?

General medical conditions
- Obesity
- Hypothyroidism
- Chronic renal failure
- Nephrotic syndrome
- Biliary atresia, biliary cirrhosis
- Hepatitis
- Diabetes mellitus
- Pregnancy
- Anorexia nervosa

Inborn errors of metabolism
- Glycogen storage disease (mostly type I)
- Congenital lactic acidosis
- Mitochondrial encephalomyopathies (some)
- Acute intermittent porphyria

Drugs
- β-Adrenergic blockers
- Alcohol
- Oral contraceptives
- Thiazide diuretics
- Anabolic steroids
- Corticosteroids
- Istretinoin (Accutane)

Genetic syndromes
- Werner syndrome
- Progeria
- Klinefelter syndrome
- Idiopathic hypercalcemia

79. Which is the most commonly encountered lipid-storage disorder in humans?

Gaucher disease, or glucosyl ceramide lipidosis, caused by a deficiency of β-glucocerebrosidase, is the most commonly diagnosed lipid-storage disorder. The incidence varies from 1/100,000 in non-Jewish populations to 1/855 in Ashkenazi Jews.

80. What lipid-storage disorder should be suspected in patients with unexplained proteinuria?

Fabry disease (α-galactosidase deficiency). Proteinuria is also a characteristic of several types of sialic acid storage disease, presenting in the newborn period with nephrotic syndrome, coarse facial features, organomegaly, bony changes (dyostosis multiplex), and neurologic abnormalities.

SCREENING

81. How frequently are the various metabolic disorders detected by newborn screening?

Disorder	**Frequency**
Tay-Sachs disease (U.S. Jews)	1/3000
Phenylketonuria	1/10,000–25,000
Galactosemia	1/40,000–60,000
Biotinidase deficiency	1/70,000
Homocystinuria	1/50,000–150,000
Maple syrup urine disease	1/250,000–300,000

82. Which common sugar does the Clinitest screen not detect?

Sucrose. Reducing sugars, such as glucose, fructose, galactose, pentoses, and lactose, are detected, but sucrose is not a reducing sugar. The test method is straightforward. Five drops of urine and 10 drops of water are mixed, and Clinitest tablet is added. Color changes are then compared to a standard chart to determine the percentage of reducing substances. Testing for sucrose can be done by substituting hydrochloric acid for the water and boiling for a few seconds. This hydrolyzes the sucrose, and a negative test will become positive.

83. What are the common causes of false-positive tests for urine-reducing substances?
- Radiologic contrast dyes
- Stool contamination

- Antibiotics, especially ampicillin, and other drugs excreted as glucuronides
- Pentosuria from pentose-enriched fruits (true-positive but nonpathologic)
- *p*-Hydroxyphenylpyruvic acid (tyrosinemias)

84. Why was the "Guthrie bacterial inhibition test" a major breakthrough?

The Guthrie was the first screening procedure that was implemented in large-scale trials. It was shown to be reliable, sensitive, specific and cost-effective in terms of diagnosing phenylketonuria before the development of irreversible mental retardation. It was this successful precedent that justified the subsequent mass screening of infants for the presence of an inborn error of metabolism.

85. Tandem mass spectrometry (MS-MS) is becoming more widely utilized for newborn screening using blood eluted from a Guthrie filter paper card. What are the two most important classes of compounds that it detects and quantitates?

1. Amino acids
2. Carnitine esters or acylcarnitines derived from organic acid and fatty acid metabolites.

86. Should all newborn infants born in the U.S. have a newborn screen using tandem mass spectrometry?

For the present, a consensus opinion in the medical community and public health system is lacking.

13. NEONATOLOGY

Philip Roth, M.D., *Ph.D.*, *Mary Catherine* Harris, M.D.,
Carlos Vega-Rich, M.D., *and* Peter *Marro*, M.D.

CLINICAL ISSUES

1. Why don't preterm infants sweat?

The failure of infants born at < 30 weeks' gestation to sweat is probably due to the incomplete development and differentiation of sweat glands. In term babies, in whom more data are available, the maximal sweat response to thermal stimuli is one-third that of adults, despite a density of sweat glands which is six times higher.

2. Do infants ever shiver?

It is uncertain whether newborns shiver. In some reports, shivering was observed only at temperatures < 22–24°C. Heat generation is mainly via nonshivering thermogenesis, consisting of muscular activity and metabolism of brown fat.

3. How does brown fat keep infants warm?

Cold-stressed infants depend principally on chemical mechanisms to maintain body temperature. When placed in a cold environment, the sympathetic nervous system is activated, and norepinephrine and thyroid hormones are released. These hormones induce the lipolysis of brown fat stores, which are located primarily in the intrascapular, axillary, perirenal, mediastinal, paraspinal, and nuchal regions. Triglycerides in the brown fat deposits are broken down into fatty acids and glycerol, which enter the abundant mitochondria and generate heat. The combustion of fatty acids in brown fat is under the control of an uncoupling protein called thermogenin.

4. What are the manifestations of neonatal cold injury?

Neonatal cold injury is primarily seen in low-birthweight infants but may also be seen in full-term infants with CNS malformations. Characteristics of this syndrome include poor feeding, lethargy, and coldness to touch associated with core temperatures of ≤ 32.2°C. Despite the presence of a bright red skin color, which is secondary to decreased dissociation of oxyhemoglobin, these infants display central cyanosis. Respirations are shallow, irregular, and sometimes associated with grunting. Bradycardia as a function of the degree of temperature depression may also be seen. Other findings include CNS depression with decreased responsiveness, abdominal distention with vomiting, and edema of the skin and face which may progress to sclerema. Concomitant metabolic disturbances include metabolic acidosis, hypoglycemia, hyperkalemia, and azotemia.

5. What are the best ways to warm a hypothermic infant?

Whether rapid or slow rewarming is preferable is a much debated issue, but no good controlled studies exist to answer this question. A general approach consists of placing the infant in a heat-gaining environment to prevent further losses. This can best be achieved by warming the infant in a convectively heated incubator at 36°C with a heat shield to reduce radiant losses and increased humidity to decrease evaporative losses. Under these conditions, the air temperature is approximately equal to the environmental temperature in the incubator. Air temperature should be monitored along with skin temperature, which should not exceed rectal temperature by > 1°C. If the patient's temperature does not stabilize or increase, the incubator temperature should be increased to 37°C and the patient's temperature observed for 15 minutes. If there is still no improvement, the temperature should be increased to 38°C. If temperatures > 38°C are necessary, an overhead warmer may need to be placed over the incubator in order to warm its walls and achieve the desired effect.

6. Should an asymptomatic infant with a single umbilical artery have a screening ultrasound done for renal anomalies?

This point has been argued for years. A single umbilical artery is a rare phenomenon. In one study of nearly 35,000 infants, examination of the placenta showed that only 112 (0.32%) had a single umbilical artery. All 112 underwent renal ultrasonography, and 17% had abnormalities (45% of which persisted). Because of the rarity of the condition and the increased association of abnormalities, patients with single umbilical arteries probably should receive a screening renal ultrasound.

Bourke WG, et al: Isolated single umbilical artery: The case for routine renal screening. Arch Dis Child 68:600–601, 1993.

7. How does the handling of the umbilical cord at birth affect neonatal hemoglobin concentrations?

At the time of birth, the placental vessels may contain up to 33% of the fetal-placental blood volume. Constriction of the umbilical arteries limits blood flow from the infant, but the umbilical vein remains dilated. The extent of drainage from the placenta to the infant via the umbilical vein is very dependent on gravity. The recommendation is to keep the baby at least 20 - 40 cm below the placenta for approximately 30 seconds before clamping the cord. More elevated positioning or rapid clamping can minimize the placental transfusion and decrease red cell volume.

Brugnara C, Platt OS: The neonatal erythrocyte and its disorders. In Nathan DG, Orkin SH (eds): Nathan and Oski's Hematology of Infancy and Childhood, 5th ed. Philadelphia, W.B. Saunders, 1998, pp 30-31.

8. What is the best method of umbilical cord care in the immediate neonatal period?

No single method of cord care has been determined to be superior in preventing colonization and infections. Antimicrobial agents, such as bacitracin or triple dye, are commonly used. Alcohol accelerates drying of the cord, but it has not been shown to reduce the rates of colonization or omphalitis.

9. Which way does the umbilical cord twist?

Usually ***counterclockwise***. Coiling of the umbilical cord occurs in approximately 95% of newborns, and most are twisted in a sinistral manner. Because this helical arrangement is absent in species in which fetuses are arranged longitudinally in a bicornuate uterus, spiraling may result from the mobility of the primate fetus. Noncoiled cords may be associated with an increased likelihood of anomalies.

Strong TH, et al: Antepartum diagnosis of noncoiled umbilical cords. Am J Obstet Gynecol 170: 1729–1733, 1994.

10. When should a parent begin to worry if an umbilical cord has not fallen off?

The umbilical cord generally dries up and sloughs by 2 weeks of life. Delayed separation can be normal up to 45 days. However, because neutrophilic and/or monocytic infiltration appears to play a major role in autodigestion, persistence of the cord beyond 30 days should prompt consideration of an underlying functional abnormality of neutrophils (leukocyte adhesion deficiency) or neutropenia.

Kemp AS, Lubitz L: Delayed cord separation in alloimmune neutropenia. Arch Dis Child 68:52–53, 1993.

11. How do you estimate the insertion distance necessary for umbilical catheters?

Measuring the distance from the umbilicus to the shoulder (lateral end of clavicle) allows an estimation of desired length.

Insertion Distance for Umbilical Catheters (cm)

SHOULDER TO UMBILICUS	AORTIC CATHETER TO DIAPHRAGM	AORTIC CATHETER TO AORTIC BIFURCATION	VENOUS CATHETER TO RIGHT ATRIUM
9	11	5	6
10	12	5	6–7
11	13	6	7
12	14	7	8
13	15	8	8–9
14	16	9	9
15	17	10	10
16	18	10–11	11
17	20	11–12	11–12

From Dunn PM: Localization of umbilical catheters by post mortem measurement. Arch Dis Child 41:69, 1966; with permission.

Alternatively, insertion distance (cm) for:

"high" umbilical ***artery*** catheter = *[3 × weight (kg)] + 9.*

umbilical ***venous*** catheter = *[1/2 × UAC insertion distance] + 1.*

12. What are the risks of umbilical catheters?

Short-term risks

- Perforation and development of retroperitoneal hemorrhage (umbilical artery [UA] catheter)
- Decreased femoral pulses and blanching of limbs and/or buttocks (UA catheter)
- Accidental hemorrhage (both UA and umbilical vein [UV] catheters)
- Infection (both UA and UV catheters)

Long-term risks

- Embolization and infarcts (both UA and UV catheters)
- Thrombosis of hepatic vein (UV catheter)
- Liver necrosis (UV catheter)
- Aortic thrombi (UA catheter)
- Renal artery thrombosis (UA catheter)
- Infection (both UA and UV catheters)

13. What are the increased risks of twin pregnancies?

- Premature delivery
- Intrauterine growth retardation, including discordant growth (which may occur in up to one-third of twin pregnancies)
- Increased perinatal mortality, especially for premature, monozygotic, and discordant twins
- Spontaneous abortion
- Birth asphyxia
- Fetal malposition
- Placental abnormalities (abruptio placentae, placenta previa)
- Polyhydramnios

14. Why are monozygotic twins considered higher risk than dizygotic twins?

Monozygotic twins (identical twins) arise from the division of a single fertilized egg.

Depending on the timing of the division of the single ovum into separate embryos, the amnionic and chorionic membranes can be either shared (if division occurs > 8 days after fertilization), separate (if < 72 hours after fertilization), or mixed (separate amnion, shared chorion if 4–8 days after fertilization). Sharing of the chorion and/or amnion is associated with potential problems of vascular anastomoses (and possible twin–twin transfusions), cord entanglements, and congenital anomalies. These problems increase the risk of intrauterine growth retardation and perinatal death. Dizygotic twins, however, result from two separately fertilized ova and, as such, usually have a separate amnion and chorion.

15. Who is at higher risk, the first- or second-born twin?

The ***second born*** twin has a 2–4-fold increased risk of developing respiratory distress syndrome and is more likely to be asphyxiated. However, the risks for sepsis and necrotizing enterocolitis may be increased in first-born twins.

16. What are the varieties of conjoined twins?

Conjoined twins are classified according to the degree and nature of their union. These are listed below in order of decreasing frequency:

Thoracopagus: Joined at the thorax
Xiphopagus: Joined at anterior abdominal wall
Joined from the xiphoid to the umbilicus
Pygopagus: Joined at buttocks or rump
Ischiopagus: Joined at ischium
Craniopagus: Joined at head

17. Who were Cheng and Eng?

The original “Siamese twins.”

18. How extensive is insensible water loss in preterm infants?

Insensible water loss is the loss of water through the lungs during respiration and from the skin by evaporation. A rough guide to the amount of insensible loss in mL/kg/d for infants in humidified isolettes is:

	BW (gm)					
Age (days)	500–750	751–1000	1001–1250	1251–1500	1501–1750	1751–2000
0-7	100	65	55	40	20	15
7-14	80	60	50	40	30	20

From Avery GB, Fletcher MA and MacDonald MG: Neonatology: Pathophysiology and Management of the Newborn, Lippincott Williams Wilkins, Philadelphia, 1999.

19. What factors affect insensible water loss?

Increase: prematurity, activity, fever, radiant warmer, phototherapy, skin breakdown/defect
Decrease: high humidity, mechanical ventilation (with humidified air)

20. How much does phototherapy increase the fluid requirements of infants?

By ***50%*** if *no heat shield* is used, or by ***10–30%*** if a *plastic heat shield* is used. The increased insensible water loss is believed to result from vasodilation secondary to a direct effect of light on the precapillary arterioles in the skin.

21. When should infection with *Malassezia furfur* be suspected in the neonate?

This dermatophyte, usually found on the skin of infants without clinical disease, can cause signs and symptoms of infection in critically ill and premature infants. Infection is almost always associated with the presence of an indwelling venous catheter. The fat emulsion administered during hyperalimentation is believed to contain fatty acids required for fungal proliferation. Although treatment with amphotericin is effective, removal of the indwelling catheter appears to eliminate the infection in most cases.

22. You are informed during sign-out rounds that a newborn is suspected to have funisitis. Where should you look for that infection?

Funisitis is inflammation of the ***umbilical cord*** vessels and Wharton jelly and has been described as either an acute exudative or subacute necrotizing process accompanying chorioamnionitis. The predominant organisms identified as etiologic agents are gram-negative bacteria, including *Escherichia coli, Klebsiella*, and *Pseudomonas*. Gram-positive organisms (e.g., streptococci, staphylococci) and candidal species are less commonly responsible.

23. Which infants require ophthalmologic evaluation for retinopathy of prematurity (ROP)?

The American Academy of Pediatrics recommends that an individual experienced in neonatal ophthalmology and indirect ophthalmoscopy examine the retinae of all premature neonates (i.e., those who are delivered at < 35 weeks' gestation or who weigh < 1800 gm) who require supplemental oxygen and/or have had an unstable clinical course. Infants who are less mature at birth (i.e., ≤ 28 weeks' gestation or < 1500 gm) should be examined regardless of oxygen exposure. The examination is best done prior to discharge or at 5–7 weeks of age if the infant is still hospitalized.

Hutchinson AK, et al: Timing of initial screen examinations for retinopathy of prematurity. *Arch Ophthalmol* 116:608-612, 1998.

24. What are the stages of ROP?

Stage I: Line of demarcation separates vascular and avascular retina

Stage II: Ridging of line of demarcation secondary to scar formation

Stage III: Extraretinal fibrovascular proliferation present (In addition, in stages II and III, the term plus disease refers to active inflammation as manifested by tortuosity of retinal vessels, which increases the risk of progression of ROP.)

Stage IV: Subtotal retinal detachment

Stage V: Complete retinal detachment

25. What are the indications for cryotherapy or laser therapy in ROP?

In a multicenter trial by the Cryotherapy for ROP Cooperative Group, "threshold" disease, defined as a level of severity at which the risk of blindness approaches 50%, was chosen for treatment. This diagnosis required the presence of at least five contiguous or eight cumulative 30° sectors (clock hours) of stage III ROP (in zone 1 or 2) and the presence of plus disease.

26. How is vitamin E used in the prevention and treatment of ROP?

Recent trials of vitamin E therapy have not shown it to be effective in preventing ROP. However, because of its activity as an antioxidant, vitamin E treatment may lessen the severity of ROP. Serum vitamin E levels should be maintained at 1–2 mg/dl. Higher levels may be associated with toxicity (necrotizing enterocolitis and/or sepsis).

27. Name the conditions associated with abnormalities in maternal serum alpha-fetoprotein concentration.

Increased

- Incorrect gestational dating
- Multiple pregnancy
- Threatened abortion
- Fetomaternal hemorrhage
- Anencephaly
- Open spina bifida
- Anterior abdominal wall defects
- Congenital nephrosis
- Acardia
- Lesions of the placenta and umbilical cord
- Turner syndrome
- Cystic hygroma
- Renal agenesis
- Polycystic kidney disease
- Epidermolysis bullosa
- Hereditary persistence (AD trait)

Decreased

- Incorrect gestational dating
- Trisomy 21
- Trisomy 18
- Intrauterine growth retardation

From Taeusch W, Ballard RA (eds): Avery's Diseases of the Newborn, 7th ed. Philadelphia, W.B. Saunders, 1998, pp 189-190; with permission.

28. If maternal drug abuse is suspected, which specimen from the infant is most accurate in detecting exposure?

Although urine has traditionally been tested when maternal drug abuse is a possibility, ***meconium*** has a greater sensitivity than urine and positive findings that persist longer. It may contain metabolites gathered over multiple weeks, compared with urine which represents more recent exposure. Of note, maternal self-reporting is notoriously inaccurate as an indicator of drug use. In addition, in some states, informed maternal consent must be given prior to drug screening of the neonate, which can hinder diagnosis and surveillance.

Ostrea EM Jr, et al: Drug screening of newborns by meconium analysis: A large-scale, prospective, epidemiologic study. Pediatrics 89:107–113, 1992.

29. What are the manifestations of drug withdrawal in the neonate?

The signs and symptoms of drug withdrawal in the neonate can be remembered by using the mnemonic "withdrawal."

W **W**akefulness
I **I**rritability
T **T**remulousness, temperature variation, tachypnea
H **H**yperactivity, high-pitched persistent cry, hyperacusis, hyperreflexia, hypertonus
D **D**iarrhea, diaphoresis, disorganized suck
R **R**ub marks, respiratory distress, rhinorrhea
A **A**pneic attacks, autonomic dysfunction
W **W**eight loss or failure to gain weight
A **A**lkalosis (respiratory)
L **L**acrimation

Committee on Drugs: Neonatal drug withdrawal. Pediatrics 72:896, 1983.

30. What bone is the most frequently fractured in the newborn?

The ***clavicle***. This injury, which stems from excessive traction during delivery, generally results in a greenstick fracture.

31. Should palpable lymph nodes in a newborn be considered pathologic?

No. Up to 25% of newborns have palpable nodes, particularly in the inguinal and cervical regions. By 1 month of age, the prevalence is nearly 40%.

Bamji M, et al: Palpable lymph nodes in healthy newborns and infants. Pediatrics 78:573–575, 1986.

32. How loud is the noise inside an infant's isolette?

The noise usually ranges from about ***55–75 db*** with a mean value of approximately 66 db. With the slamming of an isolette door, the level can approach 100 db. For comparison, room conversation is 60–70 db and louder rock music is 100–120 db. The American Academy of Pediatrics recommends no more than 58 db to avoid (1) disruption of sleep, (2) cardiovascular changes (e.g., increased heart rate), and (3) potentiation by constant loud noise of ototoxicity secondary to use of aminoglycoside antibiotics.

Beckham R, Mishoe S: Sound levels inside incubators and oxygen hoods used with nebulizaers and humidifiers. Resp Care 35:1272-78, 1990.

Committee on Environmental Hazards: Noise pollution: Neonatal aspects. Pediatrics 54:483–486, 1974.

33. In infants, why is it dangerous to use an IV flush containing benzyl alcohol as a bacteriostatic agent?

In an association first recognized in 1982, IV fluids containing benzyl alcohol can result in progressive CNS depression, increasing respiratory distress with gasps (the "gasping syndrome"), severe metabolic acidosis, thrombocytopenia, hepatic and renal failure, cardiovascular collapse, and death. Benzyl alcohol may also increase the risk of kernicterus by facilitating passage of bilirubin into the CNS. It might be said, look before you flush.

34. How valuable is the footprinting of newborns for the permanent medical record?

A time-honored tradition that is, alas, of minimal benefit. Although the AAP recommended discontinuing the practice in 1983 due to the fact that in nearly 80% the quality was so poor as to render the print useless, up to 80% of U.S. hospitals continue footprinting as a means of identification. Of note, footprinting is legally mandated only in New York State.

35. What are the most common causes of fetal death?

Chromosomal abnormalities (especially in early pregnancy) and *congenital malformations*.

36. How long should a healthy term newborn remain hospitalized?

A controversial issue. Although some neonatal problems do not appear until several days of age, most are apparent by 6 hours of life. Nevertheless, there is an increased frequency of hospital readmissions, most commonly for hyperbilirubinemia, in patients discharged at < 48 hours (some studies even suggest 72 hours) and especially in those discharged at < 24 hours.

Maisels MJ, et al: Length of stay, jaundice and hospital readmission. Pediatrics 101:995-998, 1998.

Braveman P, et al: Early discharge and evidence-based practice: Good science and good judgement. JAMA 278:334-336, 1997.

37. What are Spitzer's Laws of Neonatology?

1. The more stable a baby appears to be, the more likely he will "crump" that day.
2. The nicer the parents, the sicker the baby.
3. The likelihood of BPD (bronchopulmonary dysplasia) is directly proportional to the number of physicians involved in the care of that baby.
4. The longer a patient is discussed on rounds, the more certain it is that no one has the faintest idea of what's going on or what to do.
5. The sickest infant in the nursery can always be discerned by the fact that she is being cared for by the newest, most inexperienced nursing orientee.
6. The surest way to have an infant linger interminably is to inform the parents that death is imminent.
7. The more miraculous the "save," the more likely that you'll be sued for something totally inconsequential.
8. If they're not breathin', they may be seizin'.
9. Antibiotics should always be continued for ____ days. (Fill in the blank with any number from 1 to 21.)

10. If you can't figure out what's going on with a baby, call the surgeons. They won't figure it out either, but they'll sure as hell do something about it.

From Spitzer A: Spitzer's laws of neonatology. Clin Pediatr 20:733, 1981; with permission.

38. What is the Throgmorton sign?

Throgmorton sign is the extension of the suspensory ligament of the penis prior to micturition in newborn infants. However, thousands of house officers have come to believe that this sign relates to the radiographic finding in a male in which the penis points to the side of pathology.

THE DELIVERY ROOM

39. What is the clinical significance of fetal decelerations?

The character or pattern of decelerations often seen during fetal heart rate monitoring can be a valuable indicator of fetal well-being or need for intervention.

Early decelerations: Associated with head compression. Usually of no consequence.

Variable decelerations: Observed with cord compression. May indicate fetal distress when prolonged and associated with bradycardia.

Late decelerations: Indicate uteroplacental insufficiency and the presence of fetal distress. Both variable and late decelerations may be associated with acidosis and fetal compromise.

40. How sensitive is fetal heart rate monitoring in detecting fetal asphyxia?

Abnormal decelerations have a poor positive-predictive value, with only 15–25% being associated with a significantly compromised fetus. However, normal studies have a much higher predictive value of ongoing fetal well-being.

41. What is an acceptable scalp pH in the fetus?

Fetal scalp sampling to measure blood pH is used in conjunction with electronic fetal heart rate monitoring to assess fetal well-being during labor. The range of acceptable values for fetal pH is broad. A pH ≥ 7.25 is considered normal. Values between 7.20 and 7.25 are often referred to as pre-acidotic and may be associated with an increased incidence of depression at delivery. As labor progresses, repeat testing is warranted. A pH < 7.20 may indicate significant fetal compromise.

Normal Fetal Scalp Blood Values in Labor

	EARLY FIRST STAGE	LATE FIRST STAGE	SECOND STAGE
pH	7.33 ± 0.03	7.32 ± 0.02	7.29 ± 0.04
PCO_2 (mm Hg)	44 ± 4.05	42 ± 5.1	46.3 ± 4.2
PO_2 (mm Hg)	21.8 ± 2.6	21.3 ± 2.1	16.5 ± 1.4
Bicarbonate (mmol/L)	20.1 ± 1.2	19.1 ± 2.1	17 ± 2
Base excess (mmol/L)	3.9 ± 1.9	4.1 ± 2.5	6.4 ± 1.8

From Gilstrap LC: Fetal acid-base balance. In Creasy RK, Resnik R (eds): Maternal-Fetal Medicine, 4th ed. Philadelphia, W. B. Saunders, 1999, p 333; with permission.

42. Is length of labor the same for male and female babies?

No. Labor length for boys is about 1 hour longer than for girls.

43. How long has meconium been present in the amniotic fluid if an infant has evidence of meconium staining?

Gross staining of the infant is a surface phenomenon proportional to the length of exposure and meconium concentration. With heavy meconium, staining of the umbilical cord begins in as little as 15 minutes, and with light meconium, after 1 hour. Yellow staining of the newborn's toenails requires 4–6 hours. Yellow staining of the vernix caseosa takes about 12–14 hours.

Miller PW, et al: Dating the time interval from meconium passage to birth. Obstet Gynecol 66:459–462, 1985.

44. Is meconium staining a good marker for neonatal asphyxia?

Because 10–20% of all deliveries have in utero passage of meconium, meconium staining alone is not a good marker for neonatal asphyxia.

45. If meconium is noted prior to or at the time of delivery, what is the recommended course of action?

Regardless of the nature of the fluid, the obstetrician should suction the infant's oro- and nasopharynx prior to delivery of the shoulders. An 8- or 10-French flexible catheter is much more effective than simple bulb syringing. The next course of action depends on the clinical appearance of the baby. If the infant is crying and vigorous, visualization of the larynx and intubation is not necessary. In a depressed infant, the infant's pharynx should be suctioned followed by endotracheal intubation with suctioning below the vocal cords.

Wiswell TE, et al: Delivery room management of the apparently vigorous meconium-stained neonate: Results of the multicenter, international collaborative trial. Pediatrics 105: 1-7, 2000.

46. Name the three initial steps in resuscitation.

Thermal management, clearing the airway, tactile stimulation.

47. During asphyxia, how is primary apnea distinguished from secondary apnea?

A regular sequence of events occurs when an infant is asphyxiated. Initially, gasping respiratory efforts increase in depth and frequency for up to 3 minutes, followed by approximately 1 minute of *primary apnea*. If oxygen (along with stimulation) is provided during the apneic period, respiratory function spontaneously returns. If asphyxia continues, gasping then resumes for a variable period of time, terminating with the "last gasp" and followed by secondary apnea. During *secondary apnea*, the only way to restore respiratory function is with positive pressure ventilation and high concentrations of oxygen.

Thus, a linear relationship exists between the duration of asphyxia and the recovery of respiratory function following resuscitation. The longer the artificial ventilation is delayed after the "last gasp," the longer it will take to resuscitate the infant. However, clinically, the two conditions are indistinguishable.

48. How much pressure does it take to inflate the lungs of a normal infant at the moment of birth?

At the initiation of respiration shortly after birth, pressures of 40–70 cm H_2O are generated to inflate the neonatal lung.

49. How does one estimate the size of an endotracheal tube needed for resuscitation?

Endotracheal Tubes Needed for Resuscitation

TUBE SIZE (ID mm)	WEIGHT	GESTATIONAL AGE
2.0	500–750	< 28 wks
2.5	751–1,000 gm	< 28 wks
3.0	1,001–2,000 gm	28–34 wks
3.5	2,001–3,00 gm	34–38 wks
3.5–4.0	> 3,000 gm	> 38 wks

Adapted from Hertz D: Principles of neonatal resuscitation. In Polin RA, et al: (eds): Workbook in Practical Neonatology, 3d ed. Philadelphia, W.B. Saunders, 2001, p 13; with permission.

50. What is the "7-8-9" rule?

The "7-8-9" rule is an estimate of the length (in cm) that an oral endotracheal tube should be inserted in a 1-, 2-, or 3-kg infant, respectively. A variation of this rule is the tip-to-lip rule of adding 6 to the weight of the infant to determine the insertion distance. With good visualization, the tube should be inserted 1.0–1.5 cm below the vocal cords. Tube placement should always be verified radiographically.

51. Should infants be intubated nasally or orally?

There are studies to support both routes of intubation for newborn infants. The oral intubation school argues that since neonates are obligate nose breathers, they will demonstrate increased work of breathing as well as atelectasis following removal of nasotracheal tubes. On the other hand, the nasal intubation school suggests that orotracheal intubation results in grooving of the palate with subsequent orthodontic problems. A recent study has not confirmed the increased incidence of postextubation atelectasis in nasally intubated babies. Therefore, operator skill and institutional tradition are primary considerations in this clinical decision.

52. How is the size of the endotracheal tube related to the development of subglottic stenosis?

If the endotracheal tube size (mm)/gestational age (wks) ratio is > 0.1, there is an increased risk for development of tracheal stenosis.

53. When should epinephrine be given during a resuscitation in the delivery room?

In a depressed infant with gasping or absent respirations, 100% oxygen should be given via positive pressure ventilation (PPV). Depending on the extent of asphyxia (and depression of heart rate to below 60 bpm), cardiac compressions are usually initiated within 30 seconds. If there is no response (i.e., increased heart rate to greater than 60 bpm) after at least 30 seconds of PPV with 100% oxygen and chest compressions, epinephrine is indicated. Epinephrine, 1:10,000, can be given via IV, umbilical vein, or endotracheal tube at a dose of 0.1–0.3 ml/kg.

54. When is sodium bicarbonate administered in a resuscitation?

If there is no response to epinephrine in a severely asphyxiated infant (with continued apnea and a heart rate < 60), sodium bicarbonate (and/or a volume expander) should be considered. If an infant is being adequately ventilated, the partial correction of metabolic acidosis may improve pulmonary blood flow and improve oxygenation. Half-strength (4.2% solution or 0.5 mEq/l) bicarbonate is preferable, given in a dose of 2 mEq/kg slowly over 2–5 minutes.

55. Are there complications of sodium bicarbonate therapy in infants?

The relative risks of sodium bicarbonate therapy in infants are related to dosage (higher > lower), rapidity of administration (faster > slower), and osmolality (higher > lower). Physiologic complications include a transient increase in PaCO2 and fall in PaO2. The sudden expansion of blood volume and increase in cerebral blood flow may increase the risk of periventricular-intraventricular hemorrhage in preterm infants. Other potential complications include the development of hypernatremia and metabolic alkalosis.

56. If the newborn is stabilized and extent of acidosis determined by an arterial blood gas, how is the therapeutic correction calculated?

$$HCO_3 \text{ (mEq)} = \text{Base deficit (mEq/L)} \times 0.3 \text{ L/kg} \times \text{body wt (kg)}$$

Generally, it is safest to correct half the base deficit initially, and then reassess acid-base status to determine if further correction is necessary. Under optimal circumstances, sodium bicarbonate should be infused in small doses over 20–30 minutes as a dilute solution (0.5 mEq/ml).

57. What are the side effects of naloxone?

Naloxone has a history of being remarkably free of side effects, except for precipitating manifestations of sudden drug withdrawal in infants born to drug-addicted mothers. Other reported side effects relate to the sudden release of catecholamines, which can cause hypertension, sudden cardiac arrest, and cardiac dysrhythmias. It is important to remember that the half-life of naloxone is significantly shorter than that of narcotics.

58. Should umbilical arterial catheters be kept in a "low" or "high" position?

Umbilical catheters kept in a low position (L3–5) have a somewhat higher incidence of lower limb blanching and cyanosis compared to high lines (T6–10). However, high lines may be associated with a slightly increased risk of periventricular-intraventricular hemorrhage as well as embolization of clots to arterial vessels distal to the catheter site. No differences in the development of sepsis or necrotizing enterocolitis have been noted between infants with low or high umbilical catheters.

59. After a "traumatic" delivery, what are the commonly injured systems?

Cranial injuries: caput succedaneum, subconjunctival hemorrhage, cephalohematoma, skull fractures, intracranial hemorrhage, cerebral edema

Spinal injuries: spinal cord transection

Peripheral nerve injuries: brachial palsy (Erb-Duchenne paralysis, Klumpke paralysis), phrenic nerve and facial nerve paralysis

Visceral injuries: liver rupture or hematoma, splenic rupture, adrenal hemorrhage

Skeletal injuries: fractures of the clavicle, femur, and humerus

60. Who was Virginia Apgar?

Virginia Apgar, an anesthesiologist at Columbia Presbyterian Medical Center, introduced the Apgar scoring system in 1953 to assess the newborn infant's response to the stress of labor and delivery.

61. How does one remember the Apgar score?

A **A**ppearance (pink, mottled, or blue)
P **P**ulse (> 100, < 100, or 0 bpm)
G **G**rimace (response to suctioning of the nose and mouth)
A **A**ctivity (flexed arms and legs, extended limbs, or limp)
R **R**espiratory effort (crying, gasping, or no respiratory activity)

Each category is assigned a rating of 0, 1, or 2 points with a total score of 10 indicating the best possible condition. A score of < 3 at one minute implies possible asphyxia and the score at 5 minutes gauges the response to resuscitative efforts.

62. Is a low Apgar score alone sufficient to diagnose a neonate as asphyxiated?

No. It is not acceptable to label an infant as asphyxiated simply because of a low Apgar score. Asphyxiated neonates typically have a profound metabolic acidosis and demonstrate abnormalities in multiple organ systems. Signs referable to the CNS are often most prominent. The cardinal features of hypoxic-ischemic encephalopathy include seizures, alterations of consciousness, and abnormalities of tone. Disorders of reflexes, respiratory pattern, oculovestibular responses, and autonomic function are less significant components of this entity. Measurement of the urinary lactate:creatinine ratio is under study as a marker for early indentification of newborns at risk for hypoxic-ischemic encephalopathy.

Huang C-C, et al: Measurement of the urinary lactate:creatinine ratio for early identification of newborns at risk for hypoxic-ischemic encepalopathy. N Engl J Med 341:328-335, 1999.

Committee on Fetus and Newborn: Use and abuse of the Apgar score. Pediatrics 98:141–142, 1996.

63. When should a neonatal resuscitation be stopped?

No precise answer is possible, as clinical circumstances and responses are variable. However, in one study of 58 newborns who had an Apgar score of 0 at 10 minutes despite appropriate resuscitative efforts, only 1 of 58 survived and that infant had profound cerebral palsy. Failure of response after 10–15 minutes should prompt consideration of cessation.

Jain L: Cardiopulmonary resuscitation of apparently stillborn infants: Survival and long-term outcome. J Pediatr 118:778–782, 1991.

DEVELOPMENT AND GROWTH

64. What is the best way to assess gestational age in the fetus?

Nägele's rule, dating pregnancy from the first day of the last menstrual period, has historically been the most reliable way to assess gestational age. However, *ultrasound measurements* done between 5–20 weeks of gestation can predict gestational age quite accurately. Prior to 12 weeks' gestation, crown–rump length is the measurement of choice, and beyond 12 weeks', biparietal diameter is the preferred study. In later gestation, the accuracy of fetal age determination is improved by the assessment of multiple variables (e.g., femur length, abdominal circumference, and biparietal diameter) and by serial determinations. *Maternal dates* should always be used as the "gold standard" unless ultrasound studies are highly discrepant. Estimates of *uterine size*, which approximate gestational age from 16–38 weeks, may also be clinically useful.

65. What features constitute the biophysical profile?

The biophysical profile is a scoring system that assesses fetal well-being prior to birth. Five variables are assessed: ***fetal breathing movements, gross body movements, fetal tone, reactive fetal heart rate***, and qualitative ***amniotic fluid volume***. Normal results equate to 2 points per variable, for a possible total of 10 points.

66. How can gestational age be determined by looking at the lens of the eye?

In fetal ocular development, a web of blood vessels on the anterior lens fades as gestation progresses. Ophthalmoscopic examination of the anterior lens allows an estimation of gestational age:

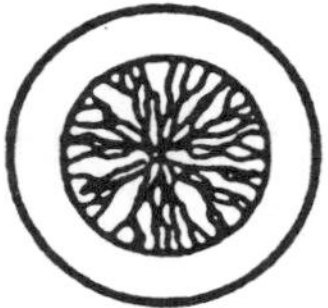
Grade 4
27 to 28 weeks

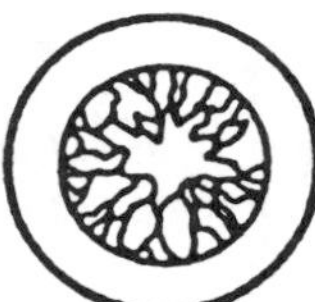
Grade 3
29 to 30 weeks

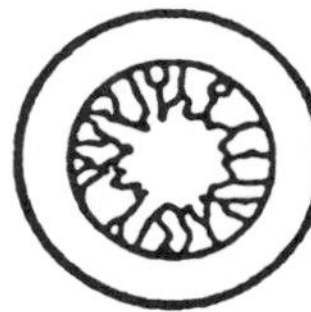
Grade 2
31 to 32 weeks

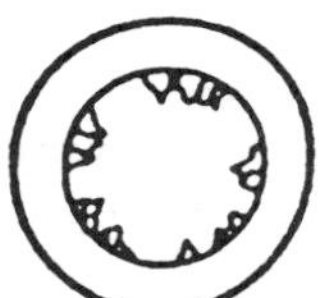
Grade 1
33 to 34 weeks

From Hittner H, et al: Assessment of gestational age by examination of the anterior capsule of the lens. J Pediatr 91:455, 1977; with permission.

67. What is the first bone in the human fetus to ossify?

The ***clavicle***. In the long bones, the process of ossification occurs in the primary centers of ossification in the diaphysis during the embryonic period of fetal development. Although the femora are the first long bones to show traces of ossification, the clavicles, which develop initially by intramembranous ossification, begin to ossify before any other bones in the body.

68. What external characteristics are useful for estimating gestational age?

External Gestational Age Characteristics

EXTERNAL CHARACTERISTICS	GESTATIONAL AGE			
	28 WKS	32 WKS	36 WKS	40 WKS
Ear cartilage	Pinna soft, remains folded	Pinna slightly harder but remains folded	Pinna harder, springs back	Pinna firm, stands erect from head
Breast tissue	None	None	1–2 mm nodule	6–7 mm nodule
External genitalia				
Male	Testes undescended, smooth scrotum	Tested in inguinal canal, few scrotal rugae	Testes high in scrotum, more scrotal rugae	Testes descended, pendulous scrotum covered with rugae
Female	Prominent clitoris, small, widely separated labia	Prominent clitoris, larger separated labia	Clitoris less prominent, labia majora cover labia minora	Clitoris covered by labia majora
Plantar surface	Smooth	1–2 anterior creases creases	2–3 anterior	Creases cover sole

From Volpe JJ: Neurology of the Newborn, 3rd ed. Philadelphia, W.B. Saunders, 1995, p 96; with permission.

69. At what gestational age does pupillary reaction to light develop?

Pupillary reaction to light may appear as early as 29 weeks' gestation but is not consistently present until approximately 32 weeks.

70. At what gestational age does a sense of smell develop?

By ***32 weeks'*** gestation, normal premature infants respond to concentrated odor.

71. When does the fetal heart begin to contract in utero?

Contractions begin by the ***22nd day*** of gestation. These contractions resemble peristaltic waves and begin in the sinus venosus. By the end of the 4th week, they result in unidirectional flow of blood.

72. How does fetal circulation differ from neonatal circulation?

- Intra- and extracardiac shunts are present: placenta, ductus venosus, foramen ovale, ductus arteriosus.
- The two ventricles work in parallel rather than in series.
- The right ventricle pumps against a higher resistance than the left ventricle.
- Blood flow to the lung is only a fraction of the right ventricular output.
- The lung extracts oxygen from the blood instead of providing oxygen for it.
- The lung continually secretes a fluid into the respiratory passages.
- The liver is the first organ to receive maternal substances, such as oxygen, glucose, amino acids, etc.
- The placenta is the major route of gas exchange, excretion, and acquisition of essential fetal chemicals.
- The placenta provides a low resistance circuit.

Allen HD, et al. (eds): Moss and Adams' Heart Disease in Infants, Children, and Adolescents, 6th ed. Baltimore, Williams & Wilkins, 2001, pp 41-63.

73. What changes occur in stroke volume, cardiac output, and heart rate after birth?

Both stroke volume (SV) and cardiac output (CO) increase into adolescence, whereas heart rate (HR) falls.

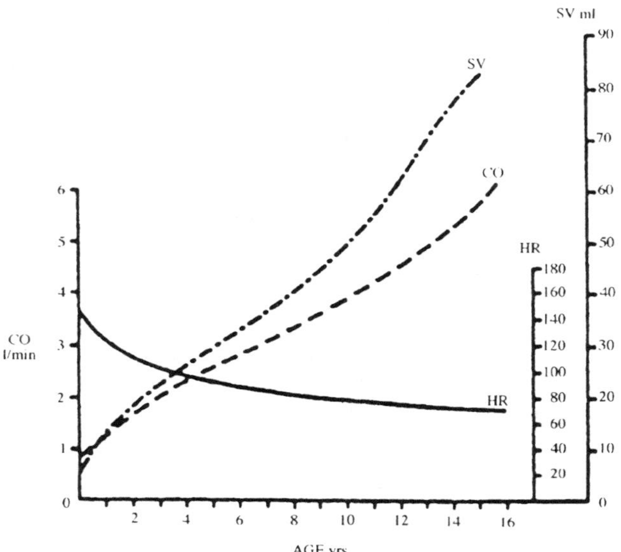

From Rudolph AM: Congenital Diseases of the Heart. Chicago, Year Book Medical Publishers, 1974; with permission.

74. Why does pulmonary vascular resistance (PVR) decline postnatally?

Within minutes after birth, the PVR drops due to rapid recruitment of peripheral arteries previously "closed." The phase of accelerated recruitment of peripheral arteries results from a combination of events, including gaseous expansion of the lung (with removal of fluid), a fall in arterial PCO_2, and a rise in arterial PO_2. PVR continues to decrease in the days following birth, principally from a gradual decrease in medial wall thickness of smaller muscular arteries (< 250 mm). Within a few months, the more proximal vessels (> 250 mm) also show a decrease in medial wall thickness. However, the specific mechanism(s) responsible for the remodeling of the pulmonary vasculature after birth are unknown.

75. How does postmaturity differ from dysmaturity?

An infant born of a postterm pregnancy (> 42 weeks' gestation) is referred to as *postmature*. The baby is *dysmature* if features of placental insufficiency are present. These include loss of subcutaneous fat and muscle mass, as well as meconium staining of the amniotic fluid, skin, and nails.

76. What is the normal rate of head growth in the preterm infant?

0.5–1.0 cm/wk during the first 2–4 months of life. An increase in the circumference of the head of ≥ 2.0 cm in 1 week should raise a suspicion of CNS pathology, such as hydrocephalus. However, some premature infants may experience rapid "catch-up" head growth following significant early stress or illness. The ratio of body length to head circumference may be used to distinguish normal from abnormal head growth. A ratio of 1.42–1.48 is reportedly normal, whereas a low ratio of 1.12–1.32 indicates relative or absolute macrocephaly.

77. How is the ponderal index used to classify growth-retarded infants?

$$\textit{Ponderal index}\ (\text{PI}) = \frac{\text{weight (gm)}}{(\text{length [cm]})^3} \times 100$$

This index has been used to estimate the adequacy of intrauterine fetal nutrition. Values < 2.0 between 29 and 37 weeks' gestation and 2.2 beyond 37 weeks' have been associated with fetal malnutrition. Growth-retarded infants with low ponderal indices also appear to be at increased risk for the development of neonatal hypoglycemia. Maternal conditions associated with a low ponderal index (fetal malnutrition) include poor maternal weight gain, lack of prenatal care, preeclampsia, and chronic maternal illness.

78. What morbidities (short- and long-term) are known to occur more frequently in growth-retarded babies?

Short-term morbidities include perinatal asphyxia, meconium aspiration, fasting hypoglycemia, alimented hypoglycemia, polycythemia-hyperviscosity, and immunodeficiency.

Long-term morbidities include poor developmental outcome and altered postnatal growth. Most studies demonstrate normal intelligence and developmental quotients in SGA infants, although there seems to be a higher incidence of behavioral and learning problems. The presence or absence of severe perinatal asphyxia is extremely important in predicting later intellectual and neurologic function.

Strauss RS: Adult functional outcome of those born small for gestational age: Twenty-six year follow-up of the 1970 British Birth Cohort. JAMA 283:625-632, 2000.

79. When do premature infants "catch-up" on growth charts?

Most catch-up growth takes place during the first 2 years of life, with maximal growth rates occurring between 36–40 weeks postconception. Little catch-up growth occurs after 3 years' chronologic age. Approximately 15% of infants born prematurely remain below normal weight at 3 years of age.

80. What is the outcome for extremely premature babies?

While outcomes differ by centers, summaries of data indicate that severe disability occurs in about 33% of 23 week babies, 25% of 24 week babies and 20% of 25 week babies. Infants born before the 29th week of gestation represent less than 1% of all births but 30% of all cases of cerebral palsy.

Woods NS, et al: Neurologic and developmental disability after extremely premature birth. N Engl J Med 343: 378-384, 2000.

Hack M, Fanaroff AA: Outcomes of children of extremely low birthweight and gestational age in the 1990s. Semin Neonatol 5:89-106, 2000.

GASTROINTESTINAL ISSUES

81. When does the newborn infant's stomach begin to secrete acid?

The pH of gastric fluid in newborns is usually neutral or slightly acidic and decreases shortly after birth. pH values are < 3 by 6–8 hours of age and then increase again during the second week of life. Preterm infants frequently demonstrate gastric pH values > 7.

82. At what rate do the disaccharidases develop prenatally?

The disaccharidases are detectable with low activity at about 12–14 weeks of gestation, and by 24 weeks, sucrase, maltase, and isomaltase generally achieve significant levels of activity. Lactase activity lags behind and is frequently not detected until 28–30 weeks of gestation. Many preterm and term infants demonstrate lactose intolerance when measured by breath hydrogen analysis; however, the significance of subclinical lactose intolerance is controversial.

83. When is meconium usually passed after birth?

Most infants pass some meconium in the first 12 hours of life. Overall, 99% of term infants and 95% of premature infants pass meconium by 48 hours of life. However, the smallest of premature infants may have delayed passage of meconium due to relative immaturity of rectal sphincteric reflexes.

84. What differentiates meconium ileus from meconium plug syndrome?

Meconium ileus: Obstruction of the distal ileum occurs secondary to thick, tenacious concretions of inspissated meconium. A barium enema may reveal a microcolon, and 25% of cases have associated intestinal atresia due to intrauterine obstruction. Meconium ileus is a common presentation of cystic fibrosis in the newborn period.

Meconium plug syndrome: This condition presents as either delayed passage of meconium or intestinal obstruction. Barium enema usually demonstrates a normal caliber colon with multiple filling defects. Small preterm infants, infants of diabetic mothers, and infants born to mothers who received magnesium sulfate are especially likely to develop meconium plug syndrome. There is also an increased frequency of cystic fibrosis in infants with meconium plug syndrome, although much less than with meconium ileus.

85. After an asphyxial event, how long should feeding be delayed?

During an asphyxial event, vasoconstriction of the mesenteric vessels can result in intestinal ischemia. Because of the relationship between ischemia and the incidence of necrotizing enterocolitis, feedings should be delayed for ***2–3 days*** to allow for repair of the intestinal mucosa.

86. List the four types of congenital diaphragmatic defects.

1. Posterolateral defect, or Bochdalek hernia
2. Parasternal defect, or Morgagni hernia
3. Septum transversum defects
4. Congenitally large esophageal orifice or hiatal hernias

87. How is gastroschisis differentiated from omphalocele in the newborn infant?

Both are ventral wall defects, yet their pathogenesis and prognosis differ markedly.

	GASTROSCHISIS	OMPHALOCELE
Incidence	1/50,000 births	1/5,000 births
Location of defect	Right paraumbilical	Central umbilical
Umbilical cord insertion	Normal	Apex of sac
Herniation of liver	Rare	Common
Extraintestinal nomalies	Rare	Common
Chromosomal abnormalities	Rare	Common

88. Which conditions are associated with intra-abdominal calcifications?

Meconium peritonitis and ***intra-abdominal tumors*** are the most common disorders associated with intra-abdominal calcifications in the neonate. The calcifications of meconium peritonitis are streaky or plaque-like and occur over the abdominal surface of the diaphragm or along the flanks. Intraintestinal calcifications appear as small round densities that follow the course of the intestine and occur in association with intestinal stenoses, atresias, and aganglionosis. Intra-abdominal calcifications have also been observed in infants with *adrenal hemorrhages* and *congenital infections*.

89. How is necrotizing enterocolitis (NEC) distinguished from volvulus?

	NEC	VOLVULUS
Pretetm infants	85–90%	30–35%
Onset by day 14 of life	85–90%	50–60%
Male:female	1:1	2:1
Associated anomalies	Rare	25–40%
Bilious emesis	Unusual	75%
Grossly bloody stools	Common	Less common
Pneumatosis intestinalis	80–90%	1–2%
Marked proximal duodenal obstruction (x-ray)	Rare	Common
Thrombocytopenia without DIC	Common	Rare

DIC, disseminated intravascular coagulation.
From Kleigman RM: Necrotizing enterocolitis: Differential diagnosis and management. In Polin RA, et al (eds): Workbook in Practical Neonatology, 2nd ed. Philadelphia, W.B. Saunders, 1993, p 456; with permission.

90. Are positive blood cultures common in babies with NEC?
Approximately 25% will have a positive blood culture at the time of diagnosis.

91. When is paracentesis indicated in a neonate with suspected NEC?
When there is a high suspicion of intestinal gangrene but no radiographic evidence of free air in the abdomen, abdominal paracentesis should be considered. A positive paracentesis, as indicated by the presence of brown fluid or bacteria on Gram stain, is diagnostic of intestinal gangrene with a specificity approaching 100%.

92. Is pneumatosis intestinalis pathognomonic for NEC?
No. Pneumatosis intestinalis can be seen in various other conditions, including Hirschsprung disease, pseudomembranous enterocolitis, neonatal ulcerative colitis, and ischemic bowel disease.

93. How long should infants with NEC be kept NPO?
Infants with *true* NEC (radiographic or surgical evidence) should remain NPO for a ***minimum of 2–3 weeks***. Infants in whom the diagnosis is *suspected but not proven* should be treated conservatively. Many of these infants may be fed ***after 3–7 days***.

94. Does the feeding of immunoglobulin to infants or the use of prophylactic antibotics prevent NEC?
Immunoglobulins: Preliminary studies show that formula fortified with immunoglobulins (IgA and IgG) may effectively reduce the incidence of NEC in very-low-birthweight infants. IgA may provide local mucosal protection, while IgG may neutralize toxins of ingested pathogenic bacteria. More definitive studies are needed to evaluate this promising therapy.

Antibiotics: In two small studies of high-risk, low-birthweight infants, the administration of oral kanamycin/gentamicin was effective in preventing NEC. However, study infants became colonized with organisms resistant to these antibiotics. More recent studies have failed to show a decreased incidence of NEC following prophylactic oral antibiotics. Therefore, antibiotic prophylaxis is not indicated for the prevention of NEC.

95. What is pig-bel?
Pig-bel is an NEC-like disease afflicting infants and adults in Papua, New Guinea. It is caused by ingestion of *Clostridium perfringens* type C enterotoxin.

96. How is the volume of gastric aspirate helpful in the diagnosis of intestinal obstruction in a newborn?

A large aspirate in the first 15 minutes after birth suggests obstruction. In normal term newborns, the mean gastric aspirate is about 5 ml. In newborns with obstruction (e.g., duodenal atresia, jejunal atresia, annular pancreas), the mean aspirate is approximately 60 ml. Any gastric aspirate > 20 ml should be viewed as suspicious.

Britton JR, Britton HL: Gastric aspirate volume at birth as an indication of congenital intestinal obstruction. Acta Pediatr 84:945–946, 1995.

HEMATOLOGIC ISSUES

97. When does the switchover from fetal to adult hemoglobin synthesis occur in the neonate?

The switch from production of hemoglobin F to hemoglobin A begins in a very programmed fashion in the fetus and neonate at approximately 32 weeks' gestation. At birth, approximately 50–65% of hemoglobin is type F.

98. How do the relative amounts of hemoglobin polypeptide chains vary in the fetus and infant?

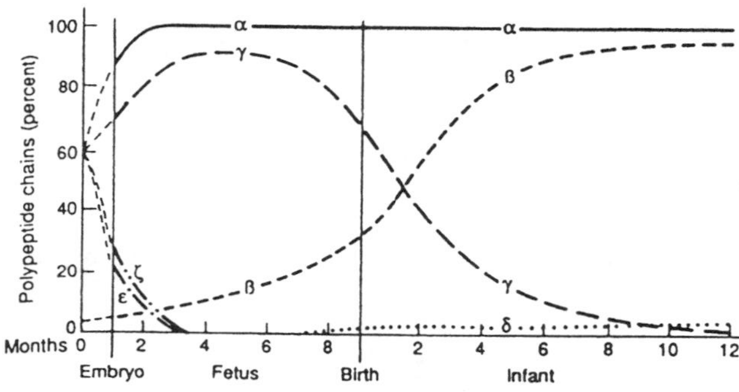

From Lane PA, et al: Hematologic disorders. In Hay WW, et al (eds): Current Pediatric Diagnosis & Treatment, 14th ed. Norwalk, CT, Appleton & Lange, 1999, p 735; with permission.

99. Does the definition of anemia vary by gestational age?

For the term infant, most authorities consider a *venous* blood hemoglobin of ***< 13.0 gm/dl*** or a *capillary* hemoglobin of ***< 14.5 gm/dl*** as consistent with anemia. In preterm infants beyond 32 weeks' gestation, hematologic values differ only minimally from those of full-term infants, and therefore the same values may be used.

100. Describe the changes in hemoglobin concentration seen during the first few days of life.

In all newborn infants, hemoglobin levels rise slightly during the first few hours of life (because of hemoconcentration) and then fall somewhat during the remainder of the first day. In healthy full-term infants, the hemoglobin concentration then stays relatively constant for the rest of the first week of life. However, appropriate-for-gestational-age infants of < 1500 gm birthweight may show a decline of 1.0–1.5 gm/day during this same period.

101. What are the indications for RBC transfusions in premature infants?

In recent years, criteria for red blood cell transfusions have become far more stringent. The following guidelines are derived from the U.S. Multicenter Trial of Erythropoietin in Treating Anemia of Prematurity.

Transfuse infants at Hct ≤ 20%:

- If asymptomatic with reticulocytes <100,000/μL

Transfuse infants at Hct ≤30%:

- If receiving <35% supplemental hood oxygen
- If on CPAP or mechanical ventilation with MAP<6 cm H_2O
- If significant apnea and bradycardia are noted (>9 episodes in 12 hours or 2 episodes requiring bag and mask ventilation) while receiving therapeutic doses of methylxanthines
- If HR >180 beats/min or RR >80 breaths/min persistently for 24 hours
- If weight gain <10 g/d over 4 days while receiving ≥100 kcal/kg/d
- If undergoing surgery

Transfuse for Hct ≤35%:

- If receiving >35% supplemental hood oxygen
- If on CPAP or mechanical ventilation with MAP ≥ 6-8 cm H_2O

Do not transfuse:

- To replace blood removed for laboratory tests alone
- For low hematocrit alone

Shannon KM, et al: Recombinant human erythropoietin stimulates erythropoiesis and reduces erythrocyte transfusions in very low birth weight preterm infants. Pediatrics 95: 1-8, 1995.

102. Which neonates should receive irradiated blood?

All premature infants and infants < 1500 gm should receive irradiated blood.

103. How does phlebotomy in a premature infant compare with that in an adult?

Withdrawing 1 ml of blood from a 1000-gm infant is equivalent to taking 70 ml of blood from an adult. It appears to be common in NICU practice to submit blood volumes for lab tests in excess of the required amount and thus iatrogenically contributing to anemia of prematurity.

Lin JC et al: Phlebotomy overdraw in the neonatal intensive care nursery. Pediatrics 106: e19, 2000.

104. Which antigens make up the Rh complex?

The Rh antigen complex is made up of six possible antigens: C, c, D, d, E, e. The vast majority of isoimmunizations causing serious neonatal disease are the result of incompatibility to the D antigen. The non-D Rh antigens (E, C, c) have been shown to cause hemolytic disease and may be associated with mild to severe hydrops fetalis.

105. How can Rh disease be prevented?

Unsensitized pregnant women who are Rh-negative should have a repeat antibody screen at approximately 28 weeks' gestation and receive 300 mg of Rh-immune globulin (RhoGAM) prophylactically. After delivery, if the infant is Rh-positive, the mother should receive an additional dose of RhoGAM. At the time of delivery, the dose of RhoGAM may be increased if the fetomaternal hemorrhage is excessively large.

106. Why is the direct Coombs' test frequently negative or weakly positive in infants with ABO incompatibility?

There are fewer A or B antigenic sites on the newborn red cell, and there is also a greater distance between antigenic sites when compared to adult red cells. There is also absorption of serum antibody by naturally occurring A and B substances scattered throughout body tissues, in foods, and gram-negative bacteria.

107. If fetomaternal hemorrhage is suspected as a cause of neonatal anemia, how is this diagnosed?

The ***Kleihauer-Betke test*** detects the presence of fetal cells in the maternal circulation. It involves an acid elution technique, which utilizes the property of fetal hemoglobin to resist elution in an acid medium. In a stained maternal blood smear, the fetal cells stain darkly, and the percentage of fetal red cells can be determined. One percent fetal cells in the maternal circulation indicates a bleed of 50 ml.

108. If a gastric aspirate contains blood shortly after birth, what test can determine if it is swallowed maternal blood or fetal hemorrhage?

The ***Apt test***. This test relies on the increased sensitivity of adult hemoglobin to alkali compared with fetal hemoglobin.

Method: Mix the specimen with an equal quantity of tap water. Centrifuge or filter. Supernatant must have pink color to proceed. To 5 parts of supernatant, add 1 part of 0.25 N (1%) NaOH.

Interpretation: A pink color persisting > 2 minutes indicates fetal hemoglobin. Adult hemoglobin gives a pink color that becomes yellow in 2 minutes or less, indicating denaturation of hemoglobin.

109. How is polycythemia defined?

Polycythemia is defined by a venous hematocrit of ≥ 65%, since this exceeds the mean hematocrit found in normal newborns by 2 standard deviations. As the central venous hematocrit rises above 65%, there is a dramatic increase in viscosity. Since direct measurements of blood viscosity are not readily available in most labs, a high hematocrit is felt to be the best indicator of hyperviscosity.

110. What are the clinical manifestations of polycythemia?

In *symptomatic* infants, the most common presentations relate to CNS abnormalities, including lethargy, hypotonia, tremulousness, and irritability. With severe CNS involvement, seizures can result. Hypoglycemia is common. Other organ systems can be involved, including the GI tract (vomiting, distension, NEC), kidneys (renal vein thrombosis and acute renal failure), and cardiopulmonary system (respiratory distress, congestive heart failure). Peripheral manifestations can include gangrene and priapism. Of note, infants with polycythemia are often *asymptomatic*.

111. In what settings is polycythemia most likely to occur?

Although the most common cause is idiopathic, identifiable causes result primarily from two mechanisms:

ACTIVE (INCREASED INTRAUTERINE ERYTHROPOIESIS)	PASSIVE (SECONDARY TO ERYTHROCYTE TRANSFUSIONS)
Intrauterine hypoxia	*Delayed cord clamping*
Placental insufficiency	Intentional
SGA infants	Unassisted delivery
Postmaturity	*Maternofetal transfusion*
Toxemia of pregnancy	*Twin-twin transfusion*
Drugs (propranolol)	
Severe maternal heart disease	
Maternal smoking	
Maternal diabetes	
Neonatal hyper- or hypothyroidism	
Congenital adrenal hyperplasia	
Chromosome abnormalities	
Trisomy 13, 18, 21	
Hyperplastic visceromegaly (Beckwith syndrome)	
Decreased fetal erythrocyte deformability	

From Oski FA, Naiman JL: Hematologic Problems in the Newborn, 3rd ed. Philadelphia, W.B. Saunders, 1982; with permission.

112. Which infants with polycythemia should be treated?

Because polycythemia results from a diverse array of etiologies, it is difficult to determine whether outcome depends more on etiology or the chronic elevation of *viscosity*. There is controversy regarding guidelines for treatment. Many authorities recommend a partial exchange transfusion, regardless of symptoms, in infants with a central venous hematocrit ≥ 70% (due to the correlation with laboratory-measured hyperviscosity) or those with a central hematocrit ≥ 65% if there are signs and symptoms attributable to polycythemia.

113. Describe the preferred method for partial exchange transfusions in polycythemic neonates.

Partial exchange transfusions can be performed through an umbilical venous catheter, umbilical arterial catheter, or peripheral venous catheter. Aliquots equal to 5% of the estimated blood volume are withdrawn and replaced by either fresh frozen plasma, Plasmanate, 5% albumin, or normal saline. The latter two solutions may be preferable since they avoid the risks of transfusion-acquired infections associated with plasma. The amount of blood volume to be exchanged with crystalloid or colloid may be calculated using the following formula:

Blood volume to be exchanged =

$$\frac{\text{Observed Hct} - \text{desired Hct (55\%)}}{\text{Observed Hct}} \times \text{Blood volume (85 – 100 ml/kg)} \times \text{Body wt (kg)}$$

114. What is the long-term morbidity of polycythemia in newborns?

Follow-up studies suggest that early polycythemia (and particularly hyperviscosity) may be associated with mild neuropsychologic handicaps, lower school achievement, fine motor abnormalities, and more speech delay in comparison with control infants in the first years of life.

Drew JH, et al: Neonatal whole blood hyperviscosity: The important factor influencing later neurologic function is the viscosity and not the polycythemia. Clin Hem & Microcirc 17:67-72, 1997.

Black VD, et al: Neonatal hyperviscosity: Association with lower achievement and IQ scores at school age. Pediatrics 83:662–667, 1989.

115. What is the definition of thrombocytopenia in the neonate?

Platelet counts ***< 100,000/mm³*** should be considered abnormal in term or preterm neonates, whereas counts in the 100,000–150,000/mm^3 range may be seen in some healthy newborns. Consequently, patients with counts in this latter category should have repeat counts as well as further studies if illness is suspected.

116. What is the differential diagnosis in a newborn with a confirmed low platelet count?

Causes of increased platelet destruction	*Causes of decreased platelet production*
Maternal idiopathic thrombocytopenic purpura	Congenital amegakaryocytic hypoplasia (e.g., (TAR)
Isoimmune thrombocytopenia	Bone marrow replacement
Infection	Pancytopenias (e.g., Fanconi anemia, trisomy 13 and 18)
Disseminated intravascular coagulation	
Drugs	
Extensive localized thrombosis	
Critically ill infants	*Undetermined mechanism*
Giant hemangiomas	Inborn errors of metabolism
Maternal lupus	Congenital thyrotoxicosis

From Andrew M, Kolton J: Neonatal thrombocytopenia. Clin Perinatol 11:363, 1984; with permission.

117. What features on physical exam suggest a specific cause for thrombocytopenia?

- ***"Blueberry muffin rash"*** (TORCH or viral infection)
- ***Absence of radii*** (TAR syndrome)
- ***Palpable flank mass*** and *hematuria* (renal vein thrombosis)
- ***Hemangioma***, large, often with bruit (Kasabach-Merritt syndrome)
- ***Abnormal thumbs*** (Fanconi syndrome, albeit thrombocytopenia less likely in newborns)
- ***Markedly dysmorphic features*** (chromosomal abnormalities, particularly Trisomy 13 or 18)

118. What are the two main types of neonatal thrombocytopenia caused by maternal antibody?

Transplacental passage of antibody from the mother to infant can be due to (1) ***maternal idiopathic thrombocytopenic purpura*** (ITP, with the newborn a secondary target) and (2) ***isoimmune thrombocytopenia*** (with the newborn a primary target). The diseases can have a similar clinical appearance. Babies are generally well-appearing, do not have hepatosplenomegaly, and have thrombocytopenia that persists for 3–12 weeks postnatally. Differences include:

	MATERNAL ITP	ISOIMMUNE NEONATAL THROMBOCYTOPENIA
Estimated incidence	Uncertain, ? in 300 births	1 in 500 births
Offending antigen	Probably part of platelet membrane glycoprotein IIb–IIIa complex: on *all* platelets	PLA[1] (Zw[a]) or HLA: on father's and neonate's platelets but not mother's
Type of antibody	Maternal autoantibody	Maternal alloantibody (isoantibody) directed against foreign platelet antigen
Maternal platelet count	Reduced (unless previous splenectomy)	Always normal
Recurrence risk	Cannot be reliably estimated from maternal platelet count	50–85% (depending on offending antigen and zygosity of father)

From Buchanan GR: Coagulation disorders in the neonate. Pediatr Cin North Am 33:212, 1986; with permission.

119. How should women known to have a previous infant with alloimmune thrombocytopenia be evaluated during pregnancy?

Fetal thrombocytopenia can usually be detected at 20–22 weeks' gestation through percutaneous umbilical blood sampling. An additional evaluation at 37 weeks' gestation is indicated to assist in directing antepartum treatments. In utero therapy includes fetal platelet transfusions with carefully washed maternal platelets and administration of intravenous immunoglobulin to the mother.

An infant with thrombocytopenia should be delivered via cesarean section to reduce the risk of intracranial hemorrhage.

120. In the mother with new-onset thrombocytopenia during pregnancy, how can one determine the risk to the fetus?

The maternal platelet count is a poor predictor of risk of thrombocytopenia in the fetus. However, an elevated maternal titer of ***circulating antiplatelet IgG*** places the infant at high risk for thrombocytopenia. When maternal thrombocytopenia is limited to late pregnancy, however, the risk for developing severe neonatal thrombocytopenia is low. In mothers who have circulating antiplatelet antibody (IgG), the infant should be delivered via cesarean section, or a cordocentesis should be performed to demonstrate a normal platelet count prior to a vaginal delivery.

121. When should a thrombocytopenic infant receive a platelet transfusion?

Infants with platelet counts of < 20,000/mm^3, or those with clinical signs of bleeding regardless of the actual count, should receive platelet transfusions. In infants at increased risk for hemorrhage (e.g., postoperative) the platelet count should be kept > 100,000/mm^3.

122. How long do transfused platelets survive?

If thrombocytopenia is not the result of increased platelet destruction, the platelet count will fall approximately *10% each day* and reach pretransfusion levels in approximately 1 week.

123. When do the prothrombin time and partial thromboplastin time "normalize" to adult values?

The *prothrombin time* reaches adult values at approximately ***1 week of age***, while the *partial thromboplastin time* does not attain adult values until ***2–9 months***.

124. How is disseminated intravascular coagulation (DIC) diagnosed in the neonate?

The laboratory findings in DIC include evidence of red cell fragmentation on peripheral smear; elevation of prothrombin time, partial thromboplastin time, and thrombin time; thrombocytopenia; decreased levels of factors V, VIII, and fibrinogen; and in some cases, the presence of fibrin split products.

125. How should newborn infants with DIC be managed?

Treatment should be directed primarily at the underlying disease rather than just at the coagulation defects. In many cases, treatment of the former makes specific treatment of the latter unnecessary. However, in cases in which stabilization of coagulopathy is not imminent, treatment with fresh frozen plasma and platelets is recommended. In cases where fluid overload is a major concern, exchange transfusion with fresh whole blood may be used. However, this second approach is not superior to the first with respect to resolution of DIC. The use of heparin in DIC is currently reserved for cases of thrombosis of major vessels or purpura fulminans.

126. What is the difference between early and late hemorrhagic disease of the newborn?

For evolutionary reasons that are unclear, a newborn has only about 50% of the normal vitamin-K-dependent cofactors, and unless vitamin K is given, these levels steadily decline in the first 3 days of life. In addition, breastmilk is low in vitamin K. *Early hemorrhagic disease* can be observed during the first few days of life in infants who are exclusively breastfed and who do not receive vitamin K prophylaxis at birth. They can present with bleeding from various sites (e.g., umbilical cord, circumcision). Infants born to mothers who have received medications that affect the metabolism of vitamin K (e.g., warfarin, antiepileptic medications, antituberculous drugs) are at risk to develop severe life-threatening intracranial hemorrhages at or shortly after delivery. *Late hemorrhagic disease* occurs most commonly between 1 and 3 months of life in infants who are exclusively breastfed and who develop diarrhea from a variety of causes. These infants typically did not receive vitamin K at birth or received it in an oral form. Although oral vitamin K supplementation should prevent late disease, the optimal oral dose, timing, and form of vitamin K required have not been clearly established.

127. Does administration of vitamin K in the newborn period increase the risk of childhood cancer?

In the early 1990s, British investigators reported an association between intramuscular vitamin K and an increased risk in childhood cancers, particularly leukemia. However, subsequent studies have refuted this claim, and perinatal use of intramuscular vitamin K is still recommended.

Klebanoff MA, et al: The risk of childhood cancer after neonatal exposure to vitamin K. N Engl J Med 329:905–908, 1993.

128. Is there a role for recombinant human erythropoietin in the treatment of the anemia of prematurity?

Since the anemia of prematurity is characterized by a relative deficiency of erythropoietin, numerous trials have been undertaken to examine the use of this growth factor and have demonstrated the development of reticulocytosis, delay in the development of anemia and modest reductions in the volume of RBC transfusions. Patients most likely to benefit are those who weigh <1300 grams at birth and are relatively stable clinically. However, the most likely factor to reduce the rate of transfusions is the adoption of strict clinical transfusion guidelines.

129. Are hematopoietic colony stimulating factors effective in the treatment and/or prevention of sepsis in the neonate?

Granulocyte-colony stimulating factor (G-CSF) and *granulocyte macrophage-colony stimulating factor* (GM-CSF) are naturally occurring glycoproteins that regulate the proliferation and differentiation of myeloid precursor cells. The rationale for the use of these factors in the treatment and/or prevention of sepsis is based on data that show:

- Reduced production of G-CSF and GM-CSF by neonatal mononuclear cells in response to inflammatory stimuli compared to adult cells
- Low levels of G-CSF in neutropenic neonates
- Good response of cultured neonatal progenitor cells to the actions of G-CSF and GM-CSF
- Improved survival in animal models of neonatal sepsis following administration of G-CSF and GM-CSF

Human studies to date have demonstrated that target cells in the bone marrow are responsive to both of these CSF's and that few adverse effects are observed following treatment. Clinical trials to date have not been large enough to prove clinical efficacy or determine the ideal strategy for use of these CSF's. Furthermore, trials are underway to assess the role of these factors in preventing nosocomial infections in neutropenic infants.

Carr R, et al: A randomized, controlled trial of prophylactic granulocyte-macrophage colony-stimulating factor in human newborns less than 32 weeks gestation. Pediatrics 103:796-802, 1999.

HYPERBILIRUBINEMIA

130. What are the normal maximum bilirubin levels for full-term healthy newborns?

The *97th percentile* for bilirubin in healthy full-term infants is ***12.4 mg/dl for bottlefed*** infants and ***14.8 mg/dl for breastfed infants***.

131. How common is extreme hyperbilirubinemia in newborns?

If untreated, at least 1-2% of newborns will develop bilirubin levels of 20 mg/dl.

Newman TB et al: Incidence of extreme hyperbilirubinemia in a large HMO. Amb Child Health 3:203A, 1997.

132. What maternal factors affect neonatal serum bilirubin levels?

	INCREASE	DECREASE
Race	East Asian Native American Greek	Black
Maternal health issues	Primipara (?) Older mothers Diabetes Hypertension Oral contraceptive use at time of conception First trimester bleeding Decreased plasma zinc level	Smoking
Drugs administered to mother	Oxytocin Diazepam Epidural anesthesia Promethazine	Phenobarbital Meperidine Reserpine Aspirin Choral hydrate Heroin Phenytoin Antipyrine Alcohol

From Maisels MJ: Neonatal jaundice. In Avery GB, et al (eds): Neonatology: Pathophysiology and Management of the Newborn, 5th ed. Philadelphia, J.B. Lippincott, 1999, p 770; with permission.

133. Which physiologic factors contribute to the rise in serum bilirubin in newborns?

Possible Mechanisms Involved in Physiologic Jaundice of the Newborn

Increased biliburin load on liver cell
- ↑ RBC volume
- ↓ RBC survival
- ↑ Early-labeled bilirubin
- ↑ Enterohepatic circulation of bilirubin

Defective hepatic uptake of bilirubin from plasma
- ↓ Ligandin (Y protein)
- Binding of Y and Z proteins by other anions
- ↓ Relative hepatic uptake deficiency (phase II)

Defective bilirubin conjugation
- ↓ UDP glucuronyl transferase activity
- ↑ UDP glucose dehydrogenase activity

Defective bilirubin excretion
- Excretion impaired but not rate-limiting

Hepatic circulation
- ↓ Oxygen supply to the liver when umbilical cord clamped
- Portal blood flow bypassing liver sinusoids if ductus venosus patent

From Maisels MJ: Neonatal jaundice. In Avery GB, et al (eds): Neonatology: Pathophysiology and Management of the Newborn, 5th ed. Philadelphia, J.B. Lippincott, 1999, p 775; with permission.

134. Why is bilirubin toxic to the brain?

Although it is well established that unconjugated bilirubin is toxic to the CNS, the exact mechanism is not known. Bilirubin is toxic/inhibitory to a wide variety of enzymatic reactions. In vitro studies have demonstrated that bilirubin impairs water and ion exchange. Furthermore, bilirubin impairs the activation of protein kinase C, decreases phosphorylation of intermediary proteins, and decreases mitochondrial functions, substrate transport, and cell viability. Bilirubin also adversely affects the conductive properties of nerve cell membranes at both the cellular and functional level. A hypothetical model for the progression of bilirubin toxicity is as follows:

SITE OF BILIRUBIN UPTAKE	EFFECT ON NEURONS	DURATION OF EFFECT
Aggregation of bilirubin at nerve terminals	Lowers membrane potentials; ↓ auditory brainstem conduction	Usually reversible
↓	↓	
Bilirubin binds to cell components	Impairs substrate transport, neurotransmitter synthesis and mitochondrial functions	Prevented or reversed by equimolar albumin
↓	↓	
Retrograde uptake of bilirubin by neuronal body	Dysfunction and death of neurons	Irreversible
↓	↓	
Pyknosis and gliosis of neurons—bilirubin staining of affected areas	Long term clinical sequelae	Irreversible

From Maisels MJ: Neonatal jaundice. In Avery GB, Fletcher MA, MacDonald MG (eds.): Neonatology: Pathophysiology and Management of the Newborn, 5th ed. Philadelphia, PA, Lippincott, Williams &Wilkins, 1999, p 790, with permission.

135. What factors suggest hemolytic disease as a cause of jaundice in the newborn?

- Family history of hemolytic disease
- Ethnicity suggestive of inherited disease (e.g., G6PD deficiency)
- Onset of jaundice before 24 hours of age
- Reticulocytosis (>8% at birth, >5% in first 2-3 days, and >2% after first week)
- Changes in peripheral smear (microspherocytosis, anisocytosis, target cells)
- Significant decrease in hemoglobin
- Bilirubin rise > 0.5 mg/dl/hr
- Pallor, hepatosplenomegaly
- Failure of phototherapy to lower bilirubin level

Provisional Committee for Quality Improvement and Subcommittee on Hyperbilirubinemia: Practice parameter: Management of hyperbilirubinemia in the healthy term newborn. Pediatrics 94:558–565, 1994.

136. Which infants are "set-ups" for ABO incompatibility?

Infants who are type A or B and whose mothers are type O. In individuals with types A or B blood, naturally occurring anti-A and anti-B isoantibodies are primarily IgM and do not cross the placenta. However, in type O individuals, isoantibodies are frequently IgG. These antibodies can cross the placenta and cause hemolysis. Although approximately 12% of maternal/infant pairs qualify as "set-ups" for ABO incompatibility, < 1% of infants have significant hemolysis.

137. Should conjugated (i.e., direct-reacting) bilirubin levels be routinely obtained in children who are being evaluated for early jaundice?

The utility of a routine measurement of conjugated bilirubin in early jaundice in healthy infants is minimal. Elevated conjugated bilirubin should be suspected in infants with dark urine or urine positive for bilirubin (conjugated bilirubin is water-soluble), light-colored stools, or jaundice that persists > 3 weeks.

138. When calculating bilirubin levels (and thus potential toxicity), should the direct component be subtracted from the total?

A traditional teaching had been to subtract the direct component from the total bilirubin to ascertain the potential neurotoxicity of indirect bilirubin (especially, it seemed, when hovering around exchange transfusion levels). However, direct bilirubin may also be neurotoxic to the newborn brain. No subtraction is warranted or substantiated.

139. What is "vigintiphobia"?

Vigintiphobia, translated from the Latin, is "fear of 20." Traditionally, it has been common to do exchange transfusions in term infants without evidence of isoimmunization or hemolysis at bilirubin levels of 20 mg/dl to prevent kernicterus. Critics argue that this practice is without scientific evidence, and support for tolerating higher levels of bilirubin (in infants without ABO incompatability or other causes of hemolysis) prior to intervention has grown.

Watchko JF, Oski FA: Bilirubin 20 mg/dL = vigintiphobia. Pediatrics 71:660–663, 1983.

140. What are the clinical features of bilirubin toxicity?

Acutely, toxicity is called *bilirubin-induced neurological dysfunction* (BIND). Chronically, the term *kernicterus* is generally used.

Acute (days to weeks): poor sucking, stupor, hypotonia, seizures; progressing to hypertonia of extensor muscles, opisthotonus and to generalized hypertonia

Chronic (months to years): active deep tendon reflexes, hypotonia, obligatory tonic neck reflexes, delayed motor skills; movement disorders (choreoathetosis, ballismus, tremor), upward gaze; sensorineural hearing loss

Dennery PA et al: Neonatal hyperbilirubinemia. N Engl J Med 344:584, 2001.

141. Can kernicterus occur at lower levels of hyperbilirubinemia?

Yes. So-called low-bilirubin kernicterus can occur for two primary pathophysiologic reasons:

1. ***Displacement of unbound bilirubin:*** Competion for albumin-binding sites by small molecules (e.g., sulfa drugs, benzyl alcohol preservative) can elevate the neurotoxic free bilirubin
2. ***Injury to the blood brain barrier:*** Various mechanisms: asphyxia, hypoxia, hyperosmolarity, seizures, meningitis, sepsis with shock, hypercapnia and respiratory acidosis, loss of cerebral blood flow autoregulation.

142. What is the value of measuring albumin levels or bilirubin:albumin ratios?

Decreases in the total amount of albumin or its ability to bind bilirubin result in increased free bilirubin, which is neurotoxic. In babies with low serum albumin (<3.4g/dl), more aggressive implementation of therapy for hyperbilirubemia may be necessary. Measuring total bilirubin and albumin permit calculation of a B:A ratio. Free bilirubin is anticipated when the B:A ratio exceeds 0.80 (7.0 mg bilirubin:1:0 gm of albumin). A molar ratio of <0.63 (5.3 mg of bilirubin:1 gm of albumin) is considered safe in term and near-term babies and may assist in equivocal cases when exchange transfusion is being considered.

143. Why should ceftriaxone and ibuprofen be avoided in very jaundiced infants?

Both displace bilirubin from the binding sites on albumin and thereby increase the levels of unbound bilirubin at a given serum bilirubin level. These drugs may also transfer to breast milk and maternal use should be discouraged, if possible.

144. When are phototherapy and exchange transfusion indicated in the term infant with hyperbilirubinemia?

This is one of the more controversial issues in pediatrics because knowledge regarding bilirubin concentration and circumstances at which CNS toxicity is likely is incomplete. Recommendations by the American Academy of Pediatrics for infants > 24 hours are as follows:

Total Serum Bilirubin (TSB) Levels (mg/dl)

AGE, HRS	CONSIDER PHOTOTHERAPY	PHOTOTHERAPY	EXCHANGE TRANSFUSION IF INTENSIVE PHOTOTHERAPY FAILS*	EXCHANGE TRANSFUSION AND INTENSIVE PHOTOTHERAPY
25–48	≥ 12	≥ 15	≥ 20	≥ 25
49–72	≥ 15	≥ 18	≥ 25	≥ 30
> 72	≥ 17	≥ 20	≥ 25	≥ 30

•Intensive phototherapy should produce a decline of TSB of 1–2 mg/dl within 4–6 hours, and the TSB level should contiue to fall and remain below the threshold level for exchange transfusion. If this does not occur, it is considered a failure of phototherapy.

From Provisional Committee for Quality Improvement and Subcommittee on Hyperbilirubinemia: Practice parameter: Management of hyperbilirubinemia in the healthy term newborn. Pediatrics 94:565, 1994; with permission.

145. What distinguishes "breast-feeding jaundice" from "breast-milk jaundice"?

Hyperbilirubinemia in breastfed infants during the first week of life is called *breast-feeding jaundice* and is thought to be secondary to poor caloric intake and/or dehydration. Hyperbilirubinemia in breastfed infants after the first week of life is known as *breast-milk jaundice*. This form of hyperbilirubinemia is believed to be caused by an increased enterohepatic circulation of bilirubin secondary to the presence of beta-glucoronidase in human milk and/or to the inhibition of the hepatic glucoronosyl transferase by a factor such as free fatty acids in some human milk samples. The incidence and duration as compared with physiologic jaundice are noted in the table.

	PHYSIOLOGIC JAUNDICE	BREAST-FEEDING JAUNDICE	BREAST-MILK JAUNDICE
Time of onset (TSB > 7 mg/dl)	After 36 hr	2–4 days	4–7 days
Usual time of peak bilirubin	3–4 days	3–6 days	5–15 days
Peak TSB	5–12 mg/dl	> 12 mg/dl	> 10 mg/dl
Age when total bilirubin < 3 g/dl	1–2 wk	> 3 wk	9 wk
Incidence in full-term neonates	56%	12–13%	2–4%

TSB = total serum bilirubin.

From Gourley G: Pathophysiology of breast milk uaundice. In Polin RA, Fox W (eds): Fetal and Neonatal Physiology. Philadelphia, W.B. Saunders, 1992; with permission.

146. Why should infants at risk for breast-feeding jaundice be fed more frequently?

Breast-feeding jaundice appears to be associated with poor feeding practices. Infants breastfed on an average of > 8 times a day in the first 3 days of life have significantly lower serum bilirubin concentrations than those less frequently breastfed. Therefore, it makes sense to encourage more frequent feedings. Supplemental feedings may be of value. However, sterile water or balanced electrolyte solutions may worsen the hyperbilirubinemia associated with breast feeding and should not be used.

147. Should breast-feeding be discontinued in an infant with hyperbilirubinemia?

Only in rare metabolic disorders (e.g., galactosemia) should breast-feeding be permanently discontinued. Breastfeeding infants do respond more slowly to phototherapy compared with formula-fed infants. In one study, Martinez et al. compared four interventions in breastfed newborns with a serum bilirubin concentration > 17 mg/dl. The authors concluded that most infants require no intervention. If phototherapy is used, there is no need to discontinue breast feeding.

	INTERVENTION	TREATMENT FAILURE*
Group I	Continued breast-feeding until TSB rose to 20 mg/dl, then breast feeding stopped and phototherapy begun	24%
Group II	Breast-feeding stopped and formula substituted; phototherapy begun at TSB of 20 mg/dl	19%
Group III	Breast-feeding stopped, formula substituted, and phototherapy begun immediately	3%
Group IV	Breast-feeding continued and phototherapy begun	14%

*Total serum bilirubin (TSB) rose to 20 mg/dl.
Martinez JC, et al: Hyperbilirubinemia in the breast-fed newborn: A controlled trial of four interventions. Pediatrics 91:470–473, 1993..

148. Where does bilirubin go when you turn on the lights?

It becomes ***lumirubin*** (through structural isomerization), which is the principal pathway of bilirubin elimination. Lumirubin is rapidly excreted in bile, with a half-life of about 2 hours. Photoisomers can also be excreted in the urine.

149. What are the contraindications to phototherapy?

Infants with a ***significantly elevated conjugated hyperbilirubinemia*** or a family history of light-sensitive ***porphyria*** should not receive phototherapy.

150. What are the common adverse effects of phototherapy?

Diarrhea, increased insensible *water loss*, *skin rashes*, *overheating*, and the potential for *burns* if the lights are placed too close to the infant's skin. If direct hyperbilirubinemia is present, the bronze baby syndrome can result.

151. A newborn who develops dark skin discoloration and dark urine after beginning phototherapy likely has what condition?

The ***bronze baby syndrome***. Infants who develop the syndrome typically have an elevated direct serum bilirubin concentration. The bronze baby syndrome results from retention of lumirubin that cannot be excreted in the bile. Most infants appear to recover without complications. However, in infants with significant conjugated hyperbilirubinemia, the use of phototherapy is controversial.

152. Why do babies receiving phototherapy develop diarrhea?

During phototherapy, unconjugated bilirubin is excreted into the gut in increased amounts, which enhances intestinal secretions. The diarrhea may be a consequence of the high concentrations of bilirubin within the intestinal lumen. Increased concentrations of bile salts also have been found in the gut of neonates during phototherapy and may be a factor in the pathogenesis of phototherapy-associated diarrhea. The diarrhea is not believed to be the result of a phototherapy-induced lactase deficiency.

153. How can the metallo-protoporphyrins assist in settings of hyperbilirubinemia?

Numerous studies have demonstrated that various metallo-protophorhyrins (such as zinc, tin, and chromium) can effectively inhibit heme oxygenase, which is the rate-limiting step in heme catabolism. These enzyme inhibitors can thus decrease bilirubin production. The potential toxicities remain under study and may include photosensitization and inhibition of cytochrome p450-drug metabolism.

Martinez JC, et al: Control of severe hyperbilirubinemia in full-term newborns with the inhibitor of bilirubin production by Sn-mesomorphyrin. Pediatrics 103:1-5, 1999.

154. What percentage of blood volume is removed in a one-, two-, and three-volume exchange transfusion?

Blood Volume Exchanged	*Blood Volume Removed and Replaced by Exchange*
1.0	63%
2.0	87%
3.0	95%

155. How quickly does the bilirubin rebound following an exchange transfusion?

Although 87% of the infant's bilirubin is removed in a two-volume exchange, the serum bilirubin concentration is only reduced to 45% of the pre-exchange level. Equilibration is complete by 30 minutes, at which time the bilirubin rises to 60% of the pre-exchange value.

156. What are the complications of exchange transfusions in the newborn?

Acute

- *Hypocalcemia* (secondary to binding of calcium by citrate)
- *Thrombocytopenia* (secondary to removal of platelets and use of stored blood that may be low in platelets)
- *Hyperkalemia* (secondary to higher potassium levels in stored blood)
- *Hypovolemia* (if blood replacement is inadequate)
- *Diminished oxygen delivery* (if blood stored > 5–7 days is used, the resultant loss of 2,3-DPG may have deleterious effects on oxygen delivery)

Late

- *Anemia* (for unknown reasons)
- *Graft vs. host disease* (secondary to introduction of donor lymphocytes into a relatively immunocompromised neonatal host)

157. How often does prolonged unconjugated hyperbilirubinemia occur?

About ***one-third*** of healthy *breastfed* infants will have persistent jaundice ≥ 14 days. In *formula-fed* infants, this prolonged jaundice occurs in **< *1%*** of neonates.

158. What are the pathologic causes of prolonged unconjugated hyperbilirubinemia?

Causes of Unconjugated Hyperbilirubinemia

- Excessive production of bilirubin (hemolysis)
  - Blood group heterospecificity (incompatibility)
    - Rh
    - ABO
    - Minor blood groups
  - Red blood cell enzyme abnormalities
    - Glucose-6-phosphate dehydrogenase
    - Pyruvate kinase
  - Sepsis
  - Red blood cell membrane defects
    - Hereditary spherocytosis, elliptocytosis, poikilocytosis
  - Extravascular blood
  - Polycythemia
- Impaired conjugation or excretion
  - Hormonal deficiency
    - Hypothyroidism
    - Hypopituitarism
  - Disorders of bilirubin metabolism
  - Crigler-Najjar syndrome: Type I
  - Crigler-Najjar syndrome: Type II (Arias disease)
  - Gilbert disease
  - Lucey-Driscoll syndrome
- Enhanced enterohepatic circulation

Intestinal obstruction, pyloric stenosis
Ileus, meconium plugs, cystic fibrosis

From McMahon JR, et al: Unconjugated hyperbilirubinemias. In Taeusch HW and Ballard RA (eds): Diseases of the Newborn, 7th ed., Philadelphia, W.B. Saunders, 1998, p. 1014; with permission.

159. How much potential bilirubin is there in meconium?

Analysis of meconium stools from preterm and term infants indicates that there is 1 mg bilirubin/gm wet weight and that 50% is unconjugated. At birth, the amount of meconium in the gut is estimated to be between 100–200 gm.

160. What is delta bilirubin?

When bilirubin is measured by high pressure lipid chromatography (HPLC), the total bilirubin includes the unconjugated fraction, conjugated fraction, and a fraction that is covalently bound to albumin—the delta bilirubin fraction. It was named delta because it is the fourth bilirubin peak on the HPLC elution curve. Most laboratories utilize the diazonium test which results in delta bilirubin being included in the conjugated fraction. At present, there is no clear clinical significance for delta bilirubin.

161. What is the relationship between delayed neonatal jaundice and urinary tract infection (UTI)?

Unexplained jaundice developing between 10–60 days of age can be associated with a UTI in infants. The typical patient is usually afebrile (in two-thirds of cases) with hepatomegaly and often minimal systemic symptoms. Hyperbilirubinemia is usually conjugated, and liver transaminases may be normal or mildly elevated. Treatment of the UTI (usually caused by *Escherichia coli*) results in reversal of the jaundice, which is felt to be caused by liver dysfunction secondary to endotoxins. Sepsis with bacterial hepatitis usually presents earlier with a more sick infant.

162. Who was Sister Ward?

In the early 1950s, Sister Ward was the nurse in charge of the unit for premature infants at Rochford General Hospital in Essex, England. On warm summer days, Sister Ward would take her infants to the courtyard to give them a little fresh air and sunshine. It was following such an afternoon of sunshine that Sister Ward observed that sunlight was able to "bleach" the skin of jaundiced neonates. The account of her discovery, as recorded by R.H. Dobbs, follows:

> One particularly fine summer's day in 1956, during a ward routine, Sister Ward diffidently showed us a premature baby, carefully undressed and with fully exposed abdomen. The infant was pale yellow except for a strongly demarcated triangle of skin very much yellower than the rest of the body. I asked her, "Sister, what did you paint it with—iodine or flavine—and why?" But she replied that she thought it must have been the sun. "What do you mean Sister? Suntan takes days to develop after the erythema has faded." Sister Ward looked increasingly uncomfortable, and explained that she thought it was a jaundiced baby, much darker where a corner of the sheet had covered the area. "It's the rest of the body that seems to have faded." We left it at that, and as the infant did well and went home, fresh air treatment of prematurity continued.

METABOLIC ISSUES

163. What is the definition of neonatal hypoglycemia?

Although there is no universally accepted definition, neonatal hypoglycemia is commonly defined as a serum glucose of ***< 35 mg/dl in a term infant*** and ***< 25 mg/dl in a preterm*** or ***low-birthweight infant*** during the first 3 days of life. However, because the fetal glucose level is typically ≥ 40 mg/dl and older children can be symptomatic with glucose levels ≤ 40 mg/dl, any glucose level < 40 mg/dl should be viewed as abnormal and treated. Other experts argue that electrophysiologic changes occur in the brains of infants when glucose levels reach 50 mg/dl and argue for more aggressive intervention at these higher levels.

164. How does glucose production compare between adults and infants?

Hepatic glucose production in infants is 3-6 times that of an adult or approximately 6 mg/kg/min. This is due to the greater glucose requirements in infants due in part to their larger brain to body size ratio. Glucose is the primary fuel for the brain and accounts for over 90% of total body oxygen consumption early in fasting.

165. When is hypoglycemia most likely to occur in a neonate?

During gestation, glucose is freely transferred across the placenta by the process of facilitated diffusion. However, after birth, the infant must adjust to the sudden withdrawal of this transplacental supply. In all infants, there is a nadir in blood sugar between 1–3 hours of life. In the first 12-24 hours of life, newborns are at increased risk for hypoglycemia because gluconeogenesis and especially keogenesis are incompletely developed. This factors are accentuated in *preterm* infants, *infants of diabetic mothers*, infants with *erythroblastosis fetalis*, *asphyxiated* infants, and infants who are *small* or *large for gestational age*.

166. How should hypoglycemia be treated?

Both symptomatic and asymptomatic hypoglycemia should be treated. If an asymptomatic infant can take oral feedings, these may suffice initially. Otherwise, the infant should receive therapy based on the response:

• Initially, the infant is given a bolus of IV glucose (200 mg/kg or 2 ml/kg of $D_{10}W$), followed by a glucose infusion of 6–8 mg/kg/min (3.6–4.8 ml/kg/hr of $D_{10}W$) with rechecking of glucose within 15 minutes, frequent glucose monitoring and increases in infusion rates and concentrations as needed.

• Glucagon, 1 mg IM, can be given as an anti-insulin measure until an IV is established, but glucagon is not as helpful in the low-birthweight infant.

• If ≥ 15–20 mg/kg/min is required, glucocorticoids (hydrocortisone, 5 mg/kg/day, or prednisone, 2 mg/kg/day) can enhance gluconeogenesis. Diazoxide (10–15 mg/kg/day) can suppress insulin secretion.

167. What is the value of a glucagon stimulation test?

A glucagon stimulation study identifies accessible hepatic glucose stores. After laboratory studies are done in search of an etiology for hypoglycemia, glucagons (1.0 mg IV or IM) is given and blood gluose is checked every 10 minutes for 40 minutes. If blood glucose increases by ≥ 30 mg/dl, the test is positive, indicating inappropriate preservation of liver glycogen. A positive test supports ***hyperinsulinemic suppression of glycogenolysis***. Exceptions to this rule are neonates with hypopituitarism who may have a positive glycemic response to glucagon.

168. In a newborn requiring a glucose infusion of ≥ 15 mg/kg/min, what condition should be suspected?

A ***marked hyperinsulinemic state***. This can be seen in a variety of conditions: nesidioblastosis (primary hyperplasia of the islets of Langerhans), islet cell adenomas, maternal diabetes mellitus, Rh incompatibility, maternal drug use (e.g., thiazide diuretics or tocolytics), or Beckwith-Wiedemann syndrome. The absence of ketone bodies in an infant with increased insulin levels, a high glucose requirement, and a low serum glucose level makes one of the islet cell disorders likely. All but the first two diagnoses are discernible by history and/or exam.

de Lonlay-Debeney, et al: Clinical features of 52 neonates with hyperinsulinism. N Engl J Med 340: 1169-1175, 1999.

169. What features on physical examination suggest the etiology of hypoglycemia?

Macrosomia: Infants of diabetic mothers, severe congenital hyperinsulinism, Beckwith-Weideman syndrome. Recall that insulin is a growth factor and hyperinsulinsm leads to macrosomia.

Midline defects: Congenital pituitary deficiency can be associated with midline defects such as cleft lip, cleft palate, single central incisor and micro-ophthalmia.

Micropenis: Congenital gonadotropin deficiency and possible pituitary abnormalities.

Hepatomegaly: Associated with glycogen storage diseases and fatty acid oxidation disorders.

170. A large-for-gestational-age newborn is noted to have a large tongue, a large umbilical hernia, ear creases, and hypoglycemia. What diagnosis should be suspected?

Beckwith-Wiedemann syndrome. This genetic overgrowth syndrome occurs in about 1 in 14,000 deliveries. Although most cases are sporadic, parentally transmitted cytogenetic abnormalities can occur on chromosome 11. In addition to the features mentioned above, other common findings include other abdominal wall defects (e.g., omphalocele, diastasis recti), infraorbital creases, visceromegaly, and GI malrotation. In the delivery room, associated features including a large and thickened placenta, polyhydramnios, and long umbilical cord may be noted.

Weng EY, et al: Beckwith-Wiedemann syndrome. Clin Pediatr 34:317–326, 1995.

171. What is the mechanism of neonatal hypoglycemia after administration of tocolytic drugs to mothers?

Beta-agonists used as tocolytics may cause beta-cell hyperplasia in the fetal pancreas, leading to elevated fetal insulin levels and hypoglycemia in the immediate postnatal period. The risk of hypoglycemia seems to be associated with long-term use of the beta-agonists, especially if therapy is discontinued < 2 days prior to delivery.

172. What are manifestations of hypocalcemia in the neonate?

The major manifestations are jitteriness and seizures. Additional signs such as high-pitched cry, laryngospasm, Chvostek sign (facial muscle twitching on tapping), and Trousseau sign (carpopedal spasm) may be present, but more commonly these are absent during the neonatal period.

173. What is the differential diagnosis of hypocalcemia in the neonate?

Early neonatal hypocalcemia (first 3 days of life)

- Premature infants
- Infants with birth asphyxia
- Infants of diabetic mothers

Late neonatal hypocalcemia (after end of first week)

- High-phosphate cow's milk formula
- Intestinal malabsorption
- Postdiarrheal acidosis
- Hypomagnesemia
- Neonatal hypoparathyroidism
- Rickets

Decreased ionized fraction of calcium

- Citrate (exchange transfusion)
- Increased free fatty acid (Intralipid)
- Alkalosis

174. When should hypocalcemia be treated in the neonate?

Hypocalcemia should be treated when it is associated with *signs or symptoms* or when the *serum calcium level is < 7.0 mg/dl*. The first line of therapy generally consists of increasing the amount of calcium in the IV infusion to achieve 75 mg of elemental Ca/kg/day and following serum levels every 6–8 hours. Once normal calcium levels are achieved, the intravenous dose can be weaned over 2-3 days. Infusion of bolus IV calcium (10% calcium gluconate, 2 ml/kg) over 10 minutes should be reserved for the infant with seizures. In the asymptomatic infant, hypocalcemia most frequently resolves spontaneously without need for further therapy.

175. In which neonates should the serum magnesium concentration be measured?

- Any *hypocalcemic* infant not responding to calcium therapy
- *Hypotonic* infants born to mothers who received magnesium sulfate therapy prior to delivery
- Infants with *seizures* of unknown etiology

176. How is hypomagnesemia treated?

Hypomagnesemic infants should be treated with 0.25 ml/kg of a 50% solution (100 mg of elemental Mg/ml) given intramuscularly. Magnesium levels are followed and the dosage repeated if necessary.

NEONATAL SEPSIS

177. What are the common clinical presentations of evolving neonatal sepsis?

Symptoms and signs of sepsis may be minimal and nonspecific. As the rap goes, "In the newborn, anything can be a sign of anything." Temperature instability (both hyper- and hypothermia), respiratory distress, apnea, cyanosis, GI changes (vomiting, distention, diarrhea, anorexia), and CNS features (irritability, lethargy, weak suck) can all be early presentations of sepsis. Of course, these can also overlap with many noninfectious processes, making the diagnosis difficult. Risk factors for sepsis (e.g., prematurity, prolonged rupture of membranes, chorioamnionitis) should increase the urgency for more detailed evaluations. While the search for the definitive screening lab test continues, cultures remain the only certain method of verifying infection.

178. Can sepsis be distinguished from other causes of respiratory distress in the neonate?

Not reliably. Diagnosis is confirmed only by a positive blood, urine, or CSF culture.

179. What laboratory tests can rule out sepsis on admission?

None. Total wbc counts, immature/total (I/T) ratios of neutrophils, and C-reactive protein are of limited value as single tests in the diagnosis of bacterial sepsis in the newborn. In one-third of infants with proven bacterial disease, total WBC counts are normal, particularly early in the course of infection. The most sensitive neutrophil index for identifying septic infants is the *immature to total (I:T) neutrophil ratio*. An I:T ratio of > 0.2 has been considered abnormal, although some studies have suggested a ratio as high as 0.27 may be seen in healthy term newborns. Neutropenia (total WBC < 5000/mm^3 or absolute neutrophil count < 1750/mm^3) is the most specific indicator. The least sensitive neutrophil index is the absolute band count (normal < 2000/mm^3). Generally, abnormal neutrophil indices have low positive-predictive values and therefore are not helpful as sole tests in clearly identifying which infants are infected. However, they have a much higher negative-predictive value, particularly if repeated 12 hours after birth, and thus can be very helpful in determining which infants do not have infection.

180. What maternal factor is most likely to result in a newborn with a *lower* than expected neutrophil count?

Maternal hypertension. The duration of this affect is approximately 72 hours.

181. What tests in combination are useful in creating a sepsis screen strategy?

A combination of diagnostic tests improves the predictive values relative to using a single test. In this strategy, negative serial sepsis screens substantially reduce the likelihood that the infant has sepsis. One suggested sepsis screen is shown below. The screen is considered positive if 2 or more points are present.

TEST	POINT VALUE
Absolute neutrophil count < 1750/mm^3	1 point
Total WBC < 7500 or > 40,000/mm^3	1 point
Immature/total neutrophil ratio ≥ 0.2	1 point
Immature/total neutrophil ratio ≥ 0.4	2 points
CRP + (≥ 1.0 mg/dl)	1 point
CRP + (≥ 5.0 mg/dl)	2 points

182. What is the role of cytokine determinations in the evaluation of possible sepsis?

A number of inflammatory mediators are being investigated as possible diagnostic tests for neonatal sepsis. Results with interleukin-6 (IL-6) have been particularly encouraging and have shown:

- IL-6 is an early mediator of inflammation that is partly responsible for the increase in acute phase reactants.
- IL-6 is elevated in most infants with systemic infection (>90% sensitivity)
- IL-6 levels fall quickly to normal during the course of therapy for sepsis.
- IL-6 is more likely than CRP to be elevated particularly when testing is done early in the course of sepsis.

Büscher U, et al: Interleukin-1 beta, interleukin-6, interleukin-8 and G-CSF in the diagnosis of early-onset neonatal infections. J Perinat Med 28:383-388, 2000.

Kuster H, et al: Interleukin-1 receptor antagonist and interleukin-6 for early diagnosis of neonatal sepsis two days before clinical manifestation. Lancet 352:1271-1277, 1998.

183. How helpful is a gastric aspirate in evaluation of infection?

Examination of gastric aspirates for leukocytes and bacteria was previously thought to be useful in identifying infants at risk for sepsis. However, the leukocytes are of maternal origin, and the bacteria represent organisms colonizing or infecting the amniotic cavity. They do not necessarily indicate fetal or neonatal infection.

184. Should a urine culture be done as part of the sepsis evaluation in the neonate?

A urine culture can be excluded as part of a sepsis evaluation in the first days of life. Urine cultures are very infrequently positive in infants < 72 hours of age, except when associated with renal anomalies.

185. Should a lumbar puncture (LP) be done on all newborns as part of the sepsis evaluation?

The need for LP in the sepsis evaluation of a newborn is controversial, with some authors suggesting its omission in asymptomatic infants. However, in symptomatic infants, an LP should be strongly considered because (1) bacterial meningitis can be present in newborns without CNS symptoms, (2) a significant number (15–30%) can have meningitis without bacteremia, and (3) meningitis can coexist in premature infants with suspected respiratory distress syndrome. The procedure should be postponed in an infant with cardiorespiratory instability or significant thrombocytopenia.

Wiswell TE, et al: No lumbar puncture in the evaluation for early neonatal sepsis: Will meningitis be missed? Pediatrics 95:803–806, 1995.

186. What is the ideal position for an infant to receive a lumbar puncture?

Infants who undergo LP in an upright position (with head support and spina flexion) exhibit less hypoxia and hypercarbia. If a lateral recumbent position is used, partial neck extension helps to minimize the respiratory stresses.

187. Are skin surface cultures helpful in the evaluation of suspected neonatal sepsis?

The theoretic value of these cultures is that they might help to identify the possible etiologic agents and thus guide therapy. However, an analysis of nearly 25,000 cultures in > 3,300 patients revealed that surface cultures correlated with urine, blood, or CSF cultures in only about 50% of cases. Most agree that surface cultures in this setting have little clinical value.

Evans ME, et al: Sensitivity, specificity, and predictive value of body surface cultures in a neonatal intensive care unit. JAMA 259:248–252, 1988.

Fulginiti VA, Ray CG: Body surface cultures in the newborn infant: An exercise in futility, wastefulness, and inappropriate practice. Am J Dis Child 142:19–20, 1988.

188. Discuss the pathogenesis of early-onset bacterial infection.

Blanc has designated the sequence of events leading to early-onset bacterial infection as the "ascending amniotic infection syndrome." Infection begins with colonization of the maternal genital tract. Pathogenic bacteria then spread upward through the cervix and into the amniotic cavity, resulting in chorioamnionitis. Susceptible infants either inhale or swallow infected amniotic fluid and develop generalized sepsis. Although chorioamnionitis increases the risk of both fetal and neonatal infection, < 5% of mothers with this condition deliver infected infants.

Blanc WA: Pathways of fetal and early neonatal infection. J Pediatr 59:473–496, 1961.

189. What are the most common pathogens responsible for sepsis in the neonate?

Gram-negative bacteria (particularly *Escherichia coli*) and ***group B streptococci***. Of note is the emergence of coagulase-negative staphylococci as the most common organisms responsible for nosocomial infections in most newborn intensive care units.

190. Compare early-onset and late-onset group B streptococcal sepsis.

Comparison of Early- and Late-Onset Group B Streptococcal Sepsis

FEATURE	EARLY ONSET (< 7 DAYS)	LATE ONSET (≥ 7 DAYS)
Median age at onset	1 hr	27 days
Incidence of prematurity	Increased	Not increased
Maternal obstetric complications	Frequent (70%)	Uncommon
Common manifestations	Septicemia (25–40% Meningitis (5–15%) Pneumonia (35–55%)	Meningitis (30–40%) Bacteremia without focus (40–50%) Osteoarthritis (5–10%)
Serotypes isolated	Ia, Ib/c, Ia/c (30%) II (30%) III (40% nonmeningeal; 80% meningeal isolates)	III (93%)
Mortality rate	10–15%	2–6%

From Baker C: Group B streptococcal infections. In Remington JS, Klein JO (eds): Infectious Diseases of the Fetus and Newborn Infant, 4th ed. Philadelphia, W.B. Saunders, 1995, p 1010; with permission.

191. What are the two strategies to determine which maternal carriers of group B streptococci (GBS) warrant prophylactic antibiotics?

Antepartum screening-based and ***risk factor-based.*** The AAP guidelines for the prevention of early onset Group B streptococcal infection proposes two strategies: one uses *prenatal cultures at 35-37 weeks* of gestation and the second using *risk factors* without prenatal culture screening. If the ***culture-based strategy*** is employed, all women identified as GBS carriers should be offered intrapartum prophylaxis *even if no risk factors are present.* If the results of culture are not available at the onset of labor or rupture of membranes, prophylaxis should be administered based on ***maternal risk factors***: gestational age <37 weeks, membranes ruptured >18 hours or maternal temperature in labor is >38°C, history of a previous baby with invasive GBS disease or urine culture positive for GBS during this pregnancy.

Committee on Infectious Diseases, Committee on Fetus and Newborn. Revised guidelines for prevention of early onset Group B Streptococcal (GBS) infection. Pediatrics 99: 489-496, 1997.

192. How successful are these screening strategies?

The incidence of early-onset GBS disease in the U.S. has fallen by 65% from 1.7 per 1000 live births (1993) to 0.6 per 1000 live births (1998) since the introduction of these strategies in the mid-1990s. Despite this impressive decline, however, *risk-factor based* strategy identifies only about 75% of affected infants' mothers and *screening-based* strategy about 85-90%. Twenty-five percent of infants with blood culture positive GBS disease are born to mothers who have received intrapartum antibiotics.

Schrag SJ, et al: Group B streptococcal disease in the era of intrapartum antibiotic prophylaxis. N Engl J Med 342:15-20, 2000.

193. In addition of early-onset GBS sepsis, what other adverse outcomes of pregnancy are associated with maternal GBS colonization?

High titer colonization is associated with:

- Early fetal loss
- Premature rupture of membranes
- Pre-term labor
- Low birth weight
- Maternal sepsis
- Maternal chorioamnionitis

194. Do intrapartum antibiotics change the clinical presentation of early-onset GBS sepsis?

No. In a study of 319 infants with early-onset GBS disease, the administration of intrapartum antibiotics to the mother did not affect the constellation and timing of clinical signs of disease. All infants born to pretreated mothers became ill in the first 24 hours (80% within the first six hours).

Bromberger P, et al: The influence of intrapartum on the clinical spectrum of early-onset Group B Streptococcal infection in term infants. Pediatrics 106:244-250, 2000.

195. In cultures positive for coagulase-negative staphylococci, what distinguishes contamination from "true" infection?

To help in differentiating a "true" coagulase-negative staphylococcal infection from blood culture contamination (especially in infants with central catheters), blood cultures should be obtained from two different sites. In infants with infections, both cultures should grow coagulase-negative staphylococci with identical sensitivity patterns. If only a single blood culture is obtained, some authors have suggested that a colony count of ≥ 50 cfu/ml is suggestive evidence of "true" bacteremia. In clinical practice, however, that number of cfus has a relatively poor predictive accuracy.

196. How is systemic candidiasis diagnosed in the neonate?

By cultures of blood, urine, and CSF or other body fluids that are generally sterile. Since cultures are only intermittently positive, multiple systemic cultures should be obtained. A urinalysis demonstrating budding yeasts or hyphae should raise suspicion of systemic infection. Gram stains of buffy coat smears may also demonstrate organisms. An ophthalomologic exam may indicate the presence of candidal endophthalmitis.

197. What is the preferred treatment of candidal sepsis and meningitis?

Systemic candidiasis is treated with amphotericin B intravenously for 4 weeks. Treatment is started at 0.1 mg/kg in a single daily dose infused over 4–6 hours. The dose is gradually increased over several days until a maximum daily dosage of 0.5–1.0 mg/kg is achieved. 5-Flucytosine (50–150 mg/kg/day) should be used to supplement amphotericin B if the infection is severe, the organism is resistant to amphotericin, or the CNS is involved.

198. Is prophylactic use of intravenous immunoglobulin (IVIG) indicated in newborns?

Data from large multicenter trials in the early 1990s showed conflicting results ranging from possible benefits for the smallest infants versus no benefits in preventing nosocomial sepsis or decreasing mortality. Additional accumulating data argue against routine use of IVIG as an efficacious preventative therapy.

Sandberg K,et al: Preterm infants with low IgG have increased risk of sepsis but do not benefit from prophylactic IgG. J Pediatr 137:623-628, 2000.

199. When is immunoglobulin therapy indicated in the acutely infected infant?

Although most studies have focused on the use of IVIG for prophylaxis, a few studies have examined its role as an adjunct to antibiotics in the acute treatment of sepsis. There appears to be a modest improvement in survival, but the numbers of patients remain too small to warrant any conclusions.

NEUROLOGIC ISSUES

200. Give the normal CSF values for healthy neonates.

In the CSF examination of a group of high-risk neonates who did not have infection, the values (mean and range) were:

	TERM	PRETERM
WBC count (cells/mm^3)	8.3 (0–32)	9.0 (0–29)
Protein (mg/dl)	90 (20–170)	115 (65–150)
Glucose (mg/dl)	52 (34–119)	50 (24–63)
CSF/blood glucose (%)	81 (44–248)	74 (55–105)

Adapted from Sarff LD, et al: Cerebrospinal fluid evaluation in neonates: Comparison of high risk infants with and without meningitis. J Pediatr 88:473, 1976; with permission.

201. Following a difficult delivery, what three major forms of extracranial hemorrhage can occur?

Caput succedaneum, cephalhematoma, and subgaleal hemorrhage.

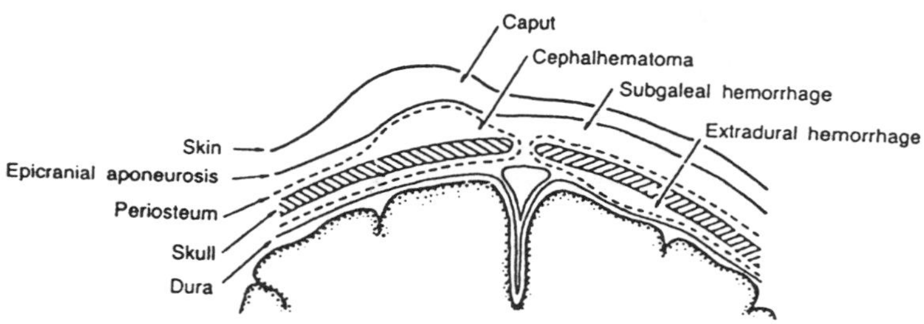

Major Varieties of Traumatic Extracranial Hemorrhage

LESION	FEATURES OF EXTERNAL SWELLING	INCREASES AFTER BIRTH	CROSSES SUTURE LINES	MARKED ACUTE BLOOD LOSS
Caput succedaneum	Soft, pitting	No	Yes	No
Subgaleal hemorrhage	Firm, fluctuant	Yes	Yes	Yes
Cephalhematoma	Firm, tense	Yes	No	No

From Volpe JJ (ed): Neurology of the Newborn, 3rd ed. Philadelphia, W.B. Saunders, 1995, p 770; with permission.

202. If a cephalhematoma is suspected, should a skull x-ray be done to evaluate for fracture?

Cephalhematomas occur in up to 2.5% of livebirths. The incidence of associated fractures ranges from 5–25% in studies. These fractures are almost always linear and nondepressed and do not require treatment. Thus, in an asymptomatic infant with a cephalhematoma over the convexity of the skull and without suspicion of a depressed fracture, x-ray is not necessary. If the exam suggests cranial depression or neurologic signs are present, radiographic imaging is warranted.

203. Should all preterm infants by examined by cranial ultrasound?

Because of the relative noninvasiveness of ultrasound, most neonatologists recommend that a single cranial ultrasonogram be obtained in the first week of life in infants born at < 35 weeks' gestational age.

204. In screening for intraventricular hemorrhage (IVH), when is the best time to perform an ultrasound?

In series of infants studied by ultrasonography, approximately 50% had the onset of hemorrhage in the first day of life, 25% on the second day, and 15% on the third day. Thus, a single scan on the fourth day of life would be expected to detect > 90% of IVHs. However, approximately 20–40% of hemorrhages show evidence of extension within 3–5 days after initial diagnosis, and thus a second scan is indicated after about 5 days after the first to determine the maximal extent of hemorrhage.

205. Describe the three clinical presentations of IVH.

1. A ***catastrophic deterioration*** characterized by an inexorable evolution in minutes to hours. Major features include stupor or coma, respiratory disturbances including apnea, generalized tonic seizures, decerebrate posturing, flaccid quadriparesis, fixed pupils, and absent "doll's eyes." Associated features include falling hematocrit, bulging anterior fontanel, hypotension, bradycardia, temperature instability, metabolic acidosis, and abnormal water homeostasis (SIADH or diabetes insipidus).

2. A ***saltatory deterioration*** that follows a stuttering evolution over hours to days. Important features include altered level of consciousness, decreased motility, decreased tone, abnormal eye movements (e.g., downward vertical drift, skew deviation), and an abnormally tight popliteal angle (< 130° for premature infants and < 110° for term infants).

3. A ***clinically silent syndrome*** often associated with an unexplained fall in hematocrit or failure of hematocrit to rise after transfusion.

206. How are IVHs classified?

Most traditional systems of classification include a grading system according to increasing severity:

Grade I Germinal matrix hemorrhage only
Grade II IVH without ventricular dilatation

Grade III IVH with ventricular dilatation
Grade IV Grade III hemorrhage plus intraparenchymal involvement

Some authorities have abandoned the grade IV classification in favor of "periventricular hemorrhagic infarction" to emphasize that these lesions have a different pathophysiology and are not simply extensions of matrix or IVH into parenchymal tissue. As such, the extent of parenchymal involvement rather than the grade of hemorrhage is more important in determining prognosis.

207. What is the cause of hydrocephalus following an intracranial hemorrhage?
The acute hydrocephalus is believed to be secondary to impairment of CSF absorption by the arachnoid membrane caused by the particulate blood clot. In subacute/chronic hydrocephalus, ventricular enlargement is due to an obliterative arachnoiditis (likely a chemical inflammatory response from the continued presence of blood) which usually causes a communicating hydrocephalus. Less commonly, obstruction of the aqueduct of Sylvius can lead to a noncommunicating hydrocephalus.

208. How common is progressive posthemorrhagic ventricular enlargement?
The likelihood of this phenomenon depends on the extent of the initial hemorrhage, ranging from only about a 5% likelihood in Grade I IVH to 80% in Grade IV IVH.

209. Can serial lumbar punctures prevent posthemorrhagic hydrocephalus?
No. Although LPs are useful in lowering increased intracranial pressure and in treating hydrocephalus once it has developed, they are of no benefit in preventing the onset. Infants with slowly progressive ventricular dilation and increasing head circumference who do not show signs of spontaneous arrest and improvement within 4 weeks should undergo a trial of serial LPs. Their effectiveness should be assessed with ultrasound. If there is no benefit, the placement of a ventriculoperitoneal shunt is necessary.

210. How much fluid should be removed by lumbar puncture in an infant with ventriculomegaly?
Because the volume of CSF in the dilated ventricles of infants with posthemorrhagic hydrocephalus is large, the removal of a significant amount (10–15 ml/kg) is usually required.

211. What causes subarachnoid hemorrhage (SAH) in the newborn?
SAH in the neonate is believed to result from traumatic or hypoxic events that increase traction on, or flow through, small fragile vascular channels, which are the remnants of anastomoses present between the leptomeningeal arteries during brain development.

212. What are the three clinical presentations of SAH?
1. ***Asymptomatic***. In most cases, only small amounts of hemorrhage have occurred, and minimal or no clinical signs are present.

2. ***Well baby with seizures***. In patients without significant hypoxic-ischemic encephalopathy, seizures secondary to SAH have their onset on the second day of life. In the interictal period, these babies appear well.

3. ***Catastrophic deterioration***. In rare instances, newborn infants with large SAHs follow a rapidly fatal course characterized by coma, respiratory disturbance, seizures, loss of brainstem reflexes, and flaccidity.

213. Which areas of the CNS are injured by hypoxia and ischemia?
Full-term infants: Asphyxia produces injury in the peripheral and dorsal aspects of the cerebral cortex. Lesions involve gyri at the depths of the sulci as well as the neuronal nuclei of the basal ganglia.

Premature infants: Injury is localized to the germinal matrix and the periventricular region, while the cortex is relatively spared.

214. What are the five major neuropathological varieties of neonatal hypoxic-ischemic encephalopathy?

1. ***Selective neuronal necrosis***: usually occurs in a characteristic, although possibly widespread, region.

2. ***Status marmoratus***: following neuronal loss, the development of gliosis and hypermyelination, often in the basal ganglia and thalamus

3. ***Parasagittal cerebral injury***: "watershed infarcts" due to ischemia

4. ***Periventricular leukomalacia***: loss of white matter in characteristic patterns due to ischemia, particularly in premature infants

5. ***Focal and multifocal ischemic brain necrosis***: infarction due to ischemia, with large areas of necrosis in the distribution of major vessels

215. How does Erb palsy differ from Klumpke palsy?

Neonatal brachial plexus injuries occur in < 0.5% of deliveries and are often associated with shoulder dystocia and breech or forceps delivery. Of the two, Erb palsy is more common.

Erb palsy

- Involves upper plexus (C5, C6, and, in 50% of cases, C7) affected
- Arm held adducted, internally rotated, and pronated with wrist flexed and fingers flexed ("waiter's tip" position)
- Biceps reflex absent, Moro reflex with hand movement but no shoulder abduction, palmar grasp present
- 5% have ipsilateral diaphragmatic involvement

Klumpke palsy

- Involves lower plexus (C8, T1)
- Small muscles of hand and wrist ("claw hand")
- Up to one-third have associated Horner syndrome

216. How is brachial plexus injury treated?

Therapy must be aimed at preventing contractures. For the first 7–10 days, the arm is gently immobilized against the abdomen to minimize further hemorrhage and/or swelling. Following this initial period, passive range of motion exercises at the shoulder, elbow, wrist, and hand are performed. In addition, wrist splints to stabilize the fingers and avoid contractures should be used. Improvements in microsurgical techniques have increased interest in this modality if recovery is delayed, particularly in cases of nerve root avulsion. Timing of intervention remains unclear. Other therapies included the use of botulinum toxin with physical therapy if severe contractions have evolved.

Noetzel MJ, Wolpaw JR: Emerging concepts in the pathophysiology of recovery from neonatal brachial plexus injury. Neurol 55:5-6, 2000.

217. What is the outcome of neonatal brachial plexus palsy?

Approximately 90% of patients have normal examinations by 12 months of age. Onset of recovery within 2 weeks and involvement of only the proximal upper extremity are both favorable prognostic signs.

Strombeck C, et al: Functional outcome at 5 years in children with obstetrical brachial plexus palsy with and without microsurgical reconstruction. Develop Med Child Neurol 42:148-157, 2000.

218. In newborns with facial paralysis, how is peripheral nerve involvement distinguished from central nerve involvement?

Peripheral: Usually results from compression of the peripheral portion of the nerve by prolonged pressure from the maternal sacral promontory. The use of forceps alone is not thought to be an important causative factor. Peripheral paralysis is unilateral. The forehead is smooth on the affected side, and the eye is persistently open.

Central: Often results from contralateral CNS injury (temporal bone fracture and/or posterior fossa hemorrhage or tissue destruction). It involves only the lower half or two-thirds of the face. The forehead and eyelids are not affected.

In both forms of paralysis, the mouth is drawn to the normal side when crying, and the nasolabial fold is obliterated on the affected side.

219. Is ankle clonus normal in the newborn infant?

Bilateral ankle clonus of 5–10 beats may be a normal finding, especially in infants who are crying, hungry, or jittery. This is particularly true if the clonus is unaccompanied by other signs of upper motor neuron dysfunction.

220. Do newborns prefer to turn their heads to the right or left?

Healthy neonates prefer to turn their heads to the right, which may reflect the normal asymmetry of cerebral function at this age. This preference has been observed as early as 28 weeks' gestation. By 39 weeks' gestation, 90% of newborn infants spend ≥ 80% of the time with their head turned to the right side.

NUTRITION

221. How many calories are required daily for growth in a healthy, growing, preterm infant?

Preterm infants need approximately 120 cal/kg/day. About 45% of the caloric intake should be carbohydrate, 45% fat, and 10% protein. Infants who expend increased calories (e.g., those with chronic lung disease, fever, cold stress, etc.) may need up to 150 cal/kg/day.

222. What are feeding strategies for the preterm infant?

The preterm infant is often started on formula feeds that are one-quarter or one-half strength. Although there are no data to support this clinical practice, many neonatologists believe that starting with dilute formula lessens the likelihood of feeding intolerance and possibly avoids serious complications such as necrotizing enterocolitis. The osmolality of the formula used may be a key determinant of the rapidity of gastric emptying. The use of GI priming (low volumes of milk) has been found to be helpful. Bolus feeding may be better tolerated than continuous feeding.

Schanler RJ, et al: Feeding strategies for premature infants: Randomized trial of gastrointestinal priming and tube-feeding method. Pediatrics 103: 434-439, 1999.

223. What are the nutritional advantages of formulas designed for preterm babies?

FEEDING COMPONENT	ADVANTAGE
Protein 60/40 whey casein	Improved digestion; increased amounts of cystine, taurine
Carbohydrate glucose polymers + lactose	Glucose polymers are better absorbed than lactose because of decreased production of intestinal lactase in the preterm infant
Fats: medium chain triglycerides (MCTs), corn/coconut	MCTs are absorbed directly into portal vein and are less dependent on bile salts for emulsification and micelle formation
Minerals: increased calcium, phosphorus	Improved bone mineralization
Calories: 24 cal/oz	Increased growth

224. How quickly can feedings be increased in preterm infants?

Feedings must be tailored to the premature infant based on the level of immaturity and current level of illness. While the average physiologic gastric capacity increases from 2 to 27 ml/kg over a course of 10 days, it is suggested that enteral feeds be advanced slowly (< 20 ml/kg/day) to decrease the risk of necrotizing enterocolitis.

225. What are the documented medical benefits of breast-feeding?

Proven benefits

- Fewer episodes of otitis media and respiratory and GI illness occur in breastfed infants.
- Human milk facilitates the growth of beneficial, nonpathogenic flora, compared with pathogenic anaerobes and coliforms that predominate in infants fed formula.
- Formula-fed infants have reduced quantities of host defense proteins in the GI tract (e.g., lactoferrin and secretory IgA).

Suggested but unproven benefits

- Decreased incidence of neonatal sepsis and necrotizing enterocolitis in preterm infants
- Enhancement of subsequent intelligence
- Reduction in incidence of atherosclerosis
- Reduction in incidence of diabetes mellitus

226. How does maternal breast milk differ for a full-term versus premature baby?

The composition of human milk for preterm infants differs from that for term infants in a number of ways. Per 100 ml, it is higher in calories (67–72 kcal vs 62–68), higher in protein (1.7–2.1 gm vs 1.2–1.7 gm), higher in lipid (3.4–4.4 gm vs 3.0–4.0 gm), lower in carbohydrates, higher in multiple minerals and trace elements (especially Na, Cl, Fe, Zn, Cu), and higher in vitamins (especially vitamins A and E).

Van Aerde J: Nutrition and metabolism in the high risk neonate. In Fanaroff AA, Martin RJ (eds): Neonatal-Perinatal Medicine, 5th ed. St. Louis, Mosby, 1992, pp 492–495.

227. How does colostrum differ from mature human breast milk?

Colostrum is the thick yellowish mammary secretion that is characteristic in the first postpartum week. It is higher in phospholipids, cholesterol, and protein concentration and lower in lactose and total fat composition than mature breast milk. Colostrum is particularly rich in immunoglobulins, especially secretory IgA.

228. In breast-feeding, how do fore milk and hind milk differ?

The caloric density of human milk increases in a nonlinear fashion while the infant is breast-feeding. *Hind* milk (produced at the end of the feeding) can have a fat content that is 50% higher than *fore* milk.

229. What are contraindications to breast-feeding?

Inborn errors of metabolism: galactosemia, phenylketonuria, urea-cycle defects

Infections: HIV, tuberculosis, HTLV-I, cytomegalovirus (in preterm infants), herpes simplex (when lesions are present on breast)

Substance abuse/use: cocaine, narcotics, stimulants

Medications: sulfonamides (in ill, stressed or preterm infants or infants with hyperbilirubinemia and G-6-PD deficiency), metronidazole, radioactive medicines, chemotherapeutic agents (alkylating agents), bromocriptine (suppresses lactation), lithium

Howard CR, Lawrence RA: Drugs and breastfeeding. Clin Perinatol 26:447-478, 1999.

230. Should breast-feeding be discontinued if the mother is on antibiotics?

In general, no. Sulfonamides have the potential to displace bilirubin from albumin and should be avoided during the first week of life. Tetracycline, which can cause tooth discoloration and enamel hypoplasia, should not be taken by lactating women. Most authorities also suggest that chloramphenicol not be administered to nursing mothers, although drug levels are unlikely to become high enough to produce the "gray baby" syndrome. Although no adverse effects have been seen in metronidazole-exposed infants, this drug is potentially mutagenic and carcinogenic. Therefore, breast-feeding should be discontinued while a mother is receiving metronidazole (Flagyl) and for a minimum of 12 hours after it has been stopped.

231. Should breastfed babies be supplemented with water?

Although a common practice, there is no basis for the supplementation of breast-feeding with water. Babies with water supplementation do not have any lesser degree of physiologic jaundice, may have more weight loss than nonsupplemented babies, and are less likely to be breastfed at 3 months than those nonsupplemented.

232. How long should infants be breastfed per feeding?

Infants nurse between 4–20 minutes per breast. Although the majority of milk volume is consumed during the first 4 minutes of nursing, the caloric density is greater during the later phase of breast feeding. If > 25 minutes is needed by an infant to empty a breast, one should suspect either poor milk production, an abnormal "let-down" response, or ineffective "latch-on."

233. What are the signs of inadequate intake in a breastfed infant?

- Irregular or nonsustained sucking at breast
- < 5 large, seedy, yellow stools each day during first month
- Failure to have a wet diaper with each feeding
- Nursing < 10 minutes/breast at each feeding
- Failure to demand to nurse at least 8 times daily
- Taking only 1 breast at each feeding
- Crying, fussing, and appearing hungry after most feedings
- Gaining < 1 oz/day

Neifert MR: Clinical aspects of lactation: Promoting breastfeeding success. Clin Perinatol 26:281-306, 1999.

234. Do breast milk and cow milk vary in lactose content?

Breast milk is 7% lactose, compared with whole or skim milk which is 4.8%.

235. What advice should be given to a mother who plans to express and save breast milk for later feedings?

Ideally, she should collect the milk as cleanly as possible and then store it rapidly at 3°–4°C or less. The milk should be used within 48 hours. If prolonged storage is necessary, the milk should be kept frozen at a temperature of at least –20°C. Once the milk has thawed, it should not be refrozen.

236. What are maternal benefits of breastfeeding?

- Increased postpartum weight loss
- More rapid uterine involution
- Postpartum amenorrhea during lactation (promotes child spacing)
- Decreased incidence of premenopausal breast cancer and ovarian cancer
- Decreased incidence of osteoporosis

Labbok MH: Health sequelae of breastfeeding for the mother. Clin Perinatol 26:491-503, 1999.

237. What are the advantages of a 60/40 whey/casein ratio in infant formulas?

The term 60/40 refers to the percentage of whey (lactalbumin) and casein in human milk or cow's milk formulas. This ratio makes for small curds and therefore easy digestibility by the infant. The 60/40 ratio is of particular advantage in the preterm infant because it is associated with lower levels of serum ammonia and a decreased incidence of metabolic acidosis. Only human milk or formulas that supply protein in this ratio provide adequate amounts of the amino acids cystine and taurine, which may be essential for the preterm infant.

238. How much formula should an average infant drink per day?

A healthy term newborn in the first 1–2 days of life may drink only 0.5–1 oz every 3–4 hours. Once feedings are well established, infants may ingest 200 ml/kg/day or more.

239. Must infant formulas be sterilized?

As a rule, ***no***. The terminal sterilization of prepared formula by boiling the bottle for 25 minutes offers no advantage over simple cleansing of the bottles and nipples in hot, soapy water and the subsequent use of unsterilized tap water in formula preparation. If bacteriologically safe tap water is used, no differences in rates of gastroenteritis occur.

Gerber MA, et al: Sterilization of infant formula. Clin Pediatr 22:344–349, 1983.

240. Among infant formulas, is low-iron or regular iron-fortified better?

Generally, low-iron formula has 1.5 mg of elemental Fe/l, while regular iron-fortified formula has 12 mg/l. Infants who are not breastfed should be placed on regular iron-fortified formula.

Although a greater percentage of iron is absorbed from the ingested low-iron formula, the quantity may not be sufficient to protect against the development of iron-deficiency anemia. In addition, despite anecdotal experiences, the incidence of colic, constipation, vomiting, and fussiness does not vary between infants fed the two formulas.

241. May milk be heated in a microwave oven?

No. Microwave heating produces uneven temperatures. Also, human milk is easily damaged by high temperatures.

242. Why are newborns who drink cow milk at risk for development of hypocalcemia?

Cow milk contains six times as much phosphorus as human milk (950 mg/l vs 162 mg/l). The neonatal kidney is unable to excrete this excessive phosphorus load, and hyperphosphatemia results. Since serum calcium and phosphorus concentrations are inversely correlated, the initial impact is increased deposition of calcium in bone and a decreased calcitriol (1,25-dihydroxyvitamin D) synthesis, which ultimately lead to hypocalcemia.

243. Is vitamin supplementation necessary in exclusively breastfed term infants?

Vitamin deficiencies are rare in breastfed infants, and as a rule, supplementation is not necessary. Exceptions include:

- Vitamin D supplementation in *black or darkly-pigmented babies* or in settings where maternal and infant *sunlight exposure is minimal*. Breast milk is low in vitamin D (approx. 22 IU/l).
- *Malnourished* mothers
- Mothers who are *strict vegetarians*. The concentration of B vitamins in their breast milk can be low.

244. Can infants with umbilical arterial catheters be fed safely?

The adequacy of GI perfusion and the risk of necrotizing enterocolitis have been major concerns in feeding infants with umbilical arterial catheters. However, no definite evidence exists that these catheters, by themselves, increase the risk of NEC when they are in place during feedings.

245. What is the mechanism of hyperalimentation-induced cholestasis?

The mechanism remains uncertain, although amino acid toxicity has been frequently implicated. Dextrose infusions may also be hepatotoxic, but Intralipid administration is probably not causative in this syndrome. Infants fed a high-protein regimen (3–6 gm/kg/day) develop a higher level of direct bilirubin at an earlier time than infants receiving a lower protein load. Other possible etiologies include (1) decreased bile flow and gut motility secondary to the lack of oral alimentation and immaturity of the enterohepatic circulation; (2) cholestasis secondary to absorption of bacterial toxins from the gut during bowel stasis; or (3) amino acid deficiency in hyperalimentation mixtures.

246. How can hyperalimentation-induced cholestasis be prevented?

Cholestasis secondary to intravenous hyperalimentation is a multifactorial disease. Newer balanced mixtures of amino acids, which include taurine, may help reduce the incidence of cholestasis. The development of cholestasis can only be prevented by establishing enteral feeds. Even minimal enteral feeds may be helpful in reducing the incidence of hyperalimentation-induced cholestasis.

247. What is the treatment for hyperalimentation-induced cholestasis?

The preferred treatment is to stop IV hyperalimentation and begin enteral feedings. If IV hyperalimentation cannot be discontinued, the amount of protein infused should be reduced to 2 gm/kg/day and the cal/N ratio kept below 200. In most infants, the condition is transient and resolves without further therapy. In infants with severe intrahepatic cholestasis, phenobarbital has been shown to stimulate bile secretion and lower serum bilirubin levels. Recent studies have also suggested that ursodeoxycholic acid, a choleretic and predominant bile acid in the polar bear, may alleviate hyperalimentation-induced cholestasis.

248. How should lipid infusions be monitored?

Intralipid infusions should be monitored by ***measuring weekly triglyceride*** and ***cholesterol levels***. Visible clearing from the serum may also be measured through a capillary tube, but this technique is probably much less reliable. Glucose levels should also be followed, as lipids cause enhanced gluconeogenesis secondary to increased fatty acid oxidation.

249. Should Intralipid usage be curtailed in the infant with hyperbilirubinemia or respiratory distress?

During lipid hydrolysis, free fatty acids are generated which may compete with bilirubin for binding to albumin. However, to date, no studies suggest a higher incidence of kernicterus in infants receiving Intralipid. Lipid deposits have been noted at autopsy in alveolar macrophages and capillaries following Intralipid administration. These adverse effects of Intralipid on pulmonary function and bilirubin binding are related both to the dose and rate of infusion. A lipid dose of 1 gm/kg administered over 15 hours is safe for any size newborn infant. Therefore, hyperbilirubinemia and respiratory distress are not contraindications to the use of Intralipid. In an infant nearing the point of exchange transfusion or receiving 100% oxygen, lipid emulsions should be used with caution.

250. If alimentation is being administered through a peripheral vein, is heparinization necessary?

The administration of heparin to premature infants in a concentration of 1 U/ml has been shown to improve the clearance of lipids. Therefore, heparin should be used whenever fats are being administered intravenously.

251. What is nonnutritive sucking?

Nonnutritive sucking is a mode of sucking unique to humans and is characterized by a highly regular, burst-pause pattern. Nonnutritive sucking occurs in all sleep and awake states, although less often during quiet sleep and crying. It assumes a recognizable rhythmic pattern after 33 weeks' gestation.

252. How do protein requirements vary with mode of nutrient delivery (intravenous vs enteral)?

Whether delivered intravenously or enterally, the protein requirements needed to achieve *in utero* accretion rates are similar. Preterm infants have slightly higher protein requirements (3.0–3.5 gm/kg/day) than term infants (2.0–2.5 gm/kg/day).

253. Which amino acids are essential for the preterm infant?

Essential

- Leucine
- Isoleucine
- Valine
- Threonine
- Methionine
- Phenylalanine
- Tryptophan
- Lysine

Conditionally Essential

- Cysteine
- Taurine
- Tyrosine
- Arginine
- Glutamine

254. Which fatty acids are essential for the neonate?

Linoleic acid and ***linolenic acid***. In infants weighing < 1750 gm who experience delay or difficulty in maintaining full enteral feedings, arachidonic and docosahexaenoic fatty acids may also be essential. These fatty acids are vital for normal brain development, myelination, cell proliferation, and retinal function. Fatty acids in human milk are composed of 12–15% linoleic acid.

255. What are the manifestations of essential-fatty-acid deficiency?

Scaly dermatitis, ***alopecia***, ***thrombocytopenia*** (and platelet dysfunction), ***failure to thrive***, and increased ***susceptibility to recurrent infection***. To prevent and treat fatty-acid deficiency, 4–5% of caloric intake should be provided as linoleic acid and 1% as linolenic acid. This requirement can be met by 0.5–1.0 gm/kg/day of intravenous lipids.

256. Why are nucleotides being added to a number of infant formulas?

Dietary nucleotides may play a role in early neonatal life in the desaturation and elongation of essential fatty acids which are necessary for brain and retinal development. The addition of nucleotides to formula, simulating the composition in breast milk, may be especially important during early development. Nucleotides are present in relatively large amounts in human milk, and several studies have suggested an important role for nucleotides in immune function, GI function, and lipoprotein metabolism.

257. What causes osteopenia of prematurity?

During the period of rapid growth, many preterm infants exhibit undermineralization of bone (rickets of prematurity). This condition results primarily from an insufficient intake of calcium and phosporus, although vitamin D insufficiency, aluminum toxicity, or liver disease can be contributing factors.

258. What tests make up a "rickets screen"?

Serum calcium, ***phosporus***, and ***alkaline phosphatase***. Infants with osteopenia of prematurity (i.e., rickets) can maintain a normal serum calcium and phosporus until late in the disease, and so increased alkaline phosphatase is usually seen first. Routine radiographs can demonstrate generalized osteopenia with widening, cupping, and fraying of the metaphyses and fractures. In research settings, adequacy of mineral status can also be followed by serial serum concentrations of osteocalcin and calciotropic hormones and by bone photon densitometry.

259. How is osteopenia of prematurity prevented?

Calcium and phosporus should be supplied in amounts that approximate the intrauterine accretion rates (120–140 mg/kg/day for calcium and 65–75 mg/kg/day for phosphorus). Since only 65% of calcium and 85% of phosporus is absorbed when preterm infants are fed enterally, the amounts must be readjusted upward in infants receiving formula.

260. What are the manifestations of vitamin E deficiency in the neonate?

Hemolytic anemia (with reticulocytosis), ***peripheral edema***, and ***thrombocytosis***. Vitamin E is important in stabilizing the red cell membrane, and a deficiency can result in a mild hemolytic anemia. The American Academy of Pediatrics recommends that 0.7 IU of vitamin E/100 kcal be present in feedings for preterm infants.

261. What are the manifestations of zinc and copper deficiency in the neonate?

Zinc deficiency: dry skin, growth retardation, hepatosplenomegaly, impaired wound healing, hair loss, perioral and perianal rashes, decreased resistance to infection

Copper deficiency: hypochromic microcytic anemia, neutropenia, bony abnormalities. respiratory issues

262. What causes infants to grunt?

Infants with respiratory disease tend to expire through closed or partially closed vocal cords in order to elevate transpulmonary pressure and therefore increase lung volume. The latter effect results in an improved ventilation/perfusion ratio with better gas exchange. It is during the last part of expiration when gas is expelled through the partially closed vocal cords that the audible grunt is produced.

263. What do hyperpnea and tachypnea signify in the neonate?

Hyperpnea refers to deep relatively unlabored respirations at mildly increased rates. It is typical of situations in which there is reduced pulmonary blood flow (e.g., pulmonary atresia) and results from ventilation of underperfused alveoli. *Tachypnea* refers to shallow, rapid, and somewhat labored respirations and is seen in the setting of low lung compliance (e.g., primary lung disease and pulmonary edema).

264. Why do newborn infants breathe faster than adults?

The total work of breathing, which is the sum of elastic and resistance work, varies with ventilatory pattern (tidal volume and rate). The respiratory centers attempt to achieve a given minute ventilation with a pattern that minimizes work. This minimum energy expenditure is achieved at higher respiratory rates in infants than in adults (35–40 breaths/min vs. 16 breaths/min).

265. Until what age are infants obligate nose breathers?

Although 30% of newborn infants breathe through their mouth or nose and mouth, the remaining 70% are obligate nose breathers until the third to sixth week of life.

266. What are the effects of severe hypercarbia ($PCO_2 \geq 100$ mm Hg) if there is no associated hypoxia?

There are few data in human newborns on the effects of isolated severe hypercarbia in the absence of hypoxia. However, results from animal studies and limited clinical observations in humans suggest that this condition can lead to a pressure-passive cerebral circulation and an increased risk of intraventricular hemorrhage. In addition, the high $PaCO_2$ may disrupt the blood–brain barrier and enhance the deposition of molecules such as bilirubin in the CNS, leading to kernicterus. Finally, on a more cellular level, data in animal model systems demonstrate alterations in brain cell membrane lipid peroxidation as well as Na^+–K^+ ATPase activity. The significance of these latter findings remains undetermined.

267. How do blood oxygen content, oxygen saturation, and PO_2 differ?

PO_2 is the partial pressure of oxygen in equilibrium with blood. The percentage of hemoglobin that is bound with oxygen at a given PO_2 is the oxygen saturation. The oxygen content, which is measured in vol %, is the total volume of oxygen bound to hemoglobin plus the volume dissolved in blood, the latter of which is generally negligible at normal values of PO_2. The oxygen content can be calculated as follows:

1.34 ml O_2/gm hemoglobin × hemoglobin (gm/dl) × oxygen saturation

268. How is mean airway pressure affected by ventilator settings?

Mean airway pressure (Pa w) is a measure of the average pressure to which the lungs are exposed during the respiratory cycle and can be calculated by dividing the area under the airway pressure curve by the duration of the cycle. Pa w is affected by changes in inspiratory flow, peak inspiratory pressure (PIP), positive end-expiratory pressure (PEEP), and ratio of inspiratory to expiratory time (I/E ratio).

269. In an infant receiving mechanical ventilation, what is an acceptable range for pH, PCO_2, and PO_2?

The goal of mechanical ventilation is to maintain the arterial PO_2 in the range of 50–80 mm Hg and arterial pH between 7.30–7.41. Earlier recommendations advocated maintenance of PCO_2 between 35–45 mm Hg. Some neonatologists now recommend that the PCO_2 be allowed to rise to levels as high as 55–60 mm Hg in order to minimize barotrauma. It is still controversial whether sustained hypercarbia has adverse side effects.

270. What mechanical ventilator settings are likely to affect PO_2 and PCO_2?

Since many ventilatory changes may affect both oxygenation and ventilation to some degree, the following table is an oversimplified but, nevertheless, useful guide:

VENTILATOR SETTING	PO_2	PCO_2
PIP	↑	↓
PEEP	↑	↑
Frequency	↑ or NE*	↓
I:E	↑	NE†
FiO2	↑	NE
Flow rate	↑	NE

NE = no consistent effect; PIP = positive inspiratory pressure; PEEP = positive en-expiratory pressure; I:E = ratio of inspiratory to expiratory time.

*At very high respiratory rates, inspiratory time may be so short as to comproise oxygenation. Furthermore, at a very high frequency, there is an increase in inadvertent PEEP which can result in CO_2 accumulation.

†CO_2 elimination may be affected at extremely low expiratory times.

271. What are the physiologic effects of positive end-expiratory pressure (PEEP)?

PEEP can prevent alveolar collapse, maintain lung volume at end expiration, and improve ventilation-perfusion mismatch. However, an increase in PEEP may decrease tidal volume and impede CO_2 elimination. Elevations in PEEP to nonphysiologic values may decrease lung compliance, impair venous return, decrease cardiac output, and reduce tissue oxygen delivery.

272. How is the optimal PEEP determined?

The "optimal PEEP" is the end-expiratory pressure at which oxygenation is maximal with minimum effect on cardiovascular function. The best way to determine optimal PEEP is controversial. In practice, the PEEP setting is generally maintained at a level equal to 10% of the inspired oxygen concentration. For example, if the inspired oxygen concentration is 60%, the PEEP should be kept in the 5–7 range; if 40%, the 4–5 range, etc.

273. When is intermittent continuous positive airway pressure (CPAP) indicated in the nonventilated infant?

Intermittent CPAP, delivered by mask, is used in nonventilated infants to reduce the incidence of segmental or lobar atelectasis following prolonged endotracheal intubation.

274. In infants with chronic lung disease receiving supplemental oxygen, what is the approximate FiO_2 delivered by nasal cannula at various flow rates?

The FiO_2 delivered by nasal cannula in an infant is dependent on the respiratory rate and minute ventilation, positioning of the cannula, and the extent of nasal versus oral breathing. Smaller infants (with lower minute ventilation) entrain less room air and thus receive more oxygen for a given flow rate. As a general rule, for infants < 3500 gm, the delivery of 100% O_2 by nasal cannula at a flow rate of 0.125 l/min corresponds to an FiO_2 of 28–30%, and at 0.5 l/min, to an FiO_2 of approximately 35%. For infants > 3500 gm, 0.5 l/min corresponds to an FiO_2 of 28 and 2.0 l/min to 35%.

Fan LL, Voyles JB: Determination of inspired oxygen delivered by nasal cannula in infants with chronic lung disease. J Pediatr 106:923–925, 1983.

275. Should newborn infants receiving mechanical ventilation be pharmacologically paralyzed?

Neuromuscular paralysis is not recommended as routine treatment for mechanically ventilated infants. However, in specific instances, such as persistence of fetal circulation, neuromuscular paralysis may benefit infants whose activity/agitation may increase right-to-left shunting and decrease oxygenation. Paralysis may also reduce the incidence of pneumothorax and intraventricular hemorrhage in infants with respiratory distress.

276. How do high-frequency oscillatory ventilation (HFOV) and high-frequency jet ventilation (HFJV) differ?

	HFOV	HFJV
Frequency	10–30 Hz	10–40 Hz
Total volume	Determined by oscillator	Increased by gas entrainment
I:E ratio	Constant*	Variable
Expiratory phase	Active	Passive
	Less risk of gas trapping	More risk of gas trapping
Airway damage	Similar to IPPV	Necrotizing tracheobronchitis†
May be used in combination with IPPV	Yes	Yes

*Some oscillators have adjustable I:E ratios.

†May be no different from conventional ventilation. IPPV = intermittent positive pressure ventilation.

In general, HFJV has been used more commonly in infants with severe pulmonary interstitial emphysema, while HFOV has been of greater value in preventing "air-leak syndrome" in infants requiring "high" settings. Neither ventilator has been proven superior to conventional ventilation in the management of infants with uncomplicated respiratory distress syndrome (RDS). Furthermore, it is controversial if either form of high-frequency ventilation lessens the incidence of bronchopulmonary dysplasia (BPD).

From Bancalari E, Goldberg RN: High-frequency ventilation in the neonate. Clin Perinatol 14:581, 1987; with permission.

277. What is the preferred method of suctioning in premature infants?

Two varieties of endotracheal tube (ETT) suctioning are used in premature infants:

1. ***"Shallow" suctioning***, in which the catheter is introduced 0.5–1 cm below the tip of the ETT.

2. ***"Deep" suctioning***, in which the catheter is introduced until resistance is felt, and then withdrawn 1 cm before suction is applied.

Shallow suctioning may be the preferred method for premature infants because of a lesser risk of traumatic injury. It should be done with a catheter no larger than two-thirds of the inner diameter of the ETT and with a negative pressure no greater than 60–100 mm Hg. Suctioning should be performed as often as necessary to maintain ETT patency, with a minimum of once every several hours. Suctioning increases intracranial pressure, slows the heart rate, and decreases lung volumes. Infants who are being suctioned commonly become hypoxemic, which may worsen ongoing pulmonary hypertension.

278. How successful are operative procedures to reverse subglottic stenosis?

Cricoid split and endoscopic excision of a subglottic lesion have been used to treat subglottic stenosis with success rates of > 75%.

279. What tests can be done to estimate lung maturity prenatally?

Most prenatal tests for lung maturity are designed to detect the presence of surfactant. The following tests are those most commonly used:

Lecithin/sphingomyelin (L/S) ratio: Since lecithin is a major component of surfactant, and sphingomyelin concentration is relatively constant during gestation, the L/S ratio can be used as a measure of lung maturity. An L/S of ≥ 2.0 carries a low risk of RDS and is generally attained at 34–35 weeks' gestation. While ratios of 1.5–2.0 carry a 40% risk of RDS, values of < 1.5 carry a risk of 75%. The L/S ratio is not reliable in pregnancies with Rh disease or maternal diabetes. Furthermore, the test cannot be performed on fluid contaminated with blood or meconium.

Phosphatidylglycerol: This surface-acting, stabilizing factor is present at > 35 weeks' gestation. Thus, its presence is indicative of lung maturity, but its absence offers no definitive help in management. The measurement can be performed on blood- or meconium-contaminated fluid and is available as a standardized latex agglutination assay. Many clinicians quantitate both the L/S ratio and phosphatidylglycerol as part of a lung profile.

Foam stability or shake test: These tests depend on the ability of surfactant-rich fluid to form stable bubbles when mixed or shaken with ethanol. The foam stability index has been developed as a standardized test using constant amounts of ethanol with different dilutions of amniotic fluid. Stable bubbles at ≥ 0.48 dilution are suggestive of mature lungs. The test is, however, limited by a high incidence of false-negative results.

Fluorescence polarimetry: This test may be used to measure microviscosity of amniotic fluid, which decreases as lung matures. This method involves expensive equipment and is not routinely available.

Optical density (OD): The OD of phospholipids in amniotic fluid peaks at 650 nm. This test is rapid and routinely available, but it may not be as reliable as other tests.

280. What is the function of surfactant?

Surfactant is a surface-active material comprised of a mixture rich in phosphatidylcholine (64%), phosphatidylglycerol (8%), and lesser amounts of proteins and other lipids. Surfactant acts as an anti-atelectasis factor in the alveolar lining by lowering surface tension at diminished lung volumes and increasing it at high volumes. This allows for maintenance of functional residual capacity, which acts as a reservoir to prevent wide fluctuation in arterial PO_2 and PCO_2 during respiration. In patients with RDS, surfactants have been shown to decrease the need for supplemental oxygen therapy, lower mortality rates, and decrease the incidence of air-leak syndromes. The incidence of BPD has also been reduced in some studies.

281. Do the kinds of surfactant used to treat infants with RDS differ in effectiveness?

Two general classes of surfactant are available for replacement therapy: ***natural surfactants*** prepared from mammalian lungs (e.g., Survanta, Infasurf, Curosurf) and ***synthetic surfactants*** (e.g., Exosurf, ALEC). Although natural surfactant extracts seem to have a better immediate effect (less supplemental oxygen required, fewer pneumothoraces), long-term clinical outcomes (e.g., chronic lung disease, death) with synthetic surfactants are comparable.

The Vermont-Oxford Neonatal Network: Comparison of surfactants in respiratory distress syndrome. Pediatrics 97:1–6, 1996.

282. In surfactant therapy, is prophylaxis or "rescue" treatment better?

When and to whom surfactant should be administered remains a heavily studied topic. Ideally, it is administered to surfactant-deficient infants as soon as possible. However, while some institutions routinely administer surfactant to all infants less than a set gestational age (e.g., 31 weeks) as soon as possible after birth, others wait for clinical signs of RDS before initiating therapy. Until precise measures are available to rapidly assess the extent of surfactant sufficiency in an infant, the debate will continue. Early administration of surfactant is more important for the very-low-birthweight infant, in whom it has been shown to reduce mortality and lower the incidence of BPD.

283. What are the adverse effects of prophylactically administering surfactant in the delivery room?

- 20–60% of healthy infants whose gestational age is ≤ 30 weeks will be treated unnecessarily.
- It imposes extra risks and unwarranted expenses.
- Use of surfactant may lead to a transient decrease in oxygen saturation.
- It delays resuscitation efforts and stabilization.
- In comparison with rescue treatment, the use of prophylactic surfactant may worsen neurodevelopmental outcome and increase the incidence of chronic lung disease (controversial).

284. When should infants with RDS be mechanically ventilated?

Mechanical ventilation is initiated when the diagnosis of respiratory failure is made.

Laboratory criteria for respiratory failure

- Respiratory acidosis with pH < 7.20 and PCO_2 > 60 mmHg
- Severe hypoxemia with PaO_2 < 50–60 mm Hg despite an FiO_2 of 0.7–1.0 and an adequate trial of continuous positive airway pressure

Clinical criteria for respiratory failure

- Severe retractions
- Cyanosis
- Intractable apnea

285. How is pulmonary interstitial emphysema (PIE) treated?

PIE is an air-leak syndrome that is usually a complication of mechanical ventilation. Thus, therapy for PIE is usually aimed at reduction of the peak inflating pressure (through jet ventilation if necessary). In cases of localized PIE, dependent positioning of the involved lung as well as selective mainstem bronchial intubation and ventilation of the uninvolved lung are beneficial. When medical management of localized PIE fails, surgical lobectomy may be considered.

286. Is the meconium aspiration syndrome a function of meconium aspirated in utero or at birth?

The *meconium aspiration syndrome* is commonly defined as respiratory distress in a meconium-stained newborn with scattered infiltrates on x-ray, no alternative explanation for the clinical findings, and a high incidence of pulmonary vasoconstriction which leads to persistent pulmonary hypertension of the newborn. Some argue that in utero gasping of meconium leads to pulmonary vascular hypertrophy demonstrable by early biopsy, while others argue that aspiration after birth with an evolving syndrome is more likely since a high proportion of infants (up to 60%) are healthy and vigorous at birth. The likely answer is that both are involved and that this syndrome is a spectrum of diseases.

Wiswell TE, Bent RC: Meconium staining and the meconium aspiration syndrome. Pediatr Clin North Am 40:955–981, 1993.

287. Where is the proper location for a chest tube?

Chest tubes should be placed in the fourth intercostal space at the midaxillary line. For evacuation of a pneumothorax, they should then be directed anteriorly toward the apex of the thorax and advanced to the midclavicular line.

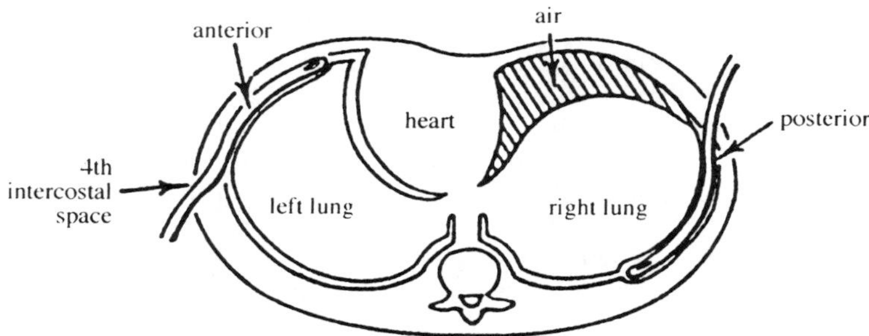

Anterior versus posterior position of the chest tube for drainage of air or fluid. Since air usually collects anteromedially in the supine neonate, the posterior tip is less appropriate.
From Fletcher MA, et al: Atlas of Procedures in Neonatology. Philadelphia, J.B. Lippincott, 1983, p 265; with permission.

288. What is the pathophysiology of pulmonary hemorrhage in the neonate?

Pulmonary hemorrhage has been associated with a number of clinical conditions, including prematurity, asphyxia, sepsis, aspiration, intrauterine growth retardation, congenital heart disease, patent ductus arteriosus, and coagulopathies. Studies have indicated that lung effluents in these patients actually represent hemorrhagic pulmonary edema and not whole blood. The unifying feature in this disorder is an elevation in pulmonary capillary pressure which results either from acute left ventricular failure or conditions favoring increased filtration of fluid, such as hypoproteinemia, hypervolemia, and lung injury.

289. Which infants benefit most from extracorporeal membrane oxygenation (ECMO)?

ECMO is prolonged cardiopulmonary bypass used as a therapy in neonates. Newborn infants (< 1 week old) with reversible pulmonary disease complicated by persistent pulmonary hypertension are most likely to benefit from ECMO therapy. The most common associated diagnoses include meconium aspiration syndrome, respiratory distress syndrome, sepsis/pneumonia, and congenital diaphragmatic hernia.

290. What are the indications for instituting ECMO therapy?

ECMO therapy is usually indicated when an infant fails to oxygenate adequately (despite maximal ventilatory support with 100% oxygen) or shows acute deterioration. Most ECMO centers use one or more of the following formulas to identify candidates with an expected mortality (80% and generally after failed therapy with high frequency ventilation and nitric oxide.

- Alveolar/arterial oxygen gradient ($AaDO_2$) > 605 for 4–12 hours.
  $AaDO_2$ (approximately) = 713 – (PaO_2 + $PaCO_2$) when the FiO_2 is 1.0 (100% inspired oxygen).
- Oxygen index (OI) (40 on three of five consecutive arterial blood gases obtained 30–60 minutes apart.
  OI = mean airway pressure x FiO_2/PaO_2 x 100.
- PaO_2 < 50 mm Hg for 4 hours.
- pH< 7.25 for 2 hours with hypotension

Other criteria include:

- Gestational age ≥ 34 weeks
- Birthweight > 2000 gm
- No evidence of bleeding, intraventricular hemorrhage or coagulopathy
- Reversible lung disease
- No major cardiac lesion

291. What percentage of infants are normal after receiving ECMO?

The overall survival of infants placed on ECMO is > 80%. The short-term outcome data suggest that approximately two-thirds of infants are normal following ECMO. It is difficult to determine if moderate to severe neurologic deficits seen in some survivors after ECMO are secondary to the infant's condition prior to bypass or to the risks of ECMO therapy.

292. What are the risks of and contraindications to ECMO?

The *risk* of thrombosis is an ever-present threat during ECMO therapy. Therefore, all infants on ECMO are heparinized. However, heparinization creates an increased risk for systemic bleeding and/or intracranial hemorrhage. Long-term morbidities are generally referable to the CNS.

Contraindications to ECMO include uncontrolled bleeding, grade II or greater intraventricular hemorrhage, irreversible pulmonary disease, and significant prematurity (birthweight < 2000 gm, gestational age < 34 weeks).

293. What characterizes the diagnosis of bronchopulmonary dysplasia (BPD)?

Since BPD was first reported in 1967, the clinical definition and diagnosis have evolved to include all patients who, after mechanical ventilation, remain oxygen-dependent at 36 weeks post-conceptional age and have persistent changes on chest radiographs. The pathologic diagnosis remains unchanged and is characterized by areas of emphysema and collapse with interstitial edema and fibrosis. The airway epithelium demonstrates hyperplasia and squamous metaplasia and the smooth muscle in the airways and vasculature frequently demonstrates hyperplasia.

294. Why is combination diuretic therapy used in infants with BPD?

Chlorothiazide/spironolactone and furosemide are used in infants with chronic lung disease to improve pulmonary compliance and decrease resistance by eliminating excess sodium and water. Furosemide produces an increase in venous capacitance and may have the added benefit of reducing right ventricular preload. Spironolactone and chlorothiazide are commonly used in combination with furosemide to minimize calcium wasting and decrease the incidence of nephrocalcinosis. In clinical practice, however, infants receiving combination therapy still waste calcium.

295. Is there a long-term benefit to diuretic therapy in BPD?

Long-term diuretic therapy in infants with BPD improves pulmonary function, decreases airway resistance, increases pulmonary compliance, and allows weaning of supplemental oxygen. However, the duration of supplemental oxygen may not be shortened. Furthermore, the long-term effect on infant mortality is not entirely clear. Diuretic therapy is not without side effects, including electrolyte imbalance, nephrocalcinosis, bone demineralization, and ototoxicity.

Kao LC, et al: Randomized trial of long-term diuretic therapy for infants with oxygen-dependent bronchopulmonary dysplasia. J Pediatr 124:772–781, 1994.

296. What is the role of vitamin A supplementation in preventing or reducing the severity of BPD?

Because vitamin A is involved in the proliferation and differentiation of epithelial cells, it is thought to play an important role in the repair process in the lung following barotrauma and oxygen exposure. While vitamin A deficiency has been associated with the development of BPD, studies examining the effects of vitamin A supplementation on the incidence of BPD have shown conflicting results. However, the most recent large multicenter trial has demonstrated a modest reduction in the incidence of chronic lung disease in extremely low birth weight infants while reducing biochemical evidence of Vitamin A deficiency.

Tyson JE, et al: Vitamin A supplementation for extremely-low-birth-weight infants. N Engl J Med 340: 1962-1968, 1999.

297. When should steroids be initiated in neonates with BPD?

Infants between 2–4 weeks of age who are infection-free, are ventilator- and oxygen-dependent, and have early radiographic signs of BPD may benefit from treatment with steroids. It remains unclear if earlier administration is beneficial. Dexamethasone clearly improves lung function and compliance in infants with BPD within 72 hours after initiation. In turn, larger numbers of infants can be weaned from assisted ventilation and extubated. The impact is less clear with regard to the duration of supplemental oxygen required, length of hospital stay, and infant mortality. Side effects can include adrenal suppression, gastroduodenal perforation, hypertension, and hyperglycemia. In addition, recent analyses suggest that steroid-treated infants may have an increased incidence of cerebral palsy and/or developmental disabilities.

Ng PC: The effectiveness and side effects of dexamethasone in preterm infants with bronchopulmonary dysplasia. Arch Dis Child 68:330–337, 1993.

298. What is a BPD spell?

BPD spells have not been well characterized. In many infants the spell is clearly due to bronchial constriction. Most of these infants are believed to have airway smooth muscle hypertrophy. Other causes of BPD spells include cor pulmonale, tracheomalacia, aspiration, and atelectasis. The frequency of spells can generally be minimized by administering bronchodilators, diuretics, and oxygen. Some infants may require increased levels of end-expiratory pressure as a treatment for tracheomalacia or the use of sedatives to decrease agitation.

299. Why are infants with BPD at increased risk for poor neurodevelopmental outcome?

- Recurrent episodes of hypoxia secondary to chronic lung disease and BPD spells
- BPD is associated with intraventricular hemorrhage and periventricular leukomalacia.
- Poor nutrition during periods of critical brain growth
- Prolonged illness and hospitalization preclude normal stimulation and parent-infant interaction

Gerdes JS: Bronchopulmonary dysplasia. In Polin RA, et al (eds): Workbook in Practical Neonatology, 3rd ed. Philadelphia, W.B. Saunders, 2001, pp 198.

300. What is the difference between apnea and periodic breathing?

Apnea is defined as periods of cessation of respiration for > 10–15 seconds with or without cyanosis, pallor, hypotonia, and/or bradycardia, or for < 10 seconds accompanied by bradycardia. *Periodic breathing*, which is commonly seen in preterm infants, is defined as a pattern of 3 or more respiratory pauses of greater than 3 seconds' duration with less than 20 seconds of respirations between pauses. Periodic breathing is not associated with bradycardia. Both apnea and periodic breathing reflect lack of maturation of respiratory control centers in the preterm infant.

301. When should apnea be treated?

In all cases of apnea, an underlying cause should be sought and treated if found. In idiopathic apnea, therapy should be initiated when episodes do not resolve with gentle tactile stimulation and require vigorous stimulation, or when patients have a frequency of > 2 episodes/8 hours.

302. What is the impact of apnea and bradycardia on cerebral blood flow in the preterm newborn?

Episodes of apnea associated with a decrease in heart rate to < 80 bpm can result in hypotension. Furthermore, these events may be accompanied by decreased diastolic and systolic cerebral blood flow velocities.

303. What methods are effective for treating apnea of prematurity?

- Use of oscillating waterbeds
- Administration of continuous positive airway pressure (CPAP) (especially helpful in apnea with an obstructive component)
- Provision of supplemental oxygen (with or without CPAP)
- Administration of respiratory stimulants (methylxanthines or doxapram).
- If supplemental oxygen is used, the PaO_2 must be carefully monitored either directly by arterial blood gases or indirectly by noninvasive oxygen monitoring devices (e.g., pulse oximetry).

304. Is caffeine or theophylline more effective in lessening apnea of prematurity?

There is no evidence to date that one methylxanthine is more effective than the other in reducing the frequency of apnea in premature infants. Caffeine, however, has become the preferred medication for several reasons: it is excreted more slowly, can be given once daily, achieves a more stable plasma level, and has fewer GI and CNS side effects.

305. When is doxapram indicated in treating apnea of prematurity?

Doxapram is a potent respiratory stimulant with predominantly peripheral chemoreceptor effects. It does not appear to be any more effective than the methylxanthines in the treatment of apnea of prematurity and has a potentially greater toxicity. However, doxapram may be helpful when used in addition to methylxanthines to avoid positive pressure therapies (i.e., CPAP or mechanical ventilation).

Brion LP, et al: Low dose doxapram for apnea unresponsive to aminophylline in VLBW infants. J Perinatol 11:359–364, 1991.

306. What are the criteria for discontinuing the use of an apnea monitor or methylxanthines?

Methylxanthines are usually discontinued after an apnea-free period of 4-8 weeks. Alternatively, 44 weeks post-conceptional age can be used as a "milestone" for the maturation of respiratory control in virtually all babies. The apnea monitor is then discontinues 4-8 weeks later if there is no recurrence of symptomatic apnea. A home pneumogram or downloading of data stored in the home "smart monitor" should be recorded before monitor discontinuance.

307. Do home apnea monitors help prevent SIDS?

The use of monitors generates considerable controversy in pediatric and neonatal circles. Infants who are usually considered for monitoring include siblings of SIDS victims, infants who have had apparent life-threatening events, infants with abnormal "predictive" studies (e.g., abnormal pneumograms, spectral cry analyses, or brainstem auditory evoked responses), or infants with apnea of prematurity. Opponents of monitors argue that no controlled studies have been done to indicate home monitoring is effective in SIDS prevention. Furthermore, monitoring is often expensive and may be anxiety-provoking (due to the false alarms). Proponents cite anecdotal data demonstrating a lower incidence of SIDS with home monitoring and a reduction in parental anxiety and stress.

Burnell RH, Beal SM: Monitoring and sudden infant death. J Paediatr Child Health 30:461–462, 1994.

308. What is the mechanism of action of inhaled nitric oxide (iNO) ?

Nitric oxide is the previously described endothelium-derived relaxation factor and is normally produced in endothelial cells via the NO synthase-catalyzed conversion of arginine and oxygen to citrulline and NO.The NO, whether endogenous or exogenously administered, diffuses to arteriolar smooth muscle cells, where it activates guanyl cyclase to convert guanosine triphospahate (GTP) to cyclic guanosine monophospahate (cGMP), which in turn causes pulmonary arteriolar smooth muscle relaxation. NO is then rapidly inactivated by binding to hemoglobin, forming nitrosohemoglobin and methemoglobin, thereby preventing any effects on the systemic circulation.

309. Does the use of inhaled nitric oxide (iNO) in the treatment of neonatal respiratory failure improve clinical outcome?

Several large multicenter trials examining the effects of iNO have been performed to date. Although they differed with respect to entry criteria, methods of randomization and dosing, to name a few, the results were fairly consistent. While there was no reduction in mortality, there was an approximately one-third reduction in the need for ECMO therapy.

310. How does liquid ventilation work?

Liquid ventilation is performed in place of gaseous ventilation via two methods, total liquid ventilation or perflurorocarbon-assisted gas exchange (partial or PAGE). Perflurorocarbon, the chemically and physiologically inert agent used, has a solubility for respiratory gases that exceeds that of blood. Instillation of this agent gradually recruits alveoli without barotrauma in part through its surfactant-like surface tension lowering properties. In addition, elimination of perflurocarbon is easily accomplished by vaporization.

311. Which infants are most likely to benefit from liquid ventilation?

- Extremely low birth weight infants failing to respond to surfactant therapy
- Infants with pulmonary hypoplasia secondary to congenital diaphragmatic hernia
- Term infants approaching need for ECMO, who have failed all other conventional and experimental therapies

14. NEPHROLOGY

Thomas Kennedy, M.D., *James Prebis*, M.D., *Stephen* J. *Wassner*, M.D., *and Michael* E. *Norman*, M.D.

ACID-BASE, FLUIDS AND ELECTROLYTES

1. What are the daily requirements for sodium for children?

Sodium intake at a level of 2-4 mEq/100 kcal (for infants this equals 2-4 mEq/kg body weight) are recommended. Salt losing states such as severe prematurity, infants with significant hydronephrosis or dysplasia, and individuals with cystic fibrosis or other abnormal causes of salt loss require more sodium. Estimated minimal daily sodium requirements for healthy individuals have been published by the National Research Council:

AGE (YRS)	WEIGHT (KG)	SODIUM (MG/MEQ)
1	11	225/10
2–5	16	300/13
6–9	25	400/17
10–18	50	500/22
>18	70	500/22

National Research Council. Recommended Dietary Allowances 10th ed. Washington, DC: National Academy Press , 1989, pp. 250-254.

2. In what situations can a child be hyponatremic but not hypotonic?

A. ***Increased extracellular osmotically active solutes***. When glucose, mannitol, glycerol, or another osmotically active substance are added to or increased in the extracellular space, the osmotic gradient pulls water from the cells and dilutes the serum sodium concentration. This dilutes the serum sodium concentration and results in hyponatremia although the presence of the other osmoles lead to hyperosmolality. This situation is most commonly encountered in diabetic ketoacidosis, and as a rule, for each 100 mg/dL increase in serum glucose, the serum sodium concentration is decreased by 1.6 mEq/L.

B. ***Elevated plasma lipids and plasma proteins***. Measurement of 100 ml of *serum* actually contains approximately 93 ml of water and 7 ml (gm) of *plasma* lipids and proteins. Since sodium is present only in plasma water, the serum sodium concentration was measured at approximately 140 mEq/L by earlier techniques (e.g., flame photometry). Increases in plasma lipids and protein decrease the amount of water (and sodium) in a fixed volume, and so the serum sodium concentration as measured per volume is artifactually decreased. This has been called *pseudohyponatremia* or *factitious hyponatremia*. Currently, within the developed world, sodium concentrations are determined using ion specific electrodes or dry chemistry methods. These methods measure the specific activity of sodium within serum and, when using undiluted specimens, should not be effected by changes in protein or lipid concentrations. If your hospital uses an ion specific electrode on a diluted sample, think about factitious hyponatremia in patients with nephrotic syndrome, diabetic ketoacidosis and other hyperlipidemic states. On average, an increase in triglyceride concentration of 1 g/dl will decrease serum Na+ concentrations by 2 mEq/L.

3. How is the cause of hyponatremia established?

Artifactual causes of hyponatremia should be ruled out. If the urine specific gravity is

<1.003, causes of water intoxication (e.g., administration of inappropriate IV fluids, use of low-solute formulas or plain water in infants, excessive use of tap water enemas or pathologic drinking behavior in psychiatric patients) should be sought by history. If none of these causes are likely, clinical evaluation based on the patient's volume status and urinary sodium concentration will help categorize the disorder.

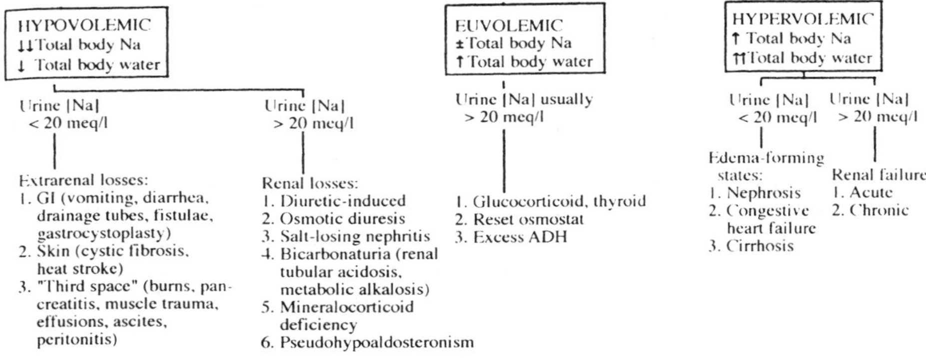

From Avner ED: Clinical disorders of water metabolism: hyponatremia and hypernatremia. Pediatr Ann 24:26, 1995; with permission.

4. What is the emergency treatment of symptomatic hyponatremia?

Symptoms of hyponatremia usually do not occur until the plasma [Na^+] is < 120 mEq/L, but they may occur at higher concentrations if the change has been sudden. Symptoms can range from GI complaints (anorexia, nausea, vomiting) to mental status changes (headaches, irritability, disorientation, cloudy sensorium) and may lead to seizures, coma, and death. If the hyponatremia is asymptomatic, treatment should either be fluid restriction or normal saline infusion based on whether the hyponatremia is due to water excess or hyponatremic dehydration. Patients with CNS symptoms should receive urgent treatment with ***hypertonic saline (3%).*** One ml/kg (= 0.513 mEq of sodium/mL) raises the serum [Na] almost 1 mEq/L. Infusions of hypertonic saline at a rate of 3 ml/kg every 10-20 minutes are generally safe. Increasing the serum sodium by only 5-10 mEq/L is usually sufficient to stop hyponatremic seizures.

5. How is the cause of hypernatremia established?

A combination of history, clinical assessment of the patient's volume status, and a urine sodium concentration measurement is helpful in establishing the diagnostic categories.

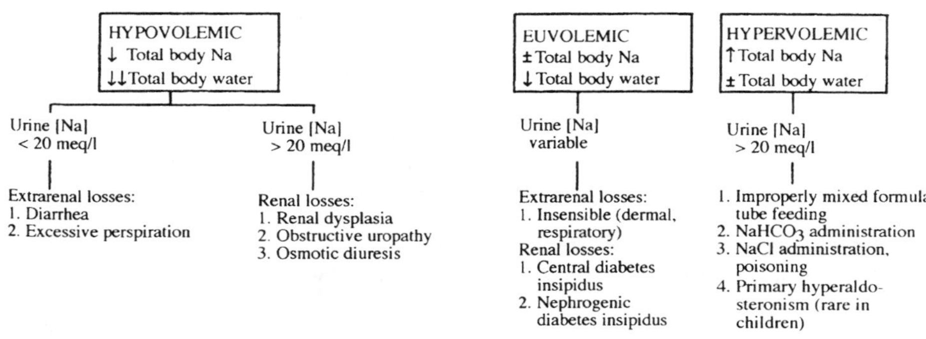

Adapted from Avner ED: Clinical disorders of water metabolism: hyponatremia and hypernatremia. Pediatr Ann 24:28, 1995.

6. Why is the treatment of hypernatremia so precarious?

Children with severe *hyponatremia* usually seize before treatment is begun, while those with hypernatremia may develop seizures in response to therapy. In *hypernatremic* dehydration, the increased extracellular tonicity draws fluid from the intracellular compartment, cell shrink in size including the brain. However, the brain can generate "idiogenic osmoles" to minimize the loss of fluids. These idiogenic osmoles are principally amino acids and other organic solutes .which cause the brain reabsorb some that water. In fact, in chronic hypernatremia, brain size is back to almost normal. It takes approximately 24 hours to begin to generate or dissipate these idiogenic. If correction of chronic (>24h duration) hypernatremia is too rapid, water flows from the extracellular compartment back into the cerebral intracellular compartment, causing cerebral edema. This can lead to seizures, cerebral hemorrhage, and even death. To prevent this situation, in chronic hypernatremia, the serum [Na] should not be allowed to fall faster than 0.5 mEq/L/hr and ideally not more than 15 mEq/L in 24 hours.

7. Why do patients with primary nephrogenic diabetes insipidus (NDI) get treated with diuretics?

Nephrogenic diabetes insipidus is defined as the inability to concentrate urine due to an abnormality in the renal medulla or collecting ducts. In contrast to patients with central diabetes insipidus in whom antidiuretic hormone (ADH) is absent, patients with NDI have adequate ADH but are unable to respond to it. Patients with primary NDI have abnormalities in either in the ADH receptor itself, or in one of the post receptor intracellular events leading to water absorption. Secondary NDI is due to inability to maintain the medullary osmolar gradient that allows water to be reabsorbed. This can be due to physical damage to the medulla such as hydronephrosis, long standing diabetes, sickle cell disease, severe chronic renal failure or even starvation where BUN concentrations are low.

Normally, about 10% of the water filtered at the glomerulus is still present within the tubule at the beginning of the collecting duct and 90% of that is reabsorbed under the influence of ADH. In adults, this amounts to about 20 liters of filtrate reaching the collecting duct each day. In NDI, the only way to avoid excreting that water is to make sure it gets absorbed in the more proximal parts of the nephron. With low salt intakes plus a thiazide diuretic NDI patients become salt depleted and mildly dehydrated. In response to this salt depletion, they have increased sodium (and water) reabsorption in both the proximal tubule and the loop of Henle. The net result is to decrease the percentage of glomerular filtrate reaching the collecting duct. So paradoxically, a diuretic can decrease daily urine output from 20 to as low as 4 or 6 liters per day.

8. How does serum potassium concentration change with alterations in serum pH?

In patients with *alkalosis*, potassium moves into cells as hydrogen moves out of cells in an effort to diminish the alkalinity. The opposite occurs in conditions of *acidosis*. For every 0.1 unit rise or fall in pH, there is a change in the opposite direction in the potassium concentration of between 0.4 and 0.6 mEq/L (i.e. lower pH leads to a higher potassium concentration). This is true in individuals and laboratory animals with acidosis due to mineral acids (e.g. HCl or NH_4Cl). The effects of organic acids on serum potassium is much less predictable.

9. If a child has anuria and acute renal failure, a potassium of 7 mEq/L in a non-hemolyzed specimen and a normal ECG, what are the ways to lower the serum potassium level?

Decrease potassium intake: *discontinue* any ongoing IV, hyperalimentation or oral potassium intakes

Increase potassium excretion: *diurectics* (IV infusion of loop diuretics are fast, effective and low risk); *dialysis* (effective, but time-consuming to initate therapy); sodium potassium polystyrene *exchange gel* (Kayexalate®). The latter is administered either orally or rectally as a 25% solution in sorbitol or water, it must be retained within the gastrointestinal tract for approximately one hour to achieve maximum benefit. This may be difficult in a young anxious child.

Shift potassium from extracellular to intracellular:

- *Insulin* increases intracellular potassium transport. To prevent hypoglycemia, insulin 0.1 U/kg and glucose 0.5 g/kg are infused together over 30 minutes. This is effective within 15-30 minutes and works for several hours.
- *Sympathomimetic* β_2 *agonists* also have a direct effect (separate from insulin) to increase cellular potassium uptake. Albuterol can be given either IV (4 ng/kg given over 20 minutes) or as a nebulizer treatment (<25 kg: 2.5 mg; otherwise, 5 mg). Nebulizer treatments work as well as IV treatments and are easier to administer.
- *Bicarbonate* infusion. Studies have shown that bicarbonate administration may not uniformly effective at lowering serum potassium and should not be a first line therapy. It is clearly important in treating significant acidosis.
- *Transfusion* of old, washed packed RBCs. Stored RBCs leak potassium into the serum. After washing to remove the potassium the transfused RBCs are "rejuvenated," reabsorb potassium and lower serum potassium concentrations.

10. When are calcium infusions indicated in a patient with elevated serum potassium?

Serum potassium >8 mEq/L or ***cardiac arrhythmia***. Calcium is the quickest way to treat an arrhythmia associated with hyperkalemia but it has no effect on serum potassium concentrations. Hyperkalemia leads to an increase in the cell's membrane potential making cells more arrythmogenic. Hypercalcemia raises the cell's threshold potential, restores the voltage difference between these two potentials and decreasing the likelihood of an arrhythmia. The effect of calcium infusion is transient while potassium concentrations remain unchanged.

11. What are the clinical and physiologic consequences of progressive hypokalemia?

- Muscle weakness and paralysis, which can lead to hypoventilation and apnea
- Constipation, ileus
- Increases susceptibility for ventricular ectopic rhythms and fibrillation, especially in children receiving digitalis
- Interferes with the ability of the kidney to concentrate urine, leading to polyuria

12. What should be the maximum rate and concentration of potassium infusions?

Ideally, if potassium supplementation or replacement is needed, the concentration of potassium in the intravenous fluids should *not* exceed ***40 mEq/L*** if given via a *peripheral vein* or ***80 mEq/L*** if given via a *central vein*. Infusion rates should not be > 0.3 mEq K^+/kg/hr. Faster delivery can lead to local irritation of the veins, paresthesias and/or weakness, and cardiac arrest because of changes in transmembrane potentials. For life-threatening conditions due to hypokalemia, such as cardiac dysrhythmias or respiratory paralysis in a patient without alkalosis or acidosis, the rate may be increased up to 1 mEq K^+/kg/hr given centrally by an infusion pump. A continuous ECG monitor should be in place.

Cronan KM, Norman ME: Renal and electrolyte emergencies. In Fleisher GR, Ludwig S (eds): Textbook of Pediatric Emergency Medicine, 4th ed. Baltimore, Lippincott Williams &Wilkins, 2001, pp. 819-820.

13. List the common causes of hypokalemia.

- Diuretics, occasionally laxatives
- Metabolic alkalosis, especially in patients with pyloric stenosis

- Severe diabetic ketoacidosis with dehydration
- Diarrhea
- Renal tubular acidosis, types I and II
- Fanconi syndrome
- Bartter and Gitelman syndromes
- Hypermineralocorticoid states: 1° hyperaldosteronism, Cushing syndrome, adrenal tumors, rare forms of congenital adrenal hyperplasia and dexamethasone suppressible hypertension
- Pituitary tumors producing ACTH
- Hyperreninemic states

14. Which foods are high in potassium?

FOOD	PORTION	POTASSIUM (MG)
Raisins	2/3 cup	751
Baked potato	1 medium	503
Cocoa	1 cup	480
Orange juice	8 oz	474
Banana	1 medium	451
French fries	3/5 cp	364
Carrot	1 raw	341

15. List the causes of hyperkalemia in children.

Increased intake
- Oral including salt substitutes
- Intravenous
- Exchange transfusion, use of aged unwashed packed RBCs •Hypovolemia

Transcellular outward movement
- Metabolic and acute respiratory acidosis
- Insulin deficiency and hyperglycemia in uncontrolled diabetes mellitus
- Increased tissue catabolism—trauma, chemotherapy, hemolysis, rhabdomyolysis
- Exercise
- Medication related: digoxin, β-blockers, succinylcholine, arginine
- Familial hyperkalemic periodic paralysis

Decreased renal excretion
- Acute oliguric renal failure—acute glomerulonephritis or acute tubular necrosis
- Oliguric end-stage renal failure
- Hypoaldosteronism
- Medications—potassium-sparing diuretics, ACE inhibitors
- Distal renal tubular acidosis, type IV
- Renal defect in potassium excretion—familial or obstructive

Pseudohyperkalemia (laboratory artifact)
- Thrombocytosis, leukocytosis, hemolysis
- Abnormal leaky RBC membrane

From McDonald RA: Disorders of potassium balance. Pediatr Ann 24:36, 1995, with permission.

16. What is the normal serum anion gap from infancy to adulthood?

The *anion gap* or *delta* is the difference between the serum [Na] and the sum of the serum [Cl^-] plus serum bicarbonate, usually measured as total CO_2. This difference represents the unmeasured anions, such as organic acids, sulfate, and phosphate. The mean anion gap in children from age 9 months to 19 years is 8 ± 2 mEq/L if the blood is assayed immediately; however, if the blood is analyzed 4 hours later, the mean is closer to 11 mEq/L, which is similar to that of adults (12 ± 2 mEq/L). An elevated anion gap, in practice, occurs when this difference is > 15–16 mEq/L.

17. What are the causes of an elevated anion gap acidosis?

The mnemonic ***MUDPILES*** is commonly used to recall these acidoses, which occur in a variety of clinical scenarios, including certain ingestions.

*M*ethanol
*U*remia (renal failure)
*D*iabetic ketoacidosis, diarrhea of infancy
*P*araldehyde, phenformin
*I*ron, isoniazid, inborn errors of metabolism
*L*actic acidosis (seen in clinical situations associated with hypoxia, severe cardiorespiratory depression, shock, prolonged seizures)
*E*thanol, ethylene glycol
*S*alicylates

18. How limited is the respiratory response to metabolic alkalosis?

Metabolic alkalosis occurs when a net gain of alkali or loss of acid leads to a rise in the serum bicarbonate concentration and pH. In metabolic alkalosis, as in metabolic acidosis, there is a measure of respiratory compensation in response to the change in pH. This response, accomplished by alveolar hypoventilation, is limited by the overriding need to maintain an adequate blood oxygen concentration. Usually the PCO_2 will not rise above ***50–55 mmHg*** despite severe alkalosis.

19. What is the differential diagnosis for a child presenting with primary metabolic alkalosis?

Metabolic alkalosis (MA) can be divided into two major categories based on the urinary Cl– concentration and the response to volume expansion with a saline infusion. The ***saline-responsive*** metabolic alkaloses usually have a urine Cl– concentration that is < 10 mEq/L and significant volume depletion. Treatment with intravenously administered normal saline usually corrects the metabolic alkalosis. The classic example is pyloric stenosis. The ***saline-resistant*** alkaloses are associated with a high urine Cl– and often hypertension. Administration of normal saline tends to aggravate, not correct the metabolic alkalosis. In most cases, mineralocorticoid excess plays the central role in the generation of the acid-base disturbance.

Causes of Saline-responsive MA

- Pyloric stenosis
- Vomiting
- Excessive upper GI suctioning
- Congenital chloride diarrhea
- Laxative abuse
- Diuretic abuse
- Cystic fibrosis
- Chloride-deficient formulas in infants
- Posthypercapnia syndrome
- Poorly reabsorbable anion administration
- Post-treatment of organic acidemias

Causes of Saline-resistant MA

- Primary hyperaldosteronism (extremely rare in children)
- Hyperreninemic hypertension
- Renal artery stenosis
- Heritable block in steroid hormone synthesis:
  17α-OH deficiency
  11β-OH deficiency
- Licorice
- Liddle syndrome
- Bartter or Gitelman syndrome
- Severe potassium deficiency

20. What is the pathophysiologic basis for "contraction alkalosis"?

Strictly speaking, contraction alkalosis refers to the loss of total body water with little or no loss of total body bicarbonate. This would "concentrate" the bicarbonate within the serum and cause alkalosis. In reality, this "contraction" cannot lead to the severe degree of alkalosis often seen in these individuals. Alkalosis is also caused by an actual increase in bicarbonate recovery whenever dehydration is accompanied by the loss of chloride. Common settings include the *loss of gastric contents* (e.g. nasogastric suction or pyloric stenosis) or *intravascular dehydration* (e.g. diarrhea or diuretic abuse).

In a normally hydrated individual, the proximal tubule reabsorbs about 50% of the filtered sodium and water. The sodium is reabsorbed primarily with chloride and secondarily by the reclamation of filtered bicarbonate. *In chloride deficient states* such as those noted above, sodium reabsorption is increased but due to a deficiency of chloride, *all the filtered bicarbonate is reabsorbed* so that none can be excreted in the urine. Furthermore, since the individual is salt (and water) depleted, *aldosterone levels are increased* and distal tubular sodium is reabsorbed (along with bicarbonate) in exchange of potassium and hydrogen ion secretion. Thus, paradoxical aciduria can be seen in the setting of systemic alkalosis.

The treatment is to provide the patient with water and chloride ion. When potassium losses are not only moderate, NaCl alone with correct the alkalosis. Otherwise, KCl must be added to the infusion since severe hypokalemia is an independent cause of alkalosis.

21. How does the "4-2-1" rule for maintenance fluid therapy work?

Infants weighing 3–10 kg have a maintenance fluid requirement of 100 ml/kg/day. For patients weighing 11–20 kg, the maintenance fluids are 1000 ml/day plus 50 ml/day for each kg of weight between 11 and 20 kg. For children weighing > 20 kg, the maintenance fluids are 1500 ml/day plus 20 ml/day for each kg of weight above 20 kg. If this daily requirement triad of 100-50-20 is divided by 24 hours to obtain an hourly rate of fluid requirements, then a rough estimate of 4-2-1 results. For example, the daily fluid requirement for a 24-kg child would be 1580 ml, or an hourly flow rate of (10 kg × 4) + (10 kg × 2) + (4 kg × 1) = 64 ml/hr. This rule is applicable up to about 80 kg.

22. Why do dieters lose so much weight during the first few days of their diet?

Rapid weight loss (and gain) is almost always due to the *loss (or gain) of water*. During dieting, two things happen. First, you eat less, including less salt. Your body takes a few days to adapt to the decrease in salt intake so that for a few days you are in negative salt balance. For every 140 mEq of salt that you excrete, you lose 1 liter of water or 2.2 pounds of weight. Secondly, many diets induce ketosis. These organic anions must be cleared in the urine along with a corresponding cation (or your urine will spark) and sodium is the predominant cation lost, again leading to water loss. Of course, over time, the body has to get back into balance and it does by increasing sodium reabsorption all along the tubule and so the rapid weight loss stops. By the way, when dieting ceases, the process reverses and water weight gain results.

CLINICAL ISSUES

23. How is enuresis categorized?

The terminology can be confusing. In an effort to standard definitions, the 1998 International Children's Continence Society recommended the following:

- *Enuresis:* A normal void occurring at a socially unacceptable time or place.
- *Nocturnal enuresis:* Voiding in bed during sleep that is socially unacceptable.
- *Primary nocturnal enuresis:* Monosymptomatic (no other urinary symptoms) bedwetting in an individual who has never been dry at night for an interrupted period of six months.
- *Dysfunctional voiding:* Functional disturbances of voiding owing to overactivity of the pelvic floor during micturition. Dysfunctional voiding is characterized by variable urinary stream, prolonged voiding and incomplete bladder emptying and may be accompanied by daytime incontinence.
- *Diurnal enuresis:* Daytime enuresis characterized by normal voiding but at a socially unacceptable time or place. Voiding is complete.

Norgaard JP, et al: Standardization and definitions in lower urinary tract dysfunction in children. BJU 81S: 1-16, 1998.

24. How common is primary nocturnal enuresis in older children?

At age 5, approximately 20% of children (boys>girls) wet the bed at least once monthly. Nightly wetting is not as common (<5%). By age 7, the overall rate is down to 10% and by age 10 to 5%. 1%-2% of teenagers and adults persist with primary nocturnal enuresis.

25. Why does bedwetting persist in some children?

Ninety-seven percent or more of the causes are nonpathologic and a number of explanations have been theorized: maturational delay of neurodevelopmental processes, small bladder capacity, genetic influence, difficulties in waking and decreased nighttime secretion of antidiurectic hormone. Genetic influences are quite strong. If both parents were enuretic, a child's likelihood is about 75% and if one parent was involved, the likelihood is about 50%, and only 3% are due to disease states. Psychological problems are an unlikely cause of nocturnal enuresis, but more commonly daytime symptoms if present.

Schmitt BD: Nocturnal enuresis. Pediatr Rev 18:183-190, 1997.

26. In what settings should a medical or surgical cause of enuresis be considered?

Medical conditions include UTI, diabetes mellitus, diabetes insipidus, fecal impaction and constipation. Suspicious symptoms include intermittent daytime wetness, polydipsia, polyuria, history of CNS trauma, or encopresis. *Surgical conditions* include ectopic ureter, neurogenic bladder, bladder calculus and foreign body and debatably adenoidal enlargement. These should be suspected if there is constant dampness, a dribbling urinary stream and abnormalities in gait or obstructive sleep apnea. A thorough history and physical exam along with urinalysis and urine culture if indicated is usually sufficient to eliminate the likelihood of any of these etiologies.

27. What are treatments available for nocturnal enuresis?

The therapeutic approach depends in large part on the age of the patient, effect of the problem on the patient and the parents' attitude. It is important to realize that 15% of patients per year will spontaneously improve.

- ***Dry bed training:*** self-awakening routines, cleanliness training, bladder training and rewards for dry nights. Generally not effective as a sole intervention.
- ***Enuresis alarms*****:** Portable alarms (audio or vibratory) worn by the child at night and designed to awaken the child to the sensation of a full bladder. Positive benefits in 70% and safe, but requires parental and child motivation.
- ***Desmopressin** (DDAVP):* the synthetic analog of vasopressin which at a renal level increases distal tubular retention of filtrate, thus diminishing nighttime bladder volume; available in oral and nasal forms; improvement noted in 12-65%; high relapse rate after discontinuation (similar to placebo); possible adverse effects, including nasal irritation; expensive.
- ***Imipramine:*** bladder effects include increasing capacity and decreasing detrusor excitability; improvement in 10% to 60%, but high relapse rate; important CNS side effects in 10% (e.g., drowsiness, agitation, sleep disturbances).
- ***Oxybutynin:*** provides an anticholinergic, antispasmodic effect that reduces unihibited detrusor muscle contractions; limited studies available on effectiveness; up to 17% with adverse reactions (e.g., dry mouth, flushing, drowsiness, constipation).

Evans JHC: Nocturnal enuresis. In Moyer VA, et al (eds): Evidence Based Pediatrics and Child Health. London, BMJ Books, 2000, p. 313-317.

Chandra M: Nocturnal enuresis in children. Curr Opin Pediatr 10:167-173, 1998.

Schmitt BD: Nocturnal enuresis. Pediatr Rev 18:183-190, 1997.

28. What are the causes of diurnal enuresis?

Organic causes account for < 5% of cases. Of these, urinary tract infections are probably the most common. An ectopic ureter should be suspected if dampness is constantly present; most children with diurnal enuresis have intermittent wetness. Rarely, a neurogenic bladder can cause this problem. Severe lower urinary tract obstruction can lead to bladder distention with overflow incontinence. Finally, pelvic masses, such as presacral teratoma, hydrocolpos, or fecal impaction, which press on the bladder, can lead to stress incontinence with running, coughing, or lifting.

Physiologic types of daytime wetting include vaginal reflux of urine, giggle incontinence, and urgency incontinence. Reflux of urine into the vagina during micturition occurs frequently; after normal voiding, when the girl stands up and walks, the urine seeps out of the vagina and wets the underpants. Giggle incontinence is a sudden, involuntary, uncontrollable, and complete emptying of the bladder when giggling or laughing. Tickling or excitement may also lead to this problem.

Urgency incontinence can be defined as an attack of intense bladder spasms that leads to abrupt voiding and wetting.

Psychogenic causes may be stress-related. Wetting can occur in any child who is significantly frightened. Chronic stress, such as the loss of a close relative, marital discord, or hospitalization, can also lead to this kind of daytime wetting. The resistant child is one who is about $2^1/_2$ years of age and refuses to be toilet trained. Seventy percent are males who are predominantly or totally wet. Often, this situation has occurred because of high-pressured attempts at toilet training. Most children with daytime wetness and nighttime dryness have a behavioral basis for the problem.

29. What simple exercises may help a child with daytime incontinence?

Kegel exercises are exercises of the pelvic muscles. The pelvic muscles can be stimulated in children by instructing them to void, then starting and stopping the urinary stream two or three times by means of pelvic contractions. These maneuvers can then be done at other times without voiding. Voluntary contracture of the pelvic floor muscles is reflexively accompanied by relaxation of the detrusor muscle. These exercises may be helpful in children with daytime incontinence.

Schneider MS, et al: Kegel exercises and childhood incontinence: A new role for an old treatment? J Pediatr 124:91–92, 1994.

30. How does relative renal blood flow differ in infants and adults?

In *adults*, about 20–25% of cardiac output is directed toward the kidney. In *full-term infants*, only about 6% is directed toward the kidney; this increases to 8–10% by the end of the first week.

31. How do you treat labial adhesions?

Labial adhesions are a relatively common gynecologic finding in girls between 4 months and 6 years of age. They may be complete or partial and are felt to be secondary to local inflammation in a low-estrogen setting with resulting skin agglutination. Treatment consists of eliminating the underlying inflammation if caused by an infection, sitz baths twice daily, maintenance of good perineal hygiene, and topical application of a 1% conjugated estrogen cream over the entire adhesion at bedtime for 3 weeks. The use of estrogen has an 80–90% cure rate and may be followed by application of a petroleum jelly for 1–2 months nightly. It should be noted that the natural history of untreated asymptomatic labial adhesions is self-resolution: 50% resolve within 6 months and nearly 100% by 18 months. Surgical correction is almost never needed.

Prasad SM: Labial adhesions. Pediatr Rev 15:87–88, 1994.

HEMATURIA

32. What distinguishes lower from upper tract bleeding?

As a general rule, brown, tea- or cola-colored urine suggests *upper tract bleeding* while bright red blood suggests *lower tract bleeding.* The darker urine has had more time to become oxidized within the urinary tract. However, exceptions occur. Rapid upper tract bleeding may be red and a dissolving clot within the bladder may produce brown urine. Establishing the source of microscopic hematuria can be difficult. *Glomerular bleeding* is said to produce red cells that are small and dysmorphic with blebs or burr cells as opposed to the normal size red cells seen in lower tract bleeding. Unfortunately, this change is best observed with phase contrast microscopy which is not readily available in most clinical settings. The presence of significant *proteinuria* also suggests upper tract (i.e., kidney) disease. The presence of even a single red blood cell or hemoglobin *cast* indicates a glomerular (or rarely tubular) etiology.

33. If a healthy 5-year-old has bright red blood at the end of a previously clear urine stream, what is the likely diagnosis?

The finding of bright red blood suggests that this is lower tract bleeding. The history that the early part of urination produced clear urine suggests that this child has a problem with his *bladder neck* or *trigone*. In the absence of pain or other symptoms, it's most likely that this child has ***benign hemorrhagic cystitis*** most often due to adenovirus. In an otherwise healthy child, the family should be reassured that hematuria will resolve within several days. Bacterial urinary tract infections almost never cause gross hematuria (certainly not bright red), the absence of pain argues against a stone or bladder calculus and the vast majority of pediatric nephrologists are still waiting to diagnose their first bladder hemangioma.

34. How common is asymptomatic hematuria?

Up to ***3%*** of all girls (and ***1.5%*** of boys) will have 2 out of 3 urines positive for >5 rbc/hpf at some time between the ages of 6 and 12 years old. This drops to only about 0.8% (0.5% for boys) if the clinician's definition of hematuria requires the presence of blood in three consecutively collected urine specimens.

35. Which children with hematuria should be evaluated?

Children who present with microscopic hematuria without proteinuria should be evaluated if the hematuria is present in essentially all tested urines over several months time. Red flags in the history and physical exam the suggest other than a benign etiology include:

History:

- *Recent illnesses* (particularly if you can associate episodes of gross hematuria with the illnesses)
- *Trauma* (particularly if there is gross bleeding after relatively minor trauma)
- *Pain*: abdominal, suprapubic, flank, or dysuria
- *Medication usage* (e.g., anticoagulants, aspirin, sulfonamide, chronic antibiotic administration)
- *Family history* of renal disease, bilateral hearing loss, hemoglobinopathies, bleeding disorders, stone disease

Physical Exam:

- *Short stature*
- *Hypertension*
- *Pallor*
- *Significant (non-functional) cardiac murmurs*
- *Abdominal mass*
- Evidence of *multi-system* disease

36. What evaluations should be considered in the evaluation of isolated hematuria?

- *BUN/creatinine*
- *Electrolytes*
- *Urine calcium/creatinine ratio*
- *Serologic evidence* of recent *streptococcal* infection (unless hematuria for several months)
- *Renal ultrasound*: evaluation for structural abnormalities (e.g. hydronephrosis, autosomal dominant or recessive polycystic kidney diseas) and for Wilms tumor in any patient less than 5 years old.
- *Hemoglobin electrophoresis*: if sickle cell trait or disease is suspected
- *C3, C4, ANA or ANCA*: However, in the absence of proteinuria or evidence of systemic involvement, these are *unlikely* to be positive.
- *Urine culture*: However, this is unnecessary for recurrent gross hematuria or in an asymptomatic child with a 6-month history due a *low likelihood* of positivity.

37. How common is hypercalciuria as a cause of hematuria?

This depends on where you live. In areas of the southeastern United States—often called "the stone belt"—this is a common cause of isolated hematuria with nearly *one third* of children with microscopic hematuria having hypercalciuria as the cause. In other parts of the United States, it is significantly less common.

38. How does hypercalciuria cause hematuria?

The mechanism is ***unknown***, but it has been hypothesized to involve *irritation* of the renal tubules by calcium-containing *microcrystals*. Since the amount of blood lost in this way is minimal, never causes anemia and only a limited number of these patients develop renal calculi, it's important to be conservative before initiating chronic therapy. If there is a history of nephrolithiasis or nephrocalcinosis, hypercalciuria can be treated by increasing fluid intake, decreasing sodium intake and if necessary, the addition of a small dose of a thiazide diuretic.

39. What causes benign familial hematuria?

In this diagnosis of exclusion, multiple family members have microscopic (and occasionally gross) hematuria without significant proteinuria, abnormal renal function, or identifiable cause (e.g., hypercalciuria). Family history is not suggestive of any other serious renal problems, including deafness (Alport disease) or macular blindness. Although renal biopsies are not usually done, the likely culprit is a ***thin glomerular basement membrane***, especially the lamina densa.

GLOMERULONEPHRITIS

40. In an evaluation of a patient with hematuria, what features suggest glomerulonephritis?

Three presentations of of glomerular involvement can occur:

Acute glomerulonephritis: Edema, proteinuria of 1+ or greater, hypertension, oliguria, dysmorphic RBCs (small, misshapen RBC with blebs) or red cells casts on urinalysis

Chronic glomerulonephritis: Minimal acute symptoms; may present with chronic fatigue, failure to thrive, or unexplained anemia with features of chronic renal failure, hypertension, abnormal urinalysis, azotemia

Nephrotic syndrome: Proteinuria > 40 $mg/m^2/hr$, edema, hypoproteinemia, hyperlipidemia

41. If glomerulonephritis is suspected, what lab tests should be considered?

- Urinalysis
- BUN/creatinine
- Serum C3 (possibly C4)
- Streptococcal serology
- Throat culture; skin culture if lesions present
- Serum albumin
- ANA, Anti-DNA antibodies (if systemic lupus erythematosus is suspected),
- Hepatitis B and C serology (in patients living in endemic areas or who have received transfusions or engage in high risk behavior),
- Anti-nuclear cytotoxic antibody (ANCA) (if rapidly progressive glomerulonephritis or vasculitis is suspected)

42. Which glomerulonephritides are associated with hypocomplementemia?

- Poststreptococcal
- Other postinfectious causes (may have normal complement)
- Subacute bacterial endocarditis
- Shunt nephritis
- Systemic lupus erythematosus
- Membranoproliferative

43. Does treatment of streptococcal skin or pharyngeal infections prevent poststreptococcal glomerulonephritis?

No study has ever demonstrated that treatment of impetigo or pharyngitis prevents renal complications in the index case. Clearly, acute rheumatic fever does not occur following the skin infections, and glomerulonephritis is limited to infections with a few serotypes, especially 49, 55, 57, and 60, which appear to be less prevalent in recent years. However, treatment lessens the likelihood of contagious spread to hosts who may be susceptible to renal complications. Serum anti-streptolysin titers, which are elevated in pharyngeal infections, are usually not elevated following skin infections. Therefore, to confirm the diagnosis of an antecedent skin infection, anti-hyaluronidase and anti-DNase B titers should be obtained.

44. What is the usual time course for poststreptococcal glomerulonephritis?

Approximately ***7–14 days*** following a pharyngitis and as long as ***6 weeks*** following a pyoderma with group A β-hemolytic streptococci, children present typically with tea-colored urine and edema. The acute phase (e.g., hypertension and gross hematuria) can last up to 3 weeks. Serum complement levels may remain depressed for up to 8 weeks, and persistence beyond this point suggests another diagnosis. Chronic microscopic hematuria can persist up to 18 months. In pediatric patients full recovery expected and progression to chronic renal insufficiency is extremely rare.

45. What percentage of children with post-streptococcal glomerulonephritis have elevated levels of serum anti-streptolysin titers?

Approximately ***80-85%*** of children with documented pharyngeal streptococcal infections develop elevated ASO titers. Streptolysin O is bound to lipids in the skin so that percentage of individuals with streptococcal impetigo who develop positive ASO titers is much lower. For this reason, a normal ASO titer does not rule out recent ASO infection. Screening for other streptococcal-associated-antigens, anti-hyaluronidase and anti-DNAase B titers or the use of the Streptozyme test which measures a variety of streptococcal antigens, will be positive in >95% of children with documented strep infection.

46. A 9-year-old boy with intermittent episodes of gross hematuria associated with febrile upper respiratory infections likely has what type of glomerular disease?

IgA nephropathy (Berger disease). This is the most common cause of chronic glomerulonephritis in persons of European or Asian descent. In children, IgA nephropathy typically causes asymptomatic microscopic hematuria with periods of gross hematuria during febrile infections. Most children are normotensive and other than the gross hematuria, have no other kidney-related findings. Previously considered a benign condition, recent studies indicate that after thirty years of follow-up approximately 30% of individuals will develop evidence of chronic renal insufficiency. Renal biopsy followed by specific treatment is generally reserved for those who develop evidence of progressive disease, (i.e., hypertension, persistent proteinuria or an elevated serum creatinine concentration). The etiology of IgA nephropathy is unclear, and diagnosis is established by renal biopsy with demonstration of IgA in the mesangium of the glomerulus.

47. What is the natural history of the hearing loss seen in children with Alport syndrome?

Alport syndrome is a combination of chronic glomerulonephritis and progressive sensorineural deafness. By far, the most common cause of Alport syndrome is a genetic defect in one of the six known collagen genes, gene 5 located on the X chromosome. Classic Alport syndrome is therefore an X-linked recessive condition where males are severely affected, most often progressing to renal failure in the late teens and early twenties while heterozygote females may demonstrate only minor urinary abnormalities and rarely progress to renal failure. In males, the hearing loss is bilateral and progressive, but hearing is normal (as is speech) in infancy and can be detected only by audiometry. Loss of high frequency hearing, begins in the second decade of life.

48. What are the most common causes of chronic glomerulonephritis in children and adolescents?

- IgA nephropathy (Berger disease)
- Diffuse proliferative glomerulonephritis
- Membranoproliferative glomerulonephritis
- Familial nephritis (primarily the sex-linked recessive form—Alport syndrome)
- Henoch-Schönlein purpura
- Crescentic glomerulonephritis (rapidly progressive GN)
- Systemic lupus erythematosus

PROTEINURIA/NEPHROTIC SYNDROME

49. How do the bedside methods for testing protein in random urine samples compare?

Dipstick assessment: This relies on the reaction of protein (primarily albumin) with tetrabromphenol blue in a citrate buffer impregnated on the dipstick patch. Mild false positive reactions can occur (1–2+) when the patient's urine is alkaline or when the dipstick is allowed to sit in the urine for too long and the buffer strength is overcome. The results are reported qualitatively as trace to 4+ which corresponds to a range of 30 to 2000 mg/dL.

Sulfosalicylic acid: Precipitates protein in the urine and allows comparison to a group of previously prepared aqueous standards and is reported in the same way. In contrast to the dipstick, all proteins, not just albumin, are precipitated. The finding of heavy proteinuria by sulfosalicylic acid testing with minimal proteinuria using the dipstick suggests the presence of large amounts of non-albumin protein most often due to multiple myeloma and the excretion of Bence-Jones proteins. Look for this on a geriatrics, not pediatrics, rotation.

50. On a routine urinalysis, an asymptomatic 7-year-old boy has 1+ protein noted on dipstick. How should this child be evaluated?

Assuming the child is otherwise healthy and without any of the subtle signs of renal disease (e.g., short stature, pallor, hypertension) and assuming that this is isolated proteinuria, it's important to determine whether this child's proteinuria is intermittent or persistent. Intermittent (transient) proteinuria is entirely benign and does not require any work up. Persistent proteinuria may or may not be benign. The presence of persistent proteinuria can be done by re-checking the urine at least three times over the two to three weeks. If one of these is done on a first morning urine specimen, the patient can be evaluated for orthostatic proteinuria at the same time. Causes of transient proteinuria include fever, vigorous exercise, dehydration, stress, cold exposure and seizures.

51. Other than a timed urine collection, what is the best "spot" method for determining the degree of proteinuria?

Urinary protein/creatinine excretion ratio. Particularly in children, a 24-hour urine collection for protein is very difficult to obtain. Although both the dipstick and sulfosalicylic testing estimate the concentration of protein in the urine, small amounts of protein in very concentrated urine will show up as more positive than the same amount of protein present in dilute urine. A number of studies have demonstrated that urinary protein/creatinine ratio more closely approximates total 24-hour urinary protein excretion. Thus, on a random sample of urine, a urine protein/creatinine ratio of < *0.2-0.25* reflects a normal daily protein excretion while values > *1* strongly suggest the presence of the nephrotic syndrome. This test has proven very effective both for the diagnosis of the nephrotic syndrome and for follow-up in children with prolonged and difficult to manage proteinuria. Of note, the test may overestimate protein excretion in individuals with abnormally low muscle mass (and hence lower creatinine excretion rates).

52. How is the diagnosis of orthostatic proteinuria established?

By definition, individuals with *orthostatic proteinuria* have normal rates of protein excretion when lying recumbent but increased excretion rates when upright. While all individuals excrete more protein when standing, some have an exaggerated response and may excrete as much as 1 gram of urinary protein/day. Protein excretion when recumbent can be assessed semiquantitatively on a first morning urine specimen immmediately upon arising, using either a urine dipstick or sulfosalicylic acid precipitation of the urine. More accurate assessment can be obtained using the urine protein/creatinine excretion ratio or as mg excreted per hour. In a reasonably concentrated first morning urine specimen (urine specific gravity (1.018) a trace or negative value by dipstick or sulfosalicylic acid precipitation is adequate to rule out proteinuria. At any urine specific gravity, a urine protein/creatinine ratio (mg/dL/mg/dL) less than 0.25 is also considered normal. Remember, even individuals with renal disease may have increased protein excretion when standing and lower protein excretion rates when recumbent. The key to orthostatic proteinuria is that protein excretion is truly normal when recumbent and the individual is otherwise entirely healthy.

53. What additional evaluation should be done for a patient with persistent proteinuria?

If the child's proteinuria is persistent and not orthostatic, protein excretion needs to determined. While the gold standard is the timed (24 hour) urine collection, this is often difficult to obtain in children. Because substantial amounts of urine are often lost, a 24-hour urinary creatinine excretion should be determined at the same time to assess for completeness. A standard definition of proteinuria was developed by the International Study for Kidney Disease in Children. They defined proteinuria as greater than 4 $mg/m^2/hr$ (or 100 mg/24h in a 30 kg child). More commonly, the urine protein/creatinine ratio is utilized.

The evaluation of a child with persistent proteinuria includes many of the same tests required to evaluate glomerulonephritis such as: BUN/creatinine; electrolytes; serum albumin; and often tests to document evidence of immunologic activation such as C3, C4, ANA, anti-DNA antibodies. Rarely, anti-cytotoxic neutrophil antibody (ANCA) may be required. Finally, renal imaging studies and renal biopsy may be necessary for diagnosis.

54. What is the natural history of orthostatic proteinuria?

Few prospective data exist on the long-term outcome of children and adolescents, but follow-up data on young adults up to 50 years after diagnosis demonstrate a *benign* clinical course. Most agree that the prognosis is excellent, although the etiology remains unclear.

55. What level constitutes "significant" proteinuria?

Protein excretion of > 4 mg/m^2/hr on a timed urine collection is considered abnormal. Children with nephrosis excrete > 40 mg/m^2/hr. The upper limit of protein excretion in adults is 150 mg/day but for some reason, adolescents may excrete as much as 250 mg/d. A urine protein/urine creatinine ratio of > 0.5 in children under 2 years of age and > 0.2 in older children is considered excessive.

56. In the presence of gross hematuria, what amount of protein excretion is considered abnormal?

500 mg/m^2/day.

57. What constellation of clinical findings defines nephrotic syndrome?

The *nephrotic syndrome* consists of ***proteinuria***, ***hypoalbuminemia***, ***edema*** and ***hyperlipidemia***. Of these, the proteinuria is primary with the development of hypoalbuminemia, edema and hyperlipidemia as secondary findings. It's not at all uncommon to find individuals with clear evidence of nephrotic range proteinuria and mild to moderate hypoalbuminemia in whom evidence of hypolipidemia and peripheral edema are minimal.

58. What distinguishes nephrosis from nephritis?

The suffix "itis" implies *evidence of inflammation* which is seen on renal biopsy as the proliferation of the cellular elements within the glomerulus and often the presence of white blood cells. Clinically, these abnormalities produce a disruption of glomerular basement structure and function leading to hematuria and proteinuria. The proteinuria may be minimal to massive, depending on the type and severity of the *nephritis*. The finding of RBC *casts* in the urine is, with rare exceptions, diagnostic of glomerulonephritis.

Nephrosis is another term for the nephrotic syndrome. "Syndrome" implies a characteristic group of findings which may have diverse causes. As noted in the previous question, the nephrotic syndrome is caused by the renal loss of protein, the development of hypoalbuminuria, edema and hyperlipidemia. This can be due to a number of renal conditions some of which demonstrate proliferative and inflammatory changes and some (e.g., minimal change nephrotic syndrome) without any evidence of nephritis. Thus, some, but not all patients with (glomerulo)nephritis may have nephrosis and some patients with the clinical syndrome called nephrosis may have evidence of nephritis on urinalysis (e.g. RBC casts) or on biopsy.

59. Which childhood diseases present primarily as glomerulonephritis or the nephrotic syndrome?

Glomerulonephritis	*Nephrotic syndrome*
Post-infectious (both streptococcal as well as other bacteria, viruses and parasites)	Minimal change nephrosis

Henoch-Schönlein nephritis	Focal segmental glomerulosclerosis
IgA nephropathy	Membranoproliferative glomerulonephritis
Membranoproliferative glomerulonephritis	Membranous nephropathy
Familial nephritis	Congenital nephrotic syndrome
Systemic lupus erythematosus	Systemic lupus erythematosus
Immune complex nephritis (Infective endocarditis or "shunt nephritis"	Henoch-Schönlein nephritis
Rapidly progressive glomerulonephritis (Wegener or polyarteritis nodosa)	IgA nephropathy
	Familial nephritis

Most of these conditions will present primarily with either a nephritic or a nephrotic picture; occasionally a mixed picture will be noted.

60. At what level of albumin do children usually start to develop edema?

When the serum albumin falls ***below 2.5 gm/dL***, edema usually *begins* to develop. ***Below 1.8 gm/dL*** edema is almost always *present* unless the child is receiving a diuretic.

61. Is urinary protein electrophoresis helpful in evaluating children with persistent proteinuria?

It is rarely useful in children because the types of proteinuria identified by electrophoresis are usually markers for diseases occurring almost exclusively in adults. When performed, results showing predominantly albumin indicate selective excretion and are suggestive of mild glomerular disease, such as minimal change disease. A wide range of proteins indicates nonselective excretion and is suggestive of more severe glomerular disease (if large molecular-weight globulins, such as immunoglobulins) or tubular disease (if small molecular-weight globulins).

62. What portion of the kidney produces Tamm-Horsfall protein?

Tamm-Horsfall protein is a large mucoprotein secreted into the urine by cells of the thick ascending limb of the ***loop of Henle***. It is the matrix of a cast.

63. Why doesn't eating more protein restore the serum albumin concentration to normal in individuals with the nephrotic syndrome?

The loss of urinary albumin is only part of the story. Under normal circumstances, very small amounts of albumin are filtered at the glomerulus. A very high percentage of what is filtered is then catabolized by the proximal tubular cells. Amino acids are reabsorbed from the tubular lumen back into the body and resynthesized into albumin within the liver. In the nephrotic syndrome, significantly more albumin is filtered. Even with increased catabolism and amino acids reabsorption at the renal tubular level, the rate of liver albumin synthesis is limited. Serum albumin levels fall. Feeding more protein would lead to increased protein absorption through the GI tract, but the rate-limiting feature of insufficient liver synthesis cannot be overcome.

64. What is the most common form of nephrotic syndrome seen in childhood?

Minimal change nephrotic syndrome (MCNS). Earlier names for this condition included lipoid nephrosis and nil disease. MCNS is a form of primary nephrotic syndrome and has most favorable therapeutic response and prognosis.. The etiology of MCNS is unknown but it appears to be a condition of abnormal T lymphocyte function. Other forms of *primary* nephrotic syndrome include conditions such as focal segmental glomerulosclerosis, membranous nephropathy and membranoproliferative glomerulonephritis. *Secondary* forms of nephrotic syndrome may also occur as a consequence of infection, as a response to some medications and as an autoimmune phenomenon.

65. What is the most important historical factor in assessing a patient for possible minimal change nephrotic syndrome?

Although the only definitive way to document the presence of minimal change nephrotic syndrome is through renal biopsy, most patients with MCNS present with a constellation of signs and a response to treatment that is characteristic. The most important characteristic for a child with minimal change nephrotic syndrome is ***age on presentation***. Seventy-five to eighty percent of all children with nephrotic syndrome have MCNS and approximately 80% of those present within the first 8 years of life. Presentation prior to one year of age is unusual and should make on suspect various forms of congenital nephrotic syndrome or a secondary etiology such as congenital syphilis.

66. What are the typical clinical features and therapeutic responses seen in MCNS?

Edema is generally present, blood pressure is normal, gross hematuria is absent, but up to 1/3 of the patients may have *microscopic hematuria* but red cell casts are not seen. In the absence of significant intravascular volume depletion, BUN, creatinine and electrolytes are all within normal limits. Children who present in this manner should be started on daily prednisone. This is often called a medical biopsy.

The standard dose recommended for the initial episode is 2 mg/kg/day with a maximum dose of 80 mg/day. A single daily dose given in the morning is as effective as split doses and may lead to fewer steroid side effects. For the initial episode, daily steroids are continued for one month regardless of how soon the patient responds. If the patient responds, then the daily prednisone is changed to alternate day dosing at the same 2 mg/kg/q.o.d. for an additional month. Thereafter, the dose is tapered over the next two months. Relapses are treated similarly except the switch to alternate day steroid is done when the urine dipstick shows a negative or trace protein reaction for 3-4 days.

After the initiation of prednisone for an initial episode, up to 93% of patients will respond in the first month, with the mean time being 10–13 days. Response is indicated by normalization of urinary protein excretion and diuresis. If therapy is prolonged for an additional month, another 4% will respond. Approximately 3% of children with biopsy proven MCNS will be steroid resistant despite two months of therapy.

67. When should secondary therapies be considered for MCNS?

- Patients who do not respond to the initial course of prednisone
- Patients who become subsequent non-responders to prednisone during relapses
- Patients who have frequent relapses
- Patients who develop significant side effects from steroids

68. What are the secondary or alternative drug therapies for MCNS?

- ***Alkylating agents*** such as chlorambucil or cyclophosphamide: Both are effective in inducing remission of the nephrotic syndrome. After an 8-12 week course of treatment remission may be permanent in up to 50% of patients.
- ***Cyclosporin***: This medication must be administered for prolonged periods before it is tapered and relapses are not uncommon when the drug is withdrawn.
- ***Levamisole***: This medication an immunomodulator which is effective in approximately 50% of children with frequently relapsing nephrotic syndrome.
- ***Angiotensin converting inhibitors*** and ***angiotensin receptor blockers***: Irrespective of the etiology, all members of these two classes of drugs effectively decrease glomerular proteinuria by up to 50% and are quite helpful in the management of patients with otherwise untreatable disease.
- ***Salt restriction*** and ***diuretics***: May help relieve the edema and improve the quality of life for children with unresponsive nephrotic syndrome.

69. When are furosemide and albumin therapy indicated in nephrotic syndrome?

Albumin is available in two forms: 5% and 25% solutions. The former is used in treatment of shock, but has no role in the treatment of nephrotic syndrome. Infusion of the 25% solution in a dose of 0.5–1 g/kg of albumin over 1-2 hours, followed by a potent diuretic such as furosemide (1-4 mg/kg), can be used to induce diuresis in a child with nephrotic syndrome unresponsive to furosemide alone. This measure is only *temporary*, since the rise in albumin will lead to increased protein excretion, returning the serum level to the previous steady-state value. However, it is useful in a child with *severe edema* leading to incapacitating ***anasarca***, ***cellulitis***, ***skin breakdown*** or respiratory embarrassment from ***pleural effusions***. Albumin alone is useful in the child with a rising BUN secondary to decreased renal perfusion, a situation most often seen after vigorous diuretic therapy.

70. What are the risks of the "albumin-Lasix sandwich"?

The administration of 25% albumin and furosemide is a serious therapy with important potential risks to the patient. The unspoken assumption in this treatment is that the fluid drawn back into the intravascular space by the albumin infusion will be excreted kidneys after the administration of furosemide. This may not be true when the nephrotic syndrome is associated with decreased renal function due to coexisting glomerulonephritis. In that situation, the interstitial fluid drawn from the periphery may lead to ***intravascular volume overload*** and ***pulmonary edema***.

71. What is the mechanism of hyperlipidemia associated with severe proteinuria?

Elevations in the plasma concentrations of cholesterol and triglycerides are characteristically seen in children with nephrotic syndrome. Low-density lipoproteins (LDL) and very-low-density lipoproteins (VLDL) are also increased, but high-density lipoproteins (HDL) may be high, normal, or low. The mechanisms underlying these lipid alterations include both ***enhanced hepatic production*** of VLDL and ***decreased peripheral catabolism/utilization*** of VLDL due to *inhibition of post-heparin lipoprotein lipase activity*. Normalization of the plasma lipids is usually the last feature of the nephrotic syndrome to resolve.

72. What is the mechanism of hypercoagulability associated with nephrotic syndrome?

Multiple factors contribute to the hypercoagulable state. ***Blood viscosity*** (in part due to hyperlipidemia) is increased. ***Platelet adhesiveness*** is increased. Nearly all ***coagulation factors*** and ***clotting inhibitors*** are altered. Fibrinogen levels are increased and anti-thrombin III levels decreased secondary to urinary losses. The overall tendency favors increased coagulation and decreased fibrinolysis.

73. Which organisms are responsible for peritonitis in children with nephrotic syndrome?

Pneumococcus remains the most important cause, although gram-negative organisms, especially ***Escherichia coli***, account for 25–50% of cases.

74. Which causes of nephrotic syndrome are likely to progress to renal impairment?

Type of Nephrotic Syndrome	*% progressing to renal failure without treatment*
Minimal change nephrotic syndrome	0%[a]
Focal segmental glomerulosclerosis	30-50%
Membranoproliferative GN	90%[b]
Membranous	30%
Systemic lupus erythematosus	30-40%
Henoch-Schönlein nephritis	1-5%
Diabetes mellitus	100%[c]
AIDS nephropathy	100%

[a] It is generally felt that patients with MCNS don't progress. Clinical deterioration (or developed—we're still arguing about this) is felt due to underlying undiagnosed focal segmental glomerulosclerosis.
[b] Treatment of membranoproliferative glomerulonephritis has been shown to be effective at decreasing the rate of progression to chronic renal failure over several years, but the long-term outcome is still unclear.
[c] Even in the absence of intensive therapy, only 40% of individuals with diabetes mellitus will develop significant proteinuria and the nephrotic syndrome. However, those that due invariably progress to chronic renal failure. Intensive treatment of the diabetes has been shown to decrease this complication by 50-70%.

75. Which chronic infections are associated with membranous glomerulopathy?

Membranous nephropathy can be divided into primary and secondary types. The etiology of primary membranous nephropathy is unknown but secondary forms are associated with chronic antigenemia. The most common infections associated with membranous nephropathy are ***hepatitis B*** and ***C***. While membranous nephropathy is unusual in pediatrics (only 2% of cases) all cases of membranous nephropathy should be serologically screened for hepatitis B and C. Other causes include ***syphilis*** (particularly with congenital nephrotic syndrome) and ***malaria***.

76. Discuss the prognostic factors in children with nephrotic syndrome.

The best prognosis is associated with the presence of *minimal change nephrosis*. For individuals with other etiologies, the two features in all categories which protend a worse prognosis are the presence of ***large amounts of urinary protein*** and the development of ***hypertension***. Thus, maintenance of normal blood pressures, including the liberal use of angiotensin converting enzyme inhibitors, is widely stressed in patients with persistent nephrotic syndrome.

77. In which children with nephrotic syndrome should renal biopsy be considered?

Since older children are more likely to have other forms of nephrotic syndrome such as focal segmental glomerulosclerosis or membranoproliferative glomerulonephritis, most pediatric nephrologists would biopsy those who present at *greater than 8 years* of age prior to beginning therapy. Certainly, the presence of significant hypertension, renal insufficiency, red cell casts, multiple organ involvement, partial lipodystrophy, or a low serum C3 level all speak against the finding of minimal change nephrotic syndrome and require a renal biopsy for definitive diagnosis. Children of any age who do not go into remission during their initial course of prednisone or who fail to respond to prednisone following relapses will also require a renal biopsy.

HYPERTENSION

78. How do you decide what is the optimum cuff size for obtaining a blood pressure?

The length of the inflatable bladder inside the cuff (easily palpated) should almost completely encircle the arm and will overestimate the blood pressure if it is too short. Additionally, the height of the cuff should be the largest that comfortably fits from the axilla to the elbow. A cuff that is too small can produce falsely elevated blood pressure readings, and one that is too large can produce falsely low blood pressure readings.

79. What were the findings of the Second Task Force regarding abnormal blood pressures in children?

In 1987, the Second Task Force on Blood Pressure Control in Children devised numerical classification of significant and severe hypertension. Other factors, such as rapidity of onset and association of end-organ damage or dysfunction, are important issues that must be considered in addition to simple numerical elevation.

Age	*Significant Hypertension (mmHg)*	*Severe Hypertension (mmHg)*
7 days	SBP ≥ 96	SBP ≥ 106
8–30 days	SBP ≥ 104	SBP ≥ 110
< 2 yr	SBP ≥ 112	SBP ≥ 118
	DBP ≥ 74	DBP ≥ 82
3–5 yr	SBP ≥ 116	SBP ≥ 124
	DBP ≥ 76	DBP ≥ 84
6–9 yr	SBP ≥ 122	SBP ≥ 130
	DBP ≥ 78	DBP ≥ 86
10–12 yr	SBP ≥ 126	SBP ≥ 134
	DBP ≥ 82	DBP ≥ 90
13–15 yr	SBP ≥ 136	SBP ≥ 144
	DBP ≥ 86	DBP ≥ 92
16–18 yr	SBP ≥ 142	SBP ≥ 150
	DBP ≥ 92	DBP ≥ 98

SBP = systolic blood pressure; DBP = diastolic blood pressure.
Task Force on Blood Pressure Control in Children: Report of the Second Task Force on Blood Pressure Control in Children—1987. Pediatrics 79:1–25, 1987.

80. What are the drawbacks of using the blood pressure norms for age as published by the Second Task Force on Blood Pressure Control in Children?

Criticism has been leveled at these normative data for several reasons. First, there is the presumption that what is normal is also usually considered to be ideal or "healthy." Normal blood pressure values in U.S. children may be neither. Second, blood pressures have a better correlation with body size (body mass index or height) than with age. Third, the normal values were obtained screening large numbers of children, but were all single blood pressure measurements. Experience shows that if a blood pressure is taken repetitively, later determinations are more likely to be lower than an initial, single reading.

81. Which Korotkoff sound best represents diastolic blood pressure?

The *Korotkoff sounds* are produced by the flow of blood as the constricting blood pressure cuff is gradually released. There are five phases of Korotkoff sounds. The first appearance of a clear, tapping sound is called *phase I* and represents the systolic pressure. As the cuff continues to be released, soft murmurs can be auscultated—*phase II*. These are followed by louder murmurs during *phase III*, as the volume of blood passing through the constricted artery increases. The sounds become abruptly muffled in *phase IV* and disappear in *phase V*, which is usually within 10 mmHg of phase IV.

In studies which compare intravascular blood pressure determinations with auscultatory readings, true diastolic pressure is most closely related to the ***5th phase*** (the disappearance of sound). However, in many young children, muffled sounds can be heard to zero and thus clearly do not always correlate with diastolic pressure. In these instances, it is best to record both the ***4th phase*** (the point where sounds become muffled) as well as the 5th (e.g., 80/45/0).

82. When should hypertension be treated in the neonate?

Hypertension is defined as a blood pressure > 90/60 mmHg in term neonates and > 80/45 in preterm infants. A sustained systolic blood pressure ***> 100 mmHg*** in the neonate should be investigated and treated.

83. In the evaluation of a child with elevated blood pressure, what risk factors should be considered for identification and/or reduction?

Important risk factors for hypertension in children include ***family history*** (if one parent has hypertension the risk is about 25%; if both parents have hypertension, the risk is 45%), other genetic factors including ***race*** (African-Americans have twice the incidence of hypertension vs. whites beginning in adolescence), ***obesity***, history of renal disease, and dietary factors (mainly salt intake). More recently, a history of ***prematurity*** has been recognized as a risk factor.

Remembering that hypertension is a critical risk factor for cardiovascular disease, the important risk factors for this largest cause of mortality should also be addressed. These include diet and its effect on serum lipids, tobacco use, and lack of exercise.

84. What is the role of ambulatory blood pressure monitoring (ABPM) in children?

ABPM has been used in adults for many years to more clearly delineate and document intermittently high and/or borderline blood pressure readings. It requires wearing a blood pressure cuff and carrying a portable monitor/recorder for 24 hours to obtain multiple, automatic measurements. ABPM is the most reliable predictor of end-organ damage in adults. It can be used for the same indications in children and adolescents. *Limitations* include (a) lack of sufficient normative data in children to permit analysis and meaningful conclusions; (b) lack of availability of small, lightweight equipment; and (c) limited ability of a small child to tolerate the cuff and its periodic inflation. As more data accumulate and equipment is further miniaturized, ABPM will gain wider use in the evaluation of children with borderline hypertension.

85. What are ways to minimize "white coat hypertension"?

White coat hypertension is the transient elevation of blood pressure which can occur in a child (or adult) due to the anxiety associated with a doctor visit. Measures to eliminate it as a cause of elevated blood pressure include any measure to make the patient relax and feel more at ease. Experienced practitioners have many creative ways to achieve this. In a young child, placing the cuff on the arm long before making the measurement and having the child sit on the parent's lap can be helpful. Also helpful is the use of another health professional, either in the office or out of the office (e.g. a school nurse) to measure the blood pressure. Multiple determinations during the course of the examination are recommended. Asking older children to take several deep breaths can help them relax. As a general rule, the true blood pressure is most likely present when the heart rate is at baseline. Traditionally, this type of transient rise has been thought to be benign. Recent studies suggest it may be a marker of sympathetic hyperactivity which persists throughout life and possibly a prelude to permanent idiopathic hypertension in adulthood.

Vaindirlis I, et al: "White coat hypertension" in adolescents: Increased values of urinary cortisol and endothelin. J Pediatr 136:359-364, 2000.

86. What constitutes a true hypertensive emergency in a child?

The glib answer is whenever there are symptoms or threat of symptoms of hypertension or when the blood pressure is very high. However, in practice the decision to treat hypertension as an emergency is not quite so simple. The term "very high" is quite subjective and may mean different things to different people. Certainly blood pressures more than 50% above the 95th %tile for age would be acceptable to most. Additionally, the clinical setting in which the hypertension is occurring will help direct the decision. For example, a child with new-onset hypertension in association with acute glomerulonephritis will not tolerate high blood pressure as well as a child with ESRD and chronic hypertension. Likewise, a child with rapidly rising blood pressure deserves more urgent therapeutic attention. Symptoms, such as headache, irritability and encephalopathy, may be very dramatic, but if not are quite non-specific and may be difficult to attribute to high blood pressure. Certainly, hypertension-induced congestive heart failure, which is very common in neonates, as well as hypertension-associated intracranial bleeding and/or sudden blindness are more straight-forward.

87. What are the advantages and limitations of four medications useful in the treatment of pediatric hypertension?

- ***Nitroprusside***, a very potent, short-acting vasodilator which is administered as a continuous intravenous infusion and gives one the ability to very effectively titrate blood pressure to a satisfactory level. Disadvantages include the time needed to prepare the medication for infusion, the need for continuous monitoring and the potential accumulation of thiocyanate as a toxic metabolite.
- ***Diazoxide***, also a vasodilator and an effective antihypertensive, is readily available and must be pushed rapidly IV. Onset of action is very rapid and duration of effect varies from 2-10 hours. It is safe to the extent that it rarely causes a precipitous fall in blood pressure or hypotension and may give temporary control of blood pressure in a critical situation until other drugs are begun. It should not be used in instances of intracranial bleeding. Side effects include tachycardia, salt retention and hyperglycemia.
- ***Labetalol*** is an adrenergic antagonist with some selective alpha$_1$- and nonselective beta-adrenergic receptor antagonist effects which can be administered intravenously with rapid onset of action (minutes) and duration for 2-4 hours. It should not be given to children with asthma or congestive heart failure and should be used with care in children with diabetes mellitus.
- ***Nifedipine***, a calcium antagonist, is very effective for the urgent reduction in blood pressure even though given orally. It is well absorbed across the mucosa whether from the sublingual area or the upper GI tract. Rapid absorption depends on getting the pharmacologically active, liquid contents of the gel caps to the mucous membrane and precise dosing, especially in small children can be a problem.

88. What are the most common causes of true hypertension in pediatric patients?

The answer(s) to this question first requires the age-old pediatric qualification of making the response based on age. The other qualifier is the definition of hypertension as systolic and/or diastolic blood pressure values consistently above the 95th percentile for age and height. By this definition, <1% of children in the general population will be defined to have hypertension.

The most common cause of clinically significant and treatable hypertension in the *newborn period* is ***renal artery occlusion***, usually by thromboembolism from an umbilical catheter. Additionally, coarctation of the aorta must always be considered. In *older infants and children*, the most common cause of secondary hypertension is ***renal*** or ***renovascular disease***. Included in the broad category of renal disease are virtually all categories of renal dysfunction including obstructive nephropathy, scarring from UTI and reflux, glomerulonephrtitis, polycystic kidney disease, and renal dysplasia.. In *adolescence*, renal disease is also very common, but ***primary*** or ***essential hypertension*** becomes the most frequent cause of high blood pressure.

89. When is it appropriate to evaluate a hypertensive child for the possibility of renal artery stenosis?

Consideration of this extremely uncommon diagnosis is very important because it is not only a potentially curable cause of hypertension, but also if unrecognized and/or untreated, can lead to major morbidity or mortality. There are several clinical conditions and/or findings which make renal artery stenosis more likely. Included are neurofibromatosis, systemic arteritis (e.g., Takayasu), Turner syndrome, Williams syndrome, previous significant renal trauma, the presence of an abdominal bruit and the finding of significant renal size discrepancy and/or decreased flow on doppler to one kidney. Less obvious situations where it is reasonable to suspect renal artery stenosis are (1) very high blood pressure, (2) blood pressure which is progressively difficult to control and (3) blood pressure resistant to usual pharmacotherapy. Despite improvement in imaging studies including ultrasound and nuclear scans, the definitive diagnostic study remains the renal arteriogram.

90. List the causes of secondary hypertension in children and adolescents.

Cause	*Acute Hypertension*	*Chronic Hypertension*	
Renal	Acute glomerulonephritis Acute renal failure Hemolytic-uremic syndrome	Congenital defects Chronic pyelonephritis Hydronephrosis	Tumors of the kidney Hypoplastic kidney Collagen vascular disease
Endocrine	—	Pheochromocytoma Hyperthyroidism (systolic)	Primary aldosteronism Neuroblastoma
Vascular	Renovascular trauma	Coarctation of the aorta Renal artery stenosis Takayasu arteritis	Renal arteriovenous fistula Neurofibromatosis Tuberous sclerosis
Neurogenic	Increased intracranial pressure Guillain-Barré syndrome	Dysautonomia	—
Metabolic	Hypercalcemia Hypernatremia	—	—
Drugs	Cocaine Phencyclidine (PCP) Amphetamines	Nonsteroidal anti-inflammatory drugs Oral contraceptives	Anabolic steroids Corticosteroids Alcohol
Miscellaneous	Burns Leg traction	Heavy metal poisons	—

Adapted from Daniels SR, Loggie JM: Essential hypertension. Adolesc Med State Art Rev 2:555, 1991; with permission.

91. What historical information suggests a secondary cause of hypertension?

History	*Suggests*
Known UTI; recurrent abdominal or flank pain with frequency, urgency, dysura; secondary enuresis	Renal disease
Joint pains, rash, fever, edema	Renal disease, vasculitis
Complicated neonatal course, umbilical artery catheter	Renal artery stenosis
Renl trauma	Renal artery stenosis
Drug use (e.g., sympathomimetics, anabolic steroids, oral contraceptives, illicit drugs)	Drug-induced hypertension
Aberrant course or timing of secondary sexual characteristics; virilization	Adrenal disorder
Muscle cramping, constipation, weakness	Hyperaldosteronism (primary or secondary)
Excessive sweating, episodes of pallor and flushing	Pheochromocytoma

Adapted from Hiner LB, Falkner B: Renovascular hypertension in children. Pediatr Clin North Am 40:128-129, 1993; with permission.

92. List the features on physical exam that suggest a secondary cause of hypertension.

Physical Finding	*Possible Secondary Cause*
Blood pressure	
> 140/100 at any age	Multiple secondary causes
Leg BP < arm BP	Coarctation of the aorta
Poor growth	Chronic renal disease
Short stature, features of Turner syndrome	Coarctation of the aorta
Multiple café-au-lait spots or neurofibromas	Renal artery stenosis, pheochromocytoma
Decreased or delayed pulse in leg	Coarctation of the aorta

Vascular bruits	
Over large vessels	Arteritis
Over upper abdomen, flank	Renal artery stenosis
Flank or upper quadrant mass	Renal malformation, renal or adrenal tumor
Excessive virilization or secondary sex characteristics inappropriate for age	Adrenal disorder
Extremities	
Edema	Renal disease
Excessive sweating	Pheochromocytoma

Adapted from Hiner LB, Falkner B: Renovascular hypertension in children. Pediatr Clin North Am 40:128-129, 1993; with permission.

93. Why shouldn't patients with hypertension and/or using diuretics eat licorice?

True licorice contains glycyrrhizic acid, which has mineralocorticoid (e.g., sodium-retaining) properties. However, most American licorice contains only licorice flavoring and thus has no mineralocorticoid properties. Some chewing tobacco also contains licorice and has been associated with an excess mineralocorticoid syndrome. Think of this if you are called to evaluate an edematous New York Yankee batboy.

RENAL FAILURE

94. What clinical tools, including laboratory studies, are useful in distinguishing pre-renal oliguria (e.g., volume depletion) from the oliguria of intrinsic acute renal failure (ARF)?

Clinical assessment of hydration, volume and perfusion status are critical, and are more likely to be impaired in a pre-renal state. In ARF, these parameters are more likely to show normal or excess volume status, including possible evidence of edema or vascular congestion. If volume status assessment suggests a volume deficit, a fluid bolus with normal saline can be both diagnostic and therapeutic.

Laboratory studies of some assistance include:

Parameter	*Prerenal*	*Renal*
U Na- random meq/L	<20	≈40–60
FE_{Na}* (%)	<1%	>3%
Urine osmolality	>500	≈300

$*FE_{Na} = (U_{Na}) \times (P_{Cr})/(P_{Na}) \times (U_{Cr}) \times 100\%$ (on a randomly collected, spot urine)

95. What is the most common cause of acute renal failure (ARF) in young children in the United States?

The answer traditionally has been the ***hemolytic-uremic syndrome***, which in most cases is associated with gastrointestinal infection with verotoxin-producing E. coli (VTEC), especially the O157:H7 serotype. However, when one considers *all* the cases of ***acute tubular necrosis*** (ATN) in childhood which most commonly result from hypoxic, hypotensive and/or hypovolemic insults or drug-induced injury, it is difficult to place this broad category of ARF in second place. If you are asked on rounds and are in an argumentative mood, answer ATN (no one knows the true answer, since statistics are not available for large populations).

96. Does the use of antibiotic therapy in children with diarrhea caused by E. coli 0157:H7 prevent hemolytic-uremic syndrome (HUS)?

On the contrary, children who received antibiotics (usually sulfa-containing or beta-lactam antibiotics) during outbreaks have had a much higher rate (50% vs. 7%) of HUS.

Wong CS, et al: Risk of hemolytic-uremic syndrome after antibiotic treatment of Eshcerichia coli 0157:H7 infections. N Engl J Med 342:1930-1936, 2000.

97. What constitutes the triad of clinical findings for the hemolytic-uremic syndrome?

- ***Acute renal failure***, usually, but not always oligo-anuric.
- ***Microangiopathic hemolytic anemia***. Examination of the smear is essential to identify RBC fragments, burr cells and schistocytes.
- ***Thrombocytopenia,*** which may vary from mild to severe.

98. What is the pathogenesis of renal osteodystrophy?

Renal osteodystrophy, also known as renal metabolic bone disease or renal rickets, is a condition affecting bone growth and development which occurs in chronic renal insufficiency. It has several etiologies. It results in both defective bone mineralization and secondary hyperparathyroidism, which can lead to poor growth, bone pain, long-bone bowing and deformities.

The pathogenesis, stated somewhat simplistically, is a combination of factors leading to hypocalcemia. These include *phosphate retention* and *hyperphosphatemia* due to decreased GFR and decreased production of 1,25 dihydroxy-vitamin D by the kidney. This leads to decreased absorption of calcium from the GI tract and decreased responsiveness of bone to parathyroid hormone (PTH). The hypocalcemia leads to increased release of PTH, which increases bone resorption. Chronic disease leads to secondary hyperparathyroidism and bone marrow fibrosis, known as osteitis fibrosis cystica. Recognition of osteodystrophy, which often has its origins when the GFR is still approximately $^1/_2$ normal, is important because early intervention with vitamin D and phosphate binders can prevent and/or heal the bone disease (although not necessarily enhance growth). Also, in states of chronic acidosis, the skeleton acts as a buffer for the net acid retained. This results in the release of calcium, contributing to osteopenia and bone disease.

99. What are indications for dialysis?

- ***Elevated BUN and creatinine***: There are no established critical levels above which dialysis needs to be instituted. However, when the creatinine reaches 10 mg/dl or the BUN 100 mg/dl, the GFR is usually markedly reduced resulting in one or more abnormalities as follows:
- ***Hyperkalemia***, either rapidly rising or stable at a dangerously high level which is not controlled by kayexalate binding resin or other measures.
- ***Volume-dependent hypertension*** or signs of ***congestive heart failure*** not responsive to diuretics.
- ***Severe metabolic acidosis*** which cannot be treated with sodium bicarbonate.
- Signs or symptoms of ***uremia*** (e.g., fatigue, encephalopathy, anorexia, pruritus, cramps, bleeding or pericarditis)
- ***Other severe electrolyte disturbances***, including symptomatic hyponatremia, hypocalcemia, hyperphosphatemia.
- The need for a ***blood transfusion*** in the presence of oligoanuria.

100. What are the cause(s) of acidosis in chronic renal failure?

The answer is *multifactorial*. Normally, the kidney acidifies the urine by (1) reclaiming all filtered bicarbonate, (2) excreting titratable acid (mainly through the excretion of hydrogen ions bound to phosphate) and (3) producing and excreting of ammonia (subsequently excreted with a hydrogen ion as an ammonium salt). In chronic renal failure, all three mechanisms may be defective. There may be a bicarbonate leak, titratable acid anions may be retained as nonvolatile acids and there may be defective hydrogen ion secretion and/or ammonium production by the kidney. Additionally, nutritional intake may be seriously compromised resulting in lipolysis, protein catabolism and acidosis.

101. What level of protein intake is reasonable in a child with chronic renal insufficiency?

The protein intake should approximate the US Department of Agriculture Recommended Dietary Allowance for age: ***1.5–2.0 gm/kg in infants*** and approximately ***1.0–1.2 gm/kg in older children***. There is no reason to severely restrict protein intake because on concerns that renal nitrogen loads will accelerate renal insufficiency. On the other hand, *very high* protein intakes do nothing to improve the health and nutrition of a child and should be avoided.

102. When should erythropoietin be started in a child with chronic renal failure?

Anemia is generally present when the ***GFR falls to about 30 ml/min/1.73m***^{2}. Recombinant erythropoietin, given as weekly or twice weekly injections, is usually begun at this time or when the ***hemoglobin falls below 9 gm/dl***. The most common side effects of therapy are iron deficiency and hypertension.

RENAL FUNCTION ASSESSMENT AND THE URINALYSIS

103. What is the simplest way to estimate GFR in the absence of a timed urine collection?

Use of the so-called *Schwartz formula* requires only a serum creatinine and the height of the child. No urine collection, timed or untimed, is necessary. The formula is:

$$\text{Creatinine Clearance (ml/min/1.73m}^2) = K \times \text{Ht. (cm)/Serum Creatinine (mg/dl)}$$

K is 0.45 in infants < 1 year, 0.55 in infants >1 year, 0.33 in low birthweight infants and 0.7 in adolescent males.

104. What are the limitations of the creatinine clearance in measuring the GFR?

Creatinine serves as a clinically useful endogenous marker of GFR because it is produced in a continuous fashion, is eliminated only by the kidney by glomerular filtration, and is neither secreted nor absorbed to a significant degree. Nevertheless, creatinine is not an "ideal solute" for measuring GFR, because there is a small component of secretion which tends to overestimate the GFR by about 10% under normal conditions. With progressive renal insufficiency, however, creatinine secretion becomes more significant and can overestimate GFR by more than two times. One way to overcome the limitation of creatinine secretion is to inhibit secretion through the concomitant use of cimetidine.

105. How can you be confident that a 24-hour urine collection (for anything) is complete?

Because creatinine is produced in a continuous fashion and eliminated only via the kidneys, there is an expectation that a given amount, determined largely by muscle mass, will be excreted daily, independent of the level of renal function. Thus, determination of total urine creatinine in a timed sample can give a reasonable estimate whether the collection approximates 24 hours. The guidelines for expected creatinine excretion applicable to children and adolescents are (1) *males*: 15-25 mg/kg/day and (2) *females*: 10-20 mg/kg/day.

106. When should routine urinalyses (UA) be performed in the pediatric age group?

There is some controversy regarding the use of the UA as a routine screening tool. It is a simple, inexpensive and non-invasive study that is quite sensitive and specific, but the yield from this test in uncovering significant, previously undiagnosed renal dysfunction is very low. However, the landscape is strewn with nephrologists who can cite from personal experience cases of significant renal disease that were first discovered on a routine UA. The American Academy of Pediatrics Guidelines for Health Supervision recommends a UA at age 5 years and another sometime between age 11 and 21 years (or annual dipstick urinalysis for leukocytes for sexually active male and female adolescents).

American Academy of Pediatrics, Committee on Practice and Ambulatory Medicine: Recommendations for Preventive Pediatric Health Care. Pediatrics 105:645-646, 2000.

107. How does Clinitest differ from typical urine dipstick testing in the evaluation of glucosuria?

The *Clinitest tablet* detects reducing substances in the urine. These include reducing sugars (e.g., glucose, galactose, lactose, pentoses and fructose), and also other compounds, including high amounts of amino acids, oxalate, ketones and uric acid. It is also positive in the presence of many drugs including high concentrations of ascorbic acid, penicillin, cephalosporins, nitrofurantoin, sulfonamides and tetracycline. The *glucose oxidase square* on the dipstick is specific for glucose. The Clinitest may be helpful as an initial screening tool for a child suspected of having galactosemia or testing the stool of a child suspected of having carbohydrate malabsorption/intolerance.

108. How are urine specific gravity and urine osmolality related?

Both tests measure the concentration or dilution of the urine, and the relationship between the two is linear and direct, although osmolality is more physiologically correct. *Maximally dilute* urine has a specific gravity of 1.001 and an osmolality of 50. *Maximally concentrated* urine has a specific gravity of about 1.032 and an osmolality of about 1200. Urine which is neither concentrated nor dilute, i.e., *isosthenuric*, has a specific gravity of approximately 1.010 and a corresponding osmolality of 300. ***Specific gravity*** is determined by the *density* (and thus weight and size) of solute in solution. ***Osmolality***, on the other hand, depends on the *numbers* of solute (independent of their size) in solution and their effect on changing its freezing point. Therefore, when there are relatively large molecular weight solutes (e.g., albumin, glucose or contrast material) in the urine, specific gravity will disproportionately increase and osmolality will be a better indicator of true urine concentration. Of note, a urine specific gravity of 1.040 is not achievable by the human kidney. In a child with nephrotic syndrome, levels that high do not represent supernormal concentrating capacity, but rather artifactual effects of heavy proteinuria.

109. What crystal, when seen in the urinary sediment, is always pathologic?

The presence of a ***cystine crystal***, which appears as a flat, simple hexagonal crystal, is never normal and is strong evidence for the amino acid transport disorder cystinuria. In classic cystinuria, the dibasic amino acids (cystine, ornithine, arginine and lysine) are affected. The condition would be of little clinical significance except for the fact that cystine is very insoluble and results in nephrolithiasis.

SURGICAL ISSUES

110. What are the risks of circumcision?

The most common complications are ***bleeding*** and ***infection***. With poor technique, injury or amputation of the glans can occur. ***Meatal stenosis*** as a consequence of meatal ulceration is another complication.

111. Is circumcision now medically indicated?

The debate continues. Data support that newborn circumcision protects males against UTIs in infancy and adulthood. Circumcision may decrease the transmission of certain sexually transmitted diseases (e.g., syphilis, chancroid, herpes simplex, human papillomavirus, HIV), but these data are not as substantial. Other benefits can include improved lifetime genital hygiene, elimination of phimosis and local foreskin infections, and a lower incidence of penile cancer. There are many proponents both for and against circumcision. The decision at present, however, still rests primarily on nonmedical issues.

Schoen EJ, et al: New policy on circumcision—cause for concern. Pediatrics 105: 620-623, 2000.

American Academy of Pediatrics, Task Force on Circumcision: Circumcision policy statement. Pediatrics 103: 686-693, 1999.

112. What is the proper method of anesthesia for neonatal circumcision?

Up to 85% of infant males in the U.S. undergo circumcision, and worldwide it remains the most commonly performed operation. Until recently, it was usually performed by most without anesthesia or analgesia. Although pacifiers, topical agents (3.0% lidocaine, EMLA cream), and parenteral analgesics (e.g, acetaminophen) help alleviate some discomfort, the most effective means of minimizing pain are a ring block or a dorsal penile nerve block. The latter consists of injecting 0.3–0.4 ml of 1% lidocaine *without* epinephrine in both sides of the dorsal penile base. The safety record of this method, when properly performed, is excellent. The addition of buffering agents to the lidocaine are of no benefit in the reduction of pain. Of note, the technique of circumcision (Plastibell vs. Gomco clamp vs. Mogen clamp) also has effects on pain. The Mogen technique appears to cause the least pain in large part because it is a faster procedure.

Kurtis PS, et al: A comparison of the Mogen and Gomco clamps in combination with dorsal penile nerve block in minimizing the pain of neonatal circumcision. Pediatrics 103:323, 1999.

Newton CW, et al: Plain and buffered lidocaine for neonatal circumcision. Obstet Gynecol 93:350-352, 1999.

Lander J, et al: Comparison of ring block, dorsal penile nerve block and topical anesthesia for neonatal circumcision: a randomized controlled trial. JAMA 278:2157-2162, 1997.

113. How are the degrees of hypospadias classified?

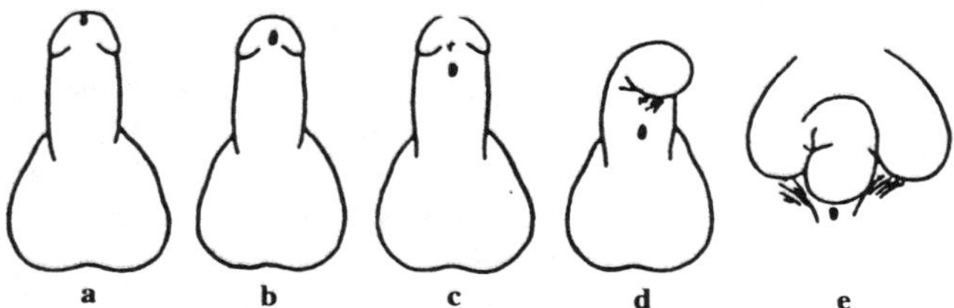

Degrees of hypospadias are classified according to the site of urethral opening:(a) normal meatus, (b) coronal or glandular, (c) distal shaft, (d) proximal shaft, and (e) perineal with bifid scrotum and penoscrotal transposition. (Penoscrotal hypospadias not depicted.)

From Perlmutter AD: Hypospadias. In Edelmann CM Jr (ed): Pediatric Kidney Disease. Boston, Little, Brown and Co., Boston, 1978, p 1235; with permission.

114. What are the consequences of hypospadias?

Hypospadias occurs in 1–2/1000 livebirths and results from failure or delay in midline fusion of the urethral folds. It is often associated with a ventral band of fibrous tissue (chordee) that causes ventral curvature of the penis, especially with an erection, making intercourse difficult or impossible. In assessing hypospadias, it is useful to describe where the urethral meatus appears—glandular, distal shaft, proximal shaft, or perineal—and also the degree and location of chordee.

A number of *associated genitourinary abnormalities* have been described with hypospadias including meatal stenosis, inguinal hernias, undescended testes, and enlarged utricle masculinus (vestigial vagina). The incidence of these abnormalities rises sharply with the more severe degrees of hypospadias. In the mild forms, which account for most cases, radiography or endoscopy of the urinary tract is unnecessary. The treatment of hypospadias is surgical repair, usually as a one-step procedure. With the advent of microsurgical techniques, the optimal time for repair appears to be 6–12 months of age.

115. What distinguishes phimosis and paraphimosis?

Phimosis is a narrowing of the distal foreskin, preventing its retraction over the glans of the penis. In newborns, retraction is difficult due to normal adhesions which gradually self-resolve. Chronic inflammation or scarring can cause true phimosis with persistent narrowing and may require circumcision.

Paraphimosis is incarceration of a retracted foreskin behind the glans. It occurs when the retracted foreskin is not repositioned. Progressive edema results, which if uncorrected, can lead to ischemic breakdown. Local anesthesia, ice, and manual reduction usually correct the problem, but if these are unsuccessful, surgical reduction is necessary.

116. How should urethral prolapse in young girls be managed?

Urethral prolapse is an uncommon problem, occurring mainly in young black girls. They present with an anterior, bleeding introital mass, perineal discomfort, and mild dysuria. Many options have been tried, from sitz baths alone to aggressive surgical fixation of the bladder neck. The recommended therapy is primary surgical excision on an outpatient basis.

Valerie E, et al: Diagnosis and treatment of urethral prolapse in children. Urology 54:1082-1084, 1999.

117. What is the most common cause of urinary tract obstruction in the newborn?

Posterior urethral valves, more commonly seen in male infants. The obstruction is frequently associated with high intravesicular pressures which may damage renal parenchyma if undetected. However, the adverse obstructive effects of the valves during intrauterine life may be associated with renal dysplasia. Thus, even with prompt recognition and treatment, renal insufficiency may progress.

118. What is the natural history of hydroceles?

Small *hydroceles* in infancy are benign and spontaneously resolve by 9–12 months of age. Large hydroceles rarely resolve and may cause vascular compromise and testicular atrophy; these should be resected. A communicating hydrocele (which changes in size) indicates a completely patent processus vaginalis and has the potential for hernia formation. This variety also should be repaired.

119. When should undescended testicles be repaired?

The optimal time for surgery on an undescended testes is ***12 months of age*** or shortly thereafter. Cryptorchidism usually resolves without intervention. 75% of full-term infants and 90% of premature cryptorchid newborns will have full testicular descent by age 9 months. Spontaneous testis descent after 9 months is unlikely. In the second year of life, ultrastructural changes in the seminiferous tubules of the undescended testes begin to appear, which may be halted by orchipexy.

Section on Urology: Timing of elective surgery on the genitalia of male children with particular reference to the risks, benefits, and psychological effects of surgery and anesthesia. Pediatrics 97:590–594, 1996.

120. How commonly are congenital genitourinary tract anomalies detected on prenatal ultrasound screening?

Approximately ***1%*** of live births.

121. What is the most common GU abnormality found on prenatal ultrasound?

Hydronephrosis. This descriptive term indicates distention of the renal pelvis and calyces which is often due to obstruction. However, it can also be seen with nonobstructing entities such as vesicoureteral reflux.

122. What are the possible causes of prenatal hydronephrosis?

- Ureteropelvic junction obstruction
- Vesicoureteral reflux
- Multicystic kidney
- Megaureter (obstructive and nonobstructive)
- Posterior urethral valves
- Prune belly syndrome
- Ectopic ureter or ureterocele
- Urethral atresia

123. If a newborn with a history of prenatal hydronephrosis has a "normal" renal ultrasound within the first two days of life, can we assume there are no GU abnormalities?

No. A normal renal ultrasound at this age does not exclude obstruction or reflux. Neonates often have transient oliguria during the first few days of life and this can result in underdistension of the renal pelvis even in an obstructed kidney. A repeat ultrasound is indicated in several weeks.

124. In patients with prenatal hydronephrosis, how commonly is vesicoureteral reflux (VUR) subsequently diagnosed?

In several studies, voiding cystourethrograms (VCUG) were performed postnatally in infants with a diagnosis of prenatal hydronephrosis based on ultrasound. The VCUG demonstrated mild to severe VUR in **18-30%** of infants with a *normal* postnatal renal ultrasound. Significant reflux was also detected in ***35-45%*** of infants with *persistent* postnatal hydronephrosis. The VCUG or nuclide cystogram are the only studies that can accurately identify VUR. Thus, even if the postnatal ultrasound is normal, antibiotic prophylaxis is recommended until VUR can be excluded by subsequent study.

Elder JS: Antenatal hydronephrosis—fetal and neonatal management. Pediatr Clin North Am 44:1299-1321, 1997.

125. What is a reasonable approach to the management of prenatally-detected hydronephrosis?

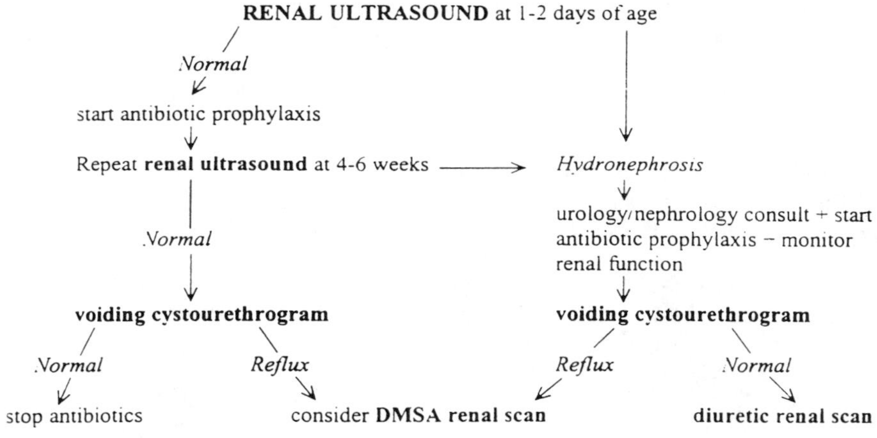

126. What physical findings should prompt a search for an underlying renal abnormality?

- Abdominal mass
- High imperforate anus
- Perineal hypospadias
- Exstrophy of the bladder
- Ambiguous genitalia
- Prune belly abdomen
- Neonatal ascites
- Oligohydramnios
- Anuria-oliguria (especially in neonate)
- Aniridia, hemihypertrophy (Wilms tumor)
- Poor urinary stream
- Persistent wetness

127. A newborn male with a distended, flabby, and wrinkled abdomen and with a greatly diminished urinary output likely has what condition?

Prune belly syndrome, or congenital absence of the abdominal musculature (also called Eagle-Barrett syndrome). Occurring predominantly in males, this condition has no known familial or genetic basis. It is associated with multiple other congenital malformations, especially urinary tract dilation with a greatly enlarged bladder and dilated and tortuous ureters. Bilateral cryptorchidism is common. Renal involvement is quite variable, ranging from complete agenesis to no involvement. It also may be unilateral. Chronic UTIs are common.

128. Which entities are known to cause renal papillary necrosis?

Diabetes, analgesic abuse, sickle cell trait and disease, pyelonephritis, urinary tract obstruction, and hypotension (usually in neonates).

129. In what settings does renal vein thrombosis occur?

Renal vein thrombosis usually occurs in the sick infant, especially in the first month of life. Dehydration, shock, septicemia, asphyxia, and cyanotic congenital heart disease (especially following angiography) are predisposing factors. The usual presenting features are a sudden change in the infant's clinical condition associated with hematuria, oliguria, proteinuria, and a flank mass. Thrombocytopenia is common, but hypertension is not. An intravenous pyelogram is often not helpful since the kidney with the thrombosis usually does not visualize. An ultrasound study, demonstrating the renal vein clot and an enlarged kidney, or a radionuclide study is usually more useful. The differential diagnoses include acute tubular or cortical necrosis, multicystic dysplasia, renal arterial thrombosis, adrenal hemorrhage, renal trauma, hydronephrosis, neuroblastoma, nephroblastomatosis, and Wilms tumor.

Zigman A, et al: Renal vein thrombosis. J Pediatr Surg 35:1540-1542, 2000.

130. What is the differential diagnosis of an abdominal mass in the neonate?

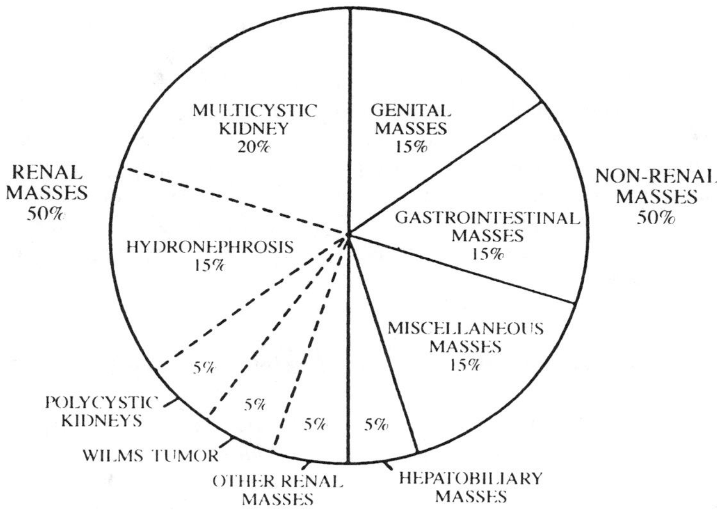

From Sunshine, et al: In Fanaroff AA, Martin RF (eds): Behrman's Neonatal–Perinatal Medicine: Diseases of the Fetus and Infant. St. Louis, Mosby, 1983, p. 531; with permission.

TUBULAR DISORDERS

131. Name the four main types of renal tubular acidosis (RTA).

Type 1—impairment in *distal* acidification

Type 2—impairment in *proximal* tubule bicarbonate reclamation

Type 3—combination of types 1 and 2

Type 4—secondary to a lack of, or insensitivity to, aldosterone

All four types are associated with a hyperchloremic, normal anion gap acidosis.

132. Describe the clinical and laboratory manifestations of the various RTAs.

	Type 1 (Classic, distal)	*Type 2 (Proximal)*	*Type 3 (Hybrid)*	*Type 4 (Aldosterone deficiency)*
Growth failure	+++	++	++	+++
Hypokalemic muscle weakness	++	+	+	Hyperkalemia
Nephrocalcinosis	Frequent	Rare	±	Rare
Low citrate excretion	+++	±	±	±
FE of filtered HCO_3 at normal serum HCO_3 levels	< 5%	> 15%	5–15%	< 15%
Daily alkali treatment (mEq/kg)	1–10	5–20	1–10	1–5
Daily potassium requirement	Decreases with correction	Increases with correction	±	
Urine pH	> 5.5	< 5.5	> 5.5	< 5.5
Presence of other tubular defects	Rare	Common	Rare	Rare
Metabolic bone disease	Rare	Common	Rare	Rare
Urine anion gap	Positive	Negative	Positive	Positive

+, Present; ++, common; +++, very common; ± variable. FE = fractional excretion.

Adapted from Chan JCM: Renal tubular acidosis. J Pediatr 103:327, 1983; and Zelikovic I: Renal tubular acidosis. Pediatr Ann 24:53, 1995; with permission.

Types 1, 2, and 3 RTA are associated with *hypokalemia*, whereas type 4 is characterized by *hyperkalemia* in addition to hyperchloremic acidosis. Hypercalciuria is typical of type 1 RTA and, in conjunction with hypocitraturia, often leads to nephrocalcinosis and renal calculi. Type 2 is often part of a more global defect of proximal tubule function, the *Fanconi syndrome* which, in addition to bicarbonaturia, is characterized by aminoaciduria, glycosuria, phosphaturia (hypophosphatemia) and rickets. Type 4 RTA is most commonly observed in pediatric patients with obstructive uropathy, tubular unresponsiveness to aldosterone (pseudoaldosteronism) which is often transient during infancy, or decreased aldosterone secretion (hypoaldosteronism). Other symptoms and signs that are common with all forms of RTA are growth failure, polyuria, polydipsia, recurrent dehydration, and vomiting.

133. How is determining the urinary anion gap helpful in the evaluation of metabolic acidosis?

Investigation of any child with a persistent metabolic acidosis must consider some form of RTA in the differential diagnosis. The *urinary anion gap* is a convenient and accurate screening test for RTA. It is an indirect estimate of urinary ammonium excretion (and thus urinary acid excretion) and is calculated by the following formula after determining *urinary* electrolyte concentrations :

$$Anion\ gap = Na^{+} + K^{+} - Cl^{-}$$

If the anion gap is *negative*, it suggests a large chloride excretion and thus adequate ammonium excretion. The urinary anion gap is negative in hyperchloremic metabolic acidosis due to diarrhea, untreated proximal RTA or prior administration of an acid load.

If the anion gap is *positive*, it suggests an acidification defect, as in distal RTA. Results are not reliable if there are large amounts of unmeasured anions such as ketoacids, penicillin or salicylates.

134. What is the primary defect in type 1 RTA?

An *inability* of the *distal tubule* to *secrete hydrogen*. Thus, in the presence of significant systemic acidosis, urine is not maximally acidified (pH < 5.5). This defect in hydrogen secretion is associated with low rates of ammonium and titratable acid excretion.

135. How is the diagnosis of type 1 RTA established?

The key to this diagnosis is the demonstration of an impaired ability of the distal tubule to secrete hydrogen (NH_4^+) in the setting of a persistent metabolic acidosis. If a patient is *acidotic*, the following urine studies are diagnostic of distal RTA: a) ***urine pH > 5.5*** (measured by meter) or b) ***diminished*** or ***absent*** NH_4^+ ***excretion*** (i.e., positive urinary anion gap).

Another test of hydrogen ion secretion involves loading the patient with bicarbonate. Normally, distally secreted hydrogen ions combine with bicarbonate to form carbonic acid, which is catalyzed to water and CO_2. In patients with distal RTA, less carbonic acid (and thus CO_2) is produced. When the difference between the urine and blood CO_2 concentration is < 20 mmHg, this indicates decreased hydrogen secretion and distal RTA is likely.

136. What disorders are associated with classic type 1 distal RTA?

Primary:

Sporadic, hereditary

Secondary:

Disorders associated with nephrocalcinosis: hypercalciuria, hyperparathyroidism, vitamin D intoxication

Autoimmune disorders: systemic lupus erythematosus, Sjögren syndrome, thyroiditis, chronic active hepatitis, polyarteritis nodosa

Drugs or toxins: amphotericin B, mercury, lithium, toluene, analgesics

Renal disorders: medullary sponge kidney, pyelonephritis, obstructive uropathy

Miscellaneous: Wilson disease, Fabry disease, hyperoxaluria

137. What is the main renal defect in type 2 RTA?

The primary defect is a ***decreased ability of the proximal tubule to reabsorb filtered*** HCO_3 at normal plasma HCO_3 concentrations—a "lowered tubular reabsorptive threshold." These patients typically present with a chronic hyperchloremic metabolic acidosis, acid urine (pH < 5.5), and a low fractional excretion of HCO_3 (FE < 5%). When plasma HCO_3 levels are increased toward normal (and thus above the lowered tubular reabsorptive threshold), patients will lose HCO_3 in the urine (FE > 15%) and the urine will be alkaline (pH > 6.0).

138. What are the causes of type 2 (proximal) RTA?

Primary

Sporadic, hereditary (autosomal dominant and autosomal recessive)

Secondary

Associated with other inherited disorders: cystinosis, tyrosinemia, galactosemia, glycogen storage diseases, Lowe syndrome, Wilson disease, idiopathic Fanconi syndrome

Drugs and toxins: acetazolamide, sulfanilamide, valproic acid, ifosamide, lead, mercury and cadmium poisoning

Miscellaneous: nephrotic syndrome, medullary cystic kidney disease, renal vein thrombosis, cyanotic congenital heart disease, hyperparathyroidism

139. What is the primary defect in type 4 RTA?

Decreased secretion of hydrogen and potassium by the collecting tubule. This is due either to *tubular resistance* to the action of *aldosterone* (pseudoaldosteronism) or to *aldos-*

terone deficiency (hypoaldosteronism). Patients typically demonstrate a hyperchloremic metabolic acidosis with hyperkalemia, a urine pH < 5.5 in response to a systemic acidosis and a decreased ability to generate and excrete NH_4^+.

140. What are the recommended therapies in the treatment of various forms of RTA?

Goals of RTA therapy: improve growth, correct metabolic bone disease, prevent nephrolithiasis/nephrocalcinosis and control any underlying disease process. Principle therapies are:

Alkali therapy (sodium citrate or sodium bicarbonate): Required in all forms of RTA with the goal of a normal plasma HCO_3 level. Patients with *distal* RTA generally require only 2-3 mEq/kg/day of alkali. However, infants may also experience some increased urinary bicarbonate wasting and require up to 10 mEq/kg/day. Patients with *proximal* RTA require large quantities of alkali (5-20 mEq/kg/day). In *Type 4* RTA, patients usually need low dose alkali therapy (1-3 mEq/kg/day) *plus* a potassium restricted diet and mineralcorticoid therapy if there is hypoaldosteronism.

Postassium supplmentation (potassium citrate): Required in distal and especially in proximal RTA.

141. How do you diagnose RTA in a patient with a hyperchloremic metabolic acidosis and normal serum anion gap?

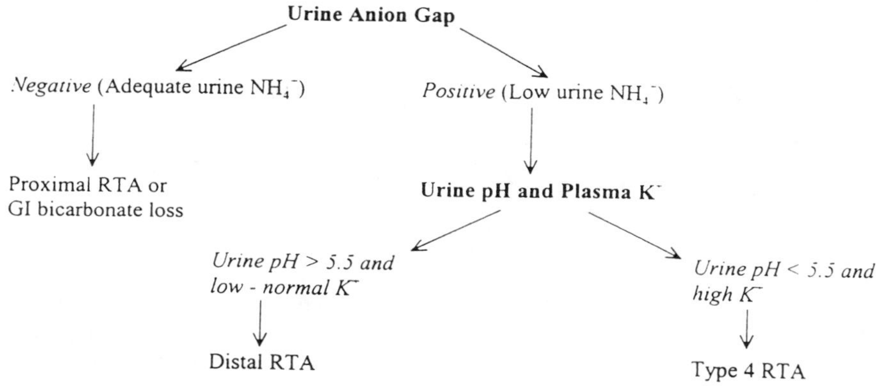

Modified from Lash JP: Laboratory evaluation of renal tubular acidosis. Clinics Lab Med 13:127, 1993.

142. What is the clinical presentation of acute interstitial nephritis (AIN)?

AIN is caused by an immune-mediated inflammatory response that initially involves the renal interstitium and tubules, usually sparing the glomeruli and vasculature. AIN has a wide array of clinical presentations ranging from isolated tubular disorders (e.g., Fanconi syndrome) to acute renal failure. Additional findings may suggest a hypersensitivity reaction (e.g., fever, rash and arthralgias).

143. What are the causes of AIN?

Drugs

Antibiotics: especially penicillin analogs, cephalosporins, sulfonamides, rifampin

Nonsteroidal anti-inflammatory drugs

Diuretics: especially thiazides and furosemide

Infections: either directly by infection of renal parenchyma or associated with systemic infection

Immonologic disorders
Systemic lupus erythematosus
Sjögren syndrome
Mixed essential cryoglobulinemia
Acute kidney transplant rejection
Idiopathic

144. What laboratory abnormalities are seen in AIN?

Urinary sediment	RBCs, leukocytes (eosinophils), leukocyte casts
Urinary protein excretion	<1 gram/day; with NSAID use, may be >1 gram/day
Fractional excretion of sodium	Usually > 1
Proximal tubular defects	Glucosuria, bicarbonaturia, phosphaturia, aminoaciduria, proximal RTA
Distal tubular defects	Hyperkalemia, sodium wasting, distal RTA
Medullary defects	Sodium wasting, urinary concentrating defects

Meyers CM: Acute interstitial nephritis. In Greenberg A (ed): Primer on Kidney Diseases. National Kidney Foundation, Academic Press, San Diego, 1998, p. 278.

145. What is the relationship of Fanconi syndrome to Fanconi anemia?

None. The *Fanconi syndrome* is synonymous with diffuse proximal tubular dysfunction. Children with this syndrome present with polyuria and polydipsia, episodes of dehydration, rickets, slow growth and failure to thrive. Evaluation for Fanconi syndrome involves identifying markers of proximal tubular dysfunction including hypokalemia, diffuse aminoaciduria, renal glycosuria, proximal renal tubular acidosis, hyperuricosuria, and decreased proximal tubular reabsorption of phosphate. Fanconi anemia is a distinct and unrelated clinical entity.

146. In what disorders can patients present with a hypokalemic, hypochloremic metabolic alkalosis?

Bartter syndrome, Gitelman syndrome and ***antenatal Bartter (hyperprostaglandin E) syndrome***.

All of these disorders are primarily due to *defects* in *sodium reabsorption*, either in the loop of Henle (Bartter syndrome) or in the distal tubule (Gitelman syndrome). Patients are normotensive and, unlike patients with primary hyperaldosteronism, have elevated plasma renin levels.

147. What renal tubular disorder mimics the chronic administration of furosemide?

Bartter syndrome, which involves abnormalities in electrolyte processing in the thick ascending limb of the Henle Loop, results in salt wasting. The laboratory profile includes: hypokalemia, metabolic alkalosis, hypomagnesemia in 30%, and high renin and aldosterone levels without hypertension.

148. What clinical features distinguish classic Bartter syndrome from the Bartter-like syndromes?

Feature	*Classic Bartter Syndrome*	*Gitelman Syndrome*	*Antenatal Bartter Syndrome*
Age at presentation	Infancy, early childhood	Childhood, adolescence	In utero, infancy
Prematurity, polyhydramnios	+/–	–	++
Delayed growth	++	–	+++
Delayed cognitive development	+/–	–	–
Polyuria, polydypsia	++	+	+++
Tetany	Rare	++	–
Serum magnesium	Low in 20%	Low in about 100%	Low-normal to normal
Urine calcium excretion	Normal to high	Low	Very high
Nephrocalcinosis	+/–	–	++
Urine prostaglandin excretion	High	Normal	Very high
Clinical response to indomethacin	+/–	–	Often life-saving

Guay-Woodford LM: Bartter syndrome: Unraveling the pathophysiologic enigma. Am J Med 105:152, 1998.

URINARY TRACT INFECTIONS

149. How helpful are dipstick testing and microscopic analysis of urine as screening tests for urinary tract infections (UTIs)?

Recalling that *sensitivity* is the probability that test results will be positive among patients who have UTIs and *specificity* is the probability that test results will be negative among patients who do not have UTIs, the value of components of the urinalysis individually and in combination as screening tools for the diagnosis of a UTI are:

Test	*Sensitivity % (Range)*	*Specificity % (Range)*
Leukocyte esterase	83 (67–94)	78 (64–92)
Nitrite	53 (15–82)	98 (90–100)
Leukocyte esterase *or* nitrite positive	93 (90–100)	72 (58–91)
Microscopy: WBCs	73 (32–100)	81 (45–98)
Microscopy: bacteria	81 (16–99)	83 (11–100)
Leukocyte esterase *or* nitrite *or* microscopy posive	99.8 (99–100)	70 (60–92)

From American Academy of Pediatrics, Committee on Quality Improvement, Subcommittee on Urinary Tract Infection: Practice parameter: the diagnosis, treatment, and evaluation of the initial urinary tract infection in febrile infants and young children. Pediatrics 103:847, 1999; with permission.

150. Can the diagnosis of UTI be made based on urinalysis alone?

No. A urine culture is the only accurate means of diagnosing a UTI. Urinalysis can be valuable in selecting individuals for prompt initiation of treatment while awaiting results of the urine culture. In older children, in whom UTI symptoms are more reliable indicators of infection, a negative nitrite test, negative leukocyte esterase test, and absence of UTI symptoms are highly correlated with the absence of infection. However, babies require a culture to exclude UTI.

151. Which children are at increased risk for bacteriuria or a symptomatic UTI?

Premature infants discharged from neonatal intensive care units

Children with:

- Immunodeficiencies or underlying systemic disease
- Urinary tract abnormalities
- Renal calculi
- Neurogenic bladder or voiding dysfunction

- Chronic severe constipation
- Family history of UTI, renal anomalies, or reflux

Girls < 5 years of age with a history of UTI

152. What are the common presenting signs and symptoms of a UTI in an infant?

The presenting findings are non-specific and can include fever, vomiting, diarrhea, irritability, and poor feeding. These same findings are often seen in infants *without* UTIs. Thus, the potential importance of cultures in febrile infants.

153. How common are UTIs in young febrile infants?

Quite. In infants and toddlers *between 2 and 24 months* with unexplained fever (>38.3° C), the prevalence is about ***5%*** with girls having twice or more as many infections as boys. The rate in circumsized boys is low (0.2% to 0.4%). In a study of 442 infants < *2 months of age,* ***7.5%*** had UTIs. Of note, in a subgroup of these infants in whom the utility of urinalysis in predicting a positive urine culture was being evaluated, 40% with UTI demonstrated by catheterization or suprapubic aspiration had no pyuria and no bacteria detectable on smears of an unspun sample.

Hoberman A, et al: Prevalence of urinary tract infections in febrile infants. J Pediatr 123:17-23, 1993.

Crain EF, Gershel JC: Urinary tract infections in febrile infants younger than eight weeks of age. Pediatrics 86:363–367, 1990.

154. In an infant or toddler who is not toilet-trained, how should urine for culture be obtained?

Suprapubic aspiration (SPA) is the gold standard (and most invasive). However, the batting average of house officers for obtaining urine by this method is only about 60% or less (increasing to over 90% with ultrasonic guidance). *Catheter specimens* have a >90% correlation with SPA (which can be increased if the first 3 ml are discarded as this is more likely to contain contaminants) and have a higher collection rate. *Sterile bag collection* has very limited accuracy with wide variations in false-positive and false-negative rates. Invasive specimen collection remains the procedure of choice in a sick febrile infant for whom rapid initiation of therapy is warranted. When time permits, allowing parents to obtain clean-catch specimens from infants and toddlers (by holding a bowl under a child's genitalia) has shown a remarkably good correlation with SPA and can be an alternative to invasive techniques.

Dayan PS, et al: A comparison of the initial to the later stream in children catherized to evaluate for urinary tract infection. Pediatr Emerg Care 16:88-90, 2000.

Ramage IJ, et al: Accuracy of clean-catch urine collection in infancy. J Pediatr 135:765-767, 1999.

155. What is a rational approach to the management of a suspected UTI in an infant?

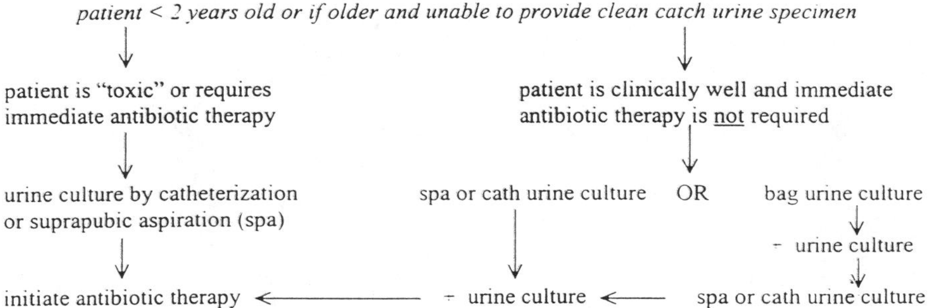

American Academy of Pediatrics, Subcommittee on Urinary Tract Infections. Practice parameters: The diagnosis, treatment, and evaluation of the initial urinary tract infection in febrile infants and young children. Pediatrics 103:813–853, 1999.

156. What is the "enhanced urinalysis"?

The *enhanced urinalysis* is a technique devised at the University of Pittsburgh as an alternative method of screening for UTIs. Traditional urinalysis has consisted of dipstick (particularly leukocyte esterase and nitrite testing) and microscopic evaluation. A positive microscopic result has been ≥5 wcb/hpf in a centrifuged specimen and any bacteria seen on an unstained specimen. The enhanced urinalysis modifies the approach as follows:

Pyuria: redefined as ≥10 wbc/mm^3 in uncentrifuged urine when viewed via a Neubauer hemocytometer

Bacteriuria: any seen on 10 oil immersion views after 2 drops of uncentrifuged urine are Gram-stained

The advantages of this method: (a) decreased variability in results caused by centrifugation and resuspension; (b) fixed volume for examination; and (c) concise visual field with uniform illumination. This technique may a higher sensivity and positive predictive value than the traditional urinalysis.

Hoberman A, Wald ER: UTI in young children: New light on old questions. Contemp Pediatr 14: 141-156, 1997.

Hoberman A, et al: Enhanced urinalysis as a screening test for urinary tract infection. Pediatrics 91:1196, 1993.

157. What bacterial counts constitute a positive urine culture?

Urine should be a sterile fluid, but the technique used to collect the specimen can introduce varying degrees of contamination. If the specimen is obtained by *suprapubic aspiration*, the presence of any bacteria indicates infection. If the specimen is obtained by *catherization*, colony counts 10,000 colonies/ml indicate infection. Infection is present 80% of the time in a *midstream clean catch* urine sample if >100,000 colonies/ml of a single species is cultured. Colony counts between 10,000-100,000 are suspicious and require reculturing, and <10,000 organisms usually indicates contamination. A "*bag*" urine culture with >100,000 colonies/ml has an *85% false-positive* result and should be repeated by suprapubic aspiration or catheterization.

158. What factors can cause low colony counts despite significant urinary infection?

- High-volume urine flow
- Recent antimicrobial therapy
- Fastidious and slow-growing organisms (e.g., enterococci, *S. saprophyticus)*
- Low urine pH (<5.0) and specific gravity (<1.003)
- Bacteriostatic agents in the urine
- Complete obstruction of a ureter
- Chronic or indolent infection
- Use of inappropriate culture techniques

From Bock GH: Urinary tract infections. In Hoekelman RA, et al (eds): Primary Pediatric Care, 4th ed. St. Louis, Mosby, 2001, p. 1896; with permission.

159. Why should urine specimens be refrigerated if they cannot be immediately processed?

The storage of urine specimens at room temperature is one of the most common causes of false-positive results. When left at room temperature, enteric organisms in specimens have a growth-doubling time of 12.5 minutes, and thus colony counts become an unreliable guide. If a urine specimen cannot be processed within 15 minutes, it should be refrigerated at < 4°C to stop *in vitro* replication.

160. What pathogens are associated with UTIs in children?

80–90% of initial UTIs are caused by ***E. coli***. Other organisms include: *Proteus* *mirabilis, Klebsiella pneumoniae, Pseudomonas, Enterobacter* and some *Staphylococcus* species.

161. What are the characteristics of complicated UTIs?

Complicated UTIs imply the presence of either an anatomic abnormality, such as obstruction or vesicoureteral reflux, or a functional abnormality, such as a neurogenic bladderor voiding dysfunction. Patients with complicated UTIs are more likely to have symptoms consistent with pyelonephritis and to have infections with more virulent organisms (e.g., *Proteus, pseudomonas*).

162. How is cystitis distinguished clinically from pyelonephritis?

Often with difficulty. *Pyelonephritis* tends to have more constitutional symptoms, such as fever, rigors, flank and back pain, while *cystitis* has more bladder symptoms, such as enuresis, dysuria, frequency, and urgency. The presence of white cell casts or impaired urinary concentrating ability is more indicative of pyelonephritis. Patients with pyelonephritis tend to have higher sedimentation rates and C-reactive proteins, but these results can also be seen in some patients with cystitis. Renal DMSA (dimercaptosuccinic acic) scintigraphy is the most accurate study for identifying acute pyelonephritis. Of note, for most children, the treatment of cystitis or pyelonephritis is essentially the same.

163. When do patients with a UTI require hospitalization and parenteral antibiotics?

- Any infant < *2 months* of age due to an increased risk for urosepsis or other serious concomitant infections.
- Any patient who is *toxic*, *dehydrated* or *unable to tolerate oral antibiotics*.

164. Should all pediatric patients with clinical pyelonephritis be hospitalized?

Traditionally, older patients with clinical evidence of pyelonephritis have been hospitalized for 24–48 hours for parenteral antibiotics and, if a good clinical response has occurred, discharged to home for additional oral antibiotic therapy. Data are emerging that the short- and long-term outcome in patients (even as young as two months) with uncomplicated pyelonephritis is the same for initial therapy either intravenously or with oral, third-generation cephalosporins. Oupatient therapy clearly mandates the ability to tolerate oral antibiotics, no concerns regarding compliance and careful and reliable follow-up.

Hoberman A, et al: Oral versus initial intravenous therapy for urinary tract infection in young febrile children. Pediatrics 104:79-86, 1999.

165. What is the duration of antibotic therapy for a UTI?

Standard duration of therapy is ***10 days*** (combined oral plus parenteral) for cystitis or pyelonephritis although shorter courses are under study or some experts lean toward 14 days for pyelonephritis. If the patient is not clinically improved within 2-3 days of starting therapy, the urine culture should be repeated and antibiotics adjusted, if indicated.

166. When are prophylactic antibiotics indicated in UTIs?

- Infants or children with their *first UTI*, who have finished their 10 day course of therapy and are *awaiting the completion of studies* (e.g., VCUG, renal ultrasound).
- Patients with *known urologic abnormalities* which place them at high risk for recurrent UTIs (e.g., vesicoureteral reflux, hydronephrosis, posterior urethral valves).
- Children and adolescents with *recurrent UTIs* and normal urinary tract anatomy. A 6-12 month course is indicated. If infections recur after stopping prophylaxis, antibiotics should be resumed.

167. Which antibiotics are commonly used for prophylaxis?

Antimicrobial	*Dosage*
TMP in combination with SMX	2 mg of TMP, 10 mg of SMX per kg as single bedtime dose *or* 5 mg of TMP, 25 mg of SMX per kg twice per week
Nitrofurantoin	1–2 mg/kg as single daily dose
Sulfisoxazole	10–20 mg/kg divided every 12 h
Nalidixic acid	30 mg/kg divided every 12 h
Methenamine mandelate	75 mg/kg divided every 12 h

From American Academy of Pediatrics, Committee on Quality Improvement, Subcommittee on Urinary Tract Infection: Practice parameter: the diagnosis, treatment, and evaluation of the initial urinary tract infection in febrile infants and young children. Pediatrics 103:849, 1999; with permission.

168. Is cranberry juice helpful in the management of UTIs in children?

The use of cranberry juice as a urine acidifying agent and treatment for UTI has been popular in adults since the 1920s, and studies in adults have shown it to be helpful in diminishing the frequency of bacteriuria, possibly due to its anti-adhesive properties against *E. coli*. Limited studies in children, primarily looking at its role as a possible prophylactic treatment for chronic bacteriuria in children who require frequent catheterization, have not shown positive benefits.

Schlager TA, et al: Effect of cranberry juice on bacteriuria in children with neurogenic bladder receiving intermittent catheterization. J Pediatr 135:698-702, 1999.

169. What is the role of DMSA scanning in the evaluation of urinary tract infections?

Injected 99mTc DMSA is taken up by renal tubular cells. Subsequent scanning provides information on renal morphology and functioning parenchyma. When carried out at the time of an acute infection, it has been touted as a reasonably rapidly available study to help in the differentiation of renal parenchymal infections from lower tract UTI. When done after the infection has been treated, the study provides assessment of renal scars. Both local inflammation and renal scars appear as 'cold' spots on the scan. Some published studies question the usefulness of the test because of a relatively high rate of false positive and equivocal scans.

170. What is the significance of a renal ultrasounds interpreted as "compatible with medical renal disease"?

Renal ultrasonography provides extremely useful information regarding anatomic abnormalities such as hydronephrosis, cystic disease, tumors, and stones. The reading of "compatible with medical renal disease" is usually applied to otherwise structurally normal kidneys which may show increased echogenicity and/or size indicative of inflammation or edema. Typically, a renal ultrasound provides no clinically useful information about renal function.

171. Which patients with a UTI warrant imaging studies of the urinary tract?

- Older girls with their first episode of pyelonephritis, history of recurrent UTIs, or UTI with a more virulent pathogen (e.g., *Proteus, Pseudomonas*)
- Any patient with evidence of diminished renal function, hypertension or persistent hematuria and/or proteinuria
- Many clinicians feel that imaging studies should be undertaken for the *first UTI* in boys of any age, or in girls through middle adolescence, especially if they have any risk factors for UTI, such as a positive family history.

172. What imaging studies are utilized for patients with UTI who warrant evaluation?

- *Voiding cystourethrogram* or *radionuclide cystogram* to evaluate for vesicoureteral reflux (the most common abnormality found in children with UTIs)

- *Renal ultrasound* to screen for urinary tract obstruction or other structural genitourinary abnormalities
- *Renal cortical DMSA scanning* is recommended by some authorities to determine if there is evidence of acute pyelonephritis or permanent renal scarring.

173. How soon after a UTI is diagnosed can imaging studies of the urinary tract be obtained?

- The voiding cystourethrogram or radionuclide cystogram can be performed as soon as the urine culture is sterile. A tradition recommendation has been to wait 3-6 weeks after a UTI for a VCUG to minimize the possibility of false positive testing due to transient reflux from inflammatory-mediated changes at the ureterovesical junction. However, most studies indicate reflux does not diminish in the interval and, in some settings, patients may be lost to follow-up so the earlier evaluation is more appropriate.
- The renal ultrasound can be done with the above studies or at the time of hospital admission if the patient appears toxic or is hypertensive or there is evidence of reduced renal function.
- A DMSA scan (if ordered to evaluate for renal scarring) should be done at least 6 months after the last acute UTI.

McDonald A, et al: Voiding cystourethrograms and urinary tract infections: How long to wait? Pediatrics 105:e50, 2000.

174. Is renal scarring a common occurrence in children with UTIs?

Renal scars are relatively uncommon (<10% in children less than age 2 years) when DMSA scanning is done 6 months following a UTI if a patient has a normal urinary tract and no bladder dysfunction. Children with recurrent UTIs and concomitant vesicoureteral reflux are at a higher risk for renal scarring. Approximately 40%–70% of children with grades II-IV reflux will have renal scarring at the time of their initial renal scan. Much recent emphasis has focused on the importance of congenital abnormalities (e.g., hypoplasia, dysplasia) rather than ongoing VUR as contributors to chronic scarring observed after UTIs in children. The potential for delayed appearance of renal scarring following normal initial studies remains controversial.

Hellerstein S: Long-term consequences of urinary tract infections. Curr Opin Pediatr 12:125-128, 2000.

Wennerstrom M, et al: Primary and acquired renal scarring in boys and girls with urinary tract infections. J Pediatr 136:30-34, 2000.

Wennerstrom M, et al: Renal function 16 to 26 years after the first urinary tract infection in children. Arch Pediatr Adolesc Med 154:339-345, 2000.

175. What factors increase the risk for permanent renal damage in children with UTIs?

- Younger age
- Obstruction
- Vesicoureteral reflux
- Recurrent infections
- Pyelonephritis
- Nephrolithasis
- Delay in diagnosis and initiation of therapy

176. Should children be screened for asymptomatic bacteriuria?

Although 1–2% of girls older than age 5 have persistent bacteriuria, mass screening at present is not recommended for the following reasons:

- In girls with radiologically demonstrable anatomic abnormalities (0.2–0.5%), most renal injury appears to occur before age 5 and may not progress.
- Older girls with asymptomatic bacteriuria and normal anatomy are unlikely to have sequelae if untreated.

Screening of infants and toddlers is technically more difficult, and the merits of screening are unclear. Infants and children at high risk should be considered for screening.

UROLITHIASIS

177. What is the composition of kidney stones in children?

Stone Composition	*North America (n = 340)*	*Europe (n = 315)*
Calcium	58%	37%
Struvite	25%	54%
Cystine	6%	3%
Uric acid/urate	9%	2%
Others	2%	4%

Modified from Polinsky MS, et al: Urolithiasis in childhood. Pediatr Clin North Am 34:683–710, 1987.

178. What disorders of childhood are known to cause calcium urolithiasis?

Normocalcemic hypercalciuria

Idiopathic hypercalciuria (absorptive, renal)
Distal renal tubular acidosis
Drug-induced (furosemide)

Hypercalcemic hypercalciuria

Immobilization
Idiopathic hypercalcemia of infancy
Hypervitaminosis D
Adrenocorticosteroid excess (Cushing syndrome, exogenous)
Primary hyperparathyroidism
Hyperthyroidism
Adrenal insufficiency
Milk-alkali syndrome

Hyperoxaluria

Enteric hyperoxaluria
Hereditary hyperoxaluria (types I and II)
Pyridoxine deficiency

Other causes

Idiopathic calcium urolithiasis
Hyperuricosuria
Hypocitraturia

179. Which disorders lead to the formation of urate stones?

- Leukemia, lymphoma
- Lesch-Nyhan syndrome
- Glycogen storage disease (type I)
- Polycythemia
- Chronic volume depletion

180. How is hypercalciuria defined in the infant and child?

The strict definition of hypercalciuria in a child is > 4 mg of urinary calcium/kg/24 hr on an unrestricted diet normal for age. Twenty-four hour urine collections can be difficult in young childen. Therefore, random urine collections have been used to *screen* for hypercalciuria. The urine ***calcium/creatinine ratio*** will vary with *age*. Morning non-fasting urine ratios that exceed the following correlate with quantitative hypercalciuria:

Patient age	*Calcium/creatinine ratio*
>7 years	>.24
5–7 years	>.30
3–5 years	>.41
1–2 years	>.56
< 1 year	>.81

181. What laboratory studies are appropriate in the initial evaluation of children with renal stones?

- Serum electrolytes, calcium, creatinine
- 24-hour urine collection for calcium, creatinine, magnesium, citrate, uric acid, oxalate, and cystine
- Urine pH (by meter), urinalysis, urine culture (if indicated)

182. How does manipulation of urine pH affect renal calculi?

Calcium oxalate stones, the most common type of renal calculi, are *unaffected* by the urine pH. These stones can be treated with thiazides diuretics, which increase renal calcium reabsorption, and thereby decrease the urinary calcium excretion. Potassium citrate can be added if the urinary citrate excretion is low. Do not restrict calcium intake uless it is excessively high. ***Calcium phosphate*** stones, which occur in distal renal tubular acidosis, respond to treatment with *alkali*. ***Uric acid*** stones form in acidic urine and also respond to *alkalinization* to a pH >6.5. Additional therapy includes a reduction in purine intake and occasionally the use allopurinol to block the formation of uric acid. High fluid intake plus urine alkalinization (pH > 7) helps to block the formation of ***cystine*** stones. Penicillamine may also be required in some of these patients. ***Struvite*** or infection stones form in extremely alkaline urine. Urine *acidification* along with antibiotics are the cornerstones of treatment for these stones.

183. When is lithotripsy or surgery indicated in children with kidney stones?

Most children with stones will spontaneously pass them. *Lithotripsy* is useful in children with large pelvic or bladder stones that are radiopaque in which fluoroscopy can be used to focus the shock waves. *Surgery* is generally reserved for children with stones causing urinary tract obstruction and for staghorn calculi that cannot be dissolved medically or fragmented by lithotripsy. Cystine stones are difficult to fragment by lithotripsy.

Cohen TD, et al: Pediatric urolithiasis: Medical and surgical management. Urology 47:292–303, 1996.

VESICOURETERAL REFLUX

184. How is vesicoureteral reflux (VUR) graded?

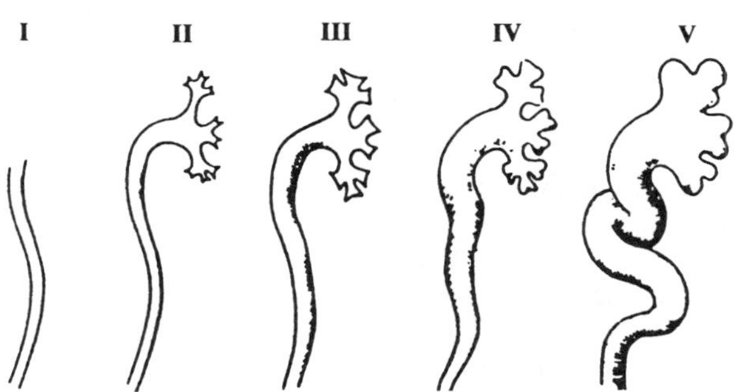

Grade I	Ureter only
Grade II	Ureter, pelvis, and calices; no dilation, normal caliceal fornices
Grade III	Mild dilation and/or tortuosity of the ureter and mild dilation of the renal pelvis; minor blunting of the fornices
Grade IV	Moderate dilation and/or tortuosity of the ureter and moderate dilation of the renal pelvis and calices; maintenance of the papillary impressions in most calices
Grade V	Significant blunting of most fornices; papillary impressions are no longer visible in most of the calices; gross dilation and tortuosity of the ureter; gross dilation of the renal pelvis and calices

From Duckett JD, Bellinger MF: A plea for standardized grading of vesicoureteral reflux. Eur Urol 8:74-77, 1982; with permission.

185. In addition to reflux, what other pathologic bladder findings may be noted on a voiding cystourethrogram?

Diverticula may be seen, especially in the presence of outflow obstruction. A ***posterior urethral valve*** or ***urethral stricture*** can be detected during the voiding phase of the study. A ***ureterocele*** may be seen and appears as a filling defect in the bladder. *Other features* to note are the bladder capacity, residual volume after voiding and thickening or trabeculation of the bladder from muscular hypertrophy.

186. What is normal bladder capacity in children?

Volume (in ounces) = *patient's age* (in years) + *2*. Normal adult bladder capacity is 12–16 oz.

187. Discuss the comparative features of a voiding cystourethrogram (VCUG) and a radionuclide cystogram (RNC) in the evaluation of reflux.

- Both studies require *catheterization* of the bladder and filling of the bladder with an imaging solution.
- The RNC allows *continuous* monitoring of the filling and emptying of the bladder versus the *intermittent* fluoroscopy which occurs with the VCUG.
- There is *less radiation exposure* with the RNC.
- The VCUG provides *greater anatomic detail* of the urethra and bladder and can aid in the evaluation of bladder dysfunction better than the RNC.
- The VCUG is *more accurate for assessing and grading* the degrees (I-V) of reflux.
- In general, the majority of authorities prefer the VCUG in the evaluation of a child with an initial UTI.

188. How does the radiation exposure differ between radionuclide cystography (RNC) and voiding cystourethrography (VCUG)?

RNC has approximately ***100 times less*** the absorbed radiation dose compared with a single x-ray VCUG. Many authorities do recommend its use for screening of siblings with reflux, evaluating the child with myelomeningocele, and for ongoing follow-up of significant reflux.

Conway JJ, Cohn RA: Evolving role of nuclear medicine for the diagnosis and management of urinary tract infection. J Pediatr 124:87–90, 1994.

189. What is the natural history of VUR?

The likelihood that reflux will resolve spontaneously is influenced by the severity of the reflux at the time of initial diagnosis. ***80-90%*** of patients with ***grade I-II reflux***, ***45%*** with ***grade III reflux*** and ***25%*** with ***grade IV reflux*** will experience spontaneous resolution *within 5 years*. Grade V reflux always requires surgical intervention. The chances for resolution are better in children with unilateral, rather than bilateral, reflux.

190. How is VUR managed: medically or surgically?

Grades I-II: Usually managed medically if the family is reliable and will comply with outpatient regimens and follow-up studies.

Grades III-IV: If followed expectantly, reflux will resolve slowly at a rate of approximately 10% per year. Surgical intervention results in elimination of this degree of reflux at least 95% of the time. Randomized studies have not shown any significant difference in long-term renal outcome (e.g., renal scarring, hypertension, reduced function) between medical vs. surgical treatment. The only major difference in outcome was a significantly lower frequency of recurrent pyelonephritis in those children managed surgically.

Grade V: Surgical intervention is indicated.

Jodal U, et al: Medical or surgical management for children with vesico-ureteric reflux? Acta Paediatrica 88S: 53-61, 1999.

Weiss R, et al: Results of a randomized clinical trial of medical versus surgical management of infants with grades III and IV primary vesioureteral reflux. J Urol 148:1667-1673, 1992.

191. What constitutes proper medical management of VUR?

- *Prophylactic night time antibiotics*. Duration of therapy is quite controversial. Some authorities recommend treatment until reflux subsides, while others stop antibiotics in boys who are free of infection for several years even if the reflux persists.
- *Surveillance urine cultures* every 2-3 months or more frequently if there are symptoms of a UTI.
- *Repeat VCUG* or *RNC* every 2 years to reevaluate VUR. A *renal ultrasound* is one biannually to evaluate renal growth. Imaging studies are continued until the reflux resolves.

192. When should a patient with vesicoureteral reflux be referred to a urologist or nephrologist?

- Recurrent UTIs despite adequate antibiotic prophylaxis
- Non-compliance with medical management
- Failure of reflux to resolve in a girl by the time of puberty
- Severity of reflux worsening over time
- History of a persistent voiding dysfunction
- Progressive renal scarring or deterioration in function of the scarred kidney as documented by renal scan

193. Should asymptomatic siblings of a patient with vesicoureteral reflux have urologic imaging done as a screen for reflux?

The incidence of reflux is thought to be <1% in normal children, but some studies have demonstrated reflux in 45% of siblings of patients with reflux. Among identical twins, the rate is 80%. Consequently, many authorities recommend screening siblings who are <7 years of age with a radionuclide cystogram. Siblings over the age of 7 who have a history of previous UTIs should also be screened for reflux.

Kaefer M, et al: Sibling vesicoureteral reflux in multiple gestation births. Pediatrics 105:800-804, 2000.

Kenda RB, Fettich JJ: Vesicoureteral reflux and renal scars in asymptomatic siblings of children with reflux. Arch Dis Child 67:506-508, 1992.

15. NEUROLOGY

Kent R. *Kelley*, M.D., *Douglas* R. *Nordli*, *Jr.*, M.D., *Peter Bingham*, M.D.,
and Robert R. *Clancy*, M.D.

ANTIEPILEPTIC DRUGS

1. Should treatment with antiepileptic drugs (AEDs) be started after the first seizure in a child?

Children with an isolated, uncomplicated seizure usually do *not* require antiepileptic drug therapy. Epidemiologic studies have shown that nearly 60% of children with an uncomplicated single seizure will not experience a second. "Delaying" treatment until after the second seizure does not adversely affect the long-term chance of epilepsy remission.

AEDs are not without risks and side effects, both dose-related and idiosyncratic.Other factors, including electroencephalogram (EEG) results, antecedent neurological history, family history, and imaging (in selective cases) influence the risk of recurrence and should be considered. Risk for recurrent seizures is sharply increased if the seizure was nocturnal, the neurologic status is not normal, there is a positive family history, if no immediate precipitating cause can be identified, and the EEG reveals epileptiform discharges.

Shinnar S, et al: The risk of seizure recurrence after a first unprovoked afebrile seizure in childhood: An extended follow-up. Pediatrics 98:216-225, 1996.

Shinnar S, Berg AT: Does antiepileptic drug therapy prevent the development of "chronic" epilepsy? Epilepsia 37:701-708, 1996.

2. Should therapy start with two agents if there are multiple seizure types?

Therapy should always begin with a **single** drug tailored to the epilepsy syndrome, even in children with more than one seizure type. Most approved antiepileptic medications are effective in treating localization-related or partial epilepsies. Some medications have broad spectra of action and are more useful than their counterparts in treating generalized epilepsies, particularly those with multiple types of seizures.

3. What are the disadvantages of polytherapy?

- Chronic toxicity is directly related to number of drugs consumed
- Compared with monotherapy, intellectual and sensorium impairment is increased for given AEDs (despite "normal" drug levels)
- Drug interactions may paradoxically lead to loss of seizure control
- Difficult to identify cause of an adverse reaction

Menkes JH, Sankar R: Paroxysmal disorders. In Menkes JH, Sarnat HB (eds): Child Neurology, 6th ed. Philadelphia, Lippincott, Williams & Wilkins, 2000, pp. 959-961.

4. What factors govern the selection of an AED for children with recurrent seizures?

A primary requirement for an AED is that it be effective for the child's seizure disorder. Once this is assured, studies in children have *not* shown statistically significant differences in the rates of seizure freedom between children randomized to carbamazepine, phenytoin, phenobarbital, and valproate. There also does not appear to be any correlation between type of medication and likelihood of remission. For these reasons, treatment selection will depend on a variety of other factors specific to the individual. These include, but are not limited to, the child's sensitivity to specific side effects, presence of other medical conditions, potential drug interactions, compliance issues, and cost of medications. By considering these factors, the medication can be matched to the patient for optimal results.

Pellock JM: Treatment of seizures and epilepsy in children and adolescents. Neurology 51(5 Suppl 4):S8-14, 1998.

5. How does the pharmacology of AEDs in children differ from adults?

Clearance rates may be several times faster than those of adults. When normalized for body weight, large dosages of phenobarbital and phenytoin are sometimes required in infants and young children. Phenytoin may be particularly difficult to regulate in infants because of the narrow margin between a therapeutic dose and a toxic one. Pharmacologic variations may contribute to suboptimal use of medications, particularly in younger children.

6. How should AEDs be adjusted in the setting of persistent seizures?

Single therapy is preferred, and the dosage of an individual AED should be gradually increased until the seizures come under control or disabling side effects present. If seizures persist and compliance is not a concern, then a second drug should be substituted. If trials of two reasonably selected drugs fail, the diagnosis should be reevaluated and consideration given to alternative forms of treatment, including surgery and the ketogenic diet. Alternatively, the patient can be prescribed two concurrent AEDs, but this is seldom satisfactory. Polypharmacy with three or more medications should always be resisted.

7. When should blood levels be obtained?

When seizures remain disabling or compliance is not assured, the physician should check ***trough*** serum drug levels to detect subtherapeutic or toxic concentrations. It is most helpful to check the serum level right before the dose, preferably in the morning before any medication is given. An inadequate serum concentration is the most common cause of persistent seizures, but drug toxicity, especially with phenytoin, may also manifest by deteriorating seizure control. There generally will be less variation in blood concentrations with tablets or capsules, rather than liquid preparations. Suspensions, in particular, result in notoriously inconsistent dosages.

Glauser TA, Pippenger CE: Controversies in blood-level monitoring: Reexamining its role in the treatment of epilepsy. Epilepsia 41:6-15, 2000.

8. Which AEDs are recommended for primary generalized tonic-clonic seizures in children?

The "traditional" AEDs (phenobarbital, primidone, phenytoin) are no longer considered the drugs of choice for grand mal seizures for many age groups, although ***phenobarbital*** remains the drug of choice for neonatal seizures. Studies have shown that most of the major anticonvulsants are comparable in reducing or eliminating seizure recurrences. However, because many children with seizures require treatment for years, the impact of chronic use of anticonvulsant drugs on the body and brain is a concern. For example, the long-term use of phenytoin may be associated with coarsened facial features, hirsutism, cerebellar atrophy, and gingival hyperplasia. Perhaps more importantly, there is a growing awareness of the neurologic side effects affecting behavior, mood, cognitive processing, memory, and attention provoked by phenobarbital and phenytoin. For these reasons, ***carbamazepine*** and ***valproate*** have emerged as the current drugs of choice for grand mal seizures.

9. What is the drug of choice for absence epilepsy?

Ethosuximide (Zarontin) and *valproate* (divalproex sodium or Depakote) are equally effective in eliminating or substantially reducing the number of absence attacks, but ethosuximide is currently the drug of choice for several reasons:

- It works well for many patients. It not only stops the clinical attacks of absence but it often normalizes the EEG by "erasing" the 3/second spike-wave discharges.
- It is well tolerated by most patients. Although rare cases of serious bone marrow, liver, or dermatologic disorders have occurred, routine or frequent blood tests are not considered obligatory by most physicians.
- It has a relatively long serum half-life (40 hrs). Thus, once or twice a day dosing is appropriate and represents a real convenience to the patient.
- It is relatively inexpensive.

Disadvantages are that ethosuximide only protects against absence seizures. Those children with coexisting generalized convulsions should be treated with valproate instead.

10. What is the first-line treatment choice for partial seizures?

Carbamazepine (Carbatrol, Tegretol) is frequently the drug of first choice for localization-related epilepsies (simple and complex partial seizures). *Oxcarbazepine* (Trileptal), a new keto-substituted analog, has a similar potency, but it has a lower incidence of side effects and may play a greater role in the treatment of children in the future.

11. What are the typical dose-related side effects of AEDs?

Dose-related side effects occur somewhat predictably and can be anticipated, particularly as the medication dose is initiated and escalated. Common dose-related side effects include: ***sedation, headache, gastrointestinal irritation, sedation, unsteadiness***, and ***dysarthria***. Management commonly consists of reducing the dose (by 25–50%) and waiting approximately 2 weeks for tolerance to develop. Behavioral and cognitive side effects can occur with some as well. These can be more subtle, and controversy exists regarding the relative effects of various AEDs.

American Academy of Pediatrics, Committee on Drugs: Behavioral and cognitive effects of anticonvulsant therapy. Pediatrics 96:538-540, 1995.

12. What idiosyncratic drug reactions are associated with antiepileptic medications?

Idiosyncratic reactions are potentially fatal, do not correlate with dose of medication, and occur unpredictably.

Carbamazepine—leukopenia, aplastic anemia, thrombocytopenia, hepatic dysfunction, rashes

Ethosuximide—leukopenia, pancytopenia, rashes

Phenobarbital—rashes, Stevens-Johnson syndrome, hepatic dysfunction

Phenytoin—hepatic dysfunction, lymphadenopathy, movement disorder, Stevens-Johnson syndrome, fulminant hepatic failure

Valproic acid—ulminant hepatic failure, hyperammonemia, pancreatitis, thrombocytopenia, rash, stupor

Freeman JM, Holmes GL: Should uncomplicated seizures be treated? Curr Probl Pediatr 24:143, 1994.

13. Which children are most susceptible to valproic acid–induced acute hepatic failure?

The highest incidences occur in ***children younger than 2 years receiving polytherapy*** (1 in 540). In children < 2 years receiving valproic acid monotherapy, the rate is reduced to about 1 in 8000. The complication is unrelated to dosage and typically occurs in the first 3 months of therapy. Up to 40% of individuals who receive valproic acid will have dose-related elevations of liver enzymes, which are transient or resolve with dosage adjustments. However, liver function test (LFT) monitoring is not helpful in prediciting acute hepatic failure.

Bryant AE, Dreifuss FE: Valproic acid hepatic fatalities. Neurology 48:465-469, 1996.

14. What can be done to minimize the potential of idiosyncratic reactions?

Routine surveillance of blood chemistries and complete blood counts (every 3–6 months) are standard practice but are unlikely to identify potentially life-threatening conditions. Symptoms often occur early, within the first months of treatment. Families need to be educated regarding the potential for drug reactions. Concerning symptoms include fever above 40ºC, protracted vomiting, lethargy, exfoliation of skin, mucosal (or palm or sole) lesions, facial edema, confluent erythema, skin pain, palpable purpura, protracted bleeding from minor cuts, lymph-node enlargment, and asthmatic symptoms. Multiple studies have shown that families fail to appreciate evolving symptoms of idiosyncratic reactions and continue to administer the offending agent.

Browne TR, Holmes GL: Epilepsy. N Engl J Med 344:1145-1151, 2001.

Stern RS: Improving the outcome of patients with toxic epidermal necrolysis and Stevens-Johnson syndrome. Arch Dermatol 136:410-411, 2000.

15. What are the suggested dosing guidelines and therapeutic ranges for AEDs?

Guidelines for Doses of Established Antiepileptic Drugs in Children

AED	TRADE NAME	STANDARD MAINTENANCE DOSE (RANGE) (mg/kg/day)	TARGET PLASMA DRUG CONCENTRATION (RANGE) (μg/ml)
Carbamazepine	Tegretol/Carbatrol	10–30	4–12
Ethosuxide	Zarontin	15–40	40–120
Gabapentin	Neurontin	30–45	5–15
Lamotrigine	Lamictal	1–5	2–20
Oxcarbazepine	Trileptal	20–40	5–50
Phenobarbital	Luminal	2–10	10–45
Phenytoin	Dilantin, Fosphenytoin	4–7	10–30
Tiagabine	Gabatril	1–2	5–70
Topiramate	Topamax	5–10	2–25
Valproate	Depakote	30–45	60–120
Zonisamide	Zonegran	4–12	10–40

Note that therapeutic ranges are somewhat arbitrary. Levels above "normal" may be maintained to control seizures if side effects do not occur. Conversely, levels in the therapeutic range may have toxic effects. It is important to treat the patient and not the number.

16. Which AEDs can be given rectally for acute management of seizures?

If intravenous or intraosseous routes are unavailable, options for rectal administration include:

Diazepam 0.5 mg/kg of parenteral solution for children 2–5 years, 0.3 mg/kg for children 6–11 years, and 0.2 mg/kg for patients 12 years and older.
Onset of action in 2–10 min and peak concentration in 5-45 min; bioavailability: 80–100%

Lorazepam 0.05–0.1 mg/kg of parenteral solution
Peak concentration in 30–120 min

Paraldehyde 0.3 ml/kg of oral solution diluted in equal volume of mineral oil
Effect in 20 min; peak concentration in 150 min
Glass syringe needed for administration (if plastic used, plunger may bond to syringe barrel)

Of note, numerous AEDs (e.g., carbamazepine, valproic acid) do not have parenteral formulations because of their poor water solubility. However, when an oral route is not feasible (e.g., due to acute gastritis) and seizures are uncontrolled, rectal administration may also be considered.

Kriel RL, et al: Rectal diazepam gel for the treatment of acute repetitive seizures. The North American Diastat Study Group. Pediatr Neurol 20:282-288, 1999.

Scott RC, et al: Buccal midazolam and rectal lorazepam for treatment of prolonged seizures in childhood and adolescence: A randomised trial. Lancet 353:623-626, 1999.

Dreifuss FE, et al: A comparison of rectal diazepam gel and placebo for acute repetitive seizures. N Engl J Med 338:1869-1875, 1998.

17. What is the possible role of intranasal midazolam in the treatment of seizures?

Midazolam is the first water-soluble benzodiazepine and has been shown to suppress epileptic activity and to improve the background of EEGs in patients with epilepsy. It has been demonstrated to be effective in control of seizures with and without fever. It may have a major future role by parents in the home treatment of children with recurrent febrile seizures. Intranasal midazolam (0.2 mg/kg) was equally as effective as intravenous diazepam (0.3 mg/kg) in controlling prolonged seizures with fever in children age 6 months to 5 years presenting to a hosptial setting.

Lahat E, et al: Comparison of intranasal midazolam with intravenous diazepam for treating febrile seizures in children: Prospective randomised study. BMJ 321:83-86, 2000.

Lahat E, et al: Intranasal midazolam for childhood seizures. Lancet 352:620, 1998.

18. After what period can AEDs be safely discontinued?

Withdrawal of antiepileptic drugs should be considered when the child is ***free of seizures for 2 years*** since well-controlled investigations have shown the risk of relapse in children whose seizures have been in remission for 2 years is low. Although there is no uniform agreement on factors predictive of outcome, the highest remission rate appears to occur in those who are otherwise neurologically normal and in whom the EEG at the time of discontinuation lacks specific epileptiform features and displays a normal background. Prognosis is worst for children with symptomatic epilepsies, persistently abnormal EEGs, and abnormal neurologic examinations.

Greenwood RS, Tennison MB: When to start and stop anticonvulsant therapy in children. Neurology 56:1073-1077, 1999.

19. When the decision is made to discontinue AEDs, should the taper period be long or short?

In practice, all AEDs should be tapered gradually rather than abruptly discontinued, even though there is no actual withdrawal state produced by a "cold turkey" reduction of most AEDs (phenytoin, carbamazepine, valproate, ethosuximide). In contrast, a withdrawal syndrome of agitation, signs of autonomic overactivity, and seizures follow the sudden elimination of habitually consumed diazepam or short-acting barbiturates (such as secobarbital). The long elimination half-life of phenobarbital lessens the risk of withdrawal symptoms following abrupt discontinuation.

In a study of over 100 children who had been seizure-free for either 2 or 4 years, the risk of seizure recurrence during tapering and after discontinuation of the AED was no different if the period of taper was 6 weeks or 9 months. Rapid tapering appears to be an acceptable means of discontinuation.

Tennison M, et al: Discontinuing antiepileptic drugs in children with epilepsy: A comparison of a six-week and a nine-month taper period. N Engl J Med 330:1407–1410, 1994.

CEREBRAL PALSY

20. How is cerebral palsy defined?

Cerebral palsy describes a heterogenous group of static motor and posture disorders of cerebral or cerebellar origin that typically manifest early in life. Note that the definition does not imply etiology. Causes include cerebral malformations, infection (both intrauterine and extrauterine), stroke, hypoxic-ischemic encephalopathy, and trauma. The process is nonprogressive and the motor function affected involves the part of the brain that is involved. Although nonprogressive, clinical manifestations often change over time as the expression of the underlying brain is modified by normal brain development and maturation.

21. What are the types of cerebral palsy?

Clinical classification is based on the nature of the movement disorder, muscle tone, and anatomic distribution. A single patient may have more than one type. Spastic cerebral is the most common, accounting for about two-thirds of cases.

- ***Pyramidal (or spastic) CP***: characterized by neurologic signs of upper motor neuron damage with increased "clasp knife" muscle tone, increased deep tendon reflexes, pathologic reflexes, and spastic weakness. Spastic CP is subclassified based on distribution:
  Hemiparesis—primarily unilateral involvement, arm usually more than leg
  Quadriparesis—all limbs involved, with legs often more involved than arms
  Diparesis—legs much more involved than arms, which may show no or only minimal impairment
- ***Extrapyramidal*** (nonspastic or dyskinetic) **CP**: characterized by prominent involuntary movements or fluctuating muscle tone with choreoathetosis the most common subtype. Distribution is usually symmetric among the four limbs.
- ***Hypotonic CP***: Generalized muscle hypotonia that persists with normal or increased deep tendon reflexes. Many develop cerebellar deficits of incoordination and ataxia. About one-third of patients have severe retardation
- ***Ataxic CP***: primarily cerebellar signs
- ***Mixed types***

22. What proportion of cerebral palsy is related to birth asphyxia?

Contrary to popular perception, large clinical epidemiologic and longitudinal studies indicate that perinatal asphyxia is an important, but relatively minor, cause. Estimates range from a low of 3% to a high of 21%. In most cases, the events leading to cerebral palsy occur in the fetus before the onset of labor or in the newborn after delivery.

MacLennan A: The International Cerebral Palsy Task Force: A template for defining a causal relationship between acute intrapartum events and cerebral palsy: International concensus statement. BMJ 319:1054-1059, 1999.

Nelson KB, Grether JK: Causes of cerebral palsy. Curr Opin Pediatr 11:487-491, 1999.

23. Why is CP difficult to diagnose clinically in the first year of life?

- Hypotonia is more common than hypertonia and spasticity in the first year, making prediction of CP difficult.
- Early abundance of primitive reflexes (with variable persistence) may confuse clinical picture.
- Infant has a limited variety of volitional movements for evaluation.
- Substantial myelination takes months to evolve and may delay the clinical picture of abnormal tone and increased deep tendon reflexes.
- Most infants who develop CP do not have identifiable risk factors. Most cases are not related to labor and delivery events.

Shapiro BK, Capute AJ: Cerebral palsy. In McMillan JA, et al (eds): Oski's Pediatrics, Principles and Practice, 3rd ed. Philadelphia, Lippincott, Williams & Wilkins, 1999, pp. 1910-1917.

24. What behavioral symptoms in the first year should arouse suspicion for the possibility of CP?

- Excessive irritability, constant crying, and sleeping difficulties. Severe colic is noted in up to 30% of babies eventually diagnosed with CP.

- Early feeding difficulties with difficulties in coordinating suck and swallow, frequent spitting up, and poor weight gain
- "Jittery" or "jumpy" behavior, especially at times other than when hungry
- Easily startled behavior
- Stiffness when handled, especially during dressing, diapering, and handwashing.
- Paradoxically "precocious" development, such as early rolling (acually a sudden, reflexive roll rather than a volitional one) or the stiff-legged "standing" with support of an infant with spastic diplegia.

Bennett FC: Diagnosing cerebral palsy—the earlier the better. Contemp Pediatr 16:67, 1999.

25. What gross motor delays are diagnostically important in the infant with possible CP?

- Inability to bring the hands together in midline while in a supine position by age 4 months
- Head lag persisting beyond 6 months
- No volitional rolling by 6 months
- Inability to independently sit straight by 8 months
- No hands-and-knees crawling by 12 months

Bennett FC: Diagnosing cerebral palsy—the earlier the better. Contemp Pediatr 16:68, 1999.

26. How well do Apgar scores correlate with the development of CP?

In a large study of 49,000 infants, a low Apgar score correlated poorly with the development of CP. Of term infants with scores of 0–3 at 1 or 5 minutes, 95% did not develop CP. Of those with scores of 0–3 at 10 minutes, 84% did not develop CP. If the 10-minute Apgar improved to 4 or more, the rate for CP was < 1%. A low Apgar score (0–3) at 20 minutes, however, had an observed CP rate of nearly 60%. Conversely, nearly 75% of patients with CP had 5-minute Apgar scores of 7–10.

Nelson KB, Ellenberg JH: Apgar scores as predictors of chronic neurologic disability. Pediatrics 68:36–44, 1981.

27. What problems are commonly associated with cerebral palsy?

- ***Mental retardation***: two-thirds of total patients; most commonly observed in children with spastic quadriplegia
- ***Learning disabilities***
- ***Ophthalmologic abnormalities*** (strabismus, amblyopia, nystagmus, refractive errors)
- ***Hearing deficits***
- ***Communication disorders***
- ***Seizures***: one-third of total patients; most commonly observed in children with spastic hemiplegia
- ***Failure to thrive***
- ***Feeding problems***
- ***Gastroesophageal reflux***
- ***Behavioral and emotional problems*** (especially attention deficit hyperactivity disorder, depression)

Eicher PS, Batshaw ML: Cerebral palsy. Pediatric Clin North Am 40:537–551, 1993.

28. What features in an infant suggest a progressive central nervous system (CNS) disorder rather than CP as the cause of a motor deficit?

- Abnormally increasing head circumference (possible hydrocephalus, tumor)
- Eye anomalies such as cataracts, retinal pigmentary degeneration, optic atrophy (possible neurodegenerative disease)
- Skin abnormalities such as vitiligo, café-au-lait spots, nevus flammeus (possible Sturge-Weber disease, neurofibromatosis)

- Hepatomegaly and/or splenomegaly (possible storage disease)
- Decreased or absent deep tendon reflexes
- Sensory abnormalities (loss of diminished sense of pain, position, vibration, or light touch)

Taft LT: Cerebral palsy. Pediatr Rev 6:41, 1984.

29. How effective is selective dorsal rhizotomy in the treatment of spasticity in CP?

Selective dorsal rhizotomy involves the cutting of lumbar spinal laminae and dura, isolating the dorsal nerve roots, and cutting selected fibers. Studies have shown benefits in reducing spasticity and improving range of motion, but the precise effects of the surgery are difficult to predict. Questions remain about which patients will benefit, which fibers should be cut, and what the long-term complications of lumbar laminotomy are.

Gul SM, et al: Long-term outcome after selective posterior rhizotomy in children with spastic cerebral palsy. Pediatr Neurosurg 31:84-95, 1999.

CEREBROSPINAL FLUID DYNAMICS

30. What is normal cerebrospinal fluid (CSF) pressure?

CSF pressure, as measured during a lumbar puncture, varies with age, positional technique, and combativeness of the patient. Normal CSF opening pressure, as measured with the patient in the **recumbent lateral** position, is up to 50 mm H_2O in neonates, up to 85–110 mm H_2O in young infants, and up to 150 mm H_2O in older children. As measured with the patient in the **flexed lateral** position, CSF pressure is higher, ranging from 100–280 mm H_2O in children. With the patient in the **sitting** position, average pressures are even higher.

Bonadio WA: The cerebrospinal fluid: Physiologic aspects and alterations associated with bacterial meningitis. Pediatr Infect Dis J 11:423–432, 1992.

Ellis RW: Lumbar cerebrospinal fluid opening pressure measured in a flexed lateral decubitus position in children. Pediatrics 93:622–623, 1994.

31. What is the normal CSF volume in an infant, child, and adolescent?

Estimates for the volume of the ventricular system are 40–50 ml in a term newborn, increasing to 65–100 ml for an older child, and 90–150 ml for a teenager and adult. The choroid plexus actively secretes a distillate of CSF at a rate of 0.3–0.4 ml/min in children and adults, which equals about 20 ml/hour or 500 ml/day. This equates to an hourly CSF volume turnover rate of approximately 15%.

32. What are the common causes of an elevated CSF protein?

Elevated CSF protein is a nonspecific finding encountered in various neurologic disorders. Several common etiologies should be considered.

- **Infection:** tuberculous meningitis, acute bacterial meningitis (pneumococcal, meningococcal, *Haemophilus influenzae*), syphilitic or viral meningitis, or encephalitis
- **Inflammation:** Guillain-Barré syndrome, multiple sclerosis, peripheral neuropathy, or postinfectious encephalopathy
- **Tumor** of the cerebral hemispheres or spinal cord
- **Vascular accidents**, such as cerebral hemorrhage (including subarachnoid hemorrhage, subdural hemorrhage, intracerebral hemorrhages) or stroke due to cranial arteritis, diabetes mellitus, or hypertension
- **Degenerative disorders** involving white matter disease (e.g., Krabbe disease).
- **Metabolic disorders** such as uremia
- **Toxins** such as lead

33. As tests of meningeal irritation, what constitutes a positive Kernig sign or Brudzinski sign?

Kernig sign or the straight-leg-raising sign: It consists of flexing the hip to 90° and attempting to extend the knee. Limitation of knee extension due to painful resistance is a positive sign.

Brudzinski sign: A positive sign is present if a reflex flexion of thighs occurs when a patient's neck is passively flexed.

34. What are the physical signs of meningeal irritation in the neonate?

In neonates, the physical signs of meningeal irritation may be overshadowed by systemic dysfunction, such as poor feeding, respiratory distress, or jaundice. Perhaps this is because meningitis commonly follows seeding of the meninges by systemic sepsis. Only a few patients present predominantly with frank neurologic signs, such as coma, seizures, or abnormal posture. Pure nuchal rigidity is rare in the newborn. More commonly, there is widespread increase of extensor tone in the neck, trunk, and limb musculature. Meningismus is not seen in every patient of any age, even with advanced purulent meningitis, and should not be considered a *sine qua non* for the diagnosis.

35. How does meningismus differ from meningism?

The term *meningismus* has various meanings. It is most commonly used to refer to the signs and symptoms of meningeal irritation associated with meningitis (abnormal CSF profile), including headache, nuchal rigidity, and positive Kernig and Brudzinski signs. Some also use this term to describe headache or stiff neck seen without meningitis, as in intracranial hypertension.

Meningism was commonly used in the older medical literature to denote the sudden onset of headache and mild meningeal signs without meningitis in the setting of an acute febrile illness. These symptoms can occur in the setting of acute systemic viral or bacterial infections, such as streptococcal pharyngitis or roseola infantum. The CSF profile is normal except for mildly increased CSF pressure.

36. How do the manifestations of increased intracranial pressure differ in an infant compared to an older child?

Infant—increasing head cirumference, delayed closure of the fontanel, suture separation, bulging fontanel, failure to thrive, macrocephaly, setting sun sign, shrill cry

Older child—headache (especially in the early morning, awakening the child from sleep or association with vomiting), nausea, persistent vomiting, personality/mood changes, lethargy, anorexia, fatigue, somnolence, diplopia secondary to sixth nerve palsy or third nerve palsy with uncal herniation, papilledema

37. What comprises the Cushing triad?

Cushing triad consists of the development of ***slow*** or ***irregular respirations, decreased heart rate***, and ***elevated blood pressure*** (particularly an increased systolic pressure with a widening pulse pressure) resulting from an increase in intracranial pressure (ICP). Cushing triad may be observed in children with increased ICP or compression of the posterior fossa, which houses the medullary circulatory control center. It is a very late finding of increased ICP.

38. How is hydrocephalus classified?

Dandy and Blackfan developed the clinically useful concept of ***communicating*** and ***noncommunicating*** hydrocephalus to describe the flow of CSF. Communicating hydrocephalus was present if a tracer dye injected into one lateral ventricle appeared in the lumbar CSF. This type of hydrocephalus is due to an inability to normally reabsorb CSF by the arachnoid granulations, which can occur from meningeal scarring due to bacterial meningitis or intraventricular hemorrhage.

Noncommunicating hydrocephalus was used to describe conditions causing intraventricular obstruction and alteration of the flow of dye into the lumbar CSF. Congenital malformations (especially aqueductal stenosis, Dandy-Walker syndrome with cystic dilatation of the fourth ventricle), and mass lesions (e.g., tumors, arteriovenous malformations) can cause noncommunicating hydrocephalus. ***Hydrocephalus ex vacuo*** describes increases in volume without increased CSF pressure, which is seen in conditions of reduced cerebral tissue as in malformation or atrophy.

39. What is the normal growth rate of head circumference in the first year of life?

Head circumference at birth is about 34 cm for the term infant. The head circumference normally grows by 2 cm/month for the first 3 months of life, 1 cm/month for months 4–6, and 0.5 cm/month up to a year of life. Measurement of head circumference should be part of the examination of any child and should be plotted at every visit. The head circumference represents brain growth, but also is influenced by hydrocephalus and subdural or epidural fluid collections.

40. What are the complications of ventricular shunts?

Ventricular shunts drain CSF from the ventricles in patients whose normal outflow or absorption has been blocked. The fluid may be drained to a variety of different locations including the peritoneum, the kidney, or the atrium. Shunts draining CSF have remarkably improved the outcome of children with hydrocephalus, but they are subject to ***obstruction, infection***, or ***mechanical malfunction***. Shunt malfunctions present with signs of increased ICP. Children with shunt infections often have a low-grade fever as well as signs of increased ICP. Because it is impossible to know the compliance properties of the ventricular system, children with shunt malfunction or infection are at risk for sudden, catastrophic decompensation. Children suspected of having shunt malfunctions or infection require urgent attention, and they should be closely observed until the shunt has been fully evaluated.

41. What are the characteristic features of pseudotumor cerebri?

Pseudotumor cerebri consists of an increased ICP in the absence of a demonstrable mass lesion and with a normal CSF formula. Characteristic features include:

- Headache, fatigue, vomiting, anorexia, stiff neck, and diplopia from increased ICP
- Normal neurologic examination except for papilledema or a third or sixth nerve palsy
- Normal computed tomography (CT) scan except sometimes for small ventricles
- Normal CSF profile with the exception of an elevated opening pressure

42. What causes pseudotumor cerebri?

Although there are multiple possible causes, over 90% of cases are idiopathic. Among the reported causes are:

- **Drugs**: tetracycline, nalidixic acid, nitrofurantoin, corticosteroids, excess vitamin A
- **Endocrine disorders**: hyperthyroidism, Cushing's syndrome, hypoparathyroidism
- **Thrombosis** of the dural venous sinuses due to head trauma, otitis media, mastoiditis, or obstruction of jugular veins in the superior vena cava syndrome

43. What morbidity is associated with pseudotumor cerebri?

Visual loss. All patients with this disorder should have periodic formal testing of visual fields. Patients with well-developed papilledema may complain of fleeting visual loss (obscurations) that may be accentuated by the Valsalva maneuver or by standing up. This sign is believed to represent reduction of optic nerve blood flow due to arterial compression. Visual obscurations do not necessarily imply imminent "stroke" of the optic nerves.

44. What treatment is recommended for severe cases of pseudotumor cerebri?

Patients with sustained visual field loss or severe refractory headache are candidates for treatment. Specific treatment depends on the presence of an identifiable precipitant, which should be removed when possible. For example, the cessation of the offending medication, such as tetracycline, or weight reduction in obese patients is recommended. Nonspecific treatment includes the administration of acetazolamide, furosemide, or hydrochlorothiazide and sometimes corticosteroids. In severe cases, surgical intervention is available in the form of the installation of a lumboperitoneal shunt or optic nerve sheath decompression.

45. Can anything be done to minimize the chance of a post–lumbar puncture headache?

- Avoid a head-up posture during the procedure
- Use the smallest possible needle (22 gauge or smaller) and advance the bevel "up" with the patient in the decubitus position

There is debate over whether maintenance of a prone position several hours following the procedure can prevent the headache.

46. Why may it be dangerous to do a lumbar puncture using a needle with the stylette removed?

The (unproven) theory is that the stylette may prevent nerve roots of the cauda equina from becoming entrapped in the needle and may cause less disruption of the dural sac. Another concern is that, without the stylette, skin cells may enter the core of the needle, where they can be introduced into the subarachnoid space and form an epidermoid tumor.

CLINICAL ISSUES

47. What distinguishes the pediatric neurologic examination?

The pediatric neurologic examination relies more on **observation** than confrontation. The most useful information is often acquired by watching the child play. The level of interaction, creativity, and degree of sustained attention can be observed and are all important components of the mental status examination. By observing eye movements, response to sounds, the child's reaction to visual stimuli introduced into the peripheral visual field, and the symmetry of facial movements, most of the cranial nerves can be tested. Persistent asymmetries of spontaneous motor activity, such as consistently reaching across midline for an object, are reliable signs of weakness. Inspection of the seated posture and gait of the child provides an assessment of the cerebellum and cerebellar outflow pathways.

48. What are the advantages and disadvantages of various imaging procedures used in pediatric neurologic evalulation?

Skull films are useful for detection of fractures, lytic lesions, and widened sutures. They have poor sensivitiy and specificity for intracranial pathology in the setting of trauma

CT scan without constrast is the best imaging technique for neurological emergencies to screen a patient with significant head trauma for skull fractures, signs of herniation, or acute intracranial hemorrhage. It can also be used to screen for acute strokes and subarachnoid hemorrhages. Midline or ventricular shifts due to masses and cerebral edema or increased ICP can be noted. It identifies bone clearly. This rapid study allows routine monitoring and is less expensive than MRI. There is a small but defined risk of radiation from CT scans.

CT scan with contrast uses radiodense contrast material to allow better identification of disruptions in the blood-brain barrier or of highly vascular structures, significantly improving detection of tumors, edema, focal inflammation, hemangiomas, and arteriovenous malformations.

Magnetic resonance imaging (MRI) without contrast is the preferred modality for most nonurgent examinations. It defines structures of brain more precisely than CT, especially within spinal cord, posterior fossa, and cisterns. It is more effective for subtle hemorrhages (especially subacute and chronic) and for tumors or masses. Different tissue-specific relaxation constants, called T1 and T2, and proton density allow for better definition of white and gray matter. It also provides an image in three dimensions. MRI is unreliable for fractures, and the longer testing time may require sedation. Also, monitoring patients is more difficult in closed units. There are no known biologic hazards from MRI, which measures the emission of radiowaves released when protons return to a lower energy state after excitation within characteristic tissue environments. MRI is contraindicated in patients with metallic implants that are ferromagnetic.

MRI with contrast is helpful in defining brain metastases and distinguishing postoperative scarring from other pathology.

Magnetic resonance angiography (MRA) is a special type of MRI that displays larger arteries and veins without the use of contrast. It is less invasive than traditional arteriograms, and it is useful in defining arterial stenosis and identifying intracranial hemangiomas, arteriovenous malformations, and vascular aneurysms.

MR spectroscopy (MRS) allows for in vivo examination of some chemical constituents of the brain including choline (NAA), a neuronal marker, and lactate (a marker of energy metabolism).

Functional MR scanning (fMRI) allows for in vivo anatomic localization of the motor strip and components of expressive and receptive language.

Altemeier WA III, et al: Imaging procedures in pediatric neurological conditions. Pediatr Ann 27:607-609, 1998.

49. A child presents with progressive left leg weakness and diplopia, especially when looking toward the left. Where is the lesion?

The above history, when combined with an examination showing upper motor neuron nerve dysfunction, long tract signs, brisk reflexes, up-going toe (Babinski sign), and a contralateral third nerve palsy (down and out), localizes the lesion to the ***right pyramidal tract before the decussation*** (crossing over) and ***involves a lesion of the right third nerve nucleus***. The progressive course suggests a slow growing lesion, such as a pontine glioma.

50. A dilated and unreactive pupil indicates compression of what structure?

The ***third cranial nerve***. This may be the result of compression anywhere along the course of the nerve. Uncal herniation is a medial displacement of the uncus of the temporal lobe and may cause this sign.

51. Pinpoint pupils and respiratory changes indicate compression of what structure?

Progressive central herniation of the brain downward through the foramen magnum causes compression of the ***pons*** and can produce this finding.

52. How does the presentation of stroke differ between infants and older children?

Infants present usually with a **seizure**, whereas older children present with ***acute hemiplegia***.

53. What is the differential diagnosis of stroke in children?

Cerebrovascular disease, or stroke, can be due to primary vascular disease, bleeding disorder (hemorrhagic stroke), or a variety of secondary problems that lead to thrombotic or embolic occlusions (most commonly the middle cerebral artery). Diagnostic possibilities include:

Cardioembolic: cyanotic congenital heart disease, atrial myxoma, endocarditis, rheumatic or other valvular heart disease

Hematologic: hemoglobinopathies (especially sickle cell disease), hypercoagulable states (antithrombin III deficiency, protein C or S deficiency), hyperviscosity (leukemia, hyperproteinemia, thrombocytosis), coagulation disorders (lupus-associated antibodies, hemophilia, thrombocytopenia, factor V abnormalities, hyperhomocysteinemia)

Circulatory: vasculitis (infectious or inflammatory), occlusive (homocystinuria, arteriosclerosis, fibromuscular dysplasia of the internal carotid artery, post-traumatic carotid scarring), carotid or vertebral artery dissection, moyamoya disease, atrioventricular malformation with steal syndrome, anomalous circulation, post-traumatic air embolism, arterial aneurysm, hemiplegic migraine

Metabolic: mitochondrial disease

54. What is the derivation of "moyamoya" in moyamoya disease?

Moyamoya, Japanese for "puff of smoke," refers to the ***cerebral angiographic appearance*** in patients with this primary vascular disease that results in stenosis of the internal carotid artery. It also occurs in a wide variety of conditions, such as neurofibromatosis type 1, sickle cell disease, Down syndrome, and tuberous sclerosis, in addition to the idiopathic condition that is endemic in Japan. Because it is a chronic condition, fine vascular collaterals can develop, and it is these collaterals that create the "puff of smoke" appearance on angiography.

55. What clinical findings are seen in cavernous sinus thrombosis?

Within the confined space of the cavernous sinus lie all three cranial nerves that move the eye (oculomotor, trochlear, and abducent nerves) and the upper two divisions of the trigeminal nerve (ophthalmic V_1 and maxillary V_2). The venous drainage of the orbit exits via the cavernous sinus. Thus, orbital infections quickly spread to these contiguous venous structures and result in an acute thrombophlebitis. Thrombosis of the venous channels of the cavernous sinus results in desperate systemic illness with fulminant constitutional signs such as fever, headache, prostration, and local signs of proptosis, prominent redness, edema of the eyelid and bulbar conjunctiva (chemosis), visual loss, papilledema, ophthalmoplegia (due to dysfunction of cranial nerves III, IV, and VI) and paresthesias, numbness, or local pain in the distribution of V_1.

56. What is the most likely diagnosis of a neonate with macrocephaly, high output heart failure, and a cranial flow murmur?

A ***vein of Galen malformation*** presents with high output cardiac failure, a cranial flow murmur, and increasing head size. This is an enlarged developmental malformation of the normal vein that limits the egress of CSF. Management includes treatment of the high output heart failure and neurosurgical and interventional radiologic repair.

57. A child who develops weakness, incontinence, and ataxia 10 days after a bout of influenza likely has what diagnosis?

Acute disseminated encephalomyelitis (ADEM) is thought to be a post- or parainfectious process targeted against central myelin. Any portion of the white matter may be affected. Multiple lesions with a perivenular lymphocytic and mononuclear cell infiltration and demyelination are seen on pathologic examination. ADEM has been associated with mumps, measles, rubella, varicella-zoster, influenza, parainfluenza, mononucleosis, and immunization. An associated transverse myelitis may be acute, developing over hours, or subacute over 1–2 weeks with both motor and sensory tract involvement. Bladder and bowel dysfunction is often early and severe. CSF examination shows mild increase of pressure and up to 250 cells/mm^3 with a lymphocyte predominance. The MRI shows an increased T2 signal intensity. Prognosis, particularly with the use of intravenous corticosteroids, is good.

58. What are the two most common types of primary brain lesions noted on MRI in the setting of head trauma?

1. ***Diffuse axonal injury*** occurs by acceleration-deceleration injury resulting in shearing or stretching of axons, especially in the brain stem or corpus callosum. On MRI, the lesions appear as small, oval, focal abnormalities in white matter tracts. In this type of injury, loss of consciousness is common, but skull fractures, increased ICP, and contusions are not.

2. ***Cortical contusion*** refers to visible injury to the brain resulting in petechial hemorrhages or more extensive hemorrhage. Contusions or lacerations are most often found in the frontal or temporal poles, where the brain may come into contact with bony structures, or in a contrecoup concussion opposite to the point of impact.

59. In acute injury to the brain, what two types of edema may occur?

1. ***Vasogenic edema*** results from increased permeability of the capillary endothelium with resulting exudation. It is more marked in cerebral white matter and is secondary to inflammation (meningitis and abscess), focal processes (hemorrhage, infarct or tumor), or vessel pathology, lead and hypertensive encephalopathy.

2. ***Cytotoxic edema*** results from rapid swelling of cells, especially astrocytes, but also neurons and endothelial cells secondary to dysfunction of the membranes and ionic pumps from energy failure, which may lead to cellular death. Hypoxia secondary to cardiac arrest, hypoxic-ischemic encephalopathy (HIE), various toxins, severe infections, status epilepticus, infarct, and increased ICP are also possible causes.

60. What are the treatments for increased intracranial pressure?

One acute but temporary measure is ***hyperventilation*** of the patient. The usual goal is to lower the pCO_2 to 25–30 mm. This causes vasoconstriction, which decreases the intracranial vascular volume. ***Fluid restriction, osmotic diuretics***, and ***hypertonic mannitol*** solution all work to shrink brain water content, provided there is an intact blood-brain barrier. Maintaining the head in a midline position with elevation to 30(maximizes venous return. External ventricular drains are sometimes placed, both to monitor pressure and to allow a minimal amount of CSF withdrawal. General supportive care with normalization of physiologic parameters is critical. It is important to avoid significant hypotension, hypoxia, hypoglycemia, and hyperthermia.

61. What are the acceptable clinical criteria for pronouncing a patient brain dead?

Brain death is defined by an irreversible absence of cortical and midbrain activity. There must be an absence of a reversible etiology (i.e., toxic-metabolic, medication, hypothermia, hypotension, or surgically remediable causes). Spinal cord, peripheral nerve, or reflex muscular activity may persist despite brain death. Decorticate or decerebrate posturing, however, is inconsistent with brain death. The examination must remain unchanged over the time. Other countries have defined brain death by absence of brain stem function alone, but in the United States, absence of cortical function also must be demonstrated. The clinical hallmark of brain death is deep, unremitting, unresponsive coma. Patients with suspected brain death should be observed over 12–24 hours for:

- Unresponsive coma and absence of eye opening, extraocular movements, vocalizations, or other cerebral-generated activity.
- Complete absence of brain stem function including nonresponsive, midposition, or fully dilated pupils, no spontaneous or reflexive eye movements on oculovestibular testing ("doll's eyes" and calorics), no bulbar muscle function (i.e., corneal, gag, cough, sucking, and rooting reflexes), and no respirations on apnea testing.
- Supportive testing, if needed, to document brain death can include absent cerebral cortical activity as evidenced by a properly recorded "flat," "isoelectric," or electrocere-

bral silence (EEG), the absence of blood flow to the hemispheres by cerebral arteriography or radionuclide study, or the presence of ICP that exceeds mean blood pressure for several hours.

The most difficult patients in whom to diagnose brain death are the neonate and infants < 2 months of age. For this age group, more stringent criteria are recommended:

1. The diagnosis of brain death should be deferred until the infant is at least 1 week old.
2. The patient should be observed in the "brain dead state" for at least 48 hours before the declaration of brain death and the termination of life support.

Wijdicks EFM: The diagnosis of brain death. N Engl J Med 344:1215-1221, 2001.

Task Force on Brain Death in Children: Guidelines for the determination of brain death in children. Pediatrics 80:298, 1987.

62. What other supportive testing is recommended in the evaluation for brain death?

- ***EEG***, performed in accordance with a standardized protocol, to document ECS. Because hypotension, hypothermia (32.2°C for adults), and medications, including a phenobarbital level > 25 μg/ml, may suppress the EEG, the patient must have a stable temperature, blood pressure, and appropriate metabolic and toxicology testing and drug levels.
- ***Four-vessel arteriography*** or radionuclide study to document absence of blood flow to the hemispheres.

Other tests that may help to confirm the diagnosis of brain death include ***transcranial Doppler***, which also may demonstrate an absence of intracranial blood flow, and ***somatosensory-evoked potentials*** (SSEPs) to demonstrate bilateral absence of cortical responses to stimulation of the median nerve.

63. How do the criteria for the determination of brain death vary by age?

The Task Force on Brain Death in Children recommends no determination of brain death be made in neonates younger than 7 days. In infants 7 days to 2 months of age, two examinations and EEGs separated by at least 48 hours are recommended. In infants 2 months to 1 year of age, two examinations and EEGs separated by at least 24 hours are recommended. A repeat examination and EEG are not required if cerebral blood flow study shows absence of flow. In children older than 1 year, if the etiology is irreversible, laboratory testing is not required, and a 12-hour period of observation is recommended. If there is a potentially reversible condition (e.g., HIE), then at least a 24-hour period of observation is recommended.

Task Force on Brain Death in Children: Guidelines for the determination of brain death in children. Pediatrics 80:298, 1987.

64. What CSF findings suggest metabolic disease as a cause of neurologic symptoms and signs?

An ***elevated CSF protein concentration*** is characteristic of metachromatic leukodystrophy and globoid-cell encephalopathy. A ***low CSF glucose concentration*** is consistent with hypoglycemia caused by a defect of gluconeogenesis or a defect in the transport of glucose across the blood-brain barrier (GLUT-1 deficiency syndrome). A ***low CSF folate concentration*** suggests a defect involving folate metabolism. The ***presence in CSF of amino acids, specifically glycine, glutamate, and gamma aminobutyric acid (GABA)*** may be diagnostic of nonketotic hyperglycinemia, pyridoxine-dependent epilepsy, or another defect in the GABA shunt. ***Lactate*** and ***pyruvate*** values are elevated in CSF disorders of cerebral energy metabolism, including pyruvate dehydrogenase deficiency, pyruvate carboxylase deficiency, numerous disturbances of the respiratory chain, and Menkes' syndrome. A ***low CSF lactate*** value may be seen in the GLUT-1 deficiency syndrome. ***Abnormal CSF biogenic amines*** suggest several disorders associated with disturbed neurotransmission.

65. What is the differential diagnosis of an intracranial bruit?

An intracranial bruit can be found in normal children. Disorders that may be associated with an intracranial bruit include:

- Fever
- Thyrotoxicosis
- Anemia
- Cardiac murmurs
- Cerebral angioma
- Cerebral aneurysm
- Cerebral arteriovenous malformations
- Intracerebral tumors
- Any cause of increased ICP
- Meningitis

Mace JW, et al: Cranial bruits in purulent meningitis in children. N Engl J Med 278:1420, 1968.

66. In a previously normal child who develops acute ataxia, what are the two most common diagnoses?

- ***Drug ingestion***, especially antiepileptic drugs and antihistamines
- ***Acute postinfectious cerebellitis***, most commonly following varicella. This is a diagnosis of exclusion if a drug screen, CT or MRI, CSF evaluation, and other testing is negative.

67. What are the causes of acute cerebellar ataxia?

An acute ataxia implicates dysfunction of the cerebellum that can be caused by an intoxication with alcohol, antiepileptic medication ingestion, heavy metal ingestion, a midline cerebellar hemorrhage, or nfectious and postinfectious process that is classically seen with varicella infection. Maple syrup urine disease can present with intermmittent ataxia precipitated by illness.

68. A 7-year-old with progressive ataxia, kyphoscoliosis, nystagmus, pes cavus (high arch), and an abnormal ECG likely has what diagnosis?

Friedreich ataxia. This heredodegenerative disease is an autosomal recessive disorder with childhood onset of gait ataxia, absent tendon reflexes, and extensor plantar responses. The spinal cord shows degeneration and sclerosis of spinocerebellar tracts, posterior column, and corticospinal tracts. The condition is rare. The gene for Friedreich ataxia has been mapped to chromosome 9, contains a trinucleotide repeating sequence (GAA), and encodes for a protein called *frataxin*. Frataxin is reduced in the disease, but how this results in the disease process is unclear.

69. What clinical features help to distinguish peripheral from central vertigo?

Peripheral vertigo implies dysfunction of the labyrinth or vestibular nerve, whereas central vertigo is associated with abnormalities of the brain stem or temporal lobe.

Peripheral

- Hearing loss, tinnitus, and otalgia may be associated.
- Past pointing and falling in direction of unilateral disease occur.
- In bilateral disease, ataxia occurs with eyes closed.
- Vestibular and positional nystagmus are present.

Central

- Cerebellar and cranial nerve dysfunction frequently associated.
- No hearing loss.
- Alteration of consciousness may be associated.

Fenichel GM: Clinical Pediatric Neurology: A Signs and Symptoms Approach, 4th ed. Philadelphia, W.B. Saunders, 2001.

70. How is the Nylen-Barany maneuver performed?

Also called the Hallpike-Barany or Hallpike-Dix maneuver, this technique is used in the evaluation of vertigo when vestibular disease is suspected; it is a method to elicit paroxysmal positional nystagmus. A seated patient is asked to lie supine with his or her head hanging off the examining table with a 45(rotation. The patient's eyes are observed for the direction and duration of nystagmus. The maneuver is repeated to the opposite side and once again with the head in midline. If the patient does not exhibit nystagmus or symptoms during the maneuver, then a vestibular problem is unlikely as the cause of vertigo.

71. Define the "persistent vegetative state."

This is "a form of eyes-open permanent unconsciousness in which the patient has periods of wakefulness and physiological sleep/wake cycles, but at no time is the patient aware of himself or herself or the environment." If this state persists for > 3 months in children, the long-term outlook is grim.

American Academy of Neurology: Position of the American Academy of Neurology on certain aspects of the care and management of the persistent vegetative state patient. Neurology 39:125, 1989.

72. What are the causes of toe-walking?

- Cerebral palsy (spastic diplegia)
- Spinal dysraphism
- Intraspinal and filum terminale tumor
- Isolated congenital shortening of the Achilles tendon
- Muscular dystrophy
- Hereditary or acquired polyneuropathies
- Equinovarus deformity
- Variation of normal in early stages of walking
- Normal development pattern in some toddlers

73. In what settings is hyperacusis noted?

Hyperacusis, or increased sensitivity to sound, is found in patients with injury to the facial nerve (CN VII), which innervates the stapedius muscle, or injury to the trigeminal nerve (CN V), which innervates the tensor tympani muscle. Exaggerated startle response to sound or vibration occurs in lysosomal storage diseases (e.g., sphingolipidoses such as Tay-Sachs disease, GM_1 gangliosidosis, Sandhoff disease), Williams syndrome, hyperkalemia, tetanus, and strychnine poisoning.

74. What is the most common cause of asymmetric crying facies?

In this entity, one side of the lower lip depresses on crying (the normal side), and the other does not. Often misdiagnosed as a facial nerve palsy secondary to forceps delivery, the most common cause is ***congenital absence of the depressor anguli oris muscle*** of the lower lip. Its occasional association with heart defects warrants electrocardiography (ECG) and chest x-ray in these patients.

75. In which condition is risus sardonicus seen?

The sardonic smile is seen in patients with **tetanus** and is due to the spasm of facial muscles.

76. What are the common causes of peripheral seventh nerve palsy?

Facial weakness due to a lesion of the facial nerve (cranial nerve VII) is common. The facial weakness involves both the upper and lower face and affects both emotional and volitional facial movements. Any part of the nerve can be disturbed: the nucleus itself, the axon as it passes through the pons, or the peripheral portion of the nerve. Common etiologies include:

- ***Trauma***
- ***Developmental hypoplasia*** or ***aplasia*** including the Möbius anomaly
- ***Bell palsy*** (usually idiopathic but may follow nonspecific viral infections)
- ***Infections*** including the Ramsay Hunt syndrome (herpes zoster invasion of the geniculate ganglion producing herpetic vesicles behind the ear and painful paralysis of facial nerve); Lyme disease; local invasion from suppurative mastoiditis or otitis media; mumps, varicella, or enterovirus neuritis; sequelae of bacterial meningitis; and parotid gland infection, inflammation, or tumor

- ***Guillain-Barré syndrome***
- ***Tumor*** of brain stem or cerebellar pontine angle tumors
- ***Inflammatory disorders*** such as sarcoidosis

77. During recovery from Bell palsy, why do the eyes water at mealtime?

These are *crocodile tears*. The facial nerve supplies autonomic motor function to the lacrimal and salivary glands. Because of aberrant reinnervation in the course of healing from a facial nerve palsy, tasting a meal can trigger tearing rather than salivation. Folklore has it that crocodiles feel compassion for their victims and weep while munching.

78. What is the significance of the Babinski response?

Stimulation of the lateral aspect of the sole of the foot to the distal metatarsals may elicit a plantar response (extension). It indicates a lack of cortical inhibition and aids in the diagnosis of central hypotonia. It is abnormal outside of the neonatal period when a flexor response develops. The stimulus elicits a numbers of sensory pathways with competing functions (including grip and withdrawal) and is somewhat dependent on the state of the infant and the examiner's technique. Its value as a localizing sign in the neonate is more controversial, but a consistent asymmetry is abnormal.

79. When is the Chaddock maneuver helpful?

The Chaddock maneuver is another means of eliciting an extensor toe response. It involves stroking the outer edge of the dorsum of the foot. It is useful for patients in whom plantar stimulation results in reflex grasping (e.g., newborns) or withdrawal.

80. How is the Hoffman reflex test performed?

Like the Babinski reflex, the Hoffman reflex is a test for corticospinal tract abnormalities. In a patient with such pathology, downward flicking of the nail (on the second or third finger) by the examiner results in flexion of the distal phalanx of the thumb. Ordinarily, there is no response or a very muted one.

81. When are "doll's eyes" movements considered normal or abnormal?

The oculovestibular reflex (also called oculocephalic, proprioceptive head-turning reflex, or doll's eyes reflex) is used most commonly as a test of brain stem function. The patient's eyelids are held open while the head is briskly rotated from side to side. A positive response is contraversive conjugate eye deviation (i.e., as the head rotates to the right, both eyes deviate to the left). Doll's eyes movements are interpreted as follows:

- In healthy awake newborn infants (who cannot inhibit or override the reflex with willful eye movements), the reflex is easy to elicit and is a normal finding. It can be used to test the range of extraocular movements of infants in the first weeks of life.
- In healthy, awake, mature individuals, normal vision overrides the reflex, which is thus normally absent, and so the eyes follow the head turning.
- In coma with preserved brain stem function, the depressed cortex does not override the reflex, and doll's eyes movements occur in rapid head rotation. Indeed, the purpose of eliciting this reflex in the comatose patient is to demonstrate that the brain stem still functions normally.
- In coma with brain stem damage, the neural circuits that carry out the reflex are impaired and the reflex is abolished.

82. How are cold calorics done?

As a test of brain stem function in an obtunded or comatose individual, 5 ml of ice cold water is placed in the external ear canal (after ensuring integrity of the tympanic membrane) with the head elevated at 30°. A normal response occurs with deviation of the eyes to the side in which the water was placed. No response indicates severe dysfunction of the brain stem and the medial longitudinal fasciculus.

83. What causes pinpoint pupils?

Pupillary size represents a dynamic balance between the constricting influence of the third nerve (representing the parasympathetic autonomic nervous system) and the dilating influence of the ciliary nerve (which conducts fibers of the sympathetic nervous system). Pinpoint pupils indicate that the constricting influence of the third cranial nerve is not balanced by opposing sympathetic dilation. This could result from a ***structural lesion in the pons*** through which descend the sympathetic pathways. Small, reactive pupils also accompany some metabolic disorders. Opiates such as heroin or morphine produce pinpoint pupils that resemble those seen in pontine lesions. Various other agents also produce constriction of the pupils including propoxyphene, organophosphates, carbamate insecticides, barbiturates, clonidine, meprobamate, pilocarpine eye drops, and mushroom or nutmeg poisoning.

84. What is the differential diagnosis of ptosis?

Ptosis is the downward displacement of the upper eyelid due to dysfunction of the muscles that elevate the eyelid. A drooping eyelid may represent pseudoptosis due to swelling of the eyelid caused by local edema or active blepharospasm. True ptosis results from weakness of the eyelid muscles or interruption of its nerve supply. Primary muscular etiologies include congenital ptosis, which may occur alone or in the setting of Turner or Smith-Lemli-Opitz syndrome, myasthenia gravis, botulism, and some muscular dystrophies. Neurologic causes include Horner syndrome, which results from the interruption of the sympathetic supply to Muller's smooth eyelid muscle, and third nerve palsy, which innervates the levator palpebral muscle.

85. What is the significance of the Marcus Gunn pupil?

The pupils are normally equal in size (except for patients with physiologic anisocoria) due to the consensual light reflex: light entering either eye produces the same strength "signal" for constriction of both the stimulated and nonstimulated pupil. Some diseases of the maculae or optic nerves affect one side more than the other. For example, a meningioma may develop on one optic nerve sheath. As a result of unilateral or asymmetric optic nerve dysfunction, a Marcus Gunn pupil (afferent pupillary defect) may result.

86. How is the swinging flashlight test done?

This tests for the Marcus Gunn pupil.

1. The patient is examined in a dim room, and fixation is directed to a distant target (this permits maximal pupillary dilation because of lack of direct light and accommodation reflexes).

2. Light presented to the "good" eye produces equal constriction of both pupils. A flashlight is swung briskly over the bridge of the nose to the eye with the "defective" optic nerve. The abnormal pupil remains momentarily constricted from the lingering effects of the consensual light response. However, the impaired eye with its reduced pupillomotor signal soon escapes the consensual reflex and actually dilates despite being directly stimulated with light. The pupil that paradoxically dilates to direct light stimulation displays the **afferent defect**.

87. A child whose eyelids elevate rather than close with yawning has what condition?

The ***Marcus Gunn reflex***, also known as the jaw-winking phenomenon, presumably arises from a congenital "miswiring" of the oculomotor and trigeminal nerves. In this anomaly, ptosis follows jaw closure, and eyelid elevation follows jaw opening.

88. What are the causes of optic atrophy in children?

Optic atrophy is characterized by disc pallor and attenuated vasculature on fundoscopy. Severe atrophy also may produce an abnormal pupillary light reflex and deficit of acuity, visual field, or color vision. It should be distinguished from optic nerve hypoplasia, in which fundoscopy shows a nerve head of diminished circumference but normal color and vasculature. The causes of optic atrophy include structural (spenoid sinus mucocele, neuroblastoma, chronic elevation of intracranial pressure, or other orbital/chiasmatic neoplasms), metabolic-toxic (hyperthyroidism, vitamin B deficiency, Leber optic atrophy, various leukodystrophies, mitochondrial diseases, methanol, chloroquine, or amiodarone exposure), and various recessive syndromes with other neurologic signs (mental retardation, paraparesis) and demyelinating (optic neuritis, multiple sclerosis) diseases.

89. Does chronic heading of the soccer ball lead to cognitive impairment in children and adolescents?

The American Academy of Pediatrics (AAP) has expressed concerns about this issue after studies in adult soccer players (who began the sport at an early age) revealed mild to severe deficits in attention, concentration, and memory in substantial numbers. However, there is insufficient published data to recommend that young players refrain from the technique, although a recent recommendation was that its use be minimized.

American Academy of Pediatrics, Committee on Sports Medicine and Fitness: Injuries in youth soccer: A subject review. Pediatrics 105:659-661, 2000.

90. What is historically the most common cause of intracranial mass lesions in India?

Tuberculomas caused by mycoplasm tuberculosis present subacutely as mass lesions. Tubercular involvement of the brain is relatively common in developing countries with 50–60% of cases seen in children younger than 3 years of age.

91. When attending a pediatric conference in London, is it prudent to avoid the meat pies?

New-variant Creutzfeldt-Jacob disease and transmissible spongiform encephalopathies (TSEs or prion diseases) have achieved some pediatric notoriety with cases having been described in adolescents. These are a group of clinical syndromes in animals and humans characterized by slowly progressive neurodegenerative disease. The increases of bovine spongiform encephalopathy (BSE) in Great Britain noted in the mid-1980s prompted successful control measures, and the U.S. Centers for Disease Control and Prevention (CDC) now characterizes the risk of exposure to BSE in Great Britain as remote.

Whitely RJ, et al: Transmissible spongiform encephalopathies: A review for pediatricians. Pediatrics 106:1160-1165, 2000.

FEBRILE SEIZURES

92. How are febrile seizures defined?

Febrile seizures are defined as a provoked convulsion secondary to fever without evidence of CNS pathology and occurring in children between the ages of 1 month to 7 years, most commonly between age 6 months and 5 years with a peak at the end of the second year of life. Children with a history of epilepsy who have exacerbation of seizures with fever are excluded. Febrile seizures occur in 2–5% of children in this country, and they are more frequent in certain populations. There is often a positive family history of febrile convulsions.

93. What is the likelihood of recurrence of a febrile seizure?

The likelihood of recurrence increases with younger age of onset with a recurrence about ***1 in 2*** if younger than 1 year of age at initial seizure and ***1 in 5*** if older than 3 years of age. About half of recurrences will occur in the first 6 months, three-fourths within a year, and 90% within 2 years. In the younger age group, there is also a 30% chance of multiple recurrences, compared to an 11% risk of multiple recurrences if the first seizure occurred after age 1 year. Overall recurrence rate in the pediatric population is about 30%.

94. What features make a febrile seizure complex rather than simple?

A **simple** febrile seizure is a generalized convulsion that is relatively brief (< 15 min) and occurs as a solitary event (1 attack/24 hrs) in the setting of fever not due to CNS infection. **Complex** (also called atypical or complicated) febrile seizures may be focal, extended in duration, or multiple occurring in 1 day. They suggest a more serious problem. For example, a focal seizure raises concern of a localized or lateralized functional disturbance of the CNS. An unusually long seizure (> 15 min) also raises the suspicion of primary CNS infectious, structural, or metabolic disease. Repeated seizures within a 24-hour period likewise imply a potentially more serious disorder or impending status epilepticus.

95. When should a lumbar puncture (LP) be done as part of the evaluation of a young child with a simple febrile seizure?

This is often a difficult question when a well-appearing infant or toddler is examined following a febrile seizure. Approaches vary by clinician and textbook. The AAP conservatively recommends that after a seizure with fever in children younger than 12 months, an LP be *strongly considered* because symptoms and signs associated with meningitis may be minimal or absent in this age group. In children between 12 and 18 months, a, LP should be *considered* because signs and symptoms can be subtle. In children older than 18 months, when meningeal signs are typically present in meningitis, an LP can be deferred if such signs are not present. In younger patients who have received prior antibiotic therapy, an LP should be strongly considered because treatment can mask the signs and symptoms of meningitis. It should be noted that a seizure as the sole manifestation of bacterial meningitis in febrile children is unusual. In one retrospective study of 503 patients with meningitis, none were noted to have bacterial meningitis manifesting solely as a simple seizure.

Green SM, et al: Can seizures be the sole manifestation of meningitis in febrile children? Pediatrics 92:527-534, 1993.

Provisional Committee on Quality Improvement: Practice parameter: The neurodiagnostic evaluation of the child with a first simple febrile seizure. Pediatrics 97:769–775, 1996.

96. What ancillary testing should be considered in a patient with a complex febrile seizure?

Most children with their first atypical febrile seizure should undergo a ***CSF exam*** to rule out intracranial infection. Children with focal motor seizures or postictal lateralized deficits (motor paresis, unilateral sensory or visual loss, sustained eye deviation, or aphasia) require a ***CT scan*** to check for a structural abnormality. The immediate performance of an ***EEG*** offers limited insight into the patient's disease. Prominent generalized postictal slowing is not unexpected. Definite focal slowing suggests a possible structural abnormality. For a simple febrile seizure, an EEG is not indicated because it is not predictive of either the risk of recurrence of febrile seizures or the development of epilepsy.

American Academy of Pediatrics: Provisional Committee on Quality Improvement: Practice parameter: The neurodiagnostic evaluation of the child with a first simple febrile seizure. Pediatrics 97:769–775, 1996.

97. What is the risk of epilepsy following a febrile seizure?

The risk depends on several variables. In otherwise normal children with a simple febrile seizure, the risk of later epilepsy is about 2%. The risk of epilepsy is higher if:

- There is a close family history of nonfebrile seizures.
- Prior neurologic or developmental abnormalities existed.

- The patient had an atypical or complex febrile seizure, defined as focal seizures, seizures lasting 15 minutes, and/or multiple attacks within 24 hours.

One risk factor increases the risk to 3%. If all three risk factors are present, the likelihood of later epilepsy increases to 5–10%.

98. What does a definite epileptiform abnormality on EEG in the setting of febrile seizure represent?

- An inherited EEG trait if a close relative has genuine epilepsy (children may inherit an "abnormal EEG" from an epileptic parent without actually inheriting clinical epilepsy)
- A sporadic, unrelated, epileptic EEG abnormality (about 2–3% of healthy children with no family history of epilepsy have an incidental unexpected epileptiform EEG abnormality but do not develop clinical seizures)
- A "lowered seizure threshold" with the implication that the febrile seizure may have been an early expression of genuine epilepsy precipitated by the stress of fever and threatens to recur without the provocation of fever

99. What is the long-term outcome for children with febrile seizures?

In a previously normal child, the risk of death, neurologic damage, or persistent cognitive impairment from a single febrile seizure is near zero. These potential complications are more likely with complex febrile seizures, but the risk is still exceedingly low. Impaired cognition in the latter group is more likely if afebrile seizures subsequently develop. Febrile status epilepticus has a very low mortality with proper treatment in recent years, and the development of mesial temporal sclerosis is less than 1 in 70,000.

Verity CM, et al: Long-term intellectual and behavioral outcomes of children with febrile convulsions. N Engl J Med 338:1723-1728, 1998.

100. Following a febrile seizure, should a child be treated with prophylactic antiepileptics?

For most children, a simple febrile seizure is an unwanted but transient disruption of their health, and treatment is not necessary. Treatment may be considered in the very young child if febrile seizures recur and in children with preexisting neurologic abnormalities or with complex febrile seizures. Long-term prophylaxis does not improve the prognosis in terms of subsequent epilepsy or motor or cognitive ability.

Knudson FU, et al: Long-term outcome of prophylaxis for febrile convulsions. Arch Dis Child 74:13–18, 1996.

101. Discuss the antiepileptic regimens that can be considered prophylactically in children with histories of complex febrile seizures.

- Continuous daily prophylactic administration of **phenobarbital** to produce a minimum serum level of 15 μg/ml. Behavioral and cognitive side effects can occur. The daily use of **primidone** is effective, but the side effect profile is similar, and it probably has little advantage over phenobarbital. Comparable protection against febrile seizures may be achieved with **valproate**, but its use is not recommended for children under age 2 because of the risk of hepatotoxicity. Neither carbamazepine nor phenytoin appears effective in preventing the recurrence of febrile seizures.
- **Oral diazepam** (0.33 mg/kg) given every 8 hours during a febrile illness reduces the risk of febrile seizures by nearly 50%. However, the side effects may obscure the clinical picture, especially in meningitis; nearly half of the children using this regimen develop ataxia, lethargy, or irritability.
- **Rectal diazepam** or **lorazepam** for administration by parents either prophylactically (controversial) or in the event of a prolonged febrile seizure.

Kriel RL, et al: Rectal diazepam gel for the treatment of acute repetitive seizures. The North American Diastat Study Group. Pediatr Neurol 20:282-288, 1999.

Rosman NP, et al: A controlled trial of diazepam administered during febrile illness to prevent recurrence of febrile seizures. N Engl J Med 329:79–84, 1993.

102. Do prolonged febrile seizures result in an increased peripheral white blood cell count?

A common clinical question in children is whether a leukocytosis, if found, can be explained on the basis of a prolonged seizure as a stress reaction. In a study of 203 children with seizures and fever, 61% had a normal peripheral white blood cell count. No association was found between blood leukocytosis and febrile seizure duration in children.

Van Stuijvenberg M, et al: The duration of febrile seizures and peripheral leukocytosis. J Pediatr 133:557-558, 1998.

HEADACHE

103. What are the emergency priorities in evaluating a child with a severe headache?

As with all common presenting symptoms, the main priority is to rule out diagnostic possibilities that may be life-threatening:

- Malignant hypertension
- Increased intracranial pressure (e.g., mass lesion or acute hydrocephalus)
- Intracranial infections (e.g., meningitis, encephalitis)
- Subarachnoid hemorrhage
- Stroke
- Acute angle closure glaucoma may present as headache but is rare in children.

104. When should neuroimaging be considered in a child with headache?

- Abnormal neurologic signs
- Headache increasing in frequency and severity
- Headache occurring in early morning or awakening child from sleep
- Headache made worse by straining or by sneezing or coughing (may be a sign of increased ICP)
- Headache associated with severe vomiting without nausea
- Headache worsened or helped significantly by a change in position
- Fall-off in linear growth rate
- Recent school failure or significant behavioral changes
- New-onset seizures, especially if seizure has a focal onset
- Migraine headache and seizure occurring in the same episode, with vascular symptoms preceding the seizure (20–50% risk of tumor or arteriovenous malformation)
- Cluster headaches in any child or teenager

Halsam RHA: Migraine headaches. In Behrman RE, et al (ed): Nelson Textbook of Pediatrics, 16th ed. Philadelphia, W.B. Saunders, 2000; pp. 1832-1834.

105. What is the origin of the word *migraine*?

Ancient Greek physicians recognized a specific type of recurring head pain that was unilateral. The modern word *migraine* is a French modification of the archaic term *hemikrania*.

106. What are the clinical presentations of migraine headaches in children?

Migraine is a periodic disorder with symptom-free periods characterized by headaches with a throbbing nature, unilateral location, relief after sleep, aura, associated abdominal pain, nausea, or vomiting. Classical migraines are uncommon in younger children and may present with a visual aura, irritability, pallor, nausea, and vomiting that last hours to days. Migraine headaches without an aura are more common in children. The prevalence of migraine in childhood is about 4% and becomes more common in teenage girls and young women. Childhood migraine may present as benign paroxysmal vertigo of childhood, ophthalmoplegic migraine, or hemiplegic, confusional, or basilar artery migraines. There may be a history of recurrent vomiting or motion sickness. There is often a family history of migraine, and the genetics may be multifactorial.

Sheveli H: A guide to migraine equivalents. Contemp Pediatr 15:71, 1998.

107. What are the diagnostic criteria for common migraine?

Common migraine is also called migraine without aura. Diagnostic criteria from the International Headache Society include:

- 5 attacks
- Duration of 4–72 hours
- Characteristics (two out of four):
  1. Unilateral
  2. Pulsating
  3. Moderate or severe
  4. Aggravated by physical activity
- Concomitant features (one out of two):
  1. Nausea and/or vomiting
  2. Photophobia/phonophobia

Singer HS: Migraine headaches in children. Pediatr Rev 15:94, 1994.

108. Which physical findings are important in the initial evaluation of possible migraine headache?

- Height and weight should be normal for age. Pituitary tumor, craniopharyngioma, or partial ornithine transcarbamylase deficiency may all result in growth failure and mimic migraine headache. Head circumference should be normal, ruling out hydrocephalus.
- Skin should be checked for abnormalities. Throbbing headaches are common in neurofibromatosis and systemic lupus erythymatosus, both of which have easily recognizable skin manifestations.
- Blood pressure should be normal.
- Check for sinus tenderness or pain with head movement (implying cervical spine disease). The patient should be examined for carious teeth, misaligned bite, or disordered chewing and jaw opening (temporomandibular joint dysfunction).
- Auscultation should reveal no cranial bruits (if present, suggest possible arteriovenous malformation or mass lesion).
- The neurologic examination should be normal.

109. When do children begin to have migraine headaches?

About 20% suffer their first headache before age 10 years.

110. Which foods have been associated with the development of migraine headaches?

Tyramine-rich foods (cheese, red wine), foods with monosodium glutamate (Chinese and Mexican food), nitrate-rich foods (smoked meats, salami), marinated foods, alcoholic beverages, caffeinated beverages, chocolate, citrus fruits, and beans.

111. What is the most common form of complex migraine in children?

Complex migraines are those migraine headaches accompanied by transient neurologic signs or symptoms. These include hemiplegic migraine, ophthalmoplegic migraine (orbital pain with third nerve palsy), acute confusional state, and the Alice-in-Wonderland syndrome (hallucinations and distortion of object size). The most common form is ***basilar artery***

migraine, which has a variety of symptoms including blurred vision, vertigo, ataxia, dysarthria, and loss of consciousness.

112. What nonpharmacologic therapy is available for the treatment of migraine?

- Migraine elimination diet
- Normalization of sleep habits
- Discontinuance of possible triggering medications (e.g., analgesic overuse, bronchodilators, oral contraceptives)
- Biofeedback
- Relaxation therapy
- Family counseling (if family stress is a trigger)
- Self-hypnosis

Van Hook E: Non-pharmacological treatment of headache—why? Clin Neuroscience 5:43-49, 1998.

113. What are the best medications to abort a severe migraine attack that has not responded to acetaminophen or nonsteroidal anti-inflammatory drugs (NSAIDs)?

Ergotamines, midrin (isometheptene mucate, dichloralphenazone, acetaminophen), and sumatriptan.

Winner P, et al: A randomized, double-blind, placebo-controlled study of sumatriptan nasal spray in the treatment of acute migraine in adolescents. Pediatrics 106:989-997, 2000.

Ueberall MA, et al: Intranasal sumatriptan for the acute treatment of migraine in children. Neurology 52:1507-1510, 1999.

114. Who should be started on prophylactic medication for migraine headaches?

There are no precise criteria, but generally prophylactic treatment should be considered if:

- Headaches with aura occur frequently
- Headaches with aura are poorly responsive to abortive medication
- School attendance is significantly affected
- Headaches, though infrequent, last for several days

115. What medications are used in children for prevention of migraine headaches?

- Beta-blockers (especially propranolol)
- Calcium channel blockers (especially verapamil)
- NSAIDs (especially naproxen)
- Tricyclic antidepressants (especially amitriptyline)
- Antiepileptics (especially divalproex sodium)
- Cyproheptadine

116. How long are the prophylactic medications continued?

The optimal duration of therapy remains unclear, but many authorities suggest a treatment duration of 4–6 months followed by an attempt at weaning. Less than 50% will require reinitiation of medication.

117. Why are migraine headaches and epilepsy thought to be linked?

- Both are familial, paroxysmal, and associated with transitory neurologic disturbances.
- There is an increased incidence of epilepsy in migraineurs and migraine in epileptics.
- Headache can be a seizure manifestation.
- Abnormal EEGs occur in both disorders (asymptomatic central spikes occur in 9% of children with migraine vs 2% of healthy children).

Fenichel GM: Clinical Pediatric Neurology: A Signs and Symptoms Approach, 4th ed. Philadelphia, W.B. Saunders, 2000.

MOVEMENT DISORDERS

118. What are the various types of pathologic hyperkinetic movements?

- ***Tremors***—rhythmic oscillatory movements, both supination-pronation and flexion-extension, seen in resting state or with activity
- ***Chorea***—quick, dancing movements of proximal and distal muscles with irregular unpredictable random jerks
- ***Athetosis***—irregular, slow, distal writhing movements
- ***Stereotypy***—repetitive, purposeless motions (e.g., body rocking, head rolling) that resemble voluntary movements often associated with akathisia (sensory and motor restlessness)
- ***Dystonia***—slow, twisting, sustained movements; may result in abnormal postures and progress to contractures
- ***Ballismus***—abrupt, random, violent, flinging movements, often proximal and unilateral
- ***Myoclonus***—abrupt, brief, jerklike contractions of one or more muscles, often stimulus-sensitive
- ***Tics***—rapid, sudden, repetitive movements or vocalizations

119. What techniques can be used to elicit abnormal movements, particularly chorea?

Methods of provocative testing include maintenance of posture in extension against gravity, hyperpronation (or "spooning," especially above the head), tongue protrusion ("trombone tongue"), squeezing the finger of the examiner ("milk-maid's grip"), poring liquid, and drawing a spiral.

120. What disorders are commonly associated with the various hyperkinetic movements?

- **Tremors, resting**—primary juvenile Parkinson disease, secondary Parkinson disease
- **Tremors, kinetic—e**ssential (familial) tremor, cerebellar disorders, brain stem tumors, hyperthyroidism, Wilson disease, electrolyte disturbance (e.g., glucose, calcium, magnesium), heavy metal intoxication (e.g., lead, mercury), multiple sclerosis
- **Chorea**—sydenham chorea (associated with rheumatic fever), Huntington disease, hyperthyroidism, infectious mononucleosis, pregnancy, anticonvulsants, neuroleptic drugs, closed head injury, systemic lupus erythematosus, carbon monoxide poisoning, Wilson disease, hypocalcemia, polycythemia, parainfectious/infectious encephalopathies (e.g., rubeola, syphilis)
- **Athetosis—c**erebral palsy, other static encephalopathies, Lesch-Nyhan syndrome, kernicterus
- **Stereotypy—a**utism, Rett syndrome, neuroleptic drugs (i.e., tardive dyskinesia), schizophrenia
- **Dystonia**—idiopathic primary dystonias (e.g., torsion dystonia), Sandifer syndrome, spasmus nutans, neuroleptic drugs, static encephalopathy, perinatal asphyxia, familial dystonia (sometimes dopa-responsive)
- **Ballismus**—encephalitis, closed-head injury
- **Myoclonus**—sleep myoclonus, benign myoclonus of infancy, postanoxic encephalopathy, uremic encephalopathy, hyperthyroidism, urea-cycle defects, side effects of tricyclic therapy, slow virus infections, Wilson disease, myoclonus-opsoclonus, neuroblastoma, epileptic encephalopathies, mitochondrial disease, prion disease, Tay-Sachs, startle disease, sialidosis

121. What constitutes a tic?

Tics are brief, sudden, repetitive, stereotyped, involuntary, and purposeless movements or vocalizations. They most commonly involve muscles of the head, neck, and respiratory tract. Their frequency can be increased by anxiety, stress, excitement, and fatigue. They are decreased during sleep and relaxation, during activities involving high concentration, and at times, through voluntary action. In some cases, premonitory feelings (e.g., irritation, tickle, temperature change) can precipitate the motor or vocal response.

122. What is the range of clinical tics?

Tics can be motor or vocal, simple or complex, clonic or dystonic.

***Motor (simple clonic)*:** Eye blinking, eye jerking, head twitching, shoulder shrugging

***Motor (simple dystonic)*:** Bruxism, abdominal tensing, shoulder rotation

***Motor (complex)*:** Grunting, barking, sniffing, snorting, throat clearing, spitting

***Vocal (complex)*:** Coprolalia (obscene words), echolalia (repeating another's words), palilalia (rapidly repeating one's own words)

123. What makes a tic tick?

Transient and chronic tic disorders usually do not have an identifiable cause. However, dyskinesias such as tics can be found in association with a number of other conditions:

Chromosomal abnormalities—Down syndrome, fragile X syndrome

Developmental syndromes—autism, pervasive developmental disorder, Rett syndrome

Drugs—anticonvulsants, stimulants (e.g., amphetamines, cocaine, methylphenidate, pemoline)

Infections—encephalitis, post-rubella syndrome

124. How should simple tics be treated?

Simple motor tics are common and occur in more than 10% of school-aged children. Simple tics generally do not require pharmacologic intervention and can be treated expectantly by developing relaxation techniques, minimizing stresses that exacerbate the problem, avoiding of punishment for tics, and decreasing fixation on the problem. Most simple tics self-resolve in 2–12 months.

125. When do tics warrant pharmacologic intervention?

Tics that have a significant disabling impact on a child's educational, social, or psychological well-being (particularly if they have been present for > 1 year) may require intervention. When the complexity of tics increases or the diagnosis of Tourette syndrome is suspected, pharmacotherapy also should be considered. Most theories point to a hyperdopaminergic state of the basal ganglia as the most likely etiology for unregulated movements. Pharmacologic management includes administration of dopamine blockers (e.g., fluphenazine, haloperidol) or clonidine (method and site of action unclear) or cessation of any stimulant drugs that can cause dopamine release. Because of the high associated incidence of obsessive-compulsive disorder and attention deficit hyperactivity disorder (ADHD), other medications may be needed, and consultation with a pediatric psychiatrist or neurologist is often warranted.

126. What are the diagnostic criteria for Tourette syndrome?

In 1885, Gilles de la Tourette described a syndrome of motor tics and vocal tics (e.g., coprolalia) with behavioral disturbances and a chronic and variable course. DSM criteria for Tourette syndrome requires :

- Multiple motor tics
- One or more vocal tics
- Onset before age 21 years
- Waxing and waning course

- Presence of tics for > 1 year (usually on a daily basis)
- No identifiable medical etiology

Coprolalia is an irresistible urge to utter profanities, occurring as a phonic tic. Only 20–40% of patients with Tourette syndrome have this phenomenon, and it is not essential for the diagnosis. Onset of Tourette syndrome is usually between age 5 and 8 years and begins in the facial muscles first and then spreads downward. It is estimated in a nonreferred sample that the prevalence of Tourette syndrome is 1% in boys and 0.1% in girls.

127. What behavioral problems are associated with Tourette syndrome?

- Obsessive-compulsive disorder
- ADHD
- Severe conduct disorders
- Learning disabilities (particularly math)
- Sleep abnormalities
- Depression, anxiety, emotional lability

128. Why is the diagnosis of Tourette syndrome commonly delayed?

- Tendency to associate unusual symptoms with attention-getting or psychologic problems
- Incorrect belief that all children with Tourette syndrome must have severe tics
- Attributing vocal tics to upper respiratory infections, allergies, sinus or bronchial problems
- Diagnosing eye blinking or ocular tics as ophthalmologic problems
- Mistaken belief that coprolalia is an essential diagnostic feature

Singer HS: Tic disorders. Pediatric Ann 22:22–29, 1993.

129. What is the cause of tardive dyskinesia?

Tardive dyskinesia is a hyperkinetic disorder of abnormal movements, most commonly involving the face (e.g., lip smacking or pursing, chewing, grimacing, tongue protruding). Tardive dyskinesia occurs during treatment with neuroleptics (e.g., chlorpromazine, haloperidol, metoclopramide) or within 6 months of their discontinuance. This disorder is thought to be secondary to dopaminergic dysfunction of the basal ganglia, because these drugs act as dopamine receptor blockers.

130. For a patient on neuroleptic medication, how long must therapy last before symptoms of tardive dyskinesia can develop?

About ***3 months*** of continuous or intermittent treatment with neuroleptics is needed before the risk of tardive dyskinesia increases.

131. Which movement disorder in children presents with "dancing eyes and dancing feet"?

Opsoclonus-myoclonus (infantile polymyoclonus syndrome or acute myoclonic encephalopathy of infants) is a rare but distinctive movement disorder in children in the first 1–3 years of life. Opsoclonus is characterized by wild, chaotic, fluttering, irregular, rapid, conjugate bursts of eye movements (saccadomania). Myoclonus is sudden, shock-like muscular twitches of the face, limbs, or trunk. The anatomic site of pathology is the cerebellar outflow tracts. The etiology may be direct viral invasion, postinfectious encephalopathy, or neuroblastoma.

132. A 10-month-old child with head tilt, head nodding, and nystagmus is likely to have what condition?

Spasmus nutans is a rare, acquired movement disorder of unknown etiology beginning between ages 4 and 14 months. The full triad consists of head tilt (torticollis), head nodding, and nystagmus. The condition often presents first with the head nodding, which is out of synchrony with the speed, direction, and tempo of the nystagmus. The condition lasts several months to years and usually fades by age 5 years. The nystagmus is present in the primary position (with the patient looking straight ahead) but is characteristically unilateral or markedly asymmetrical. The nystagmus has a pendular quality (a pendulum arm sweeps arcs of equal magnitude and velocity). The direction of the nystagmus can be horizontal, vertical, or rotatory and may vary with the direction of gaze. Spasmus nutans occasionally has been associated with developmental abnormalities or optic chiasmal gliomas. Congenital or sensory nystagmus also should be considered. Therefore, a CT scan should be obtained before reassuring the parents of the benign nature and favorable outcome of the disorder.

NEONATAL SEIZURES

133. How are neonatal seizures classified?

Although there is no universally accepted standard classification system, one based on clinical criteria is commonly used. It divides neonatal seizures into four types:

1. ***Subtle***
2. ***Tonic*** (partial or generalized)
3. ***Clonic*** (partial or multifocal)
4. ***Myoclonic*** (partial, multifocal, or generalized)

All seizure types are recognized as paroxysmal alterations in behavioral, motor, or autonomic function. Not all clinically observed phenomena, however, are accompanied by associated epileptic surface-EEG activity. Partial clonic, tonic, and myoclonic seizures have been shown to have the most consistent EEG ictal correlate.

134. What are the causes of neonatal seizures?

- Hypoxic-ischemic encephalopathy due to asphyxia
- Infection
- Toxins (e.g., inadvertent fetal injection with local anesthetic; cocaine, including withdrawal)
- Metabolic abnormalities (e.g., hypoglycemia, hypocalcemia, hypomagnesemia, pyridoxine deficiency, inborn errors)
- CNS malformations
- Cerebrovascular lesions (e.g., intraventricular, periventricular hemorrhage, subarachnoid hemorrhage, infarction, arterial cerebral occlusion)

135. What is an acceptable workup in a newborn with seizures?

The workup should include a careful prenatal and natal history as well as a complete physical examination. Laboratory studies should include blood for glucose, electrolytes, calcium, phosphorus, and magnesium. A lumbar puncture should be performed to rule out meningitis. Neuroimaging studies (cranial ultrasound, CT scan, or MRI) are mandatory. Additional studies, where warranted, include blood levels for ammonia, lactate, and pyruvate, additional CSF studies (e.g., lactate, pyruvate, glycine if metabolic disease is suspected), and urine studies for organic and amino acid analysis for possible inborn errors of metabolism. Serial use of EEG-polygraphy can document persistent of seizures.

136. In what settings should an inborn error of metabolism be suspected as a cause of neonatal seizures?

- Onset of seizures is beyond day 1 of life (exception is pyridoxine deficiency)
- Infants becomes symptomatic following introduction of enteral or parenteral nutrition
- Seizures are intractable and do not respond to conventional AEDs

Scher MS: Neonatal seizures. In Polin RA, et al (eds): Workbook in Practical Neonatology, 3rd ed. Philadelphia, W.B. Saunders, 2001, p. 359.

137. In premature and full-term infants, how do the causes of seizures vary in relative frequency and time of onset?

Variance in Relative Frequency and Time of Onset of Causes of Seizures

	POSTNATAL TIME OF ONSET		RELATIVE FREQUENCY	
ETIOLOGY	0–3 DAYS	> 3 DAYS	PREMATURE	FULL-TERM
Hypoxic-ischemic	+		+++	+++
Intracranial hemorrhage*	+	+	++	+
Hypoglycemia	+		+	+
Hypocalcemia	+	+	+	+
Intracranial infection†	+	+	++	+
Developmental defects	+	+	++	++
Drug withdrawal	+	+	+	+

*Hemorrhages are principally germinal matrix-intraventricular in the premature infant and subarachnoid or subdural in the term infant.

†Early seizures occur usually after intrauterine nonbacterial infections (e.g., toxoplasmosis, CMV infection), and later seizures usually occur with herpes simplex encephalitis or bacterial meningitis.

Adapted from Volpe JJ (ed): Neurology of the Newborn, 3rd ed. Philadelphia, W.B. Saunders, 1995, p 184.

138. Why are focal seizures in the neonate not necessarily indicative of a focal brain abnormality?

The immature CNS cannot sustain a synchronized, well-orchestrated, generalized seizure. The anatomic basis for this observation is the paucity of myelination in the newborn brain. More extensive myelination is required for conduction of discharges throughout the brain in generalized seizures. Focal seizures in newborns often arise from diffuse, toxic, or metabolic conditions, whose epileptogenic influence affects those cortical areas of the brain mature enough to produce a seizure. On the other hand, stroke, localized hemorrhage, and trauma do occur in infants and should be included in the differential diagnosis of seizures in this age group.

Painter MJ, Gaus RN: Neonatal seizures: Diagnosis and treatment. J Child Neurol 6:101–108, 1991.

139. What is the most common type of clinical seizure in the neonatal period?

The so-called ***subtle seizure***. Rather than arising as an abrupt dramatic "convulsion" with obvious forceful twitching or posturing of the muscles, the subtle seizure appears as an unnatural, repetitive, stereotyped choreography, featuring oral-buccal-lingual movements, eye blinking, nystagmus, lip smacking, or complex integrated limb movements (swimming, pedaling, or rowing) and other fragments of activity drawn from the limited repertoire of normal infant activity.

140. What behavioral states may be confused with seizures in neonates?

A variety of "seizure-like" behaviors, which show no evidence of simultaneous EEG discharges consistent with seizures, are believed to originate in the brain stem and spinal cord without superimposed inhibitory cortical influences. These include jitteriness, movements during REM sleep, "rowing" and "bicycling" movements, decorticate and decerebrate posturing, and autonomic dysfunctions.

141. How are seizures differentiated from tremors in the neonate?

Clinical Feature	Jitteriness	Seizure
Abnormality of gaze or eye movement	0	+
Movements exquisitely stimulus-sensitive	+	0
Predominant movement	Tremor	Clonic jerking
Movements cease with passive flexion	+	0
Autonomic changes	0	+

Adapted from Volpe JJ (ed): Neurology of the Newborn, 3rd ed. Philadelphia, W.B. Saunders, 1995, p 182.

142. Does tonic posturing require treatment?

Generalized tonic posturing and subtle clinical phenomena not associated with concurrent autonomic disturbance or EEG seizure activity are nonepileptic events that should not be treated with anticonvulsant medication. Such events rarely affect ventilatory or cardiovascular function and require high levels of anticonvulsant drug therapy for suppression.

143. What are the treatment options for neonatal seizures?

Neonatal seizures may be treated with phenobarbital. Studies of the pharmacokinetics of phenobarbital in neonates have indicated that it is most appropriate to load with a full 20 mg/kg rather than smaller fractions. If seizures persist, additional increments of phenobarbital to total loading doses of 40 mg/kg can be given. Continued seizures may be treated with a loading dose of 20 mg/kg of phenytoin, or phenytoin equivalents in the case of fosphenytoin. The usual maintenance dose for phenobarbital is between 3 and 6 mg/kg/day and between 3 to 4 mg/kg/day for phenytoin. Efficacy from either of these two agents is low, with only one-third showing an immediate complete response. Even after apparently successful intravenous treatment with phenobarbital and phenytoin with resolution of clinical seizures, electrographic seizures may continue unabated. The significance of this finding is unclear, and the need to suppress electrographic seizures without clinical accompaniments is controversial.

Painter M, et al: Phenobarbital compared with phenytoin for the treatment of neonatal seizures. N Engl J Med 341:485-489, 1999.

144. What is the treatment for refractory seizures in the neonate?

Frequent and recurrent seizures are not uncommon in newborns and are especially common in the setting of asphyxia. If seizures are refractory to full dosing of phenobarbital and phenytoin, addition of drugs in the benzodiazepine family (e.g., diazepam, lorazepam) or paraldehyde is generally effective. It is important to ensure that no underlying biochemical disturbance is present before the serum levels of anticonvulsants are raised to maximal concentrations. Although pyridoxine-dependent seizures are rare, a trial dose of pyridoxine should be administered intravenously to infants with recurrent seizures of uncertain etiology. If possible, simultaneous EEG recording should be performed to document the cessation of seizure activity and the normalization of the EEG within minutes of pyridoxine treatment.

145. After an infant has recovered from a seizure, how long should medication be continued?

Maintenance therapy typically involves the use of phenobarbital, because it is difficult to achieve therapeutic levels of phenytoin with oral administration in infancy, and other medications are (e.g., carbamazepine) are less well-studied. Although phenobarbital is generally well tolerated, it may have deleterious effects on behavior, attention span, and possibly brain development. It does not prevent the later development of epilepsy. Many authorities recommend discontinuing therapy if the neurologic exam has normalized. In addition, if the neurologic exam is abnormal but an EEG by age 3 months reveals no seizure activity, consideration also can be given to stopping phenobarbital.

146. Are seizures without concurrent hypoxia or acidosis harmful in a neonate?

Although the hypoxemia and hypercarbia that accompany seizures may result in brain injury, CNS damage can be produced by other associated events as well:

- Increased cerebral blood flow accompanying seizures may result in hemorrhagic injury of vulnerable vascular beds (e.g., the germinal matrix in premature infants).
- Changes in the concentrations of critical high-energy phosphate compounds (e.g., adenosine triphosphate [ATP], phosphocreatinine) may lead to irreparable injury.
- Brain substrates such as glucose are depleted despite increased cerebral blood flow.
- Excessive release of synaptic excitatory amino acids, such as glutamate, exerts a toxic effect at sites where they would otherwise serve as neurotransmitters (experimental animal data).

147. In neonatal seizures, how does the cause affect the prognosis?

Relationship between Cause and Prognosis of Neonatal Seizure

ETIOLOGY	FAVORABLE OUTCOME*	MIXED OUTCOME	UNFAVORABLE OUTCOME*
Toxic-metabolic	Sample late-onset hypocalcemia Hypomagnesemia Hyponatremia Mepivacaine toxicity	Hypoglycemia Early-onset complicated hypocalcemia Pyridoxine dependency	Some aminoacidurias
Asphyxia	—	Mild hypoxic-ischemic encephalopathy	Severe hypoxic-ischemic encephalopathy
Hemorrhage	Uncomplicated subarachnoid hemorrhage	Subdural hematoma Intraventricular hemorrhage (grades I and II)	Intraventricular hemorrhage (grades III and IV)
Infection	—	Aseptic meningoencephalitis; some bacterial meningitides	Herpes simplex encephalitis; some bacterial meningitides
Structural		Simple traumatic contusion	Malformations of CNS

*Favorable prognosis implies at least an 85–90% chance of survival and subsequent normal development. Unfavorable prognosis implies a high likelihood (85–90% of death or serious handicap in survivors.

From Scher MS: Neonatal seizures. In Polin RA, et al (eds): Workbook in Practical Neonatology, 3rd ed. Philadelphia, W.B. Saunders, 2001, p 366; with permission.

148. Of what prognostic value is the interictal EEG in a neonate with seizures?

It can have significant prognostic value. Severe interictal EEG abnormalities (e.g., burst-suppression, marked voltage suppression, flat or isoelectric) are highly predictive (90%) of a fatal outcome or severe neurologic sequelae. Conversely, a normal interictal EEG in a term infant with seizures confers a very low (10%) likelihood of significant neurologic impairment. Moderate abnormalities (e.g., voltage asymmetries, immature patterns) have a mixed outcome.

NEUROCUTANEOUS SYNDROMES

149. What are the three most common neurocutaneous syndromes?

- Neurofibromatosis
- Tuberous sclerosis complex
- Sturge-Weber syndrome

150. What are the inheritance patterns of the various neurocutaneous syndromes?

Neurofibromatosis	Autosomal dominant
Tuberous sclerosis complex	Autosomal dominant

von Hippel-Lindau syndrome	Autosomal dominant
Incontinentia pigmenti	X-linked dominant
Sturge-Weber syndrome	Sporadic
Klippel-Trenaunay-Weber syndrome	Sporadic

151. What is the derivation of the term *phakomatosis*?

The term *phakomatosis* is derived from the Greek *phakos*, meaning "lentil" or "lens-shaped," and refers to patchy, circumscribed dermatologic lesions that are the hallmark of this group of disorders. In addition to dermatologic features, these syndromes have hamartomatous involvement of multiple tissues, especially the CNS and eye. More commonly, the term *neurocutaneous syndrome* is used.

152. What are the diagnostic criteria for neurofibromatosis-1 (NF1)?

Two or more of the following:

- Café-au-lait spots (6 or more > 5 mm in diameter before puberty; 6 or more > 15 mm in diameter after puberty)
- Skinfold freckling (axillary or inguinal region)
- Neurofibromas (2 or more) of any type or 1 plexiform neurofibroma
- Optic glioma
- Iris hamartomas, also called Lisch nodules (2 or more)
- Characteristic bony lesion (i.e., sphenoid dysplasia, thinning of cortex of long bones, with or without pseudoarthrosis)
- First-degree relative(s) with NF1

North K: Neurofibromatosis type I. Am J Med Genet 97:119-127, 2000.

153. How does NF1 differ from NF2?

NF1, classic von Recklinghausen disease, is much more common (1:3000–4000 births) and accounts for up to 90% of cases of neurofibromatosis. NF2 (1:50,000 births) is characterized by bilateral acoustic neuromas, intracranial and intraspinal tumors, and affected first-degree relatives. NF1 has been linked to alterations on chromosome 17, whereas NF2 is linked to alterations on chromosome 22. Dermatologic findings and peripheral neuromas are rare in NF2. Other rarer subtypes of neurofibromatoses (e.g., segmental distribution) have been described.

154. How common are café-au-lait spots at birth?

Up to 2% of black infants will have three café-au-lait spots at birth, whereas one café-au-lait spot occurs in only 0.3% of white infants. White infants with multiple café-au-lait spots at birth are more likely than black infants to develop neurofibromatosis. In older children, a single café-au-lait spot > 5 mm can be found in 10% of white and 25% of black children.

Hurwitz S: Neurofibromatosis. In Clinical Pediatric Dermatology, 2nd ed. Philadelphia, W.B. Saunders, 1993, pp 624–629.

155. If a 2-year-old has seven café-au-lait spots > 5 mm in diameter, what is the likelihood that neurofibromatosis will develop and how will it evolve?

Up to 75% of these children, if followed sequentially, will develop one of the varieties of neurofibromatosis, most commonly type 1. NF1 evolves. In a study of nearly 1900 patients, 46% of patients with sporadic NF1 did not meet criteria by age 1. By age 8, 97% met the criteria and by age 20 years, 100% did. The typical order of appearance of features is café-au-lait spots, axillary freckling, Lisch nodules, and neurofibromas. Yearly follow-up of patients with suspicious findings should include a careful skin examination, ophthalmologic evaluation, and blood pressure measurement.

Debella K, et al: Use of the National Institutes of Health criteria for the diagnosis of neurofibromatosis 1 in children. Pediatrics 105:608-614, 2000.

Korf BR: Diagnostic outcome in children with multiple café-au-lait spots. Pediatrics 90:924–927, 1992.

156. How common is a positive family history in cases of NF1?

Because of the high spontaneous mutation rate for this autosomal dominant disease, only ***about 50%*** of newly diagnosed cases are associated with a positive family history.

157. What are the primary diagnostic criteria for tuberous sclerosis complex (TSC)?

TSC is characterized by hamartomatous growths that occur in multiple tissues. The National Institutes of Health Consensus Conference in 1998 revised diagnostic criteria for TSC based on major or minor features. Definite TSC consisted of 2 major features *or* 1 major and 2 minor features. Probable and possible TSC had fewer features. No single finding was considered pathognomonic for TSC. Two gene site abnormalities, *TSC1* (chromosome 9) and *TSC2* (chromosome 16), have been identified, but genetic testing is not yet available.

Major features include:
Facial angiofibromas
Nontraumatic ungual or periungual fibroma
Hypomelanotic macules (more than 3)
Shagreen patch
Multiple retinal nodular hamartomas
Cortical tuber
Subependymal nodule or giant cell astrocytoma
Cardiac rhabdomyoma, single or multiple

Minor features include:
Dental enamel pits
Bone cysts
Hamartomatous rectal polyps
Gingival fibromas
Cerebral white matter migration tracts

Hyman MH, Whittemore VH: National Institutes of Health Concensus Conference: Tuberous sclerosis complex. Arch Neurol 57:662-665, 2000.

158. What is the classic triad of TSC?

Seizures, mental retardation, and ***facial angiofibroma*** (adenoma sebaceum). Less than one-third of patients, however, will develop these classic features.

159. What is the most common presenting symptom of TSC?

Seizures. About 85% of patients have generalized seizures, and infantile spasms are the most common. Tonic and atonic seizures are also seen. Complex partial seizures are frequently seen in conjunction with other seizure types. Mental retardation is especially common with onset of seizures before 2 years of age. Autism and other behavioral disturbances are also frequently seen in children with TSC.

160. What are Lisch nodules?

Pigmented iris hamartomas. Of note, although these are not usually present at birth in patients with NF1, up to 90% will develop multiple Lisch nodules by age 6. Hamartomas are focal malformations, microscopically composed of multiple tissue types, which can resemble neoplasms but (unlike neoplasms) grow at similar rates as normal components and are unlikely to pathologically compress adjacent tissue.

161. What are skin findings in tuberous sclerosis?

Skin Findings in Tuberous Sclerosis

AGE AT ONSET	SKIN FINDINGS	INCIDENCE
Birth or later	Hypopigmented macules	80%
2–5 years	Angiofibromas	70%
2–5 years	Shagreen patches	35%
Puberty	Periungual and gingival fibromas	20–50%
Birth or later	Café-au-lait spots	25%

162. Why is the term *adenoma sebaceum* a misnomer when used to describe patients with tuberous sclerosis?

On biopsy, these papules are actually angiofibromas. They have no connection to sebaceous units or adenomas. This rash occurs in about 75% of patients with tuberous sclerosis, usually developing on the nose and face between ages 5 and 13 years. It is red, papular, and monomorphous and is often mistaken for acne. The diagnosis of TSC should be entertained in children who develop a rash suggestive of acne well before puberty.

163. What is the "tuber" of tuberous sclerosis?

These 1–2-cm lesions consist of small stellate neurons and astroglial elements thought to be primitive cell lines resulting from abnormal differentiation. They may be located in various cortical regions. They are firm to the touch, like a small potato or tuber.

164. What is the tissue type of a shagreen patch?

A shagreen patch is an area of cutaneous thickening with a pebbled surface that, on biopsy, is a ***connective tissue nevus***. The term *shagreen* derives from a type of leather that is embossed by knobs in the course of processing.

165. Which types of facial port-wine stains are most strongly associated with ophthalmic or CNS complications?

Port-wine stains can occur as isolated cutaneous birthmarks or, particularly in the areas underlying the birthmark, in association with structural abnormalities in (1) choroidal vessels of the eye leading to glaucoma, (2) leptomeningeal vessels in the the brain leading to seizures (Sturge-Weber syndrome), and (3) hemangiomas in the spinal cord (Cobb syndrome). In a study by Tallman et al., glaucoma or seizures were most associated with port-wine stains in children demonstrating:

- Involvement of the eyelids
- Bilateral distribution of the birthmark
- Unilateral involvement of all three branches (V_1, V_2, V_3) of the trigeminal nerve

Ophthalmologic assessment and radiologic studies (CT or MRI) are indicated for children exhibiting these findings.

Tallman B, et al: Location of port-wine stains and the likelihood of ophthalmic and/or central nervous system complications. Pediatrics 87:323–327, 1991.

166. What is unique to the genetics of epidermal nevus syndrome?

The ***complete absence of vertical transmission*** and the ***exclusively partial character*** of the epidermal nevus syndrome support the hypothesis that the epidermal nevus syndrome is due to an autosomal dominant lethal mutation with expression from a partial somatic mutation. It involves eye, bone, and brain. The central nervous system abnormalities consist of hemimegencephaly, mental retardation, seizures, and stroke due to cerebrovascular dysplasia. Dermatologic findings include verrucous, hyperkeratotic papules in a linear array (often widespread), hemangiomas, café-au-lait spots, and areas of hypopigmentation.

167. What are the three stages of incontinentia pigmenti?

Incontinentia pigmenti is an X-linked dominant disorder associated with seizures and mental retardation. The condition is presumed lethal to boys in utero because nearly 100% of cases are female.

Stage 1—***Vesicular stage***. Lines of blisters on the trunk and extremities in the newborn that disappear in weeks or months. They may resemble herpetic vesicles. Microscopic examination of the vesicular fluid demonstrates eosinophils.

Stage 2—***Verrucous stage***. Lesions develop around age 3–7 months that are brown and hyperkeratotic, resembling warts. These disappear over 1–2 years.

*Stage 3—**Pigmented stage***. Whorled, swirling (marble cake-like) macular hyperpigmented lines develop. These may fade over time, leaving only remnant hypopigmentation in late adolescence or adulthood (which is sometimes considered a fourth stage).

NEUROMUSCULAR DISORDERS

168. What constitutes the motor unit?

The anatomic unit of histologic organization of striated skeletal muscle is the fiber, microscopically visible as a long cylindrical cell with numerous nuclei dispersed along its length. Numerous parallel fibers are grouped together into fascicles, visible to the naked eye. The functional unit of organization of skeletal muscle is the motor unit, which includes (1) the ***anterior horn cell or alpha motor neuron***, whose cell body lies in the ventral gray mass of the spinal cord; (2) its ***axon***, which leaves the cord in the ventral root and courses in the peripheral nerve wrapped in its myelin sheath; and (3) ***several target muscle fibers*** within the same fascicle. Thus, the smallest natural amount of muscle activity is the firing of one motor neuron, producing contraction of its multiple target fibers.

169. How do muscle fibrillation and fasciculation differ?

A **fibrillation** is the spontaneous contraction of an individual muscle fiber. It produces no shortening of the muscle and cannot be observed through the skin but may rarely be visible in the tongue. Fibrillations are detected by an electromyographic (EMG) examination and recognized as irregular, asynchronous, brief (1–5 msec), low-voltage (20–300 μV), electrical discharges of the muscle fiber that recur with a frequency of 1–30/second. They usually arise in the setting of denervation from injury to the cell body or axon but also may occur in primary disorders such as myopathy.

A **fasciculation** is the spontaneous, relatively synchronous contraction of numerous fibers within a fascicle that belong to the same motor unit. The contraction may produce a visible movement of the muscle and can be seen through the skin. On EMG examination, the electrical discharge of the fasciculation is distinctly longer (8–20 msec) and has a higher voltage (2–6 mV) than the fibrillation potential. Fasciculations recur at irregular intervals with a frequency of 1–50/minute. Benign fasciculations in the calf and small muscles of the hands or feet can be seen in some healthy people. Fasciculations are not characteristic of primary muscle diseases. They are usually associated with denervation of any cause but are especially prominent in disorders of anterior horn cells such as Werdnig-Hoffman disease.

170. How is tone defined?

Tone is the ***resistance to passive stretch***. Abnormalities of tone are hypertonia, caused by upper motor neuron dysfunction, and hypotonia, which can result from damage to any part of the nervous system, although it is classically associated with lower motor neuron dysfunction. The upper motor neuron has its cell body in the cerebral cortex. Its axon terminates in either the brain stem (to innervate a cranial nerve) or the spinal cord (to innervate the lower motor neurons of the rest of the body). The cell body of the lower motor neuron is in the anterior portion of the spinal cord; its axon extends to the neuromuscular junction, where it innervates the muscle.

171. Why are tendon (stretch) reflexes important?

Gently tapping the tendon insertions of muscles and palpating the muscle and observing its contraction tests a reflex arc from the sensory input to the cord and back to the muscle as modified by a cortical inhibition feedback loop. The biceps and patellar reflexes are most reliably testable in term neonates. An asymmetry of reflexes suggests a unilateral process and a spread of reflexes to the contralateral muscle group to that tested indicates

CNS involvement. A decrease or absence of reflexes indicates involvement of the peripheral nervous system and an increase in tendon reflexes dysfunction of upper motor neurons.

172. What are signs of upper and lower motor nerve dysfunction?

Hypotonia and weakness can result from a myriad of causes. Lesions of the upper motor neuron may show normal to slightly decreased bulk, increased tone, and increased tendon reflexes and extensor plantar responses. Lesions of the lower motor neuron show decreased muscle bulk, decreased tone, decreased or absent reflexes, and nonreactive or flexor plantar responses. Fasciculations are fine, irregular, trembling, twitching movements of small lower motor neuron groups, and they usually indicate an abnormality of the anterior horn cell. They are difficult to detect in the infant and are best seen in the tongue of the infant when comfortable and quiet. They may be seen normally in the muscles of individuals who are tired or under stress.

173. When are nerve conduction studies (NCS) and EMG useful?

The examination of nerve conduction velocities and muscle potentials is an extension of the neurologic examination and is useful in distinguishing nerve from muscle disorders and for examination of the neuromuscular junction. Nerve conduction may be slowed in processes affecting the large diameter fibers, or there may be a decrease in amplitude as seen in a demyelinating neuropathy. Needle EMG may show abnormal spontaneous activity and the recruitment pattern seen in activation of motor units. Performance of needle EMG may be somewhat painful, is difficult to perform well in children and infants, and should be done by those familiar with the interpretation of findings in children.

174. How can the anatomic site responsible for muscle weakness be determined clinically?

Clinical Determination of Anatomic Site Responsible for Muscle Weakness

	UPPER MOTOR NEURON	ANTERIOR HORN CELL	NEUROMUSCULAR JUNCTION	PERIPHERAL NERVE	MUSCLE
Tone	Increased (may be decreased acutely)	Decreased	Normal, variable	Decreased	Decreased
Distribution	Pattern (hemiparesis, paraparesis, etc.) Distal > proximal	Variable, asymmetric	Fluctuating, cranial nerve involvement	Nerve distribution	Proximal > distal
Reflexes	Increased (may be decreased early)	Decreased to absent	Normal (unless severely involved)	Decreased to absent	Decreased
Babinski	Extensor	Flexor	Flexor	Flexor	Flexor
Other	Cognitive dysfunction, atrophy only very late	Fasciculations, atrophy, no sensory involvement	Fluctuating course	Sensory nerve involvement, atrophy, rare fasciculations	No sensory deficits; may be tenderness and signs of inflammation

Adapted from Packer RJ, Berman PH: Neurologic emergencies. In Fleisher GR, Ludwig S (eds): Textbook of Pediatric Emergency Medicine, 3rd ed. Baltimore, Williams & Wilkins, 1993, p 584.

175. What are the causes of acute generalized weakness?

- ***Infectious/postinfectious conditions*****:** acute infectious myositis, Guillain-Barré syndrome, enteroviral infection

- ***Metabolic disorders*:** acute intermittent porphyria, hereditary tyrosinemia
- ***Neuromuscular blockade*:** botulism, tick paralysis
- ***Periodic paralysis*:** familial (hyperkalemic, hypokalemic, normokalemic)

Fenichel GM: Clinical Pediatric Neurology: A Signs and Symptoms Approach, 4th ed. Philadelphia, W.B. Saunders, 2001.

176. If a child presents with weakness, what aspects of the history and physical exam suggest a myopathic process?

History

- Onset gradual rather than sudden
- Proximal weakness predominates (e.g., climbing stairs, running) rather than distal weakness (more characteristic of neuropathy)
- Absence of sensory abnormalities, such as “pins-and-needles” sensations
- No bowel and bladder abnormalities

Physical exam

- Proximal weakness > distal weakness (except in myotonic dystrophy)
- Positive Gower sign (patient arises from sitting position by pushing the trunk erect by bracing arms against anterior thigh, due to weakness of the pelvic girdle and lower extremities)
- Neck flexion weaker than neck extension
- In early stages, reflexes normal or only slightly decreased
- Normal sensory exam
- Muscle wasting, but no fasciculations
- Muscle hypertrophy seen in some dystrophies

Weiner HL, Urion DK, Levitt LP: Pediatric Neurology for the House Officer. Baltimore, William & Wilkins, 1988.

177. How does EMG help differentiate between myopathic and neurogenic disorders?

EMG measures the electrical activity of resting and voluntary muscle activity. Normally, the action potentials are of standardized duration and amplitude with 2–4 distinguishable phases. In **myopathic** conditions, the durations and amplitudes are shorter than expected. In **neuropathies**, they are longer. In both conditions, extra phases (i.e., polyphasic units) are usually noted.

178. How is pseudoparalysis distinguished from true neuromuscular disease?

Pseudoparalysis (hysterical paralysis) or weakness may be seen in conversion reactions (i.e., emotional conflicts presenting as symptoms). In conversion reactions, sensation, deep tendon reflexes, and the Babinski response are normal. Movement may also be noted during sleep. The *Hoover test* is helpful in unilateral paralysis. With the patient lying supine on the table, the examiner places a hand under the heel of the unaffected limb and asks the patient to raise the plegic limb. In pseudoparalysis, no pressure is felt under the heel on the unaffected side.

179. Why is localization of the cause of hypotonia important?

Hypotonia is a common but nonspecific sign in neonates and young infants. Localization of the level of the lesion is critical in determining the nature of the pathologic process. In the absence of an acute encephalopathy, the differential diagnosis of hypotonia is best approached by asking the question: Does the patient have normal strength despite the hypotonia, or is the patient weak and hypotonic? The combination of weakness and hypotonia usually points to an abnormality of the anterior horn cell or the peripheral neuromuscular apparatus, whereas hypotonia with normal strength is more characteristic of brain or spinal cord disturbances.

- **Systemic causes** include any acute serious medical illness, such as sepsis, shock, dehydration, hypoglycemia and electrolyte abnormalities.
- **Cerebral disorders** include genetic abnormalities (e.g., trisomy 21, Turner syndrome, Prader-Willi syndrome); congenital structural malformations of the brain (e.g., lissencephaly or Miller-Dieker syndrome); acute infectious or traumatic insults; and metabolic encephalopathies (e.g., hypothyroidism, Lowe syndrome, Canavan disease).
- **Brain stem, spinal cord lesions**, and **motor neuron disorders** include spinal muscular atrophy, glycogen storage disease type II (Pompe), and polio.
- **Peripheral nerve** causes include familial dysautonomia (Riley Day syndrome) and, acutely, in Guillain-Barré syndrome.
- **Neuromuscular junction** conditions include myasthenia gravis and infantile botulism.
- **Muscle** causes include dystrophies and myopathies.

In the absence of other causes and with normal development, benign congenital hypotonia may be tentatively diagnosed.

180. How can you detect myotonia clinically?

Myotonia is the painless tonic spasm of muscle following voluntary contraction, involuntary failure of relaxation, or delayed muscle relaxation following a contraction. It can be elicited by grip (e.g., handshake), forced eyelid closure (or delayed eye opening in crying infants), lid lag after upward gaze, or percussion over various sites (e.g., thenar eminence or tongue).

181. How do the presentations of the two forms of myotonic dystrophy differ?

***Congenital*:** Presentation is in the immediate newborn period. Symptoms include hypotonia, facial diplegia with "tenting" of the upper lip, and frequently severe respiratory distress secondary to intercostal and diaphragmatic weakness, especially the right hemidiaphragm. Feeding problems due to poor suck and gastrointestinal dysmotility are also present.

***Juvenile*:** Presentation is in the first decade of life. This form is characterized by progressive weakness and atrophy of facial and sternocleidocmastoid muscles and shoulder girdle, impaired hearing and speech, and excessive daytime sleepiness. Clinical myotonia is more likely, and there may be mental retardation.

182. In a newborn with weakness and hypotonia, what obstetric and delivery features suggest a diagnosis of congenital myotonic dystrophy?

History of spontaneous abortions, polyhydramnios, decreased fetal movements, delays in second-stage labor, retained placenta, and postpartum hemorrhage all raise the concern for congenital myotonic dystrophy. Because the mother is nearly always affected in congenital myotonic dystrophy (although previously diagnosed in only half the cases), a careful clinical and EMG evaluation of the mother is essential.

183. Why is myotonic dystrophy an example of the phenomenon of "anticipation"?

Genetic studies have shown that the defect in myotonic dystrophy is an expansion of a trinucleotide (CTG) in a gene on the long arm of chromosome 19 that codes for a protein kinase. The gene product was named myotonin-protein kinase (MT-PK), and it is thought to be involved in sodium and chloride channel function. In successive generations, this repeating sequence has a tendency to increase, sometimes into the thousands (normal is < 40 CTG repeats), and the extent of repetition correlates with the severity of the disease. Thus, each succeeding generation is likely to get more extensive manifestations and earlier presentations of the disease (i.e., the phenomenon of *anticipation*).

184. How does the pathophysiology of infant botulism differ from that of food-borne botulism?

Infant botulism results from the ingestion of *Clostridium botulinum* spores that germinate, multiply, and produce toxin in the infant's intestine. The source of the spores is often unknown, but it has been linked to honey in some cases, and spores have been found in corn syrups. Therefore, these foods are not advised for infants < 1 year of age. In **food-borne botulism**, preformed toxin is already present in the food. Improper canning and anaerobic storage permits spore germination, growth, and toxin formation, which results in symptoms if the toxin is not destroyed by proper heating. **Wound botulism**, which is rare, occurs if spores enter a deep wound and germinate.

185. What is the earliest indication for intubation in an infant with botulism?

Intubation is indicated is there is loss of protective airway reflexes. This occurs before respiratory compromise or failure because diaphragmatic function is not impaired until 90–95% of the synaptic receptors are occupied. Indeed, an infant with hypercarbia or hypoxia is at very high risk for imminent respiratory failure.

Schreiner MS, et al: Infant botulism: A review of 12 years' experience at the Children's Hospital of Philadelphia. Pediatrics 87:159–165, 1991.

186. What is so big about BIG in the treatment of infant botulism?

BIG is botulinum immune globulin or now more properly called human-derived botulinum antitoxin. Antitoxins have traditionally not been used in cases of infant botulism because of delayed diagnosis, concerns about serum sickness and anaphylaxis, erroneous beliefs that circulating toxins were not found in ongoing disease and questions of efficacy. However, a 5-year randomized study has shown that the early use of this antitoxin (even before laboratory confirmation of the disease) has safely resulted in fewer hospital days, lessened the need for mechanical ventilation and tube feedings and significantly reduced hospital costs. At present, the product is available through the California Department of Health Services.

187. In an infant with severe weakness and suspected botulism, why is the use of aminoglycosides relatively contraindicated?

The botulism toxin acts by irreversibly blocking acetylcholine release from the presynaptic nerve terminals. Aminoglycosides, as well as tetracyclines, clindamycin, and trimethoprim, also interfere with acetylcholine release. Therefore, they have the potential to act synergistically with the botulinum toxin to worsen or prolong neuromuscular paralysis.

188. Why does botulism occur more commonly in mountain locales?

Most cases of food-borne botulism result from ingestion of improperly canned or cooked food. Usually, boiling for 10 minutes destroys the botulinum toxin if it is present in food. However, in the higher altitudes of mountainous areas, water boils at a lower temperature, which may be insufficient for exotoxin destruction.

189. What are the two most common symptoms in children presenting with juvenile myasthenia gravis?

Ptosis and ***diplopia***. Myasthenia gravis is characterized by a highly variable clinical course of fluctuating weakness (characteristically with increasing contractions) initially involving muscles innervated by cranial nerves. It is caused by a defect in neuromuscular transmission due to an autoimmune antibody–mediated attack on the acetylcholine receptors.

190. How is congenital myasthenia gravis differentiated from infant botulism?

Very few cases of **botulism** have been reported in neonates. Symptoms have always occurred after discharge from the neonatal nursery. Botulism is usually heralded by constipation, followed by early facial and pharyngeal weakness, ptosis, and dilated, sluggishly reactive pupils with diminished deep tendon reflexes. The injection of edrophonium does not improve muscle strength. EMG examination demonstrates distinctive abnormalities such as brief small-amplitude polyphasic potentials (BSAPs) and an incremental response in the amplitude of evoked muscle potentials to repetitive nerve stimulation. Stool cultures may be positive for the toxin or clostridia organism.

Congenital myasthenia gravis usually presents at birth or within the first few days of life. There may be a family history of myasthenia in the mother or siblings. The distribution of weakness depends on the specific subtype of myasthenia, but pupils and deep tendon reflexes are spared. The EMG examination shows a distinctive progressive decline in the amplitude of compound motor action potentials with repetitive stimulation of the nerve. Edrophonium temporarily improves the patient's clinical strength and abolishes the pathologic EMG response to repetitive stimulation.

191. What are the risks to a neonate born to a mother with myasthenia gravis?

Passively acquired neonatal myasthenia develops in about 10% of infants born to myasthenic mothers because of the transplacental transfer of antibody directed against acetylcholine receptors (AChR) in striated muscle. Signs and symptoms of weakness typically arise within the first hours or days of life. Pathologic muscle fatigability commonly causes feeding difficulty, generalized weakness, hypotonia, and respiratory depression. Ptosis and impaired eye movements occur in only 15% of cases. The weakness virtually always resolves as the body burden of anti-AChR immunoglobulin diminishes. Symptoms typically persist about 2 weeks but may require several months to disappear entirely. General supportive treatment is usually adequate, but oral or intramuscular neostigmine may help to diminish symptoms.

192. How does the pathophysiology differ in juvenile versus congenital myasthenia gravis?

Juvenile (and adult) myasthenia gravis is caused by ***circulating antibodies*** to the AChR of the postsynaptic neuromuscular junction. Occurrence is rare before age 2 years. *Congenital myasthenia gravis* is a ***nonimmunologic process***. It is caused by morphologic or physiologic features affecting the pre- and postsynaptic junctions, including defects in ACh synthesis, endplate acetylcholinesterase deficiency, and endplate AChR deficiency. *Neonatal myasthenia gravis* refers to the transient weakness occurring in infants of mothers with myasthenia gravis.

193. How is the edrophonium (Tensilon) test done?

Edrophonium is a rapid-acting anticholinesterase drug of short duration that improves symptoms of myasthenia gravis by inhibiting the breakdown of ACh and increasing its concentration in the neuromuscular junction. A test dose of 0.015 mg/kg is given intravenously, and if tolerated, the full dose of 0.15 mg/kg (up to 10 mg) is given. If measurable improvement in ocular muscle or extremity strength occurs, myasthenia gravis is likely. Because edrophonium may precipitate a cholinergic crisis (e.g., bradycardia, hypotension, vomiting, bronchospasm), atropine and resuscitation equipment should be available.

194. Does a negative antibody test exclude the diagnosis of juvenile myasthenia gravis?

No. Up to 90% of children with juvenile myasthenia have measurable anti-AChR antibodies, but in the other 10%, continued clinical suspicion is necessary because their symptoms are usually milder (e.g., ocular muscle weakness or minimal generalized weakness). In these children, other tests (e.g., edrophonium, electrophysiologic studies, single-fiber EMG) may be needed to make the diagnosis.

195. What are the four characteristic features of damage to the anterior horn cells?
Weakness, fasciculations, atrophy, and ***hyporeflexia***.

196. What processes can damage the anterior horn cells?

- ***Degenerative*** (spinal muscular atrophy): Werdnig-Hoffman, Kugelberg-Welander, Pena-Shokeir, and Manden-Walker syndromes
- ***Metabolic*:** Tay-Sachs disease (hexosaminidase deficiency), Pompe disease, Batten disease (ceroid-lipofuscinosis), hyperglycinemia, neonatal adrenoleukodystrophy
- ***Infectious*:** poliovirus, coxsackievirus, ECHO viruses

197. How are the inherited progressive spinal muscular atrophies distinguished?

Recessive spinal muscular atrophy (SMA) of both early (type 1) and late (type 3) onset have been linked to the same region chromosome 5. A diagnostic test using polymerase chain reaction technology that has high sensitivity and specificity is available.

Progressive Spinal Muscular Atrophies

DISORDER	INHERITANCE	AGE OF ONSET	CLINICAL FEATURES
Acute infantile SMA (Werdnig-Hoffmann disease, SMA type 1)	Autosomal recessive	In utero–6 mos	Frog-leg posture; areflexia; tongue atrophy and fasciculations; progressive swallowing and respiratory problems; survival < 4 yrs
Intermediate SMA chronic Werdnig-Hoffmann disease,	Autosomal recessive; rarely autosomal dominant SMA type 2)	3 mos–15 yrs	Proximal weakness; most sit unsupported; decreased or absent reflexes; high incidence of scoliosis, contractures; survival may be up to 30 years
Kugelberg-Welander disease (SMA type 3)	Autosomal recessive; rarely autosomal dominant	5 yrs–15 yrs	May be part of spectrum of SMA 2; hip girdle weakness; calf hypertrophy; decreased or absent reflexes; may be ambulatory until fourth decade

Adapted from Parke JT: Disorders of the anterior horn cell. In McMillan JA, et al (eds): Oski's Pediatrics. Principles and Practice, 3rd ed. Philadelphia, J.B. Lippincott, 1999, p 1959.

198. What are muscular dystrophies?

A *muscular dystrophy* is an inheritable myopathy affecting limbs or facial muscles that are progressive with pathologic evidence of degeneration or regeneration without any abnormal storage material.

199. What is the clinical importance of dystrophin?

Dystrophin is a muscle protein that is presumed to be involved in anchoring the contractile apparatus of striated and cardiac muscle to the cell membrane. Due to a gene mutation, this protein is completely missing in patients with Duchenne muscular dystrophy. On the other hand, muscle tissue from patients with Becker muscular dystrophy contains reduced amounts of dystrophin or, occasionally, a protein of abnormal size.

200. How are Duchenne and Becker muscular dystrophy distinguished?

	GENETICS	DIAGNOSIS	MANIFESTATIONS
Duchenne	1:3,500 male births X-linked Several different deletions/ point mutations in dystrophin gene result in a completely nonfunctional protein New mutations occur Carrier females may have mild weakness or cardiomyopathy	Whole blood DNA may reveal a deletion in ~ 65%. Otherwise, EMG and muscle biopsy studies are definitive	Clinically evident at 3-5 years of age Regular, stereotyped course of progressive Proximal weakness Calf hypertrophy Loss of ambulation by 9–12 years Worsening scoliosis and contractures Eventual dilated cardiomyopathy and/or respiratory failure Life expectancy of 16–19 years
Becker	1:20,000 male births X-linked Various mutations in dystrophin gene result in reduced amount or partially functional protein	More benign clinical course Reduced dystrophin levels in muscle cells (by immunostaining) or abnormal dystrophin	Clinically evident in early second decade Milder, slower course compared to Duchenne Calf pseudohypertrophy Pes cavus Cardiac and CNS involvement unusual Ambulatory until 18 years or beyond Life expectancy twice as long compared to Duchenne

Adapted from Tsao VY, Mendell JR: The childhood muscular dystrophies: Making order out of chaos. Semin Neurol 19:9-23, 1999.

201. Is corticosteroid therapy effective in Duchenne muscular dystrophy?

Several studies have documented an improvement in strength with an optimal dose of prednisone of 0.75 mg/kg/day. The strengthening effect lasts for up to 3 years while the steroid is continued. Appropriate timing and duration of treatment have not been established, and side effects (weight gain and increased susceptibility to infection) may outweigh the benefits in many cases.

202. What are the hereditary neuropathies?

Some disorders of the peripheral nerve result from an inherited molecular or biochemical disturbance. Although relatively uncommon, they collectively account for a substantial percentage of neuropathies that are supposedly "idiopathic." Inheritance is most commonly dominant (e.g., type 1 or demyelinating Charcot-Marie-Tooth disease) but may be recessive or X-linked. They present as a chronic, slowly progressive, noninflammatory degeneration of the nerve cell body, peripheral axon, or Schwann cells (myelin). The neurologic consequences may be predominantly sensory (e.g., congenital insensitivity to pain) or mixed motor and sensory abnormalities (e.g., Charcot-Marie-Tooth). Deafness, optic neuropathy, and autonomic neuropathy are occasionally associated.

203. In an individual infected with poliovirus, how likely is the development of paralysis?

In immunocompetent hosts, up to 95% of poliovirus infections in susceptible individuals are asymptomatic. About 4–8% of patients experience a minor illness of low-grade fever, sore throat, and malaise. Less than 1–2% of patients experience CNS involvement, which can include aseptic meningitis (nonparalytic poliomyelitis) and paralytic poliomyelitis. Only 0.1% of patients have residual paralysis.

204. What is the most likely diagnosis in a child with progressive walking difficulties evolving over several days?

Guillain-Barré syndrome (GBS) is an acute demyelinating neuropathy characterized by ascending, acute, progressive peripheral and cranial nerve dysfunction and paresthesias. In younger children (< 6 years), it may be heralded by pain. It is frequently preceded by a viral respiratory or gastrointestinal illness, immunizations, or surgery. The disease is characterized by the presence of multifocal areas of inflammatory demyelination of nerve roots and peripheral nerves. As a result of the loss of the healthy myelin covering, the conduction of nerve impulses (action potentials) may be blocked or dispersed. The resulting clinical effects are predominantly motor—the evolution of flaccid, areflexic paralysis. There is a variable degree of motor weakness. Some individuals have mild brief weakness, whereas fulminant paralysis occurs in others. Autonomic signs (e.g., tachycardia, hypertension) or sensory symptoms such as painful dysesthesias are not uncommon but are overshadowed by the motor signs. More than half of patients develop facial involvement, and mechanical ventilation may be required. The ***Miller-Fisher variant*** is characterized by gait ataxia, areflexia, and ophthalmoparesis.

Nguyen DK, et al: Pain and the Guillain-Barré syndrome in children under 6 years old. J Pediatr 134:773-776, 1999.

205. What CSF findings are characteristic of GBS?

The classic CSF finding is the ***albuminocytologic dissociation***. Most common infections or inflammatory processes generate an elevation of white blood cell count *and* protein. The CSF profile in GBS includes a normal cell count with elevated protein, usually in the range of 50–100 mg/dl, but at the onset of disease, the CSF protein concentration may be normal.

206. Outline the management of acute Guillain-Barré syndrome.

Early clinical monitoring is focused on the development of bulbar or respiratory insufficiency. Bulbar weakness manifests as unilateral or bilateral facial weakness, diplopia, hoarseness, drooling, depressed gag reflex, or dysphagia. Frank respiratory insufficiency may be preceded by air hunger, dyspnea, or a soft muffled voice (hypophonia). The autonomic nervous system is occasionally involved, as signified by the presence of labile blood pressure and body temperature. The management of GBS includes:

- Observation in an intensive care unit with frequent monitoring of vital signs.
- The early institution of plasmapheresis or intravenous immunoglobulin shortens the clinical course and lessens long-term morbidity. The value of corticosteroid therpy is controversial.
- If bulbar signs are present, the patient should receive nothing orally (NPO), and the mouth is suctioned frequently. Hydration is maintained intravenously, and nutritional support is rovided by nasogastric feedings.
- The vital capacity (VC) is measured frequently. In children, the normal VC may be calculated as VC = 200 ml × age (in yrs). If the VC falls below 25% of normal, endotracheal intubation is done. Careful pulmonary toilet is conducted to minimize atelectasis, aspiration, and pneumonia.
- Meticulous nursing care includes careful patient positioning to prevent pressure sores, compression of peripheral nerves, and venous thrombosis.
- Physical therapy is conducted to prevent the development of contractures by passive range of movement exercises and splinting to maintain physiologic hand and limb postures until muscle strength returns.

207. What is the prognosis for children with GBS?

Children seem to recover more quickly and more fully than adults. Fewer than 10% have significant residual deficits. In rare cases, the neuropathy may recur as a chronic inflammatory demyelinating polyneuropathy.

208. How do syndromes of ascending paralysis compare in the clinical presentation?

Features of Four Similar Syndromes of Ascending Paralysis

FEATURE	TICK PARALYSIS	GUILLAIN-BARRÉ SYNDROME	SPINAL CORD LESION	POLIOMYELITIS
Ataxia	Present	Absent	Absent	Absent
Rate of progression	Hours to days	Days to weeks	Gradual or abrupt	Days to weeks
Muscle-stretch reflexes	Absent	Absent	Variable	Absent
Babinski sign	Absent	Absent	Present	Absent
Sensory loss	None	Mild	Present	None
Meningeal signs	Absent	Rare	Absent	Present
Fever	Absent	Rare	Absent	Present
Cerebrospinal fluid findings				
Protein level	Normal	High	Normal or high	High
White-cell count (per mm^3)	< 10	< 10	Variable	> 10
Time to recovery	< 24 hr after tick removal	Weeks to months	Variable, dependind on cause	Months to years or no recovery (permanent paresis)

From Felz MW, et al: A six-year-old girl with tick paralysis. N Engl J Med 342:90–94, 2000; with permission.

209. How does multiple sclerosis (MS) present in childhood?

MS is extremely rare in childhood (0.2–2.0% of all cases). Studies of affected children demonstrate a variable predominance of boys in early childhood and females during adolescence. Ataxia, muscle weakness, and transient visual or sensory symptoms are relatively common presentations. CSF examination may demonstrate mild (< 25 cells/mm^3) mononuclear pleocytosis with an increasing probability of oligoclonal bands with each recurrence. MRI is the single most useful diagnostic test: the presence of multiple, periventricular white matter plaques (bright areas on T2 images) confirms the diagnosis.

Duquette P, et al: Clinical profiles of 125 children with multiple sclerosis. J Pediatr 111:359, 1987.

SEIZURE DISORDERS

210. What is epilepsy?

Epilepsy is a word that describes a syndrome of recurrent, unprovoked, seizures. It is derived from the Greek verb meaning "to seize upon" or "take hold of." The early Greeks referred to it as the sacred disease, but Hippocrates debunked this notion and argued from clinical evidence that it arose from the brain. Epilepsy is not an entity, or even a syndrome, but rather a symptom complex arising from disordered brain function that itself may be secondary to a variety of pathologic processes.

211. How common is epilepsy in the U.S.?

Approximately 2 million Americans have epilepsy, and about one-third are children. Over 4% of white middle-class populations can be expected to have a seizure by age 20, and people living in socioeconomically deprived areas are at double the risk. The cumulative incidence of epilepsy is 1.2% through age 24 years. Seizures and epilepsy occur most frequently in infants and the elderly. The annual incidence of epilepsy per 100,000 population is 86 in the first year of life; 62 at ages 1–5 years, 50 at 5–9 years, and 39 at 10–14 years. In over 65% of patients, epilepsy begins in childhood.

Annegers JF: Epidemiology and genetics of epilepsy. Neurol Clin 12:15-29, 1994.

212. What is the long-term outcome for children with epilepsy?

There are many different causes of epilepsy, and, in large part, the outcome relates to the underlying etiology. Children with idiopathic or genetically determined epilepsy have the best prognosis, whereas children with antecedent neurologic abnormalities fare less well. Nearly 75% of children will enter into a sustained remission 3–5 years after onset of their epilepsy. There is no evidence that antiepileptic medications, as they are currently used in clinical practice, are neuroprotective or that they alter the long-term outcome of our patients. Even though there is a favorable prognosis for remission of seizures, children with epilepsy are at an increased risk for having other long-term challenges, including difficulties achieving social, educational, and vocational goals. Treatment with antiepileptic medications is one important part of the management of the child, but other critical aspects of the physician-patient interaction, including educating, counseling, and advocacy, are equally important.

213. How often are EEGs abnormal in healthy children?

Approximately 10% of "normal" children have mild, nonspecific abnormalities in background activity. About 2–3% of healthy children have unexpected incidental epileptiform (i.e., spikes or sharp wave) patterns. Some may have heritable, familial EEG abnormalities without a clinical seizure disorder.

214. Should an EEG be done on all children who have a first afebrile seizure?

This is a major, controversial issue. Of new-onset seizures in children, about one-third do not involve fever. The American Academy of Neurology has recommended that all children with a first seizure without fever undergo an EEG in effort to better classify the epilepsy syndrome. Others argue that the quantity of expected information from obtaining EEGs on all cases is too low to affect treatment recommendations in most patients. They suggest a selective approach to EEG use should be pursued, particularly for children with a seizure of focal onset, children under the age of 1 year, and any child with unexplained cognitive or motor dysfunction or abnormalities on neurologic exam.

Gilbert DL, et al: An EEG should not be routinely obtained after first unprovoked seizure in childhood. Neurology 54:635-641, 2000.

Hirtz D, et al: Practice parameter: evaluating a first nonfebrile seizure in children: Report of the Quality Standards Subcommittee of the American Academy of Neurology, the Child Neurology Society, and the American Epilepsy Society. Neurology 55:616-623, 2000.

215. Which disorders commonly mimic epilepsy?

Many conditions are characterized by the sudden onset of abnormal consciousness, awareness, reactivity, behavior, posture, tone, sensation, or autonomic function. Syncope, breath-holding spells, migraine, hypoglycemia, narcolepsy, cataplexy, sleep apnea, gastroesophageal reflux, and parasomnias (night terrors, sleep walking, sleep talking, nocturnal enuresis) feature an abrupt or "paroxysmal" alteration of brain function and suggest the possibility of epilepsy. Perhaps one of the most difficult attacks to distinguish is the "pseudoseizure," also called a pseudoepileptic seizure or hysterical seizure. These attacks are outwardly modeled after the patient's subconscious or conscious perception of a seizure and occur without abnormal electrical discharges of neurons in the CNS.

216. What are two key questions in the initial classification of seizures in children?

1. ***Where does the seizure begin?*** If it appears to begin in part of the brain, the seizure

is partial or "localization related." Partial seizures (formerly termed *focal*) are divided into simple and complex types. **Simple partial seizures** occur in the presence of a normal level of consciousness. **Complex partial** (formerly termed *psychomotor*) **seizures** produce an impairment of consciousness. If it appears to be a diffuse process involving the entire brain from the outset, it is a generalized seizure. Generalized seizures entail simultaneous, synchronous EEG discharges in both cerebral hemispheres. There may be complete loss of consciousness from the onset. **Primary generalized seizures** include some of the familial and sporadic epilepsy syndromes such as childhood absence (formerly termed *petit mal*) seizures, while **secondary generalized seizures** arise from localized lesions of the cortex. Generalized seizures of both types may involve a variety of motor patterns: tonic-clonic (formerly termed grand mal), myoclonic, atonic, clonic, and tonic.

2. ***Is brain development normal?*** Is it primary or idiopathic epilepsy or does it arise from a developmentally abnormal brain that is a secondary or symptomatic epilepsy. *Cryptogenic* is the term used to describe seizures in a child who has not had normal neurologic development in whom the etiology can not be found.

The EEG provides much additional information in classifying the seizure and syndrome as generalized or localization related and is also useful in guiding treatment and prognosis.

217. What are the categories of seizures in children?

The syndrome classification, as codified by the International League Against Epilepsy, distinguishes seizure on the basis of type rather than etiology. Combinations of seizure categories may occur in an individual patient.

International League Against Epilepsy Seizure Classification

Partial (focal, local) seizures	Generalized seizures
Simple partial seizures	Absence seizures, with impairment of consciousness, with clonic, atonic, tonic, or autonomic components, or with automatisms occurring alone or in combination
With motor signs: focal motor, Jacksonian, versive, postural, phonatory	Atypical absences, more pronounced changes of tone than in absence seizures; onset and/or cessation not abrupt
With somatosensory or special sensory symptoms (simple hallucinations, e.g., tingling, light flashes, buzzing): somatosensory, visual, auditory, olfactory, gustatory, vertiginous	Monoclonic seizures (single or multiple)
With autonomic symptoms and signs	Clonic seizures
With psychic symptoms (disturbances of higher cerebral functions): dysphasic, dysmnesic, cognitive, affective, illusions, structured hallucinations	Tonic seizures
Complex partial seizures (with impairment of consciousness)	Tonic–clonic seizures
Simple partial onset followed by impairment of consciousness	Atonic seizures
With no other features	***Unclassified epileptic seizures***
With simple partial features as in A1–A4	
With automatisms	
Partial seizures evolving to secondarily generalized tonic–clonic seizures	

Adapted from Vedanarayanan VV: Diagnosis of epilepsy in children. Pediatr Ann 28:219, 1999.

218. What are the causes of "symptomatic" seizures?

Symptomatic seizures are those that are caused by an identifiable injury to the brain (as opposed to idiopathic or cryptogenic epilepsy in which recurrent seizures are unprovoked).

The seizures are a sign of underlying disease or pathology that must be managed, if possible, independently of the seizure itself.

Causes of Symptomatic Seizures

Fever	**Toxins**
Simple febrile seizures	Drugs
Complicated febrile seizures	Drug withdrawal
Trauma	Biologic toxins
Impact seizures	**Stroke**
Early posttraumatic seizures	Ischemic stroke
Late posttraumatic seizures	Embolic stroke
Hypoxia	Hemorrhagic stroke
Complicated breath-holding spells	**Intracranial hemorrhage**
Hypoxic seizures	Subdural hemorrhage
Metabolic	Subarachnoid hemorrhage
Acquired metabolic disorders	Intracerebral hemorrhage
Neurologic effects of systemic disease	Intraventricular hemorrhage
Inborn errors of metabolism	

Adapted from Evans OB: Symptomatic seizures. Pediatr Ann 28:232, 1999.

219. If a previously normal child has an afebrile, generalized tonic-clonic seizure, what should parents be told about the risk of recurrence?

Studies indicate that the recurrence rate is *between 25% and 50%*. The EEG is an important predictor of recurrence. A subsequent normal EEG reduces the 5-year recurrence risk to 25%. Occurrence of the seizure during sleep increases the risk to 50%. Half of recurrences will occur in the first 6 months following the seizure, two-thirds by one year, and 90% or more by 2 years. The child's age at the time of first seizure or the duration of the seizure do not affect the recurrence risk.

Shinnar S, et al: The risk of seizure recurrence after a first unprovoked afebrile seizure in childhood: An extended follow-up. Pediatrics 98:216-225, 1996.

220. What characterizes generalized seizures in children?

A generalized seizure represents a diffuse process, and it is characterized by an abrupt onset with loss or alteration of consciousness and variable bilaterally symmetrical motor activity often associated with changes in muscle tone. The patient has no warning of an attack. Likewise, the EEG expression in this group of seizures is epileptiform activity that is generalized and bilaterally synchronous. Historically, seizures were of two types: "grand mal" and "petit mal." The tonic-clonic seizure (grand mal seizure) is the classic epileptic attack known since antiquity. Consciousness is lost immediately and completely in conjunction with massive sustained contractions of the entire musculature. As air is forcibly expressed through contracted vocal cords, the characteristic "epileptic cry" results. The eyes deviate conjugately upward. This tonic phase lasts 10–20 seconds and is followed by the clonic phase, which lasts about 30 seconds. This is a series of relaxations that simultaneously affects all muscle groups and rhythmically interrupts the sustained tonic muscular spasm. During the tonic phase, marked autonomic phenomena are evident. The interictal EEGs of children with idiopathic generalized convulsive seizures are similar and show generalized bursts of spikes and runs of irregular 4–6 Hz spike-wave complexes. Generalized epileptic seizures occur with greater frequency in children than in adults, representing about 55% of all seizures of childhood.

221. How does the etiology of partial seizures in children compare with adults?

The specific behavioral manifestations of partial or focal seizures relate to the region of brain involved in the epileptogenic discharge. In marked contrast to adults, most focal seizures in children are ***idiopathic***. Focal seizures are less frequent in children than in adults, accounting for about 45% of all childhood seizure disorders. As in adults, they may imply localized cerebral dysfunction, although in children this is unlikely to be caused by a definable lesion. Furthermore, there are several age-related focal epilepsy syndromes of childhood. All partial seizures have the potential for becoming secondarily generalized.

222. A previously healthy 6-year-old who develops sudden, intractable unilateral seizures likely has what condition?

Rasmussen syndrome involves the cataclysmic onset of partial (focal) seizures associated with cerebral inflammation evolving into epilepsia partialis continua and progressive loss of motor function on the affected side. There is progressive atrophy of the brain, and although immunosuppression has been tried with limited success, surgical resection is curative. It is thought to result from an autoimmune process against glutamate receptors of the cerebral cortex initiated by a focal break in the blood-brain barrier.

223. What is the clinical picture of children with complex partial seizures?

Complex partial seizures (formerly called *psychomotor seizures*) have only recently been well studied in children using modern monitoring techniques. Typical clinical and EEG manifestations seem to be uncommon in the very young child but are similar to those observed in adults after 8–10 years of age. The symptoms are varied, but they usually include alterations in consciousness, unresponsiveness, and automatisms. Complex partial seizures have now been well described in infants and young children and are characterized by an interruption of activity that has been described as a "behavioral arrest" or as a "hypomotor" seizure. Autonomic changes, hypopnea, and subtle "baby" automatisms have also been described. Eye deviation does not have the localizing value that is seen in older children and adults. Automatisms are repetitive complex motor activities that are purposeless, undirected, and inappropriate to the situation. Examples include lip smacking, repetitious swallowing or chewing, fidgeting movements of the fingers or hands, and clumsy preservation of a preceding motor act. Psychic phenomena may be reported at the onset of an attack, including a sense of detachment or depersonalization, forced thinking, visual distortions and formed hallucinations, visceral sensations, and a feeling of intense emotion such as fear. Postictally, patients are confused and recover full consciousness slowly. Postictally during a time of incomplete awareness, a child may resist restraint and react aggressively or angrily to objects and persons in their way. Nevertheless, rage attacks or temper tantrums do not occur as manifestations of epilepsy.

224. What are the treatment options for complex partial seizures?

Treatment of complex partial seizures is often frustrating, and seizures stop completely in less than one third of affected children. Carbamazepine and phenytoin are first-line medications. Gabapentin has recently been studied in younger children. Temporal lobectomy should be considered for a carefully selected number of children with refractory complex partial seizures arising exclusively from the anterior temporal lobe on one side with mesial temporal sclerosis or a structural lesion. Surgical results for focal epilepsy arising from other brain areas are not as good.

225. A 5-year-old with previously normal language development develops progressive aphasia and seizures and has an abnormal sleep EEG. He likely has what condition?

Landau-Kleffner syndrome. This is a syndrome of an acquired aphasia, seizures, and behavioral disorder that develops before age 7 years in children with early normal language acquisition. It is characterized by verbal and auditory agnosia and a progressive decline in language. Seizures are usually simple partial or generalized tonic-clonic. They typically appear between age 5 and 10 years, disappear between 10 and 15 years of age, and are usually responsive to AEDs. The EEG shows diffuse or multifocal spike wave discharges and focal spike wave discharges that are most prominent in the anterior and midtemporal regions. It is one of the syndromes characterized by continuous spike and wave discharges and can occur in up to 90% of the sleeping state. Etiology remains unknown.

226. What distinguishes atonic and akinetic seizures?

Atonic and akinetic seizures, astatic seizures, epileptic drop attacks, and "minor motor seizures" are all used interchangeably to encompass a variety of behavioral and clinical seizure manifestations. An **atonic** seizure is manifested by sudden and usually complete loss of tone in the limb, neck, and trunk muscles. An **akinetic** seizure is one in which movement is arrested without significant loss of muscle tone; this is very rare. In atonic seizures, muscular control is lost without warning, and the child may be seriously injured. This situation is often aggravated by the occurrence of one or more myoclonic jerks immediately before muscle tone is lost, so that the fall is associated with an element of propulsion. Atonic seizures are particularly common in children with static encephalopathies and may prove refractory to therapy.

227. What are the four most common inherited seizure syndromes?

1. Febrile convulsions
2. Benign rolandic epilepsy
3. Absence seizures
4. Juvenile myoclonic epilepsy (of Janz)

228. What are the diagnostic criteria for benign rolandic epilepsy?

Benign rolandic epilepsy is an idiopathic localization-related epilepsy with characteristic EEG and clinical features that occurs in previously healthy children ages 4–13 years. It represents 10–15% of all childhood seizure disorders. The following criteria help to establish the diagnosis:

- It begins during school age in otherwise healthy and neurologically normal children.
- The seizures are idiopathic or familial (rolandic epilepsy may be inherited in an autosomal dominant fashion).
- The clinical seizures may be simple or complex, partial or generalized. During wakefulness, the seizures have a clearly focal onset, with twitching of one side of the face, anarthria, drooling, and paresthesias of the face, gums, tongue, or inner cheeks that may be followed by hemiclonic movements or hemitonic posturing. Consciousness is typically preserved. These may become secondarily generalized, so that parents report only tonic-clonic convulsions. During sleep, generalized seizures seem to predominate, and as many as 75% of children have seizures principally or only at night.
- The EEG shows a distinctive type of sharp-slow wave discharges localized to the rolandic (central, midtemporal, central-temporal, or sylvian) regions.
- Ancillary neurodiagnostic tests are normal.

Rolandic epilepsy is often referred to as a benign syndrome because (1) the individual is otherwise normal; (2) the seizures are usually easily controlled with low doses of a single anticonvulsant (usually carbamazepine); and (3) the seizures virtually always abate after puberty.

229. Should all children with a new-onset afebrile generalized seizure have a CT or MRI evaluation?

While most adults with new-onset seizures should have a head imaging study (preferably MRI), the relatively high frequency of idiopathic seizure disorders in children often obviates a scan in those with generalized seizures, nonfocal EEGs, and normal neurologic exams. Consider obtaining a cranial imaging study for:

- Any seizure with focal components (other than mere eye deviation)
- Newborns and young infants with seizures
- Status epilepticus at any age
- Focal slowing or focal paroxysmal activity on EEG

230. What is the classic triad of infantile spasms?

Spasms, hypsarrhythmia, and ***developmental delay or regression.*** The condition is also called West syndrome, named for the physician who first described the condition (in his own son) in 1841:

> As the only case I have witnessed is in my own child . . . was a remarkably fine, healthy child when born, and continued to thrive till he was four months old. It was at this time that I first observed slight bobbings . . . increased in frequency, and at length became so frequent and powerful, these bowings and relaxings would be repeated alternatively at intervals of a few seconds, and repeated from ten to twenty or more times at each attack . . . he sometimes two, three, or more attacks in the day; just before they come on he is all alive and in motion, making a strange noise, and then all of a sudden down goes his head and upwards his knees; he then appears frightened and screams out.

West WJ: On a peculiar form of infantile convulsions. Lancet 1:724-725, 1841.

231. What characterizes hypsarhythmia?

The term means "mountainous slowing." It describes the classic interictal EEG of infantile spasms and is characterized by extremely high-voltage, slowed, disorganized brain waves with multifocal spike activity. Hypsarhythmia may either precede or follow the onset of infantile spasms. This EEG configuration may appear first or most obviously in non-REM sleep and confirms the clinical diagnosis of infantile spasms.

232. What are the proposed three main types of infantile spasms?

Infantile spasms are a unique epileptic syndrome of infancy and childhood characterized by clusters of spasms, usually beginning between 3 and 9 months of age. Traditionally classified as a myoclonic epilepsy, a phenomenologic division of infantile spasms into ***flexor, extensor***, and ***mixed-type*** spasms has been proposed on the basis of detailed video-EEG monitoring. However, such a division has no etiologic or prognostic significance.

Commission on Pediatric Epilepsy, International League Against Epilepsy: Workshop on infantile spasms. Epilepsia 33:195, 1992.

233. How commonly is a cause identified in infantile spasms?

A cause can be identified in up to 75% of children with infantile spasms, usually in those symptomatic at the time of the initial seizure. Of identifiable causes, three-fourths are prenatal/perinatal and one-fourth are postnatal. All patients with infantile spasms should have detailed neuroimaging and metabolic and genetic studies.

- **Prenatal/perinatal:** hypoxic-ischemic encephalopathy, tuberous sclerosis, neurofibromatosis, intrauterine infection (e.g., cytomegalovirus), brain malformations (e.g., lissencephaly, agenesis of the corpus callosum), inborn metabolic errors (e.g., nonketotic hyperglycinemia, phenylkenouria, maple syrup urine disease, pyridoxine dependency)
- **Postnatal:** infectious (e.g., herpes encephalitis), hypoxic-ischemic encephalopathy, head trauma

234. What is the prognosis for infants with infantile spasms?

Prognosis in large part depends on the clinical state at the time of the first seizure. In the cryptogenic or idiopathic group (10–15% of total), development and the neurologic exam and studies are normal at the onset. With adrenocorticoltropic hormone (ACTH) treatment, 40–65% will have a complete or near-complete recovery. In the symptomatic group (85–90% of total), neurologic deficits or cranial abnormalities are present before the first seizure. In this group, complete or near-complete recovery is achieved by only 5–15%.

235. What is the treatment of choice for infantile spasms?

Currently, in the United States, most children with infantile spasms are treated with ACTH as the first treatment option. The majority of patients will respond to this medication. American and Japanese data indicate that low-dose ACTH (10–20 IU of ACTH gel per day or less), given intramuscularly, can be effective. Some clinicians use doses as high as 150 IU/m^2 /day. The optimal dose, length of treatment, and schedule for weaning ACTH remain controversial. Vigabatrin, particularly in infants with tuberous sclerosis and those under 3 months of age, has been found useful in some studies. Vigabatrin is not approved for use by the FDA in the U.S., in part because of the possible side effects of constriction of peripheral visual fields.

Wong M, Trevathan E: Infantile spasms. Pediatr Neurol 24:89-98, 2001.

236. What is the rationale for administering ACTH or corticosteroids to children with infantile spasms?

There is believed to be a disturbance in the cortical-brain stem-adrenal axis, resulting in elevated levels of an endogenous epileptogenic substance (i.e., corticotropin-releasing factor [CRF]). Although the precise method of action is unclear, the administration of ACTH or steroids may serve as a negative feedback inhibitor of CRF. Studies suggest that even short-term ACTH therapy may be more efficacious than corticosteroids and is particularly useful in cryptogenic infantile spasms of recent onset.

Baram TZ, et al: High-dose corticosteroids (ACTH) versus prednisone for infantile spasms: A prospective, randomized, blinded study. Pediatrics 97:375–378, 1996.

237. What are the side effects associated with ACTH?

The potential side effects of ACTH are prodigious. The treatment is associated with approximately 5% mortality in some series due to massive ***gastric hemorrhage*** from ulceration of the mucosa, ***sepsis*** due to immunolgic compromise, or ***cardiac failure*** caused by a dilated cardiomyopathy. Echocardiography can reveal changes in advance of the clinical hypertension and may be a useful screening tool for the latter complication. Routine testing of stool for occult blood, regular monitoring of blood pressure, screening of urine for glucose, and institution of a low-salt diet are other appropriate precautions. In addition to these short-term side effects of ACTH, there are other complications related to prolonged use as with other steroid treatments.

238. What is the most likely diagnosis in a child of Ashkenazi descent with stimulus-sensitive seizures, cognitive deterioration, and slightly enlarged head?

The classic lysosomal lipid storage disorder presenting as a progressive encephalopathy in infancy is ***Tay-Sachs disease***. The infantile forms of GM_2 gangliosidosis includes Tay-Sachs disease, caused by deficiency of hexosaminidase A, and Sandhoff disease, caused by deficiency of hexosaminidase A and B. Tay-Sachs is an autosomal recessive disorder localized to chromosome 15 with an incidence of 1:3900 in the Ashkenazi Jewish population of Eastern or Central European descent. The enzymatic defect leads to intraneuronal accumulation of GM_2 ganglioside. Normal development is seen until 4–6 months when hypotonia and a loss of motor skills occur. Within the next 1–2 years, spasticity, blindness, and macrocephaly develop. At this stage, seizures become prominent with frequent partial motor, complex partial, and atypical absence seizures that respond poorly to medications. Myoclonic jerks are frequent and are often triggered by the exaggerated startle response to noise. The classic cherry red spot is present in the ocular fundi of more than 90% of patients.

239. A teenager, like his father, develops brief, bilateral, intermittent jerking of his arms. What seizure disorder is he likely to have?

Juvenile myoclonic epilepsy (JME), also called myoclonic epilepsy of Janz, is a familial form of primary idiopathic generalized epilepsy typically with "fast" 3–5-Hz spike and wave discharges on EEG ("impulsive petit mal") and autosomal dominant inheritance. The distinctive clinical features of JME include morning myoclonic jerks, generalized tonic-clonic seizures upon awakening, normal intelligence, a family history of similar seizures, and onset between 8 and 20 years of age. About one-third have a history of absence seizures presenting in the preteen period. Although linkage studies have mapped JME to the short arm of chromosome 6, it is unclear if this locus is for JME specifically, for the spike-wave EEG abnormality, or for some other feature of idiopathic generalized epilepsy. Seizures are precipitated by sleep deprivation or disruption and by alcohol. Absence or tonic-clonic seizures may precede the characteristic myoclonic jerks, which usually begin in adolescence. Valproate is the drug of choice, with some studies suggesting that seizures stop completely in 95% of patients. The probability of lifelong remission is small.

240. What are myoclonic seizures?

Myoclonic seizures are characterized by rapid, bilateral, symmetric muscle contractions of short duration: "quick jerks." They may be isolated or may occur repetitively. Myoclonic seizures may be the sole manifestation of epilepsy, or more commonly, they may be associated with absence attacks or tonic-clonic attacks. Juvenile myoclonic epilepsy is seen in children with nonprogressive static encephalopathies due to a variety of causes and rarely in the progressive myoclonic epilepsies. Myoclonic seizures respond best to valproate or benzodiazepines and in some cases a ketogenic diet.

241. A patient with seizures, a normal serum glucose, and a low CSF glucose without pleocytosis has what likely condition?

The ***GLUT-1 deficiency syndrome***, previously referred to as the **glu**cose **t**ransporter protein deficiency syndrome, was first described in 1991. The clinical phenotype is variable, but the child usually presents in the first years of life with seizures and delays of motor and mental development. The diagnosis should be suspected if CSF reveals low glucose (and lactate) concentrations without evidence of inflammation, and blood sugars are normal. Diagnosis can be furthered by assays of glucose transport in erythrocytes, which is diminished. Seizures tend to be refractory to anticonvulsant agents, and initiation of the ketogenic diet is effective in the treatment of seizures as well as of the overall disease process because it provides an alternative cerebral energy source.

242. What is the clinical triad of the Lennox-Gastaut syndrome?

Disorganized ***slow spike and wave activity*** on an EEG, ***mental retardation***, and ***seizures*** of various types. The seizures usually begin in the first 3 years of life and are characteristically severe and refractory to anticonvulsant drugs. Atonic, tonic, and atypical absences are the most common types in younger children. In older children and adolescents, tonic-clonic convulsions are also frequent. The majority of children suffer from two or more kinds of seizures, usually on a daily basis. Mental retardation is present in 80–90% of these patients and is severe in half this number. One-half to two-thirds of children show other abnormalities on neurologic examination, most commonly motor signs such as quadriparesis, spastic diplegia, and hemiparesis. Prognosis is poor, with over 80% of children continuing to have seizures into adulthood.

243. What are the causes of the Lennox-Gastaut syndrome?

The name Lennox-Gastaut syndrome (also called childhood epileptic encephalopathy) is applied to a heterogenous group of children. The clinical and EEG features are the result of a diffuse encephalopathy with diverse causes as cerebral malformation, perinatal asphyxia, severe head injury, anoxic encephalopathy from cardiopulmonary arrest, and CNS infection. There is no pathologic entity peculiar to the syndrome. A presumptive cause cannot be determined in 30–35% of children with Lennox-Gastaut syndrome.

244. What are the treatment options for Lennox-Gastaut syndrome?

Treatment is often difficult, and a variety of approaches, both individually and in combination, are tried including valproate, lamotrigine, and topiramate. Zonisamide and levetiracetam may be other alternatives, but there is less experience with these agents at the current time. Felbamate is effective at controlling many different seizure types. Unfortunately, it is associated with potentially life-threatening liver toxicity and bone marrow failure; as a consequence, it generally is not used until other options are exhausted. Benzodiazepines may be effective, but often the patient becomes tolerant to the medication and escalating doses (with accompanying side effects) are required to achieve efficacy. The ketogenic diet, vagal nerve stimulator, and epileptic surgery are other options when pharmacologic management is failing.

245. What are the symptomatic and cryptogenic age-related epilepsy syndromes?

Early infantile epileptic encephalopathy (EIEE) and ***early myoclonic epilepsy*** (EME). For fixed metabolic or structural abnormalities (e.g., hemimegalencephaly), the clinical expression and types of partial and generalized seizures can change by age. Both are characterized by early onset of spasms, a burst-suppression EEG pattern, poor response to treatment, and poor prognosis. These syndromes represent the early onset of the spectrum of severe age-dependent epilepsies, including infantile spasms and Lennox-Gastaut syndromes.

246. What are the varieties of partial epilepsy of childhood?

Simple partial seizures (without alteration in consciousness):

- Motor (e.g., clonic jerking of facial muscles)
- Somatosensory (e.g., numbness of a leg)
- Special sensory (e.g., visual or auditory sensations)
- Autonomic (e.g., piloerection, sweating, pupillary dilatation)
- Combinations of the above

Complex partial seizures: any signs included in simple partial seizures but involving alteration or loss of consciousness. In addition, all seizures are categorized by etiology as either idiopathic or symptomatic, the latter occurring in association with some other brain abnormality.

247. What are the types of absence seizures?

Typical Absence

- EEG: 3-Hz spike and wave
- Observations: Abrupt onset and ending (typically 5-10 seconds)
- Subtypes: Simple—unresponsiveness with no other associated features except minor movements (e.g., lip-smacking or eyelid twitching)

  Complex—unresponsiveness with more prolonged mild atonic, myoclonic, or tonic features or automatisms

Atypical Absence (most common in Lennox-Gastaut syndrome)

- EEG: 2-Hz (or slower) spike and wave
- Observations: gradual onset and ending; frequency more cyclic; unresponsive with more prolonged and pronounced atonic, tonic, myoclonic, or tonic activity

248. What is the prognosis for children with absence epilepsy?

The prognosis for patients with childhood absence epilepsy has been studied prospectively; nearly 90% of patients who have normal intelligence, normal neurologic examination, normal EEG background activity, no family history of convulsive epilepsy, and no history of tonic-clonic convulsions will become seizure free. Conversely, complete absence of favorable factors is associated with a poor prognosis for cessation of seizures. It may be that absence seizures are expressed on a spectrum from typical childhood absence epilepsy that is genetic in origin to the Lennox-Gastaut syndrome that is symptomatic of brain injury.

249. When a parent reports a child has been having staring spells, what features help distinguish epileptic and nonepileptic events?

In a study of 40 children, the staring spells were likely nonepileptic when reports indicated the child had preserved responsiveness to touch, body rocking, and intitial identification by a teacher or health professional. Epileptic events were more common when limb twitches, upward eye movement, interruption of play, or urinary incontinence were present.

Rosenow F, et al: Staring spells in children: Descriptive features distinguishing epileptic and nonepileptic events. J Pediatr 133:660-663, 1998.

250. In a child suspected of having absence seizures, how can a seizure be elicited during an exam?

Hyperventilation for at least 3 minutes is a useful provocative maneuver to precipitate an absence seizure. Young patients may be coaxed into overbreathing by making a game of it. Hold a tissue paper in front of the child's mouth. Instruct the patient to keep breathing fast enough to keep the tissue aloft.

251. What percentage of patients with absence seizures also have occasional grand mal seizures?

About 30–50%.

252. How is status epilepticus defined?

- More than 30 minutes of continuous seizure activity
- Recurrent seizures without full recovery of consciousness between seizures

253. What are the most common precipitants of status epilepticus in children?

- Fever/infection (36%)
- Medication change (20%)
- Unknown (9%)
- Metabolic (8%)
- Congenital (7%)
- Anoxia (5%)
- CNS infection (5%)
- Trauma (4%)
- Cerebrovascular (3%)
- Ethanol/drug-related (2%)
- Tumor (1%)

Dodson WE, et al: Treatment of convulsive status epilepticus: Recommendations of the Epilepsy Foundation of America's Working Group on Status Epilepticus. JAMA 270:855, 1993.

254. How should a child who presents with status epilepticus be managed?

0–5 minutes: Confirm the diagnosis. Maintain airway by head positioning or oropharyngeal airway. Administer nasal oxygen. Suction as needed. Obtain and frequently monitor vital signs, also utilizing pulse oximetry and ECG. Establish an intravenous line. Obtain venous blood for laboratory determinations (e.g., glucose, serum chemistries, hematology studies, toxicology screen, culture, anticonvulsant levels if known epileptic).

6–9 minutes: If hypoglycemic (or if a rapid reagent strip for glucose testing is not available), administer 2 ml/kg of $D_{25}W$ or 5 ml/kg of $D_{10}W$. In an infant with no known seizure disorder, give pyridoxine, 100 mg IV. Monitor oxygenation by pulse oximetry.

10–20 minutes: Administer lorazepam, 0.1 mg/kg (up to 4 mg) at 2 mg/min IV, *or* (2) diazepam, 0.2 mg/kg (up to 10 mg) at 5 mg/min IV. Repeat diazepam in 5 minutes if seizure persists. If IV access cannot be established, given diazepam, 0.5 mg/kg PR. Intramuscular therapy is not recommended.

21–60 minutes: If seizures persist, administer fosphenytoin (preferred for children), IV, at 15-20 mg phenytoin equivalents (PE)/kg loading dose at 150 mg PE/min or 3 mg PE/kg/min. If phenytoin is used, the dose is 15–20 mg/kg at 1 mg/kg/min IV while monitoring ECG and blood pressure. The infusion should be slowed if dysrhythmia or QT-interval widening develops.

> 60 minutes: If seizures persist for 15 minutes after use of phenytoin, additional doses of fosphenytoin/phenytoin, 5 mg/kg to maximum of 30 mg/kg total. If seizures persist, give phenobarbital (20 mg/kg), IV at 100 mg/min. With use of phenobarbital following benzodiazepines, the risk of respiratory depression is increased, and the likely need for intubation increases and should be anticipated. If phenobarbital fails to stop the seizure, other measures, such as general anesthesia, are usually necessary.

Rivera RF, Laureta E: Emergency management of seizures. Contemp Pediatr 16:52, 1999.

Dodson WE, et al: Treatment of convulsive status epilepticus: Recommendations of the Epilepsy Foundation of America's Working Group on Status Epilepticus. JAMA 270:855, 1993.

255. What is non-convulsive status epilepticus?

Lennox described "petit mal status" in 1945, and focal nonconvulsive status epilepticus was recognized by Gastaut in 1956. It has been estimated to account for a small proportion to approximately 25% of all cases of status epilepticus (SE). It has been defined as a state characterized by slowness in behavior and mentation, confusion, and sometimes stupor (or coma), accompanied by generalized epileptiform continuous or nearly continuous activity in the form of spike waves, polyspike waves, or more complex discharges on the EEG. The types essentially reflect all seizure types and may be partial or generalized (absence status). Absence status is also known as petit mal status, spike-wave stupor, prolonged petit mal automatism, epilepsia minoris continua, and epileptic twilight state. Partial nonconvulsive status is clinically characterized by a prolonged confusional state or clouding of consciousness ranging from slowing of thinking to complete loss of awareness and responsiveness. The typical ictal behavior is drowsiness and confusion, but patients may continue to function normally except for subtle changes in coordination or alertness. While convulsive SE is a medical emergency, absence nonconvulsive status epilepticus is not life threatening. The potential for neurologic morbidity, however, is not known.

256. What is the significance of a burst-suppression pattern in an EEG?

The burst-suppression EEG pattern in the full-term neonate and infant is characterized by periods of marked voltage *suppression* of the background activity that usually lasts longer than 10 seconds, alternating with briefer high-voltage (75–250 μV) paroxysmal *bursts* of theta and delta activity with intermixed spikes. It is distinguished from trace alternant by its persistence (i.e., it does not change with the state of the patient) and its lack of reactivity to external stimuli. It was first used to describe an alternating pattern of "burst" and "blackouts" seen in barbiturate anesthesia and then in hypothalamic lesions. It is an age-related pattern that was initially described in a child with infantile spasms and hypsarrhythmia during sleep. This pattern has also been found in infants with brain malformations, in infants with dentato-olivary dysplasia, and in association with the Aicardi syndrome. The burst-suppression EEG pattern has also been associated with metabolic diseases, classically with nonketotic hyperglycinemia. Thus, the burst-suppression EEG pattern is a nonspecific pattern that may be secondary to the effects of medications, hypoxic-ischemic injury, structural lesions, and metabolic disease.

257. Why is the role of the ketogenic diet in the treatment of seizures?

The *ketogenic diet* is effective in treating all seizure types, particularly in children with myoclonic forms of epilepsy. In children with refractory seizures, the ketogenic diet offers an effective alternate to medications without bothersome sedative side effects. The diet involves supplying the majority of calories through fats with concurrent limitation of carbohydrates and protein. The mechanism of seizure control is unclear, perhaps related to a switch from cerebral metabolism from utilization of glucose to β-hydroxybutyrate. After 24 hours of fasting, the child is place on a high-fat diet in which the ratio of fats to carbohydrates and protein combined is 3-4:1. Anticonvulsant drugs may be reduced or eliminated entirely if the diet is effective. The regimen must be followed closely and parents must understand the demands of close adherence to the diet. A skilled dietitian is instrumental in providing variety and palatability to the diet. It is important to recall that the diet may have adverse effects, including serious, potentially, life-threatening complications, including hypoproteinemia, lipemia and hemolytic anemia and disturbances in liver function.

Lefevre F, Aronson N: Ketogenic diet for the treatment of refractory epilepsy in children: A systematic review of efficacy. Pediatrics 106:e46, 2000.

Ballaban-Gil K, et al: Complications of the ketogenic diet. Epilepsia 39:744-748, 1998.

258. When should treatment be begun if a seizure episode cannot be categorized?

Sometimes information regarding the seizure semiology is lacking and the EEG is not sufficiently informative to allow an accurate epilepsy syndrome classification. In these circumstances, one must make an empiric decision regarding the risk of recurrent seizures versus treating a poorly characterized epilepsy. Carbamazepine is often used, recognizing that there is a small risk of increasing the frequency of generalized seizures in some patients with generalized epilepsies. This risk is small, and the favorable side-effect profile of carbamazepine makes this a reasonable option. An alternative is valproate, which can effectively treat almost any type of epilepsy, but the disadvantage is the risk of an idiosyncratic hepatic reaction. This risk is increased with polypharmacy and in those children younger than 2 years.

259. If a patient with a known seizure disorder has another seizure, what should be discussed with the family in a telephone conversation?

When a family calls to report a seizure and to discuss their child's care, there is a strong urge to do something. On some occasions, the appropriate thing to do is to adjust the medication, particularly if the child is not experiencing dose-related side effects and the seizures are occurring at a disabling rate. However, as important as knowing when to escalate treatment is knowing when to exercise restraint. The phone call could present opportunities for discussing other important items: reviewing the implications of a single seizure, discussing ways to reduce the risk of recurrent events, and working out strategies for dealing with emergencies. Possible aggravating factors include concurrent illnesses, sleep deprivation, concurrent medications, and other specific precipitants (photic activation). Many times, seizures flare during an acute infectious illness, and the best remedy is to provide antipyretics, treat the underlying source of irritation, and provide a back-up emergency plan, such as rectal diazepam for severe clusters.

260. What is the most common cause of refractory seizures?

An ***inadequate serum concentration*** of antiepileptic mediction is the most common cause of persistent seizures, but other causes should be considered:

- *Drug toxicity*, especially with phenytoin, may manifest by deteriorating seizure control.
- *Metabolic abnormalities*, particularly in patients with inborn errors of metabolism
- *Medications* may have a paradoxic reaction and exacerbate certain types of seizures, particularly in children with mixed seizure disorders. For example, carbamazepine or phenytoin may control generalized tonic-clonic seizures in patients with juvenile myoclonic epilepsy, but aggravate myoclonic and absence seizures.
- *Incorrect identification* of the epilepsy syndrome. Partial seizures may masquerade as a generalized form of epilepsy in the very young child (bilateral symmetric tonic posturing may be seen in partial seizures). Conversely, generalized forms of epilepsy may first present with partial seizures (severe infantile myoclonic epilepsy). Treatment based on an epilepsy syndrome rather than ictal semiology usually improves control in these circumstances.

261. When is surgery for epilepsy indicated?

Surgery is considered in children with medically intractable epilepsy or declining neurologic function or for syndromes for which medical treatment is known to be ineffective. These determinations require accurate epilepsy syndrome classification, knowledge of the natural history, response to antiepileptic drug trials, and serial assessments of development. Many types of infantile and early childhood epilepsies are difficult to classify and of uncertain prognosis. Thus, surgical outcome is best with older children and adolescents who have focal cerebral lesions or mesial temporal sclerosis. There is growing interest, however, in operating earlier, especially in selected patients who have catastrophic epilepsy. Children in whom surgery is considered should have a reasonable expectation either of seizure elimination or substantially fewer disabling seizures that translates into improved quality of life and perhaps development. There should be minimal risk of losing neurologic function. The definition of *intractable* is not fixed and must be individualized. In practical terms, this may be a failure to adequately respond to three well-selected antiepileptic medications, used in isolation, or in combination. Because the frequency of seizures in children is often high, this determination need not take years and, often, can be established within a year of onset of the epilepsy.

Saneto RP, Wyllie E: Epilepsy surgery in infancy. Semin Pediatr Neurol 7:187-193, 2000.
Engel J: Surgery for seizures. N Engl JMed 334:647–652, 1996.

262. Which children have the highest likelihood of success with epilepsy surgery?

Those children with ***complete resections of focal structural MRI lesions*** fare best, with seizure-free rates as high as 90%. Many of these lesions are congenital low-growing tumors or cerebral dysgenesis. Mesial temporal sclerosis (a common condition in adult epilepsy surgery) is infrequent in young children and adolescents. Without a clear MRI focus, complete long-term seizure freedom is achieved in less than half of patients.

263. What is the role of the vagal nerve stimulator in seizure control?

The *vagal nerve stimulator* (VNS) is a surgically implanted device that intermittently stimulates the left vagus nerve. Why this decreases seizure frequency is not well understood. It is a palliative, not curative, procedure that has been performed in adults and in some children with intractable complex partial seizures or generalized tonic seizures who were thought not to be candidates for definitive surgical cure. The VNS has been placed in children as young as 2–3 years, but most of the experience is in older children. It is generally well tolerated and relatively safe. The response in children is similar to that of adults. There is a median reduction of seizure frequency of about a third at 1 year that increases to over 40% at 18 months. The use of the VNS in younger children with other seizure types, especially, those who would previously have been considered for corpus callostomy, awaits further study.

264. What should a teenager with a seizure disorder be told about the potential to obtain a driver's license?

State requirements vary regarding individuals with epilepsy and the right to drive. The most common requirement is a specified seizure-free period and submission of a physician's evaluation of the patient's ability to drive safely. Many states require periodic submission of medical reports while the license is active. Many states also allow exceptions under which a license may be issued for a shorter seizure-free period (e.g., if a seizure occurred in isolation due to medication change or intercurrent illness) as well as the issuance of licenses with restrictions (e.g., daytime driving only). A summary of requirements for each state is available from the Epilepsy Foundation (http://www.efa.org).

265. In addition to the seizures themselves, what are other important issues to discuss with families during follow-up sessions?

Children with epilepsy are at risk for not achieving their long-term education, vocational, and social goals. At the office visit, the parents should be asked about sensitive indicators of AED toxicity including behavioral changes, difficulty with cognitive tasks, and problems maintaining attention. Many factors could be causing these complaints. Too often, seizure control is achieved at the expense of multiple intoxicating medications, making the child incapable of performing optimally. Monotherapy with a single effective agent is superior to the use of multiple medications at inadequate doses. In addition, education about the underlying condition, goals of treatment, and potential side effects of medicine helps to ensure proper responses to emergencies and minimizes adverse consequences. Attention problems, difficulties at school, and problems with behavior all should receive prompt attention, evaluation, and intervention, where appropriate. These issues may play a more important role in determining long-term outcome and, ironically, too often receive inadequate professional attention. The health care professional must strive to balance these concerns and to ensure that the entire professional interaction is not relegated to a discussion of the seizure themselves, but that it incorporates consideration of these other issues as well.

SPINAL CORD DISORDERS

266. Which spinal segments do each of the common reflexes test?

DEEP TENDON REFLEX	SUPERFICIAL REFLEX	PERIPHERAL NERVE	SEGMENTAL ORGANIZATION
	Pupillary	Optic/oculomotor	CN II–III
Jaw jerk		Trigeminal	CN V
	Corneal	Trigeminal/facial	CN V–VII
	Gag	Glossopharyngeal/vagal	CN IX–X
Biceps		Musculocutaneous	C5–6
Brachioradialis		Radial	C5–6
Triceps		Radial	C6–8
Finger flexion		Median/ulnar	C7–T1
Abdominal reflex		Thoracic	T8–12
	Umbilical	Thoracic	T8–12
	Cremasteric	Genitofemoral	L1–2
Adductor		Femoral/obturator	L2–4
Quadriceps		Femoral	L2–4
	Plantar reflex	Sciatic	S1–2
	Anal wink	Pudendal	S3–5

267. What are early signs of spinal cord compression?

Early spinal cord compression may be easily overlooked before flagrant motor or sensory signs are prominent. Some early clinical clues that may be helpful in detecting this compression promptly include:

- Scoliosis producing sustained poor posture
- Back pain or abdominal pain that begins abruptly or paroxysmally during sleep
- Increased sensitivity of the spinal column to local pressure or percussion
- In extramedullary tumors that compress the cord, prodromal pains of radicular distribution are common because such tumors often arise from the posterior nerve roots themselves.
- Bowel or bladder dysfunction may be a presenting feature of sacral or conus medullaris compression.
- Because the somatotopic organization of sensory fibers places the sacral and lumbar dermatomes nearest to the cord surface, extrinsic compression commonly results first in diminished sensation in the anogenital region and lower limbs.

268. How common are asymptomatic spinal anomalies in normal children?

Up to 5% of children have spina bifida occulta, an incomplete fusion of the posterior vertebral arches, usually noted as a radiographic incidental finding. The defect most commonly involves the lower lumbar lamina of L5 and S1.

269. When should an occult spinal dysraphism be suspected?

Occult spinal dysraphism (or malformation) should be suspected in children who have the following dorsal midline features:

- An abnormal collection of hair
- Cutaneous abnormalities (e.g., hemangioma, pigmented nevi)
- Cutaneous dimples or tracts, abnormal gluteal folds
- Subcutaneous mass (lipoma, fluid or bone) on the lower back

In 80–90% of cases, there is an associated vertebral abnormality. Almost all the symptoms and signs of spinal cord malformation involve the lower extremities, bowel and bladder, and spine. In older individuals, sexual function may be affected. The diagnosis should also be suspected in patients with symptoms of progressive lower extremity weakness or sensory loss, atrophy, gait abnormalities, foot deformities, pressure sores, incontinence and urinary tract infections, and scoliosis.

270. What is the recurrence rate for open neural tube defects?

Open neural tube defects (myelomeningocele or spina bifida and anencephaly) are usually multifactorial, but in some cases may have Mendelian recessive inheritance. The general recurrence rate is 2.5% for mothers of affected children, sisters of mothers and the child and female children born to individuals with spina bifida. Daily folic acid of 400 μg reduces the risk of spina bifida by as much as 70%. Serum and amniotic alpha-fetoprotein can detect open neural tube defects, and ultrasound is also a useful tool.

271. What is the Chiari II malformation?

The *Chiari II malformation* is a complex malformation that involves the entire brain. Features include a small posterior fossa with herniation of the cerebellar vermis, fourth ventricle, and medulla into the cervical canal; deformities of the quadrageminal plates, massa intermedia, and corpus callosum; and cortical gyral abnormalities and migrational defects. The impaired egress of CSF caused by aqueductal stenosis commonly results in hydrocephalus (80–90%).

272. What differentiates the various Chiari malformations?

Chiari malformations are characterized by cerebellar elongation and protrusion of the foramen magnum into the cervical spinal cord. Anatomic anomalies of the hindbrain and skeletal structure result in different positioning of the various structures relative to the upper cervical canal and foramen magnum with different clinical features.

Type I is clinically the least severe and generally asymptomatic in childhood. The presentation of a Chiari I may be insidious and is associated with mental retardation. Epilepsy is found in a small minority. There may be paroxysmal vertigo, drop attacks, vague dizziness, and headache, which may be increased by Valsalva. Occipital headache precipitated by exertion may progress to torticollis, downgaze nystagmus, periodic nystagmus, and oscillopsia. MRI findings in Chiari I include malformations of the base of the skull and upper cervical spine including hydromyelia, syringomyelia, or syrinx.

Type II is the most common of those diagnosed in childhood. Medulla and cerebellum, together with part or all of the fourth ventricle, are displaced into spinal canal. A variety of cerebellar, brain stem and cortical defects can occur. It is strongly associated with noncommunicating hydrocephalus and lumbosacral myelomeningocele.

Type III comprises any of the features of types I and II, but the entire cerebellum is herniated throught the foramen magnum with a cervical spina bifida cystica. Hydrocephalus a common feature.

Type IV is cerebellar hypoplasia without connect to the other malformations (designation was made by Chiari).

Menkes JH, Sarnat HB: Malformations of the central nervous system. In Menkes JH, Sarnat HB (eds): Child Neurology, 6th ed. Philadelphia, Lippincott, Williams & Wilkins, 2000, pp 324-326.

273. What is the full anatomic expression of myelomeningocele?

Children with myelomeningocele have a complex, multifaceted, congenital disorder of structure that represents a dysraphic state—a defective closure of the embryonic neural groove. In its full expression, it is typified anatomically by:

- The presence of unfused or excessively separated vertebral arches of the bony spine (spina bifida)
- Cystic dilation of the meninges that surround the spinal cord (meningocele)
- Cystic dilation of the spinal cord itself (myelocele)
- Hydrocephalus and spectrum of congenital cerebral abnormalities

274. If the diagnosis of myelomeningocele is made prenatally, should delivery be done by cesarean section?

This remains controversial. A 1991 study of infants delivered by cesarean section prior to the onset of labor had significantly less paralysis at age 2 years than did infants with comparable lesions who were delivered vaginally following a period of labor. On the basis of this study, many centers adopted a policy of elective cesarean section for uncomplicated fetal myelomeningocele. Others have criticized this study and continued vaginal deliveries without detecting any differences in short-term and long-term outcomes for these infants. A multicenter, randomized trial may be required to provide a more definitive answer.

Merrill DC, et al: The optimal route of delivery for fetal meningomyelocele. Am J Obstet Gynecol 179:235-240, 1998.

Luthy DA, et al: Cesarean section before the onset of labor and subsequent motor function in infants with meningocele diagnosed antenatally. N Engl J Med 324:662–666, 1991.

275. What is the likelihood that a patient with myelomeningocele will have hydrocephalus?

Hydrocephalus is seen in 95% of children with thoracic or high lumbar myelomeningocele. The incidence decreases progressively with more caudal spinal defects to a minimum of 60% if the myelomeningocele is located in the sacrum.

276. What is the usual cause of stridor in a child with myelomeningocele?

The stridor is usually due to ***dysfunction of the vagus nerve***, which innervates the muscles of the vocal cords. In their resting position, the edges of the cords meet in the midline; in speech, they move apart. Hence, in bilateral vagal nerve palsies, the free edges of the vocal cords are closely opposed and obstruct air flow, resulting in stridor. In symptomatic patients, the motor nucleus of the vagus nerve may be congenitally hypoplastic or aplastic. More commonly, the vagal dysfunction is believed to arise from a mechanical traction injury secondary to hydrocephalus, which produces progressive herniation and inferior displacement of the abnormal hindbrain. Shunting the hydrocephalus may alleviate the traction and improve the stridor. Sometimes, the later recurrence of stridor indicates reaccumulation of hydrocephalus due to ventriculoperitoneal shunt failure.

277. What are the four principal options for managing urinary incontinence in patients with myelomeningocele?

About 80% of patients have a neurogenic bladder, most commonly a small, poorly compliant bladder and an open and fixed sphincter. Options include:

1. Clean intermittent catheterization, which results in more complete emptying than simple Credé maneuvers
2. Artificial urinary sphincter to increase outlet resistance
3. Surgical urinary diversion (e.g., suprapubic vesicostomy), which is uncommonly used
4. Augmentation cystoplasty to increase bladder capacity in combination with the use of oxybutynin (a smooth muscle antispasmodic)

Blum RW, Pfaffinger K: Myelodysplasia in childhood and adolescence. Pediatr Rev 15:480-488, 1994.

278. How frequently is myelomeningocele associated with mental retardation?

Only ***15–20%*** of patients have associated mental retardation. Hydrocephalus per se does not cause the mental retardation associated with this syndrome. (Recall that children with appropriately treated congenital hydrocephalus due to simple aqueductal stenosis usually have normal psychomotor development.) Only severe hydrocephalus with a very thick cortical mantle predicts lower intelligence. Mental retardation is usually attributed to acquired secondary CNS infection or subtle microscopic anomalies of neuronal migration and differentiation, which may coexist with the macroscopically visible malformation of the hindbrain.

279. In an infant born with myelomeningocele, how does the initial evaluation predict long-term ambulation potential?

The level of motor function and not the level of the defect is most predictive of ambulation.

Thoracic**:** No hip flexion is noted. Almost no younger children will ambulate, and only about a third of adolescents will ambulate with the aid of extensive braces and crutches.

High lumbar **(L1, L2):** Able to flex hips but no knee extension. About a third of children and adolescents will ambulate, but with extensive assistive devices

Mid lumbar **(L3):** Able to flex hips and extend knee. The percentage of ambulators is midway between those with high and low lumbar lesions.

Low lumbar **(L4, L5):** Able to flex knee and dorsiflex ankle. Nearly half of younger children and nearly all adolescents will ambulate with varying degrees of braces or crutches.

Sacral **(S1–S4):** Able to plantar flex ankles and move toes. Nearly all children and adolescents will ambulate with minimal or no assistive devices.

16. ONCOLOGY

Peter Langmuir, M.D., Richard Aplenc, M.D., and Peter C. Adamson, M.D.

CHEMOTHERAPY/RADIATION THERAPY

1. What are the four phases of a cancer clinical trial?

Phase I: *The dose determination phase.* Investigates the toxicities and maximum tolerated dose (MTD) of different schedules and routes of administration in an effort to determine the recommended dose for future studies and to evaluate the pharmacokinetics of the drug. Preliminary evidence of antitumor efficacy is collected.

Phase II: *The efficacy phase.* Evaluates in greater numbers the agent's activity against various tumor types.

Phase III: *The comparative phase.* Assesses the agent against standard therapies and anticipated disease progression.

Phase IV: *The post-commercialization phase.* Verifies the clinical utility of drugs in conditions of daily practice.

Shah S, et al: Phase I trials in children with cancer. J Pediatr Hematol Oncol 20:431-438, 1998.

2. Where are the sites of action of various anticancer drugs?

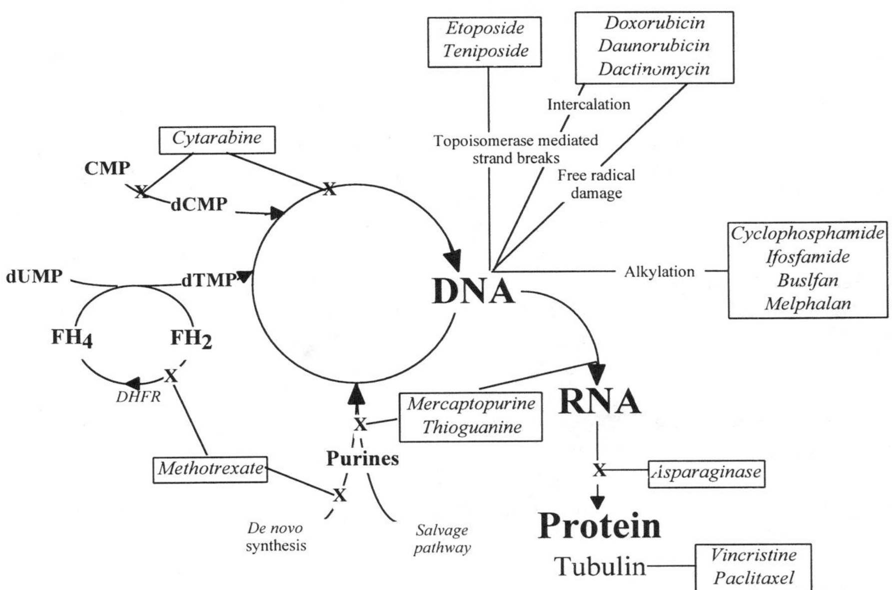

Sites of action drugs used in the treatment of childhood leukemia. Drugs may directly inhibit critical steps in the cell cycle, or may incorporate as fraudulent substrates into DNA and less commonly RNA. *DHFR* = dihydrofolate reductase; FH_2/FH_4 = dihydro/tetrahydrofolate; dUMP/dTMP = deoxyuridine/deoxythymidine monophosphate. (Adapted from Balis FM, Holcenberg JS, Poplack DG: General principles of chemotherapy. In: Pizzo PA, Poplack DG, eds. Principles and Practice of Pediatric Oncology. Philadelphia, J.B. Lippincott, 1997, pp 215-272.)

3. What is the difference between adjuvant and neo-adjuvant chemotherapy?

Adjuvant chemotherapy is therapy that is administered following the primary treatment of a tumor (usually surgical resection or radiation therapy). As such, adjuvant therapy is administered in the setting where there is no remaining gross tumor that can be assessed for response to the chemotherapy. *Neo-adjuvant chemotherapy* is administered beginning prior to delivery of definitive local treatment. Several cycles of neo-adjuvant chemotherapy may be administered to improve the chances of achieving complete surgical resection of a primary tumor; this therapy is then continued post-resection in the adjuvant setting.

4. What is the most widely used antimetabolite in pediatric oncology?

Methotrexate. Antimetabolites are structural analogs of compounds critical in the formation of nucleic acids and proteins. Antimetabolites serve as enzymatic competitors, blocking production, or may be incorporated, resulting in defective metabolic products. Methotrexate is an analog of folic acid, a cofactor for purine and thymidine synthesis, and its excess leads to deficiency of DNA precursors and thus DNA synthesis. Others include the purine analogs, mercaptopurine and thioguanine, and the pyrimidine analogs, cytarabine and fluorouracil.

5. What are the common presenting signs of a patient with methotrexate toxicity?

The toxicity of methotrexate is dependent upon the duration of time patients are exposed to concentrations above the toxicity threshold. ***Mucositis*** (potentially involving the entire oro-gastro-intestinal mucosa), ***hepatitis*** and ***myelosuppression*** are the most common complications. Nephrotoxicity is primarily a complication of *high dose* methotrexate.

6. From what does leucovorin rescue?

Leucovorin is a reduced folate, which can rescue cells from the ***toxicity of methotrexate***. Methotrexate inhibits the enzyme dihydrofolate reductase, thus depleting cells of a major pathway which synthesizes reduced folates. To avoid toxicity, leucovorin, which replenishes cells with an alternative reduced folate, must be administered to patients receiving intermediate (100 to 1000 mg/m^2) or high (> 1 gm/m^2) doses of methotrexate.

7. What is the major dose-limiting toxicity for the alkylating agents?

Myelosuppression. Alkylating agents are chemically reactive compounds which covalently add a alkyl group, most importantly to macromolecules involved in DNA synthesis, damaging templates and inhibiting synthesis. Agents include the nitrogen mustards, oxazaphosphorines (including cyclophosphamide and ifosfamide), busulfan and cisplatin.

8. What are the most effective antiemetics for the prevention and treatment of chemotherapy-induced vomiting?

The serotonin-receptor antagonists ***ondansetron*** and ***granisetron*** (and potentially ***dolasetron)*** are the most effective agents for chemotherapy-associated emesis. They work less well for delayed emesis, for which combinations of antihistamines and phenothiazines may be used. Dexamethasone is a useful adjunct when administering highly emetogenic chemotherapy.

Coppes MJ, et al: Safety, tolerability, antiemetic efficacy, and pharmacokinetics of oral dolasetron mesylate in pediatric cancer patients receiving moderately to highly emetogenic chemotherapy. J Pediatr Hematol Oncol 21:274-281, 1999.

9. Which children are most vulnerable to long-term central nervous system radiation-induced side effects?

The long-term neurotoxicity of cranial radiation, manifested by a range of symptoms ranging from learning disabilities to profound decreases in IQ, impacts the developing brain to a greater extent than the mature brain. By the age of 3 years, brain size is approximately 80% of adult values. ***Children less than 3 years of age*** are the most vulnerable to severe neurotoxic effects of cranial radiation.

10. If it were not for guinea pigs, which anti-leukemic drug might we not have today?

In 1953, Kidd noted that guinea pig serum, but not sera from other species, could cause *in vivo* regression of transplanted mouse and rat lymphomas. Ten years later, in 1963, Broome demonstrated that the fraction of guinea pig serum responsible for this effect contained ***L-asparaginase***. Lymphoblasts are asparagine autotrophs and thus must rely on exogenous sources of asparagine for their survival. Asparaginase rapidly depletes plasma asparagine, resulting in leukemic cell cytotoxicity.

11. What did Capizzi teach us about how to administer methotrexate and L-asparaginase to children with leukemia?

Asparaginase will antagonize the effects of methotrexate, and thus asparaginase must not be administered either immediately prior to or concomitantly with methotrexate. Capizzi demonstrated that asparaginase could rescue patients from the toxicity of methotrexate, and by administering asparaginase 24 hours following methotrexate, one could increase the dose and efficacy of methotrexate. The combination of 10-day cycles of increasing IV doses of methotrexate followed 24 hours later by asparaginase is referred to as the *Capizzi regimen*.

12. Which commonly used anti-cancer drugs are vesicants?

A *vesicant* is an agent that produces a vesicle; in oncology, it is a chemotherapeutic drug that can cause a severe burn if the drug infiltrates around the intravenous catheter. The ***anthracyclines*** (doxorubicin, daunorubicin), ***dactinomycin***, and the ***vinca alkaloids*** (vincristine, vinblastine) are all vesicants. These drugs must be administered either through a central venous catheter or through a newly placed, free-flowing intravenous catheter that does not cross over a joint space.

13. If one had to choose a single laboratory test prior to administering high dose methotrexate, what would it be?

Determination of a ***serum creatinine*** is essential prior to administering high dose methotrexate. More than 90% of methotrexate is eliminated by the kidneys. In the presence of abnormal renal function, high dose methotrexate carries a high risk of severe to fatal toxicity.

14. In a child receiving chemotherapy, what conditions can produce acute abdominal signs?

- *Esophageal varices*, especially after hepatotoxic therapy (e.g., daunorubicin, 6-thioguanine)
- *Gastric or duodenal ulcers* (especially with high-dose corticorsteroids, increased intracranial pressure, following high-dose irradiation)
- *Small intestinal intussusception*, primarily ileoileal, usually without intramural intestinal tumor involvement but may be led by tumor nodule
- *Intestinal-wall tumor lysis* with necrosis, perforation, or hemorrhage associated with chemotherapy response
- *Typhlitis* (often with agranulocytic necrosis), *enterocolitis* (nonspecific), *leukemic cecal infiltration*
- *Small bowel hemorrhage*, due to fungal ulceration (aspergillosis or mucormycosis)
- *Lower-lobe pneumonia*
- *Hepatic* or *splenic abscesses*; subdiaphragmatic, subhepatic, or pelvic septic collections; portal vein thrombosis

- *Hemorrhagic pancreatitis* (especially with L-asparaginase, corticosteroids, or increased intracranial pressure)
- *Splenic infarcts*
- *Hemoperitoneum* or *retroperitoneal hematoma* secondary to coagulation defects or tumor rupture
- *Primary peritonitis*
- Diseases common to children without neoplasms (e.g., acute appendicitis, although this is quite rare)

Lange B, et al: Oncologic emergencies. In Pizzo PA, Poplack DG (eds): Principles and Practice of Pediatric Oncology, 3rd ed. Philadelphia, Lippincott-Raven, 1997, pp 1030-1033.

15. Which chemotherapeutic agent, sometimes used in the treatment of Hodgkin disease, is known to cause pulmonary toxicity?

Bleomycin, a mixture of low molecular weight peptides isolated form the fungus *Streptomyces verticullus*, is part of the ABVD (adriamycin, bleomycin, vinblastine and dacarbazine) regimen that has been used in the treatment of Hodgkin disease. Sub-acute or chronic pneumonitis progressing to interstitial fibrosis is its primary toxicity. Exposure to high concentrations of oxygen, such as might occur in the operating room, can exacerbate bleomycin's pulmonary toxicity, and should be avoided.

16. What chemotherapeutic agents are derived from leaf extracts of the periwinkle plant?

Vinca alkaloids, *vincristine and vinblastine.* The exert their effect by binding to tubulin and interfering with its role in mitosis, cell cytostructure and solute transport.

17. Which class of drugs is a cause of long-term cardiotoxicity?

Cardiac toxicity is usually associated with the ***anthracyclines***, doxorubicin and daunorubicin. The risk of cardiotoxicity increases with increasing cumulative doses, with clinically apparent congestive heart failure increasing after cumulative doxorubicin doses of 450 mg/m^2. Sub-clinical cardiac injury can occur at lower doses, and thus it is generally recommended to perform cardiac function evaluations (echocardiogram or MUGA) prior to and at cumulative doses of 200, 300 and 400 mg/m^2, and then at each 50 mg/m^2 thereafter. Heart failure may occur many years after the completion of therapy; therefore, every-other-year evaluations should be continued. Myocardial damage appears to result from the generation of free radicals by the anthracyclines, and may be increased by concurrent radiation therapy to the heart. Co-administration of the cardio-protectant drug Zinecard may be beneficial; prolonged infusions, which avoid high peak concentrations, may also diminish the risk of cardiotoxicity.

18. Which anti-leukemic drugs can produce hyperglycemia as a side effect?

Corticosteroids and ***asparaginase*** can both result in hyperglycemia. During induction chemotherapy, if hyperglycemia develops, these drugs are not stopped; rather, low doses of insulin can be administered, thus providing the patient with the necessary exposure to these highly effective remission inducing drugs.

19. What drug must always be administered with ifosfamide, and what laboratory abnormality will always result from its administration?

Ifosfamide is a nitrogen mustard analog and a major urinary metabolite is acrolein, the causative agent of hemorrhagic cystitis. This invariably occurs if ifosfamide is not administered with the uroprotector, ***mesna*** (2-mercaptoethanesulfonate). A dipstick of urine from a patient receiving mesna will reveal the drug's presence by being positive for ketones. Mesna is also administered with high dose cyclophosphamide.

20. What drug, made famous in Frank Capra's 1944 film of two sweet old ladies, is making a dramatic comeback in the treatment of one form of leukemia ?

The remedy used by the ladies in "Arsenic and Old Lace" is making an encore performance. In the early 1990s, investigators in China reported that ***arsenic***, an ancient remedy, was found to be highly effective in the treatment of patients with *acute promyelocytic leukemia*. Arsenic appears to trigger an apoptotic response in promyeloblasts, but its precise mechanism of action is still under investigation.

21. What vitamin derivative is now used as a highly effective treatment for acute promyelocytic leukemia?

Retinoic acid, a vitamin A derivative, can induce remission in more than 85% of patients with newly diagnosed APL. The translocation found in APL involves the retinoic acid receptor alpha (RAR-α) gene on chromosome 17 and the PML gene on chromosome 15. Pharmacological concentrations of the RAR-α ligand all-*trans*-retinoic acid can overcome the block in differentiation found in APL. When retinoic acid is combined with chemotherapy, more than 70% of patients are cured of their disease.

22. What drug used in the treatment of Wilms tumor has been associated with the development of veno-occlusive disease (VOD)?

Dactinomycin administered as a single day bolus dose appears to carry a higher risk of VOD than when it is administered on the more common daily times 5 schedule.

23. How do the toxicities of carboplatin and cisplatin differ?

Cisplatin's primary toxicities are nephrotoxicity and ototoxicity. In contrast, *carboplatin's* primary toxicity is myelosuppression, usually in the form of thrombocytopenia.

24. When is "radiation recall" likely?

Radiation recall, a phenomenon that occurs when certain anti-cancer drugs are administered following completion of radiation therapy (XRT), results in a flare of radiation-like reactions within the radiation field. This phenomenon can occur as late as 2 years following completion of XRT, and has been observed with dactinomycin, doxorubicin and daunomycin.

25. Who develops the "somnolence syndrome"?

Transient symptoms attributed to *temporary demyelination* have been observed 6 to 8 weeks following completion of ***CNS radiation***, most commonly CNS prophylaxis for ALL. Children who develop the "somnolence syndrome" have lethargy, headache and anorexia that last for about 2 weeks. CT and CSF studies show no consistent abnormality, but an EEG will often reveal a slow-wave activity consistent with diffuse cerebral disturbance. The use of steroids during irradiation appears to minimize the occurrence of the syndrome.

26. Should children receiving chemotherapy be given routine immunizations?

Children who are receiving chemotherapy can be given routine diphtheria/tetanus/pertussis (DTaP) immunization when they have discontinued the intensive part of treatment. They should not be given live-virus vaccines (measles, mumps, rubella, polio) until at least three months after all immunosuppressive therapy has been completed. An exception may be the measles vaccine. They can receive the Salk vaccine for polio protection, but the response may be suboptimal. Patients with severe pulmonary disease secondary to malignancy or cancer treatment should receive influenza immunization. They can receive pneumococcal, Hib, and DTaP vaccines if clinically indicated. The response is likely to be suboptimal, particularly if treatment includes steroid, cyclophosphamide, or radiation therapy. However, there is no evidence that tolerance is induced with immunization.

27. Should patients receiving chemotherapy receive the varicella vaccine?

The answer to this is controversial. As the varicella vaccine is a live viral vaccine, some specialists recommend that it not be given to patients who are receiving chemotherapy. However, the vaccine was initially studied in patients with ALL, in whom it was found to be both safe and effective. It is not yet approved for this patient population, however.

28. What do you do for a chemotherapy patient whose sister develops chickenpox?

Immunocompromised patients are at high risk for disseminated varicella infections. Exposed seronegative patients (or patients with low titer anti-varicella antibody) should receive varicella zoster immune globulin (VZIG) within 96 hours of the exposure. Patients who develop an active varicella infection should be treated with intravenous acyclovir. All exposed patients, even if they receive VZIG, should be isolated from other immunocompromised patients for 28 days after exposure.

29. Why does drug resistance develop during the course of chemotherapy?

Resistance to chemotherapeutic agents probably has several mechanisms, only a few of which are understood. A genetic basis is strongly suggested with tumor cells spontaneously generating resistant clones through mutation and chromosomal rearrangements. Gene products then alter cellular metabolism in ways that foil the intended chemotherapeutic effect. The *mdr-1* (multiple drug resistance) gene is associated with resistance to chemotherapy in a number of tumors. The protein product of the *mdr-1* gene, P-glycoprotein, is responsible for pumping toxic substances out of cells. It may be responsible for resistance to vinca alkaloids, epipodophyllotoxins, and antitumor antibiotics, all of which can be actively excluded from cells by the *mdr-1* protein. Presumably, the gene is induced by exposure to chemotherapy. Resistance to methotrexate occurs by a different mechanism. Exposure to methotrexate results in the amplification of genes that encode enzymes which circumvent the block in dihydrofolate reductase activity caused by the drug.

30. How is body surface area calculated in children?

Body surface area (BSA) is most commonly used in chemotherapy calculations and is usually derived from nomograms after height and weight are measured. A rapid (and reasonably reliable) estimate is as follows:

$$BSA\ (m^2) = (weight\ [lbs]/60) + 0.1$$

Barton DH: Quick calculation for body surface area in children. Consultant 34:907, 1994.

CLINICAL ISSUES

31. How is the DNA content useful in assessing the prognosis of tumors?

With flow cytometric analysis, the content of DNA per cell (i.e., tumor DNA index) can be calculated. The *DNA index* correlates with cell *ploidy* (i.e., the number of chromosome sets in a cell) and can be compared with that of normal cells. In various neoplasms (e.g., leukemia, neuroblastoma) DNA indexes > 1.16 (or cell ploidy > 50 chromosomes) are associated with a better prognosis.

32. What is the triad of tumor lysis syndrome?

Hyperuricemia, hyperkalemia, and ***hyperphosphatemia***. These metabolic complications occur as a result of the rapid lysis of a large tumor burden, especially in Burkitt lymphoma and in T-cell leukemia/lymphoma. Secondary renal failure and symptomatic hypocalcemia can also occur.

33. What are the laboratory findings in the tumor lysis syndrome?

Tumor lysis syndrome results from the lysis of malignant cells due to their inherent fragility or as a result of chemotherapy. The electrolyte abnormalities include *hyperkalemia*, *hyperphosphatemia*, and *hyperuricemia*. *Hypocalcemia* may result from hyperphosphatemia.

34. Which patients are at highest risk for tumor lysis syndrome?

The patients at highest risk are those with the most rapidly dividing tumors. The highest risk is with ***Burkitt lymphoma/leukemia***, followed by T-lineage acute lymphoblastic leukemia.

35. What factors can contribute to renal failure in tumor lysis syndrome?

- ***Uric acid nephropathy*:** The degradation of nucleic acids leads to increases in serum uric acid, which is soluble at physiologic pH but can precipitate in the acid milieu of the collecting tubules.
- ***Calcium-phosphate crystallization*:** Lymphoblasts (which contain four times the phosphate of lymphocytes) release phosphate, and if the calcium-phosphate product exceeds 60, crystals can form in the renal microvasculature.
- ***Tumor burden*:** The tumor itself may contribute to preexisting renal problems by parenchymal involvement, obstructive uropathy, and venous stasis.

36. How is the tumor lysis syndrome best managed?

- *Hydration*, at 2-4x maintenance, to maintain high urine output and excretion of electrolytes. Potassium should not be given in the intravenous fluids unless significant hypokalemia develops. Diuretics may need to be administered.
- *Allopurinol*, to prevent uric acid crystals from forming in the urine. Allopurinol inhibits xanthine oxidase, which is involved in the formation of uric acid from hypoxanthine and xanthine (nucleic acid degradation products).
- *Alkalinization*, with sodium bicarbonate, to maintain the urine pH at 7-7.5. A more acidic urine promotes uric acid crystals, while too alkaline an urine promotes hypoxanthine and calcium phosphate precipitation.
- *Dialysis* may be necessary in severe cases.

37. What is superior mediastinal syndrome, and how is it managed?

Superior mediastinal syndrome results from the presence of an anterior mediastinal mass that compresses the trachea and superior vena cava. Patients present with cough and dyspnea, particularly when supine, and have swelling of the head and upper extremities due to venous compression. Patients with a large mediastinal mass must not be anesthetized because of the risk of complete airway obstruction and vascular collapse. The optimal management of a mediastinal mass is prompt diagnosis and the initiation of appropriate treatment. Irradiation of the mass may provide emergent relief while the diagnosis is being made.

38. Which tumors most commonly cause SVC syndrome?

In childhood, the most common primary cause is ***non-Hodgkin lymphoma***. Less frequent causes are Hodgkin disease, neuroblastoma, and sarcomas. Nonmalignant infectious causes are unusual but can include histoplasmosis or tuberculosis. The *most frequent cause* in children, however, is ***iatrogenic***, resulting from vascular thrombosis following surgeries for congenital heart disease, shunting procedures for hydrocephalus, or central catheterization for venous access.

39. How do the superior vena cava (SVC) syndrome and superior mediastinal syndrome (SMS) differ?

SVC syndrome generally refers to symptoms that develop from obstruction of a major vessel, while *SMS* is the designation when tracheal impingement is also present. In adults, the respiratory problems are less common. In children, however, because vascular and tracheal problems frequently occur concurrently, the terms SVC syndrome and SMS are used synonymously. SVC syndrome is the more frequently used term.

40. Why is a generous mediastinal shadow on x-ray much more worrisome in a teenager compared with an infant?

The incidence of Hodgkin disease in infants is extremely low. The thymus normally has a distinctive shape associated with it, flaring at the base with indentations from the ribcage ("sail sign"), which can usually be delineated on plain film. In teenagers with Hodgkin disease, thymic enlargement has a higher likelihood of malignancy, which is usually accompanied by lymphadenopathy in other areas of the mediastinum, particularly the paratracheal, tracheobronchial and hilar regions.

41. Which neoplasms are associated with hemihypertrophy?

Wilms tumor, ***hepatoblastoma***, and ***adrenal cortical carcinoma*** are associated with hemihypertrophy either as part of Beckwith-Wiedemann syndrome or in isolation. 1–3% of Wilms tumor patients have hemihypertrophy.

42. Virilization may be associated with which childhood cancer?

Tumors that cause virilism are most commonly those producing large quantities of dehydroepiandrosterone (DHEA), a 17-ketosteroid. Tumors producing testosterone may also cause virilization. Most commonly these are benign tumors of the adrenal; rarely they are malignant. However, the distinction between carcinoma and benign adenoma frequently is difficult. Occasionally males with primary hepatic neoplasms may become virilized because of production of androgens by the tumor.

43. What can cause stroke in children with cancer?

Malignancy-related
Leptomeningeal disease
Metastatic disease
Disseminated intravascular coagulation

Chemotherapy-related
L-Asparaginase
Methotrexate

Radiation-related
Large-vessel occlusion
Mineralizing microangiopathy

Infection-related
Bacterial meningitis
Fungal meningitis

Packer RJ, et al: Cerebrovascular accidents in children with cancer. Pediatrics 76:194–201, 1985.

44. Which cancers are often associated with splenomegaly?

Acute leukemia, chronic myeloid leukemia, chronic myelomonocytic leukemia, Hodgkin disease, and ***non-Hodgkin lymphoma***. Solid tumors rarely metastasize to the spleen to the point of causing splenomegaly.

45. What are the predictors of malignancy in the pediatric patient with peripheral lymphadenopathy?

A common clinical problem is which patients with enlarged lymph nodes require biopsy for diagnosis. In a study of 60 patients, risk of malignancy increased with increasing size (>1 cm), increasing number of adenopathy sites and ages (8 years of age or older). Supraclavicular location, abnormal CXR and fixed nodes were also significantly predictive of malignancy.

Soldes OS, et al: Predictors of malignancy in childhood peripheral lymphadenopathy. J Pediatr Surg 34:1447-1452, 1999.

46. What paraneoplastic signs can occur in childhood?

Paraneoplastic signs or symptoms are those unrelated to a malignancy, but which can herald cancer. They occur more commonly in adults than children. However, an unexplained high calcium, watery diarrhea, polymyositis, dermatomyositis, unexplained high hemoglobins, hypertension, precocious puberty, and opsoclonus/myoclonus can be associated with childhood malignancies.

Shuper A, et al: Myopathic changes as a paraneoplastic sign in childhood acute lymphoblastic leukemia. Clin Pediatr 37:565-568, 1998.

de Graaf JH, et al: Paraneoplastic manifestations in children. Eur J Pediatr 153:784-791, 1994.

47. Which cancers and chemotherapeutic agents are associated with the syndrome of inappropriate secretion of antidiuretic hormone (SIADH)?

SIADH occurs with ***CNS tumors***, ***lung tumors*** (especially small cell carcinoma in adults), ***lymphoma***, or ***GI carcinoma***. It is also associated with vincristine or cyclophosphamide therapy.

48. A patient receiving chemotherapy has known bone marrow failure and a platelet count of 15,000/mm^3 but no symptoms. Should prophylactic platelet transfusions be given?

A controversial matter. Many institutions empirically give platelets when the count falls below 20,000/mm^3.

Reasons for	*Reasons against*
Hemorrhage from all sites reduced by maintaining platelet count > 20,000/mm^3	Unnecessary since life-threatening bleeding rarely occurs without warning in a stable afebrile thrombocytopenic host
Risk of fatal intracranial hemorrhage practically eliminated	Fatal intracranial hemorrhage is extremely rare unless platelet count is < 5,000/mm^3
Psychological benefit of preventing minor hemorrhage rather than treating it after it occurs	Platelets administered therapeutically for mucosal or internal bleeding just as effective as platelets given prophylactically
Alloimmunization, hepatitis, and other side effects not increased appreciably because most affected patients are heavily transfused anyway; leukocyte depletion filters and improved donor screening have reduced frequency of these complications	Lack of controlled studies proving efficacy
	Expense
	Greater likelihood of alloimmunization and allergic reactions
	Increased incidence of infectious complications, especially viral hepatitis

From Buchanan GR: Hematologic supportive care of the pediatric cancer patient. In Pizzo PA, Poplack DG (eds): Principles and Practice of Pediatric Oncology, 3rd ed. Philadelphia, Lippincott-Raven, 1997, p. 1057; with permission.

49. Does "reverse isolation" help prevent infection in neutropenic patients?

Reverse isolation is the placement of a patient in a single room with all medical staff and visitors wearing gowns, masks, and gloves. It is ineffective in preventing illness in neutropenic patients because most infections arise from the patient's endogenous microbial flora. Other measures that have been shown to have little value are (1) the patient's wearing of a surgical mask outside his or her room and (2) avoidance of fresh fruits and vegetables to minimize acquisition of bacteria, particularly gram-negative organisms.

50. How is fever and neutropenia defined and managed?

In most centers, a ***temperature of at least 38.5°C*** and ***an absolute neutrophil count less than 500/mm^3*** (or 1000/mm^3 and rapidly falling) comprise *febrile neutropenia*. Most centers also include patients with neutropenia and three temperatures of 38.0°C taken 4 hours apart.

Febrile neutropenia is a *medical emergency* because of the high risk of life-threatening bacterial infections. Blood cultures should be obtained, and broad-spectrum antibiotics administered promptly. Patients who have persistent or recurrent fever and continued neutropenia after 5 to 7 days of anti-bacterial treatment should receive empiric antifungal therapy.

Pizzo PA: Fever in immunocompromised patients. N Engl J Med 341:893-900,1999.

51. Can patients with fever and neutropenia be managed as outpatients?

These patients have traditionally been managed with hospitalization for parenteral antibiotics. As criteria for possible outpatient treatment have been developed in other pediatric patients with high-risk fevers (e.g., infants less than 2 months of age, children with sickle cell disease), outpatient approaches to fever and neutropenia are being evaluated as well. In limited studies, low risk patients with fever and neutropenia, defined as older than 2 years, adequate venous access, ability to take oral meds, access to a telephone and no more than one hour from the hospital, have done well after receiving one dose of IV ceftazidime and subsequent oral ciprofloxacin.

Mullen CA, et al: Outpatient treatment of fever and neutropenia for low risk pediatric cancer patients. Cancer 86:126-134, 1999.

52. Following broad-spectrum antibiotics therapy for four days for fever and neutropenia, a patient on day 4 develops a new fever associated with abdominal cramps and bloody diarrhea. What is the most likely diagnosis?

The patient most likely has ***Clostridium difficile colitis***, brought on by treatment with broad-spectrum antibiotics. The diagnosis should be confirmed by detection of the *C. difficile* toxins in the stool, and either metronidazole or oral vancomycin should be initiated promptly.

53. In a granulocytopenic patient receiving antibiotics who develops symptoms of esophagitis, what are the two most common infectious causes?

Candidiasis and ***herpes simplex***. If examination of the oropharynx does not reveal signs of infection, this does not exclude the diagnosis because 50% of patients can have esophageal candidiasis without oral lesions. Controversy exists about whether to treat empirically (e.g., amphotericin, acyclovir, or both) or to perform esophagoscopy for a more definitive diagnosis (but with the risk of inducing bacteremia).

54. What is the best way to prevent nosocomial infections?

Hand-washing is the most effective means to prevent the spread of infections within the hospital.

55. What is typhlitis?

Typhlitis (from the Greek *typhlon* for cecum) is an inflammation of the cecum that occurs in neutropenic patients. It is usually associated with infection by anaerobic bacteria, and treatment is with bowel rest and broad-spectrum antibiotics. Surgery should be avoided, except in cases of perforation, because of the high risks of surgery in a neutropenic patient.

56. When are transfusions necessary?

Although there are no absolute criteria, packed red blood cells are given for a hemoglobin less than 8.0 g/dl in most centers. Platelets are empirically administered for a platelet count less than 10,000-20,000/mm^{3-} in an otherwise well patient; a higher threshold may be used if there is active bleeding, DIC, or a planned procedure. Granulocyte transfusions may be effective in neutropenic patients with a refractory infection secondary to a gram negative organism. Transfusions with plasma may be used in the treatment of coagulopathies.

57. Why are blood products irradiated and leukocyte-depleted?

Irradiation of blood products prevents transfusion-associated graft-versus-host disease, which occurs when small numbers of T cells in the blood product are transferred into an immunocompromised patient. Leukocyte-depletion removes other white blood cells that would increase the risk of febrile transfusion reactions, allo-immunization, and transmission of CMV.

58. Why do patients on chemotherapy receive trimethoprim-sulfimethoxazole?

Trimethoprim-sulfimethoxazole is used to prevent *Pneumocystis carinii* pneumonia. Prophylaxis can be obtained with 2 to 3 days of consecutive day dosing per week.

59. Which hematopoietic growth factors are in common use?

Granulocyte-colony stimulating factor (G-CSF) promotes the production of granulocytes by the bone marrow, and is widely used for the treatment of neutropenia. However, while it effectively shortens the duration of neutropenia, most studies have shown minimal effect on the incidence of febrile neutropenia or bacterial infections. ***Granulocyte-macrophage colony stimulating factor*** (GM-CSF) also reduces the duration of neutropenia, but it has more side-effects than G-CSF. It has been an effective adjunct to anti-fungal therapy in severe fungal infections. ***Interleukin-11*** is used in the treatment of thrombocytopenia and mucositis, but it has not been fully evaluated in pediatric patients.

Pui CH, et al: Human granulocyte colony-stimulating factor after induction chemotherapy in children with acute lymphoblastic leukemia. N Engl J Med 336:1781-1787, 1997.

60. What are the most common symptoms experienced by oncology patients who are receiving only palliative care at the end of life?

Fatigue, ***pain*** and ***dyspnea***. Parents report that these symptoms are managed effectively in less than one-third of children. Compared with adults, twice as many children die in hospitals in the final stages, half of them on a ventilator. Insufficient attention to palliative care is a large problem.

Wolfe J, et al: Symptoms and suffering at the end of life in children with cancer. N Engl J Med 342:326-333, 2000.

61. How common is the use of alternative medical practices in the treatment of cancer in children?

In some studies, 25-50% of families utilize alternative therapies. The three most widely used in children appear to be the use of ***faith healers, megavitamin therapy*** and ***metabolic therapy. ****Faith healing* involves prayer, the laying on of hands and a combination of spirituality and psychology in part seeking divine restorative intervention. *Megavitamin therapy* utilizes high doses of vitamins B and/or C. *Metabolic therapy* includes special diets, detoxification by enemas and enzymatic supplements aimed at purifying the body of accumulated toxins. Their benefits remain unproven.

Lerner JJ, Kennedy BJ: The prevalence of questionable methods of cancer treatment in the United States. Cancer 42:181, 1992.

62. What Internet sites are helpful for parents of children with cancer?

The National Cancer Institute maintains the Cancer Information Service website (http://cis.nci.nih.gov/contact/faqform.html) and the PDQ website (http://cancernet.nci.nih.gov/pdq.html). The Cancer Information Service website provides current scientific information on cancers in layman's language. The PDQ website provides a searchable database of cancer treatments, screening, supportive care and ongoing clinical trials. The pediatric cancer cooperative groups also have a website that provides information about various protocols (http://www.nccf.org/). OncoLink, maintained by the University of Pennsylvania, is another useful resource (http://www.oncolink.com).

EPIDEMIOLOGY

63. Is cancer the most common cause of death in children less than age 15 years?

Cancer ranks a distant second, accounting for 10% of deaths in children < age 15. Accidents account for nearly 45% of deaths. Congenital anomalies rank third with 8%, and homicide ranks fourth with 5%.

64. What is the most common neoplasm of childhood?

Acute lymphoblastic leukemia. Approximately 4/100,00 children aged <15 years develop this neoplasm annually, or about 2000 cases/year in the United States.

Pui C: Childhood leukemias. N Engl J Med 332:1618–1630, 1995.

65. What are the relative risks for children to develop leukemia?

Population at Risk	*Estimate Risk*	*Time Interval (yrs)*
U.S. white children	1:2800	10
Siblings of child with leukemia	1:700	10
Identical twin of child with leukemia	1:5	Wks to mos
Children with		
Down syndrome	1:75	10
Fanconi syndrome	1:12	21
Bloom syndrome	1:8	26
Ataxia-telangiectasia	1:8	25
Exposures		
Atom bomb within 100 m	1:60	12
Ionizing radiation	?	10–25
Benzene	1:960	12
Alkylating agents	1:2000?	10–20

From Mahoney DH Jr: Neoplastic diseases. In McMillan JA, et al (eds): Oski's Pediatrics, Principles and Practice, 3rd ed. Philadelphia, J.B. Lippincott, 1999, p 1494; with permission.

66. What is the relative incidence of the childhood cancers in the U.S.?

Leukemias	27%	*Soft tissue tumors*	6%
CNS tumors	21%	*Bone tumors*	5%
Lymphomas	11%	*Retinoblastoma*	3%
Neuroblastoma	7%	*Other tumors*	14%
Wilms tumor	6%		

Gurney JG, et al: Incidence of cancer in children in the United States. Cancer 75:2186, 1995.

67. How does the types of malignancies compare between infants and adolescents?

Infants
(approximate incidence)

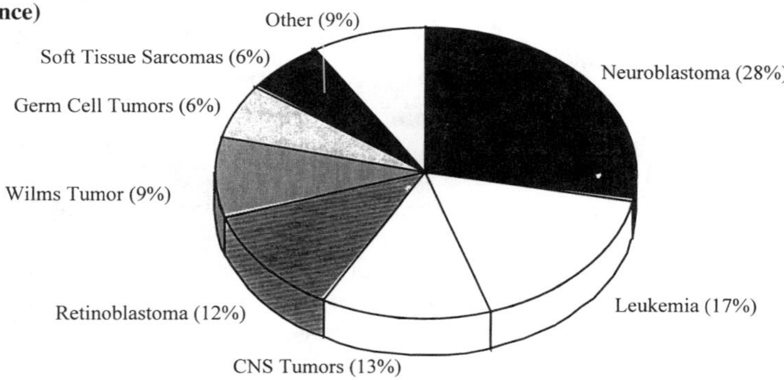

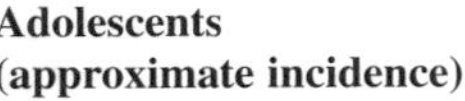

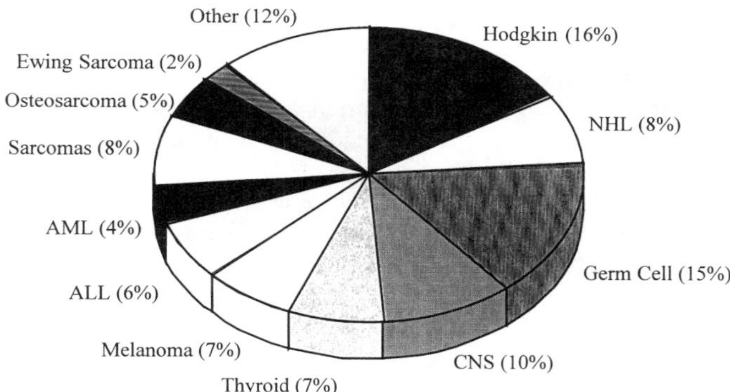

68. Which childhood cancers can be congenital?

In a 30-year period at the M.D. Anderson Hospital, there were 423 infant neoplasms, of which 24 (5%) occurred in neonates and could be considered congenital. These included 8 fibrosarcomas, 6 neuroblastomas, 3 CNS tumors, 3 leukemias, 2 retinoblastomas, 1 Langerhans cell histiocytosis, and 1 malignant melanoma.

Cangir A, et al: Malignant neoplasms in the neonatal period. Proc Am Soc Clin Oncol 6:A847, 1987.

69. What are the risks of the Li-Fraumeni syndrome?

Li-Fraumeni syndrome is an autosomal dominant condition caused by heritable mutations in the *p53* tumor suppressor gene. The *p53* gene is located on chromosome 17 and plays a central role in controlling progression through the cell cycle. Patients with a heritable mutation in one *p53* allele are at high risk of malignancy if they develop a spontaneous mutation in the second allele. Patients with Li-Fraumeni syndrome are predisposed to many cancers, including rhabdomyosarcoma, brain tumors, acute leukemia, adrenocortical cell carcinoma, and premenopausal breast cancer. Members of such families have an estimated ***50% probability of developing an invasive cancer*** by the age of 30.

70. Which cancers have a significant racial predilection?

Wilms tumor has a higher incidence in black female infants. Ewing tumor is about 30 times more common in whites than in blacks. Hodgkin disease is rare in those of East Asian descent.

71. What cancers are most commonly associated with a second neoplasm?

Primary Tumors	*Secondary Tumors*
Retinoblastoma	Osteosarcoma Pinealoblastoma
Hodgkin disease	Acute nonlymphoblastic leukemia Non-Hodgkin lymphoma Sarcoma (in radiation field) Thyroid carcinoma Breast carcinoma (in radiation field)
Acute lymphoblastic leukemia	Brain tumors Non-Hodgkin lymphoma
Sarcomas	Sarcomas

72. Are any childhood cancers associated with an increased alpha-fetoprotein?

Increased *alpha-fetoprotein* is associated with germ cell tumors, including endodermal sinus tumors of the ovary and testicular yolk sac carcinoma, hepatocellular tumors, and retinoblastoma. Normally, alpha-fetoprotein is synthesized in the liver, yolk sac, and GI tract of the fetus. Synthesis usually stops at birth; it disappears with a half-life of 3.5 days. Elevated serum levels are most commonly seen with nonmalignant liver disease. Levels remain elevated for 5–7 weeks after resection of the tumor but persistence beyond that time is suggestive of residual disease.

73. Are there any known transplacental carcinogens?

Diethylstilbestrol, which was used to prevent spontaneous abortion, has been associated with an increased risk of vaginal cancer in the female offspring. It has also been reported that there is a 10-fold increased risk of monoblastic leukemia in the infants of mothers who smoke marijuana. It has been suggested that sedatives and a number of nonhormonal drugs are transplacental carcinogens, but this is not proven. It also has not been proved that cigarette smoke or the use of oral contraceptives are transplacental carcinogens.

74. If an expectant mother admits to smoking, drinking, and illicit drug use during pregnancy, is there an increased risk of malignancy for the unborn child?

Several studies have shown weak associations (odds ratios of approximately 2) between acute lymphoblastic leukemia (ALL) and maternal smoking, alcohol intake, and drug use. However, the baseline risk of ALL is so small, that the additional risk of ALL conferred by maternal smoking, alcohol intake, and drug use is not substantial. Moreover, the risk of other congenital anomalies and health problems from maternal smoking, alcohol, and drug use is far greater than any additional risk of ALL.

75. Is prenatal ultrasound associated with a risk of leukemia later in childhood?

No. *In vitro*, ultrasound has been shown to cause cell membrane changes and thus concern has been expressed regarding potential effects on embryogenesis and pre- and postnatal development. However, in a study of all deaths due to leukemia in Swedish children over a 16 year period, no association with prenatal ultrsound was found. Of note, the only known association of prenatal ultrasound to alterations in development has been a preference to non-righthandedness.

Naumburg E, et al: Prenatal ultrasound examinations and risk of childhood leukaemia: Case-control study. BMJ 320:282-283, 2000.

Kieler H, et al: Routine ultrasound screening in pregnancy and aspects of the children's subsequent neurological development. Obstet Gynecol 91:750-756, 1998.

76. Do children living near electrical power lines have an increased risk of developing cancer?

Although a few small studies have suggested an association between power lines and an increased risk of ALL, the largest and best designed study as reported by Linet did ***not*** find evidence to support this hypothesis. Since that time, additional overseas studies have not demonstrated a significant risk.

UK Childhood Study Investigators: Exposure to power-frequency magnetic fields and the risk of childhood cancer. Lancet 354:1925-1931, 1999.

Linet MS, et al: Residential exposure to magnetic fields and acute lymphoblastic leukemia in children. N Engl J Med 337:1-7, 1997.

77. What should be the surveillance strategy for malignancy for children with trisomy 21?

While children with trisomy 21 have an increased risk of leukemia, they appear to have a lower risk of solid tumors than children with normal karyotypes. Thus any surveillance schema for solid tumors is inappropriate. Presently, no screening schema for leukemia is recommended for patients with trisomy 21.

LEUKEMIA

78. What is the normal lymphoblast concentration in bone marrow?

5%. At least 25% of the bone marrow should be occupied by lymphoblasts to confirm the diagnosis of leukemia. In most cases, the marrow is very hypercellular, with 60–100% of the contents being lymphoblastic.

79. What are the most common clinical findings in the initial presentation of acute lymphoblastic leukemia (ALL)?

- *Hepatosplenomegaly:* 70% (10–15% of children have marked enlargement of the liver or spleen to a level below the umbilicus)
- *Fever*: 40–60%
- *Lymphadenopathy*: 25–50% with moderate or marked enlargement
- *Bleeding*: 25–50% with petechiae or purpura
- *Bone/joint pain*: 25–40%
- *Fatigue*: 30%
- *Anorexia*: 20–35%

80. What are the typical hematologic findings noted on presentation of ALL?

Leukocyte count (mm^3)	
<10,000	45–55%
10,000–50,000	30–35%
> 50,000	20%
Hemoglobin (gm/dl)	
< 7.5	45%
7.5–10.0	30%
> 10	25%
Platelet count (mm^3)	
<20,000	25%
20,000–99,000	50%
> 100,000	25%

81. Why do children with acute leukemia under 1 year of age have a poorer prognosis?

The great majority of infants with ALL under age 1 year often have a full complement of ***unfavorable features***: high WBC count, CNS leukemia, bulky extramedullary disease, and t(4;11) (a translocation associated with poor response to therapy). In contrast, the prognosis for infants with AML is not necessarily less favorable than for older children (except for those with monoblastic leukemia, who fare poorly).

82. 55. Why do boys with ALL fare more poorly than girls?

The precise answer is unclear, but two factors may be important:

1. In boys who are in remission after a full course of chemotherapy, testicular involvement is a common site of relapse, occurring in up to 10% of cases. In girls, ovarian relapse is very rare, though difficult to diagnose after bone marrow relapse.

2. In older boys and teenage males, there is a higher incidence of T-cell disease than in girls. T-cell disease is associated with adverse prognostic factors (high WBC count, hepatosplenomegaly, and mediastinal masses) and alone carries a poorer prognosis.

83. Although the cause of the majority of leukemias remains unknown, what are known risk factors for the development of childhood leukemia?

	ALL	AML
Congenital	Down syndrome Ataxia telangiectasia	Down syndrome Neurofibromatosis type I Fanconi anemia Severe congenital neutropenia
Acquired	Radiation (high-dose)	Radiation (high-dose) Pesticide exposure Maternal ethanol use Epipodophyllotoxins Alkylating agents

84. In addition to leukemia, what other diagnoses should be considered in evaluating a child presenting with pancytopenia?

- Aplastic anemia
- Viral-induced suppression
- Drug-induced suppression
- Metastatic disease to the bone marrow
- Hemophagocytic syndromes
- Disseminated histoplasmosis
- Transfusion-associated graft-versus-host disease

85. Athough many prognostic factors have come and gone for childhood ALL, which two have remained significant for the past 40 years?

The two most consistent prognostic factors are ***age*** and ***elevation of presenting white blood cell count***. Children less than 1 year old or greater than 10 years old have a worse prognosis, as do those with a presenting white blood cell count ≥ 50,000/mm^3. Prognostic factors are important because although 95% of ALL patients achieve remission (less than 5% lymphoblasts in bone marrow), 25% relapse. Identifying patients at higher risk is important so that more aggressive or novel therapy can be considered.

86. Other than age at diagnosis and white blood count, what other factor that has the greatest prognostic impact on long term survival?

A better prognosis is seen in patients who have a ***brisk initial response to therapy***. This has been defined differently in separate studies. The Children's Cancer Group found an improved prognosis in patients with less than 5% blasts in the bone marrow after seven days of chemotherapy. The Berlin-Frankfurt-Münster group found a similar prognosis in patients who had <1000 blasts/mm^3 in the peripheral blood after seven days of prednisone.

87. What is the prognostic value of minimal residual disease?

PCR technology can identify children with *minimal residual disease* after completion of induction therapy by identifying residual leukemic cells (beyond detection of conventional microscopic evaluation) in patients in remission. Leukemia-associated immunophenotyping is another technique that can detect their presence. In a study of 174 patients using PCR technology, the presence of minimal residual disease was associated with much higher and faster rates of relapse. Other studies using PCR-based qualitative and quantitative methods have been developed to detect clonal rearrangement of the immunoglobulin or T-cell receptor gene in the leukemic cell. Clonal rearrangement is also associated with a poorer prognosis.

Cave H, et al: Clinical significance of minimal residual disease in childhood acute lymphoblastic leukemia. N Engl J Med 339:591-598, 1998.

Evans PAS, et al: Residual disease detection using fluorescent polymerase chain reaction at 20 weeks of therapy predicts clinical outcome in childhood acute lymphoblastic leukemia. J Clin Oncol 16:3616-3627, 1998.

88. What is the optimal duration for maintenance chemotherapy in ALL?

While this may ultimately be shown to vary by prognostic factors (e.g., sex), most centers treat between 2.5–3 years. The optimal duration remains a question for ongoing study.

89. What are the more common cytogenetic abnormalities observed in ALL?

Immunophenotype Translocation	*Features*	*Affected Genes*		*% of Leukemias*
All				
t(9;22)(q34;q11)	Ph[1] chromosome	ABL	BCR	3–5%
B lineage				
t(12;21)(p12;q22)	Favorable	TEL	AML1	16–22%
t(1;19)(q23;p13)	High WBC	PBX	E2A	5–6%
t(4;11)(q21;q23)	Infant ALL	AF-4	MLL	2%
t(11;19)(q23;p13)		MLL	ENL	< 1%
T lineage				
t(11;14)(p13;q11)	High WBC/CNS disease		TTG2	GCR∂
t(8;14)(q24;q32.3)	L3 morphology	MYC	Ig locus	1–2%

90. What is the acute risk of a very elevated blast count noted at the time of the initial diagnosis of leukemia?

An elevated blast count at diagnosis may cause ***CNS leukostasis and stroke***. The risk is higher in patients with AML, because myeloblasts are larger in size and may have procoagulant activity that increases the risk of stroke or hemorrhage. Leukocytapheresis is sometimes used to reduce the blast count prior to initiating therapy, but its impact on improving outcome remains unproven.

91. What are the most common sites of extramedullary relapse of ALL?

The most common is the ***central nervous system***, followed by ***testicular*** relapse. Testicular disease presents with painless testicular swelling (usually unilateral). The diagnosis must be confirmed by biopsy. Patients with testicular disease require irradiation in addition to intensive re-treatment with chemotherapy.

92. What role did Nobel Prize winners Gertrude Elion and George Hitchings play in the treatment of childhood leukemia?

Both won the Nobel Prize for physiology and medicine for their extensive work on purine biochemistry and goals of creating medicines to target DNA synthesis. They designed 6-mercaptopurine, the first rationally synthesized anti-leukemic drug. The other drugs that emerged from their laboratory included 6-thioguanine, allopurinol, azathioprine, and acyclovir.

93. What clinical intervention did Donald Pinkel and colleagues at St. Jude Children's Research Hospital pioneer in the 1960s that resulted in the largest incremental improvement in the survival rates of children with ALL?

Cranial radiation combined with intrathecal methotrexate. This regimen was incorporated for the prevention of CNS disease in ALL, which markedly improved survival rates. Prior to this, up to 75% of children with ALL suffered a CNS relapse, despite having no evidence if CNS disease at diagnosis. Because of the long-term side effects associated with cranial radiation, intrathecal chemotherapy combined with appropriate systemic chemotherapy is used more commonly for CNS preventive therapy today.

94. What are the long-term side effects of cranial radiation administered for the prevention of CNS leukemia?

A number of endocrinologic complications can occur, including growth hormone deficiency, hypothyroidism, hypogonadism, impaired fertility and premature ovarian failure. Children are also at risk for deficits in attention, memory and IQ. Less commonly, leukoencephalopathy may occur. Finally, children receiving cranial radiation are at risk of developing a second malignant neoplasm.

95. When evaluating a new patient with suspected acute leukemia, what diagnostic studies performed with cells obtained from a bone marrow aspirate help to differentiate ALL and AML?

	ALL	*AML**
Morphology		
Cell size	Usually smaller	Usually larger
Nuclear:cytoplasmic ratio	High	Low
Nucleoli	<2	2–5
Granules	Absent	May be present
Auer rods	Absent	May be present
Histochemistry		
Periodic acid–Schiff	Positive	Negative
Sudan black	Negative	Positive
Peroxidase	Negative	Positive
TdT	Present	Absent
Immunophenotype	CD10, CD19, HLA-DR (pre-B) CD2, CD7 (pre-T)	CD13, CD14, CD33, CD38

*There is considerable variability between different AML subtypes

96. How do remission and relapse rates vary in ALL and AML?

Most children with ALL survive relapse-free, and so the median duration of first remission has not been reached. If relapse occurs in the CNS or testes, many children can still be cured with irradiation and additional chemotherapy. If relapse occurs in the marrow within 18 months of diagnosis, the chance of cure with either chemotherapy or stem cell transplant is <10%. If marrow relapse occur > 18 months from diagnosis, and especially if it occurs after treatment has been stopped, intense chemotherapy or stem cell transplant may offer prolonged second remission and possible cure in > 25% of patients.

Between 75–80% of children with AML achieve remission, with median remission duration of about 14 months. About 10% of the patients die from infectious or hemorrhagic complications during induction, and another 10–20% fail to respond to the initial therapy. Of the children who achieve remission, between 40–50% survive 5 years. If disease recurs, it is usually fatal. Transplant may cure some patients who relapse.

Chessells JM: Recent advances in management of acute leukaemia. Arch Dis Child 82:438-442, 2000.

97. How do survival rates in children vary by leukemia type?

- Chemotherapeutic regimens cure as many as 70-80% of children with ALL, ranging from approximately 40% with multiple high-risk factors to 90% with lower risk.
- AML is associated with a cure rate of 30–40%.
- CML requires allogenic stem cell transplantation and has a 5-year survival rate of 80–90% for the adult form of the disease and 40–50% for the juvenile form.

Stiller CA, et al: Patterns of care and survival for children with acute lymphoblastic leukaemia diagnosed between 1980 and 1994. Arch Dis Child 81:202-208, 1999.

Pui C-H: Childhood leukemias. N Engl J Med 332:1618–1630, 1995.

98. What distinguishes leukemia from lymphoma?

The distinction is often difficult because ALL can resemble non-Hodgkin lymphoma.

Cytomorphologically, there is little difference between T-cell lymphoblastic lymphoma and ALL or between the B-cells of Burkitt lymphoma and mature B-cell ALL. As a rule, the presence of a significant number of blasts cells in the bone marrow (in most centers, > 25%) indicates leukemia.

99. Besides leukemia, what childhood malignancies can present with significant bone marrow involvement?

Neuroblastoma, rhabdomyosarcoma, retinoblastoma, non-Hodgkin lymphoma

100. What types of leukemia are common in patients with Down syndrome?

Down syndrome patients are more likely (18x) to develop both ***AML*** and ***ALL*** than other children. AML predominates in children less than 3 years old, while ALL is more common in older children. The most common subtype of AML in Down syndrome is acute megakaryoblastic leukemia, which is otherwise very rare. Neonates with Down syndrome may also develop a transient myeloproliferative disorder that closely resembles AML, but that resolves without treatment within a few months.

Hasle H, et al: Risks of leukemia and solid tumors in individuals with Down's syndrome. Lancet 355:15-169, 2000.

101. What are the common cytogenetic abnormalities observed in myeloid leukemias?

Translocation	*Features*	*Affected Genes*	
AML			
t(8;21)	M2	AML1	ETO
Inv (16)	M4	CBFβ	MYH11
t(15;17)	M3	RARα	PML
11q23 rearrangements	Infant leukemias M5 Therapy induced leukemia	MLL	Multiple partners
CML			
t(9;22)(q34;q11)		ABL	BCR

102. What factors are associated with an increased incidence of AML?

Genetic factors: Down syndrome, Fanconi anemia, Bloom syndrome, Kostmann syndrome, Diamond Blackman syndrome, paroxysmal nocturnal hemoglobinemia, Li-Fraumeni syndrome, neurofibromatosis

Drugs: benzene, alkylating agents, nitrosoureas, epipodophyllotoxins

Ionizing radiation

Myelodysplastic syndromes

Golub TR, et al: Acute myelogenous leukemia. In Pizzo PA, Poplack DG (eds): Principles and Practice of Pediatric Oncology, 3rd ed. Philadelphia, Lippincott-Raven, 1997, p 464.

103. What is a chloroma?

A *chloroma* is a tumor formed by a coalescence of AML blasts. It may present in bones, skin, soft tissue or other sites. Its name derives from its green appearance on its cut surface.

104. What is the survival rate of pediatric patients with AML?

Overall survival of children with AML is approximately ***40%***. Survival may be improved to 60% if an HLA-matched sibling is available for bone marrow transplant, but unrelated donors are not used in first remission because of a high risk of graft-versus host disease. About 15% of patients will fail induction because of regimen-related toxicity or failure to achieve remission. Monosomy 7 carries a particularly poor prognosis in AML.

Downing JR, Burnett A: Acute myeloid leukemia. N Engl J Med 341:1051-1062, 1999.

105. What is the significance of the Philadephia chromosome?

The *Philadelphia chromosome*, discovered in Philadelphia in 1960 by Nowell and Hungerford, was the first clonal cytogenetic abnormality (a balanced translocation between chromosomes 9 and 22) described in leukemia. The result is a new fusion gene that codes for a tyrosine kinase with increased enzymatic activity. The Philadelphia chromosome is seen in > 90% of patients with CML, but also in up to 5% of children with ALL (20% of adult ALL) and in up to 2% with AML. Different isoforms of the fusion gene may be present in ALL. Ph^+ ALL has a poor prognosis with overall survival about one third of those without it.

Arico M, et al: Outcome of treatment in children with Philadelphia chromosome-positive acute lymphoblastic leukemia. N Engl J Med 342:998-1006, 2000.

106. What is the appropriate treatment for chronic myelogenous leukemia (CML)?

The *definitive* treatment for CML is ***allogeneic stem cell transplantation***. However, for patients who do not have an appropriate stem cell donor, treatment with interferon-α may reduce the white blood cell count, and may occasionally result in a cytogenetic remission. Hydroxyurea may also be employed to reduce the peripheral white blood cell count, but it is not curative. A new drug, STI-571, appears highly effective in inducing remission.

107. What are the differences between CML and juvenile CML (JCML)?

	CML	*JCML*
Philadelphia chromosome	Present	Absent
Facial rash	Absent	Present
Lymphadenopathy	Absent	Present
Presenting WBC/mm^3	>100,000	<100,000
Monocytosis	Absent	Present
Thrombocytopenia	Absent	Present
Fetal hemoglobin	Absent	Elevated
Ineffective erythropoiesis	Absent	Present
Immunoglobulins	Normal	Elevated
Response to therapy	Good	Poor

108. In children who have very elevated WBC counts, why are CNS hemorrhagic complications more likely in AML than ALL?

Compared with lymphocytes, leukocytes (especially promyelocytes and monoblasts) contain compounds with procoagulant activity that are released as the cells lyse and may led to microthrombi formation, disseminated intravascular coagulation, and hemorrhage.

LYMPHOMA

109. Which tumor has the shortest doubling time?

Burkitt lymphoma. The generation time of the Burkitt cell is 24–36 hours. However, the actual doubling time is less than that because there is a very high spontaneous cell death rate. Some T-lymphoblastic leukemia/lymphomas have a doubling time similar to that of Burkitt cells.

110. What is the malignant cell of Hodgkin disease?

Reed-Sternberg cell. Its normal cell of origin remains unclear, with the predominance of evidence indicating a B or T lymphocyte. However, the cells alone are not pathognomonic of Hodgkin disease and may be seen in infectious mononucleosis, non-Hodgkin lymphoma, carcinomas and sarcomas.

111. How is Hodgkin disease "staged"?

Hodgkin lymphoma, like non-Hodgkin lymphoma, is classified according to ***stage of disease*** and ***histology***, as in the Ann Arbor System. It is also staged according to whether there are ***symptoms***. Patients with no symptoms are referred to as having *A* disease. Patients with documented fever, involuntary weight loss > 10%, or night sweats are considered to have *B* disease. Intractable pruritus may also be a symptom but is not among the B symptoms used for staging.

Stage is determined both *clinically* and *pathologically*. Location of lymph node regions is the critical factor: *I* (single region), *II (*regions on same side of diaphragm), *III* (regions on both sides of diagphragm) or *IV* (diffuse disease). ***Clinical staging*** refers to staging that is done without histologic proof. ***Pathologic staging*** refers to biopsy-proven disease in a given region and usually involves a staging laparotomy and splenectomy to determine the extent of disease.

112. What is the histologic classification of Hodgkin disease?

*The Rye, New York, Histologic Classification**

	LYMPHOCYTES	R/S CELLS	OTHER	INCIDENCE
Lymphocyte predominant	Many	Few	Histiocytes	10–15%
Nodular sclerosing	Many	Few or many	Bands of refractile fibrosis	40–70%
Mixed cellularity	Many	Few or many	Eosinophils, histiocytes	20–30%
Lymphocyte depletion	Few	Many	No refractile fibrosis	< 5%

•Based on the relative number of lymphocytes and Reed-Sternberg (R/S) cells.

113. What is the prognosis for the various stages of Hodgkin disease?

The prognosis for children with Hodgkin disease is excellent in that most are cured. For stages I and IIA, the 5-year relapse-free survival is > 80% for patients treated with radiation only and may be > 90% for patients given radiation and chemotherapy. For stage IIB, prognosis is less good, especially if there is a massive mediastinal tumor, but 5-year survival is still >80%. The same survival figures pertain to stage IIIA disease, but treatment generally is more extensive than that for a limited stage II disease. For stage IV disease, 5-year relapse-free survival is 70–90%.

114. How are non-Hodgkin lymphomas classified?

Non-Hodgkin lymphomas (NHLs) include a heterogeneous group of malignant solid tumors that are of lymphoid origin. Their classification is still disputed. In general, NHLs are divided according to the ***extent of spread*** in the body and histology. The disease is either localized or disseminated. Localized tumors are limited to either a node or an area, such as the appendix or a tonsil, and may include some regional surrounding nodes. It can also originate in bone. The tumor cells may spread to the bone marrow or spinal fluid much like leukemia or disseminate throughout the abdomen and pleural space.

Histology is divided into *lymphoblastic* and *nonlymphoblastic* types. The most common type of lymphoblastic lymphoma occurs in the mediastinum and probably originates in the thymus. Disease is virtually always disseminated at diagnosis. Nonlymphoblastic lymphomas include Burkitt lymphoma or peripheral T-cell lymphomas. Burkitt lymphoma often occurs in the retroperitoneum and is usually disseminated. The classification of NHLs of childhood is very different from that of adults.

Sandlund JT, et al: Non-Hodgkin's lymphoma in childhood. N Engl J Med 334:1238–1248, 1996.

115. What are the common types of lymphoma in children?

Compared to adults, aggressive, high-grade lymphomas occur more frequently in children. The three most common types are ***Burkitt lymphoma***, ***lymphoblastic lymphoma*** and ***large-cell lymphoma***.

116. What is the difference between sporadic and endemic Burkitt lymphoma?

Endemic Burkitt lymphoma, associated with the Epstein-Barr virus, is the most common form in Africa, and often presents as a jaw tumor. The *sporadic* form, less frequently associated with EBV, is the more common form in developed countries, and often presents as rapidly enlarging abdominal tumor.

Shad A, Magrath I: Non-Hodgkin's lymphoma. Pediatr Clin North Am 44:863-890, 1997.

117. What is the common cytogenetic abnormality in Burkitt lymphoma?

t(8;14) fuses the c-myc oncogene to the immunoglobulin heavy chain gene. This ***translocation*** is found in both endemic and sporadic forms, though the breakpoints differ.

118. What are B symptoms?

Fever, ***night sweats***, and ***weight loss***. Their presence carries a poorer prognosis in patients with Hodgkin disease.

119. What second malignancies are common in patients treated for Hodgkin disease?

The type of second malignancy depends in part on the treatment used for the primary tumor. Depending on the field included in primary treatment, *radiation* increases the risk of skin, bone and breast cancer. *Chemotherapy* with alkylating agents increases the risk of AML.

Hudson MM, Donaldson SS: Hodgkin's disease. Pediatr Clin North Am 44:891-906, 1997.

120. What is an eosinophilic granuloma?

Eosinophilic granuloma is a lytic tumor of bone that presents with pain and sometimes swelling. Its histology is identical to that of Langerhans cell histiocytosis, with which it is now classified. Biopsy of an isolated eosinophilic granuloma is often curative, though lesions may also regress spontaneously.

121. What are the features of Langerhans cell histiocytosis (LCH)?

LCH is a multifaceted disorder and replaces the diseases grouped under the term histiocytosis X. LCH may present with isolated bone lesions (*eosinophilic granuloma*), bone lesions together with exophthalmos and diabetes insipidus (*Hand-Schüller-Christian disease*), or with disseminated disease (*Letterer-Siwe*). Other features include skin rashes that resemble seborrheic dermatitis, chronic otitis externa, lymphadenopathy, hepatosplenomegaly, pancytopenia, neurologic deficits, and pulmonary disease. Mild forms of the disease tend to wax and wane, even without treatment, while disseminated disease is often resistant to therapy.

122. What is FEL?

Familial erythrophagocytic lymphohistiocytosis. As its name suggests, it is a familial disorder that occurs in young children, in which abnormal histiocytes engulf normal hematopoietic cells. Expansion of the histiocytes causes massive hepatosplenomegaly and pancytopenia, and the disorder is rapidly fatal. Bone marrow transplant may be curative if performed early in the course of the disease. A related disorder, viral-associated hemophagocytic syndrome occurs in older children and may have a better prognosis.

NERVOUS SYSTEM TUMORS

123. With regard to the primary site of origin, how do childhood brain tumors contrast with those of an adult?

Approximately 50% of brain tumors in children are ***infratentorial***, with three fourths of these located in the cerebellum or fourth ventricle. In contrast, the majority of brain tumors in adult patients are ***supratentorial*** in location.

124. What are the four most common infratentorial tumors diagnosed in children?

1. *Cerebellar astrocytoma*, which is usually pilocytic but occasionally may be invasive or high-grade
2. *Medulloblastoma*, also referred to as primitive neuroectodermal tumor
3. *Ependymoma*
4. *Brain stem glioma*, which is usually diagnosed on MRI without biopsy

Packer RJ: Brain tumors in children. Arch Neurol 56:421-5, 1999.

125. Which three types of childhood brain tumors occur in the sellar/suprasellar region?

Sellar/suprasellar tumors comprise approximately 20% of childhood brain tumors and include ***craniopharyngiomas***, low-grade ***gliomas*** (chiasmic, hypothalamic, and/or thalamic) and ***germinomas***.

126. What are the key evaluations for a child with a newly-diagnosed medulloblastoma?

Medulloblastomas may spread contiguously to the cerebellar peduncle, to floor of the fourth ventricle, into the cervical spine, or above the tentorium. In addition, medulloblastomas may disseminate via the cerebrospinal fluid. Every patient should thus be evaluated with diagnostic imaging (MRI) of the spinal cord and whole brain. Examination of CSF should be performed following resection of the primary tumor.

127. Which cranial nerve abnormality is most common in children presenting with increased intracranial pressure secondary to a posterior fossa tumor?

Inability to *abduct* one or both eyes (***cranial nerve VI palsy***) may result from an elevation in ICP and can be a false localizing sign for the primary brain tumor.

128. What factors predict poor prognosis for children with medulloblastoma?

Children ***younger than 3 years*** of age, those with ***metastatic disease***, or those with ***subtotal resection*** (>1.5 cm^3 of residual disease) are at highest risk of treatment failure.

129. What is the prognosis for children with brainstem gliomas?

The outlook for children with intrinsic brainstem gliomas remains ***extremely poor***, as radiation therapy and chemotherapy to date have not proven curative. In a small number of children with low-grade dorsally exophytic tumors, surgical resection may prove beneficial. Patients with small tectal lesions and hydrocephalus can be treated with a venticulo-peritoneal shunt, as these tumors tend to be low-grade and progress slowly.

130. Children with neurofibromatosis type 1 are at increased risk for which intracranial neoplasm?

Children with neurofibromatosis type 1 are at increased risk for ***visual pathway*** and ***hypothalamic gliomas***, which may occur anywhere along the optic tracts and are usually low-grade astrocytomas that grow slowly.

131. What CNS tumor might be suspected in an apparently euphoric young child with severe failure to thrive?

Hypothalamic gliomas may result in the ***diencephalic syndrome***. Such children may have little in the way of other neurologic findings, but can have macrocephaly, intermittent lethargy, and visual impairment.

132. Should a child with a completely resected low grade astrocytoma of the occipital lobe receive radiation therapy?

There is ***no*** evidence that radiation therapy is of benefit for children with completely resected low grade astrocytomas. For patients with incomplete resections, treatment options include observation, re-resection, radiation, and/or chemotherapy.

133. Where do germ cell tumors of the central nervous system tend to arise?

Germ cell brain tumors usually arise in the ***pineal*** or ***suprasellar regions***. Histologic subtypes include teratoma, germinoma, and the more malignant embryonal cell carcinoma, choriocarcinoma, and endodermal sinus tumor. Every patient with a germinoma or malignant germ cell tumor should be evaluated with an MRI of the spinal cord and whole brain, as these tumors have a propensity for subarachnoid spread.

134. What's the difference between an astrocytoma, a glioma and glioblastoma multiforme?

A *glioma* (from the Greek word glia for glue and the suffix -oma for tumor) is a neoplasm derived from one of the various types of cells that form the interstitial tissue of the central nervous system, such as astrocytes, oligodendria and ependymal cells. Of the gliomas, astrocytomas of variable malignancy are the most prevalent. Cerebral *astrocytomas* are subdivided into categories (grades) based on the degree of tumor anaplasia and the presence or absence of necrosis. The juvenile pilocytic and subependymal astrocytoma are low grade gliomas. Anaplastic astrocytomas (grade 3) grows more rapidly than the more differentiated astrocytomas. The highest grade astrocytoma (grade 4) is termed *glioblastoma multiforme*.

135. What is the Cushing Triad?

The *Cushing response* or *triad* represents the brainstem's effort to maintain cerebral perfusion in the face of markedly elevated intracranial pressure (ICP). The trio of manifestations include ***increased blood pressure***, ***decreased respiration*** and ***bradycardia***.

136. What is a "dropped met"?

Most brain tumors do not metastasize. They are fatal because of local invasion. A *dropped metastases* is the term used when a primary brain tumor spreads via CSF pathways resulting in meningeal deposits along the spinal cord. These metastases have "dropped" from their original site down to the spinal cord or cauda equina.

137. Which posterior fossa tumor is commonly associated with erythrocytosis?

Cerebellar hemangioblastoma. This tumor can secrete erythropoietin.

138. How does the pathophysiology of spinal cord compression differ in children compared with adults?

In *children*, spinal cord compression most commonly is due to primary or metastatic disease in the epidural space, especially with sarcoma, neuroblastoma, lymphoma, and leukemia. In *adults*, metastatic disease is likely to involve the vertebral body, with compression caused by tumor growth extending through the intervertebral foramina. This event rarely occurs in children.

139. How can the site of spinal cord compression be clinically localized?

Spinal tenderness on percussion correlates with localization in up to 80% of patients. In addition, neurologic evaluation of strength, sensory level changes, reflexes, and anal tone can help to pinpoint the location in the spinal cord, conus medullaris (terminal neural portion of the spinal cord), or cauda equina.

Clinical Localization of Site of Spinal Cord Compression

SIGN	SPINAL CORD	CONUS MEDULLARIS	CAUDA EQUINA
Weakness	Symmetric, profound	Symmetric, variable	Asymmetric, may be mild
Tendon reflexes	Increased or absent	Increased knee, decreased ankle	Decreased, asymmetric
Babinski reflex	Extensor	Extensor	Plntar
Sensory	Symmetric, sensory level	Symmetric, saddle	Asymmetric, radicular
Sphincter abnormality	Spared until late	Early involvement	May be spared
Progression	Rapid	Variable, may be rapid	Variable, may be rapid

From Lange B, et al: Oncologic emergencies. In Pizzo PA, Poplack DG (eds): Principles and Practice of Pediatric Oncology, 3rd ed. Philadelphia, Lippincott-Raven, 1997, p 1039; with permission.

140. In addition to retinoblastoma, what diseases can present with leukokoria?

Leukokoria, or white pupil, can be obvious or can be a subtle asymmetry on pupillary red reflex evaluation. Of note, 20–30% of cases of retinoblastoma are bilateral. A pediatric ophthalmologist familiar with the disease is usually able to distinguish retinoblastoma from other causes of leukokoria, which include:

- *Toxocara canis* infection
- Persistent hyperplastic primary vitreous
- Coats disease
- Large chorioretinal coloboma
- Retinopathy of prematurity (retrolental fibroplasia)
- Congenital cataract
- Retinal dysplasia
- Medulloepithelioma (dictyoma)
- Congenital retinal fold
- Uveitis

French-Howard GL, Ellsworth RM: Differential diagnosis of retinoblastoma: A statistical survey of 500 children. Am J Ophthalmol 60:610, 1965.

141. What is the heredity of retinoblastoma?

Although the majority of cases are sporadic, retinoblastoma can be inherited as an autosomal dominant trait with nearly complete penetrance. Of all cases, 60% are nonhereditary and unilateral, 15% are hereditary and unilateral, and 25% are hereditary and bilateral. Families of patients with retinoblastoma should have genetic counseling.

142. How are tumor-suppressor genes involved in retinoblastoma?

Tumor-suppressor genes encode for proteins necessary in the control of cell growth and differentiation. The *RB1* gene belongs to a group of tumor-suppressor genes located on chromosome 13. In some cases of retinoblastoma, there appears to be loss of one allele of the *RB1* gene in the germline followed by the loss of the other allele in the tumor. This loss of heterozygosity leaves the tumor cells without the regulatory function of the gene and is thought to contribute to oncogenesis. A similar situation is thought to occur with the p53 tumor-suppressor gene in the Li-Fraumeni syndrome.

143. In what age group does retinoblastoma usually occur?

Retinoblastoma most often occurs in younger children, with 80% of cases diagnosed before the age of 5 years. Retinoblastoma is usually confined to the eye, with greater than 80% of children being cured with current therapy.

Shields CL, Shields JA: Recent developments in the management of retinoblastoma. J Pediatr Ophthalmol Strabismus 36:8-18, 1999.

144. What is trilateral retinoblastoma?

Trilateral retinoblastoma consists of unilateral or bilateral hereditary retinoblastoma associated with an intracranial neuroblastic tumor (an ectopic retinoblastoma). It has been observed that 5% to 15% of children with either familial, multiple, or bilateral retinoblastoma may develop an intracranial neuroblastic tumor as well. Intracranial neuroblastic tumor is a major cause of death among children with retinoblastoma.

145. For what other tumors are retinoblastoma patients at increased risk?

Patients with the hereditary type of retinoblastoma have a markedly increased frequency of second malignant neoplasms. The cumulative incidence is about 26±10% in non-irradiated and 58±10% in irradiated patients by 50 years after diagnosis of retinoblastoma. Most of the second malignant neoplasms are ***osteosarcomas***, ***soft tissue sarcomas***, or ***melanomas***.

146. What urinary test aids in the diagnosis of neuroblastoma?

Urinary concentrations of ***catecholamines*** and ***metabolites***, including dopamine, homovanillic acid (HVA), and vanillylmandelic acid (VMA), are often increased (> 3 standard deviations above the mean per milligram creatinine for age) in children with neuroblastoma.

147. Should all children under the age of one year be tested for elevated urinary catecholamines as a screen for the presence of neuroblastoma?

This ongoing controversy surrounding the utility of screening infants for neuroblastoma is nearing an end. Although Japan and Canada have had routine screening programs in place, the United States has not. Screening programs identify more children with neuroblastoma at earlier stages, but this increase in earlier detection has not resulted in a decrease in the number of high-stage neuroblastoma cases in subsequent years of life. Cases detected in the first year of life are more likely to be localized tumors with favorable biology, a substantial portion of which will spontaneously regress without treatment.

Suita S, et al: Mass screening for neuroblastoma at 6 months of age: Difficult to justify. J Pediatr Surg 33:1674-1678, 1998.

148. What are the most common presentations of neuroblastoma?

The most common presentation is ***generalized disease*** in a child < 5 years of age (88%). 55% of children with generalized disease are under age 2. Most children with neuroblastoma are irritable and ill, and they often have exquisite bone pain, proptosis, and periorbital ecchymoses. 70% of neuroblastomas arise in the abdomen; half of these arise in the adrenal, and the other half in the parasympathetic ganglia distributed throughout the retroperitoneum and the paravertebral area in the chest and neck. The tumor produces and excretes catecholamines, which can cause systemic symptoms such as sweating, hypertension, diarrhea, and irritability. Children with localized neuroblastoma may have symptoms referable to a mass such as Horner syndrome. Some may have no symptoms, but the condition may be detected on a routine newborn examination when an adrenal mass is felt, or on a chest radiograph taken for other reasons where an incidental posterior mediastinal mass is seen.

149. What percentage of neuroblastoma tumors do not produce catecholamines?

5–10%. About 70% of the neuroblastomas secrete vanillylmandelic acid (VMA) which is excreted in the urine. If all catecholamines and their metabolites (e.g,. norepinephrine, epinephrine, dopamine, homovanillic acid [HVA], and VMA) are measured, 90–95% of patients will have elevated values. A high ratio of HVA to VMA and the absence of any catecholamine excretion are considered unfavorable prognostic factors.

150. What characterizes patients with stage IV-S neuroblastoma?

Described by Drs. Evans and D'Angio in 1971, this a sub-group of infants with metastases limited to the liver, skin and bone marrow who fare astonishly well. These children are cured of their disease with minimal or no cytotoxic therapy.

151. What are the common biologic variables that carry prognostic significance in children with neuroblastoma?

Hyperdiploid tumor DNA is associated with a *favorable* prognosis, especially in infants. ***Increased expression of N-myc***, a proto-oncogene, is associated with *poor* outcome in children over 1 year of age. Expression of the gene encoding the ***high-affinity nerve growth factor receptor***, Trk-A, is associated with a *good* outcome.

Matthay KK: Neuroblastoma: Biology and therapy. Oncology 11:1857-66, 1997.

152. Where does neuroblastoma metastasize?

Regional lymph node involvement occurs in approximately 35% of patients with apparently localized disease. Hematogenous spread occurs most frequently to ***bone***, ***bone marrow***, ***liver*** and ***skin***. Rarely, disease may spread to the lung and brain, usually as a manifestation of relapsing or end-stage disease.

153. A cerebral neuroblastoma correlates with more commonly used tumor designation?

A *cerebral neuroblastoma* is an older term for a ***supratentorial primitive neuroectodermal tumor (PNET)***. Histologically, these tumors are similar to medulloblastomas with varying proportions of features that suggest astrocytic or ependymal differentiation. A PNET that arises in the pineal body classically has been referred to as a pineoblastoma.

154. A child who presents with eyes that are "dancing" and other abnormal movements, including truncal ataxia, is most likely to have what neoplasm?

Neuroblastoma can present with a syndrome of *opsoclonus-myoclonus*, most likely the result of an autoimmune response against cerebellar and other neuronal tissues. These children often have localized, low-stage disease that responds well to current therapy. However, opsoclonus-myoclonus can persist despite treatment of the primary disease. ACTH is thought to be the most effective treatment for opsoclonus-myoclonus, but other modalities including intravenous immunoglobulin have been used. The long-term neurologic outcome may be superior in patients treated with chemotherapy.

155. Although Zukerkandl sounds like a ski resort in Austria, where and why is it anatomically important?

Emil Zukerkandl, an Austrian anatomist, described this ***para-aortic sympathetic ganglion*** located in the ***presacral pelvis***. It, similar to any other sympathetic ganglion, can be the primary location of a neuroblastoma.

156. How is neuroblastoma classified?

International Classification of Neuroblastoma

Stage I	Localized tumor grossly excised with or without microscopic residual disease; lymph nodes negative microscopically
Stage IIA	Unilateral tumor incompletely excised with lymph nodes negative microscopically
Stage IIB	Unilateral tumor completely or incompletely excised with positive ipsilateral regional lymph nodes; identifiable contralateral lymph nodes negative microscopically
Stage III	Tumor infiltrating across the midline incompletely excised with or without lymph node involvement; or unilateral tumor with contralateral regional lymph node involvement
Stage IV	Dissemination of tumor to distant lymph nodes; bone marrow, bone, liver, and/or other organs
Stage IV-S	Localized primary tumor as defined for Stage I or IIA with dissemination limited to liver, skin, or bone marrow in an infant ≤ 12 months of age

157. How does the prognosis for patients with neuroblastoma vary by stage?

***Stage I or II*:** 90% chance of cure with surgery alone. Children whose disease is not controlled with surgery frequently have unfavorable biologic features, such as unfavorable histology (i.e., many mitotic figures and/or karyorrhexis) and elevated serum ferritin, amplified N-*myc* cellular oncogene, or both.

***Stage III*:** 50% chance of cure with surgery, radiation, and chemotherapy. Their prognosis is also determined by biologic features at diagnosis.

***Stage IV*:** 20% chance of long-term survival. Age is an especially important prognostic variable in that those < 1 year have a considerably better outlook.

Stage IV-S : > 80% chance of long-term survival with supportive care alone. Infants under age 6 weeks may die of liver failure or mechanical problems related to a big liver. Few patients with stage IV-S disease actually progress to typical Stage IVdisease with bone and extensive marrow involvement.

SOLID TUMORS

158. What is the most common solid malignancy of childhood?

As a group, ***brain tumors*** are most common. *Medulloblastoma*, a primitive neuroectodermal tumor arising in the cerebellum or vermis, is the single most common type of this tumor.

159. What are the peak ages of incidence of the most common solid tumors of childhood?

Neuroblastoma and Wilms tumor are tumors of *early* childhood. Ewing sarcoma and osteosarcoma are more prevalent during *adolescence*. Rhabdomyosarcoma occurs throughout childhood and the teenage years.

160. What are the factors contributing to relapse of solid tumors?

Even in the best centers with treatment delivered in an optimal manner for very curable tumors, relapses occur for reasons that remain unexplained and are probably intrinsic to the biology of the tumor. However, the following variables may contribute to treatment failure:

- Suboptimal treatment not according to a recognized protocol or administered by an inexperienced physician
- Failure to control the primary tumor with surgery and irradiation
- Metastatic spread of tumor at presentation
- Tumor resistant to chemotherapy

Poor patient compliance with the treatment regimen has been documented, but its contribution to outcome remains unclear.

161. How is Wilms tumor distinguished radiographically from neuroblastoma?

In Wilms tumor, CT images will show *intrinsic* distortion of the kidney parenchyma and collecting system. Neuroblastoma is almost always *extrarenal* and causes displacement, not distortion, of the renal parenchyma and collecting system. In addition, *calcifications* are seen in >50% of children with abdominal neuroblastoma, but in only 10% of children with Wilms tumor.

162. Who was Wilms?

Max Wilms was a German surgeon who described the most common type of renal tumor occurring in childhood. Wilms tumor has its peak incidence in the second and third year of life. The development of its treatment, which now cures approximately 90% of children, serves as a model for the cooperative approach of pediatric oncologists, surgeons, radiation therapists, and pathologists in rationally organizing, introducing new therapies, and critically evaluating outcome for treatment of this disease.

163. Why can congestive heart failure develop in some patients

Heart failure in uncommon in this disease, but if it develops, and most commonly caused by a combination of irradiation and drugs, such as doxorubicin and dactinomycin. Radiation alone is ur ure, but the addition of the cardiotoxic doxorubicin may add to my omycin is not cardiotoxic but can contribute to heart damage b Heart failure can also be caused by the upward spread of a renal vein tumor thro heart, causing tamponade. Rarely, long-standing hypertension may result in dilated cardiomyopathy and congestive heart failure.

164. What are unfavorable prognostic factors in Wilms tumor?

The most important prognostic factors include the presence of metastases and tumor histology. In the National Wilms Tumor Study, patients with no metastatic disease had an actuarial survival of 83%, but only 31% of those with liver metastases and 5% of children with pulmonary metastases survived. Anaplastic, sarcomatous, or clear cell histology are all unfavorable prognostic factors. Additional unfavorable factors include age > 2 years, positive regional lymph nodes, operative spillage of tumor, large tumor size, direct extension within the abdomen, and invasion of extrarenal vessels.

165. Which congenital syndromes have an increased risk of Wilms tumor?

Mutations in the first Wilms tumor gene described, WT1, are associated with a variety of genitourinary abnormalities including cryptorchidism, hypospadias, and the rare Denys-Drash syndrome (intersexual disorders, nephropathy). A gene that causes aniridia is located near the WT1 gene on chromosome 11p13, and deletions encompassing the WT1 and aniridia genes may explain the association between aniridia and Wilms tumor. A second Wilms tumor gene is located at or near the Beckwith-Wiedemann gene locus (11p15), and children with Beckwith-Wiedemann syndrome are at increased risk for developing Wilms tumor.

Petruzzi MJ, Green DM: Wilms' tumor. Pediatr Clin North Am 44:939-52, 1997.

166. Where does Wilms tumor metastasize?

Locally, Wilms tumor can grow through the renal capsule, invade the renal veins, extend into the vena cava, and even progress into the chambers of the heart. The lungs are a common site of metastasis. Spread also occurs into the regional lymph nodes.

167. What is the most common kidney tumor in neonates?

In newborns and young infants, the infantile congener of Wilms tumor, most commonly ***congenital mesoblastic nephroma***, is the most common renal tumor. Mesoblastic nephroma is not encapsulated and infiltrates into normal renal parenchyma. Complete surgical resection with a meticulously performed nephrectomy is curative. The risk of metastasis is minimal.

168. "Small round blue cell tumor" is often used in the description of which childhood tumors?

Neuroblastoma, rhabdomyosarcoma, Ewing sarcoma, lymphoblastic leukemia and ***lymphoma***. All appear as small round blue cells on low power microscopic examination. High power microscopic examination, usually combined with a panel of immunohistochemical stains and molecular diagnostics, are required for definitive diagnosis.

169. Which solid tumors metastasize to the bone marrow?

Neuroblastoma, lymphoma, alveolar rhabdomyosarcoma, Ewing sarcoma/PNET, retinoblastoma.

hat is the cell of origin of Ewing sarcoma?

Until the 1980s, it was believed that this tumor was of endothelial origin. More ently, evidence suggests that it arises from the neural crest and specifically ***postganglionic parasympathetic cholinergic neurons***. This contrasts with classic neuroblastoma, which arises from adrenergic or mixed neurons of the adrenal medulla and sympathetic nervous system.

171. What are the two most common sites of metastases for patients with Ewing sarcoma?

Ewing sarcoma often metastasizes to the ***lungs***, and somewhat less frequently to other ***bones***. In general, lymph nodes are not involved, suggesting that dissemination of this tumor is primarily hematogenous.

172. What molecular diagnostic test distinguishes Ewing sarcoma/PNET from other tumors?

Polymerase chain reaction to detect the ***(11;22) translocation*** is the molecular diagnostic test for this tumor. A pathologically distinct tumor, the *peripheral* primitive neuroectodermal tumor (PNET), shares this translocation, suggesting that these tumors represent different phenotypic expressions of the same underlying malignancy. The treatment approach for both Ewing sarcomas and peripheral PNETs is identical.

173. Do all patients with Ewing sarcoma require surgical resection of the primary tumor?

No. Surgery should be limited to patients with tumors arising in an expendable bone (e.g. fibula), or when surgical resection is neither mutilating nor debilitating. As control of distant spread of the disease is essential for cure of patients with Ewing sarcoma, long delays in chemotherapy for surgical interventions should be minimized. For tumors which are not readily amenable to resection, a combination of external beam radiation and chemotherapy provides very good local control.

Arndt CA, Crist WM: Common musculoskeletal tumors of childhood and adolescence. N Engl J Med 341:342-52, 1999.

174. Osteosarcoma is generally located in which part of the bone?

The ***metaphyses*** of long bones of the extremities. Sixty to eighty percent of tumors are located in the metaphyses of the knee, i.e., the proximal tibia or distal femur.

175. Do all patients with osteosarcoma require surgical resection of the primary tumor?

Surgical resection of the primary tumor is a requirement for curative treatment of osteosarcoma. In contrast to Ewing sarcoma, osteosarcoma is a relatively radiation resistant tumor, and thus surgical resection following neo-adjuvant chemotherapy is a mainstay of treatment.

176. What is the prognosis for children with osteosarcoma?

Between ***40–70%*** of children with osteosarcoma will be alive without evidence of metastatic disease 2 years after diagnosis if they are treated with amputation or limb-salvage procedure plus multiagent chemotherapy. Some of these children will develop pulmonary metastases at a later time, and a proportion of these can be saved with thoracotomy. Without the use of chemotherapy, only 20% of the children will be free of metastatic disease 1 year after diagnosis.

177. For patients with localized osteosarcoma, what factor is most predictive of a favorable outcome?

Patients with greater than 95% necrosis of the primary tumor, determined by pathological examination, following neo-adjuvant chemotherapy have a better prognosis than those with lesser amounts of necrosis.

178. Why is surgical intervention (i.e., amputation) alone insufficient in the treatment of osteosarcoma?

Up to 80–90% of patients have ***silent pulmonary micrometastases*** at the time of diagnosis. The micrometastases are not apparent on imaging studies but will become radiographically evident in 6–9 months if not treated with adjuvant chemotherapy. Surgical treatment alone is associated with only a 10–20% survival rate.

179. In what solid tumor has surgical resection of pulmonary metastases been shown to result in long-term cure?

Although many pediatric sarcomas metastasize to the lungs, only surgical resection of pulmonary metastases from ***osteosarcoma*** has been definitively shown to contribute to cure, and only, in general, when the metastases are few in number. The role of surgical resection of pulmonary metastases arising from other sarcomas (rhabdomyosarcoma, Ewing sarcoma) is less clear and is only undertaken is select circumstances.

180. Embryonal and alveolar refer to the histology of which pediatric solid tumor?

Rhabdomyosarcoma. Rhabdomyosarcoma accounts for approximately 3.5% of the cases of cancer among children 0 to 14 years of age. The embryonal subtype is the most frequently observed, accounting for approximately 60% to 70% of rhabdomyosarcomas of childhood. Embryonal tumors typically arise in the head and neck region or in the genitourinary tract. The alveolar subtype is more prevalent among older patients who often present with extremity tumors and metastatic disease, all less favorable clinical features. Unique translocations between the FKHR gene on chromosome 13 and either the PAX3 gene on chromosome 2 or the PAX7 gene on chromosome 1 are characteristic of alveolar rhabdomyosarcoma. Embryonal tumors often show loss of specific genomic material from chromosome 11p15.

Pappo AS, et al: Soft tissue sarcomas in children. Semin Surg Oncol 16:121-43, 1999.

181. What are the three most common sites of metastases for patients with rhabdomyosarcoma?

In contrast to Ewing sarcoma, the ***regional lymph nodes*** are often involved in patients with rhabdomyosarcoma. Metastases to ***lungs*** and ***bone marrow*** also frequently occur.

182. Which primary sites of tumor carry the most favorable prognosis for children with rhabdomyosarcoma?

Primary sites with more favorable prognoses include tumors that arise in the orbit, in other non-parameningeal head and neck sites, and tumors that arise in non-bladder, non-prostate genitourinary (especially paratesticular and vaginal) region.

183. What are the two most common liver tumors in children?

Liver cancer, a rare malignancy in children and adolescents, is divided into 2 major histologic subgroups: ***hepatoblastoma*** and ***hepatocellular carcinoma***. Hepatoblastomas usually occur before 3 years of age, whereas the incidence of hepatocellular carcinoma in the United States varies little throughout childhood and adolescence. The overall survival rate is only 25% for children with hepatocellular carcinoma but at 70% is significantly better for children with hepatoblastoma.

Gerber GA: Use of intrahepatic chemotherapy to treat advanced pediatric malignancies. J Pediatr Gastroenterol Nutr 30:137-144, 2000.

184. Which tumor marker is most likely to be elevated in children with hepatic tumors?

The majority of patients with either hepatoblastoma or hepatocellular carcinoma have an elevated concentration of ***alpha-fetoprotein (AFP)*** that parallels disease activity. Lack of a significant decrease of AFP with treatment may signify a poor response to therapy. Occasionally hepatoblastomas produce beta human chorionic gonadotropin (β-HCG) and can result in isosexual precocity.

185. What factors predispose children to the development of hepatocellular carcinoma?

Hepatocellular carcinoma is associated with ***hepatitis B*** and ***C infection***, especially in children with perinatally-acquired virus. In contrast to adults, the incubation period from hepatitis virus infection to the development of hepatocellular carcinoma may be extremely short in children.

186. Which germ cell tumor usually presents in young children?

The majority of germ cell tumors that present in young children are ***benign teratomas*** occurring in the sacrococcygeal region. In general, patients with mature teratomas are managed by surgical resection, with care taken for sacrococcygeal tumors that the entire coccyx is removed.

187. Where do rhabdomyosarcomas usually develop?

The four most common areas are the ***head*** and ***neck***, ***genitourinary region***, ***extremities***, and ***orbit***. Survival of patients with orbital disease is nearly 100%. The survival rate for those with tumors in other areas is dependent on the amount, if any, of tumor left after resection and the presence or absence of metastatic disease.

188. What is the most common ovarian tumor of childhood?

Germ cell tumors. In contrast, women more commonly develop stromal tumors. The most frequent ovarian germ cell tumors are dysgerminomas, followed by endodermal sinus tumors, teratomas, and mixed germ cell tumors. Stromal tumors are rare.

189. Which germ cell tumors occur in children?

The most common germ cell tumor is a histologically benign, mature ***cystic teratoma*** occurring in the sacrococcygeal area. Germ cell tumors can occur outside the gonads in brain, kidneys, mediastinum, lung, liver, or stomach. Malignant germ cell tumors include embryocarcinomas, choriocarcinomas, teratocarcinomas, endodermal sinus tumors (yolk sac tumors), dysgerminomas, seminomas, and mixed germ cell tumors.

190. List the risk factors for testicular cancer.

Cryptorchidism, ***atrophic testes***, ***prenatal exposure to diethylstilbestrol (DES)***, history of ***viral orchitis***, and ***positive family history*** of testicular cancer. Because testicular cancer is the most common solid tumor in males aged 15–34 years and because prognosis is clearly related to early diagnosis, testicular self-examination should be taught to all male adolescents.

191. How great is the risk of malignant transformation in undescended testes?

The risk of malignancy may be ***5–10 times higher*** in the undescended testis than in a normal testis. The risk in the contralateral testis may also be increased. Orchidopexy decreases, but does not eliminate, the risk of subsequent malignant transformation.

192. In evaluating an 8-month-old with constipation, you feel a firm, discrete mass on rectal exam. What is the likely diagnosis?

If the mass is *posterior* in the presacral area, it is most likely a ***sacrococcygeal germ cell tumor*** or a ***neuroblastoma***. If the mass is *anterior*, a ***rhabdomyosarcoma*** is likely.

STEM CELL TRANSPLANTATION

193. Identify the three types of stem cell transplantation.

1. ***Allogenic*:** transfer of bone marrow, peripheral blood stem cells, or umbilical cord blood from a donor to another individual
2. ***Autologous*:** use of a person's own bone marrow or peripheral blood stem cells
3. ***Syngeneic*:** transfer of bone marrow, peripheral blood stem cells, or umbilical cord blood from a genetically identical donor (i.e., identical twins)

194. What is the chance of siblings having the same HLA type?

The human leukocyte antigens (HLA), located on chromosome 6, approximate simple mendelian inheritance, with two siblings having a 1:4 chance of same typing. A 1% crossover of material may also occur during meiosis. The larger the family, the more likely a match becomes, as shown by the formula $[1 - (0.75)^n]$, with n being the number of siblings. Thus, a child with five brothers and sisters has a 76% chance of having a sibling with an HLA match.

195. What is the chance of finding an HLA-matched unrelated donor?

Although in theory the number of possibilities would equal or even exceed the world's population, making a match astonishingly unlikely, HLA types cluster in individuals of similar genetic and racial backgrounds. In one estimate of persons of European ancestry, approximately 200,000 individuals would need to be screened to reach a 50% chance of finding a match.

Gahrton G: Bone marrow transplantation with unrelated volunteer donors. Eur J Cancer 27:1537–1539, 1991.

196. What is the survival rate for children with solid tumors receiving autologous stem cell transplantation?

The cure rate for most solid tumors is still well below 50% because stem cell transplantation is being used for patients with relapsed or high-risk disease. The best results in children are in those with otherwise fatal neuroblastoma, in whom a cure rate of about 30% has been achieved.

197. How are tumor cells purged from a marrow or peripheral blood stem cell specimen?

- Immunologic methods using monoclonal antibodies
- *Ex vivo* use of chemotherapy
- Selective binding of tumor cells to lectins
- Treatment of marrow with anti-sense cDNA
- Selective culture of normal cells
- Selection of normal hematopoietic progenitor cells (e.g., CD34+ cells)

198. What are the indications for G-CSF and GM-CSF in stem cell transplant and cancer patients?

Granulocyte–colony-stimulating factor (G-CSF) and *granulocyte/macrophage–colony-stimulating factor* (GM-CSF) are used to shorten the period of neutropenia, and hence the associated risk of infection, after stem cell transplantation and myelosuppressive chemotherapy. They have been effective at shortening the period of isolation after transplantation and in allowing for more intensive chemotherapy regimens. Thus far, no effect on disease progression or survival has been demonstrated. The use of these growth factors in patients with myeloid leukemia is controversial because receptors for these factors are present on the surface of myeloid leukemia cells.

199. What are the different sources of stem cells for transplantation?

Stem cells may be obtained either from the peripheral blood, the bone marrow itself, or from the umbilical cord blood of a newborn. Peripheral blood stem cells are collected by leukocytopheresis while bone marrow stem cells are collected by multiple bone marrow aspirates. Cord blood is harvested from the placenta at the time of delivery. Stored placental/cord blood is a useful source for patients without a related histocompatible donor because of less GVH disease. Studies have shown random cord blood engrafts well, so storing an infant's own blood for potential future use has become less urgent.

Rubenstein P, et al: Outcome among 562 recipients of placental-blood transplants from unrelated donors. N Engl J Med 1565-1577, 1998.

200. Is a stem cell transplantation most commonly performed to replace dysfunctional hematopoietic stem cells?

Although transplantation has a major role in the treatment of aplastic anemia, most transplants are performed to allow for the delivery of otherwise lethal doses of chemotherapy. In children with hematologic malignancies, stem cell transplantation may also provide a graft-versus-leukemia effect that contributes to the control of the disease. Worldwide, the most common reason for which hematopoetic transplantation has been used is beta thalassemia.

201. Which prophylactic measures should be taken following stem cell transplantation?

Patients receive antibiotics for gut decontamination. An oral antifungal agent, such as fluconazole, is also administered. Patients should receive *Pneumocystis carinii* prophylaxis and replacement of immunoglobulins with IVIG. Acyclovir may also be administered.

202. How does the risk of infection vary over the months following stem cell transplantation?

	0-2 weeks	*1-2 months*	*> 2 months*
Bacterial	Gram positive (esp. coagulase-negative *Staphylococcus, Strep. viridans*); Gram negative		Encapsulated bacteria (chronic GVHD)
Viral	HSV	CMV	VZV
Fungal	*Candida* *Aspergillus*	*Pneumocystis carinii*	

Engelhard D: Bacterial and fungal infections in children undergoing bone marrow transplantation. Bone Marrow Transplant 21: S78-80, 1998.

203. What are the major features of acute graft-versus-host disease (GVHD)?

Acute GVHD typically begins with a ***fever*** followed by a salmon colored ***rash*** on the palms of the hands and the soles of the feet. The rash may be pruritic and may desquamate. ***Hepatitis***, with jaundice and transaminase elevation, and ***gastroenteritis***, with diarrhea, weight loss and abdominal pain, may also occur.

204. How does the pathophysiology of acute and chronic graft-versus-host disease differ?

Acute GVHD is characterized by an attack by cytotoxic donor T-cells on various tissues in the transplant recipient, whereas *chronic GVHD* resembles an autoimmune disorder. While chronic GVHD often follows acute GVHD, chronic GVHD may occur without acute

GVHD. Although the pathophysiology of chronic GVHD is incompletely understood, dysregulated development of precursor donor T-cells and secondary host thymic damage are thought to be central to the development of chronic GVHD. Like other autoimmune diseases such as scleroderma, chronic GVHD often involves dermatologic changes, kerato-conjunctivitis, arthritis, polymyositis, serositis, bronchiolitis obliterans and pulmonary fibrosis.

Klingebiel T, Schlegel PG: GVHD: Overview on pathophysiology, incidence, clinical and biological features. Bone Marrow Transplant 21:S45-9 1998.

205. How is graft-versus-host disease managed?

Doses of methotrexate or cyclosporine in the immediate post transplant period may be given in an attempt to prevent the development of acute GVHD. T-cell depletion of the bone marrow graft also decreases the incidence of GVDH. For the treatment of acute GVHD, steroids, cyclosporine, or FK506 may be used alone or in combination depending on the extent of donor-recipient mismatch and the severity of GVHD.

206. What are the advantages and disadvantages of T-cell depletion of donor bone marrow?

The primary advantage of T-cell depletion is a decrease in the risk of acute and chronic GVHD. As GVHD accounts for a substantial portion of transplant related morbidity and mortality, this reduction may be of significant benefit. However, T-cell depletion decreases the extent of the graft-versus-leukemia effect. Thus T-depleted transplant recipients are more likely to relapse from their primary leukemia than T-replete graft recipients. Additionally, graft rejection can occur more frequently in T-depleted grafts. Patients with T-replete grafts reconstitute their T-cell function more rapidly and are therefore at lower risk for lymphoproliferative disorders. No randomized trials have been performed to fully compare the risks and benefits of T-cell depletion.

207. What is lymphoproliferative disease (LPD)?

Lymphoproliferative disease is a heterogenous group of diseases that arise from unregulated and often clonal proliferation of lymphocytes, typically B-cells. Several risk factors predispose transplant patients to LPD: donor-recipient mismatch, severe GVHD with intensive immunosuppression, T-cell depletion of the graft, and use of anti-thymocyte globulin. LPD is often triggered by re-activation of Epstein-Barr virus in B cells. Infected B-cells are transformed into a state of continuous proliferation that may be unchecked by the suppressed immune system. Transformed lymphocytes may undergo clonal expansion (i.e. become malignant). Therapy for LPD centers on carefully withdrawing immune suppression to allow the immune system to regain control over the expanding lymphocyte population. Despite this, LPD can be rapidly progressive and fatal.

208. When the oncology fellow on the transplant service declares a patient to have a "full house match," what does the term mean?

Compatibility between donor and recipient is evaluated by comparing HLA genotypes between the donor and recipient. The HLA system is found on chromosome 6 and encodes a series of cell surface proteins that regulate recognition of foreign antigens. A *"full house match"* means that the donor and recipient match at all HLA loci evaluated. In the case of a related transplant, the donor and patient may not match at minor loci not explicitly evaluated in the HLA typing. However, an unrelated donor transplant would not match at all minor HLA loci even when matched at the major HLA loci.

209. Following stem cell infusion, what is the expected time course of engraftment and return of normal hematopoiesis?

Patients generally recover leukocytes first, followed by red cells and then platelets. Evidence of white cell engraftment generally occurs 8 to 14 days after the infusion of donor cells. Red cell transfusion independence typically occurs in the first 6 weeks post transplant. Complete recovery may take up to six months, although chronic GVHD may significantly impair recovery.

210. Seven days following a matched unrelated T-depleted transplant for relapsed AML, a patient develops progressive weight gain, right upper quadrant pain, ascites and jaundice. What is the likely diagnosis?

This patient likely has ***veno-occlusive disease***, which is characterized by weight gain from fluid retention, hepatic tenderness, and jaundice in the first 60 days post-transplant. Unfortunately, a substantial proportion of patients progress to hepatic and renal failure. The diagnosis is made primarily on clinical grounds. Doppler ultrasound of the liver may demonstrate reversal of portal venous blood flow due to increased intrahepatic pressure. The therapy for veno-occlusive disease is primarily supportive. Anti-fibrinolytics have been used with some success.

211. A patient who received a matched related BMT five weeks ago with busulfan and cyclophosphamide conditioning presents with red urine and increasing difficulty in voiding. What is the likely diagnosis and initial management plan?

Hemorrhagic cystitis, which may be a side effect of cyclophosphamide, although this usually occurs in closer proximity to drug administration. She may also have an adenoviral or BK viral infection. In either case, the patient should be admitted for hydration and close observation for signs of urinary obstruction. A CBC should be obtained and platelet transfusion given for significant thrombocytopenia. If the patient develops urinary obstruction, a three-way irrigating Foley catheter should be placed.

212. What are the major side effects from total body irradiation used in pre-transplant conditioning for bone marrow transplant?

In the *short term*, total body irradiation may cause interstitial pneumonitis and nephritis. Over the *long term*, total body irradiation may lead to cataracts, growth retardation, hypothyroidism, other endocrine dysfunction, infertility and secondary malignancies. The long-term effects of total body irradiation on pulmonary, cardiac, and neuropsychiatric function continue to be studied.

213. Why do patients conditioned with thiotepa require sponge baths every 4 to 6 hours after administration of thiotepa?

Thiotepa or its metabolites are excreted in the sweat and in high concentrations may be caustic to skin. If patients are not bathed every 4 to 6 hours in the first few days after thiotepa administration, they may develop chemical skin burns.

214. How are skin, gut, and liver acute GVHD graded?

	Grade I	*Grade II*	*Grade III*	*Grade IV*
Skin (area involved)	< 25%	25-50%	>50%	Desquamation or blood loss
Gut (diarrhea L/d)	< 0.5	0.5-1.0	1.0-1.5	Ileus, bloody diarrhea
Liver (bilirubin mg/dl)	< 3	3-6	6-15	> 15 or ↑ ALT or AST

215. What is the clinical grading of chronic GVHD?

The clinical grading schema divides chronic GVHD into “limited” and “extensive.” Limited chronic GVHD is localized skin involvement (loss of elasticity, pigmentation changes, loss of sweat gland or hair follicles) or hepatic dysfunction. Limited chronic GVHD is usually controlled with immunosuppressive agents. Extensive chronic GVHD has either generalized skin involvement or local skin involvement with other organ system damage including hepatic dysfunction, eye involvement (keratoconjunctivitis) mucosal involvement (sicca syndrome) or involvement of any other organ. Extensive chronic GVHD is more difficult to control than limited chronic GVHD. Patients with extensive chronic GVHD are at high risk for infectious complications, the leading cause of morbidity and mortality for these patients.

216. How is GVHD prevented?

The best means of prevention is use of identical HLA-matched stem cells, but this is often not possible. Multiple immunosuppressive regimens are utilized involving cyclosporine, methotrexate, corticosteroids, and antithymocyte globulin. One promising method had been the removal of T cells from the stem cell product by various means (e.g., lectins, sheep RBC agglutination, monoclonal antibodies) prior to transplant. However, for reasons unclear, T-cell-depleted marrow has resulted in increased rates of nonengraftment of the marrow and increased relapse rates in patients with CML. The best method(s) of prevention of GVHD remains under investigation.

217. A 3-year-old patient who was given cyclophosphamide prior to receiving a bone marrow transplant seven days ago and is now receiving cyclosporine for GVHD prophylaxis develops a seizure. What is the likely cause?

While high dose cyclophosphamide may cause fluid retention resulting in hyponatremia and seizures, this more commonly occurs during or immediately after cyclophosphamide administration. Seven days following transplant, ***cyclosporine*** is the more likely etiology of the seizures. Appropriate laboratory studies include a cyclosporine level and serum sodium, calcium, magnesium, and glucose. Toxic levels of cyclosporine would require decreases in the cyclosporine dose.

218. An uncle of a patient asks you about the risks associated with transplants. What general information do you give him?

Transplant related morbidity and mortality vary substantially depending on the underlying disease process, type of transplant, intensity of prior therapy, and extent of prior end organ damage. Transplantation for certain diseases, such as Fanconi anemia (a syndrome of increased chromosomal fragility) carries a significantly higher risk of morbidity and mortality than other transplants. In general, allogenic transplants have higher morbidity and mortality than autologous transplants because of GVHD. The risk of GVHD is proportional to the extent of donor-recipient mismatch, with matched related donors having less GVHD than matched unrelated donors. Prior intense therapy increases the likelihood of pre-transplant end organ damage; transplant related morbidity and mortality increase in proportion to underlying end organ dysfunction.

219. What is the long term survival rates for allogenic bone marrow transplantation?

In a study of 6691 patients of all ages who received transplants for a variety of diseases, patients who were disease-free after two years were likely cured. Survival for five additional years was 89%. However, for many years after transplantation, the mortality rate exceeded that of a normal population.

Socie G et al: Long term survival and late deaths after allogenic bone marrow transplantation. N Engl J Med 31:14-21, 1999.

Thomas ED: Does bone marrow transplantation confer a normal life span? N Engl J Med 341:50-51, 1999.

17. ORTHOPEDICS

Joshua E. Hyman, M.D., Francis Y. Lee, M.D., John P. Dormans, M.D., Richard S. Davidson, M.D., Mark Magnusson, M.D., and David P. Roye, M.D.

CLINICAL ISSUES

1. What causes a Sprengel deformity?

Sprengel deformity (congenital elevation of the scapula) is a failure of normal scapular descent during fetal life, resulting in an elevated, hypoplastic scapula. The affected side of the neck appears shorter and broader and may give the appearance of torticollis. A fibrocartilaginous band or omovertebral bone may bridge the space between the medial upper scapula and the spinous process of a cervical vertebra. Abduction of the ipsilateral arm is usually limited, but this limitation may not be clinically significant. Sprengel deformity may be associated with congenital scoliosis and renal anomalies.

2. How does a joint form?

The region in which a joint will form is initially made up of a single mesenchymal anlagen. Cell death, or apoptosis, leads to the development of a cleft within this anlagen. Early fetal movement leads to further development of the joint. Failure to cavitate leads to synchondrosis. Examples are congenital radioulnar synostosis and tarsal coalition.

3. What is torticollis?

Combined head tilt and ***rotatory deformity***.

4. What is the differential diagnosis for torticollis?

Osseous: Atlanto-occipital anomalies, unilateral absence of C1, Klippel-Feil syndrome (fusion of cervical vertebrae), atlantoaxial rotatory displacement, basilar impression

Nonosseous: Congenital muscular torticollis, Sandifer syndrome (severe gastroesophageal reflux), CNS tumors, syringomyelia, Arnold-Chiari malformation, ocular dysfunction (strabismus, oculogyric crisis), infections (cervical adenitis, retropharyngeal abscess), abnormal skin webs (pterygium colli)

5. When does the mass of congenital muscular torticollis disappear?

In the presence of congenital muscular torticollis, a soft nontender mass may appear in the sternocleidomastoid muscle on the affected side. The mass reaches its maximal size at 1 month and usually disappears by 4–6 months. Histologically, it consists of dense fibrous tissue and may represent prenatal venous obstruction and muscle damage to the sternocleidomastoid muscle. Congenital muscular torticollis may be associated with developmental dysplasia of the hips.

6. Are stretching excerises helpful for congenital muscular torticollis?

Studies have shown that conservative management with strectching, particularly when intiated at an early age, is very advantageous and lessens the potential need for surgical correction.

Demirbilek S, Atayurt HF: Congenital muscular torticollis and sternomastoid tumor: Results of nonoperative treatment. J Pediatr Surg 34:540-551, 1999.

7. Which tests can be used to distinguish between ocular and orthopedic torticollis?

Abnormal head tilt caused by extraocular muscle imbalance is **ocular** torticollis, while that caused by sternocleidomastoid muscle imbalance is **orthopedic** torticollis. If the torticollis vanishes when one of the patient's eyes is covered (i.e., changing from binocular to monocular vision), the likely culprit is ocular. If the torticollis vanishes when the patient goes from sitting to supine, ocular pathology is also likely. If the cause remains uncertain, ophthalmologic testing of ocular deviation in various fields of gaze may be needed.

Caputo AR:The sit-up test:Alternate clinical tests for evaluating pediatric torticollis. Pediatrics 90:612–615, 1992.

8. What is infantile cortical hyperostosis?

Caffey disease (or syndrome), which usually occurs before 6 months of age, is a condition of unknown etiology that consists of tender, nonsuppurative, cortical swellings of the shafts of bone, most commonly the mandible and clavicle. It remits spontaneously, but exacerbations may persist for several years. In severe cases, corticosteroids may be helpful. Infantile cortical hyperostosis is a rare condition. The presence of periosteal reaction, especially if asymmetric, should raise the suspicion of battered child syndrome.

9. What are four entities associated with an absent or hypoplastic radius?

1. Congenital thrombocytopenia–absent radius (TAR) syndrome
2. VACTERL (formerly VATER) syndrome (anomalies of vertebrae, imperforate anus, cardiac origin, tracheoesophageal fistula, absent radii, renal origin and limbs)
3. Fanconi anemia
4. Holt-Oram syndrome (associated with a secundum atrioseptal defect)

10. What are the causes of osteoporosis in children?

In *osteoporosis,* bone is normal in structure and appearance but reduced in quantity. Susceptibility to fractures may result. *Osteopenia* is a nonspecific term indicating a reduction in bone mass, usually noted radiographically. Inability to mineralize osteoid for whatever reason is termed osteomalacia or rickets in children. Osteoporosis is fortunately rare in children. It is usually secondary to other problems, such as immobilization, chronic renal or liver failure, renal tubular acidosis, malabsorption, or medications (e.g., steroids, heparin). Osteoporosis may be associated with Turner syndrome, osteogenesis imperfecta, or homocystinuria and may also be seen in a primary juvenile idiopathic form. The vertebrae and ends of long bones are usually affected.

11. What are the physical signs suggestive of rickets?

The anatomic abnormalities of rickets result primarily from the inability to normally mineralize osteoid. The bones become weak and subsequently distorted. Signs of rickets include:

- Craniotabes
- Delayed suture and fontanel closure
- Frontal thickening and bossing
- Defective tooth enamel
- Palpably widened physes at wrists and ankles
- Femoral and tibial bowing
- "Pigeon breast," or sternal protrusion secondary to use of accessory muscles
- Harrison's groove, a rim of rib indentation at insertion of the diaphragm
- "Rachitic rosary"(enlarged costochondral junctions)

12. Which growth sites are known to develop aseptic necrosis?

The ***osteochondroses*** are a group of disorders in which aseptic necrosis of growth centers (epiphyses and apophyses) occurs with subsequent fragmentation and repair. The exact cause is unknown. The patient usually presents with pain at the affected site.

Location	*Eponym*	*Typical Age of Onset (yrs)*
Tarsal navicular bone	Köhler disease	6
Capitellum of distal humerus	Panner disease	9–11
Carpal lunate	Keinböck disease	16–20
Distal lunar epiphysis	Burn disease	13–20
Head of femur	Legg-Calvé-Perthes disease	3–5
Second metatarsal head	Freiberg disease	12–14
Calcaneal Achilles tendon insertion	Sever disease	8–9

13. What are the skeletal dysplasias?

The *skeletal dysplasias* are a group of disorders characterized by an intrinsic abnormality in the growth and remodeling of cartilage and bone. These generalized disturbances in the development of the skeleton affect the skull, spine, and extremities in varying degrees. These children frequently have disproportionate short stature and dysmorphic facial features.

14. Discuss the inheritance pattern and clinical features of osteogenesis imperfecta (OI).

Of the several types of OI, the most common is type IV, which occurs in 1:30,000 live births. The clinical features vary and depend on the severity of the condition.

Type	*Inheritance*	*Clinical Features*
I	Autosomal dominant	Bone fragility, blue sclerae, onset of fractures after birth (most at preschool age Type A, without dentinogenesis imperfecta Type B, with dentinogenesis imperfecta
II	Autosomal recessive	Lethal in perinatal period, dark blue sclerae, concertina femurs, beaded ribs
III	Autosomal recessive	Fractures at birth, progressive deformity, normal sclerae and hearing
IV	Autosomal dominant	Bone fragility, normal sclerae, normal hearing Type A, without dentinogenesis imperfecta Type B, with dentinogenesis imperfecta

15. McCune-Albright syndrome is associated with what skeletal abnormalities?

Polyostotic fibrous dysplasia (i.e., fibrous tissue replacing bones). The fibrous dysplasia occurs most commonly in long bones and pelvis and may result in deformity and/or increased thickness of bone. There is associated precocious puberty and café-au-lait spots.

16. What are the causes of in-toeing gait (pigeon-toeing)?

The condition may be due to problems anywhere in the lower extremity.

Foot: metatarsus adductus
metatasus varus
talipes equinovarus (clubfoot)
pes planus (flat feet)

Leg: tibial torsion (internal)
genu valgum (knock knees)
tibia vara (Blount disease)
bow legs

Hip: femoral anteversion (medial femoral torsion)
paralysis (polio, myelomeningocele)

spasticity (cerebral palsy)
maldirected acetabulum

Tunnessen WW Jr: Signs and Symptoms in Pediatrics, 3rd ed. Philadelphia, Lippincott Williams & Wilkins, 1999, pp. 693-695.

17. A 15-year-old with tibial pain (which is worse at night and relieved by aspirin) has a small hypodense area surrounded by reactive bone formation on x-ray. What is the likely diagnosis?

Osteoid osteoma, which is a benign bone-forming tumor. It is typically seen in older children and adolescents and exhibits a male predominance (M:F 2:1). Most children complain of localized pain, usually in the femur and tibia; however, arms and vertebrae may also be involved. Radiographs and CT scans demonstrate an osteolytic area surrounded by densely sclerotic reactive bone. Bone scans reveal "hot spots." The site is usually <1 cm in diameter and arises at the junction of old and new cortex. Pathologically, the lesion is highly vascularized fibrous tissue with an osteoid matrix and poorly calcified bone spicules surrounded by a dense zone of sclerotic bone. Treatment is surgical excision.

18. What is the clinical significance of limb-length discrepancy?

A significant portion of the population has mild limb-length discrepancy. Limb-length discrepancies of <2 cm in a skeletally mature individual usually require no treatment. In addition to quantitating leg discrepancy in a skeletally immature child, it is important to estimate what the limb-length discrepancy will be at skeletal maturity. This can be done by periodically measuring leg-length discrepancy radiographically and using charts, such as the Green and Anderson "growth remaining graph" or the Moseley "straight line graph," to calculate anticipated leg-length discrepancy at skeletal maturity. Assessment of skeletal age is based on the bone age from an anteroposterior hand and wrist radiograph,

19. What are the possible causes of a limb-length discrepancy?

Congenital anomalies: congenital short femur, proximal femoral focal deficiency, congenital absence of fibula, posteromedial bowing of tibia, tibial hypoplasia, congenital hemihypertrophy

Tumors: neurofibromatosis, fibrous dysplasia, enchondromatosis, hereditary multiple exostosis, Klippel-Trenaunay-Weber syndrome

Trauma: physeal injuries, fracture

Infection: septic arthritis, osteomyelitis

Inflammation: juvenile rheumatoid arthritis

20. What are the long-term effects of uncorrected limb-length discrepancy?

Equinus contracture of the ankle, scoliosis, low-back problems, and ***late degenerative arthritis*** of the hip.

21. What are the general management principles for a limb-length discrepancy?

0–2 cm:	No treatment
2–6 cm:	Shoe lift, epiphysiodesis
6–20 cm:	Limb lengthening
>20 cm:	Prosthetic fitting

There is flexibility in these guidelines to account for factors such as environment, motivation, intelligence, compliance, emotional stability, patient and parent wishes, and associated pathology in the limbs.

Guidera KJ, et al: Management of pediatric limb length inequality. Adv Pediatr 42:501–543, 1995.

22. What is a *nursemaid's elbow*?

Also known as a "pulled elbow," a nursemaid's elbow is a subluxation of the radial head resulting from axial traction applied the extended arm of a young child. The child typically presents unwilling to move the affected limb with tenderness directly over their radial head. Radiographs are normal in this condition. The diagnosis is made by history and physical exam. Discomfort is relieved by reducing the subluxation. This is accomplished by forcefully supinating the extended forearm followed by flexion of the forearm. An audible and palpable click are occasionally present. Following successful reduction the child begins to use the arm spontaneously. If symptoms persist, the child should be reassessed for a possible fracture.

23. Why have many Little Leagues banned the throwing of a curve ball?

To minimize the cases of Little League elbow, which is a medial epicondylitis that results from overuse and flexor-pronator strain. The throwing of a curve ball puts extra stress on the ulnar collateral ligament of the medial aspect of the elbow. Severe strain can result in partial separation of the apophysis. Occasionally bony avulsions can occur.

24. What signs and symptoms suggest a serious cause of back pain in children that warrants further evaluation?

Symptoms: Pain in children <4 years of age; interference with daily activities in school, play, or athletics; pain persistence > 4 weeks; night pain (associationn with tumor); radiation down the leg (suggests herniated disc or apophysis)

Signs: Concurrent fever; postural changes; neurologic abnormalities; reproducible point tenderness; limitation of motion on forward bending

Thompson GH: Back pain in children. J Bone Joint Surg Am 75:928–937, 1993.

25. What is the differential diagnosis of back pain in children?

Infectious: discitis, vertebral osteomyelitis, vertebral tuberculosis

Developmental: Scheuermann kyphosis, scoliosis, spondylolysis, spondylolisthesis

Traumatic: herniated disc, muscle strain, fractures, slipped vertebral apophysis

Inflammatory: juvenile rheumatoid arthritis, ankylosing spondylitis

Neoplastic: eosinophilic granuloma, osteoid osteoma, aneurysmal bone cyst, leukemia, lymphoma, Ewing sarcoma, osteosarcoma

Visceral: urinary tract infection, hydronephrosis, ovarian cysts, inflammatory bowel disease

26. Do school backpacks contribute to back pain?

This is controversial, but some experts suggest that the limits of maximum loads lifted by children should be 10-15% of body weight. In one study from Italy, over 1/3 of students carried more than 30% of their bodyweight at least once during the school week. With an apparent increasing incidence of back pain in children ((particularly those with open ephiphyses), the bulging back pack may be one contributing cause.

Negrini S, et al: Backpack as a daily load for schoolchildren. Lancet 354:1974, 1999.

27. Which sports injuries are the most common in school-aged children and adolescents?

Some 75% of injuries in school-aged children involve the lower extremities, and a majority of injuries to the knee and ankle are reinjuries due to incomplete healing from a previous problem. Contusions and sprains are the most common types of injury, with fractures and dislocations accounting for an additional 10 – 20%. Cranial injuries are the most common cause of sports fatality.

Adolescent boys who participate in contact team sports, particularly football and wrestling, are at highest risk for injuries. Among girls, softball and gymnastics have the highest injury rate.

Only 10%of sports injuries are caused by an opponent. Most injuries are caused by stumbling, falling, or misstepping. The latter finding suggests that improving intrinsic factors, such as raising the level of physical fitness, avoidance of overuse, and strengthening joint stability, may be more important factors in prevention of injuries than external factors such as the choice of equipment.

28. What entities most commonly constitute orthopedic emergencies?

Open fracture, impending compartment syndrome, dislocation of major joints (i.e., knee, hip, spine), ***septic arthritis, major arterial injury***.

FOOT DISORDERS

29. Do infants and children need shoes?

Barefoot is the natural state of the foot. Individuals who spend most of their lives unshod have stronger feet and fewer foot deformities than those who wear shoes. Prior to walking, infants do not need foot coverings other than to keep their feet warm. Once the child begins to walk, shoes will offer protection from the cold and sharp objects.

30. What features should be given to a parent about buying shoes for a toddler?

The best shoe is one that simulates the barefoot, including:

- The shoe should easily flex.
- The bottom of the shoe should be flat. Heels should be avoided because they tend to force the foot forward and cramp the toes.
- The shoe should be foot-shaped and generously fitted. The toe box should be wide and high to properly accommodate the toddler's pudgy feet.
- The sole should have the same friction as the skin on the bottom of the child's foot.

31. When are x-rays needed in the evaluation of the newborn foot?

X-rays offer limited information in the immature foot. Use of x-rays should be limited to situations in which there is a clinical suspicion of a more complex foot deformity.

32. What is the most common congenital foot abnormality?

Metatarsus adductus. In this condition, the front part of the foot (forefoot) is turned inward due to adduction of the metatarsi at the tarsometatarsal joints associated with normal alignment of the hindfoot and midfoot. Most cases are mild and flexible, with the foot easily dorsiflexed and the lateral aspect easily straightened by passive stretching. A simple test to determine if the kidney-shaped curvature is within normal limits is to draw a line that bisects the heel. When extended, this line normally falls between the second and third toe space. If it falls more laterally, metatarsus adductus is present. *In utero* positioning is the suspected cause of the condition. It is seen more frequently in first-born children, presumably because primagravida mothers have stronger muscle tone in the uterine and abdominal walls.

33. How is metatarsus adductus treated?

If the foot can be passively abducted beyond neutral, the prognosis is excellent for a spontaneous correction without any therapeutic intervention. In those feet that are stiffer, a program of passive stretching is in order. The parents are taught to hold the heel in neutral position and manually abduct the forefoot using their thumb placed over the cuboid as a fulcrum. This exaggerated position should be held for a few seconds and the stretching repeated 10 times each session. These sessions should occur with bathing and diaper changing.

34. How do congenital metatarsus adductus and congenital metatarsus varus differ?

Both deformities are types of kidney-shaped feet in which the forefoot becomes adducted secondary to varying degrees of intrauterine compression. In *metatarsus adductus*, there is no bone abnormality, and the curvature can be readily corrected by passive stretch. In *metatarsus varus*, there is subluxation of the tarsometatarsal joints when the foot is dorsiflexed. Physical exam usually reveals a deep medial cleft, prominence of the base of the fifth metatarsal, and an inability to correct the forefoot passively to align with the heel. Making the distinction is important because metatarsus adductus usually resolves spontaneously while metatarsus varus gradually worsens without treatment.

Craig CL, Goldberg MJ: Foot and leg problems. Pediatr Rev 14:395 400, 1993.

35. How is clubfoot distinguished from severe metatarsus varus?

Clubfoot, or talipes equinovarus congenita, is distinguished pathologically by a combination of forefoot and hindfoot abnormalities (e.g., malrotation of the talus under the calcaneus and plantar flexion or equinus of the ankle). As a rule, clubfoot is a rigid deformity, while metatarsus is more flexible. If the ankle can be dorsiflexed to neutral or beyond, metatarsus is a much more likely diagnosis.

36. Clubfoot is associated with which syndromes?

- Arthrogryposis
- Caudal regression syndrome
- Cerebral palsy
- Craniocarpotarsal dystrophy
- Diastrophic dwarfism
- Larsen syndrome
- Meningomyelocele
- Progressive muscle atrophy (peroneal type)
- Spinal cord tumor
- Myotonic dystrophy

37. How are clubfeet treated?

Many clubfeet respond well to serial casting. The casts should be applied as soon after birth as possible and are changed weekly. Over the course of 2-3 months significant improvement in the shape of the foot can be seen. About 80% of the feet that are corrected with casting will require an Achilles tenotomy to correct the equinus deformity. Those feet that are not adequately corrected with casting will require surgical release.

38. What is a calcaneovalgus foot?

This common deformity is the result of an *in utero* "packaging defect" and is considered a normal variant. The foot lies in an acutely dorsiflexed position, with the top of the foot in contact with the anterolateral surface of the leg. The heel is in severe valgus and the forefoot is markedly abducted. Overall, the foot is flexible and both the heel and the forefoot can be corrected into varus. Spontaneous correction is the norm. However, having parents passively stretch the foot is often beneficial.

39. What foot abnormality results in the appearance of a "Persian slipper" foot?

Also called "rocker bottom foot," this abnormality is due to ***congenital vertical talus***. Lateral radiographs reveal a vertically oriented talus with dislocation of the talonavicular joint. On exam, the forefoot is markedly dorsiflexed, and the heel is rigid and points downward, giving the sole the characteristic convex or boat-shaped appearance. Serial casting and subsequent surgical reversion are the usual treatments. The syndrome most commonly associated with this deformity is trisomy 18.

40. What should be suspected when pes cavus is noted on exam?

Pes cavus, or high-arched feet (often associated with claw toes), can result from contractures or disturbed muscle balance. A neurologic cause should be suspected. The differential diagnosis includes normal familial variant, Charcot-Marie-Tooth disease, spina bifida, cauda equina lesion, peroneal muscle atrophy, Friedreich ataxia, Hurler syndrome, and polio.

41. Should children with flexible flat feet be given corrective shoes?

Flexible flat feet (*pes plenovalgus*) is a common finding in infants and children and up to 15% of adults. On weight-bearing, the medial longitudinal arch is depressed toward the ground formation, and the heel is in valgus (outward) position. There are no radiographic parameters that define a flatfoot. It is felt to be a normal variant due to ligamentous laxity. Children do not complain of pain, and an arch can be created easily by having the child stand on his/her toes or by dorsiflexing the great toe. This condition is distinguished from pathologic flat feet in which lack of weight-bearing does not lessen the flatness and rigidity is present on physical examination. Prospective studies have shown that corrective shoes or plastic insets (orthotics) are not necessary in children with flexible flat feet, as the arch spontaneously develops during the first 8 years of life.

Wenger DR, et al: Corrective shoes and inserts as treatment for flexible flat feet in infants and children. J Bone Joint Surg 71:800–810, 1989.

42. How does the cause of foot pain vary by age?

Probable Causes of Foot Pain by Age

0–6 YEARS	6–12 YEARS	12–19 YEARS
Ill-fitting shoes	Ill-fitting shoes	Ill-fitting shoes
Foreign body	Foreign body	Foreign body
Occult fracture	Accessory navicular bone	Ingrown toenail
Osteomyeoitis	Occult fracture	Pes cavus
JRA (if other joints involved)	Tarsal coalition (peroneal spastic flat foot)	Hypermobile flat foot with tight Achilles tendon
Rheumatic fever	Ingrown toenail	Ankle sprains
(Hypermobile flat foot)	Ewing sarcoma	Stress fracture
	(Hypermobile flat foot)	Ewing sarcoma
		Synovial sarcoma

From Gross RH: Foot pain in children. Pediatr Clin North Am 33:1397, 1986; with permission.

43. A 10-year-old boy with recurrent ankle sprains and painful flat feet should be evaluated for what possible diagnosis?

Tarsal coalition. Fusion of various tarsal bones via fibrous or bony bridges can result in a stiff foot which inverts with difficulty. When inversion of the foot is done during an exam, tenderness occurs on the lateral aspect of the foot, and peroneal tendons become very prominent. Thus, the condition is also referred to as "peroneal spastic flat foot." Unless the condition is very severe warranting surgery, corrective shoes are usually adequate treatment. Other possible causes of a rigid flatfoot include rheumatoid arthritis, septic arthritis, post-traumatic arthritis, neuromuscular conditions, and congenital vertical talus.

44. What radiographic studies are used to evaluate tarsal coalitions?

Calcaneonavicular coalitions can be diagnosed with plain radiographs; typically the coalition may be seen on the oblique view. Talocalcaneal coalitions are more difficult to visualize with plain radiographs. Frequently, a CT scan is necessary. If the coalition is fibrous, then an MRI may be needed.

45. What is a curly toe?

A toe whose distal portion is flexed, medially deviated, and externally rotated. Such toes may underlie or, less commonly, overlie the adjacent toe(s). Curly toes are usually familial, bilateral, symmetric, and asymptomatic. They rarely interfere normal foot function.

46. Is treatment necessary for the curly toe?

25% of children have spontaneous improvement. The majority are asymptomatic. Strapping or taping of the toes has not been shown to be effective. For the rare child who has pain, release of the long toe flexor alone or with release of the short toe flexor has proven to be effective treatment.

FRACTURES

47. What are the four developmental regions of a bone?

1. *Diaphysis*—the shaft of the bone.
2. *Metaphysis*—the flared region of the bone at the end of the diaphysis.
3. *Physis*—the region of growth cartilage.
4. *Epiphysis*—the end of the bone that was initially cartilaginous.

48. What are the most common types of fractures in children?

Unique to pediatrics, ***physeal*** and ***metaphyseal*** fractures are the most common in children. These are sites where children's bones are weakest and ossification is not yet complete. Buckle (compression) and greenstick (incomplete) fractures are also common.

49. Where are the most frequent sites for fractures in children?

- The clavicle
- Distal radius
- Distal ulna

50. What is an open fracture?

The fracture site is communicated with the external environment. Open fractures have higher incidence of developing infection and higher degree of soft tissue damage when compared to closed fractures.

51. What is a toddler fracture?

A toddler fracture is a fracture of the tibia in a child 9 months to 3 years of age due to low-energy forces. Typically these fractures have a spiral appearance and are non-displaced. The fibula is rarely fractured. The child will present with a limp or inability to bear weight. Immobilization in a splint or cast for three weeks is the usual treatment.

52. How are growth plate fractures classified?

The *Salter-Harris classification* of growth plate (physis) injuries was devised in 1963:

Type I: Epiphysis and metaphysis separate; usually no displacement occurs due to the strong periosteum; radiograph may be normal; tenderness over the physis may be the only sign; normal growth after 2–3 week cast immobilization.

Type II: Fragment of metaphysis splits with epiphysis; usually closed reduction; casting is for 3–6 weeks (longer for lower extremity than upper extremity); growth usually not affected, except distal femur and tibia

Type III: Partial plate fracture involving a physeal and epiphyseal fracture to the joint surface; occurs when growth plate is partially fused; closed reduction more difficult to achieve

Type IV: Extensive fracture involving epiphysis, physis, metaphysis, and joint surface; high risk for growth disruption unless proper reduction (usually done operatively) is obtained

Type V: Crush injury to the physis; high risk for growth disruption

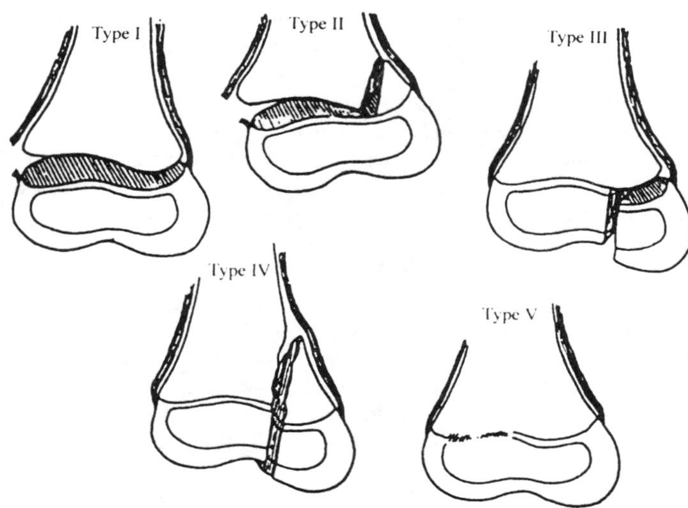

From Bachman D, Santora S: Orthopedic trauma. In Fleisher G, Ludwig S (eds): Textbook of Pediatric Emergency Medicine, 4th ed. Baltimore, Lippincott, Williams & Wilkins, 2000, p 1437; with permission.

53. What are the sequelae of growth plate fractures?

Most growth plate fractures heal without incidence. If there is an injury to the growth plate, a growth disturbance may occur. These are caused by the formation of a bony bridge or bar at the site of physeal damage. If there is damage to the entire physis, premature physeal closure occurs with resulting longitudinal growth arrest. Asymmetric closure leads to angular deformity of the limb.

54. What is the Thurston-Holland sign?

The small section of metaphyseal bone that remains attached to the epiphysis in a type II fracture. It is diagnostic of injury to the growth plate.

55. What is the difference between subluxation and dislocation?

Subluxation is an incomplete or partial dislocation.

56. What is the most common cause of a pathologic fracture?

Also called *secondary fractures*, these are fractures through a bone that is weakened by a pathologic process. The most common such fracture is through unicameral bone cysts (simple bone cysts). These cysts usually occur in the metaphysis of a long bone, most frequently the humerus. They occur predominantly in males, are usually asymptomatic (until a fracture occurs), are centrally located in the bone, and are often quite large.

57. In a patient with suspected fracture, what are the key points on physical examination?

Assess "the five P's" in the affected extremity:

1. ***P***ain and point tenderness
2. ***P***ulse (distal to the fracture)
3. ***P***allor
4. ***P***aresthesia (distal to the fracture)
5. ***P***aralysis (distal to the fracture)

Examine for pain above and below the suspected injury site; multiple fractures are known to occur. The involved extremity also should be carefully examined for deformity, swelling, crepitus, discoloration, and open wounds. A primary concern in any evaluation is a distal neurovascular compromise, which may require immediate surgical intervention.

58. What are the signs of a compartment syndrome?

The 5 Ps noted above (pain, paresthesia, paralysis, pulselessness and pallor) are seen in impending or established compartment syndrome in which swelling is causing distal ischemia. Among these signs, significant pain with passive stretching of the digits (either flexion or extension) raises suspicion. Once the nerve is severely damaged, the patient does not complain of pain. Compartment syndrome is often unrecognized in unconscious patients. A high index of suspicion must be maintained in patients with severe injuries and an altered mental status. In addition, a frightened young child or infant may be very difficult to examine. If there is any concern regarding a compartment syndrome, the compartment pressures must be measured.

59. What is the treatment of a compartment syndrome?

A compartment syndrome is an emergency. Compartment pressures can be lowered by incision of the skin and fascia of the involved compartments (e.g., anterior, lateral, deep posterior, superficial posterior in the leg). The wound is left open and covered with sterile dressing until swelling decreases. Dressing changes and partial wound closure are usually done in the operating room. Skin grafts may be necessary.

60. How do you treat a simple clavicular fracture?

These fractures are best managed with a sling and activity restriction. Union occurs in 2-4 weeks, but the sling may be removed once the child is comfortable. The residual bump (fracture callus) may take up to 2 years to smooth out (remodel). Surgery is only necessary if the fracture is open, there is a neurovascular injury, or the vascularity of the skin is compromised from significant displacement.

61. A teenager who punches a wall in anger typically incurs what fracture?

Boxer fracture. This is a a fracture of the distal fifth metacarpal, usually with apical dorsal angulation. Up to 35% of dorsal angulation can be accepted without compromise of function. Reduction often requires pin fixation.

62. Children who fall on outstretched arms often suffer what type of fracture?

Colles fracture. This is a group of complete fractures of the distal radius with varying displacement of the distal fragment. The fall, with the hand outstretched, wrist dorsiflexed, and forearm pronated, often results in a classic "dinner-fork" deformity of the wrist on exam.

63. Compare Monteggia and Galleazzi fractures.

These fractures occur at opposite ends of the lower arm. In the various types of *Monteggia fractures*, there is dislocation of the radial head with an angulated diaphyseal fracture of the ulna. In *Galleazzi fractures*, the distal radioulnar joint is dislocated with a distal radial diaphyseal fracture.

64. How is the anterior humeral line helpful in evaluating an elbow fracture?

On a lateral x-ray, a line drawn along the anterior edge of the humerus ordinarily intersects the middle third of the capitellum. In acute elbow trauma, especially with hyperextension, the distal humerus can be displaced posteriorly when a fracture occurs. On an x-ray in this setting, the anterior line will intersect the capitellum in the anterior third or beyond. If this occurs, a fracture should be suspected. In children < $2\frac{1}{2}$ years of age, this sign becomes less helpful because of variations in the rates of ossification of the capitellum.

65. What does the presence of the posterior fat pad on an elbow x-ray suggest?

Of the two fat pads that overlie the elbow joint, only the anterior one is visible on a lateral x-ray. If fluid accumulates in the joint space, as in bleeding, inflammation, or fracture, the fat pads are displaced upward and outward. The position of the anterior pad changes, and the posterior pad becomes visible. If acute trauma has occurred, a fracture should be suspected, and immobilization continued with follow-up studies as needed.

66. In a teenager with wrist trauma, why is palpation of the anatomic "snuff box" a critical part of the physical sign?

The anatomic snuff box, the inpouching formed by the tendons of the abductor pollicis longus and extensor pollicis longus when the thumb is abducted (in hitchhiker fashion), sits just above the scaphoid (carpal navicular) bone. The scaphoid is the carpal bone most commonly fractured, and these fractures are at higher risk for nonunion or avascular necrosis. Snuff box tenderness, pain on supination with resistance, and pain on longitudinal compression of the thumb should increase suspicion for fracture of the scaphoid bone. Even when an x-ray is negative, if there is significant snuff box tenderness, a fracture should be suspected and the wrist and thumb immobilized. A repeat x-ray in 2–3 weeks may better reveal a fracture. If very high clinical suspicion exists, MRIcan identify a fracture when the plain film is negative.

67. Name the eight carpal bones of the wrist.

Disdaining some of the classic (mostly obscene) mnemonics, remember what will happen if a wrist fracture is missed:

Sinister **L**awyers **T**ake **P**hysicians **T**o **T**he **C**ourt **H**ouse

In order of proximal to distal, lateral to medial: ***scaphoid, lunate, triquetrum, pisiform, trapezium, trapezoid, capitate, hamate.***

68. In pediatric fractures, what amount of angulation is acceptable before reduction is recommended?

Acceptable angulation or displacement varies with a child's age. Younger children have remarkable healing potential to remodel with minimal to no residual deformity or limitation of rotation. As a rule, in children up to 8 years, as much as 30° of angulation will heal satisfactorily without reduction. In older children, percentages are lower. In general, fractures that are in the metaphysis or growth plate remodel more completely than midshaft factures. Rotational malalignment will not remodel.

69. In which fractures will remodeling of bone *not* occur?

Bony deformities in children (angulation, displacement, or shortening) can remodel as bone is removed from the tension side and placed on the compression side of the deformity by redirection of physeal growth. Factors that favor remodeling include young age, proximity of the fracture to the physis, and angulation in the plane of motion of the adjacent joint. The following fractures have a low chance of remodeling and may require closed or open reduction:intra-articular fractures; fractures with excessive shortening, angulation, or rotation; displaced epiphyseal plate fractures; and midshaft or diaphyseal fractures.

70. How long should fractures be immobilized?

Children's fractures generally heal more quickly than their counterparts in adults. The length of immobilization, however, depends on several variables, including the child's age, location of fracture, type of treatment, etc. As a rule of thumb, physeal, epiphyseal, and metaphyseal fractures heal more rapidly than diaphyseal fractures. On average, epiphyseal, physeal, and metaphyseal fractures heal in children within 3–5 weeks, whereas diaphyseal fractures may heal in 4–6 weeks.

71. How long do fractured clavicles and femurs take to heal?

	Newborn	*16-Year-Old*
Clavicle	10–14 days	6 wks
Femur	3 wks	6–10 wks

72. When is open reduction of a fracture indicated?

An open reduction is an operative reduction of a fracture. Open reduction may be combined with internal fixation with pins, plates, or screws. Indications include:

- Failed closed reduction (often in older children with displaced fractures)
- Displaced intra-articular fractures
- Displaced Salter-Harris III and IV fractures (to prevent premature growth plate closure)
- Unstable fractures in patients with head trauma
- Open fractures (for irrigation and debridement)

HIP DISORDERS

73. Why has DDH replaced CHD?

The term *developmental dysplasia of the hip* (DDH) has replaced congenital hip dislocation (CHD) to reflect the evolutionary nature of hip problems in infants in the first months of life. About 2.5–6.5 infants per 1000 livebirths develop problems, and a significant percentage of these are not present on neonatal screening examinations. Clearly, the overt pathologic process may not be present at birth, and periodic examination of the infant's hip is recommended at each routine well-baby exam until the age of 1 year.

DDH also refers to the entire spectrum of abnormalities involving the growing hip ranging from dysplasia to subluxation to dislocation of the hip joint. Unlike CHD, DDH refers to alterations in the hip growth and stability *in utero*, in the newborn period, and in the infant period. DDH also refers to hip disorders associated with neurologic disorders (e.g., myelomeningocele), connective tissue disorders (e.g., Ehlers-Danlos syndrome), myopathic disorders (e.g., arthrogryposis multiplex congenital) and syndromic conditions (e.g., Larson syndrome).

Bauchner H: Developmental dysplasia of the hip (DDH): an evolving science. Arch Dis Child 83:202, 2000.

74. What signs are indicative of DDH in the newborn?

The most reliable clinical methods of detection remain the ***Ortolani*** reduction and the ***Barlow*** provocative maneuvers. The infant should be lying quietly supine. Both examinations begin with the hips flexed to 90°. To perform the *Ortolani* maneuver, the hip is abducted and the trochanter is gently elevated. This allows a dislocated femoral head to glide back into the acetabulum. The *Barlow* test is performed by adducting the flexed hip and gently pushing the thigh posteriorly in an effort to dislocate the femoral head.

75. What is the significance of a "hip click" in a newborn?

A hip click is the high-pitched sensation felt at the very end of abduction when testing for development dysplasia of the hip with Barlow and Ortolani maneuvers. It occurs in up to 10% of newborns. Classically, it is differentiated from a hip "clunk" which is heard and felt as the hip goes in and out of joint. Although a debatable point, the hip click is felt to be benign. Its cause is unclear and may be due to movement of the ligamentum teres between the femoral head and acetabulum or the hip adductors as they slide over the cartilaginous greater trochanter. Worrisome features that might warrant evaluation (e.g., hip ultrasound, hip x-ray) include late-onset of click, associated orthopedic abnormalities, or other clinical features suggestive of developmental dysplasia (e.g., asymmetric skin folds/creases, unequal leg length).

76. What is the most reliable physical finding for DDH in the older child?

Limited hip abduction. This is due to shortening of the adductor muscles.

77. What other diagnostic signs are suggestive of DDH?

- ***Asymmetry*** of thigh and gluteal folds. However, these may be present in up to 10% of normal infants.
- ***Galleazzi test***. With the hips flexed at 90°, the knees may be at different levels due to apparent femoral shortening on one side in asymmetrical dislocation.
- ***Allis test***. With the hips flexed and the heels on the table, uneven knee level suggests hip dislocation.
- ***Waddling gait, hyperlordosis of lumbar spine.*** Seen in older patients with bilateral dislocations.

78. What radiographic studies are most valuable in diagnosing DDH in the newborn period?

In infants <6 months of age, the acetabulum and proximal femur are predominantly cartilaginous and thus not visible on plain x-ray. In this age group, these structures are best visualized with ***ultrasound***. In addition to morphologic information, ultrasound provides dynamic information regarding the stability of the hip joint.

Weintroub S, Grill F: Ultrasonography in developmental dysplasia of the hip. J Bone Joint Surg 82-A(7):1004-1018, 2000.

79. Should all infants be routinely screened by ultrasound for DDH?

Because physical exam is not completely reliable and the incidence of late-diagnosed DDH has not declined, some investigators have recommended routine ultrasonographic screening. However, others argue that ultrasonography can lead to overdiagnosis and treatment. At present, the issue remains controversial. Universal screening is more commonly done in Europe, whereas in the U.S. selective screening based on risk factors and physical exam findings is more the norm.

American Academy of Pediatrics: Clinical practice guideline: Early detection of developmental dysplasia of the hip. Pediatrics 105: 896-905, 2000.

80. Who is at higher risk for DDH?

Dislocated, dislocatable, and subluxable hip problems occur in about 1–5% of infants. However, 70% of dislocated hips occur in girls, and 20% occur in infants born in breech position. Other risk associations include:

- Congenital torticollis
- Skull or facial abnormalities
- First pregnancy
- Positive family history of dislocation
- Metatarsus adductus
- Calcaneovalgus foot deformities in infants < 2500 gm
- Amniotic fluid abnormalities (especially oligohydramnios)
- Prolonged rupture of membranes
- Large birthweight

MacEwen GD: Congenital dislocation of the hip. Pediatr Rev 11:249–252, 1990.

81. What other orthopedic conditions are associated with DDH?

Skull or ***facial abnormalities***, ***torticollis***, ***congenital hyperextension of the knee***, ***club-foot***, and ***metatarsus adductus***. If any of these deformities are present at birth, there should be increased suspicion that DDH may be present.

82. How is DDH treated?

The first goal is to obtain a reduction and maintain that reduction to provide an optimal environment for the femoral head and acetabular development. This is accomplished by keeping the legs abducted and the hips and knees flexed. The most commonly used devices are the Pavlik harness, Frejka pillow and the van Rosen splint. Triple diapers have no role in the treatment of DDH. They provide the parents with a false sense of security and do not provide reliable stabilization or positioning.

83. What is the natural history of untreated DDH?

A child with *unilateral* DDH may have a leg-length discrepancy and painless (Trendelenburg) limp throughout childhood and young adulthood. Osteoarthritis of the hip joint may develop in the fifth decade of life. Hip fusion and total hip arthroplasty are surgical treatment options for the symptomatic hip in young adults. Children with *bilateral* DDH often have no leg length inequality and no appreciable limp. They tend to walk with hyper-extension of the lumbar spine (hyperlordosis) and have a waddling gait. As with patients with unilateral DDH, these patients tend to develop early osteoarthritis. Total hip arthroplasty is the treatment of choice for adults with symptomatic bilateral DDH.

Some recent studies suggest that a high percentage of newborns with DDH may spontaneously improve without treatment.

Bialik V, et al: Developmental dysplasia of the hip: a new approach to incidence. Pediatrics 103:93-99, 1999.

84. What is the significance of a positive Trendelenburg test?

If a normal individual stands on one leg, ipsilateral hip abductors (primarily the gluteus medius) prevent the pelvis from tilting, and balance is maintained. Children over 4 years of age can usually stand this way for at least 30 seconds. If the opposite side of the pelvis does tilt or the trunk lurches to maintain balance, this is a positive Trendelenburg sign. It may be an indicator of muscle weakness (due to muscular or neurologic pathology) or of hip instability (such as acetabular dysplasia).

85. What is a Trendelenburg gait?

A *Trendelenburg gait* results from functionally weakened hip abductor muscles. It is commonly seen in children with a dislocated hip. With a dislocated hip, the abductor muscles area at a mechanical disadvantage and are effectively weakened, which makes it difficult for them to support the child's body weight. As a result, the pelvis tilts away from the affected hip. In an effort to minimize this imbalance during the stance phase of gait, children lean over the affected hip.

86. What is the most common cause of a painful hip in a child less than age 10 years?

***Acute transient synovitis* (ATS).** It has also been called toxic synovitis, irritable hip, and coxitis fugax.

This is a self-limited inflammatory condition that occurs before adolescence, has no known cause, and generally has a benign clinical outcome. However, it can cause considerable anxiety among physicians and family members during its clinical course because it can mimic other more sinister conditions such septic arthritis, soft tissue injury, osteomyelitis, Legg-Calve-Perthes disorder, juvenile rheumatoid arthritis, slipped capital femoral epiphysis or tumor. It may occur anytime from the toddler age group to the late juvenile years, but the peak age is between 3 and 6 years of age. It is more common in boys. ATS remains a diagnosis of exclusion. Treatment consists of rest and reduction of the synovitis with anti-inflammatory agents. Most patients experience complete resolution of their symptoms within 2 weeks of onset. The remainder may have symptoms of lesser severity for several weeks.

Do TT: Transient synovitis as a cause of painful limps in children. Curr Opin Pediatr 12:48-51, 2000.

87. How can transient synovitis be differentiated from septic arthritis?

	Transient Synovitis	*Septic rthritis*
History	Preceding URI ± low-grade fever Hip or referred knee pain Limp	Fever Usually large joint involvement (hip, ankle, knee, shoulder, elbow)
Physical	Refusal to bear weight Can delicately elicit range of motion in affected hip joint	Exquisite pain, swelling, warmth Marked resistance to mobility
Laboratory	ESR normal or mildly elevated Mild peripheral leukocytosis Negative blood culture Joint fluid cloudy Negative Gram stain	ESR markedly elevated Leukocytosis with "left shift" Often positive blood culture Joint fluid purulent Often positive Gram stain
Radiographs	Occasionally shows fluid in joint space)	Possible associated bony findings (early osteomyelitis)

88. What is Legg-Calvé-Perthes (LCP) disease?

LCP disease is a disorder of the femoral head of unknown etiology that is characterized by ischemic necrosis, collapse and subsequent repair. Children typically present with pain and/or a limp. The pain may be localized to the groin or may be referred to the thigh or knee.

89. What are the pathologic stages in Legg-Calvé-Perthes (LCP) disease?

LCP is a condition of aseptic necrosis of the femoral head involving children primarily ages 4–10.

1. ***Incipient or synovitis stage***. Lasting 1–3 weeks, this first stage is characterized by an increase in hip-joint fluid and a swollen synovium associated with reduced movement.

2. ***Avascular necrosis***. Lasting 6 months to 1 year, the blood supply stops to part (or all) of the head of the femur. That portion of the bone essentially dies, but the contour of the femoral head remains unchanged.

3. ***Fragmentation or regeneration and revascularization***. In the last and longest pathologic stage of LCP, lasting 1–3 years, the blood supply returns and causes both resorption of necrotic bone and laying down of new immature bone. Permanent hip deformity can occur in this last stage.

It is important to note that plain radiographs may lag behind the progression of the disorder by as much as 3–6 months. Radionuclide bone scans are much better because early ischemia and avascular necrosis are depicted as decreased localizations of isotope.

90. What is the prognosis for children with Legg-Calvé-Perthes disease?

The two main prognostic factors for LCP disease include the age of the child and the amount of epiphyseal involvement. Children < 6 years of age tend to have a more favorable prognosis. Those with less epiphyseal involvement also tend to have a better prognosis. Epiphyseal involvement has been classified by Salter into Type A (those with < 50% epiphyseal involvement) and Type B (those with > 50% head involvement).

91. Which conditions are associated with coxa vara?

Coxa vara is a conditon of a decreased femur shaft-neck angle. The three most common associations: ***developmental coxa vara***, ***avascular necrosis*** of the femoral head, ***cleidocranial dysostosis***.

92. What condition does this child have?

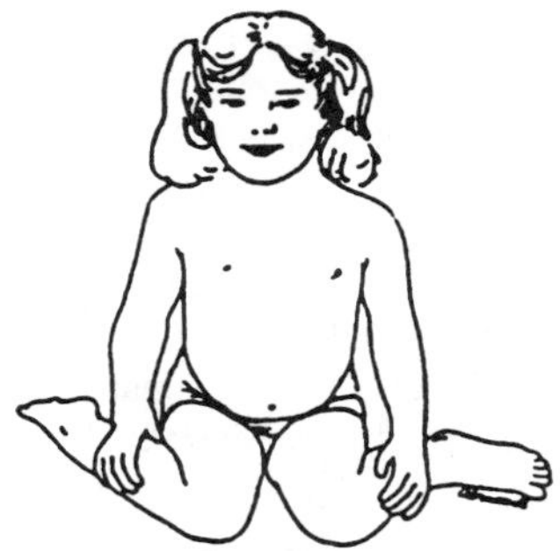

This is ***femoral anteversion*** (or medial femoral torsion), which is a common cause of in-toeing in younger children. The child is demonstrating the reverse tailor position, a sign of the internally rotated hip.

From Staheli LT: Torsional deformity. Pediatr Clin North Am 33:1382, 1986; with permission.

93. How is the extent of femoral anteversion measured?

With the child lying prone and knees flexed at 90°, the hip normally cannot be rotated internally (i.e., feet pushed outward) more than 60° (angle *A* in diagram A). In addition, external rotation (angle *B* in diagram B) should exceed 20°. A normal child averages approximately 35°. Abnormal results indicate that the cause of in-toeing is likely due to physiologic femoral anteversion (or less commonly, hip capsular contractions such as in cerebral palsy).

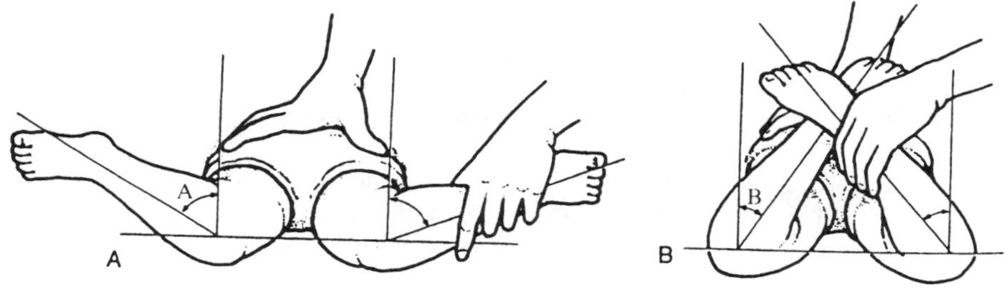

From Dormans JP: Orthopedic management of children with cerebral palsy. Pediatr Clin North Am 40:650, 1993; with permission.

94. How do children with slipped capital femoral epiphysis (SCFE) present?

SCFE involves progressive displacement with external rotation of the femur on the epiphyseal growth plate. The patient presents with intermittent or constant hip, thigh, or knee pain which has often lasted weeks to months. In 25%, the pain is bilateral. A limp, lack of internal rotation, and a hip flexion contracture may be noted. If the patient's hip is flexed, the thigh tends to fall into external rotation. It is important to realize that any patient presenting with knee pain may have underlying hip pathology.

95. What systemic conditions are associated with SCFE?

Children with SCFE tend to have delayed skeletal maturation and obesity and usually present between the ages of 8–14 years. This suggests that hormonal factors may lessen the bone's ability to resist shearing forces, resulting in a pathologic fracture through the proximal femoral physis. Systemic factors associated with SCFE include hypothyroidism, panhypopituitarism, hypogonadism, rickets, and irradiation.

INFECTIOUS DISEASES

96. Which patients with septic arthritis warrant open drainage?

There is debate as to the relative merits of open surgical drainage versus repeated needle aspiration. Three settings warrant consideration for surgical intervention:

1. Septic arthritis of the hip (and possibly shoulder)
2. Large amounts of fibrin, debris, or loculation within the involved joint space
3. Lack of improvement in 3 days by medical treatment alone

Dagan R: Management of acute hematogenous osteomyelitis and septic arthritis in the pediatric patient. Pediatr Infect Dis J 12:88–93, 1993.

97. Where does acute hematogenous osteomyelitis most commonly localize in children?

Lower extremity (femur, tibia, fibula)	70%
Upper extremity (humerus, radius, ulna)	15%
Foot	4%
Pelvis	4%
Vertebrae, skull, ribs, sternum, scapulae	2%

Gold R: Diagnosis of osteomyelitis. Pediatr Rev 12:293, 1991.

98. What are the most common bacterial agents in osteomyelitis?

Neonates
- *Staphylococcus aureus*
- Group B streptococci
- Enterobacteriaceae (*Salmonella, Escherichia coli, Pseudomonas, Klebsiella*)

Children
- *Staphylococcus aureus*
- Group A streptococci
- *Haemophilus influenzae*

The incidence of *H. influenzae* osteomyelitis has significantly declined due to immunization.

99. How helpful is a screening white blood count (WBC) in the diagnosis of osteomyelitis?

Not very. In two-thirds of patients, the total WBC is normal (although in half of these, the differential is left-shifted). In the other one-third, the WBC is elevated, usually with a left shift. The erythrocyte sedimentation rate (ESR) is more sensitive, as 95% of cases have an ESR >15 mm/hr with an average rate of 70 mm/hr.

100. How often are blood cultures positive in osteomyelitis?

Only 50% or less. Because this rate is relatively low, direct bone aspiration should be strongly considered. Aspiration raises the yield to 70 – 80% and greatly facilitates antibiotic therapy.

101. As osteomyelitis progresses, how soon do x-ray changes occur?

3–4 days: deep-muscle plane shifted away from periosteal surface
4–10 days: blurring of deep tissue muscle planes
10 – 15 days: changes in bone occur (e.g, osseous lucencies, punched-out lytic lesions, periosteal elevation)

102. Intreatment of osteomyelitis, which serum bactericidal level is a better indicator of successful outcome:peak or trough?

Both may be important. Peak titers (approx. 20–30 min after infusion) are associated with successful treatment in acute osteomyelitis if ≥ 1:8 and in chronic osteomyelitis if ≥ 1:16. Trough titers are predictive of a good outcome if ≥ 1:2 in acute osteomyelitis and if ≥ 1:4 in chronic osteomyelitis.

103. When is treatment of osteomyelitis with oral antibiotic agents appropriate?

- An identified organism
- Available oral antibiotic against the organism
- Adequate surgical debridement
- Improving clinical course on IV antibiotics
- Patient without vomiting or diarrhea
- Adequate serum levels can be obtained on oral therapy
- Reliable parents and/or patient

Nelson J: Skeletal infections in children. Adv Pediatr Infect Dis 6:59, 1991.

104. How long should antibiotics be continued in osteomyelitis and septic arthritis?

The precise answer is unclear, but infections caused by *Staphylococcus aureus* or enteric gram-negative bacteria must be treated for longer periods than those caused by *Haemophilus influenzae, Neisseria meningitidis,* or *Streptococcus pneumoniae.* A minimum of 4–6 weeks is likely necessary for the former group and 2–3 weeks for the latter. If diagnosis has been delayed, initial clinical response is poor, or ESR remains elevated, longer durations may be needed.

105. When is open surgical drainage indicated in cases of osteomyelitis?

- Abscess formation in the bone, subperiosteum, or adjacent soft tissue
- Bacteremia persisting > 49–72 hours after initiation of antibiotic treatment
- Continued clinical symptoms (e.g., fever, pain, swelling) after 72 hours of therapy
- Development of a sinus tract
- Presence of a sequestrum (i.e., detached piece of necrotic bone)

Dagan R: Management of acute hematogenous osteomyelitis and septic arthritis in the pediatric patient. Pediatr Infect Dis J 12:88–93, 1993.

106. Why are treatment failures more common in osteomyelitis than in septic arthritis?

- Antibiotic concentrations are much greater in joint fluid than in inflamed bone. Concentration in joint fluid may actually exceed peak serum concentrations, while those in bone may be significantly less than serum concentration.
- Devitalized bone may serve as an ongoing nidus for infection.
- Diagnosis of osteomyelitis is more likely to be delayed than that of septic arthritis.

107. How do the features of osteomyelitis in the neonate differ from those in the older child and adult?

- Neonatal osteomyelitis almost invariably follows hematogenous dissemination.
- Multiple foci of infection are frequently seen.
- Septic arthritis is a frequent association, probably reflecting the spread of infection via blood vessels penetrating the epiphyseal plates.
- Chronic osteomyelitis is infrequent.
- The pathogens causing neonatal osteomyelitis are the same as those responsible for sepsis neonatorum.

108. Why are young children more susceptible to infectious discitis than adolescents or adults?

Increased susceptibility in younger children is due to the differing anatomy of the spine. In children < 12, blood vessels extend from the vertebral body through hyaline cartilage to supply nutrition directly to the intervertebral disc and nucleus pulposus. These vessels slowly regress until the adult picture is reached (age 12), at which time nutrition to the nucleus pulposus is supplied primarily by diffusion. The extra blood vessels in early life may facilitate hematogenous spread of infection or direct extension of early vertebral osteomyelitis.

109. How is the diagnosis of discitis established?

Discitis, which is infection and/or inflammation of the intervertebral disc, most commonly occurs in children between ages 4–10. The etiology is often unclear, but a bacterial cause, particularly *Staphylococcus aureus*, is identified by blood cultures in about 50%of cases. The diagnosis can be difficult because of varied presentations, including generalized back pain with or without localized tenderness, refusal to stand or walk, back stiffness with loss of lumbar lordosis, abdominal pain, and unexplained low-grade fever.

As with osteomyelitis, a most helpful laboratory test is an elevated ESR. WBC counts may often be normal, and early x-rays (< 2–4 weeks of symptoms) may not show changes. Technetium-99 bone scans will demonstrate abnormalities early in the course of illness. MRI studies can help distinguish between discitis and vertebral osteomyelitis.

Treatment consists of 3–6 weeks of antistaphylococcal antibiotics, with variable amounts of immobilization and bracing depending on severity of symptoms. Persistent or atypical cases may require biopsy to identify the etiology.

Cushing AH: Diskitis in children. Clin Infect Dis 17:126, 1993.

110. When is bone scintigraphy used in the evaluation of children with obscure skeletal pain?

When correlated with clinical findings, the results of bone scintigraphy can help localize an abnormality in the bones, joints, or soft tissues. Additional unrelated asymptomatic lesions also may be identified. The bone scan is very sensitive but not very specific. Often, other diagnostic tests are needed to establish the exact etiology of the pain. A bone scan should only be considered after a careful history and physical exam have been performed and plain x-rays of the abnormal area are obtained. The scan is most useful in establishing or ruling out occult infection or bone tumor.

111. What are the phases of a bone scan?

The phases are generally demarcated by the time elapsed since injection of the radionuclide dye.

Phase I—angiographic phase. In the first few seconds, the dye passes through the large blood vessels and provides early assessment of regional vascularity and perfusion.

Phase II—blood pool phase. Usually obtained in the first minutes after an injection, this phase highlights the movement of the dye into extracellular spaces of soft tissue and bone.

Phase III—delayed phase. By 1.5–3 hours after injection, the dye localizes in the bone with minimal soft tissue imaging.

The three-phase process is used to differentiate soft tissue from bony abnormalities. At times a ***Phase IV*** study may be done by rescanning for the same dye at 24 hours, which further minimizes soft tissue background activity.

KNEE, TIBIA, AND ANKLE DISORDERS

112. What is the difference between valgus and varus deformities?

Some things seem to be destined to be learned, forgotten, and relearned many times as a rite of passage. The Krebs cycle is one. This is another. The terms refer to angular deformities in the musculoskeletal system. If the distal part of the deformity points toward the midline, the term is **varus**. If the distal part points away from the midline, it is **valgus**. For example, in knock-knees, the lower portion of the deformity points away, so the term is genu valgum.

Another method is to consider the body in the supine (anatomic) position. Draw a circle around the body. All angles conforming to the curve of the circle are varus; all angles going against the circle are valgus. Bowleggedness conforms to the circle around the body and is, therefore, genu varum.

113. Are children normally knock-kneed or bowlegged?

It varies by age. If you use the angle formed by the tibia and femur as a guide, most children at birth are bowlegged (genu varum) up to 20°, but this tendency progressively diminishes until about 24 months, when the trend toward knock-knees (genu valgum) begins. Knock-knees continue to age 3 (up to 15°) and then begin to diminish. At about age 8, most children are, and will remain, knock-kneed at about 7–9°.

114. Which bowlegged infants or toddlers require evaluation?

Radiographs should be considered if bowleggedness is:

- Present after 24 months (the time of normal progression to physiologic genu valgum)
- Worse after age 1 as the infant begins to bear weight and walk
- Unilateral
- Visually > 20° (tibiofemoral angle)

115. Which children are more likely to develop Blount disease?

Tibia vara, or Blount disease, is a medial angulation of the tibia in the proximal metaphyseal region due to a growth disturbance in the medial aspect of the proximal tibial epiphysis. In the infantile type, the child is usually obese and an early walker and develops pronounced bowlegs during the first year of life. Black females are particularly at risk for severe deformity. In the adolescent variety, the onset occurs during late childhood or early adolescence, and the deformity is usually unilateral and mild. Correction of severe deformity often requires surgical intervention.

116. How does tibial torsion change with age?

Tibial torsion, the most common cause of in-toeing in children aged 1–3, gradually rotates externally with age. For excessive internal rotation, bracing was used extensively in the past, but its efficacy is questionable as the natural history of the condition is self-resolution. Measurement is done by noting the thigh–foot angle with the knee flexed to 90°.

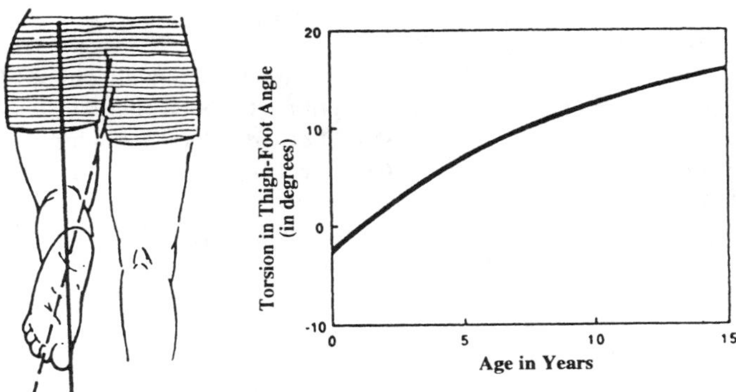

From Sponseller PD: Bone, joint, and muscle problems. In Macmillan JA, et al (eds): Oski's Pediatrics Principles and Practice, 3rd ed. Philadelphia, J.B. Lippincott, 1999, p 2112; with permission.

117. How effective is the Denis Browne splint in the treatment of tibial torsion?

The splint consists of a metal bar connected to shoes or strings about the feet. The bar provides varying degrees of external rotation. The splint has been used in children with tibial torsion in whom spontaneous correction is not occurring. However, there is no scientific evidence that this device alters the natural history of tibial torsion.

118. What is the most likely diagnosis if a 15-year-old basketball player presents with painful swelling below both knees?

Osgood-Schlatter disease. A *traction apophysitis,* the condition results from repetitive microtrauma to the immature tibial tubercle, which is the site of the insertion of the knee extensor mechanism on the proximal tibia. It is related to the adolescent growth spurt and the level of physical activity. Physical exam reveals tenderness to palpation and swelling over the tibial tubercle. The pain is exacerbated with resisted knee extension.
Appropriate clinical mangement includes the judicious use of anti-inflammatory medications, restricted activities, quadriceps stretching and strengthening, and cross-training. The condition is usually self-limited and resolves with skeletal maturity. Immobilization, which may lead to disuse atrophy, is rarely necessary.

119. What painful condition is snowshoeing likely to produce?

Shin splints. This term describes the pain and cramping felt in the compartments of the lower leg after strenuous exercise. It is rare in children but may be seen in teenagers who exercise (especially running on hard surfaces) after extended periods of inactivity. The pain results from muscle strain and inflammation of the musculotendinous units. Swelling and cramping occur, particularly in the flexor digitorum longus muscle, which flexes the lateral four toes and plantar-flexes the foot at the ankle joint. The muscle swelling may contribute to ischemia. Snowshoeing may be the ultimate test of the anterior tibial muscles.

120. Which long bone is most frequently absent congenitally?

The ***fibula***. Absence of the fibula may be partial or complete and is usually unilateral. The involved leg is shortened and commonly demonstrates bowing of the tibia and slight shortening of the femur. The foot usually shows a severe deformity with equinus and valgus deformities with absence or abnormal development of lateral toes.

121. Why are ligamentous injuries unusual in children?

In children, ligaments are stronger than growth plates and thus the growth plate will fail (i.e., fracture) before the ligament tears.

122. How are ankle sprains graded?

80–90% of ankle sprains are the result of excessive inversion and/or plantar-flexion resulting in injury to the lateral ligaments (anterior talofibular and calcaneofibular). The anterior ankle drawer sign is a test of ankle stability (particularly the anterior talofibular ligament). It is accomplished by immobilizing the lower tibia with one hand and, with the ankle at 90°, moving the heel and foot forward with the other hand. If there is marked laxity with a poor endpoint, a complete tear or ***third-degree sprain*** is likely. Moderately increased laxity compared with the other ankle indicates a partial tear or ***second-degree sprain***. No laxity indicates a ***first-degree sprain***.

123. Which ankle sprains should be evaluated with an x-ray?

More than 5 million radiographs are estimated to be taken annually in children and adults for ankle injuries, yet there are no widely accepted guidelines. One set of guidelines suggests obtaining an x-ray if there is malleolar pain and one or both of the following conditions is present: (1) inability to bear weight for 4 steps immediately following the injury and on office or ER evaluation, and/or (2) bone tenderness at the posterior edge or tip of either malleolus. When these simple criteria were used in studies involving children and adults, no fractures were missed and unnecessary x-rays were reduced by 25%.

Chande VT: Decision rules for roentgenography of children with acute ankle injuries. Arch Pediatr Adolesc Med 149:255–258, 1995.

Stiell IG, et al: Decision rules for the use of radiography in acute ankle injuries. JAMA 269:1127–1132, 1993.

124. Should ankle sprains be casted?

If inversion ankle sprains are not complicated by a fracture or peroneal tendon dislocation, casting is not warranted. It has no benefit over early immobilization with a wrap, such as a commercially available air stirrups. Additionally, complete immobilization may delay rehabilitation.

125. What is the most common risk factor for an ankle sprain?

A previous ankle sprain. This highlights the importance of a rehabilitation program and, if the previous sprain has been moderate or severe, the potential use of an orthosis for at least 6 months.

Thacker SB, et al: The prevention of ankle sprains in sports: a systematic review of the literature. Am J Sports Med 27:753-760, 1999.

126. How should knee pain be evaluated?

Evaluation by history and physical exam should focus not only on the offending knee but also the hip and contralateral knee. The history should seek information regarding the mechanism of injury, the onset and duration of pain, the change in pain with activities and rest, and the presence of night pain. The precise location of the pain is crucial to making the correct diagnosis. The effect of previous treatments, presence of swelling, locking, or giving way are also pertinent points. For the examination, the patient should be in shorts or a gown. Always examine both knees; the uninjured knee will serve as a normal control. Begin with an evaluation of gait, lower-extremity weight-bearing alignment, muscle definition, leg lengths, swelling and ligament. Next test for range of motion (active/passive), effusion, tenderness (joint line, physis, patella, tibial tubercle, collateral ligaments), strength, patella tracking, and stability.

127. What is the most significant mistake made in the evaluation of knee pain?

Failure to evaluate the hip as a source of the pain. Hip pathology frequently masquerades as knee pain as in the conditions Perthe's disease and slipped capital femoral epiphysis.

128. If a ninth-grade soccer player with knee swelling "felt a pop" while scoring a goal, what are three possible diagnoses?

A pop or snap sensation in the setting of acute knee injury is usually associated with:

1. Anterior cruciate ligament injury
2. Meniscal injury
3. Patellar subluxation

129. In acute injury, what are the main causes of blood in the knee joint?

Acute hemarthrosis is most commonly due to:

- Rupture of the anterior or posterior cruciate ligaments
- Peripheral meniscal tears
- Intratrabecular fracture
- Major disruption or tear in the joint capsule

130. How common are meniscal tears in younger children?

Meniscal tears rarely occur before the age of 12 years. A discoid meniscus is a congenitally abnormal meniscus and can present at almost any age. Meniscal tears in youths are typically associated with significant injuries that arise from a memorable event. They produce pain, swelling, and limping. There is often an associated injury to the anterior cruciate ligament.

131. A 5-year-old boy with a painless swelling in the back of his knee has what likely condition?

Popliteal cyst. Also called Baker cysts, these are occur more frequently in boys, are usually found on the medial side of the popliteal fossa, and are painless. In children, the cysts are rarely associated with intraarticular pathology. The natural history is for the cyst to disappear spontaneously after 6 to 24 months. A prolonged period of observation is recommended prior to considering surgical excision. Atypical findings such as tenderness or firmness or a history of rapid enlargement and/or pain are justification for further diagnostic evaluation.

Seil R, et al: Popliteal cysts in children. A sonographic study and review of the literature. Arch Ortho Trauma Surg 119:73-75, 1999.

132. A teenager presents with chronic knee pain, swelling, and occasional "locking" of the knee joint, and his x-ray reveals increased density and fragmentation at the medial femoral condyle. What condition does he likely have?

Osteochondritis dissecans. In this avascular necrosis syndrome, focal necrosis of articular cartilage and underlying bone occurs. The cause is unknown, but antecedent trauma is common. The section of bone may detach and lodge in the contiguous joint. Males are more commonly affected, and pain occurs especially with strenuous activity. Associated findings may include stiffness, swelling, clicking, and occasional locking. A plain radiograph can reveal the diagnosis, but MRI is more sensitive when findings are equivocal. Extended immobilization is the primary treatment. Continued pain or locking of the joint warrants consideration of arthroscopy to search for intra-articular fragments. Long-term complications can include degenerative arthritis.

133. What predisposes a child or teenager to recurrent dislocation of the patella?

Orthopedic conditions: genu valgum, patella alta, hypoplasia of the lateral femoral condyle, laterally located tibial tubercle, vastus medialis insufficiency, abnormal attachment of the iliotibial tract

Syndromes of generalized ligamentous laxity: Down syndrome, Ehlers-Danlos syndrome, Marfan syndrome, Turner syndrome

Mizuta H, et al: Recurrent dislocation of the patella in Turner syndrome. J Pediatr Orthop 14:74–77, 1994.

134. Who manifests the *apprehension sign*?

Individuals with acute or subacute ***subluxation*** or ***dislocation of the patella.*** With the patient's knee supported at 30°, the examiner applies pressure to the medial border of the patella. If the patient displays impending distress or apprehension, the test is positive. No discomfort makes patellar pathology less likely. The apprehension sign is also seen in individuals with ***shoulder instability*** (especially glenohumeral problems) who fear dislocation when certain maneuvers are performed. For anterior instability, the arm is placed in maximal external rotation and abduction (similar to an overhand throw position). For posterior instability, the shoulder is placed at 90° of forward flexion and internal rotation.

135. How does patellofemoral stress syndrome occur?

This major cause of chronic knee pain in teenagers results from malalignment of the extensor mechanism of the knee due to a variety of causes. It is most commonly seen as an "overuse" entity in sports that involve running and full-knee flexion, such as track or soccer. It has been inappropriately called chondromalacia patella, which is a specific pathologic diagnosis of an abnormal articular surface that occurs in a minority of these patients. The patella serves as the fulcrum on which the various muscles of the quadriceps extend the knee. Forces may act asymmetrically, causing greater stress on lateral aspect of the patella, especially in individuals with anteversion of the femur, external torsion of the patella, high (alta) patella, abnormally developed quadriceps, excessive flattening of the femoral groove, or wide Q angle. Treatment consists of ice, rest, nonsteroidal anti-inflammatory drugs, quadriceps strengthening, hamstring stretching, and possibly patellar-stabilizing braces.

136. What is the Q angle?

Draw a line from the anterior-superior iliac spine through the center of the patella, and then draw a line from the center of the patella to the tibial tubercle. The resultant angle is the Q angle, or quadriceps angle. For teenage males, the average Q angle is 14°, and for females, 17°. Angles >20° predispose to chronic knee pain (particularly in runners) because of patellar strain.

SPINAL DISORDERS

137. What conditions are associated with congenital scoliosis?

Congenital scoliosis results from either failure of vertebral formation or segmentation usually in the first eight weeks of prenatal development. The embryologic development of the spine and intra-abdominal organs occurs at the same time. Structural abnormalities of the urinary tract such as renal agenesis, duplication, and ectopia can occur in up to one-third of patients. VATER syndrome includes *V*erterbral anomalies, *A*nal anomalies, *T*racheo-*E*sophageal fistula and *R*adial limb deficiencies. The incidence of congenital heart disease is also increased. Congenital scoliosis is strongly associated with occult intraspinal anomalies, such as tethering of the cord, diastematomyelia, lipoma and lipomeningocele, teratomas and syringomyelia. In a recent study, nearly half of infants with congenital scoliosis undergoing MRI had abnormalities. Identification of associated intraspinal anomalies is important because these conditions may limit movement of the cord within the canal, placing the infant at increased risk for neurologic deficits with progession of the scoliosis.

Prahinski JR, et al: Occult intraspinal anomalies in congenital scoliosis. J Pediatr Orthoped 20:59-63, 2000.

138. What is the differential diagnosis for scoliosis?

Scoliosis is a lateral curvature of the spine (i.e., coronal plane deformity). *Kyphosis* and *lordosis* are posterior and anterior curvatures, respectively (i.e., sagittal plane deformity). About 1–2% of the pediatric population have a spinal deformity, but very few are severe enough to require treatment: 85% of cases are idiopathic; 5% are congenital (including hemivertebrae and vertebral fusions); 5% neuromuscular (cerebral palsy, polio, spinal muscular atrophy, muscular dystrophy); and 5% miscellaneous (Marfan syndrome, Ehlers-Danlos syndrome, tumors).

139. How is screening for spinal deformity performed?

The child should be undressed or dressed only in underwear or a gown (open from the back). From the back and side, the child is examined standing, flexed forward at the hips, and sitting (to eliminate leg-length inequality). The head and arms hang down unsupported. The contour of the back is observed from the side, the rear, and the front for the following signs which can suggest scoliosis:

- Shoulder or scapular asymmetry.
- Visible deformity of spinous processes.
- Asymmetry of paraspinal muscles or rib cage in the thoracic spine while bending (> 0.5 cm in lumbar region and > 1.0 cm in thoracic region). A scoliometer may be used for this determination.
- Sagittal plane deformity when viewed from the side.
- Waist crease asymmetry that does not disappear on sitting. Most waist crease asymmetries are due to minor leg-length discrepancies.
- Excessive thoracic kyphosis in forward-bending when viewed from the side.

140. What constitutes an abnormal scoliometric measurement?

The *scoliometer*, also called an inclinometer, is a type of protractor used to measure the vertebral rotation and rib-humping that is seen in scoliosis with the forward-bending test. An angle of 5° or less is usually insignificant; 7° or more warrants consideration of standing posteroanterior and lateral radiographs for more precise assessment of curvature.

141. Are males or females more likely to have scoliosis?

Females are 5 times more likely than males.

142. How valuable are school-based screening programs for scoliosis?

This is controversial. About 26 states in the U.S. mandate school scoliosis screening. Experts in favor of these programs contend that reliable screening procedures exist and that early identification will lead to earlier non-operative care and prevention of progression and need for surgical intervention. Opponents argue that the low incidence of children requiring treatment, the low positive predictive value of screening programs and high numbers of children unnecessary referred do not justify the programs. Others suggest that the expense of screening (and follow-up x-rays if needed) can be minimized by screening only girls in two grades—5th and 7th.

Yawn BP, et al: A population-based study of school scoliosis screening. JAMA 282:1427-1432, 1999.

143. How is scoliosis measured by the Cobb method?

This is the standard technique used to quantify scoliosis in posteroanterior or lateral radiographs. One line is drawn along the vertebra tilted the most at the top of the curve, and another at the bottom of the curve. The curvature is represented by angle a, which can be measured in the two ways illustrated:

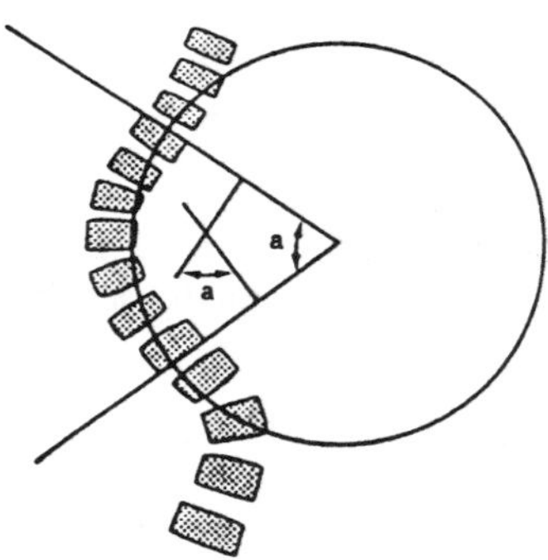

From Tolo VT, Wood B: Pediatric Orthopaedics in Primary Care. Baltimore, Williams & Wilkins, 1993, p. 88; with permission.

144. Why is Risser staging important in following patients with scc

Risser staging is a method of estimating bone growth potential ł ance of the iliac crest on radiographs taken for scoliosis. Scoliosis pr the rapid growth phase of adolescence. The **iliac apophysis** is the s center which develops laterally to the iliac crest and can be used to quantify growth potential. Stage I begins shortly after puberty, and stage IV indicates spinal growth is nearly complete. Stage V, seen in adults, indicates complete fusion. If a patient has entered stage IV or V, progression of scoliosis is unlikely. Earlier stages indicate that careful follow-up must be done because of increased risk of progression.

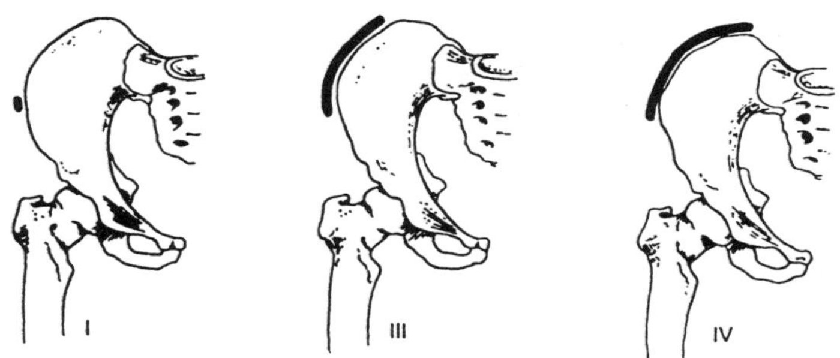

From Tolo VT, Wood B: Pediatric Orthopaedics in Primary Care. Baltimore, Williams & Wilkins, 1993, p. 90; with permission.

145. What is the recommended treatment for scoliosis?

- Observation with serial exams every 4-6 months if the patient is mature and the curvature is <25°.
- Bracing if the curvature is 25–40° with >2 years of growth remaining.
- Surgery if the curvature is > 40°.

146. What is the differential diagnosis of disc space narrowing seen on a radiograph?

Disc space infection, posttraumatic changes, congenital abnormalities, and tumor. If the patient presents with disc space narrowing and a history of pain, the diagnosis of acute disc space infection is likely. Asymptomatic patients with isolated findings of disc space infection may have congenital abnormalities (such as congenital kyphosis or a failure of segmentation).

147. What diagnosis should you consider in a teenage male with very poor posture that is not self-correctable?

Scheuermann kyphosis. This is a wedge-shaped deformity of vertebral bodies of unclear etiology that causes juvenile kyphosis (abnormally large dorsal thoracic or lumber curves). Common in teenagers (up to 5–8%), it is distinguished from simple bad posture ("postural round-back deformity") by its sharp angulation and lack of correction by active or passive maneuvers. X-ray studies reveal anterior vertebral body wedging and irregular erosions of the vertebral endplate. Treatment consists of exercise, bracing, and, rarely, surgical correction (for severe deformities).

148. How does spondylolysis differ from spondylolisthesis?

Spondylolysis is a condition in which there is a defect in the pars interarticularis (vertebral arch) of a vertebra that is most common at L5 in children and adolescents. **Spondylolisthesis** is a condition (usually resulting from spondylolysis) characterized by slippage of vertebra forward on the lower vertebra. Pain is the most common presenting symptom ɟr both conditions. The etiology is unclear, but various theories relate it to hereditary factors, congenital predisposition, trauma, posture, growth and biomechanical factors. Treatment includes watchful waiting, limitation of activity, exercise therapy, bracing, casting and surgery depending on the patient's age, magnitude of the slippage, extent of pain and predicted likelihood of progression of the deformity.

18. PULMONOLOGY

Robert W. Wilmott, M.D., Ellen B. Kaplan, M.D., Carlos R. Perez, M.D., William D. Hardie, M.D., Barbara A. Chini, M.D., and Cori L. Daines, M.D.

ALLERGIC RHINITIS

1. What conditions should be considered in the differential diagnosis of chronic nasal stuffiness in children?

- *Allergic rhinitis*
- *Infection* (e.g., sinusitis)
- *Anatomic obstruction* (e.g, adenoidal hypertrophy, nasal polyps, deviated nasal septum, foreign body, tumor)
- *Drugs* (legal and illegal): aspirin, nonsteroidal anti-inflammatory drugs, oral contraceptive pills, cocaine)
- *Endocrinologic* (hypothyroidism, pregnancy, diabetes mellitus, oral contraceptive pills, premenstrual congestion)
- Associated with *systemic immunologic* disease (e.g., Wegener granulomatosis)
- *Rhinitis medicamentosa*
- *Nonallergic rhinitis* (a subset of which is nonallergic rhinitis with eosinophilia [NARES])
- *Idiopathic rhinitis*
- *Reflux associated*
- *Choanal atresia*

Rajakulasingam K, Anderson DF, Holgate ST: Allergic rhinitis, nonallergic rhinitis, and ocular allergy. In: Kaplan AP: Allergy. Philadelphia, W.B. Saunders, 1997. pp 421-448.

Druce HM: Allergic and nonallergic rhinitis. In: Middleton E, et al: Allergy: Principles and Practice. St. Louis, Mosby, 1998, pp 1005-1016.

Naclerio R, Solomon W: Rhinitis and inhalant allergens. JAMA 278:1842-1848, 1997.

2. How does the time of year help identify the potential cause of allergic rhinitis?

Tree pollen is usually associated with the onset of the growing season. After local tree pollenation, *grass* pollens appear. This may occur earlier in locales where there are short winters. *Weed* pollen is associated with the late summer pollen peak, and ragweed is the primary weed pollen in eastern and central North America. *Fungal* aeroallergens span the growing season. Relative concentrations of household *animal* allergen, *dust mites*, and *indoor fungi* generally increase when doors and windows are closed. However, dust mites proliferate in areas of high humidity and may cause perennial symptoms.

Naclerio R, Solomon W: Rhinitis and inhalant allergens. JAMA 278:1842-1848, 1997.

3. How do the RAST and ELISA tests differ?

RAST (*radioallergosorbent test*): An *in vitro* laboratory method to quantify the amount of allergen-specific IgE. The test allergen is bound to solid-phase particles, with which the patient's serum is then incubated. If the patient's serum contains the antigen-specific IgE, then the RAST antigen will bind to the patient's IgE. Nonspecific IgE is removed by washing. Radiolabeled anti-IgE is then added and binds to the IgE-antigen complex. Quantification of radioactivity (which correlates with the quantity of antigen-specific IgE) is determined using a gamma counter.

ELISA (*enzyme-linked immunosorbent assay*): A variation of the RAST that uses enzyme-conjugated, rather than radiolabeled, anti-IgE. The amount of the enzyme bound (and, hence, antigen-specific IgE) is determined by adding the appropriate substrate and measuring the colored product of the reaction spectrophotometrically.

4. Discuss the pros and cons of skin testing versus *in vitro* (e.g., RAST) testing for allergies.

In vitro tests:
- No risk of anaphylaxis
- Results not influenced by medications, dermatographism, extensive dermatologic disease
- More costly

Skin testing:
- Less costly
- More sensitive than *in vitro* tests such as RAST
- Results immediately available

5. Which variables affect allergy skin testing in children?

Test site: The forearm is less reactive than the back. The lower back is less reactive than the mid- and upper back.

Patient age: Wheals on skin testing increase in size from infancy on and, then, often decline after 50 years of age. Infants react primarily with a small wheal and a large erythematous flare.

Seasonality: There is increased allergen skin test sensitivity after the pollen season that then declines until the next season.

Medications: Can inhibit allergen skin test response for various lengths of time: Cetirizine (3-10 days), loratadine (3-10 days), diphenhyramine (1-3 days), chlorpheniramine (1-3 days), hydroxyzine (1-10 days).

Test technique: Prick skin tests are more specific than intradermal skin tests.

Demoly P, Michel FB, Bousquet J: In vivo methods for study of allergy skin tests, techniques, and interpretation. In: Middleton E, et al: Allergy, Principles and Practice. St. Louis, Mosby, 1998, pp 430-439.

6. What is the recommended treatment for children with chronic allergic rhinitis?

Optimally, *allergen avoidance* or limiting allergen exposure by environmental control measures is the first line of treatment. However, adjunctive *pharmacotherapy* is often necessary. These include topical and/or systemic medications. Topical intranasal corticosteroids appear to be more affective than oral antihistamines in controlling nasal blockage and discharge. Oral antihistamines are better at treating nasal itching, sneezing and eye symptoms. Allergen *immunotherapy* is considered in those individuals with allergic rhinitis in which the above measures provide suboptimal control.

Weiner JM, et al: Intranasal steroids versus oral H1 receptor antagonists in allergic rhinitis: Systematic review of randomised controlled trials. BMJ 317:1624-1629, 1998.

7. How can you get rid of cat allergen?

- Reduce cat allergen harbors such as carpets, sofas, etc.
- Vacuum with appliances with effective filtration systems.
- Improve ventilation or use HEPA filters to remove small airborne particles.
- Bathe the cat on a regular basis.

After felinectomy, which is the ultimate solution, it will take months to remove the cat allergen from the house. Even with banishing the cat from the house, passive transfer of cat allergen from playing with the cat outside this environment, will introduce cat allergen into the home.

Solomon W, Platts-Mills TAE: Aerobiology and inhalant allergens. In: Middleton E et al: Allergy, Principles and Practice. St. Louis, Mosby 1998, pp 367-403.

8. How can house dust mite (HDM) concentrations be minimized?

Allergens from HDM are extremely important triggers of allergic rhinitis and asthma. They are airborne during and immediately after disturbance. Individuals often sleep or sit on surfaces containing high concentrations of HDM, such as the bed, pillow, or sofa.

To decrease HDM concentrations in the bedroom:

- Encase mattresses and pillows with airtight covers.
- Wash bedding at very high temperatures (> 130ºF) weekly.
- Remove carpeting
- Eliminate stuffed animals, books, and toys from the bedroom.
- Weekly vacuuming with a unit with a double-thickness bag or high-efficiency filter.

To decrease HDM concentrations in the remainder of the house:

- Use as little carpeting and upholstered furniture as possible.
- Decrease humidity <45% relative humidity.
- Treat carpets with chemicals such as benzyl benzoate or tannic acid that degrade the HDM allergen.

Solomon W, Platts-Mills TAE: Aerobiology and inhalant allergens. In: Middleton E, et al: Allergy, Principles and Practice. St. Louis, Mosby, 1998, pp 367-403.

9. Which children should be considered for immunotherapy?

Allergen immunotherapy can be helpful for many children with IgE-mediated sensitivities including allergic rhinitis, asthma, and hymenoptera venom hypersensitivity. In general, indications for the latter in children include life-threatening systemic reactions. Whole body extracts (in contrast to venom) have been effective for individuals with fire ant hypersensitivity. Immunotherapy for IgE-mediated disease, specifically allergic rhinitis and allergic-based asthma, should be considered when allergen avoidance and adjunctive pharmacotherapy have produced supoptimal results.

Weber RW: Immunotherapy with allergens. JAMA 278:1881-1887, 1997.

10. How common is exercise-induced bronchospasm in children with allergic rhinitis?

Up to 40% of patients with allergic rhinitis but no history of asthma have abnormal pulmonary function tests in response to exercise.

Bierman EW: Incidence of exercise-induced asthma in children. Pediatrics 56:847-850, 1975.

ASTHMA

11. When does asthma usually have its onset of symptoms?

Approximately 50% of childhood asthma develops before 3 years of age and nearly all by age 7 years. The signs and symptoms of asthma, including chronic cough, may be evident much earlier than the actual diagnosis but may be erroneously attributed to recurrent pneumonia or "wheezy bronchitis."

12. Is asthma more common in males or females?

Asthma is two to three times more common in boys than girls until the onset of puberty. It equalizes in adolescence. When onset is in adulthood, it is more common in females.

13. What historical points suggest that a child's asthma may have an allergic trigger?

- Seasonal nature with concurrent rhinitis (suggesting *pollen*)
- Symptoms worsen when visiting a family with pets (suggesting *animal dander*)
- Wheezing occurs when carpets are vacuumed or bed is made (suggesting *mites*)
- Symptoms develop in damp basements or barns (suggesting *molds*)

14. What types of challenge testing are given to children to test for airway hyperreactivity?

Pharmacologic:	Methacholine (stimulates muscarinic receptors on bronchial smooth muscle)
	Histamine (direct bronchoconstrictive effect and reflex vagal stimulation)
Physiologic:	Exercise
	Cold air hyperventilation
	Ultrasonically nebulized distilled water inhalation
Allergenic:	Cat dander or ragweed

15. What is the "88% saturation test"?

A test that can be performed in young, uncooperative, or developmentally delayed children who cannot adequately perform standard spirometry. The patient breathes a nonhumidified 12% oxygen and nitrogen mixture for 10 minutes or until oxygen saturation as measured by pulse oximetry falls to 88%. The dry, hypoxic air acts as a bronchial challenge, and the inability to complete 10 minutes may indicate reactive airways disease.

Wagner CL, et al: The "88% saturation test": A simple lung function test for young children. Pediatrics 93:63-67, 1994.

16. How common is exercise-induced bronchospasm (EIB)?

Very common, and often overlooked. In asthmatic children, significant symptoms (e.g., cough, chest tightness, wheezing, dyspnea) are noted following exercise in approximately 80%, although abnormal pulmonary function tests can be found in nearly 100%. In atopic children, the incidence of EIB has been estimated to be as high as 40%.

17. How is exercise-induced bronchospasm diagnosed?

EIB is likely if the peak flow rate or FEV_1 drops by 15% after 6 minutes of vigorous exercise. This exercise can include jogging on a motor-driven treadmill (15% grade at 3–4 mph), riding a stationary bicycle, or running up and down a hallway. Peak flow can then be measured with simple peak flow meters or a spirometer every 2–3 minutes, although peak flows are not as reliable as spirometry. The greatest reduction in EIB is seen usually 5–10 minutes after exercise. As further verification of the diagnosis, if the patient has developed a decreased peak flow (and possibly wheezing), two puffs of a β_2-agonist should be administered to reverse the bronchospasm.

18. What mechanisms lead to airway obstruction during an acute asthma attack?

The main causes of airflow obstruction in acute asthma are *airway inflammation*, including edema, *bronchospasm*, and increased *mucus* production. Chronic inflammation often results in airway remodeling, which may not be clinically apparent.

Bousquet J, et al: Asthma, from airway bronchoconstriction to airways inflammation and remodeling. Am J Respir Crit Care Med 161:1720-45, 2000.

19. Can you get rid of cockroach allergen?

Cockroach allergen has been identified as a major trigger for asthma, but ridding the home of cockroach allergen is difficult. Avoidance measures await further study. Baits such as boric acid or Hydromethanon have been shown to kill cockroaches but have not been shown to control allergen. Spraying with substances that generate irritant fumes should be avoided. Sealing of food and immaculate cleaning are imperative.

Solomon W, Platts-Mills TAE. Aerobiology and inhalant allergens. In: Middleton E et al: Allergy, Principles and Practice. St. Louis, Mosby, 1998, pp 367-403.

20. Which other noninfectious diseases besides asthma should be considered in an infant who wheezes?

- *Aspiration pneumonitis*, especially in a neurologically impaired infant or an infant with gastroesophageal reflux, especially if there is coughing, choking, or gagging with feedings. If there is a clear association with feedings, consider the possibility of tracheoesophageal fistula.
- *Bronchiolitis obliterans* (chronic wheezing often following adenoviral infection)
- *Bronchopulmonary dysplasia* (especially if prolonged oxygen therapy/ventilatory requirement in the neonatal period)
- *Ciliary dyskinesia* (especially if recurrent otitis media, sinusitis, or situs inversus is present)
- *Congenital malformations* (including tracheobronchial anomalies and malacia, lung cysts, and mediastinal lesions)
- *Cystic fibrosis* (if associated with recurrent wheezing, failure to thrive, chronic diarrhea, or recurrent pneumonia)
- *Congenital cardiac anomalies* (especially lesions with large left-to-right shunts)
- *Foreign-body aspiration* (if associated with acute choking episode in infant > 6 months of age)
- *Vascular rings, slings, or compression*

21. What clinical signs correlate best with severity of respiratory disease during an acute asthmatic attack?

- *Markedly increased respiratory rate*
- *Pronounced retractions* (especially sternocleidomastoid retractions) or respiratory muscle fatigue
- *Altered mental state* (agitation, drowsiness)
- *Diminished breath sounds* (wheezing may be absent if flow rates are very low)
- *Increased pulsus paradoxus* (This is performed by measuring the blood pressure and noting the difference in pressure between the point at which the systolic pressure is initially heard intermittently and the point at which the systolic pressure is heard with every heart beat. Normally, this is < 10 mmHg.)

22. What is the Hoover sign?

The ***paradoxical inward motion*** (retraction) of the costal margins with ***inspiration***. It is seen in children with significant asthma, bronchiolitis, or other conditions in which the lungs are overinflated and the diaphragm is flattened. This mechanical change in the contour of the diaphragm results in costal margin retraction rather than elevation with diaphragmatic contraction.

Klein M: Hoover sign and peripheral airways obstruction. J Pediatr 120:495, 1992.

23. Is a chest x-ray necessary for all children who wheeze for the first time?

"To get a chest x-ray, or not to get a chest x-ray? That is the question." In children > 2 years of age who wheeze for the first time, the most likely diagnosis is asthma. Whereas in children < 2, bronchiolitis is the most likely cause. A chest x-ray is often recommended for evaluation of an initial episode of wheezing to rule out other diagnoses such as pneumonia or foreign-body aspiration, but the vast majority will not add any new information for diagnosis or treatment if the clinical picture is consistent with bronchiolitis or asthma. A chest x-ray should be considered for a first-time wheezing patient in the following situations:

- *Findings on physical exam* that suggest other diagnoses (e.g, marked adenopathy suggesting mediastinal mass, digital clubbing suggesting a chronic respiratory problem, hyperresonance to percussion suggesting pneumothorax, or supraclavicular crepitance suggesting pneumomediastinum)

- Marked *asymmetry* of breath sounds
- Suspected *pneumonia* (e.g., high fever, localized rales, or locally diminished breath sounds)
- Suspected *foreign-body* aspiration
- *Hypoxemia* or *marked respiratory distress*
- *Older* child with *no family history* of asthma or atopy
- Suspected *congestive heart failure*
- History of *trauma* (e.g., burns, scalds, blunt or penetrating injury)

24. What are the usual findings on arterial blood gas sampling during acute asthma attacks?

The most common finding is ***hypocapnia*** (i.e., low CO_2) because of hyperventilation. Hypoxemia may also be present unless the child is being treated with oxygen. Therefore, hypercapnia is a serious sign, which suggests that the child is tiring or becoming severely obstructed. This finding should prompt reevaluation and consideration of admission to a high acuity unit.

25. Which asthmatics should be admitted to the hospital?

After therapy, admission is advisable if a child has:

- Depressed level of consciousness
- Incomplete response with moderate retractions, wheezing, peak flow $< 60\%$ predicted, pulsus paradoxus >15 mmHg, $SaO_2 \leq 90\%$, $pCO_2 \geq 42$ mmHg
- Breath sounds significantly diminished
- Evidence of dehydration
- Pneumothorax
- Residual symptoms and history of severe attacks involving prolonged hospitalization (especially if intubation was required)
- Parental unreliability

An equally difficult (and very unpredictable) challenge relates to which patients will relapse after responding to therapy and subsequently require hospitalization. This is a major problem, as rates of relapse can approach 20-30%.

26. How has management for an acute asthma attack changed in the past decade?

While there remains variability in approach, certain trends have emerged:

- Use of subcutaneous epinephrine, intravenous theophylline, and aggressive hydration in initial management has greatly diminished.
- Aerosolized β_2-adrenergic agents (especially albuterol), including frequent miniboluses or continuous aerosol therapy, have become the first-line therapy.
- More aggressive use of oral and intravenous corticosteroids.
- Use of combination β_2-agonist/anticholinergic therapy.

27. What is the advantage of the "minibolus" aerosolized treatment of acute asthmatic exacerbations?

Although the most beneficial dosing regimen of β_2-agonists remains unclear, studies have shown that in acute exacerbations, the dose-response curve of bronchial smooth muscle is shifted to the right. Thus, higher doses may be needed to obtain a response. In addition, the duration of action of the aerosolized agent is significantly shorter in an acute episode compared with chronic asthma. Thus, a common recommendation is to administer albuterol, 0.15 mg/kg/dose (max 5 mg/dose) by nebulizer or four to eight puffs by metered-dose inhaler every 20 minutes up to 1 hour for initial management.

28. How much medication reaches the lungs in metered-dose inhaler or nebulizer therapy?

On average, about ***10-15%*** of the total dose, if proper technique is used. The percentage is usually lower in children than adults due to differences in delivery techniques.

29. Is a nebulizer more effective than a metered-dose inhaler (MDI) with a spacer in the treatment of asthma?

In the treatment of exacerbations of asthma, nebulizers are used almost exclusively in children < 2 years because of the ease of administration. While an MDI with a spacer is used more commonly in older children, some studies indicate that they are equally or more effective to nebulizers in young children, even those with moderate or severe acute asthma. Furthermore, the MDI with spacer requires less treatment time and has fewer side effects. They are often preferred by patients and parents.

Leversha AM, et al: Cost and effectiveness of spacer versus nebulizer in young children with moderate and severe acute asthma. J Pediatr 136:497-502, 2000.

Ploin D, et al: High-dose albuterol by metered-dose inhaler plus a spacer device versus nebulization in preschool children with recurrent wheezing: A double-blind randomized equivalence trial. Pediatrics 106:311-317, 2000.

30. List the possible acute side effects of albuterol.

General: hypoxemia, tachyphylaxis

Renal: hypokalemia

Cardiovascular: tachycardia, palpitations, premature ventricular contractions, atrial fibrillation

Neurologic: headache, irritability, insomnia, tremor, weaknness

Gastrointestinal: nausea, heartburn, vomiting

31. How significant is the risk of death with use of β-agonists?

In the mid-1960s, several Western countries experienced a dramatic increase in the number of asthma deaths (England and Wales, Scotland, Ireland, New Zealand, Australia, and Norway). Subsequent analysis indicated that the increase in asthma deaths was temporarily related to the introduction of a high-dose formulation of isoproterenol. In the mid-1970s, a similar epidemic was observed in New Zealand, and was attributed to a high potency formulation of fenoterol. There appears to be no risk of mortality related to the use of short-acting, lower potency beta-agonists such as albuterol and terbutaline. The possible mechanisms whereby high potency beta-agonists can lead to increased morbidity and instability from asthma are by increasing bronchial hyperresponsiveness, by inducing tolerance, and by masking evidence of deteriorating asthma control, leading to a delay in seeking medical attention.

Beasley R, et al : Beta-agonists: What is the evidence that their use increases the risk of asthma morbidity and mortality? J Allergy Clin Immunol 103:518-30, 1999.

Mullen M, et al: The association between beta-agonist use and death from asthma. JAMA. 270:1842, 1993.

32. Do inhaled steroids suppress the hypothalamic-pituitary axis?

Not to the same extent as systemic steroids, but they do impair nocturnal cortisol secretion. However, the response to stimulation with ACTH is normal in children receiving up to 800 mg/day of beclomethasone or budesonide. It is possible that the suppression of nocturnal cortisol secretion is of little clinical significance, but diminished pulmonary function and asthmatic attacks are common at night.

Wagener JS: Inhaled steroids in children: Risks versus rewards. J Pediatr 132:381-383, 1998.

33. Do inhaled steroids affect growth in children?

For children who require frequent courses of oral steroids, inhaled corticosteroids are indicated, particularly if inhaled cromolyn sodium has been of no benefit. The data on side effects of inhaled steroids continue to emerge. Results are conflicting but tend to indicate that mild growth suppression occurs on moderate to high doses, particularly in more severe asthmatics, primarily during the first year of therapy. However, asthma per se can also inhibit growth, and inhaled steroid therapy does not appear to affect eventual adult height. There is recent evidence that treatment of children with asthma before puberty, using inhaled steroids, leads to altered collagen metabolism. It is important that accurate growth measurements are made with a stadiometer on children requiring extended use of inhaled steroids and that they are monitored for height and height velocity.

Agertoft L, Pedersen S: Effect of long-term treatment with inhaled budesonide on adult height in children with asthma. N Engl J Med 343:1064-1069, 2000.

Crowley S, et al: Collagen metabolism and growth in prepubertal children with asthma treated with inhaled steroids. J Pediatr 132:409-413, 1998.

34. Do children on inhaled steroids for asthma need regular slit-lamp examinations?

Children on inhaled corticosteroids for asthma are at *increased risk* for developing posterior subcapsular and nuclear cataracts, especially if they are on higher doses for a prolonged duration. The clinician can screen for such cataracts in the office using a direct ophthalmoscope at a distance of six to eight inches from the eye with a +4.00 diopter lens. In children who receive systemic, as well as inhaled, steroids an annual slit-lamp examination by an ophthalmologist should be considered.

Chylack LT: Cataracts and inhaled corticosteroids. N Eng J Med 337:46-48, 1997.

Cumming RG, et al: Use of inhaled corticosteroids and the risk of cataracts. N Eng J Med 337:8-14, 1997.

35. Why has theophylline fallen from grace as a treatment for asthma?

Due to concerns about its potential toxicity (e.g., vomiting, tachycardia, seizures), side effects (e.g., behavioral changes, impaired school performance), and questionable efficacy, it is no longer considered part of routine therapy. Its use may be considered in an acute setting if a patient is becoming fatigued and developing respiratory failure. Some practitioners still use it in chronic settings, particularly for nocturnal asthma.

Weinberger M, Hendeles L: Drug therapy: Theophylline in asthma. N Engl J Med 334:1380-1388, 1996.

Szefler ST, et al: Evolving role of theophylline for treatment of chronic childhood asthma. J Pediatr 127:176-185, 1995.

36. What daily medications are used in the treatment of chronic asthma in children?

Cromolyn inhibits mast-cell degranulation (blocking mediator release) and reduces airway hyperreactivity by unknown mechanisms. It has no bronchodilator properties and is thus not useful in acute settings. However, when used by inhalation on a regular basis, it is helpful in treating allergic (extrinsic) asthma and exercise-induced bronchospasm. ***Leukotriene-receptor antagonists***, such as montelukast (Singulair) and zafirlukast (Accolate), are non-steroidal anti-inflammatory agents. Their precise role (i.e., primary therapy vs. "sparing" drug for steroid use) remains under evaluation, particularly in such areas as exercise-induced bronchospasm. The role of ***nedocromil***, a nonsteroidal anti-inflammatory medication with mechanisms of action similar to those of cromolyn, also remains to be elucidated in children. ***Inhaled glucocorticoids*** have largely replaced cromolyn as a first-line anti-inflammatory treatment for chronic asthma.

37. Are anticholinergics useful in the treatment of pediatric asthma?

The precise role of anticholinergics (including ipratropium bromide and atropine sulfate) in pediatrics remains ill-defined due to potential side effects and the paucity of studies on their efficacy in both acute and chronic asthma management. However, some evidence suggests that multiple doses of anticholinergics may be of value in the initial management of pediatric patients with severe exacerbations of asthma ($\leq$ 55% of predicted FEV_1). For mild to moderate disease, evidence does not suggest a benefit.

Plotnick LH, Ducharme FM: Should inhaled anticholinergics be added to β_2 agonists for treating acute childhood and adolescent asthma? A systematic review. BMJ 317:971-977, 1998.

Qureshi F, et al: Effect of nebulized ipratropium on the hospitalization rates of children with asthma. N Engl J Med 339:1013-1020, 1998.

38. Is high dose magnesium therapy in children helpful in moderate to severe asthma exacerbations?

The jury is still out. Magnesium has been shown to relax smooth muscle in bronchoconstriction and to stabilize mast cells. Clinical results in children are conflicting.

Ciarallo L, et al: Higher-dose intravenous magnesium therapy for children with moderate to severe acute asthma. Arch Pediatr Adolesc Med 154:979-983, 2000.

Scarfone RJ, et al: A randomized trial of magnesium in the emergency department treatment of children with asthma. Ann Emerg Med 36:572-578, 2000.

39. What is the theoretic value of the use of helium-oxygen mixtures in asthma attacks?

When airway diameter narrows (as in bronchoconstriction or edema), airflow turbulence increases. The density of the flowing gas has a greater effect on airway resistance under turbulent conditions, with less dense gases resulting in less resistance. The use of lower density gas mixtures (helium-oxygen or heliox) has been used in the past during the preoperative treatment of upper airway obstruction (e.g, epiglottitis). Beyond the third-generation bronchial airways in normal individuals, gas density is felt not to affect resistance substantially because the airway cross-sectional area (due to the proliferation of airways) is increased. Thus, the value of helium-oxygen has not been expected to be substantial in primarily lower airway disease. However, in adult studies, total airway resistance was much improved on this therapy and preliminary studies in children have shown benefit. It is an evolving area of research.

Kudukis TM et al: Inhaled helium-oxygen revisited: Effect of helium-oxygen during the treatment of status asthmaticus in children. J Pediatr 130:217-224, 1997.

40. Is there a role for alternative medicine therapies in the treatment of asthma?

A comparison study of active versus simulated chiropractic manipulation revealed no benefits for asthma care. However, massage and relaxation therapy in children ages 4-14 years did demonstrate substantial improvements in pulmonary function. Other alternative therapies that have shown benefit include hypnosis, acupuncture and yoga.

Field T, et al: Children with asthma have improved pulmonary functions after massage therapy. J Pediatr 132:854-858, 1998.

Balon J, et al: A comparison of active and simulated chiropractic manipulation as adjunctive treatment for childhood asthma. N Engl J Med 339:1013-1020, 1998.

41. In chronic asthma, how do mild, moderate, and severe types differ?

	Mild	*Moderate*	*Severe*
Episodes of cough or wheeze	Brief, < 2/wk	≥ 2/wk	Almost daily, continuous
Symptoms between episodes	No	Occasional	Present
Exercise tolerance	EIB with strenuous exercise	EIB with most exercise	Activity limited even with medication
Nocturnal cough or wheezing	< 2/mo	Weekly	Frequent
School loss	None	> 7 days/yr	> 21 days/yr
ER, office visits for acute asthma	None	≤ 3/yr	> 3/yr
Hospitalization	None	None	1/yr
PEFR % reference	≥ 80%	60–80%	< 60%
PEFR variability	20%	20–30%	> 30% episodes while medicated
Response to optimal medication	Symptoms controlled with prn inhaler	Regular medication required to control	Symptoms even with regular medication

EIB—exercise-induced bronchospasm; PEFR—peak expiratory flow rate.

From Eggleston PA: Asthma. In: Oski FA, et al (eds): Principles and Practice of Pediatrics, 2nd ed. Philadelphia, J.B. Lippincott, 1994, p 220; with permission.

42. How useful are pulmonary function tests (PFTs) in evaluating and following children with asthma?

PFTs are very useful in the longitudinal evaluation of outpatients with asthma, in demonstrating a satisfactory response to therapy, and for identifying the severely obstructed, hyperinflated asymptomatic patient who has a poor prognosis if unrecognized. The use of home peak flow meters to measure the peak expiratory flow rate (PEFR) on a daily or as-needed basis can also be helpful. A baseline predicted or personal-best value can be obtained and home therapy initiated when the PEFR falls. PFTs may be particularly helpful in cough-variant asthma to distinguish between upper and lower airway disease.

43. What proportion of childhood asthmatics "outgrow" their symptoms?

Popular pediatric teaching has been that most children with asthma outgrow their symptoms. However, studies suggest that this is erroneous and that only 30-50% become symptom-free, primarily those with milder disease. Many children who "outgrow" symptoms have recurrences in adulthood. Studies also indicate that many infants who wheeze with viral infections and are asymptomatic between illnesses tend to "outgrow" their asthma, but that children whose initial wheezing occurs later in life, with allergen sensitization as a major factor, tend to have more persistence of recurrent bronchospasm. Although the overall trend is for asthma to become more muted, a large percentage of adults have persistent obstructive disease, both recognized and unrecognized.

Godden DJ, et al: Outcome of wheeze in childhood: Symptoms and pulmonary function 25 years later. Am J Respir Crit Care Med 149:106-112, 1994.

Silverman M: Out of the mouths of babes and sucklings: Lessons from early childhood asthma. Thorax 48:1200-1204, 1993.

44. Can asthma be prevented?

Asthma is an environmentally-induced lung disease with genetic predispositions. Since the prevalence of asthma has increased substantially over the past three decades, genetic mutation is unlikely. A variety of specific preventative interventions—extended breastfeeding, avoidance of allergens (e.g., food, dust-mite, pets) and tobacco smoke, use of hypoallergenic partially hydrolyzed—have been attempted to reduce this prevalence. Results have been contradictory and even positive benefits quite modest.

Chan-Yeung M, et al: A randomized controlled study of the effectiveness of a multifaceted intervention program in the primary prevention of asthma in high-risk infants. Arch Pediatr Adolesc Med 154:700-705, 2000.

BRONCHIOLITIS

45. What is the most important cause of lower respiratory tract disease in infants and young children?

Respiratory syncytial virus (RSV). Up to 100,000 children are hospitalized annually in the U.S. due to this pneumovirus (different from, but closely related to, the paramyxoviruses). Disease most commonly occurs during outbreaks in winter or spring in the U.S. and in the winter months of July and August in the Southern Hemisphere.

46. What other agents cause bronchiolitis?

Although RSV is estimated to cause 50–90% of cases, other agents responsible for bronchiolitis include *parainfluenza* viruses (second most common cause), *influenza* virus types A and B, *adenovirus, enterovirus, rhinovirus, Chlamydia trachomatis, Chlamydia pneumoniae,* and *Mycoplasma pneumoniae.*

47. What are the best predictors of the severity of bronchiolitis?

The single best predictor at an initial assessment appears to be ***oxygen saturation***, which can be determined by pulse oximetry. $SaO_2 < 95\%$ correlates with more severe disease. Of note, low SaO_2 is often not clinically apparent, and objective measurements are necessary. An arterial blood gas with PaO_2 of ≤ 65 or $PaCO_2 > 40$ mmHg is particularly worrisome. Other predictors of more severity include:

- An ill or "toxic" appearance
- History of prematurity (gestational age < 34 wks)
- Atelectasis on chest x-ray
- Respiratory rate > 70/min
- Infant < 3 months old

48. What are the typical findings on chest x-ray in a child with bronchiolitis?

The picture is varied. Most commonly, there is ***hyperinflation*** of the lungs. Bilateral interstitial abnormalities with ***peribronchial thickening*** are common. Up to 20% of children may have lobar, segmental, or subsegmental consolidation which can mimic bacterial pneumonia. Of note, with the possible exception of atelectasis, the chest x-ray findings do not correlate well with the severity of the disease.

49. How common is apnea in RSV bronchiolitis?

About 20% of hospitalized infants develop apnea. Infants at highest risk include former premature infants, particularly those who are < 44 weeks postconception, the very young (1-4 months), and those with chronic lung disease. Infants may first have apnea and progress to bronchiolitis, or show signs of bronchiolitis and then develop apneas, or have apnea as the sole sign of RSV infection. A large number of infants with RSV infection, who require assisted ventilation, do so because of severe recurrent apnea rather than respiratory failure. The mechanisms leading to apnea are unclear, but they tend to resolve within a few days. Monitoring should be done for hospitalized high-risk infants. Of note, SIDS has not been clearly associated with RSV infection.

50. Is the use of steroids justified for bronchiolitis?

Although corticosteroids have been utilized by clinicians for many years in the treatment of bronchiolitis, the preponderance of multiple controlled studies has shown no immediate or long-term advantage with their use, either by the systemic or inhaled route. However, their value or lack thereof continues to be debated.

Garrison MM, et al: Systemic corticosteroids in infant bronchiolitis: A meta-analysis. Pediatrics 105:e44, 2000.

Bulow SM, et al: Prednisolone treatment of respiratory syncytial virus: A randomized controlled trial of 147 infants. Pediatrics 104:377, 1999.

51. Are bronchodilators such as albuterol effective as a therapy for bronchiolitis?

The use of bronchodilator therapy for bronchiolitis is controversial. 30-50% of infants with RSV bronchiolitis will have a positive response to inhalation therapy, and infants with a strong family history of asthma are most likely to respond. In infants with significant wheezing, a trial of albuterol may be indicated with continuation if benefits are noted.

52. Is there a vaccine to prevent RSV infection?

No, there is not yet a safe and effective vaccine against RSV. However, Palivizumab (Synagis), a monoclonal antibody directed against RSV, is effective for prophylaxis of RSV infection in premature infants. It is given intramuscularly and must be given once per month during the RSV season. This drug is not indicated for the treatment of RSV infection.

53. Does infection with RSV confer lifelong protection?

No. In fact, reinfection is very common. In day-care centers, up to 75% of infants who acquire RSV infections in the first year of life are reinfected during the subsequent 2 years. Primary infections tend to be the most severe episodes, with subsequent illnesses being more muted. In older children and adults, RSV infections present as "colds," and reinfection is also common.

54. If a 5-month-old is hospitalized due to RSV bronchiolitis, what should the parents be told about the likelihood of future episodes of wheezing?

In follow-up studies, ***40-50%*** of these infants have subsequent ***recurrent episodes*** of wheezing, usually in the first year after illness. Subclinical pulmonary abnormalities may also persist. The question of whether the pulmonary sequelae are due to the bronchiolitis or a genetic predisposition to asthma remains unclear. Host factors, including pulmonary abnormalities prior to the illness, passive cigarette smoke exposure, atopic diathesis, and immunologic responses of virus-specific IgE, may be involved in recurrent problems.

55. How is bronchiolitis distinguished from asthma in a wheezing infant?

Asthma is a clinical diagnosis in all age groups that is characterized by reversible airway obstruction with hyperresponsiveness to various stimuli, including viral infections. However, the viral infections themselves, rather than underlying bronchial pathology, can be responsible for the wheezing in an infant with acute symptoms. Differentiating between the two diseases at the time of presentation can be virtually impossible. The infant wheezing from bronchiolitis generally has other symptoms, such as fever and rhinorrhea, and RSV antigen testing may be positive. If repeated episodes of reversible wheezing occur, especially out of the RSV season, asthma is likely. Other diagnoses, such as cystic fibrosis and gastroesophageal reflux, must also be considered.

CLINICAL ISSUES

56. How is hemoptysis differentiated from hematemesis?

	Hemoptysis	***Hematemesis***
Color	Bright red and frothy	Dark red or brown
pH	Alkaline	Acid
Consistency	May be mixed with sputum	May contain food particles
Symptoms	Preceded by gurgling	Preceded by nausea
	Accompanied by coughing	Accompanied by retching

Rosenstein BJ: Hemoptysis. In: Hilman BC (ed): Pediatric Respiratory Disease. Philadelphia, W.B. Saunders, 1993, p 533.

57. What are the indications for surgical repair of pectus excavatum?

This is still an area of considerable controversy. Children with pectus excavatum tend to have reduced total lung capacity, reduced vital capacity, increased residual volume, and reduced stroke volume during maximum exercise. However, most patients are still in the normal range for these values. The most common complaints relate to poor self-image and decreased exercise tolerance. Counseling is often sufficient for the cosmetic aspects, but most older patients will report an improvement in exercise tolerance following repair, despite what seems to be minor changes in stroke volume. Whether for cosmetic reasons or to improve maximum exercise, operative repair should be delayed until the child is older than 6 years of age to decrease risk of recurrence during the pubertal growth spurt.

Haller JA, Loughlin GM: Cardiorespiratory function is significantly improved following corrective surgery for severe pectus excavatum. J Cardiovasc Surg 41:125-130, 2000.

58. What's all the fuss about Nuss?

The traditional repair of pectus excavatum has been the Ravitch procedure. This repair requires sternal osteotomy and extensive dissection with resection of all of the deformed costal cartilages and anterior fixation of the sternum. A new minimally invasive operation—the Nuss procedure—involves inserting a convex steel bar under the sternum through a small lateral incision without rib incision or resection. Once in place, the bar is rotated and the convex surface pushes against the sternum. Utilizing the principles of orthopedic remodeling, the bar is left in place. After two years, the bar is removed in an outpatient procedure and results demonstrating sternal expansion have been very positive. Indications for surgical repair remain controversial, but the Nuss procedure, if prospective and long-term studies are positive, would certainly be a less traumatic surgical option.

Molik KA, et al: Pectus excavatum repair: Experience with standard and minimal invasive technique. Pediatr Surg 36:324-328, 2001.

Nuss D, et al: A 10-year review of a minimally-invasive technique for the repair of pectus excavatum. J Pediatr Surg 33:545-552, 1998.

59. How is the "slipping rib syndrome" diagnosed?

The *slipping rib syndrome* is a cause of upper abdominal or chest pain during which a patient will often experience a slipping sensation of the ribs with a pop or click upon heavy lifting. Anatomically, the tip of one of the lower "floating" (not joined directly to the sternum) ribs overrides a rib above. This condition may follow trauma. Diagnosis is likely if the pain can be reproduced by grasping the affected rib and pulling it anteriorly.

Porter GE: Slipping rib syndrome: An infrequently recognized entity in children: A report of three cases and review of the literature. Pediatrics 76:810-813, 1985.

60. How do the possible causes of chronic cough vary by age group?

Infancy	***Preschool***	***School Age and Up***
Infectious	*Infectious*	*Infectious*
RSV	Viral	Viral
Chlamydia	Rhinitis	Mycoplasma
Pertussis	Sinusitis	Sinusitis
Tuberculosis	Tuberculosis	? Pertussis
Other viral illnesses	Acute pneumonia	
Irritative	*Irritative*	*Irritative*
Smoke exposure	Smoke exposure	Smoke exposure
Wood burning stoves	Hydrocarbon ingestion	Cigarette smoking
	GER	GER
		? Pollution
Aspiration	*Aspiration*	*Aspiration*
Oropharyngeal	Oropharyngeal	Oropharyngeal
Foreign body	Foreign body	
Congenital	*Congenital*	*Congenital*
Cystic fibrosis	Cystic fibrosis	Cystic fibrosis
Laryngomalacia		
Innominate artery compression		
Reactive	*Reactive*	*Reactive*
Post-infectious	Post-infectious	Post-infectious
Asthma	Asthma	Asthma
Post-nasal drip	Post-nasal drip	Post-nasal drip
		Psychogenic

61. Which specific infectious agents have most prominently been identified as a cause of severe persistent pertussis-like coughs?

Bordetella pertussis, Bordetella parapertusssis, Chlamydia pneumoniae, adenovirus, human parainfluenza virus, RSV, influenza A and B, *Mycoplasma pneumoniae.*

Hagiwara K, et al: An epidemic of pertussis-like illness caused by Chlamydia pneumoniae. Pediatr Infect Dis J 18:271-275, 1999.

Von Konig, et al: A serologic study of organisms possibly associated with pertussis-like coughing. Pediatr Infect Dis J 17:645-649, 1998.

62. When should the diagnosis of psychogenic cough be considered?

A psychogenic cough should be considered in those children with a dry, barky, explosive daytime cough that disappears with sleep or pleasant activity. It often starts after a URI. The patient complains of a tickle or something in their throat. Physical exam and lab work are normal, and conventional therapies are ineffective. Behavior management is the preferred treatment, although, in some cases, psychological intervention is required.

63. Which is more effective as a cough medicine in children, dextromethorphan or codeine?

Multiple studies have failed to show that either agent is superior to placebo in the treatment of cough due to URI.

Committee on Drugs: Use of codeine- and dextromethorphan-containing cough remedies in children. Pediatrics 99:918-919, 1997.

64. What are the risks of passive smoking in children?

Passive cigarette smoke exposure, which consists of the inhalation of both the smoker's exhalation (mainstream smoke, about 15% of total) and the more noxious sidestream (the unfiltered burning end of the cigarette, about 85% of total), has been the subject of much study. While the extent of effect is debated, risks include:

- Decreased fetal growth
- Increased incidence of SIDS
- Increased incidence of middle ear effusions
- Increased frequency of upper and lower respiratory tract infections
- Presentation of asthma at an earlier age with more frequent exacerbations
- Impaired lung function

Longer-term issues of increased cancer rates and cardiovascular disease remain under study. Of note, if a parent smokes, a child is twice as likely to become a smoker.

DiFranza JR, Lew RA: Morbidity and mortality in children associated with the use of tobacco products by other people. Pediatrics 97:560-568, 1996.

65. How is clubbing diagnosed?

Digital *clubbing* is caused by the presence of increased amounts of connective tissue under the base of the fingernail. This may be determined by:

1. ***Rocking the nail*** on its bed between the examiner's finger and thumb. In clubbing, the nail seems to be floating.

2. ***Visual inspection*** reveals that the distal phalangeal depth (DPD), which is the distance from the top of the base of the nail to the finger pad, exceeds the interphalangeal depth (IPD), which is the distance from the top of the distal phalangeal joint to the underside of the joint. Normally, the DPD/IPD ratio is < 1, but in clubbing it is > 1. If the abnormality is not readily apparent, precise measurements can be made from a plaster cast of the finger.

3. The ***diamond (or Schamroth) sign***. Normally, if the nails of both index fingers or any other two identical fingers are opposed, there is a diamond-shaped window present between the nail bases (see figure). This window disappears in clubbing.

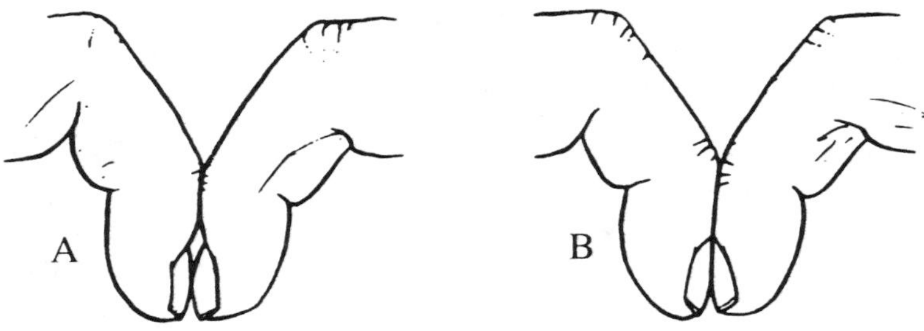

A, A normal child with a diamond-shaped window present between the nail bases when the fingers are opposed. *B*, The appearance of digital clubbing where the diamond-shaped window has been obliterated by the increased amount of soft tissue under the base of the nail.

66. Clubbing is associated with which diseases?

Pulmonary: Bronchiectasis (as in cystic fibrosis, bronchiolitis obliterans, ciliary dyskinesia), pulmonary abscess, empyema, interstitial fibrosis, malignancy, pulmonary atrioventricular fistula

Cardiac:	Cyanotic congenital heart disease, chronic congestive heart failure, subacute bacterial endocarditis
Hepatic:	Biliary cirrhosis, biliary atresia, alpha1-antitrypsin deficiency
Gastrointestinal:	Crohn disease, ulcerative colitis, chronic amebic and bacillary diarrhea, polyposis coli, small bowel lymphoma
Endocrine:	Thyrotoxicosis, thyroid deficiency
Hematologic:	Thalassemia, congenital methemoglobinemia (rare)
Idiopathic:	May be variation of normal and not indicative of underlying disease
Hereditary:	May be variation of normal and not indicative of underlying disease

Modified from Hilman BC: Clinical assessment of pulmonary disease in infants and children. In: Hilman BC (ed): Pediatric Respiratory Disease. Philadelphia, W.B. Saunders, 1993, p 61.

67. What is the pathophysiology of clubbing?

The answer is unclear. The increased connective tissue under the nailbeds that causes digital clubbing may be caused by the presence of vasoactive substances that are increased because of hypoxia or increased production in chronic inflammatory disease or by decreased lung clearance. Another theory proposes that digital clubbing is caused by local release of platelet-derived growth factor. Ordinarily, platelet-emboli containing this factor are trapped by the pulmonary circulation, but in cases of pulmonary shunting they may become trapped in the digital vessels.

68. Nasal polyps are associated with which conditions?

Pediatric: Nasal polyps are very rare in children except as a manifestation of cystic fibrosis. Approximately 3% of children with cystic fibrosis present with nasal polyps, which are often a recurrent problem. A sweat test is essential in these patients.

Adolescents: There is a wider range of possible diagnoses, including cystic fibrosis, allergic rhinitis, chronic sinusitis, malignancy, "triad asthma" (asthma, nasal polyps, aspirin sensitivity), and ciliary dyskinesia syndrome (e.g., Kartagener syndrome).

69. A 13-year-old with chronic sinusitis and recurrent pulmonary infections has a chest x-ray demonstrating a right-sided cardiac silhouette. What diagnostic test should be considered next?

Bronchial or nasal turbinate mucosal biopsy for electron microscopic evaluation of cilia. *Kartagener syndrome* is one of the ciliary dyskinesia (or immotile cilia) syndromes. It presents with a constellation of recurrent pulmonary infections, chronic sinusitis, recurrent otitis media, situs inversus, and infertility (in males). Structural ciliary abnormalities (most commonly absent dynein arms) result in abnormal ciliary beat and decreased clearance of respiratory secretions, predisposing to infection. In addition, since spermatozoa have tails with the same ultrastructural abnormalities as respiratory cilia, they move less well. The cause of the situs inversus is not fully understood, but it occurs in approximately 50% of individuals with primary ciliary dyskinesia. It has been suggested that cilia are important for proper organ orientation during embryonic development and that dysfunctional cilia make organ orientation a random event, possibly leading to situs inversus.

70. If a teenager presents with hemoptysis, frequent nosebleeds, and mucosal telangiectasia (just like his father), what condition should you suspect?

Hereditary hemorrhagic telangiectasia (also called Osler-Weber-Rendu syndrome). This autosomal dominant condition is characterized by increasing numbers of telangiectasias as the patient ages (often on the lips, tongue, ears, fingers, and toes). The development of AV fistulas and AV malformations in multiple organs is common.

71. In which children who snore should obstructive sleep apnea (OSA) be suspected?

At *night*, the child with OSA may have persistent snoring interrupted by periods of silence during which respiratory efforts are made, but there is no air movement; increased work of breathing with retractions; prominent mouth breathing; unusual sleep postures; frequent nighttime awakenings; enuresis; and night sweats. In the *day*, there may be excessive daytime sleepiness, learning problems, morning headaches, or personality change.

72. What evaluations should be done in a child with suspected OSA?

Examination, looking for mouth breathing while awake, dysphagia, midface or mandibular hypoplasia, tonsillar hypertrophy, cleft palate, palatal deformity caused by adenoidal hypertrophy, FTT, or obesity. A lateral airway radiograph is one of the easiest and most direct means of assessing upper airway caliber. Nasal endoscopy is useful for a dynamic assessment of the upper airway and larynx. But, until consistent clinical correlates can be found, the gold standard for the definitive diagnosis of OSA is detailed nocturnal polysomnography (overnight sleep study or PSG). Nocturnal pulse oximetry testing is being evaluated as a less costly and more readily available alternative, especially for uncomplicated OSA attributable to adenotonsillar hypertrophy in children older than 12 months. Compared with PSG, positive oximetry testing has a positive predictive value of 97% while negative testing does not exclude OSA and further follow-up with a PSG is needed. Cardiologic assessment is recommended (CXR, ECG, and echocardiography) in children with documented OSA and severe or sustained oxygen desaturation.

Brouillette RT. et al: Nocturnal pulse oximetry as an abbreviated testing modality for pediatric obstructive sleep apnea. Pediatrics 105:405-412, 2000.

73. What are the potential long-term consequences of OSA?

The most severe complications of OSA in children are right ventricular hypertrophy, hypertension, polycythemia, compensatory metabolic alkalosis, life-threatening cor pulmonale, and respiratory failure.

74. What is the natural history of laryngomalacia?

Congenital *laryngomalacia* is the most common cause of infantile stridor and generally has an excellent prognosis. Even children with mild laryngomalacia have increased episodes of brief desaturation and hypercapnia, but they are usually otherwise asymptomatic and the symptoms resolve by 2 years of age. However, close follow-up is mandatory. Symptoms generally worsen until approximately four months of age, and then gradually begin to improve. An occasional child has failure to thrive, difficulty in feeding, and significant obstruction. This may require surgical correction or tracheostomy to relieve the obstruction.

75. How can you clinically distinguish bilateral from unilateral vocal cord paralysis in an infant?

Normally, the vocal cords are tonically abducted, with voluntary adduction resulting in speech. With unilateral paralysis, one cord is ineffective in speech and hoarseness results. The infant's cry may be weak or absent. Stridor is usually minimal but may be positional (e.g., sleeping on the side with the paralyzed cord up may allow it to fall to midline and produce obstructive sounds). With bilateral paralysis, hoarseness is less apparent, the cry remains weak, but stridor (both inspiratory and expiratory) is usually quite prominent. Also with bilateral paralysis, the infant is more likely to have symptoms of frank pulmonary aspiration.

76. What is the most common cause of chronic hoarseness in children?

Screamer nodes. These are vocal cord nodules caused by vocal abuse, such as repetitive screaming, throat-clearing, and coughing. They are the cause of a hoarse voice in > 50% of children when hoarseness persists for > 2 weeks.

77. A 3-month-old who wheezes loudly while active, but not while sleeping, should be suspected of having what condition?

Congenital intrathoracic tracheomalacia or ***bronchomalacia***. In these infants, the underlying weakness of the airways may not be evident in the newborn period, but it becomes manifest later when the larger infant is able to generate greater expiratory pressure during periods of activity. This increased intrathoracic pressure results in airway collapse. Fluoroscopy or bronchoscopy will confirm the diagnosis.

78. Which clinical features are suggestive of foreign-body aspiration?

Symptoms and history
- Child < 4 years old
- Boys twice as common as girls
- Coughing
- Hemoptysis
- Respiratory infection not resolving with treatment
- History of choking
- Difficulty in breathing

Signs
- Fixed, localized wheeze
- Generalized wheezing in child with no prior history of asthma
- Reduced breath sounds over one lung, one lobe, or one segment
- Mediastinal shift
- One nipple higher than other
- Stridor

79. Are chest x-rays useful in evaluating a foreign-body aspiration?

Unfortunately, only about *10–15%* of aspirated foreign bodies are radiopaque. Thus, inspiratory films are often normal. Features suggesting a foreign-body aspiration are:
- Expiratory chest x-ray showing asymmetry in lung aeration due to obstructive emphysema (the foreign body often acts as a ball-valve mechanism, allowing air in but not out)
- Decubitus films that show the same asymmetry (these views are often used in uncooperative children who cannot or will not exhale on command)
- Obstructive atelectasis

80. What characterizes the acute respiratory distress syndrome (ARDS)?

This entity was previously known as the *adult* respiratory distress syndrome, but it is a significant cause of morbidity in critically ill children. Most typically, a patient with previously normal lungs has an acute insult with subsequent deterioration in pulmonary function characterized by:

- Hypoxemia with a PaO_2/FiO_2 ratio less than 200 regardless of positive end-expiratory pressure (PEEP) administered
- Bilateral densities on the chest radiograph
- No clinical evidence of left atrial hypertension and/or a pulmonary artery wedge occlusion pressure <18 mm Hg

Redding GJ: ARDS in the pediatric patient. In: Chernick V, Boat TF, Kendig EL (eds): Disorders of the Respiratory Tract in Children. Philadelphia, W.B. Saunders, 1998, p 641.

81. In what settings can children develop ARDS?

Direct pulmonary injury

- Smoke or chemical inhalation
- Gastric aspiration
- Near-drowning
- Fat embolism
- Trauma
- Infection

Indirect pulmonary injury

- Septic or hypovolemic shock
- Burns
- Multiple trauma
- Pancreatitis
- Drug overdoses (e.g., aspirin, barbiturates, tricyclic antidepressants)

82. Is surfactant an efficacious therapy in ARDS?

An important clinical manifestation of ARDS is stiff lungs due to surfactant deficiency. The protein leak into the lungs of patients with ARDS inhibits the normal function of surfactant, with a resulting increase in surface tension of the alveolar air-liquid interface. This inhibition can be overcome by providing exogenous surfactant proteins and phospholipid. So far, only limited data address the role of surfactant in the clinical management of ARDS. Anecdotal reports of individuals treated with large doses of surfactant show a positive response in lung compliance and oxygenation. One potential drawback is the high cost of the large doses that would be required.

Paulson TE, et al: New concepts in the treatment of children with acute respiratory distress syndrome. J Pediatr 127:163-175, 1995.

83. What four types of disease can be produced by pulmonary aspergillosis?

Aspergillus fumigatus is a mold that produces four different types of disease in humans:

1. ***Invasive*** infection in ***immunocompromised*** hosts (e.g., chronic granulomatous disease, T-cell deficiencies, chemotherapy patients).

2. ***Allergic*** disease–sensitized individuals with ***asthma*** may simply react to *A. fumigatus* as an allergen in the same way that they might react to ragweed.

3. ***Mycetoma***: the mold fills an old cavity in the lung (e.g., tuberculosis).

4. ***Allergic bronchopulmonary aspergillosis***. This is a hypersensitivity response to saprophytic colonization of diseased airways. A significant component of the disease is produced by the immune response to *A. fumigatus* and not by the organism itself. This disease tends to affect children with abnormal airways, especially those with cystic fibrosis. In adults, it is usually associated with asthma, but this association is uncommon in childhood.

84. List the characteristic features of allergic bronchopulmonary aspergillosis.

- Hyphae in the sputum
- Sputum eosinophilia
- Peripheral blood eosinophilia
- Increased serum IgE
- Positive IgE antibody test (RAST)
- Positive serum precipitins
- Positive immediate and delayed skin tests
- Transient infiltrates on chest x-ray
- Proximal, cylindrical bronchiectasis

85. When should bronchiolitis obliterans be suspected?

Bronchiolitis obliterans is a condition of diffuse fibrosis and scarring of the bronchioles and alveolar ducts following a lower respiratory insult (e.g., infection, aspiration, toxic inhalation). It has also been associated with connective tissue diseases and transplantation, but many times a cause is not determined. The diagnosis should be suspected in patients with prolonged respiratory symptoms (including exercise intolerance) or auscultatory findings following infection. Often, the radiographic findings are disproportionately minor compared with the severity of respiratory impairment and clinical findings. In some cases, a unilateral hyperlucent lung is noted (Swyer-James syndrome).

86. What are the possible mechanisms for the development of lung abscesses in children?

- ***Following pneumonia***, particularly *Staphylococcus aureus, Haemophilus influenzae, Streptococcus pneumoniae*, and *Klebsiella pneumoniae*
- ***Hematogenous*** spread, especially if an indwelling central catheter or right-sided endocarditis is present
- ***Direct extension*** from a liver abscess or rib osteomyelitis
- Penetrating ***trauma***
- ***Aspiration***, especially in neurologically compromised patients
- Secondary to ***infection*** of an underlying pulmonary ***anomaly***, such as a bronchogenic cyst

Campbell PW: Lung abscess. In: Hilman BC (ed): Pediatric Respiratory Disease. Philadelphia, W.B. Saunders, 1993, pp 257-262.

87. What are the typical clinical findings in bronchiectasis?

Bronchiectasis is the progressive dilation and possible eventual destruction of bronchi most likely from acute and/or recurrent obstruction and infection. It may result from a variety of infections (e.g., adenoviral, rubeola, pertussis, tuberculosis) and is often associated with underlying pulmonary susceptibility (e.g., cystic fibrosis, ciliary dyskinesia syndromes, immunodeficiencies). Clinical findings can be variable but usually include persistent cough, production of purulent sputum, recurrent fevers, and digital clubbing. Inspiratory crackles and coarsening of breath sounds are often heard over the affected area. Hemoptysis and wheezing can occur but are uncommon.

88. What are the most common finding in childhood sarcoidosis?

The findings in childhood sarcoidosis vary with age of presentation. Children younger than 4 years of age tend to present with a triad of rash, uveitis, and arthritis that may be confused with juvenile rheumatoid arthritis. Older children present similarly to adults. Weight loss, dry cough, and fatigue are the most common symptoms. Lymphadenopathy, eye, and skin changes are the most common signs. An ***abnormal chest radiograph*** is present from 60 to 90% of the time with ***hilar adenopathy*** the most common finding.

89. A novice teenage mountain-climber develops headache, marked cough, and orthopnea at the end of a rapid, second-day climb. What is the likely diagnosis?

Acute mountain sickness with high-altitude pulmonary edema. This condition results from insufficient time to adapt to altitude changes with resultant alveolar and tissue hypoxia, increased pulmonary vascular permeability, and possible pulmonary hypertension. In severe cases, cerebral edema can result. Treatment consists of returning to lower altitude, administration of oxygen, and use of medications to lessen cerebral edema (e.g., diuretics, acetazolamide, corticosteroids). Unfortunately, the effectiveness of these medications is highly variable.

Dumont L: Efficacy and harm of pharmacological prevention of acute mountain sickness: Quantitative systematic review. BMJ 321:267-272, 2000.

90. What are the two forms of pulmonary sequestration?

Pulmonary sequestration is a portion of lung tissue that has become isolated from the rest of the lung during morphogenesis and has a systemic blood supply without the normal connections to the airways and pulmonary circulation. There are two forms: ***Intrapulmonary*** sequestrations, which are the more common, often become infected and may be discovered during evaluation for recurrent pneumonia.

Extrapulmonary sequestrations, which are separated from the lung by a pleural reflection, are often asymptomatic but may come to light because of associated congenital malformations such as diaphragmatic hernia.

91. What is the likely diagnosis in a child with diffuse lung disease, microcytic anemia, and sputum containing hemosiderin-laden macrophages?

Pulmonary hemosiderosis. This condition, which can present with chronic respiratory problems or acute hemoptysis, is characterized by alveolar hemorrhage and microcytic hypochromic anemia with a low serum iron level. Hemosiderin ingested by alveolar macrophages can often be detected in sputum or gastric aspirates after staining with Prussian blue. Most commonly, the condition is idiopathic and isolated, but it can be associated with cow's milk hypersensitivity (Heiner syndrome), glomerulonephritis with basement membrane antibodies (Goodpasture syndrome), collagen vascular disease, or pancreatitis.

92. How should a child with a spontaneous pneumothorax be managed?

If the pneumothorax is *small* and the child *asymptomatic*, observation alone is appropriate. Administration of 100% oxygen may speed resorption of the free air, but this technique is less effective in older age groups. If the pneumothorax is > *20%* [as measured by the (diameter of pneumothorax)^3/(diameter of hemithorax)^3] and/or the patient has *evolving respiratory symptoms*, insertion of a thoracotomy tube and application of negative pressure should be considered. Signs of *tension* pneumothorax (e.g., marked dyspnea, tachypnea and tachycardia, unilateral thoracic hyperresonance with negligible breath sounds, tracheal shift) necessitate emergent aspiration and tube placement. Of note, children and adolescents with spontaneous pneumothoraces have a high recurrence rate because of the common association with subpleural blebs. Many authorities recommend chest CT with contrast as a follow-up, because significant blebs can be treated with surgical pleurodesis.

93. In children with pleural effusions, how are exudates distinguished from transudates?

The identification of transudates or exudates is determined by analyzing the levels of protein and lactate dehydrogenase (LDH) in the pleural fluid and the serum. Exudative pleural effusions meet a least one of the following criteria:

- Pleural fluid protein/serum protein ratio >0.5
- Pleural fluid LDH/serum LDH >0.6
- Pleural fluid LDH >2/3 of the upper normal limit for serum

If none of these criteria are met, then the patient has a transudative pleural effusion.

94. What pediatric diseases are associated with exudative and transudative pleural effusions?

Exudative	*Transudative*
• Pneumonia	• Congestive heart failure
• Tuberculosis	• Cirrhosis
• Malignancy	• Nephrotic syndrome
• Chylothorax	• Upper airway obstruction

In children, the most common cause for a pleural effusion is pneumonia ("parapneumonic") while, in adults, the most common etiology is congestive heart failure.

95. What are the most common infectious agents associated with an empyema?

An *empyema* is a term that is not specific for the lung, and it is Greek for "pus in a cavity." In the pleural cavity, an empyema develops when pneumonia progresses and the infectious agent and the inflammation spread from the lung into the pleural space. In developed countries, *Streptococcus pneumoniae* is the most common cause for an empyema with group A strep, *Staphylococcus aureus* and *Haemophilus influenzae* occasionally reported. It is important to note that while pleural effusions are seen commonly in pediatric pneumonias, most parapneumonic effusions are *not* empyemas. Empyemas occur in less than 2% of pediatric pneumonias.

96. What is the value of chest physiotherapy in pediatric pulmonary disease?

The main function of chest PT is to assist in the removal of tracheobronchial secretions in order to lessen obstruction, reduce airway resistance, enhance gas exchange and reduce the work of breathing. Its use has been advocated in disorders of chronic sputum production (e.g. cystic fibrosis), primary pneumonia, bronchiolitis, asthma, atelectasis, intubated neonate, postextubation, and postoperatively. Clinical benefits in each category, with the exception of diseases of chronic sputum production, remain highly anecdotal and understudied. Limited evidence does not support a role in bronchiolitis and asthma.

Prasad SA, et al: Physiotherapy in cystic fibrosis. J Roy Soc Med 93S: 37-39, 2000.

Wallis C, Prasad A: Who needs chest physiotherapy? Moving from anecdote to evidence. Arch Dis Child 80:393-397, 1999.

97. Who was Ondine, and what was her curse?

Ondine was a legendary water nymph who fell in love with Hans, a mortal, and put a curse on him that, should he ever betray her, he would suffocate by not breathing when he fell asleep. Unfortunately, Hans fell for the greater charms of Bertha, and he eventually succumbed while dozing. The term Ondine curse has been used to describe the syndrome of sleep apnea secondary to reduced respiratory drive, although the term central hypoventilation syndrome (CHS) is used more commonly. This rare condition is often associated with other abnormalities of brainstem function. CHS can be idiopathic or a complication of an earlier insult to the developing brain. In some families, it is genetic. Children with CHS are treated by tracheostomy and mechanical ventilation during sleep. Recent results with phrenic nerve pacing have been good.

CYSTIC FIBROSIS

98. How has the survival rate for CF changed since the 1960s?

In 1969, the median survival for patients with CF in the U.S. was age 14 years. By 1999, the rate had increased to 29.1 years (95% confidence interval 27.5–31.6 yr).

99. What is the importance of the CFTR protein in cystic fibrosis (CF)?

Cystic fibrosis transmembrane conductance regulator (CFTR) protein is a key ion channel that regulates chloride and sodium transfer across the apical membrane of epithelial cells. In CF patients, chloride is poorly secreted, and there is increased absorption of sodium from the luminal surface of the airway or duct, resulting in respiratory and pancreatic secretions that are relatively dehydrated and viscid. These hyperviscous secretions obstruct pancreatic ducts and interfere with pulmonary mucociliary clearance, resulting in steatorrhoea from exocrine pancreatic insufficiency and chronic respiratory disease.

100. What is the incidence of cystic fibrosis in various ethnic groups?

Whites	1:3,300 live births
Hispanic	1:9,500 live births

Native Americans (U.S.)	1:11,200 live births
Blacks (U.S.)	1:15,300 live births
Asians	1:32,100 live births

North American CF Registry, Cystic Fibrosis Foundation, Bethesda, Maryland, 1996.

101. List the indications for sweat testing.

Pulmonary/Upper Respiratory	*Gastrointestinal*	*Metabolic/Other*
Atelectasis, chronic/recurrent (especially RUL)	Cirrhosis and portal hypertension	Acrodermatitis enteropathica
Bronchiectasis	Intestinal atresia	Aspermia/absent vas deferens
Bronchiolitis, chronic/recurrent	Meconium ileus	Edema, hypoproteinemia
Chronic cough	Meconium plug syndrome	Failure to thrive
Digital clubbing	Mucoid-impacted appendix	Hypoprothrombinemia beyond newborn period
Hemoptysis	Recurrent intussusception	Metabolic alkalosis, hypochloremia
Mucoid *Pseudomonas* colonization	Recurrent pancreatitis	Positive family history
Nasal polyps	Rectal prolapse	Salt depletion syndrome
Pansinusitis	Steatorrhea, malabsorption	Salty taste/salt crystals
Pneumonia, chronic/recurrent		Vitamin A deficiency (bulging fontanel)

Adapted from Rosenstein BJ: Cystic fibrosis. In: Loughlin GM, Eigen H (eds): Respiratory Disease in Children. Baltimore, Williams & Wilkins, 1994, p 275; with permission.

102. What constitutes an abnormal sweat test?

Sweat gland secretions should be obtained by pilocarpine iontophoresis. A level of sweat chloride **> *60 mEq/L*** is *abnormal*, ***40-60 mEq/L*** is *borderline*, and **< *40 mEq/L*** is *normal*.

103. What is the pathophysiology of rectal prolapse in CF?

Rectal prolapse is a common complication of CF—up to 20% of patients may be affected. Possible explanations include:

- Poor nutrition with weakened connective tissue supporting structures
- Chronic coughing increases intra-abdominal pressure
- Abnormal bowel movements (increased volume of stools with abnormal consistency)
- Redundant colonic mucosa

104. Explain the mechanisms of action of amiloride, recombinant human DNase, and alpha1-antitrypsin in the treatment of CF.

1. *Amiloride* is a sodium channel blocker that was shown to decrease sputum viscosity in patients with CF and delay the rate of respiratory deterioration in a pilot study. The use of medications that alter electrolyte transport at the membrane level is a major focus of current research, although amiloride itself was not sufficiently effective in a double-blind placebo-controlled follow-up trial to be an active candidate for a therapeutic role.

2. The sputum of patients with CF has a very high DNA content due to degenerating host neutrophils, and this contributes greatly to its increased viscosity. Aerosolized *recombinant DNase* (Dornase alpha) degrades this DNA, reduces viscosity, and has proven beneficial in clinical trials.

3. Recurrent pulmonary infections with marked neutrophil accumulation lead to lysosomal release of hydrolytic enzymes, such as elastase, often in excess of natural inhibitors such as α1-*antitrypsin*. This imbalance can lead to airway destruction and bronchiectasis. Aerosolized treatment with α1-antitrypsin or other antiproteases may lessen the damage.

Zeitlin PL: Future pharmacological treatment of cystic fibrosis. Respiration 67:351-351, 2000.

105. How is hemoptysis managed in CF?

Minor to moderate bleeding (< 1 to 6 oz blood/24 hrs)

- See the patient if hemoptysis represents a new problem.
- Consider coagulation studies, hemoglobin, and sputum culture.
- Start antibiotics if the patient has infection.
- Stop medications which can exacerbate bleeding (e.g., aspirin, Mucomyst, nonsteroidal anti-inflammatory agents).
- Stop percussion temporarily and substitute vibration and postural drainage. (The need to stop percussion is of some debate.)

Major bleeding (> 6 oz blood/24 hrs)

- All of the above.
- Admit to hospital.
- IV antibiotics (avoid ones which cause platelet dysfunction such as ticarcillin)
- Transfuse if necessary.
- Consider vitamin K even if coagulation studies are normal.
- Consider IV premarin or pitressin.
- Consider bronchoscopy to define bleeding site.
- Consider embolization of bronchial artery or partial pneumonectomy.

106. How are recurrent pneumothoraces in CF managed?

Medical treatment includes chemical pleurodesis with intrapleural instillation of tetracycline or quinacrine. Surgical treatment includes parietal pleurectomy (also known as pleural stripping) or pleural abrasion with dry gauze/abrasive pads. The morbidity and efficacy of medical and surgical therapy appear to be similar. Thoracoscopic evaluation and talc pleurodesis are a growing trend in adult pulmonology that may have application in the treatment of CF.

107. What are the complications of pediatric lung transplantation?

Mortality in the early post-transplant period is associated mostly with acute pulmonary rejection, perioperative hemorrhage, infection, and multisystem organ failure. After the first three months, morbidity and mortality are due principally to obliterative bronchiolitis. Another complication is tracheal stenosis at the anastomotic site, which is sometimes associated with generalized bronchomalacia that may proceed to obliterative bronchiolitis. The side effects of immunosuppressants sometimes create difficulties, and diabetes mellitus may be precipitated by the use of steroids. With longer use of immunosuppressants, there is concern about the increased incidence of lymphoma and other malignancies related to Epstein-Barr virus and and post-transplant lymphoproliferative disorder (PTLD).

108. Which features of CF have prognostic significance?

• ***Gender***. Males have better survival rates than females, although the gap is narrowing.

• ***Colonization with virulent bacteria***. *Pseudomonas aeruginosa* and *Burkholderia* (formerly *Pseudomonas*) *cepacia* are more serious pathogens, which are often multi-resistant and difficult to clear once the patient is persistently infected. *Stenotrophomonas mualtophilia* also appears to be an emerging problem. Patients who are chronically colonized with these organisms have significantly poorer survival rates than other patients with CF.

• ***Nasal polyps*** appear to be a positive prognostic indicator. Patients with polyps appear to have milder pulmonary disease. This is a surprising observation with no obvious explanation.

• ***Cor pulmonale*** is one of the late complications of CF because progressive obstructive airway disease leads to the development of pulmonary hypertension and respiratory failure. The prognosis after developing cor pulmonale is poor.

• ***Pneumothorax*** is associated with moderate to advanced lung disease in patients with CF. Therefore, air leak has traditionally been regarded as a poor prognostic sign. The prognosis has been improving now that pneumothoraces are being managed aggressively.

• ***Worsening pulmonary function tests***. Patients with an FEV_1 < 30% of predicted have an increased 2-year mortality rate.

109. What are the barriers to widespread screening for CF?

The CFTR gene was identified in 1989 on the long arm of chromosome 7. Although the most common mutation was found to be a deletion of phenylalanine at position 508 (delta F508), this mutation accounts for only 75% of the total mutations. More than 900 mutations to date have been identified. Although the more common mutations could be included in screening, the potential for false-negative testing is significant. The largest barrier to screening is the lack of data demonstrating improved clinical outcomes in patients identified by screening.

PNEUMONIA

110. What agents cause pneumonia in children?

The etiology of community-acquired pneumonia in pediatrics is highly dependent on the *age* of the child. Most studies cannot determine an etiology in about 50% of patients. Determining an infective organism can be very difficult, especially in younger children. From the newborn period to three months of age, group B streptococcus, gram-negative bacilli, *Chlamydia trachomatis* and *Ureaplasma urealyticum* are common as well as RSV and other viruses. For children over three months of age, the table below summarizes two recent prospective studies that examined the etiology of community-acquired pneumonia by culture and serology in largely outpatient populations.

	3 mos.-5 yrs.	*5-10 yrs.*	*10-15 yrs.*
Bacterial	33%	30%	31%
Viral	33%	16%	3%
Mycoplasma pneumoniae	5%	19%	40%
Chlamydia pneumoniae	2%	8%	26%

111. What are the important trends in the etiology of infectious pneumonia?

Three important trends are evident:

1. A bacterial etiology remains prevalent in all three age groups studied and does not change from infancy to adolescence. The most common bacterial etiology after three months of age is *Streptococcus pneumoniae*.
2. A viral etiology is more common in younger age groups, and it is most commonly RSV. Viruses can be associated with pneumonia in school-age children but become less common with age. In older children, influenza is one of the more common etiologies, especially during epidemics.
3. "Atypical pneumoniae" caused by *Mycoplasma pneumoniae* and *Chlamydia pneumoniae* are uncommon in preschool children. Both mycoplasma and chlamydia become more prevalent in school-age children and are the most common etiology for pneumonia in the older child.

Wubbel L, et al.: Etiology and treatment of community-acquired pneumonia in ambulatory children. Pediatr Infect Dis J 18:98-104, 1999.

Heiskanen-Kosma T, et al.: Etiology of childhood pneumonia: Serologic results of a prospective, population-based study. Pediatr Infect Dis J 17:986-991,1998.

112. Are throat or nasopharyngeal cultures helpful in the diagnosis of pneumonia?

As a rule, the correlation between throat and nasopharyngeal bacterial cultures and lower respiratory tract pathogens is poor and of limited value. Healthy children may be colonized with a wide variety of potentially pathologic bacteria (e.g., *Staphylococcus aureus, Haemophilus influenzae*) which can be considered part of the normal flora. *Bordetella pertussis* is an exception. Cultures or antigen detection systems to identify respiratory viruses or chlamydia, however, are highly informative, because these organisms are rarely carried asymptomatically.

113. How often are blood cultures positive in children with suspected bacterial pneumonia?

10% or less. This number is an estimate because the true denominator in the equation (the number of true bacterial pneumonias) is difficult to ascertain due to the difficulty in making a definitive diagnosis. The low rate of positive blood cultures does suggest that most bacterial pneumonias are not acquired through hematogenous spread.

114. How often are pleural fluid cultures positive in children with suspected bacterial pneumonia?

60-85% are positive if antibiotics have not already been initiated. This high yield emphasizes the importance of recognizing a pleural effusion in patients with pneumonia and the value of early thoracentesis before starting antibiotic therapy.

115. How common is an occult pneumonia in a febrile child with leukocytosis?

In a search for a focus of infection, the chest is always a suspect. In a study of children less than age 5 years without clinical evidence of pneumonia but a temperature ≥39°C and a total WBC of ≥ 20,000, a CXR was positive in 19%.

Bachur R, et al: Occult pneumonia in febrile children with leukocytosis. Ann Emerg Med 33:166-173, 1999.

116. Can a chest x-ray reliably distinguish between viral and bacterial pneumonia?

No. Although viral infections more commonly have perihilar, peribronchial, or interstitial infiltrates, hyperinflation, segmental atelectasis, and hilar adenopathy, there can be considerable overlap with bacterial (and chlamydial and mycoplasmal) pneumonia. Bacterial pneumonia more commonly results in an alveolar infiltrate, but the sensitivity and specificity of this finding are not very high.

Swingler GH, et al: Radiologic differentiation between bacterial and viral lower respiratory infection in children: A systematic literature review. Clin Pediatr 39:627-633, 2000.

Donnelly LF: Maximizing the usefulness of imaging in children with community-acquired pneumonia. Am J Roentgenol 172:505-512, 1999.

117. Which children with pneumonia should be hospitalized?

This question becomes more difficult to answer all the time. Prospective studies in children are nonexistent. Thus, this becomes a matter of clinical judgement based on recommendations colored by previous bad experiences. Features that strongly suggest a need for hospitalization include:

- All who appear *toxic*, *dyspneic*, or *hypoxic*
- Suspected *staphylococcal* pneumonia (e.g., pneumatocele on chest x-ray)
- Significant pleural *effusion*
- Suspected *aspiration* pneumonia (because of the higher likelihood of progression)
- Children who *cannot tolerate oral medications* or who are at significant risk for *dehydration*
- Suspected bacterial pneumonia in *very young* infants, especially with *multilobar* involvement
- *Poor response* to outpatient therapy after *48 hours*
- Those whose family situation is *unsupportive*

118. What clinical clues suggest atypical pneumonia?

These infections tend to start gradually, have minimal or a nonproductive cough, and have frequent constitutional signs such as headache, rash, or pharyngitis. Chest radiographs tend to show patchy, peribronchial infiltrates with only occasional lobar consolidation.

119. What are the causes of "afebrile infant pneumonia" syndrome?

The syndrome is usually due to *Chlamydia trachomatis*, CMV, *Ureaplasma urealyticum*, or *Mycoplasma hominis*. Affected infants develop progressive respiratory distress over several days to a few weeks, along with failure to thrive. A maternal history of a sexually transmitted disease is common. Chest x-rays reveal bilateral diffuse infiltrates with hyperinflation. There may be eosinophilia and elevated quantitative immunoglobulins (IgG, IgA, IgM). The causes overlap clinically, although a history of conjunctivitis suggests chlamydia.

120. How likely is an infant to develop infection if born to a mother with positive cervical cultures for *Chlamydia trachomatis*?

Up to ***50%*** of infants demonstrate an ***inclusion conjunctivitis***, and ***5-20%*** develop ***pneumonia***. Prevalence of the organism in pregnant women varies from 6-12% but can be as low as 2% or as high as 37% in adolescents. Up to 30,000 infants annually may develop chlamydial pneumonia, making it the most common cause of pneumonia in children under 6 months of age.

121. What are the clinical characteristics of chlamydial pneumonia in infants?

- Illness occurs between *2 and 19 weeks* after birth. Most infants present by 8 weeks of age.
- Onset is *gradual* with upper respiratory prodromal symptoms lasting > 1 week.
- Nearly 100% are *afebrile.*
- Less than half have *inclusion conjunctivitis.*
- Respiratory signs and symptoms: staccato cough, tachypnea, diffuse crackles, little wheezing.
- Chest x-ray: bilateral hyperexpansion, symmetric interstitial infiltrates
- 70% have an *elevated absolute eosinophil count* (> 400/mm^3).
- Over 90% have *elevated quantitative immunoglobulins* (IgG, IgM).

122. What is the best method for diagnosing chlamydial pneumonia?

Definitive diagnosis can be made by isolating the organism in tissue culture. Because chlamydia are obligate intracellular organisms, culture specimens must contain epithelial cells, not just exudate. Nucleic acid amplification methods, e.g. PCR, are more sensitive than cell culture and more specific and sensitive than DNA probe, direct fluorescent antibody (DFA) tests, or enzyme immunoassays (EIAs). PCR is useful for evaluating conjunctival specimens from infants, but has not been evaluated adequately for detection of *C. trachomatis* in nasopharyngeal specimens. Positive DFA, EIA, or DNA probe tests should be verified. Confirmation can be accomplished by culture, a second nonculture test different from the first test, or use of a blocking antibody or competitive probe. Serum antibody determinations are difficult to perform and available in only a few clinical laboratories.

123. What is the most common auscultatory finding in mycoplasmal pneumonia?

Fine crackles (80%), which may persist for 2 weeks or more along with cough and sputum production. Wheezing is heard in < 50% of patients.

124. How characteristic is the radiologic picture of mycoplasmal pneumonia?

The chest x-ray is variable and nonspecific. Most findings are unilateral (up to 85%) and occur in the lower lobes. Early in the course of illness, the picture is one of increased interstitial markings with a reticulonodular pattern. Frequently, this progresses to patchy, segmental, or even lobar areas of consolidation. Hilar adenopathy occurs in up to one-third of patients. Pleural effusions, as demonstrated by lateral decubitus views, may occur in up to 20% of children.

125. How helpful are cold agglutinins in the diagnosis of *Mycoplasma pneumoniae* infections?

Cold agglutinins are IgM autoantibodies that agglutinate red cells at 4°C by reacting with the I antigen. Up to 75% of patients with mycoplasmal infections will develop them, usually toward the end of the first week of illness with a peak at 4 weeks. A titer of 1:64 supports the diagnosis. Other infectious agents, including adenovirus, cytomegalovirus, Epstein-Barr virus, influenza, rubella, *Chlamydia*, and *Listeria*, can also give a positive result. A single cold agglutinin titer of 1:64 is therefore suggestive but not conclusive evidence of infection with *M. pneumoniae*.

126. How is the bedside test for cold agglutinins done?

In a tube containing sodium citrate, blood of equal volume (usually about 4-5 drops) is added. The tube is immersed in ice for 30-60 seconds, and the fluid is observed by rolling the tube on its side. Coarsely flocculating red blood cells constitute a positive test, which correlates with a cold agglutinin titer of 1:64.

127. When do the radiologic findings with pneumonia resolve?

Although there is a wide range, as a rule, most infiltrates due to *Streptococcus pneumoniae* resolve in 6-8 weeks and those due to RSV in 2-3 weeks. However, with some viral infections (e.g., adenovirus), it may take up to 1 year for x-rays to normalize. Unfortunately, in most instances, the underlying etiology is not known. If significant radiologic abnormalities persist > 6 weeks, there should be a high index of suspicion for a possible underlying problem (e.g., unusual infection, anatomic abnormality, immunologic deficiency).

Regelmann WE: Diagnosing the cause of recurrent and persistent pneumonia in children. Pediatr Ann 22:561-568, 1993.

128. Do children with pneumonia need follow-up x-rays to verify resolution?

Generally, no. The exceptions would include children with pleural effusions, those with persistent or recurrent signs and symptoms, and those with significant comorbid conditions such as immunodeficiencies.

129. What factors can contribute to recurrent pneumonia?

- ***Aspiration susceptibility*** (oropharyngeal incoordination, vocal cord paralysis, and gastroesophageal reflux)
- ***Immunodeficiency*** (congenital and acquired)
- ***Congenital cardiac defects*** (ASD, VSD, PDA)
- ***Abnormal secretions*** or ***reduced clearance of secretions*** (asthma, cystic fibrosis, ciliary dyskinesia
- ***Pulmonary anomalies*** (sequestration, cystic adenomatoid malformation, tracheoesophageal fistula, tracheal stenosis)
- ***Airway compression*** or ***obstruction*** (foreign body, vascular ring, enlarged lymph node, malignancy)
- ***Miscellaneous*** (e.g., sickle cell disease, sarcoidosis)

Owayed AF, et al: Underlying causes of recurrent pneumonia in children. Arch Pediatr Adolesc Med 154:190-194, 2000.

130. How does the pH of a substance affect the severity of disease in aspiration pneumonia?

A ***low pH is more harmful*** than a slightly alkaline or neutral pH and is more likely to be associated with bronchospasm and pneumonia. The most severe form of pneumonia is seen when gastric contents are aspirated; symptoms may develop in a matter of seconds. If the volume of aspirate is sufficiently large and the pH is < 2.5, the mortality may exceed 70%. The radiographic picture may be that of an infiltrate or pulmonary edema. Unilateral pulmonary edema may occur if the child is lying on one side.

131. How should children with aspiration pneumonia be managed?

Acute aspiration can often be treated supportively without antibiotics because the initial process is a chemical pneumonitis. If secondary signs of infection occur, then antibiotics should be started after appropriate cultures. For community-acquired pneumonia, either penicillin or clindamycin is a reasonable choice to cover anaerobes which predominate. If the aspiration is nosocomial, then antibiotic coverage should be extended to include gram-negative organisms as well.

PULMONARY PRINCIPLES

132. In addition to underlying immunologic immaturity, why are infants more susceptible to an increased severity of respiratory disease?

- Very compliant chest wall (allows passage through birth canal, but limits inspiratory effort)
- Respiratory muscles more easily fatigued due to decreased muscle mass
- Chest wall elastic recoil is low in infancy (airway closure occurs at a higher relative lung volume)
- High airway compliance facilitates airway collapse and air trapping
- Collateral ventilation poorly developed, increasing likelihood of atelectasis during illness
- Higher airway mucous gland concentration in infants than adults

133. At what age do alveoli stop increasing in number?

Although extraacinar airway development is complete by 16 weeks of gestation, alveolar multiplication continues after birth. Early studies suggested that postnatal alveolar multiplication ends at 8 years of age. However, more recent studies have shown that it is terminated by 2 years of age, possibly between 1 and 2 years of age. After the end of alveolar multiplication, the alveoli continue to increase in size until thoracic growth is completed.

134. What is the normal respiratory rate in a child?

Rates in an awake child can be widely variable depending on the state of anxiety or agitation. Rates while sleeping are much more reliable and are a good indicator of pulmonary health. As a general rule, the sleeping rate in *infants* is usually ***< 35/min***; in *toddlers*, ***< 30/min***; in *older children*, ***< 25/min***; and in *adolescents*, ***< 20/min***. However, fever and metabolic acidosis can lead to an increased respiratory rate in the absence of pulmonary disease.

135. What is normal oxygen saturation in healthy infants less than six months of age?

In a longitudinal study using pulse oximetry, baseline saturation is >95% (normal is 98% with lower 10th percentile at 95.2%). However, acute desaturations are common. Almost all are associated with brief episodes of apnea while sleeping.

Hunt CE et al: Longitudinal assessment of hemoglobin saturation in healthy infants during the first six months of life. J Pediatr 134:580-586, 1999.

136. What is the difference between Kussmaul, Cheyne-Stokes, and Biot types of breathing patterns?

Kussmaul: Deep, slow, regular respirations with prolonged exhalation. Seen in diabetic ketoacidosis.

Cheyne-Stokes: Crescendo-decrescendo respirations alternating with periods of apnea (no breathing). Causes include heart failure, uremia, CNS trauma, increased intracranial pressure, and coma.

Biot: Also known as ataxic breathing. Characterized by unpredictable irregularity. Breaths may be shallow or deep and stop for short periods. Causes include respiratory depression, meningitis, encephalitis, and other central nervous system lesions involving the respiratory centers.

137. Why a sigh?

A sigh is just a sigh in Casablanca, but it is also a very effective anti-atelectatic maneuver. By definition, it is a breath more than three times the tidal volume.

138. Is there a respiratory basis for yawning?

Although a respiratory function for yawning is frequently suggested, scientific support for this belief is minimal. Increasing the concentration of CO_2 in inspired air increases the respiratory rate but does not change the rate of yawning. Relief of hypoxia and opening areas of microatelectasis are other theories that are not supported by scientific studies. Some studies hypothesize that yawning may be an arousal reflex.

139. What are "coarse" breath sounds?

In coarse breath sounds the loudness of expiration equals the loudness of inspiration on auscultation. In large airways, expiratory breath sounds are louder than inspiratory breath sounds due to turbulence. Coarse breath sounds can be physiologic (as when listening just below the center of the clavicle to primarily bronchial sounds) or pathologic (if interposed fluid allows transmission of large airway sounds or if airways are widened such as in bronchiectasis).

140. At what concentration is inspired oxygen toxic?

In addition to atelectasis, high oxygen concentration can cause alveolar injury with edema, inflammation, fibrin deposition, and hyalinization. The precise level of hyperoxia that results in injury is unclear and subject to variance by age and underlying lung pathology, but a reasonable rule is to assume that a concentration of > 80% for > 36 hours is likely to result in significant ongoing damage; 60-80% is likely to be associated with more slowly progressive injury. An inspired oxygen concentration of 50%, even when administered for extended periods of time, is unlikely to cause pulmonary toxicity.

Jenkinson SG: Oxygen toxicity. J Intens Care Med 3:137-152, 1988.

141. Why is a child receiving 100% oxygen more likely to develop atelectasis than one breathing room air?

Nitrogen is more slowly absorbed than oxygen by alveoli. In room air (with its 78% nitrogen), alveolar collapse is minimized by continued presence and pressure of nitrogen gas. In 100% oxygen, however, the more rapid absorption of oxygen can lead to absorption atelectasis with intrapulmonary shunting.

142. At what PaO_2 does cyanosis develop?

Cyanosis develops when the concentration of desaturated (i.e., reduced) hemoglobin is at least 3 gm/dl centrally or 4-6 gm/dl peripherally. However, multiple factors affect the likelihood that a given PaO_2 will result in clinically apparent cyanosis: anemia (less likely), polycythemia (more likely), reduced systemic perfusion or cardiac output (more likely), and hypothermia (more likely). Cyanosis is generally a sign of significant hypoxia. In a patient with adequate perfusion and a normal hemoglobin, central cyanosis is commonly noted when the PaO_2 is approximately 50 mmHg.

143. How is the A-a gradient calculated?

The *alveolar-arterial oxygen difference* or *gradient* (A-aDO_2) is a measure of the efficiency of gas exchange and can be especially useful in critical care settings to monitor changes in disease severity. It is the difference between the theoretical PO_2 in the alveoli (PAO_2) and the measured oxygen tension (PaO_2) and is calculated according to the following formula:

$$A\text{-}aDO_2 = FiO_2\,(PB - 47) - (PaCO_2/RQ) - PaO_2$$

where PB = barometric pressure, FiO_2 = inspiratory oxygen concentration, 47 = saturated water vapor pressure at 37°C, RQ = respiratory quotient (usually 0.8), and $PaCO_2$ = measured arterial CO_2 tension. The normal A-aDO_2 is usually < 15 mmHg, rising up to 30 mmHg in older adults. Of note, in a healthy individual breathing 100% oxygen, the A-aDO_2 increases significantly (up to 100 mmHg) for reasons that are not fully understood but that probably reflect oxygen toxicity.

144. What are the causes of a reduced PaO_2 associated with an increased A-aDO_2?

- ***Right-to-left shunting***: intracardiac, abnormal arteriovenous connections; intrapulmonary shunts which result from perfusion of airless alveoli (e.g., pneumonia, atelectasis), often referred to as ventilation-perfusion mismatching
- ***Maldistribution of ventilation***: as in asthma, bronchiolitis, atelectasis
- ***Impaired diffusion***: an uncommon mechanism, as many of the conditions previously thought to have a "diffusion block," such as respiratory distress syndrome, also have a major component of shunting; may be seen when interstitial edema affects the septal walls (e.g., in early pulmonary edema and interstitial pneumonia)
- ***Decreased central venous oxygen content***: secondary to a sluggish circulation (e.g., shock) or increased tissue oxygen demands (e.g., sepsis)

145. What are the causes of a reduced PaO_2 associated with a normal A-a DO_2?

- Breathing hypoxic gas mixtures
- High altitude
- Hypoventilation (e.g., narcotic overdose, neuromuscular disease)

146. How does the pulse oximeter work?

The key principle behind pulse oximetry is that oxygenated hemoglobin allows more transmission of red light than does reduced hemoglobin. In contrast, transmission of infrared light is unaffected by the amount of oxyhemoglobin present. A light source of red and infrared wavelengths is applied to an area of the body thin enough that the light can transverse a pulsating capillary bed and be detected by a light detector on the other side. Each pulsation increases the distance the light has to travel, which increases the amount of light absorption. A microprocessor derives the arterial oxygen saturation by comparing absorbencies at baseline and during the peak of a transmitted pulse.

147. What are the disadvantages or limitations of pulse oximetry?

- Patient movement disturbs measurements
- Poor perfusion states affect accuracy

- Fluorescent or high-intensity light or sunlight can interfere with results
- Unreliable if abnormal hemoglobins present (e.g., methemoglobin)
- Unable to detect hypoxia until the PaO_2 decreases below 80 mmHg
- Accuracy diminishes with arterial saturations below 70-80%

148. What are the advantages of rigid versus flexible bronchoscopy in children?

Flexible

- No requirement for general anesthesia; may be done with sedation and topical anesthetics
- Possible to examine more distal airways
- Assessment of airway dynamics is improved
- Ability to examine airways through an existing endotracheal tube or tracheostomy
- Possible aid to intubation
- Ability to perform guided bronchoalveolar lavage

Rigid

- Easier removal of foreign bodies
- Better airway control, allowing patient to be ventilated through the bronchoscope
- Superior optics
- Better view of posterior airway structures
- Facilitates surgical procedures

149. What symptoms and physical findings would make you suspect a foreign body in the lower airway?

- Asymmetric breath sounds/wheezing
- Persistent cough
- Persistent localized air trapping on chest radiographs

150. Why is the determination of "leak pressure" important in intubated children?

The leak pressure is important to insure that the endotracheal tube chosen is not producing too much pressure at the level of the cricoid cartilage. Tubes that are too tight will have high leak pressures that are above tissue perfusion pressure. Acutely, this pressure predisposes to post-extubation stridor; while chronically, it predisposes to subglottic narrowing. Problems with inter-observer agreement make it difficult to provide absolute numbers, but levels greater than 35 cm H_2O have been associated with airway complications.

DiCarlo JV, Steven JM: Respiratory failure in congenital heart disease. Pediatr Clin North Am 41: 525-542, 1994.

Schwartz RE, Stayer SA, Pasquariello CA: Tracheal tube leak test—is there inter-observer agreement? Can J Anaesth 40:1049-1052, 1993.

151. What features on pulmonary function testing distinguish obstructive from restrictive lung disease?

Obstructive

- Impaired airflow during expiration with decreased flow rates (decreased FEV_1, decreased $FEF_{25-75\%}$).
- FEV_1/FVC ratio is decreased.
- Air trapping with increased residual volume (RV)/total lung capacity (TLC) ratio.

Restrictive

- Decreased FVC and TLC
- Decreased expiratory flow rates; however, the FEV_1/FVC ratio is normal or slightly increased.

152. In infants with unilateral lung disease, should the good lung be up or down?

The ***good*** lung should be ***up***. This is another example of why children are not simply small adults. It is well established that adults with unilateral lung disease treated in a decubitus position will have an increase in oxygen saturation when the good lung is placed down; this occurs because of an increase in ventilation to the dependent lung. Studies have shown that the opposite occurs in infants and children because ventilation is preferentially distributed toward the uppermost lung. This positional redistribution of ventilation seems to change to an adult pattern during the late teenage years.

Davies H, et al: Effect of posture on regional ventilation in children. Pediatr Pulmonol 12:227-232, 1992.

153. Are home vaporizers of proven scientific value for treatment of respiratory tract infections?

Home vaporizers are one of the most frequently prescribed home remedies by grandmothers and physicians alike. One small problem: There are few data to support their utility for most of their currently prescribed indications. First, deposition data show that only 5% of the actively nebulized fluid in a mist tent enters the body. The percentage from a home vaporizer would be significantly less, and most of the mist is trapped in the nasopharynx or GI tract. Thus, vaporizing liquid to help with lower airway secretions is of dubious value. However, warmed mist does help improve nasal patency in adults with colds or allergic rhinitis. In young infants, where respiration is primarily nasal, any improvement in nasal patency during colds is likely to produce some symptomatic relief. With regards to laryngotracheitis, no prospective, placebo-controlled trial evaluating the benefit of mist therapy has ever documented an improvement in obstruction. As always, the benefits from warmed mist need to be weighed against the risk of burns, infections, and mold allergy from improper cleaning of humidifiers. Now, what are the data on chicken soup?

Szilagyi PG: Humidifiers and other symptomatic therapy for children with respiratory tract infections. Pediatr Infect Dis J 10:478-479, 1991.

19. RHEUMATOLOGY

Balu H. Athreya, M.D., Carlos D. Rose, M.D., Andrew Eichenfield, M.D., and Elizabeth Chalom, M.D.

CLINICAL ISSUES

1. What are the common ocular manifestations seen in pediatric rheumatic diseases?

The eyes have it! Eye problems, especially various types of conjunctivitis, uveitis and retinopathy, are common in pediatric rheumuatic diseases. The most well-known is the chronic uveitis of JRA.

Ocular Disease and Rheumatic Syndromes

Conjunctivitis	Kawasaki disease Stevens-Johnson syndrome Reiter syndrome
Keratitis	JRA Lyme disease
Scleritis	RF positive JRA Polychondritis Sjögren syndrome
Uveitis (anterior)—*acute*	Kawasaki disease Spondyloarthropathy
(anterior)—*chronic*	JRA Sarcoid TINU syndrome (see below)
Uveitis (posterior)	Sarcoid Behçet disease
Panuveitis	Sarcoid Toxoplasmosis Behçet disease
Retinal vasculitis	SLE Behcet disease

2. Who knew about TINU?

TINU, as mentioned in the above table, is an acronym for **T**ubular **I**nterstitial **N**ephritis with **U**veitis syndrome. This relatively rare disorder is charecterized by nonspecific illness (e.g., fever, weight loss) followed by signs of interstititial nephritis (e.g., concentration defect, proteinuria and glycosuria). Biopsy of the kidney at this stage shows interstitial infiltration with predominantly T cells. Later progression is to fibrosis. At the earlier stage, evidence of inflammation is present with an elevated sedimentation rate and anemia. The uveitis typically manifests itself when the kidney disease subsides. It is most often an anterior uveitis. The kidney disease has a good prognosis, whereas the eye disease has a tendency for relapse and chronicity.

Vanhaesebrouck P, et al: Acute tubulo-interstitial nephritis and uveitis syndrome. Nephron 40: 418, 1985.

3. What is an ANA profile?

Antinuclear antibody (ANA) is made up of circulating gammaglobulins directed against several known and unknown nuclear proteins. At last count, ANA is directed against at least 33 different proteins. Since it is measured by immunofluorescent technique, it is also called FANA. It is now possible to identify several of the specific antigens against which this antibody is directed by using ELISA, immunodiffusion and immunoelectrophoresis. This is the *ANA profile*.

4. What is the significance of various antibodies included in the ANA profile?

Antibody	*Associated illness*
Anti-double stranded DNA (ds DNA)	SLE
Anti-histone	Drug-induced lupus
Anti Ro (also called anti-SS A)	Sjögren syndrome neonatal lupus
Anti La (also called anti-SS B)	Sjögren syndrome neonatal lupus

5. What is the significance of a positive ANA test?

ANA is a sensitive but non-specific test for the recognition of autoimmune diseases in general, and systemic lupus erythematosus in particular. It is used as a screening diagnostic test when SLE is suspected. In the case of SLE, this has to be followed by a specific test—anti ds DNA antibody—to confirm this diagnosis. ANA is very helpful as a test to determine the prognosis of pauciarticular JRA (pJRA). The risk of future uveitis is over 80% in children with pJRA and positive ANA.

6. A 6-year-old girl with a 2 month history of joint pain (onset following a viral illness) has a normal PE, CBC and ESR, but a positive ANA titer of 1:60. What are some of the possible explanations for this positive ANA?

- Laboratory variation
- Nonspecific response to viral illness
- Pre-clinical state of SLE (*least* likely)
- Normal population frequency
- Other autoimmune/paraneoplastic conditions

Tan EM, et al: Range of antinuclear antibodies in "healthy" individuals. Arthritis Rheum 40:1601, 1997.

7. What distinguishes dermatomyositis and polymyositis in children?

The clinical criteria of Bohan and Peter were developed to aid in diagnosis. A definitive diagnosis of dermatomyositis or polymyositis is made in the presence of 4 criteria:

1. Symmetrical proximal muscle weakness (Gowers sign, etc.)
2. Elevated serum enzymes in muscle (CK, LDH, AST, and/or aldolase)
3. Abnormal EMG (increased insertional activity; bizarre high-frequency discharges)
4. Inflammation and/or necrosis on muscle biopsy
5. Characteristic skin eruption

Presence of the rash distinguishes dermatomyositis from polymyositis. Thus, a child who has the rash and 3 of the other 4 criteria (biopsy is not necessary if you know what the rash looks like) has definite juvenile dermatomyositis and if the rash and 2 criteria are fulfilled, possible dermatomyositis. If there is no rash, there is no dermatomyositis, so definite polymyositis requires a muscle biopsy for diagnosis.

Pachman LM, et al: Juvenile dermatomyositis at diagnosis: Clinical characteristics of 79 children. J Rheumatol 25:1198-1204, 1998.

Bohan A, Peter JB: Polymyositis and dermatomyositis. N Engl J Med 292:344–347, 1975.

8. What are some of the newer tests used in the investigation of suspected dermatomyositis/ polymyositis?

- *MRI* of the proximal or affected muscles. In T2 weighted images, edema of the inflamed muscle is seen as bright signal (white).

- *Myositis-specific antibodies* (MSA). This group includes anti-Jo1, anti-PL 12, anti-P7, anti MI 2 and anti SRP.
- *Myositis- associated antibodies* (MAA). This group includes anti-U1 RNP, anti-U2 RNP, anti- U3 RNP and anti-PM/Scl.
- *vWF (von Willebrand factor) antigen* as evidence of endothelial damage from vascultis
- *Magnetic resonance spectroscopy* (MRS), which measures metabolic changes in the muscle

9. What skin changes are pathognomonic for dermatomyositis?

Gottron patches. They begin as inflammatory papules over the dorsal aspect of interphalangeal joints and extensor aspect of the elbows and knee joints. The papules become violaceous and flat-topped and may coalesce to become patches. Eventually the lesions show atrophic changes and become hypopigmented.

10. What are the other classic cutaneous findings in dermatomyositis in children?

- Periorbital edema and erythema with violaceous color of the upper eyelid (heliotrope rash)
- Rash over the upper chest in the shawl distribution
- Photosensitivity
- Cutaneous vasculitis with ulceration
- Nailfold capillary abnormailities

11. Which infectious agents are known to cause myositis?

Viral: Notably Coxsackie (named after Coxsackie, NY), influenza A and B
Bacterial: *Staphylococcus* and *Yersinia* (causing pyomyositis)
Protozoal: Toxoplasma and trichinosis
Spirochetal: *Borrelia*

12. What are some of the drugs associated with myopathy?

Glucocorticoids, hydroxychloroquine, diuretics, amphotericin B, d-penicillamine, cimetidine, vincristine and clofibrate.

13. Is Raynaud phenomenon a disease?

In 1874 Maurice Raynaud, while still a medical student, described a triad of episodic *pallor*, *cyanosis* and *erythema* following exposure to cold stress. The term ***Raynaud phenomenon*** describes this clinical triad. When this phenomenon is associated with a disease such as scleroderma or lupus, it is called ***Raynaud syndrome***. When the phenomenon is seen as an isolated condition without any other rheumatic disorder, it is called ***Raynaud disease,*** although some patients on long-term follow up may develop a disease (e.g, CREST syndrome, a limited form of systemic sclerosis).

14. What is CREST syndrome?

It is a subset of systemic sclerosis characterized by the following clinical features: ***C****alcinosis*, ***R****aynaud phenomenon*, ***E****sophageal dysmotility*, ***S****clerodactyly,* ***T****elangiectasia*. It is now known that patients with this condition may start with Raynaud phenomenon and develop other features after several years or decades. This variety is now known as limited form of systemic sclerosis and is serologically defined by the presence of anticentromere (kinetochore) antibody.

15. Name the varieties of localized scleroderma.

Localized scleroderma is also called morphea or linear scleroderma depending on the type of lesion and distribution. One proposed classification suggests the name morphea for the entire group of localized scleroderma (i.e., no systemic features) and subdivides it into several categories.

Morphea is a patch (or patches) of plaque-like, hidebound skin, with violaceous border when active. It subsequently hardens and becomes waxy. It is generally a superficial lesion. Depending on the morphology this may be called plaque morphea , guttate morphea, etc. If there are several patches affecting more than two anatomical sites or if individual lesions become confluent it is called generalized morphea. Of note, skin lesions of Lyme disease may mimic morphea and some authors have suggested that certain cases of morphea may be due to *Borrelia burgdorferi*.

Linear scleroderma occurs in bands, involves deeper structures, seen often in the extremities, crossing joint lines but without dermatome distribution.

En coup de sabre is linear slceroderma involving the face and scalp, may involve deeper structures resulting in hemifacial atrophy.

Peterson LS, et al: Classification of morphea (localized scleroderma). Mayo Clinic Proc 70:1068, 1995.

16. Which systems are commonly involved in systemic scleroderma in children?

Systemic scleroderma, also called systemic sclerosis, is charecterized by excess deposition of abnormal collagen and fibrosis of the skin and several internal organs. In children, the most commonly involved organs are the ***GI tract*** (abnormal motility), ***lung*** (interstitial fibrosis), and the ***heart*** (fibrosis and conduction defects). Renal disease is less common in children compared to adults.

17. Which conditions with thickening of the skin can mimic scleroderma?

- Eosinophilic fasciitis
- Vinyl chloride toxicity
- Bleomycin toxicity
- Phenylketonuria
- Graft-versus-host disease
- Werner syndrome
- Scleredema

18. When is a child considered to have hypermobile joints?

There are wide variations in the range of movements of joints. Young children have greater flexibility than older children. Girls have greater range than boys. There may be racial differences also. True hypermobility should be demonstrable in both upper and lower extremities.

Rheumatologists often use Cater-Wilkerson's criteria as modified by Beighton. According to this criteria, the presence of three of the following features suggests true hypermobility:

1. Apposition of the thumb to the flexor aspect of the forearm.
2. Hyperextension of the fingers so that they lie parallel to the dorsum of the forearm.
3. Hyperextension at the elbow of greater than 10 degrees
4. Knee hyperextension of greater then 10 degrees
5. Ability to touch the floor with the heel and palm of the hands from a standing position without flexing the knee.

19. What children can demostrate a Gorlin sign?

Gorlin sign is the ability to touch the tip of the nose with the tongue. It is seen in conditions associated with hypermobility syndromes such as Ehlers-Danlos.

20. Describe the rheumatologic manifestations of parvoviral infection in children.

Although joint symptoms are present in up to 80% of adults with parvovirus B19 infection, these are rare in children. Nocton and colleagues identified 22 children with joint complaints associated with parvoviral infection, 20 of whom had arthritis and 2 had arthralgia. Ten children presented with polyarthralgia/arthritis, and 12 had oligoarticular course (2 with monarticular disease). Larger joints were affected more than small joints, and the knee was the most commonly affected joint. While the duration of symptoms was usually brief, 8 children had persistent symptoms and fulfilled the criteria for juvenile rheumatoid arthritis.

Naides SJ: Rheumatic manifestations of parvo virus 19 infection: Rheum Dis Clinic North Am 24: 375, 1998.

Nocton JJ, et al: Human parvovirus B19–associated arthritis in children. J Pediatr 122:186-190, 1993.

21. In what settings can reactive arthritis occur?

Reactive arthritis in its broadest sense refers to a pattern of arthritis associated with a non-articular infection. By definition, it is an inflammatory arthritis, but a live organism cannot be isolated by culture of synovial fluid or synovial biopsy. A restricted definition of the syndrome includes arthritis following enteric infections (e.g., *Salmonella, Shigella, Yersinia, Campylobacter* and *Giardia*) or genitourinary infections(e.g., chlamydia). Some cases of polyarthritis following gonococcal and meningococcal infections may be reactive in origin, as is polyarthritis associated with mycoplasma and tuberculosis (Poncet disease). Some consider rheumatic fever an example of reactive arthritis . So-called post-streptococcal reactive arthritis is probably rheumatic fever with a new name. Reiter syndrome is a specific syndrome of reactive arthritis defined by the triad of arthritis, urethritis and conjunctivitis. It is often seen following enteritis or non-gonococcal urethritis.

Arthritis is often acute, involving larger joints of the lower extremities, with tendency for spontaneous recovery over several months. Other common features include skin lesions, enthesitis, tendonitis and association with HLA-B27.

Schumacher HR: Reactive arthritis. Rheum Dis Clinic North Am 24:261, 1998.

22. What conditions are associated with gastroenteritis and arthritis?

Noninfectious:
- Ulcerative colitis
- Crohn disease
- Behçet disease
- Henoch-Schönlein purpura
- Celiac disease

Infectious:
- *Salmonella*
- *Shigella*
- *Yersinia*
- Campylobacter
- Tuberculosis
- Whipple disease
- Giardiasis

23. Is Beaver fever a cause of reactive arthritis?

Yes! But what is Beaver fever? An epidemic of giardiasis was reported in Canada following ingestion of contaminated untreated water from a reservoir habitated by infected beavers. Hence the name.

Dykes AC, et al: Municipal water-borne giardiasis: Epidemiological investigation. Ann Intern Med 92:165, 1980.

24. How do synovial fluid charecteristics help in determining the diagnosis of arthritis?

Synovial Fluid Characteristics in Various Arthridites

GROUP/CONDITION	SYNOVIAL COMPLEMENT	COLOR/ CLARITY	VISCOSITY	MUCIN CLOT	WBC COUNT (μl)	PMN (%)	MISCELLANEOUS FINDINGS
Noninflammatory							
Normal	N	Yellow Clear	↑↑	G	< 200	< 25	
Traumatic arthritis	N	Yellow Turbid	↑	F–G	< 2,000	< 25	Debris
Osteroarthritis	N	Yellow Clear	↑	F–G	1,000	< 25	
Inflammatory							
SLE	↓ Clear	Yellow	N	N	5,000	10	LE cells
Rheumatic fever	N–↑	Yellow Cloudy	↓	F	5,000	10–50	
JRA	N–↓	Yellow Cloudy	↓	Poor	15,000–20,000	75	
Reiter syndrome	↑	Yellow Opaque	↓	Poor	20,000	80	Reiter cells
Pyogenic							
Tuberculous arthritis	N–↑	Yellow-white Cloudy	↓	Poor	25,000	50–60	Acid-fast bacteria
Septic arthritis	↑	Serosanguinous Turbid	↓	Poor	50,000–30,000	> 75	Low glucose, bacteria

25. An 8-year-old girl presents one week after mild trauma with pain and tenderness in the right foot and leg, which are both cold to the touch. What is the likely diagnosis?

Complex regional pain syndrome*, type 1.* More commonly called *reflex sympathetic dystrophy (RSD),* this poorly understood entity is often confused with arthritis because of localized severe pain in one of the extremities. However, there are several features which separate it from arthritis. The pain is not confined to a single joint. It is a regional in nature, involving portions of an extremity, and often follows minor trauma. The pain is very severe, and even light touch causes pain (i.e., hyperesthesia). Several dysautonomic changes such as mottling, color changes and sweating may occur. Laboratory findings are normal. Autonomic dysfunction can be confirmed by thermography or by technetium scan which demonstrates reduced blood flow. Regional osteopenia secondary to disuse may develop.

Because the role of the sympathetic nervous system is unclear and dystrophy may not occur in all cases, the terminology change has been advised by the International Association for the Study of Pain. In type 1, all the features of the complex are present without definable nerve injury. In type 2, a definable nerve injury is present.

Murray CS: Morbidity in reflex sympathetic dystrophy. Arch Dis Child 82:231-233, 2000.

26. How is complex regional pain syndrome managed?

Although many children are casted because of suspected hairline fractures, immobilization is *contraindicated.* Treatment is aimed at providing pain relief using analgesics and other non-medical modalities. A good explanation of the mechanism of pain and assurance that this condition is controllable are essential in managing these children and their families. A physical therapy program should be started immediately with emphasis on passive and active range of motion and maintenance of function. Aquatherapy is particularly useful in these children to initiate therapy. Desensitization of the painful area using one of several modalities such as biofeedback, TENS, visualization and acupuncture should be part of the program. A positive attitude on the part of physicians and therapists is essential. In extreme situations, sympathetic blockade may be needed. Newer therapies also include electrical stimulation of the spinal cord and the use of intrathecal baclofen (a GABA receptor agonist which inhibits sensory input to the neurons of the spinal cord).

van Hilten BJ, et al: Intrathecal baclofen for the treatment of dystonia in patients with reflex sympathetic dystrophy. N Engl J Med 343:625-630, 2000.

Kemler MA, et al: Spinal cord stimulation in patients with chronic reflex sympathetic dystrophy. N Engl J Med 343:618-624, 2000.

27. Can this syndrome (complex regional pain or RSD) also have a psychological basis?

There is a psychological profile associated with this syndrome in children. Children with RSD are often highly motivated, overachieving individuals and are involved in an extensive array of school and extracurricular activities. Psychotherapy may be required if the RSD is resistant or prolonged.

Sherry DD, Weisman R Psychological aspects of childhood reflex neurovascular dystrophy. Pediatrics 81:572, 1988.

28. Do children develop fibromyalgia?

Children as young as 9 years of age have been described with this syndrome. *Fibromyalgia* is a condition characterized by musculoskeletal aches and pains, fatigue, disturbed sleep pattern and tenderness over various parts of the body. These tender points are specific for the diagnosis (see diagram below). There should be tenderness over at least 4 of these 11 points for proper classification of individuals. In addition there should be no tenderness over non-specific sites such as the forehead or the pretibial region.

Aches and pains are extremely common in children and may be due to serious medical diseases such as leukemia, mental illness such as depression and psychosocial stress. Differentiation of chronic musculoskeletal pain of nonorganic origin may be difficult in children and adolescents.

Criteria for diagnosis of fibromyalgia (American College of Rheumatology)

1. History of widespread pain
Pain is considered widespread when it occurs on both sides of the body above and below the waist. Axial skeletal pain must be present.

2. Pain in 11 of 18 bilateral tender point sites on digital palpation
(using about 4 kg of pressure)

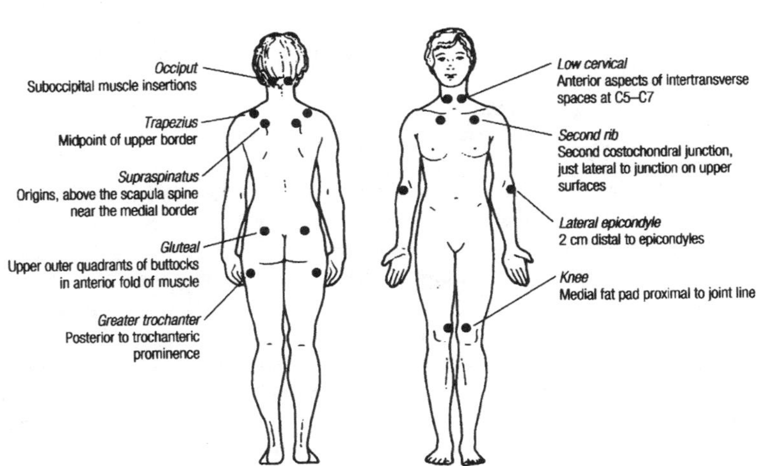

From Ballinger S, Bowyer S: Fibromyalgia: The latest "great" imitator. Contemp Pediatr 14:147, 1997; with permission.

29. How is chronic fatigue syndrome defined?

The clinical definition of chronic fatigue syndrome (as defined by the CDC) is a patient with ***persistent or relapsing fatigue of 6 months' duration*** with at least ***4 minor*** criteria including *impaired cognition, sore throat, adenopathy, muscle pain, joint pain, headache, unrefreshing sleep,* and/or *postexertional malaise*. Although the symptomatology is similar to adults, the outlook in children and adolescents is brighter, with 95% improvement with medical and psychosocial care.

Franklin A: How I manage chronic fatigue syndrome. Arch Dis Child 79:375-378, 1998.

Krilov LR, et al: Course and outcome of chronic fatigue in children and adolescents. Pediatrics 102:360-366, 1998.

30. What should be considered prior to the diagnosis of chronic fatigue syndrome in children?

Although fatigue is a common symptom in children, chronic fatigue syndrome is not. Since fatigue can be a manifestation of psychosocial and developmental issues including depression, substance abuse, school failure and learning disability, one should think of these possibilities whenever a label of chronic fatigue syndrome is contemplated. Marshall has suggested that this syndrome be considered an illness rather than a disease. Current evidence points to a combination of biological and psychosocial factors in the initiation of this illness. Of particular interest is the high prevalence of abnormal hemodynamic responses to prolonged upright posture noted on tilt-table testing (similar to that seen in neurocardiogenic syncope).

Marshall GS: Report of a workshop on the epidemiology, natural history, and pathogenesis of chronic fatigue syndrome in adolescents. J Pediatr 134: 395, 1999.

Stewart JM, et al: Orthostatic intolerance in adolescent chronic fatigue syndrome. Pediatrics 103:116-121, 1999.

31. What therapies are effective in patients given the diagnosis of chronic fatigue syndrome?

As with any condition with controversies about its nature and pathophysiology (and even its existence), a wide variety of therapies are attempted. A review of proposed or attempted therapies found:

Beneficial:	Exercise, cognitive behavioral therapy
Unknown effectiveness:	Corticosteroids, antidepressants, dietary supplements, nicotinamide
Unlikely to beneficial:	Immunotherapy
Likely to be ineffective or harmful:	Prolonged rest

Reid S, et al: Chronic fatigue syndrome. BMJ 320:292-296, 2000.

32. What are the agents associated with true serum sickness in the modern era?

Now that there is no need for the treatment of or prophylaxis against tetanus or diphtheria, true serum sickness is not common. When seen, it is associated with the use of serum in the treatment of botulism, snake bite, gas gangrene, rabies and the use of antithymocyte globulin.

33. What is the difference between complementary and alternative medicine?

Complementary medicine generally refers to treatments used in addition to or in conjunction with traditional medicine, whereas *alternative* medicine refers to therapies used in place of traditional medicine.

34. What is the role of acupuncture for the pediatric patient?

An NIH consensus conference regarding acupuncture and adults found it to be effective in treating some types of nausea and pain, particularly dental pain, migraine headaches, back pain and dysmenorrhea. In children, the data are more limited. Acupuncture has been used to treat post-extubation laryngospasm, asthma, allergies, postoperative nausea and pain. The Pain Treatment Service at Boston Children's Hospital refers adolescents with chronic and refractory pain to a licensed acupuncturist primarily for migraine headache, endometriosis, and complex regional pain syndrome (reflex sympathetic dystrophy). 70% of patients reported relief.

Kemper KI, et al: On pins and needles? Pediatric pain patients' experience with acupuncture. Pediatrics 105:941-947, 2000.

Lee C, et al: The effect of acupuncture on the incidence of postextubation laryngospasm in children. Anaesthesia 53:910-924, 1998.

JUVENILE RHEUMATOID ARTHRITIS

35. At what point is a synovitis considered chronic?

At 6 weeks in the U.S., 3 months in Europe.

36. Which is the most common chronic arthritis in children?

Juvenile rheumatoid arthritis (JRA).

37. What are the diagnostic criteria for the classification of JRA?

JRA is a diagnosis of exclusion. Features include:

- Onset < 16 years of age
- Clinical arthritis with joint swelling or effusion, increased heat, and limitation of range of motion with tenderness
- Duration of disease ≥ 6 weeks
- Major subgroups (systemic-onset, pauciarticular or oligoarticular, polyarticular, polyarticular) determined by:
  a. Presence or absence of fever at presentation
  b. Number of joints involved in the first 6 months of illness
  c. No other known etiology for arthritis

38. What are the main subsets of JRA and their characteristics?

Subset Frequency	*# of Joints*	*Gender*	*Age*	*+ANA*	*+RF*	*Uveitis*	*Outcome*
Pauciarticular	1–4	F	2yrs	++	–	Yes	Good 50%
Polyarticular RF-	≥5	F	3&9	+	–	Yes	Poor 25%
Polyarticular RF+	≥5	F	Teens	+	+	No	Very poor 5%
Systemic	Any	Either	0–16	–	–	No	Very poor(*) 20%

(*)Intriguingly, it is excellent in some patients.

39. Describe the pattern of fever and rash of the systemic subset.

Systemic-onset JRA (Still disease) accounts for approximately 20% of children with JRA. Affected individuals typically present with fevers of unknown origin with single or twice daily (i.e., quotidian) spikes, often > 40°C. Shaking chills often precede the fever. The temperature characteristically returns to 37° or lower. Continuous fever should suggest other diagnoses.

A blotchy, light pink, evanescent rash, which blanches on compression and which may show perimacular pallor, accompanies the fever in over 90% cases. The rash of systemic

JRA is diagnostic only *after* the diagnosis is made (by exclusion). Of note, arthritis may not be present for the first several weeks of illness.

40. Why is it sometimes difficult to distinguish systemic JRA from leukemia?

Up to 20% of patients with leukemia present with some degree of musculoskeletal symptoms including joint pain and occasional swelling. In both diseases there is anemia, fever, and weight loss. Both can present with hepatosplenomegaly and lymphadenopathy. In leukemia, however, the fever usually is not usually spiking. Platelets tend to be low to low normal. A good exam of a peripheral smear is crucial. A high LDH is very suggestive of leukemia, and the Tc_{99} bone scan shows a different pattern of uptake. More than one bone marrow biopsy may be necessary.

Tuten HR, et al: The limping child: A manifestation of acute leukemia. J Pediatr Orthop 18:625-629, 1998.

Ostrov BE, Goldsmith DP, Athreya BH: Differentiation of systemic juvenile rheumatoid arthritis from acute leukemia near the onset of disease. J Pediatr 122:595-8, 1993.

41. In a patient with suspected rheumatologic disease, what clinical features are more suggestive of malignancy?

Particularly concerning are ***nonarticular bone pain, back pain*** as the principal presenting feature, ***bone tenderness*** and ***severe constitutional symptoms***. Children with rheumatic joint problems are typically are stiff, but rarely complain about pain. The pain in malignancy is out of proportion to the amount of swelling around the joint. Pain of malignancy tends to be worse at night. It is vital to think about the possibilities of malignancy in children presenting with rheumatic complaints.

Cabral DA, Tucker LB: Malignancies in children who initially present with rheumatic complaints. J Pediatr 134:53-57, 1999.

42. What is the value of measuring ANA and RF in JRA?

Once JRA has been diagnosed on clinical grounds, results of these tests help assign the patient to the appropriate category (e.g., pauciarticular or RF positive polyarticular). Because ANA can be present in up to 10% of normal children, this test should not be used as a screening test to diagnose JRA in children who experience non-inflammatory pain. These tests are also useful as prognostic indicators. The presence of ANA increases the risk of uveitis, making ophthalmologic surveillance more important. RF is valuable as a marker of poor prognosis in adolescents with polyarticular arthritis.

43. What other laboratory tests are diagnostic for JRA?

None. Complete blood count, liver function tests and renal function tests are important for monitoring purposes. Quantitative immunoglobulins are commonly measured at disease onset to rule out arthritis associated with immunoglobulin deficiency which can be clinically identical to JRA.

44. Are x-rays helpful in the diagnosis of JRA?

No, there are no characteristic x-ray changes at onset. The value of radiology is to rule out of other skeletal conditions and to provide a documented baseline status.

45. What has been the traditional approach to JRA medical management?

The goal of therapy in JRA is to provide the best possible control of inflammation with minimum side effects. Because the natural history of the disease cannot be modified with our current knowledge, the basic goal is to minimize joint damage and hope for spontaneous remission. In unremitting disease, the goal is to keep inflammation under the best possible control.

The so-called ***first line therapy*** consists of non-steroidal anti-inflammatories (NSAIDs). Given at the correct dose, they exert pain relief and suppress inflammation (decrease in morning stiffness) with a peak action at 4-6 weeks. The classic representatives of this group are aspirin, ibuprofen, naproxen, tolmetin and indomethacin. Choice among them is based upon availability in liquid form, half-life, side effect profile, individual doctor preferences and results of an individual trial. Most of their action is through inhibition of cyclo-oxygenase (COX). About 1/3 of patients will have their symptoms controlled through the use of NSAIDs; 2/3 require more aggressive drug therapy.

46. What newer modalities may be useful in JRA management?

There are two isoenzymes with cyclooxygenase (COX) activity, COX-1 and COX-2, which are involved in prostaglandin synthesis. COX-1 is a ubiquitous constitutive enzyme present in the GI tract, renal parenchyma and platelets and responsible for multiple physiologic functions COX-2 is inducible by pro-inflammatory cytokines and present at sites of inflammation. NSAIDs inhibit both COX species and therefore responsible for various adverse effects related to the GI tract, kidneys and platelets. A new generation of drugs with preferential inhibitory effects on COX-2 with little or no effect on COX-1 have become available recently. These COX-2 inhibitors have been associated with significantly less mucosal damage compared to NSAIDs, but they have not been well tested in children. The level of COX-2 specificity varies, and the two most specific are Rofecoxib (Vioxx®) and Celecoxib (Celebrex®).

For refractory polyarticular, extended pauciarticular and systemic disease, azulfidine and methotrexate are widely used. They and other disease modifying antirheumatic drugs (DMARDs) have side effects that require monitoring. A newly developed family of biological agents—etanercept and infliximab—are effective inhibitors of the pro-inflammatory actions of TNF (tumor necrosis factor). The first has been investigated in clinical trials in JRA with excellent results. Finally, intra-articular steroids are useful in selected clinical situations. For severe refractory JRA unresponsive to conventional therapy, stem-cell transplantations have been done. Limited early results have been positive.

Lovell DJ, et al: Etanercept in children with polyarticular juvenile rheumatoid arthritis. N Engl J Med 342:763-769, 2000.

Hawkey CJ: COX-2 inhibitors. Lancet 307-314, 1999.

Wulffraat N, et al: Autologous haematopoetic stem-cell transplantation in four patients with refractory juvenile chronic arthritis. Lancet 353:550-553, 1999.

47. When are corticosteroids indicated in children with JRA?

- *Life threatening disease* (e.g., carditis or myocarditis)
- *Unremitting fever* unresponsive to NSAIDs
- *Unrelenting polyarthritis* with severe limitations requiring intensive physical therapy to achieve ambulatory status
- Topical therapy for *uveitis* (rarely, systemic steroids are needed for children with aggressive uveitis unresponsive to topical therapy)
- Intra-articular administration for a *single severely symptomatic joint*

48. What are the most common side effects of prolonged cortiscosteroid therapy?

A trip to Stockholm awaits the individual who can synthesize an anti-inflammatory steroid without untoward side effects. These effects can be minimized by alternate-day therapy, but some times the treatment is worse than the disease. Commonly encountered problems associated with high-dose corticosteroid use in children can be remembered by referring to the "Cushingoid map":

C Cataracts
U Ulcers
S Striae
H Hypertension
I nfectious complications
N Necrosis of bone (avascular)
G Growth retardation
O Osteoporosis
I Increased intracranial pressure (pseudotumor cerebri)
D Diabetes mellitus

M Myopathy
A Adipose tissue hypertrophy (obesity, "buffalo hump")
P Pancreatitis

49. Which children with JRA require the most frequent monitoring for uveitis?

Uveitis (also called iridocyclitis) is inflammation of the iris and ciliary body. It occurs on average in 20% of patients with pauciarticular JRA and in 5% with polyarticular disease, but those in either group with positive ANA are at higher risk. ***Patients less than 7 years of age with ANA-positivity*** should be seen every 3-4 months for ophthalmologic evaluation. Fewer than 2% of patients with systemic JRA will develop ocular inflammation. These children require eye examinations only once a year. Periodic examinations are critical because most patients with ocular inflammation are asymptomatic.

Nguyen QD, Foster CS: Saving the vision of children with juvenile rheumatoid arthritis-associated uveitis. JAMA 1133-1134, 1998.

50. What is the earliest sign of uveitis among patients with JRA?

When the anterior chamber of the eye is examined with a slit lamp, a ***"flare"*** is the earliest sign. This is a hazy appearance due to an increased concentration of protein and inflammatory cells. Later signs can include a speckled appearance of the posterior cornea (secondary to keratic precipitates), an irregular or poorly reactive pupil (secondary to synechiae between the iris and lens), band keratopathy, and cataracts.

51. What do we know about etiology and pathogenesis of JRA?

Sibling and family studies suggest that JRA has an important genetic determinant, 50% of which links to the short arm of chromosome 6, the HLA coding region. The same studies, however, suggest that the disease is polygenic, requiring a combination of genes both neighboring and remote. This latter explains why familial cases are so rare. The primary defect, however, could lie anywhere in the inflammatory cascade or in the very central antigen presentation process. In addition, the effect of the gene(s) is time limited with age windows at which the effect is more or less notable. Most authors agree that an environmental (infectious) triggering event is necessary as well.

Glass DN, Giannini EH: Juvenile rheumatoid arthritis as a complex genetic trait. Arthritis Rheum 42: 2261-2268, 1999.

52. What is the value of HLA-B27 test?

In the presence of higher clinical probability (e.g., 8-18 year old male with synovitis and enthesitis), the presence of HLA-B27 is very useful to make a diagnosis of spondyloarthropathy. However, it should be recalled that approximately *8%* of normal whites carry this marker. Also, only a small percent of individuals with HLA-B27 develop a spondyloarthropathy syndrome. Therefore, this is not a test with good positive predictive value.

LYME DISEASE

53. Where in the world is Lyme disease prevalent?

Lyme disease is a zoonosis caused by the spirochete *Borrelia burgdorferi* that populates the midgut of the deer tick (mainly *Ixodes scapularis*). Human cases, as expected, parallel the rate of tick infestation and the abundance of ticks. The former in turn is highly dependent on the abundance of parasitized white-footed mice (reservoir) and the latter on the abundance of deer (main support of the adult female ticks). Favorable climatic conditions are found in a wide belt of temperate woodlands around the world which in the U.S. includes mid-Atlantic states, New England, West Coast states (California, Oregon and Washington State) and upper Midwest (Wisconsin, Minnesota, Michigan). Other areas of the world with high prevalence of this disease include northern Spain and France, Austria, Germany, Russia and Japan. Vectors and reservoirs vary by region. So does the strain of *Borrelia*.

54. Is the time of year important to suspect the diagnosis of Lyme disease?

Depends upon the area and the stage of the disease. In areas where ticks can be found year around, the seasonality is less marked. In general, most cases of skin rash and acute neuroborreliosis (cranial neuropathies and aseptic meningitis) occur between April and November, while arthritis is seen year around.

55. What criteria are needed to diagnose Lyme disease?

Classification criteria (i.e., case definition) by the CDC include:

A. ***Erythema migrans***: enlarging circular erythematous lesion (minimum size 5 cm; ***or***
B. At least ***one clinical*** manifestation (arthritis, cranial neuropathy, atrioventricular block, aseptic meningitis, radiculoneuritis) and ***isolation or serologic evidence*** of *B. burgdorferi* infection.

56. How is Lyme disease confirmed in the laboratory?

Although attempts to demonstrate borrelial DNA in infected tissues by PCR has met with some success and cultures occasionally render positive results, the main diagnostic tool continues to be serology. IgM peaks about 4 weeks after infection, and IgG does so at 6 weeks. This is the main reason why antibodies may not be detected during the early dermatologic and neurologic stages.

There are two detection techniques: ***ELISA*** and ***Western blot***. Both are available for IgG and IgM. Initial disagreements on the criteria (cutoff) for the interpretation of Western blot were settled in Dearborn, Michigan, in 1996. Basically, a negative ELISA requires no further investigation at a given time. Sero-conversion can be sought in situations of high suspicion in 2 or 3 weeks. Enhancement of test sensitivity by ELISA has led to high rates of false positivity resulting in over-diagnosis. All positive ELISAs, particularly those with borderline positivity, should be confirmed by Western blot.

The main problem with serology results from the tendency of sera from patients with EBV infection, parvovirus infection and syphilis to react positively in *Borrelia* assays by the ELISA method. Sera from patients with autoimmune diseases (SLE, JRA) may also cross-react. However, most of these will be negative when tested by Western blot.

57. Describe the classic rash of Lyme disease.

Erythema migrans (EM, previously known as erythema chronicum migrans or ECM) is the distinctive cutaneous lesion of Lyme disease. The lesion begins as a small red maculae or papule and enlarges in an annular centrifugal fashion to approximately 10–15 cm or more in diameter. The lesions may have varying intensities of redness within the plaque, partial central clearing, or a ring-within-a-ring configuration. Occasionally, the central area may become indurated, vesicular, or crusted. EM lesions usually appear within 14 days of the bite of an infected *Ixodes* tick (range 2-28 days). Multiple lesions are present in only about 20% of cases.

58. After a tick bite has occurred, how does Lyme disease progress?

***1-2 weeks*:** Following the bite of an infected *Ixodes* deer tick, EM develops in two-thirds of cases. The skin lesion may be associated with constitutional symptoms (fever, arthralgia, myalgia, severe headache, and profound fatigue), especially in patients in whom secondary lesions occur. The rash and other symptoms are self-limited, even without antibiotic treatment.

***Weeks to months*:** If treatment has not been given, early-disseminated Lyme disease occurs, characterized by neurologic and/or cardiac involvement. Neuroborreliosis occurs in up to 20% of patients and presents mostly commonly as facial palsy, lymphocytic meningitis, or peripheral radiculoneuropathy. Up to 8% of patients develop cardiac involvement (most commonly fluctuating atrioventricular block or, more rarely, myopericarditis).

***Months to years*:** The most common late manifestation of Lyme disease is a self-limited oligoarthritis, most often affecting the knees. Late neurologic disease does occur and, like tertiary syphilis, usually presents as a subacute encephalopathy, although it can mimic multiple sclerosis. In Europe, a morphea-like eruption termed acrodermatitis chronica atrophicans is a late dermatological sequela.

59. How is the diagnosis of Lyme meningitis established?

The diagnosis is often inexact and is commonly based on the finding of CSF pleocytosis and the presence of erythema migrans and/or positive serology. Both ELISA and Western blot testing may be negative or indeterminate early in the course of infection when dissemination to the CNS has occurred. Specific testing of the CSF fluid for intrathecal production of specific antibody or demonstration of *Borrelia burgdorferi* DNA by PCR testing is not readily available, and the latter is relatively insensitive.

60. How are Lyme and viral meningitis clinically distinguished?

Both are predominantly summertime illnesses, but the distinction is critical because Lyme meningitis requires weeks of intravenous antibiotics. In addition to the possible presence of erythema migrans, other areas of clinical distinction in patients with symptoms and signs of meningitis include:

- ***Cranial neuropathy***, especially periperal 7th nerve palsy (i.e., Bell palsy) is strongly suggestive of Lyme meningitis.
- ***Papilledema*** is more commonly seen in Lyme meningitis.
- A ***longer duration of symptoms*** prior to lumbar puncture is more typical of Lyme.
- ***Fever*** at the time of diagnosis is more likely viral meningitis.
- ***CSF pleocytosis***, especially the neutrophilic component, is less pronounced in Lyme meningitis.

Eppes SC, et al: Characterization of Lyme meningitis and comparison with viral meningitis. Pediatrics 103:957-960, 1999.

61. What is the prognosis for children diagnosed with Lyme arthritis?

Multiple studies have shown the long-term prognosis for treated patients is excellent with little morbidity.

Gerber MA, et al: Lyme arthritis in children: Clinical epidemiology and long-term outcome. Pediatrics 102:905-908, 1998.

Wang TJ, et al: Outcomes of children treated for Lyme disease. J Rheumatology 25:2249-2253, 1998.

62. What should be suspected if a patient with Lyme disease develops fever and chills after starting antibiotic treatment?

The ***Jarisch-Herxheimer reaction***. This reaction consists of fever, chills, arthralgia, myalgia, and vasodilation and follows the initiation of antibiotic therapy in certain illnesses, most typically syphilis. It is thought to be mediated by endotoxin release as the organism is destroyed. A similar reaction occurs in up to 40% of patients treated with Lyme disease and may be mistaken for an allergic reaction to the antibiotic.

63. Is antibiotic prophylaxis indicated for all tick bites?

All controlled studies have shown ***no benefit*** from antibiotic prophylaxis. In most regions the rate of tick infestation is low, making the likelihood of transmission below 10%. Treating all tick bites with antibiotics is impractical (some children will be on oral antibiotics throughout the summer). In areas where infestation rates approach 60 or 90%, the story may be different.

Nymphs (responsible for 85% of disease transmission) are very small (2 mm) and tan colored and smart (they do not hang around after a meal). The attachment has to be for at least 24 to 48 hours before transmission of infection occurs and is the theoretical basis for the efficacy of the daily tick check. If a tick is found, it should carefully be removed and the area observed for the development of a rash for 1-2 weeks.

If a rash suggestive of EM develops, prompt treatment with appropriate antibiotic has to be instituted. In an endemic area, if an individual develops flu-like symptoms without EM following documented tick bite, it will be necessary to perform tests for *Borrelia* antibody (IgM and IgG) by ELISA and Western blot and treat.

Shapiro ED, Gerber MA: Lyme disease. Clin Infect Dis 31:533-542, 2000.

Wormser GP et al: Practice guidelines for the treatment of Lyme disease. Clin Infect Dis 31S: 1-14, 2000.

64. What is the status of the vaccine for Lyme disease?

Because of the concerns about severe reactions to whole-cell vaccines, a recombinant immunogenic *B. burdorferi* protein (outer surface protein A [Osp A]) was used in human trials. In 1998, results indicating positive protection (76% efficacy) were published and in 1999 the vaccine was licensed for use in patients 15-70 years. Follow-up studies in younger children have indicated beneficial immunogenicity, tolerability and efficacy. Questions remain about long-term safety and efficacy.

Feder HM Jr: Lyme disease vaccine: Good for dogs, adults and children? J Pediatr 105:1333-1334, 2000.

Feder HM Jr, et al: Immunogenicity of a recombinant Borrelia burdorferi outer surface protein A vaccine against Lyme disease in children. J Pediatr 135:575-579, 1999.

RHEUMATIC FEVER

65. What is acceptable proof of antecedent streptococcal pharyngitis in diagnosing acute rheumatic fever?

Evidence of preceding streptococcal infection is a *sine qua non* for establishing a diagnosis of acute rheumatic fever. A history of sore throat alone is not sufficient, inasmuch as it is not possible to differentiate viral from group A streptococcal (GAS) pharyngitis clinically. Acceptable proof is limited to the following:

1. ***Throat culture***: A positive result from a swab of secretions from the posterior pharynx cultured on sheep blood agar remains the gold standard for diagnosis of GAS. False negative tests occur less than 10% of the time. Positive cultures, however, do not distinguish GAS pharyngitis from a carrier state. Attempts should be made to obtain cultures in all children at the time of presentation with acute rheumatic fever before treatment with antibiotic is instituted.

2. ***Streptococcal antigen tests***: Rapid diagnostic tests for the detection of GAS antigens in pharyngeal secretions are acceptable evidence of infection, as they are highly specific. Depending on the quality of the specimen obtained and the skill of the person performing them, such

tests may lack sensitivity, and negative results should be confirmed with a conventional throat culture. Again, positive tests do not distinguish true infection from a carrier state.

3. ***Antistreptococcal antibodies***: At the time of clinical presentation with rheumatic fever, throat cultures are usually negative. It is reasonable to assess the levels of antistreptococcal antibodies in all cases of putative rheumatic fever, as the antibodies should be elevated at the time of presentation. They will thereby provide confirmation of actual infection in those children with documented positive cultures and antigen tests, and are the only evidence of infection in children without such histories.

66. Which antistreptococcal antibodies are most commonly measured?

The most commonly employed test measures antibodies to ***anti-streptolysin* O** (ASO). The cut-off for a positive test in a school-aged child is 320 Todd units (240 in an adult); levels peak from 3 to 6 weeks after infection. If the test is negative, as may be the case in up to 20% of patients with ARF (and 40% of those with isolated chorea), other antistreptococcal antibodies may be detected. The most practically available of these identifies antibodies to ***deoxyribonuclease B*** (positive cut-off: 240 units in children, 120 in adults). Kits for the determination of anti-hyaluronidase antibodies are not available at present, and the Streptozyme slide agglutination test is unreliable in this setting. Alternatively, subsequent convalescent samples run simultaneously with the acute sample may detect rising titers of either ASO or anti-deoxyribonuclease B.

67. What are the common manifestations of carditis in acute rheumatic fever (ARF)?

In his *Etudes Médicales; du rhumatisme,* Lasègue remarked that "rheumatic fever licks the joints . . . and bites the heart," meaning that the severity of the two manifestations tends to be inversely related. In the more recent outbreaks of ARF, up to 80% of patients have had evidence of carditis. ARF causes a pancarditis, potentially affecting all layers from the pericardium through the endocardium. Carditis is most frequently heralded by a new or changing murmur of valvulitis. The most common manifestation is ***isolated mitral regurgitation***, followed in frequency by a mid-diastolic rumble of unclear pathophysiology (Carey-Coombs murmur), and then aortic insufficiency in the presence of mitral regurgitation. Isolated aortic insufficiency is uncommon, as are stenotic lesions. Electrocardiographic abnormalities typically involve some degree of *heart block*.

Pericarditis and myocarditis virtually never occur in isolation. Mild myocarditis may manifest itself as resting tachycardia out of proportion to fever, but when clinically more severe, and in combination with valvular damage, may lead to congestive heart failure. Heart failure should be managed aggressively, as it is potentially life-threatening.

Messeloff CR: Historical aspects of rheumatism. Medical Life 37:3-56, 1930.

68. How quickly can valvular lesions occur in children with ARF?

New murmurs appear within the first two weeks in 80% of patients and rarely occur after the second month of illness.

69. What is the "silent carditis" of rheumatic fever?

"Doppler echocardiography was performed in selected patients to detect possible regurgitant mitral or aortic flow that was not audible." With that statement in their 1987 report on the resurgence of rheumatic fever in Salt Lake City, Veasy and colleagues inadvertently opened Pandora's box by introducing the notion of "silent carditis." They documented *inaudible* mitral regurgitation in 19% of their subjects, in 9/19 (47%) of children with chorea and carditis and in 5/31 (16%) of children with arthritis and carditis.

This would at first appear to be quite reasonable; Doppler echocardiography is a much more sensitive tool for detecting valvular insufficiency than even the most astute clinician's ears. The problem is that substantial numbers of healthy, asymptomatic children can be documented to have some degree of regurgitant mitral flow and that this can vary based on the settings used. The current revision of the Jones criteria specifically states that Doppler echocardiography should not be employed as the only evidence of carditis.

Rancorous debate has ensued, and the jury is still out. Many pediatric cardiologists allow that they have encountered children with silent carditis, usually because they have seen occasional patients with Doppler evidence of inaudible regurgitation involving both mitral and aortic valves, but do not believe it to be common. A child with more than two minor, but no major Jones criteria who is found to have a significantly leaky valve on echocardiogram, but nothing on auscultation, might well be considered to have rheumatic fever until the situation is further clarified.

Veasy LG, et al: Resurgence of acute rheumatic fever in the intermountain area of the United States. N Engl J Med 316:421-427, 1987.

70. Describe the clinical characteristics of arthritis in ARF.

> The Disease comes at any time, but especially in the Autumn, and chiefly seizes those that are in the Flower of their Age. . . . It begins with shivering and shaking, and presently heat, restlessness, and thirst; and other symptoms which accompany a Fever. After a day or two, and sometimes sooner, the Patient is troubled with a violent Pain, sometimes in this, sometimes in that Joint, in the Wrist and Shoulders, but most commonly in the Knees; it now and then changes places, and seizes elsewhere, leaving redness and swelling in the Part it last possessed. . . . When this Disease is not accompanied with a Fever it is often taken for the Gout though it differs essentially from that as plainly appears to anyone that well considers both Diseases. —Thomas Sydenham, 1676

This classical description of the ***migratory polyarthritis*** of acute rheumatic fever has withstood the test of time. It is usually the earliest symptom of the disease and typically affects the large joints, the knees, ankles, elbows, and wrists (although hips are uncommonly involved). The joints are extraordinarily painful; weight-bearing may not be possible. Physical examination discloses warmth, erythema, and exquisite tenderness, such that the weight of even bedclothes and sheets may not be tolerable. This tenderness is typically is out of proportion to the degree of swelling.

Messeloff CR: Historical aspects of rheumatism. Medical Life 37:3-56, 1930.

71. What is the effect of aspirin therapy on the arthritis of rheumatic fever?

The arthritis of rheumatic fever is exquisitely sensitive to even modest doses of salicylates, effectively arresting the process within 12-24 hours. If aspirin or other nonsteroidal anti-inflammatory drugs (NSAIDs) are employed early in the course, the arthritis will not migrate, and a delay in diagnosis may result. Such medications should be withheld until the clinical course of the illness has clarified itself. Conversely, if there is not a dramatic response to aspirin, a diagnosis other than rheumatic fever should be considered.

72. How long does the arthritis associated with ARF usually persist?

In untreated cases of ARF, arthritis affects a number of joints sequentially for less than a week each. The entire process rarely lasts more than one month. Treatment with aspirin or NSAIDs will shorten the clinical course.

73. What is Jaccoud arthropathy?

Jaccoud syndrome is a periarticular fibrosis, which results in severe, reducible articular subluxations in the absence of radiographic signs of joint erosion. It results in ulnar deviation of the wrist and metacarpophalangeal joints. Initially described as a chronic manifestation of rheumatic fever, most cases are now thought to be related to lupus and other connective tissue diseases.

74. How is post-streptococcal arthritis differentiated from rheumatic fever?

Often with difficulty. Children occasionally develop arthritis following GAS pharyngitis that does not fulfill Jones criteria. In some cases a monarthritis is noted, most commonly an artifact due to the premature administration of salicylates or other NSAIDs. The prompt response of such monarthritis to anti-inflammatory therapy should serve to confirm that the child has bona fide rheumatic fever. Post-streptococcal reactive arthritis has emerged in the literature as a somewhat confusing entity distinct from the arthritis of acute rheumatic fever. Some reports include children who have migratory polyarthritis but do not fulfill two minor Jones criteria, i.e., they lack fever or acute phase reactants. Many clinicians consider these to be rheumatic fever variants and advise prophylaxis accordingly.

There is another group of patients whose post-streptococcal arthritis appears to be quite different from that of patients with rheumatic fever. In these patients, the period between pharyngitis and onset of arthritis is shorter (1-2 weeks) and the response to salicylates and NSAIDs is not dramatic. Silent and clinical carditis have developed in such patients; antibiotic prophylaxis is warranted, although there is no agreed upon duration for such therapy.

75. How common is erythema marginatum in rheumatic fever?

You probably don't know anyone who has seen this rash, occurring in less than 5% of cases of ARF, but if you do and you call them to the bedside to confirm it, it is likely to have disappeared in the meantime. An evanescent, pink to slightly red, non-pruritic eruption with pale centers and serpiginous borders, it may be induced by the application of heat and always blanches upon palpation. The outer edges of the lesion are sharp, while the inner borders are diffuse. It is most often found on the trunk and proximal extremities, but not the face. Erythema marginatum is seen almost solely in patients with carditis.

76. Are corticosteroids of benefit in the treatment of ARF?

Controlled studies in the 1950s failed to show any definite benefit of corticosteroids in the treatment of rheumatic carditis. Nonetheless, it is generally recommended that patients with *severe carditis* (e.g.,congestive heart failure, cardiomegaly, third-degree heart block) receive prednisone (2 mg/kg/day) in addition to conventional therapy for their heart failure. The unusual patient with well-documented rheumatic arthritis that does not respond to salicylates or NSAIDs will benefit symptomatically from prednisone.

77. What are appropriate regimens of prophylaxis for patients who have had ARF?

The goal of prophylaxis is to prevent GAS pharyngitis, thereby preventing recurrences of ARF. Recurrences can happen at any time, but the greatest risk is in the two years following the initial attack. Appropriate regimens include:

- Intramuscular benzathine penicillin G 600,000-1,200,000 units every 3-4 weeks
- Oral penicillin V potassium 250 mg twice daily
- Oral sulfadiazine 500-1000 mg once daily
- Oral erythromycin 250 mg twice daily, if allergic to the above

The cut-off for larger doses is 27 kg. (Dosing is not linear; a child just under the cut-off will receive benzathine penicillin ~23,000 units/kg, whereas a child just over it will receive ~44,000/kg.) In areas in which rheumatic fever is endemic or in other high-risk situations, the 3-week intramuscular regimen is preferable.

78. Can antibiotic prophylaxis for rheumatic fever ever be discontinued?

The optimal duration of anti-streptococcal prophylaxis following documented ARF is the subject of some debate. It is clear that the risk of recurrence decreases after five years have elapsed from the most recent attack. Most clinicians therefore recommend discontinuing prophylaxis in patients who have not had carditis *after five years* or on the *21st birthday* (whichever comes later). Those at high risk for contracting streptococcal pharyngitis (e.g., school teachers, health care professionals, military recruits and others living in crowded conditions) and anyone with a history of carditis should receive antibiotic prophylaxis for longer periods of time. Recommendations vary, ranging from ten years to the 40th birthday (whichever is longer) to lifelong prophylaxis, depending on the extent of residual heart disease.

79. Is the incidence of rheumatic fever increasing or decreasing?

The epidemiology of rheumatic fever parallels that of streptococcal pharyngitis. Early in the 20th century cases of rheumatic fever were linked to poverty, overcrowding, and poor sanitation. The general decrease in the number of cases in the last 60 years preceded the introduction of antibiotics and no doubt reflected a general improvement in public health. The resurgence of acute rheumatic fever in 25 states in the 1980s was attributed to changes in the virulence of the organism, as it occurred primarily in suburban locales, affecting middle- to high-income families. Nationwide, however, the incidence of rheumatic fever remained largely unchanged during this time.

80. Where do PANDAS live in the world of pediatric rheumatology?

In 1989 Swedo and colleagues characterized the psychiatric abnormalities found in children with Sydenham chorea, noting a high prevalence of obsessive-compulsive (OCD) behaviors. They went on to describe a syndrome which they dubbed ***PANDAS*** (**P**ediatric **A**utoimmune **N**europsychiatric **D**isorders **A**ssociated with **S**treptococcal infection), in which OCD and Tourette syndrome in some children appeared to be triggered or exacerbated by streptococcal infections in the absence of classical chorea or other manifestation of rheumatic fever.

The existence of PANDAS remains controversial. There has been no prospective study of GAS infection to confirm the association of streptococcal pharyngitis with these behavioral abnormalities. The symptoms of tic disorders and OCD tend to fluctuate spontaneously and may be nonspecifically exacerbated by illness. In some cases, the only link to streptococcal infection has been a single throat culture or serological test, bringing the specificity of the condition into question.

Swedo SE, Leonard HL, Garvey M, et al: Pediatric autoimmune neuropsychiatric disorders associated with streptococcal infections: Clinical description of the first 50 cases. Am J Psychiatry 155:264-71, 1998.

Swedo SE, Rapoport JL, Cheslow DL, et al: High prevalence of obsessive-compulsive symptoms in patients with Sydenham's chorea. Am J Psychiatry 146:246-9, 1989.

81. Who was Saint Vitus?

Saint Vitus was a Sicilian youth martyred in the year 303. In the Middle Ages, individuals with chorea would worship at shrines dedicated to this saint. Accordingly, Sydenham chorea is also known as Saint Vitus' dance. Saint Vitus is now known as the patron saint of dancers and comedians.

SPONDYLOARTHROPATHIES

82. How are the juvenile spondyloarthropathies distinguished from juvenile rheumatoid arthritis?

Under the rubric juvenile spondyloarthropathies (JSA) are subserved the following conditions: *juvenile ankylosing spondylitis, juvenile psoriatic arthritis, post-dysenteric reactive arthritis, Reiter syndrome,* and *the arthritis of inflammatory bowel disease*. They are distinguished from JRA by the following features:

- Age of onset in early adolescence.
- They are the only rheumatic diseases with a clear male predominance.

- Enthesitis (inflammation of tendon and ligament insertion sites) is characteristic.
- Prodromal oligoarthritis involving large joints of the lower extremities may resemble JRA, but hip involvement points to JSA. Episodes of arthritis tend to be briefer than in JRA.
- Involvement of the sacroiliac joints and of the back, manifested as pain and stiffness and reduced range of motion.
- Association with HLA-B27 (up to 90% in children with ankylosing spondylitis and 60% of other spondyloarthropathies vs. 15% of JRA).
- Seronegativity: ANA and rheumatoid factors typically negative.

83. How is enthesitis diagnosed clinically?

The *enthesis* is the site of attachment of ligaments, tendons, or fascia to bone. Enthesopathy is unique to the spondyloarthropathies and presents as painful localized tenderness at the tibial tubercle (which may be mistaken for Osgood-Schlatter disease), the peripheral patella, and at the calcaneal insertion of the Achilles tendon and plantar fascia (which may be mistaken for Sever disease). Thickening of the Achilles tendon and tenderness of the metatarsophalangeal joints are associated findings.

84. Why is the diagnosis of ankylosing spondylitis difficult to make in children?

A child may have undifferentiated spondyloarthritis characterized by enthesitis and recurrent episodes of lower extremity oligoarthritis for several years before he develops back symptoms. In order to fulfill criteria for ankylosing spondylitis, clinical features of lumbar spine pain, limitation of lumbar motion, and radiographic signs of sacroiliitis must be present. The average time from onset of symptoms to diagnosis in an adult with ankylosing spondylitis is five years; many adolescents are adults before they fulfill criteria.

85. What is the connection between young men and the SEA?

No apologies to Hemingway needed here. The syndrome of seronegative enthesopathy and arthropathy (SEA) was described in 1982 in a group of children, mostly boys, with enthesitis and arthralgia or arthritis who were seronegative for ANA and rheumatoid factor. Many were HLA-B27-positive, but did not fulfill criteria for definite spondyloarthritis. Long-term follow-up disclosed that about half went on to develop definite ankylosing spondylitis.

86. Where are the dimples of Venus?

The *dimples of Venus* are prominent paravertebral indentations in the lower back of some individuals. A line drawn between the dimples marks the lumbosacral junction, the midpoint for the Schober test, a measure of anterior flexion of the lumbosacral spine.

SYSTEMIC LUPUS ERYTHEMATOSUS

87. What are the most common manifestations of systemic lupus erythematosus (SLE) in children?

Arthritis	80–90%
Rash/fever	70%
Re*nal disease (proteinuria, casts)**	70%
Serositis	50%
Hypertension	50%
CNS disease (psychosis/seizures)	20–40%
Anemia, leukopenia, thrombocytopenia	30% each

*Every patient with SLE is likely to have some abnormality demonstrated on renal biopsy.

Iqbal S, et al: Diversity in presenting manifestations of systemic lupus erythematosus in children. J Pediatr 135:500-505, 1999.

88. Describe the neurologic manifestations of SLE.

Lupus cerebritis is a term that implies an inflammatory etiology of CNS disease. Microscopically, however, widely scattered areas of microinfarction and noninflammatory vasculopathy are seen in brain tissue; actual CNS vasculitis is rarely observed. A lumbar puncture may reveal CSF pleocytosis or an increased protein concentration, but it can be normal as well. Neuropsychiatric manifestations (psychoses, behavorial changes, depression, emotional lability) or seizures are most commonly observed. An organic brain syndrome with progressive disorientation and intellectual deterioration can be seen. Cranial or peripheral neuropathies, chorea and cerebellar ataxia are less common manifestations of CNS lupus. Severe headaches and cerebral ischemic events have also been seen.

Steinlein MJ, et al: Neurological manifestations of pediatric systemic lupus erythematosus. Pediatr Neurol 13:191, 1995.

89. What laboratory tests should be ordered in a child suspected of having SLE?

A useful screening test for SLE is the ***fluorescent antinuclear antibody (FANA) test***. Up to 97% of patients with SLE have positive ANAs at some point in their illness (although not necessarily at the time of diagnosis). In a patient with characteristic signs and symptoms, a positive ANA may help confirm suspicions of SLE. Unfortunately, however, up to *10%* of the normal childhood population may also have a positive ANA. Therefore, a positive ANA in the absence of any objective findings of SLE means very little. Other autoantibodies are much more specific, but less sensitive for SLE. These include antibodies to double-stranded DNA and the extractable nuclear antigen Sm. Complement levels are often depressed in active SLE, and sedimentation rates are often elevated. The combination of a *positive anti-double stranded DNA Ab* and a *low* C_3 is nearly 100% specific for SLE. Anemia, leukopenia, lymphopenia, and/or thrombocytopenia may also be seen.

90. Which diseases should be considered in the differential diagnosis of children with a butterfly rash?

A malar rash is present in 50% of children with SLE. The typical butterfly rash involves the malar areas and crosses the nasal bridge, but spares the nasolabial folds. Occasionally it is difficult to distinguish from the rash of dermatomyositis. (Accompanying erythematous papules on the extensor surfaces of the MCP and PIP joints are common in dermatomyositis, but are not generally seen in SLE.) Seborrheic dermatitis or a contact dermatitis may be similar to the rash of SLE. Vesiculation should suggest another disease, such as pemphigus erythematosus. A malar flush is clinically distinct and may be seen in children with mitral stenosis or hypothyroidism.

91. Should children with SLE undergo a renal biopsy?

This is an area of controversy, as nearly all children with SLE will have some evidence of renal involvement. Usually, clinical disease (e.g., abnormal urine sediment, proteinuria, renal function changes) correlates with the severity of renal disease on biopsy, but this is not always the case. Extensive glomerular abnormalities can be found on biopsy with minimal concurrent clinical manifestations. For this reason, many authorities are aggressive with early biopsy. Three circumstances in particular warrant biopsy:

1. A child with SLE and nephrotic syndrome: to distinguish membranous glomerulonephritis from diffuse proliferative glomerulonephritis (which would warrant more aggressive therapy)

2. Failure of high-dose corticosteroids to reverse deteriorating renal function: to determine the likelihood of benefit from cytotoxic therapy
3. A prerequisite to entry into clinical therapeutic trials

Cassidy JT, Petty RE: Textbook of Pediatric Rheumatology, 3rd ed. Philadelphia, WB Saunders, 1995, pp 260-322.

92. How can the result of renal biopsy affect treatment in SLE?

Biopsy can reveal a spectrum of renal pathology, ranging from a normal kidney (rare) to mesangial nephritis or glomerulonephritis (focal or diffuse, proliferative or membranous). Histologic transformation from one group to another over time is not unusual. Treatment of lupus nephritis is based on the severity of the lesion. Mesangial disease may require little or no intervention. Patients with membranous nephropathy commonly present with nephrotic syndrome and usually respond to prednisone. Focal proliferative glomerulonephritis is often controlled with corticosteroids alone, but diffuse proliferative glomerulonephritis often requires corticosteroids, intravenous pulse cyclophosphamide and possibly other immunosuppressives.

93. When should high-dose corticosteroid therapy be considered in SLE management?

High dose corticosteroids usually consists of either IV pulse methylprednisolone (30 mg/kg/dose with a maximum dose of 1 gram, given daily or on alternate days given as an IV bolus for up to 3 doses) or oral prednisone (1-2 mg/kg/day). Often IV pulses are then followed by high dose oral steroids. The main indications for high-dose steroids in SLE are:

- Lupus crisis (widespread acute multisystem vasculitic involvement)
- Worsening CNS disease (as long as steroid psychosis in not thought to be the etiology)
- Severe lupus nephritis
- Acute hemolytic anemia
- Acute pleuropulmonary disease

94. What is the prognosis for children with confirmed SLE?

The prognosis for survival has improved remarkably in the last 20 years. Survival rates at 10 years are close to 90%. 20-year survival, however, drops down to approximately 75%. Most pediatric lupus deaths are due to infections. About half of patients with childhood lupus still have active disease as adults.

95. What is the association of antiphospholipid antibodies and lupus?

Antiphospholipid antibodies (aPL) can cause recurrent arterial and/or venous thromboses (e.g., stroke, phlebitis, renal vein thrombosis, placental thrombosis leading to fetal demise). Antiphospholipid antibodies are usually detected as anticardiolipin antibodies (aCL) or lupus anticoagulant (LA). These antibodies are often seen in SLE, but their prevalence in pediatric lupus varies widely (30-87% for aCL and 6-65% for LA), depending on the study cited. The pathogenesis of thromboses in patients with aPL antibodies remains unclear.

Ravelli A, Martini A: Antiphospholipid antibody syndrome in pediatric patients. Rheum Dis Clin North Am 23:657-676, 1997.

96. In addition to SLE, which other clinical situations are associated with the presence of antiphospholipid antibodies?

- Primary antiphospholipid syndrome
- Idiopathic thrombocytopenia purpura
- Juvenile rheumatoid arthritis
- Rheumatic fever
- Juvenile diabetes mellitus
- Juvenile dermatomyositis
- HIV infection

97. Which laboratory tests are useful in monitoring the effectiveness of therapy in SLE?

Serologic studies can provide useful information regarding the activity of SLE. The ANA titer does not correlate with disease activity. However, anti-double stranded DNA titers (if present) often drop and complement levels may increase and return to normal with effective therapy. Sedimentation rates usually decrease and CBCs may return to normal (or at least improve) with effective therapy and decreased disease activity.

98. What are the most common manifestations of neonatal lupus?

The syndrome of neonatal lupus erythematosus (NLE) was first described in babies born to mothers with SLE or Sjögren syndrome. However, it has now been found that 70-80% of mothers are asymptomatic. NLE is most likely caused by the transmission of maternal IgG autoantibodies. The main manifestations are:

- ***Cutaneous***: Skin lesions are found in about 50% babies with NLE. Although the rash may be present at birth, it usually develops within the first two or three months of life. The lesions include macules, papules, and annular plaques, and may be precipitated by exposure to sunlight. The lesions are usually transient and non-scarring.
- ***Cardiac***: Complete congenital heart block (CCHB) is the classic cardiac lesion of NLE and 90% of all CCHB is due to neonatal lupus. Most cases of CCHB present after the neonatal period, and 40–100% of these patients will eventually require a pacemaker, usually before 18 years of age. The average mortality from CCHB in the neonatal period is 15%.
- ***Hepatic***: Hepatic involvement is seen in at least 15% of babies NLE. Hepatomegaly +/- splenomegaly is usually seen. Hepatic transaminases are either mild-moderately elevated or normal. Clinically and histologically, the presentation is often one of idiopathic neonatal giant cell hepatitis.
- ***Hematologic***: Thrombocytopenia, hemolytic anemia, and/or neutropenia may be seen.

Silverman ED, Laxer RM: Neonatal lupus erythematosus. Rheum Dis Clin North Am 23:599-618, 1997.

99. What is the pathophysiology of the complete congenital heart block (CCHB) in neonatal lupus?

CCHB is caused by maternal autoantibodies that cross the placenta and deposit in the conducting system, usually the AV node, of the fetal heart. This leads to a localized inflammatory lesion, which may then be followed by scarring with fibrosis and calcification. The autoantibodies are usually anti-Ro (SS-A) antibodies (particularly to the 52 kd protein), but anti-La (SS-B) antibodies can also be the etiologic agents.

Silverman ED, Laxer RM: Neonatal lupus erythematosus. Rheum Dis Clin North Am 23:599-618, 1997.

100. What are the common features of drug-induced lupus?

Fever, *arthralgias/arthritis*, and *serositis* can be seen in drug induced lupus. *ANA* and *anti-histone antibodies* are often positive, but antibodies to double-stranded DNA are usually negative and complements remain normal. Renal involvement, CNS disease, malar rash, alopecia and oral ulcers are not usually seen in drug induced lupus, and their presence should raise suspicions of SLE.

101. What are the most common causes of drug-induced lupus in children?

Antiepileptic medications (especially ethosuximide, phenytoin, and primidone) are the most common and up to 20% children on antiepileptic drugs will develop a positive ANA. Minocycline, hydralazine, isoniazid, alpha-methyldopa, and chlorpromazine are also associated with drug-induced lupus, as are a variety of anti-thyroid medications and beta-blockers.

VASCULITIS

102. What clinical features suggest a vasculitic syndrome?

A multisystem disease with fever, weight loss and rash is often the presenting picture in a vasculitic disorder. Many different types of rashes may be seen, the more common of which are palpable purpura, vasculitic urticaria, or dermal necrosis. CNS involvement, arthritis, myositis and/ or serositis may be seen.

Blanco R, et al: Cutaneous vasculitis in children and adults: Associated diseases and etiologic factors in 303 patients. Medicine 77:403-418, 1998.

103. How are the primary systemic vasculitides classified?

One scheme proposed by an international consensus classifies vasculitides on the basis of the size of the vessels predominantly affected.

Small Vessel Vasculitis

ANCA-associated small vessel vasculitis
Microscopic polyangiitis
Wegener granulomatosis
Churg-Strauss syndrome
Drug-induced ANCA-associated vasculitis
Immune complex small-vessel vasculitis

- Henoch-Schönlein purpura
- Cryoglobulinemic vasculitis
- Lupus vasculitis
- Rheumatoid vasculitis
- Sjögren syndrome vasculitis
- Hypocomplementemic urticarial vasculitis
- Behçet disease
- Goodpasture syndrome
- Serum-sickness vasculitis
- Drug-induced immune-complex vasculitis
- Infection-induced immune-complex vasculitis

Paraneoplastic small-vessel vasculitis
Inflammatory bowel disease vasculitis

Large Vessel Vasculitis

Giant-cell arteritis
Takayasu arteritis

Medium-sized Vessel Vasculitis

Polyarteritis nodosa
Kawasaki disease
Primary granulomatous
CNS vasculitis

Jennette JC, Falk RJ, Andrassy K, et al: Nomenclature of systemic vasculitides: Proposal of an international consensus conference. Arthritis Rheum 37:187-92,1994.

104. Which infectious agents are associated with vasculitis?

Viral:	HIV, hepatitis B and C
	CMV, EBV, varicella
	Rubella and parvovirus B19
Rickettsial:	Rocky Mountain spotted fever
	Typhus, rickettsialpox
Bacterial:	Meningococcus
	Disseminated sepsis due to any organism
	Subacute bacterial endocarditis
Spirochete:	Syphilis
Mycobacterial:	Tuberculosis

105. What are the conditions grouped under the term "pulmonary-renal syndromes"?

- Wegener granulomatosis
- Goodpasture syndrome

- Churg-Strauss syndrome
- Henoch-Schönlein purpura
- Systemic lupus erythematosus

106. What is the clinical triad of Behçet disease?

Aphthous stomatitis, ***genital ulcerations***, and ***uveitis***. Behçet disease is a vasculitis of unclear etiology. In two-thirds of cases in children, polyarthritis and inflammatory GI lesions occur, which can confuse the diagnosis with inflammatory bowel disease.

107. Should it be Henoch-Schönlein or Schönlein-Henoch purpura?

In 1837 Johann Schönlein described the association of purpura and arthralgia. Edward Henoch later added the additional clinical features of GI symptoms in 1874 and renal involvement in 1899. Purists would say more properly the term should be Schönlein-Henoch. However, in 1801, William Heberden described a 5-year-old boy with joint and abdominal pains, petechiae, hematochezia, and gross hematuria in his *Commentaries on the History and Cure of Disease*. Purists might say most properly it should be Heberden syndrome.

108. What are the characteristic laboratory findings in Henoch-Schönlein purpura (HSP)?

Acute phase reactants, including the ESR, are commonly elevated, and there is frequently a mild leukocytosis. Thrombocytopenia is *never* seen. Microscopic hematuria and proteinuria are indicators of renal involvement. HSP appears to be an IgA-mediated illness; elevated serum IgA has been noted and has been demonstrated by immunofluroscence in skin and renal biopsies. (The latter are indistinguishable from Berger disease.) Circulating immune complexes and cryoglobulins containing IgA are also commonly seen.

109. What kind of skin lesions are noted in HSP?

HSP is one of the hypersensitivity vasculitides and, as such, is characterized by leukocytoclastic inflammation of arterioles, capillaries and venules. Initially, *urticarial lesions* predominate, which may itch or burn. These develop into pink maculopapules. With damage to the vessel walls, there is bleeding into the skin, resulting in nonthrombotic petechiae and palpable purpura. A migrating soft-tissue edema is also commonly seen in younger children.

110. In additions to the skin, what other organ systems are typically involved in HSP?

Classically, HSP involves the ***musculoskeletal*** system, ***GI tract***, and/or ***kidneys***.

- The most common abdominal finding is GI colic (70%), frequently associated with nausea, vomiting, and GI bleeding. These findings may precede the skin rash in up to 30% cases. Intussusception occurs in up to 5% cases.
- Renal involvement occurs in about 50% reported cases, and is usually apparent early in the course of the illness. It ranges in severity from microscopic hematuria to nephrotic syndrome.
- Joint involvement is very common (80%), and can be quite painful. Periarticular swelling of the knees, ankles, wrists and elbows, rather than a true arthritis, is usually seen.
- Up to 15% males can have scrotal involvement with epididymitis, orchitis, testicular torsion, and scrotal bleeding.
- Pulmonary hemorrhage is a rare complication of HSP, mainly seen in adolescents and adults. It is associated with significant mortality.

111. How often does chronic renal disease develop in children with HSP?

The long-term prognosis in HSP mainly depends on the initial renal involvement. Overall <5% patients with HSP develop end-stage renal disease. However, up to two-thirds of children who have severe cresentric glomerulonephritis documented on biopsy will develop terminal renal failure within one year. Of those with nephritis or nephrotic syndrome at the onset of illness, almost half may have long-term problems with hypertension or impaired renal function as adults. Microscopic hematuria as the sole manifestation of HSP is common and is associated with a good long-term outcome.

Scharer K, et al: Clinical outcome of Schönlein-Henoch purpura nephritis in children. Pediatr Nephrol 13:816-823, 1999.

112. Why is the diagnosis of intussusception often difficult in patients with HSP?

- Intussusception can occur suddenly, without preceding abdominal symptoms.
- Nearly half the cases of HSP intussusception are ileoileal (compared to non-HSP intussusceptions of which 75% are ileocolic). This increases the likelihood of a false-negative barium enema.
- The variety of possible GI complications in HSP (e.g., pancreatitis, cholecystitis, gastritis) can confuse the clinical picture.
- The common occurrence (50-75%) of melena, guaiac-positive stools, and abdominal pain in HSP without intussusception may lead to a lowered index of suspicion.

113. When are corticosteroids indicated in the treatment of HSP?

The precise indication for corticosteroids in HSP remains controversial. Prednisone, 1-2 mg/kg/day for 5-7 days, is often used for severe intestinal symptoms and may decrease the likelihood of intussusception. Corticosteroids may be helpful in the settings of significant pulmonary, scrotal, or CNS manifestations to minimize vasculitic inflammation. They are sometimes used if severe joint pain is present and NSAIDS are contraindicated. Steroids do not prevent recurrences of symptoms, and symptoms may flare when steroids are discontinued. There is a great deal of controversy whether or not the early use of corticosteroids (oral or intravenous pulses) in renal disease improves long-term outcome.

Saulsbury FT: Henoch-Schönlein purpura in children: Report of 100 patients and review of the literature. Medicine 78:395-409, 1999.

114. Which etiologic agents are thought to cause HSP?

HSP is probably mediated by *immune complexes* that require the participation of an inciting antigen. Any number of infectious agents or drugs can fit the bill. The vast majority of children with HSP have a history of a prodromal illness, usually an upper respiratory tract infection. Serologic evidence of antecedent streptococcal infection is present in up to 50% of cases. Drugs associated with HSP include penicillin, tetracycline, sulfonamides, thiazides, and aspirin.

INDEX

Page numbers in **boldface type** indicate complete chapters.